Fear

- Related to severity of condition, family distress, or threat of death (Chap. 11, The Person with Congestive Heart Failure and Cardiogenic Shock, p. 347)
- Related to inadequate knowledge of disease process or to chest wall pain (Chap. 15, The Person with Pericarditis, Pericardial Effusion, and Cardiac Tamponade, p. 475)

MOVING PATTERN
Impaired Physical Mobility

- Related to decreased cardiac output (Chap. 11, The Person with Congestive Heart Failure and Cardiogenic Shock, p. 324)
- Related to chest pain, dyspnea, and fatigue (Chap. 12, The Person with Valvular Heart Disease, p. 386)
- Related to prolonged intravenous therapy and restricted activities (Chap. 13, The Person with Infective Endocarditis, p. 417)
- Related to activity restriction (Chap. 16, The Person with an Artificial Cardiac Pacemaker, p. 502)
- Related to restricted activity and incisional discomfort (of the affected extremity with permanent pacemaker) (Chap. 16, The Person with an Artificial Cardiac Pacemaker, p. 533)

Activity Intolerance

- Related to inadequate myocardial tissue perfusion (Chap. 9, The Person with Angina Pectoris, p. 234)
- Related to inadequate myocardial tissue perfusion (Chap. 10, The Person with Myocardial Infarction, p. 266)
- Related to acute or chronic illness (Chap. 14, The Person with Cardiomyopathy or Myocarditis, p. 442)

Fatigue

- Related to limited cardiac reserve (Chap. 11, The Person with Congestive Heart Failure and Cardiogenic Shock, p. 325)

Sleep Pattern Disturbance

- (Discussion, Chap. 10, The Person with Myocardial Infarction, p. 268)
- Related to invasive monitoring procedures (Chap. 7, Hemodynamic Monitoring, p. 190)
- Related to environmental factors, nursing care demands, and medications (Chap. 17, The Person Undergoing Cardiac Surgery, p. 579)

PERCEIVING PATTERN
Body Image Disturbance

- Related to side effects of corticosteroids (Chap. 18, The Person Undergoing Cardiac Transplant Surgery, p. 621)

Hopelessness

- Related to unpredictable outcome of acute or chronic illness (Chap. 14, The Person with Cardiomyopathy or Myocarditis, p. 443)

Powerlessness

- Related to lifestyle cha[nges] with Coronary Artery [...]
- Related to perceived in[...] disease process (Chap. 14, The Person with Cardiomyopathy or Myocarditis, p. 445)

EXCHANGING PATTERN
High Risk for Impaired Neurologic Function

- Related to surgery, drugs, and environment (Chap. 17, The Person Undergoing Cardiac Surgery, p. 573)

Altered Peripheral Perfusion

- Related to compromised circulation associated with invasive monitoring (Chap. 7, Hemodynamic Monitoring, p. 187)

Fluid Volume Deficit

- Related to bleeding due to the transvenous epicardial, or transthoracic lead insertion (Chap. 16, The Person with an Artificial Cardiac Pacemaker, p. 501)

Fluid Volume Excess

- (Discussion, Chap. 11, The Person with Congestive Heart Failure and Cardiogenic Shock, p. 569)

High Risk for Altered Fluid and Electrolyte Balance

- Related to the stress response of surgical trauma, the physiologic effects of cardiopulmonary bypass, and extravascular fluid shifts (Chap. 17, The Person Undergoing Cardiac Surgery, p. 574)
- Related to corticosteroid therapy (Chap. 18, The Person Undergoing Cardiac Transplant Surgery, p. 617)

High Risk for Bleeding

- Related to the removal of the temporary pacing leads (Chap. 16, The Person with an Artificial Cardiac Pacemaker, p. 512)

High Risk for Ventricular Tachydysrhythmia

- Related to the insertion of temporary cardiac pacing lead (Chap. 16, The Person with an Artificial Cardiac Pacemaker, p. 497)

High Risk for Bradydysrhythmia or Tachydysrhythmia

- Related to (state cause necessitating temporary cardiac pacing) (Chap. 16, The Person with an Artificial Cardiac Pacemaker, p. 498)
- Related to (state cause necessitating permanent cardiac pacing) (Chap. 16, The Person with an Artificial Cardiac Pacemaker, p. 523)

High Risk for Pacemaker Malfunction

- Related to (state cause of temporary pacemaker malfunction) (Chap. 16, The Person with an Artificial Cardiac Pacemaker, p. 505)
- Related to the newly implanted pacing lead and pulse generator (for permanent pacemakers) (Chap. 16, The Person with an Artificial Cardiac Pacemaker, p. 528)

(Continued on back cover).

CARDIOVASCULAR NURSING

Holistic Practice

CARDIOVASCULAR NURSING
Holistic Practice

CATHIE E. GUZZETTA, PhD, RN, FAAN

Director, Holistic Nursing Consultants,
Bethesda, Maryland;
Formerly, Associate Professor and Chairperson,
Cardiovascular Nursing,
The Catholic University of America,
Washington, D.C.

BARBARA MONTGOMERY DOSSEY, MS, RN

Director, Holistic Nursing Consultants,
Santa Fe, New Mexico;
Director, Bodymind Systems,
Temple, Texas

With 255 illustrations

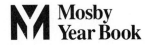 **Mosby**
Year Book

St. Louis Baltimore Boston Chicago London Philadelphia Sydney Toronto

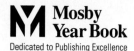
Mosby
Year Book
Dedicated to Publishing Excellence

Executive Editor: Don Ladig
Developmental Editor: Robin Carter
Project Manager: Carol Sullivan Wiseman
Production Editors: Florence Achenbach and Pat Joiner
Book and Cover Design: Gail Morey Hudson

Printed in the United States of America

Mosby–Year Book, Inc.
11830 Westline Industrial Drive, St. Louis, MO 63146

Library of Congress Cataloging in Publication Data

Guzzetta, Cathie E.
    Cardiovascular nursing : holistic practice / Cathie E. Guzzetta,
Barbara Montgomery Dossey.
        p.   cm.
    Includes bibliographical references and index.
    ISBN 0-8016-2784-2
    1. Cardiovascular system—Diseases—Nursing. 2. Holistic
medicine. I. Dossey, Barbara Montgomery. II. Title.
    [DNLM: 1. Cardiovascular Diseases—nursing. 2. Holistic Health.
WY 152.5 G993c]
RC674.G89 1992
610.73′691—dc20
DNLM/DLC
for Library of Congress   91-42123
                                                                          CIP

92 93 94 95 96 GW/VH 9 8 7 6 5 4 3 2 1

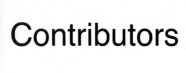

Contributors

URSULA K. ANDERSON, MSN, RN, ANP, CCRN

Adult Nurse Practitioner, Fairfax Hospital,
Falls Church, Virginia

SUZETTE CARDIN, MS, RN, CCRN,

Nurse Manager, Cardiac Care Unit/Cardiac Observation Unit,
Assistant Clinical Professor,
University of California at Los Angeles Medical Center,
Los Angeles, California

GAIL A. OSWALD CAVALLO, MSN, RN

Nurse Specialist and Research Coordinator,
Division of Cardiology,
George Washington University Medical Center,
Washington, D.C.

MARY SUE CRAFT, MSN, RN

Cardiovascular Clinical Nurse Specialist,
University of Alabama Hospital,
Birmingham, Alabama

ELAINE KIESS DAILY, BS, RN

Consultant, Cardiovascular Clinical Research,
Madison, Wisconsin;
Formerly, Clinical Cardiovascular Research Nurse,
University of California at San Diego Medical Center,
San Diego, California

DIANE K. DRESSLER, MSN, RN, CCRN, CCTC

Clinical Transplant Coordinator,
Midwest Heart Surgery Institute,
St. Luke's Medical Center,
Milwaukee, Wisconsin

MARY KAY FEENEY, MN, RN

Medical Specialist,
Underwriting Standards and Services,
Northwestern Mutual Life Insurance Company
Milwaukee, Wisconsin

SANDRA W. HAAK, MS, RN

Clinical Assistant Professor, College of Nursing,
University of Utah,
Salt Lake City, Utah

CAROLYN D. HENSON, BS, MA, RN

President, Wellness Communications, Inc.;
Editor, "RX: Live Well,"
Dallas, Texas

SUE E. HUETHER, PhD, RN

Associate Professor, College of Nursing,
University of Utah,
Salt Lake City, Utah

VIRGINIA BURKE KARB, PhD, RN

Assistant Dean and Associate Professor,
School of Nursing, University of North Carolina at
Greensboro, Greensboro, North Carolina

MARGUERITE R. KINNEY, DNSc, RN, FAAN

Professor and Coordinator of Cardiovascular Nursing,
University of Alabama at Birmingham,
Birmingham, Alabama

LESLIE KOLKMEIER, BS, RN

Private practice,
Psychophysiologic Self-Regulation,
Plano, Texas

CAROLYN L. MURDAUGH, PhD, RN, FAAN

Professor, College of Nursing,
University of Arizona,
Tucson, Arizona

LINDA A. PRINKEY, MSN, RN, CCRN, FNS

Cardiovascular Program Coordinator,
Prince George's Hospital Center,
Cheverly, Maryland

SUSAN J. QUAAL, MS, PhD (c), RN, CVS, CCRN

Cardiovascular Clinical Specialist,
Associate Clinical Professor,
Veterans Administration Hospital Medical Center,
University of Utah Health Sciences,
Salt Lake City, Utah

DIANE PROCTOR SAGER, MSN, RN

Nursing Pacemaker Consultant,
Olney, Maryland

ANITA P. SHERER, MSN, RN, CCRN

Clinical Nurse Specialist, Cardiology Unit,
Moses H. Cone Memorial Hospital,
Greensboro, North Carolina

SUE WINGATE, MSN, RN, CCRN, CS

Cardiology Clinical Nurse Specialist,
National Institutes of Health,
Bethesda, Maryland;
Doctoral Candidate, The Catholic University of America,
Washington, D.C.

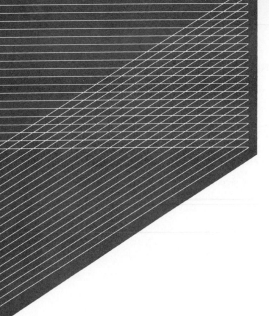

Consultants

JEANNE ACHTERBERG, PhD

Chairperson, Department of Research,
Institute of Transpersonal Psychology,
Menlo Park, California

ANNE ACKERMAN, MSN, RN

Cardiac Rehabilitation Coordinator,
Washington Hospital Center,
Washington, D.C.

VIRGINIA BECKWORTH, MSN, RN

Cardiovascular Clinical Nurse Specialist,
Baptist Medical Center, Birmingham, Alabama

SHELIA BUNTON, LTC, AN, MSN, RN

Head Nurse, Surgical Intensive Care Unit,
Tripler Army Medical Center,
Honolulu, Hawaii

LAURA J. BURKE, MSN, RN

Cardiovascular Clinical Nurse Specialist,
Sinai Samaritan Medical Center,
Milwaukee, Wisconsin

PATRICIA A. BURKE, MS, RN, CCRN

Clinical Nurse Specialist, Transplant Coordinator,
Midwest Heart Surgery Institute,
Milwaukee, Wisconsin

TONI CASCIO, MN, RN, CCRN

Clinical Educator—Critical Care,
Ochsner Foundation Hospital,
New Orleans, Louisiana

PATRICIA E. CASEY, MSN, RN

Education Coordinator, Cardiovascular Nursing,
Fairfax Hospital, Falls Church, Virginia;
Clinical Educator,
The Catholic University of America,
Washington, D.C.

NANCY F. COURTS, MSN, PhD (c), RN

Assistant Professor, School of Nursing,
University of North Carolina at Greensboro,
Greensboro, North Carolina

MARGARET CARTY FARRELL, MSN, RN, CCRN, CNS

Clinical Nurse Specialist,
Critical Care Department of Nursing Education,
Lawrence Hospital, Bronxville, New York

ZINA G. FIRMAGE, MS, RN

Senior Research Nurse, Division of Cardiology,
University of Utah Medical Center,
Salt Lake City, Utah

ROSS D. FLETCHER, MD, FACC

Chief, Cardiology Section,
Veterans Administration Medical Center,
Washington, D.C.

TERRY MATTHEW FOSTER, BSN, RN, CEN, CCRN

Clinical Director,
Mercy Hospital–Anderson,
Cincinnati, Ohio

ANNA GAWLINSKI, MSN, RN, CCRN

Cardiovascular Clinical Specialist, Assistant Professor,
University of California at Los Angeles Medical Center,
Los Angeles, California

KATHLEEN A. GRESK, BSN, RN

Head Nurse, Telemetry Unit,
St. Joseph's Hospital,
Milwaukee, Wisconsin

PHILIP C. GUZZETTA, Jr., MD

Professor of Surgery and Child Health and Development,
George Washington University; Attending Surgeon,
Children's Hospital National Medical Center,
Washington, D.C.

GAIL HANDYSIDES, MS, RN

Lecturer,
Department of Nursing,
San Diego State University,
San Diego, California

WILLIAM L. HOLMAN, MD

Assistant Professor of Surgery, Cardiothoracic Surgery,
University of Alabama at Birmingham,
Birmingham, Alabama

SANDRA G. KANE, MPH, RN, CCRN

Associate Nurse Manager, Cardiac Observation Unit,
University of California at Los Angeles Medical Center,
Los Angeles, California

RICHARD J. KATZ, MD

Professor and Director, Non-Invasive Cardiology,
George Washington University Medical Center,
Washington, D.C.

LESLIE S. KERN, MN, RN

Cardiovascular Clinical Nurse Specialist,
University of California at Los Angeles Medical Center,
Los Angeles, California

PARRY J. KNAUSS, MA, RN

Assistant Director, Nursing Education Department,
Yale New Haven Hospital,
New Haven, Connecticut

LESLIE KOLKMEIER, BS, RN

Private Practice,
Psychophysiologic Self-Regulation,
Plano, Texas

CHRISTINE KRUSKAMP, MSc, RN, CCRN

Staff Nurse, Intensive Care,
Holy Cross Hospital,
Salt Lake City, Utah

BARBARA LEEPER, MN, RN, CCRN

Cardiovascular Clinical Nurse Specialist,
Humana Hospital, Medical City Dallas Hospital,
Dallas, Texas

ROY LEIBOFF, MD, FACC

Associate Clinical Professor,
George Washington University Hospital,
Washington, D.C.

ANNE NICHOLSON MACDONALD, MS, RN

Cardiac Transplant Clinical Specialist,
Department of Surgery, University of Arizona Medical Center,
Tucson, Arizona

ROBERT O'ROURKE, MD

Director, Division of Cardiology,
The University of Texas Health Science Center
at San Antonio,
San Antonio, Texas

SUSAN G. OSGUTHORPE, MS, RN, CCRN, CNA

Assistant Chief Nursing Service/Surgery,
Veterans Administration Medical Center,
Salt Lake City, Utah

EDWARD V. PLATIA, MD

Director, Cardiac Arrhythmia Center,
Washington Hospital Center,
Washington, D.C.

JOYCE POWERS, MSN, RN, CS

Clinical Nurse Specialist,
Cardiology Consultants,
Albuquerque, New Mexico

LINDA A. PRINKEY, MSN, RN, CCRN, FNS

Cardiovascular Program Coordinator,
Prince George's Hospital Center,
Cheverly, Maryland

ALLAN M. ROSS, MD

Professor and Director, Division of Cardiology,
George Washington University Medical Center,
Washington, D.C.

JENNIFER B. SANDOVAL, MN, RN

Lecturer, School of Nursing,
University of North Carolina at Greensboro,
Greensboro, North Carolina

LINDA H. SCHAKENBACH, MSN, RN, CCRN

Clinical Nurse Specialist,
Cardiovascular Critical Care,
Fairfax Hospital,
Falls Church, Virginia

TERENCE M. SCHMAHL, MD

Thoracic and Cardiovascular Surgeon,
Midwest Heart Surgery Institute,
Milwaukee, Wisconsin

JOHN S. SCHROEDER, MD

Professor of Medicine, Cardiology Division,
Stanford University Medical Center,
Stanford, California

PATRICIA C. SEIFERT, MSN, RN, CNOR

Operating Room Coordinator, Cardiac Surgery,
The Arlington Hospital,
Arlington, Virginia

NANCY URBAN, MSN, RN, CCRN

Cardiovascular Clinical Nurse Specialist,
Waukesha Memorial Hospital,
Waukesha, Wisconson

P. JACOB VARGHESE, MD

Professor and Director of Coronary Care,
George Washington University Medical Center,
Washington, D.C.

JOAN VITELLO-CICCU, MSN, RN, CCRN, CS

Clinical Nurse Specialist, Surgical Critical Care,
Co-Editor, Journal of Cardiovascular Nursing,
Boston University Medical Center,
Boston, Massachusetts

SUE WINGATE, MSN, RN, CCRN, CS

Cardiology Clinical Nurse Specialist,
National Institutes of Health,
Bethesda, Maryland;
Doctoral Candidate,
The Catholic University of America,
Washington, D.C.

KIMBERLY WOODS-McCORMICK, BSN, RN, CCRN

Staff Education Coordinator, Cardiovascular Services,
Poudre Valley Hospital,
Fort Collins, Colorado

COVER: "Early Spring," the tapestry on the cover, is by Silvia Heyden, a North Carolina artist whose inspiration she describes as follows: "During my daily violin practice, I have a silent companion outside of my window, a little tree with a circular outline of branches. I watch the changes year round, especially in early spring, when new life is about to burst into that familiar design. One day I could not resist drawing it into the notes of my Mozart sonata. Several springtimes later, I felt like playing the same music again, but there was that drawing in Mozart's phrase. It seemed to be waiting for yet another transformation, this time into a tapestry called 'Early Spring.'" Tapestry courtesy Style Works, St. Louis, Mo.

Throughout history, master weavers have described the weaving of a tapestry as healing, as transforming, as a calling, or as sacred work. Weaving a great tapestry is usually a collective effort involving others; it is not done in isolation. All of nursing is like a tapestry in which the single threads of our experiences become incorporated into the fabric of life. As nurses weave their technologic and intuitive skills—of knowing, doing, being—into their work, facilitating healing in self and others, they recognize that they are co-learners and co-walkers with patients and families and friends in a healing journey. This is the spirit of healing—the urge toward wholeness, oneness, and interaction—that has always been the essence of nursing. It is the eternal human quest for meaning and unity.

To our colleagues in cardiovascular nursing:

When a nurse
Encounters a patient
Something happens
What occurs
Is never a neutral event

A pulse taken
Words exchanged
A touch
Resuscitation
Two persons
Are never
The same

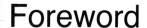

Foreword

Guzzetta and Dossey have extended their thought process and vision of nursing in ways that seek to recover healing and wholeness. This is not just an update of their earlier remarkable book; it is a conversation continued in practice about how we can heal ourselves and become more healing in our practice. They seek nothing less than a transformation of health care "from a disease management industry to a healing system."

Holism is a cover term that they now seek to further explicate in practice. They would have the healer's imagination and relational ethic be skilled in the ways of Western Medicine and the most advanced nursing techniques. However, in the midst of the nursing techniques and "lasing, lysing, ballooning, bypassing, scraping, stenting and transplanting," they call the reader to a larger vision of healing and recovery. They would move the nurse to healing relationships with themselves, colleagues, and those for whom they care. This text makes public a private dialogue among the most advanced cardiovascular nurse clinicians.

No cardiovascular nurse can practice long before seeing the limited use of techniques without attentiveness to social and personal causes. Heart transplantation, for example, is a brief moment with a past and a future. Persons with new hearts do not receive a new world to match the new hearts. They must return to the old world with new pressures. New demands created by living with a transformed internal milieu of medications require attending to signs of rejection and infection. There is no cure without care. There is a limit to our technical magic. We are finite and vul-

nerable but not helpless and hopeless and therein lies the quest for more realistic approaches to self-care and care of others found in this work.

Guzzetta and Dossey call for a new dialogue between practice and technology—a weaving of "the tapestry of the interconnectedness of all human beings." Implicit throughout the work is the notion that healers are not technical experts separate from those whom they would heal. One finds a lively connection between Florence Nightingale's plea to place the person in an environment conducive to healing (*Notes on Nursing*) and the call for a more healing environment in this work. I am also reminded of Virginia Henderson's plea for attending the patients' and families' spiritual resources for health. I look forward to the lively dialogues that this work will create in practice. I applaud the permission it gives for us to be public about our healing arts. The vision in this book gathers what is already embedded in the best of nursing practice. The book will raise questions in the practice about how we can become more responsible for our health without blaming ourselves for illness. How can we exercise choice while recognizing the limits of control? Let the dialogue continue as practitioners work out what it means to care for the whole person with empowering respect and attentiveness.

Patricia Benner

Patricia Benner, RN, PhD, FAAN
Professor, Department of Physiological Nursing,
University of California Medical Center, San Francisco,
San Francisco, California

Preface

HOLISM AND CARDIOVASCULAR NURSING

Cardiovascular Nursing: Holistic Practice was written in response to requests for us to put together our teaching on cardiovascular nursing with a focus on holistic concepts. Portions of this book first appeared in *Cardiovascular Nursing: Bodymind Tapestry* in 1984. From the responses we received from our readers and from the well-worn book pages that we have seen, we have been led to believe that this book was useful in helping nurses define and practice cardiovascular nursing from a holistic approach.

Bodymind Tapestry was written when there was a decisive move away from the biomedical model to a more holistic approach to nursing practice. During this time, each of us struggled to understand holism. We wrestled to unravel the assumptions of the holistic model so that we could translate them into concrete nursing implications. In doing so, our direction in nursing became increasingly more clear. Our clarity, in turn, altered the way we practice nursing. For example, we are emphasizing not only illness prevention but also health promotion and high-level wellness. Likewise, we are replacing the traditional biomedical physical assessment with a bio-psycho-social-spiritual approach to evaluate holistic patterns and processes. Our nursing diagnoses focus on human responses of not only the body but also the mind and spirit in both illness and wellness. Nurses are gaining expertise not only in technology but also in biobehavioral techniques. We are using rational and intuitive ways of knowing when prescribing interventions and administering care to facilitate body-mind-spirit healing.

Thus we are witnessing enormous changes within the profession. Most nurses value and subscribe to a holistic philosophy. Many are able to explain what holistic nursing is. More than ever, we believe that nurses are ready and willing to incorporate holism into their practice and are becoming united about the need to do so. We also believe, however, that the total impact of the holistic movement on nursing has not yet been fully realized.

Our early ideas of holism, like a single thread, have taken on new meaning over the past several years as we have interwoven the many diverse threads of knowledge from other disciplines. These new threads have engendered a more vivid, dynamic, and diverse understanding about the nature of holism and its implications for nursing. Thus we have taken the ideas and threads of *Bodymind Tapestry* to its next level: holism is no longer a nursing *approach*—rather it is the essence of *practice*. We have attempted to capture this essence in *Cardiovascular Nursing: Holistic Practice*.

The text is intended for all nurses, students, educators, and researchers who are interested in gaining an in-depth knowledge of the cardiovascular patient. Nurses will find the book particularly useful because of the development of autonomous biobehavioral nursing interventions and the emphasis on the scientific data to support technologic advances and holistic concepts.

FOCUS

This book focuses on adult patients with medical and surgical cardiovascular dysfunctions. It presents the most up-to-date, in-depth, and comprehensive coverage of the causes of cardiovascular dysfunction and ways to assess, diagnose, and treat such dysfunctions. It transforms advances in medical science into tangible implications for advanced nursing practice by solidly integrating the nursing process. Perhaps more important, this book examines how cardiovascular dysfunctions have an impact on patients' minds and spirits. It incorporates the belief that total healing can occur only when patients' emotional and spiritual needs are addressed with their physical needs. Scientific knowledge and research are used to explain the interrelationship of body-mind-spirit in all matters of health and illness; interventions are included for promoting patient healing in all three dimensions. Thus the theme of this book involves holism and healing of the cardiovascular patient. To achieve this focus, we have included the following areas:

1. Nursing practice guided from a holistic (bio-psycho-social-spiritual) model
2. The American Association of Critical-Care Nurses' *Process Standards for Nursing Care of the Critically Ill* and the American Heart Association's *Standards of Cardiovascular Nursing Practice*
3. Comprehensive coverage of all major cardiovascular dysfunctions, addressing the stages of prevention, critical illness, rehabilitation, and health promotion
4. Recent advances in pathophysiologic, pharmacologic, technologic, and biobehavioral interventions to provide state-of-the-art content
5. Concepts of holism and body-mind-spirit relatedness, the psychophysiology of bodymind healing, and the scientific data to support the critical link between mind and body
6. Common trends in the biobehavioral treatment of cardiovascular patients, including self-regulation techniques (e.g., relaxation, imagery, and music) as interventions for common nursing diagnoses
7. Ways that cardiovascular nurses can care for themselves, enhance their own wellness, and integrate self-care in their lives

Each chapter is preceded by an Interchapter discussion to translate theoretical notions of holism and healing into understandable nursing actions. These discussions were written by us and include topics such as right- and left-brain thinking, intuition, placebo effect, touch, and bringing healing into technology. Each chapter incorporates Learning Objectives that are linked to Key Concept Reviews, or study questions, that appear at the end of each chapter and can be used as a formal or informal evaluation of the learner's progress.

ORGANIZATION

The text is divided into four units. *Unit I* presents the holistic framework for cardiovascular nursing practice. It investigates the psychophysiologic effects of bodymind healing and qualities of a nurse healer. It addresses the merging crossroads of technology, consciousness, and spirituality and discusses the reasons that nurses must blend these dimensions to achieve holistic patient care to move from a *disease-management industry* to a *healing system*. This unit also includes information on how nurses can assess and care for themselves to facilitate healing in patients. In addition, it introduces a new holistic assessment format, which is integrated throughout the book, and helps to validate the application of nursing diagnoses in practice. Up-to-date information on nursing diagnoses and critical issues on implementation are included. Biobehavioral interventions also are discussed with step-by-step procedures

and scripts for integrating these techniques into practice.

Unit II includes selected cardiovascular testing and monitoring techniques. The comprehensive discussion on diagnostic testing presents common noninvasive and invasive tests, including implications for patient teaching. The content on hemodynamic monitoring addresses patients undergoing central venous, pulmonary artery, intra-arterial, and SVO_2 monitoring. Patient teaching, troubleshooting of problems, and nursing care plans are included.

Units III and IV contain clinical chapters related to nursing care of patients with common cardiovascular dysfunctions and those undergoing selected cardiovascular therapies. Each chapter is divided into two well-defined sections: the knowledge base (i.e., anatomy and physiology, significance, incidence, etiology, risk factors, and pathophysiology) and the nursing process. Within the nursing process section, medical knowledge is rendered into advanced nursing practice and presented in a consistent, clinically functional format to facilitate application of content. For example, patient case studies are presented to exemplify the application of theory in real day-to-day situations. After the case studies, a nursing assessment format based on the nine human response patterns of Taxonomy I (from the North American Nursing Diagnosis Association [NANDA]) is included. This format promotes a nursing rather than a medical patient assessment. Then common human responses anticipated for patients with specific cardiovascular dysfunctions are outlined based on NANDA's list of accepted nursing diagnoses (i.e., Taxonomy I). The nursing care plan format that follows is driven by the specific nursing diagnosis and includes patient outcomes, nursing prescriptions, and evaluation of the outcomes. For each nursing diagnosis, a discussion about the factual information that supports the plan and implementation of care is included to demonstrate how nursing standards are applied to practice.

Five appendixes are included to augment the reader's knowledge base. Appendix A presents four different cardiovascular assessment tools (Holistic Cardiovascular Assessment Tool, Cardiovascular Rehabilitation Assessment Tool, Transplant Assessment Tool, and Cardiovascular Screening Tool); all are based on a format used to evaluate the nine human responses and are illustrated with data from case studies to exemplify the process of a holistic nursing assessment. Appendix B presents an overview of the major cardiac dysrhythmias and nursing interventions. Appendix C outlines the major cardiovascular drugs and possible nursing diagnoses for each drug category. Appendix D includes updated information on defibrillation, cardioversion, and the automatic implantable cardioverter-defibrillator. Finally, Appendix E presents information related to survivors of a cardiac arrest who have had a near-death experience.

ESSENCE OF HOLISTIC PRACTICE

As we were preparing this Preface, we both reflected on the tremendous advances that have occured not only in nursing but also in medicine within the past decade. We have seen the advent of laser and thrombolytic therapy, percutaneous transluminal coronary angioplasty, coronary artery atherectomies and stents, ventricular assist devices, total artificial hearts, and cardiac transplantation occurring as standard practice at most major medical centers. Many of the advances in medicine have occurred because of a more focused investigation on the cellular and molecular mechanisms underlying cardiovascular diagnosis and treatment. This focus is entirely consistent with the molecular theory of disease causation and the biomedical model that guides the practice of medicine.

Despite these advances, however, the cause and cure for many cardiovascular problems still have not been discovered. So we are painfully aware that lasing, lysing, ballooning, bypassing, scraping, stenting, and transplanting really do not provide the answers in preventing, reversing, and treating cardiovascular illness. Also, we are aware that the biomedical model does not explain the psychologic, social, or spiritual causes of disease. Why then are medical outcomes still falling short of predicted criteria? Could it be that after all these centuries we now realize that the biomedical model can never provide us with complete answers in treating heart disease because it has taken into account neither the profound devastating affects nor the enormous healing effects of the mind and spirit on the body?

This insight and our intuitive experiences have driven us to seek, adopt, and expand our understanding of holism. We now find ourselves living within a profession that ascribes to the holistic model. Because this model offers a philosophic revolution so different from the traditional biomedical model, it has been called a *paradigm shift*.[1] Such a shift not only brings with it a new philosophic reposturing of the profession but also the realization of its monumental implications that are certain to change the profession forever. This paradigm makes us realize that identifying and treating pathophysiologic problems exclusively with medical therapies is only half the answer. It weaves the tapestry of the interconnectedness of all human beings and proposes the presence of an undefined and powerful healing energy that remains to be harnessed. It challenges us to entertain new ideas that may conflict with logic and science. It forces us to move away from a purely mechanistic view of the way that human beings function. Thus this paradigm fashions a new portrait of ourselves and our profession, altering our image of who we are and who we can become.

This new paradigm is destined also to alter the way we practice nursing. Our challenge is to actualize the implications and determine the course of this destiny. This book suggests that our goal as nurse healers is to help patients find their own pathways to wellness. It is intended to provide the essence of holistic practice as nurses embark on this caring-healing journey. The boundaries by which we can assist patients to achieve wellness and help them to realize their own healing potential still remain to be defined. Nonetheless, as we help patients facilitate their inner healing, we discover our own and begin our journey as nurse healers. Each of us, however, must discover the path.

ACKNOWLEDGMENTS

For sharing their knowledge and expertise, we are indebted to our current contributors and to those who were involved in *Cardiovascualr Nursing: Bodymind Tapestry:* Mike Riley, Nursing Editor, Donald A. Bille, Larry L. Burden, Zandra (Zee) Clark, Susan G. Davis, Joan Marie Bowen DiBianco, Larry Dossey, Jeanne E. Doyle, Jeanne Fitzpatrick, Philip C. Guzzetta, Janet M. Lauer, Maureen T. McElligott, Barbara B. Ott, Barry Silverman, and Jean C. Toth.

For their assistance, counsel, and guidance in directing the development of this book, we thank Don Ladig and Robin Carter. For keeping our writing consistent, clean, and honest, we thank Florence Achenbach, Pat Joiner, and Carol Wiseman. For spending hours developing a smart design that is pleasing to the eye, we thank Gail Morey Hudson.

Most of all, for all their love, understanding, and encouragement in seeing us through one more book, we thank our families—Philip, Angela, and P.C. Guzzetta; and Larry Dossey—who share our tapestry of interconnectedness and are a part of our caring-healing journey.

Cathie E. Guzzetta

Barbara Dossey

REFERENCES

1. Weber R: Foreword. In Dossey BM, Keegan L, Guzzetta CE, and Kolkmeier L: Holistic nursing: a handbook for practice, Gaithersburg, Md, 1988, Aspen.

Contents

xix

Detailed Contents

UNIT III
THE PERSON WITH CARDIOVASCULAR DYSFUNCTION

Interchapter 8 Risk Factors and Coronary Artery Disease, 196

8 The Person with Coronary Artery Disease Risk Factors, 197

Carolyn L. Murdaugh

Interchapter 9 Killer Mondays, 220

9 The Person with Angina Pectoris, 221

Sandra W. Haak
Sue E. Huether

Interchapter 10 The Value of Denial and Illusion, 250

10 The Person with Myocardial Infarction, 252

Sandra W. Haak
Sue E. Huether

Interchapter 11 Stressors and Cardiac Illness, 300

11 The Person with Heart Failure and Cardiogenic Shock, 302

Susan J. Quaal

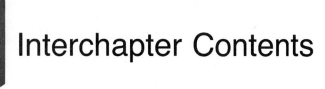

Interchapter Contents

Barbara Montgomery Dossey
Cathie E. Guzzetta

UNIT 1

HOLISTIC CARDIOVASCULAR FRAMEWORK

Interchapter 1

Wisdom, Meaning, and Health

T.S. Eliot once said,

Where's the wisdom we have lost in knowledge?

Where's the knowledge we have lost in information?[2]

Our profession—our entire society—has been swept along this century by a progressive movement toward technology and specialization. Archibald MacLeish[6] observed that ". . . we are deluged with facts, but we have lost, or are losing, our human ability to *feel* them."

At the patient's bedside we may sometimes feel overwhelmed with technical information and an avalanche of numbers. There is a tendency to lose sight of what all this information means—that it is connected to a living individual with feelings, emotions, and sensitivities that can never be fully represented by "data." We must devise ways to avoid being crushed by the deadening effects of technology. To do this we must remain open to those once-honored concepts of "caring" and "healing." This can help us cultivate wisdom—something that comes from inside us, not from the outside, and which has nothing to do with "the numbers."

Nursing wisdom is our antidote to the effects of technology, our way of transforming it from a threat into an ally. Wisdom alone can prevent us from becoming a robot at the bedside. We must find meaning in what we do and what illness and disease mean to our patients, as well as to us. Nikos Kazantzakis in *Zorba the Greek*[4] expresses this notion of meaning:

Everything in this world has a hidden meaning. . . . Men, animals, trees, stars, they are all hieroglyphics. . . . When you see them, you do not understand. You think they are really men, animals, trees, stars. It is only later . . . that you understand. . . .

Modern medical science, rooted in molecular biology and the "laws of nature," portray illness and disease as meaning nothing, simply an expression of what the atoms and molecules in our body are doing. Looking at illness as a purely physical event has proved helpful and led to stunning technical advances. But it is arbitrary and a limited way of viewing illness.

Our task as nurses is to go behind the obvious. We must seek the hidden meanings that Kazantzakis spoke about. To do this with our patients, we must be open, sensitive, and ask new questions. We must actively listen to the stories that our patients tell us. Life stories assign meaning to life's experiences and help shape one's world view. Learning to listen in a new way to our patients' stories or the stories we tell ourselves creates the potential for opening new dialogue for meaning. What does the illness *mean?* (That is, what does it symbolize, represent, or stand for to the person experiencing it or to us as we hear it?) When we can "catch the meaning" of our patients' illnesses, we can become "meaning therapists," as well as technical experts. This can revolutionize how we deal with our patients, and it can make our task as nurses immensely more fulfilling as well. Consider for example, a cardiac rehabilitation nurse who was able to "catch the meaning" of her patient's acute myocardial infarction (AMI). She was able to use this insight to help the patient explore the meaning of his job dissatisfaction and its possible link to his illness. On his return visit to the cardiac rehabilitation program, he related the following story to the nurse:

After talking to you last week, I came home and reflected on my continuing recovery from my heart attack. I was sitting in my back yard watching the birds flitting and chattering. It was Mon-

day. Ordinarily I would have been very unhappy on Monday—the first day of the week back at the office with the whole week ahead of me. But the birds didn't know it was Monday; they're just as happy on Monday as on Friday. Suddenly I wondered if the dread I have of Mondays had something to do with my health. I had my heart attack on Monday.[1]

Why Monday morning? Evidence suggests that job dissatisfaction may be the best predictor of AMI.[7,8] Going to a job that one despises, year after year, may be one of the most uniquely stressful events we can experience.[9] (See *Killer Mondays*, Interchapter 9, for details).

The issue of job satisfaction poses important questions not only for those patients we serve but for ourselves as well. What does our job mean to us? Does it challenge us? Does it offer us the chance to contribute, grow, and become wiser? These issues should be taken quite seriously, since the evidence suggests they are as important to our health as our blood pressure and cholesterol level. Some people in high-stress jobs seem to thrive and never get sick, while others break under the strain. What makes the difference?

Robert Krasek[3] and a team of researchers at the University of Southern California investigated the AMI rate in nearly 5,000 men. Correcting for age, smoking, and other factors, they found that the occupations with the highest incidence of AMI were those that combined high job stress with little control over the work load. Waiters in busy restaurants, gasoline service station attendants, certain data processors, cashiers, and assembly line workers were among those hit hardest—all occupations involving mindless, rushed work. When confronted with a high volume of work, they could only "peddle faster" to keep up. They were approxi-

2

mately four times more likely to have AMIs than persons in occupations who could control their work load and have a say in job tasks.[3]

Psychologist Suzanne C. Kobasa[5] has described the "three Cs" as factors preventing job-related illness. These are *control* (having a say in one's work), *challenge* (believing one's job is inherently worthwhile and that it offers one a chance to grow and become wiser), and *commitment* (not just to the job but to life off the job as well—to family, community, friends, and life in general). Without these factors, the incidence of illness is significantly increased in high-stress occupations.[5]

Nursing is a stressful profession, and being a nurse frequently involves life-or-death decisions. But although stressful, our opportunities to cultivate the "three Cs" are immense. We can work creatively with administrators to control our work load and keep it at a manageable level. We can recognize the unique challenge of patient care contributions we can make daily to the welfare of other persons, and the enrichment and wisdom that we gain in the process. The sense of personal fulfillment that comes from the nursing experience can enhance our commitment to life off the job. Our profession contains many built-in potentials for wisdom, meaning, and good health. For this we should be grateful.

REFERENCES

1. Dossey L: Meaning and medicine: a doctor's tales of breakthrough and healing, New York, 1991, Bantam.
2. Eliot TS: Choruses from the rock. In Eliot TS: Selected poems: the centenary edition, New York, 1988, Harcourt-Brace-Jovanovich.
3. Karasek R and others: Job characteristics in relation to the prevalence of myocardial infarction in the US health examination survey and the health and nutrition survey, Am J Pub Health 78(8):910, 1988.
4. Kazantzakis N: Zorba the greek, New York, 1952, Simon & Schuster.
5. Kobasa SC and others: Hardiness and health: a prospective study, J Personal Soc Psych 42(1):168, 1982.
6. MacLeish A: In May R and Paulus: Tillich as spiritual teacher, Dallas, 1988, Saybrook Press.
7. Muller JE: Circadian variation in the frequency of sudden death, Circ 75(1):131, 1987.
8. Rabkin SW and others: Chronobiology of cardiac sudden death in men, JAMA 244(12):1357, 1980.
9. Work in America: report of a special task force to the secretary of health, education and welfare, Cambridge, Mass, 1973, MIT Press.

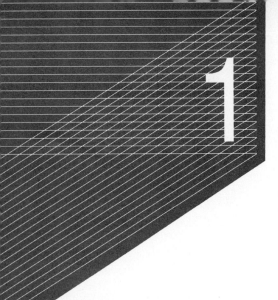

1

Holistic Cardiovascular Nursing

Barbara Montgomery Dossey
Cathie E. Guzzetta

LEARNING OBJECTIVES

1. Synthesize the components of a bio-psycho-social-spiritual model.
2. Discuss the difference between curing and healing.
3. Discuss the concept of holism.
4. Examine the components of a healing system.
5. Compare and contrast the different components and states of consciousness in Era I, Era II, and Era III medicine.
6. Analyze the different elements of holistic nursing practice.

As we approach the twenty-first century, two major challenges are emerging in cardiovascular nursing. The first is to integrate the concepts of technology, mind, and spirit into nursing practice; the second is to create models of health care that guide healing of the self and others. The following quotation from Patricia Benner and Judith Wrubel[4] highlights the predicament of technology and nursing today:

The dominant view of knowledge in the Western tradition emphasizes abstract, general, theoretical knowledge while overlooking and devaluing local, specific, practical knowledge and expert skillful clinical judgments about particular clinical situations. The way that involvement is central to expert knowledge is overlooked, reinforcing the myth that the expert must stand outside the situation, aloof and detached, to pronounce expert judgment.

Nursing and other caring practices have become paradoxical in a highly technical culture that seeks sweeping technologic breakthroughs to provide liberation and disburdenment. For example, American health care emphasizes the heroics of trauma centers while overlooking and underfunding programs for nutrition and prenatal care. Heart transplants receive tremendous funding and attention, whereas preventive measures are not funded as much because they are less exciting and culturally appealing. People typically focus on the dramatic transplant of a transplanted heart as the "breakthrough." Few notice that the intensive medical and nursing follow-up—solving the day-to-day problems of living with a transplanted organ, treating sores in the mouth resulting from immunosuppression, coping with a

new hormonal milieu, promptly recognizing and responding to infection and rejection—were all caring "breakthroughs" that led to the eventual success of heart transplantation. These essential day-to-day nursing care issues had to be solved. Yet they were overlooked in the scientific and popular media coverage of the transplant story.

Despite the significant technologic breakthroughs that have occurred in the treatment and management of patients with coronary artery disease, many problems remain. Technologic interventions, which include thrombolysis, percutaneous transluminal coronary angioplasty (PTCA), lasers, intracoronary stents, atherectomy devices, myocardial revascularization, and cardiac transplantation, are the major treatment and research foci for cardiovascular disease. Lesser significance is given to the role of the patient's attitudes, perceptions, emotions, and lifestyle, which contribute to risk factors leading to coronary artery disease.

Thrombus recanalization or lysis by thrombolytic agents such as t-PA, streptokinase, and urokinase is being widely incorporated. To date, t-PA appears to have the best reperfusion rates, but the reocclusion rate of 9% to 13% is equal among the agents.[33]

Research with a wide variety of cutters, grinders, shavers, and extractors are in clinical trials and close to approval for general usage. The principle common to all of these devices is the actual removal of atheromatous plaque and thrombus from the artery. Research has demonstrated that vascular smooth muscle cell proliferation in response to mechanical intervention in atheromatous disease causes a rate of recurring stenosis of about 30%.[33] The vascular smooth muscle cell remains the nemesis of percutaneous interventions in coronary disease.

Although patients may have a successful recovery from myocardial revascularization with patent jump grafts, the rate of vein graft occlusion varies from 5% to 20% within the first year after surgery; there is a yearly occlusion rate of 2.2% between 1 and 6 years.[43] Recurrent angina pectoris after the first year of surgery is probably caused by progressive atherosclerotic changes within the vein grafts or the native coronary arteries; this leads to direct stenosis and occlusion.[43] Atherosclerotic progression in the native circulation can decrease the outflow from the graft, and this low velocity can lead to thrombus formation. Also, competition between the bypass graft and the coronary artery after surgery may occur because of the reduced blood flow in the artery proximal to the graft. Thus if a partially occluded coronary artery becomes completely obstructed after bypass, later graft occlusion can be dangerous because the patient has less coronary blood flow than before surgery. This is a major problem and drawback to aortocoronary bypass surgery.[43]

Patients with angina pectoris after surgery can be taught to significantly reduce or eliminate chest pain and the associated anxiety with biobehavioral interventions, as well as make alterations in lifestyle that lead to coronary artery disease.[43] Clinical experience suggests that patients may be less adherent to lifestyle modifications after PTCA than after myocardial revascularization, perhaps because PTCA is less traumatic.[33]

Even after the use of technology such as surgery, the problem of coronary artery disease remains unless patients learn new strategies to reverse it. Health care professionals must address healing rather than just curing of symptoms and formulate steps to lead patients to a healthy lifestyle.

It is debatable whether real healing takes place in our modern hospitals, clinics, ambulatory care centers, cardiac rehabilitation programs, and home health care programs because much of the health care system functions as a disease-management industry. Many patients are asking how they can stabilize or reverse heart disease and thereby improve the quality of their lives.

In 1990, cardiologist Dr. Dean Ornish[29] published a landmark prospective, randomized, and controlled study demonstrating for the first time that it is possible for patients with supposedly fixed coronary artery lesions to reverse the disease through lifestyle changes. During this 1-year study, patients in the experimental group were asked to change to a vegetarian diet, stop smoking, and engage in stress-management techniques and moderate exercise.

The low-fat diet was nutritionally adequate and met the recommended daily allowances for all nutrients except vitamin B_{12}, which was supplemented. The diet included fruits, vegetables, grains, legumes, and soybean products without caloric restriction, no animal products except egg whites, and 1 cup of nonfat milk or yogurt. The diet contained approximately 10% of calories as fat (a polyunsaturated/saturated ratio greater than 1), 15% to 20% protein, and 70% to 75% predominately complex carbohydrates. Cholesterol intake was limited to 5 mg a day or less. Salt was restricted only for hypertensive patients. Caffeine was eliminated, and alcohol was limited to no more than 2 ounces per day. Alcohol was excluded for anyone with a history of alcoholism, and no one was encouraged to drink.

Exercise prescriptions were given based on baseline treadmill results. Patients were asked to reach target training heart rates of 50% to 80% of the heart rate at which 1 mm ST depression occurred during the baseline treadmill testing or, if the patient was not ischemic, to 50% to 80% of their age-adjusted maximum heart rate based on conditioning. Patients were also taught to evaluate exertion levels based on the Borg rating of perceived exertion. Patients were asked to exercise for at least 3 hours a week and to spend a minimum of 30 minutes per session exercising within their target heart rates.

Only one person in the experimental group was smoking at baseline. She agreed to quit smoking when she entered into the study.

The stress-management component included yoga, stretching exercises, breathing, progressive relaxation exercises, imagery, and meditation. The purpose of each intervention was to increase patients' sense of relaxation, concentration, and awareness about psychophysiologic self-regulation. Patients were asked to practice at least 1 hour each day and were given a 1-hour audiocassette tape to assist them in learning these skills.

Patients met twice a week for group discussion and social support. Each session was led by a clinical psychologist who helped the group to discuss increasing adherence to the lifestyle change program, to understand the meaning of their illness, and to connect emotionally and spiritually.

After 1 year, the patients in the experimental group demonstrated significant regression in their coronary artery disease, whereas the control group, who followed more standard medical recommendations, demonstrated a significant progession of their disease. The experimental group had an 82% overall change toward regression. Until this study, researchers had been unable to demonstrate regression of coronary artery disease.

This study was different because it considered the biologic, physiologic, sociologic, and spiritual aspects of the patient to be as important as the disease. It demonstrated the difference between "curing," which implies *intervention* (or medical, technologic intervening on the patients' behalf) and "healing," which implies *interaction* (or helping patients to act in their own behalf). It also demonstrated the effects possible when the health care team views the patient as a whole person, or holistically.

BIO-PSYCHO-SOCIAL-SPIRITUAL MODEL

The biopsychosocial model of health and illness represents the most comprehensive model available in health care. The assumptions of the biopsychosocial model suggest that all disease has a psychosomatic component and that biologic, psychologic, and sociologic factors are always involved in a patient's symptoms, disease, or illness. If these components are not addressed and treated properly, suboptimal therapeutic results occur.

The sociobiologic research that emerged in the 1960s demonstrated that lifestyles and life events could predict how and when a person might become ill.[32] The impact of these studies led to the introduction in 1977 of the biopsychosocial model of health and illness by George Engel,[20] which is based on the general-systems theory by Ludvig von Bertalanffy.[40] This dynamic model, which considers the integration of biologic, psychologic, and sociologic factors, was developed as a hierarchical structure or a continuum from the smaller, less complex units of life, (i.e., quarks, atoms, molecules, organelles, cells, tissues, and organ systems) to the level of person.[26] The individual is the lowest unit of the social hierarchy, which also includes family, culture, community, society, nation, and biosphere. Because no system is isolated and the hierarchy is part of the dynamic whole, a disturbance in one part of the system can affect other levels of the hierarchy. The implications of this biopsychosocial model for nursing are enormous.

In the quest for understanding the healing process, nurses have come to realize that even this biopsychosocial model falls short in characterizing the whole person. To facilitate healing, spirituality must be included. This new model illustrates all four dimensions as interdependent and interrelated (Figure 1-1).

Although many nurses recognize the importance of the human spirit, the spiritual dimension does not lend itself easily to objective measurement and is therefore often not addressed with the same relevance as the biopsychosocial dimensions.

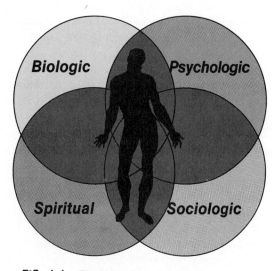

FIG. 1-1 The bio-psycho-social-spiritual model.

Human spirit and physiology

Spirituality is a broad concept that encompasses a person's values, meaning, and purpose in life. The human spirit involves traits of caring, love, honesty, wisdom, and imagination. It may be evidence of a higher power or existence or a guiding spirit. Others may believe spirit is a quality of transcendence, a guiding force, or something outside the self and beyond the individual nurse or patient. This may include the concept of organized religion or group worship with other people with similar belief systems. To others, spirit may suggest a purely mystical feeling or a flowing dynamic quality of unity. From this viewpoint, spirit is ineffable and undefinable.

The scientific physiologic data of mind modulation of the autonomic nervous system explains how the human spirit is transduced to the cellular level. Spirit, emotions, love, attitudes, meaning, and purpose literally leave their "tracks" in the body. The mind modulates the biochemical functions within the major organ systems of the autonomic nervous system (Figure 1-2). Mind modulation of cellular activities by the autonomic nervous system has three stages:[34]

1. Images, thoughts, attitudes, and feelings are generated in the frontal cortex (preverbal imagery).[1]
2. Images and thoughts are transmitted through state-dependent memory-learning, and emotional areas of the limbic-hypothalamic system by neurotransmitters that regulate the organ systems of the autonomic nervous system branches.
3. The neurotransmitters, norepinephrine (sympathetic branch) and acetylcholine (parasympathetic branch), initiate the information transduction that activates the biochemical changes within the different tissues down to the cellular level. Neurotransmitters act as messenger molecules. They cross the nerve cell junction gap and fit onto receptor sites in the cell walls, thus changing the receptor molecule structure. This causes a change in cell wall permeability and a shift of ions such as sodium, potassium, and calcium. The basic metabolism of each cell is also changed by activating hundreds of complex cell enzymes, which are the second-messenger system.

Biochemical changes occur simultaneously in the endocrine, immune, and neuropeptide systems in relation to emotions, attitudes, and thoughts. These biochemical changes are "tracks" of the spirit in the body. For example, if anatomic locations in the limbic system are traced down the nerve pathways and into the extremities and organs, these emotions, attitudes, and images correlate with physiologic changes in these brain structures and pathways. Likewise, neurotransmitters carry sensations and impressions back to the brain, providing it with further expressions and dimensions of our spirituality.

There is also a powerful physiologic component in the quality of being human, the concept of treating another with loving kindness. When people respond humanely,

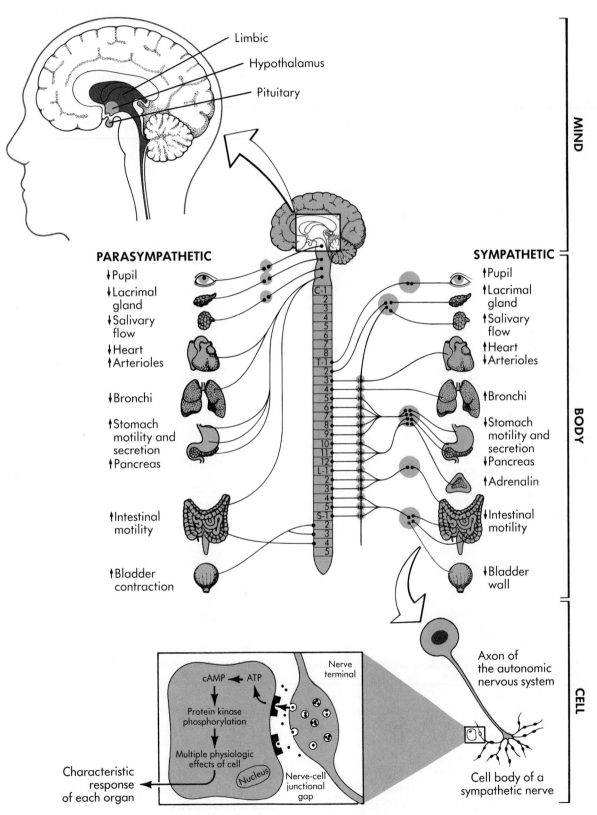

FIG. 1-2 Bodymind communication: mind modulation of the autonomic nervous system and its two branches, the sympathetic and parasympathetic, down to the cellular level.

Adapted from Rossi EL: The psychobiology of mind-body healing, New York, 1986, WW Norton & Co.

part of their autonomic nervous system produces positive physiologic changes. On the other hand, if they behave inhumanely, negative physiologic alterations occur. The state of humaneness exerts a powerful, yet frequently overlooked effect on physiologic well-being.

When nurses use biobehavioral interventions for themselves or teach patients how to use modulators such as relaxation, imagery, music, prayer, affirmations, or meditation, the sympathetic responses to stress are reduced and calming effects of the parasympathetic nervous system take over.[12] Anxiety, fear, pain, and grief, which occur in the patient with specific cardiovascular dysfunction, can be translated into physiologic and pathophysiologic changes such as chaotic dysrhythmias.[21,28] Chaotic QRS complexes reflect the patient's pathophysiologic state and simultaneous limbic-hypothalamic flow of anxiety and fear about cardiac symptoms. Patients' images, thoughts, and feelings are part of the "concrete QRS complexes" that are seen on the cardiac monitor or electrocardiogram. These same images also create and change the "unconscious complexes" of self-perception, which also plays a significant role in the healing process.[38]

Psychologic versus spiritual elements

With advancing technology, spiritual concerns have been little understood or confused with psychologic elements, organized religion, or personal religious beliefs. However, the spiritual component is a crucial cornerstone of healing. Psychologic elements must be distinguished from spiritual elements for an understanding of spirituality to occur.

Psychologic elements are characterized by language, perception, cognition, mood, thought, symbolic images, memory, intellect, and the ability to analyze and synthesize data.[24] *Spiritual elements* are characterized by the ability to seek purpose and meaning in the struggle and challenge of life. These elements include the ability to love, forgive, pray, worship; to transcend or move above ordinary circumstances; and to seek out the unfolding mystery, connectedness, and harmony of human existence. In summary, spiritual elements are capacities that enable a person to rise above or transcend the circumstances at hand.[24]

Joan Borysenko,[6] a psychologist and scientist, has written about *psychological pessimism,* which is the state of learned helplessness associated with physical illness and mental distress. She believes that psychological pessimism must be extended to include *spiritual pessimism,* or the idea that a person will somehow be punished unless they are "good enough." This notion is often associated with Judeo-Christian thought and has recently been coined "new-age guilt" by Ken Wilbur.[44] An important role of nurses is to be aware of these issues and help facilitate a shift within patients from spiritual pessimism and the underlying psychological pessimism to *spiritual optimism.*[6] Spiritual optimism presupposes the intrinsic goodness and the poten-

tial within each person and views mistakes and problems as teachers of compassion and wisdom rather than as evidence of unworthiness. A shift in these fundamental attitudes heals not only the physical body but leads to a recovery of the soul where a person becomes spirit filled.[17]

Dr. Clifford Kuhn,[24] a psychiatrist, has integrated a "bio-psycho-social-spiritual" model within the Division of Behavioral Medicine at the University of Louisville School of Medicine. He has developed a list of objective inquiries about meaning, belief and faith, love, forgiveness, prayer, capacity for quiet and meditation, and worship to help distinguish psychologic from the spiritual elements. His research shows that the role of the psychologic elements are to work or manipulate the data at hand, whereas the function of spirit is to rise above the manifest data. He further states that the mind brings a person into a problem, whereas the spirit lifts the person above it. The prototype of a healthy spirit is as follows:[24]

A healthy spirit is demonstrated by the ability to attach a meaning and purpose to life events, reflecting hope, faith, and a relative absence of guilt. A healthy spirit enables a person to love and forgive self and others, and to participate in laughter and celebration. The spiritually healthy person is involved in a community of faith and exercises his or her spirit in worship, prayer, and meditation as broadly defined in our inventory. If such attributes cannot be observed in a person, it is likely there is a spiritual illness present that should be addressed if the treatment plan is to be a thorough one.

Characteristics of spirituality

Margaret Burchardt[8] synthesized 109 nursing research studies and articles on the concept of spirit and spirituality. Her synthesis reveals that this concept falls into the following categories:
  1. Spirit/spirituality
  2. Spiritual dimension
  3. Spiritual well-being
  4. Spiritual needs

From these categories, three defining characteristics of spirituality evolved: unfolding mystery, harmonious interconnectedness, and inner strengths. *Unfolding mystery* refers to a person's experience about life's purpose and meaning, mystery, uncertainty, and struggles. *Harmonious interconnectedness* includes relatedness, connectedness, and harmony with the self, others, environment, and higher power or God. *Inner strengths* refers to a sense of awareness, self, consciousness, inner resources, sacred source, unifying force, inner core, and transcendence. The box, p. 10, provides reflective questions for assessing, evaluating, and increasing awareness of the spirituality in the self and others. This tool is based on the three defining characteristics of spirituality.

From the synthesis of the current literature, spirit and spirituality are frequently linked to religiosity. Thus the

ASSESSING THE SPIRITING PROCESS

To facilitate the healing process in patients, families, significant others, and yourself, the following reflective questions assist in assessing, evaluating, and increasing awareness of the spiriting process in yourself and others.

UNFOLDING MYSTERY

These questions assess a person's ability to seek meaning and fulfillment in life, manifest hope, and accept ambiguity and uncertainty.
- What gives your life meaning?
- Do you have a sense of purpose in life?
- Does your illness interfere with your life goals?
- Why do you want to get well?
- How hopeful are you about obtaining a better degree of health?
- Do you feel that you have a responsibility in maintaining your health?
- Will you be able to make changes in your life to maintain your health?
- Are you motivated to get well?
- What is the most important or powerful thing in your life?

INNER STRENGTHS

These questions assess a person's ability to manifest joy and recognize strengths, choices, goals, and faith.
- What brings you joy and peace in your life?
- What can you do to feel alive and full of spirit?
- What traits do you like about yourself?
- What are your personal strengths?
- What choices are available to you to enhance your healing?
- What life goals have you set for yourself?
- Do you think that stress in any way caused your illness?
- How aware were you of your body before you became sick?
- What do you believe in?
- Is faith important in your life?
- How has your illness influenced your faith?
- Does faith play a role in regaining your health?

HARMONIOUS INTERCONNECTEDNESS

These questions assess a person's positive self-concept, self-esteem, and sense of self; sense of belonging in the world with others; capacity to pursue personal interests; and ability to demonstrate love of self and self-forgiveness.
- How do you feel about yourself right now?
- How do you feel when you have a true sense of yourself?
- Do you pursue things of personal interest?
- What do you do to show love for yourself?
- Can you forgive yourself?
- What do you do to heal your spirit?

These questions assess a person's ability to connect in life-giving ways with family, friends, and social groups and to engage in the forgiveness of others.
- Who are the significant people in your life?
- Do you have friends or family in town who are available to help you?
- Who are the people to whom you are closest?
- Do you belong to any groups?
- Can you ask people for help when you need it?
- Can you share your feelings with others?
- What are some of the most loving things that others have done for you?
- What are the loving things that you do for other people?
- Are you able to forgive others?

These questions assess a person's capacity for finding meaning in worship or religious activities and a connectedness with a divinity or universe.
- Is worship important for you?
- What do you consider the most significant act of worship in your life?
- Do you participate in any religious activities?
- Do you believe in God or a higher power?
- Do you think that prayer is powerful?
- Have you ever tried to empty your mind of all thoughts to see what the experience might be like?
- Do you use relaxation or imagery skills?
- Do you meditate?
- Do you pray?
- What is your prayer?
- How are your prayers answered?
- Do you have a sense of belonging in this world?

These questions assess a person's ability to experience a sense of connection with all of life and nature; an awareness of the effects of the environment on life and well-being; and a capacity or concern for the health of the environment.
- Do you ever feel at some level a connection with the world or universe?
- How does your environment have an impact on your state of well-being?
- What are your environmental stressors at work and at home?
- Do you incorporate strategies to reduce your environmental stressors?
- Do you have any concerns for the state of your immediate environment?
- Are you involved with environmental issues such as recycling environmental resources at home, work, or in your community?
- Are you concerned about the survival of the planet?

Based on Burkhardt M: Spirituality: an analysis of the concept, Holistic Nurs Pract 3(3):69, 1989.

use of the participle, *spiriting,* is more representative of the concept of spirit,[8] and it reflects the concept of spirit in its broadest sense. The reflective questions in the box also facilitate healing because they can stimulate spontaneous, independent, and meaningful initiatives to improve the patient's capacity for recovery and healing.

Spirit has been documented as the healing force in the reversal of cardiovascular disease, as well as in the remission of other diseases. The human spirit influences inner life and perceptions about purpose and meaning, which can make the difference between life and death.*

Meaning

Nurses play a key role in helping patients recognize the impact of perceived meaning surrounding all aspects of their heart disease. In Ornish's study,[29] a major component for the regression of coronary artery disease was the new insights gained by patients about their perceived meaning of their illness (see p. 5). Thus meaning, reasons for seeking it, reactions to it, and ways to retain it are important factors to consider when assessing a patient.

When a person is faced with crisis or illness, the ascribed meaning is one of the most important factors in that person's state of well-being. The basis for illness can be viewed from at least eight points of reference: illness as (1) challenge, (2) enemy, (3) punishment, (4) weakness, (5) relief, (6) strategy, (7) irreparable loss or damage, and (8) value.[27]

Meaning can be viewed in two ways.[18] One is the meaning of patients' illness—their interpretation of the event, the significance it holds, and what they believe it may symbolize or represent. The second type of meaning is the impact of "life meanings" on health and illness—the capacity of the perceived meaning and experiences of a lifetime to affect bodies. In both usages, meaning is inseparable from actual thoughts, feelings, and emotions. Because "meaning" and "emotions" occupy a continuum, the nurse must be aware of both types of meaning to help facilitate healing.

Meaning is seen as differences—contrast, novelty, and heterogeneity—and it is necessary for the healthy function of human beings. People seek meaning because life seems fuller and richer when it represents something positive for them. The more they understand about meaning in life, the more they empower themselves to recognize more effective ways to cope with life and to learn more effective methods of handling issues. In doing this, they create richer meaning in their daily lives. This attention to meaning also allows nurses to be more effective with patients in teaching about meaning.

When people believe meaning is absent, their bodies become bored; boredom can develop into depression, disease, and death.[18] At times, it seems that meaning may be absent from life and the universe; in fact, it is only a matter

of the meaning chosen. The choices are crucial. Nowhere is this more important or apparent than in health and illness. Much scientific data supports that it is impossible to separate the mental and physical parts of being. The importance of meaning is directly linked with mind modulation of all body systems, which influence states of wellness or illness. The following true case study is an example of how meaning can surface in the life of an individual and be a matter of life or death.

A 50-year-old man has had multiple abscesses of his right breast for 1 year.[22] These had required incision and drainage over 8 months, which kept him out of work for an appreciable amount of time. He finally agreed to go to the hospital and had a mastectomy in August. He had no previous history of cardiovascular disease, but the evening after his surgery and recovery from anesthesia, he developed a myocardial infarction. After this he did quite well in recovery from his infarction in the hospital and at home. According to his wife, however, he was increasingly depressed and particularly upset that he was not able to return to work. In late October, he had become "not angry," she said, but just "feeling he couldn't do anything about it" when a group of local youngsters blew up a firecracker, damaging their mailbox on the night of Halloween. Three days later his wife persuaded him to take their first stroll of his convalescence into the garden of their home. They walked into the back garden and noted for the first time that an arborway, which he had built early that summer and of which he was very proud, had been sprayed with tar paint. While his wife expressed anger, the patient said he did not feel good and wanted to return to the house. He got 20 yards, as far as the kitchen door, and collapsed. His wife asked him whether he was having any pain. He replied, "No." He died within 5 minutes.

Because it was unusual for a man to have a mastectomy, I asked the patient's wife whether having a mastectomy was of any particular significance to this man. She stated that her sister had died 2 years before, on November 12, with a carcinoma of the breast after a mastectomy. This man's death occurred on November 3. His wife then indicated that on November 3, 1 year before, the patient's sister, who had a carcinoma of the breast and a mastectomy, had also died. Also on November 12, 1 year before, his older and favorite brother had died instantly of a myocardial infarction.*

This man's plight illustrates how meaning can disrupt physical health. He was overwhelmed with a sense of failure and helplessness, all the feelings that make up the "no-exit" syndrome. He could not express his outrage but kept those feelings inside. It is possible, of course, for persons to have an inner acceptance of life's events, but that is not what this man felt. He was simply overpowered and beaten down, and as his world continued to collapse, he relented. Meaning was gone, and all emotions were absent so there was no reason to live any longer.

His death is also a classic example of the "anniversary phenomenon," in which something dreadful occurs at some yearly increment from the death of a significant person in someone's life.[19] It seems that this man was living out the fate of others about whom he cared—two women

---

*References 10, 16-18, 35, 37, and 39.

*Adapted from Green WA, Goldstein S, and Moss A: Psychosocial aspects of sudden death, Archives Intern Med 129:725, 1972.

who had mastectomies at the same time of year and his favorite brother who had died a year earlier, also from a heart attack.

Specific meaning is also illustrated in the following situations involving two different individuals.[15] One healthy woman, when told that her husband was suing for a divorce, experienced immediate emotional shock, suffered a cardiac arrest, and died abruptly. Another woman with severe heart disease and incapacitating angina was also told that her husband was suing for a divorce. Having endured a miserable marriage for decades, she was delighted and experienced an amazing clinical improvement. Her angina disappeared, her physician stopped her cardiac medication, and she took up jogging. These life events were the same, but the meaning they held for each person differed. The difference in meaning was a difference between life and death.

Because meaning and emotions go hand in hand, the meanings that a person perceives can affect the body, as well as emotions. These connections are so intimate that a person must think of the body and mind as a single, integrated unit, or bodymind.

To keep meaning in life, a person should pay more attention to the meaning of life. This is difficult to do. It may be easier to concentrate on cholesterol level, blood pressure, diet, vitamin intake, body weight, and annual physical examinations, but if people really believe that death is possible not only from heart failure but from "meaning failure," perhaps they would be more attentive to the meanings they create in their lives.

Wellness and illness are linked. Wellness is not simply physical health because there is no clear separation of the physical, mental, and spiritual. This recognition places much more responsibility on the individual and less on the health care providers for health. As a result, nurses should routinely assess and evaluate their patient's human potential to keep meaning in his or her life.

Nurses should be leary of proclamations that any particular problem is "all physical, mental, or spiritual." These simplistic statements cannot be defended any longer in modern medical science. Those who make such claims cannot define "physical," "mental," or "spiritual" because the dividing line between them has become increasingly thin.

Nurses as learners of meaning

Nurses continually learn about meaning. Their meaning is influenced by what they read, hear, and feel. Em Bevis[5] states that a person's meanings are individual and personal and that they must have congruence with the person's experience, belief systems, expectations, and the context of the event. Context assumes significance in uncovering meaning and involves past and present life, as well as beliefs about the future. Interpretation and meaning also are part of the "syntactical category of learning."[5] In syntax, a per-

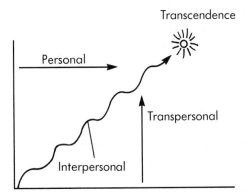

FIG. 1-3 Dimensions of individual growth. Personal growth is represented on the left, transpersonal on the right. The curved line is life's path, which is never linear but fluctuates as it incorporates aspects of each as a person grows. The star is the point where individuality (personal dimension) and universality (transpersonal dimension) join.
Adapted from Brown M: The unfolding self, Los Angeles, 1983, Intermountain Associates for Psychosynthesis Press.

TABLE 1-1
Dimensions of Individual Growth

Dimension	Characteristics
Personal dimension	Sense of meaning; reasoning skills and logic; self-motivation; goal-oriented focus
Interpersonal dimension	Communication and social skills; friendship and relationships with family and community; development of self-reflection and biobehavioral skills to evoke more transcendental moments that lead to transpersonal understanding
Transpersonal dimension	Understanding of belonging to humanity; acceptance of a universal existence

son looks at insights, patterns, and processes and finds or seeks the meanings.

Nurses can become more aware of meaning in themselves and can help patients explore their meaning when purpose and dimensions of individual growth are explored.[7,13] Purpose implies a conscious attempt toward maximizing potential. Increasing purpose can be achieved along three dimensions of growth, the *personal, interpersonal,* and *transpersonal* (Figure 1-3 and Table 1-1).

The personal dimension of growth concerns meaning and integration of personal life. This dimension—possessing logical and analytical thought and being self-motivated and goal oriented in personal and professional life—is highly valued in Western culture. The transpersonal dimension is traditionally less valued in Western culture; yet it is equally important. This dimension concerns the ultimate meaning and purpose of the universal existence of humanity.

A third dimension of human growth, the interpersonal dimension, which is part of the other dimensions, should also be considered. This is life's path, which weaves between the personal and transpersonal. In the interpersonal dimension, people develop the basic social skills of communication, courtesy, and friendship that are necessary for survival with others. When beginning to develop along the transpersonal dimension, these persons become aware of the basic interdependency of the self merging with others.[31] The interpersonal dimension allows them to have balanced and supportive relationships with family, friends, community, and patients. It allows the depth necessary in meaningful relationships. As patients and nurses integrate their personal and transpersonal dimensions, the following identifiable characteristics emerge:[7,13]

1. The capacity for responsibility and choice for the moment and throughout life
2. A preference for living in accordance with personal purpose and regarding as less valuable any conflicting aspects of life
3. The capacity to accept the limitations of life and a responsibility and willingness to be in the world just as it is
4. A sense of having a destiny, meaning, or overall purpose in life

Nurses must be sensitive to the effects of meaning. Words intended as innocent can carry powerful meanings for a patient and can have unanticipated effects.[11,12] Nurses must strive to develop a "sixth sense" or sensitivity to the needs of patients and intuition about their emotional requirements and responses. This is not as difficult as it might seem. When nurses remember the importance of being fully present with patients or family, giving them undivided attention, and caring genuinely for them, higher levels of meaning evolve and healing occurs.

HOLISM

With holism, a person must consider the integrated whole to understand an object, person, or situation. Holism is a way of viewing everything in terms of patterns and processes that combine to form a whole, instead of seeing things as fragments, pieces, or parts.

Cartesian dualism

In the 1700s, Rene Descartes, a French philosopher, developed ideas that greatly influenced the modern approach to illness and disease. He contended that humans were composed of two parts: mind and body. It was thought that ordinarily these two parts did not interact. This body-mind split is referred to as *cartesian dualism.*

Descartes believed that, because the body and mind did not interact, disease must be a body process. Thus science was given a rationale for investigating the body without considering the soul. As the scientific era dawned, more research was done. With the invention of the microscope and development of histology, the effect of disease on the body was further established.

In this century the level of scientific investigation has gone deeper. Modern techniques of biochemistry and molecular biology have made it possible to identify molecular abnormalities that cause certain diseases. A tenet of modern medicine states that it should be possible to identify the molecular abnormality for every disease. Thus the modern theory of disease has come to be known as the *molecular theory of disease causation.*

Developments in molecular theory have given rise to the philosophy of *reductionism,* or the idea that all the workings of humans are accounted for by the behavior of the parts of the body—the atoms and electrons that make up the substance. Currently our philosophy is one of *determinism,* where mental life—our consciousness—is determined by molecules. However, this framework of modern molecular medicine, when examined more carefully, is not entirely complete.

Allopathy versus holistic models

Allopathy is the method of combating disease with techniques that produce effects different from those produced by the disease. The primary assertion of the holistic framework is that consciousness is real. Holistic concepts do not explain how consciousness and spirit arise, and reductionist concepts do not explain how the brain generates consciousness. Table 1-2 provides a comparision of the allopathic versus holistic models.

Many diseases can be explained at the molecular level, but this is only one level. The holistic framework asserts that any explanation about the cause of disease must include consciousness and spirit as central factors. Holism is at the root of the debate that has occupied philosophers for the past 300 years: the relationship between the body, mind, and spirit and how they are connected.

Holistic nursing

A working description of holistic nursing is seen in the box, p. 13. Nurses who practice from a holistic perspective feel more satisfied with their professional life because the holistic model is truer to the value systems of the patient and the nurse. Thus it meets more of the nurse's needs. As the health care profession has become more humanized, nurses have learned to be more humane to themselves, not

TABLE 1-2

Assumptions of Allopathic and Holistic Models of Health Care

Allopathic model	Holistic model
Treatment of symptoms	Search for patterns, causes
Specialized	Integrated; concerned with the whole patient
Emphasis on efficiency	Emphasis on human values
Professional should be emotionally neutral	Professional's caring is a component of healing
Pain and disease are wholly negative	Pain and disease may be valuable signals of internal conflicts
Primary intervention with drugs, surgery	Minimal intervention with appropriate technology, complemented with a range of noninvasive techniques (psycho-technologies, diet, exercise)
Body seen as a machine in good or bad repair	Body seen as dynamic system, a complex energy field within fields (family, workplace, environment, culture, life history)
Disease or disability seen as an entity	Disease or disability seen as a process
Emphasis on eliminating symptoms and disease	Emphasis on achieving maximum bodymind health
Patient is dependent	Patient is autonomous
Professional is authority	Professional is therapeutic partner
Body and mind are separate; psychosomatic illnesses seen as mental; may refer (patient) to psychiatrist	Bodymind perspective, psychosomatic illness is the province of all health care professionals
Mind is secondary factor in organic illness	Mind is primary or co-equal factor in all illness
Placebo effect is evidence of power of suggestion	Placebo effect is evidence of mind's role in disease and healing
Primary reliance on quantitative information (charts, tests, and dates)	Primary reliance on qualitative information, including patient reports and professional's intuition; quantitative data an adjunct
"Prevention" seen as largely environmental; vitamins, rest, exercise, immunization, not smoking	"Prevention" synonymous with wholeness: in work, relationships, goals, body-mind-spirit

From Ferguson M: Aquarian conspiracy, Los Angeles, 1980, JP Tarcher.

WORKING DESCRIPTION OF HOLISTIC NURSING

Holistic nursing embraces all nursing practice, which has healing the whole person as its goal. Holistic nursing requires that the nurse integrate self-care/self-responsibility in his or her life to help facilitate healing and caring for others. Self-care/self-responsibility leads the nurse to a greater awareness of the interconnectedness of all individuals and their relationships to the human and global community.

Holistic nursing is both an art and a science. Holistic nursing allows dichotomies to be affirmed and acknowledged. Therefore holistic nursing involves analyzing and synthesizing the interrelationships of the bio-psycho-social-spiritual dimensions of the person, understanding that the whole is greater than the sum of its parts. Holistic nursing also involves understanding an individual as an integral totality interacting with and being acted on by both internal and external environments. Holistic practice draws on nursing knowledge, theories, expertise, and intuition to guide the nurse in becoming a therapeutic partner with the individual in strengthening the individual's responses to facilitate the healing process and achieve wholeness.

From American Holistic Nurses' Association, July, 1991. Address: 4101 Lake Boone Trail, Suite 201, Raleigh, NC 27607. (919) 787-5181.

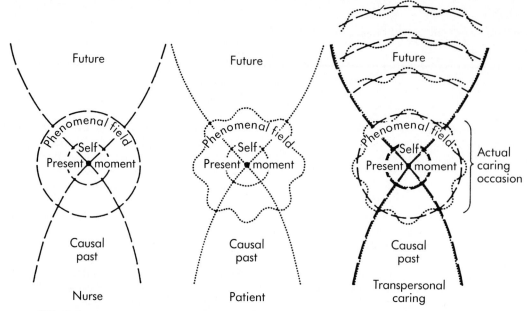

FIG. 1-4   Dynamics of the human caring process.
From Watson J: Nursing: human science and human care: a theory of nursing, East Norwalk, Conn, 1985, Appleton & Lange. Illustration by Melvin L. Gabel, University of Colorado Health Sciences Center, Biomedical Communications Department.

just to their patients. They are learning to say as professionals, "I have needs, too. I must honor these needs, even as I respect your needs."

HEALING SYSTEM
Human science and transpersonal caring

Jean Watson,[42] the visionary nurse theorist, views nursing as a human science, which must be based on the following:

1. A philosophy of human freedom, choices, and responsibility
2. A biology and psychology of holism
3. A theory of origins, methods, and limits of knowledge (epistemology) that allows not only for practical experiences (empirics) but also for advancement of ethestics, ethical values, intuition, and the process of discovery
4. A branch of metaphysics that deals with the nature of being/reality (ontology) of space and time
5. A context of interhuman events, processes, and relationships
6. A scientific world view that is open

Watson[42] believes that transpersonal human caring and caring transactions are the giving-receiving behaviors and responses between two people (nurse and other) that allow for contact within the subjective world of persons (through physical, mental, and spiritual routes). The nurse and pa-

tient share their individual uniqueness, which creates an event of caring (Figure 1-4).[42]

The dynamics of the human caring process are mutually interdependent; patient, nurse, and family are a part of one another. This experience is an *intersubjective*, human-to-human relationship in which the nurse affects and is affected by the patient.[42] They become co-participants. This involves actions and choices by both; it also involves the integration of the feminine and masculine principles.

Integrating masculine and feminine principles

Over the last 25 years the focus of health care has been on curing symptoms, as in an allopathic model. Curing is associated with power, analysis of data, and technology, which are typically associated with masculine values. Caring, which is more typically associated with feminine values, has had little status and fewer financial rewards.[2]

Jeanne Achterberg,[1,2] a leading psychophysiologist and authority on the psychophysiology of healing and the history of woman in the healing profession, suggests that men and women health care professionals should learn to recognize masculine and feminine qualities. Examples of these qualities are listed in Table 1-3.

As nurses learn to integrate their masculine and feminine qualities, they can motivate each other and learn to honor and talk about their healing interactions. Within the context of community, nurses honoring each other facili-

TABLE 1-3

Examples of Masculine and Feminine Qualities

Masculine	Feminine
Intellect	Intuition
Linear	Nonlinear
How	Why
Knowledge	Wisdom
Power	Compassion
Analysis	Synthesis
Expansive	Contained
Proactive	Reactive
Giving	Receiving
External/public	Internal/private
Technical	Natural
Form	Process
Competition	Collaboration
Objective	Subjective
Doing to	Being with
Curing	Caring
Fixing	Nurturing
Reason	Feelings
Physical world	Invisible world
Decisive	Flexible

Adapted from Achterberg J: Woman as healer, Boston, 1990, Shambhala Publications, Inc.

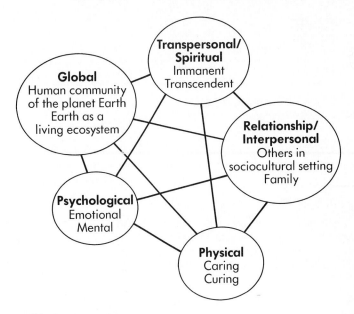

FIG. 1-5   The healing system.

From Achterberg J: Woman as healer, Boston, 1990, Shambhala Publications, Inc.

tate empowerment and inner peace. Achterberg[2,3] calls for a redefinition of healing, which includes the following concepts that incorporate masculine and feminine qualities:

1. Healing is a lifelong journey toward wholeness.
2. Healing is remembering what has been forgotten about connections, unity, and interdependency among all living and nonliving things.
3. Healing is embracing what is feared most.
4. Healing is opening what has been closed and softening what has hardened into obstruction.
5. Healing is entering into the transcendent, timeless moments when a person experiences the divine.
6. Healing is creativity, passion, and love.
7. Healing is seeking and expressing the self in its fullness, its light and shadow, and its male and female.
8. Healing is learning to trust life.

Achterberg[2] views a more effective healing system as interconnected with feminine energy compared with the more traditional model of linear, hierarchical relationships, which has its origins in a masculine order of thought. This healing system (Figure 1-5) has a complexly interwoven set of bonds at various levels. These bonds are the healing forces of the human spirit: Love, compassion, motivation, conscious and unconscious thought, purpose, and will. Achterberg[2] states the following:

Each level of the healing system demands a technology and a data base. True meaning comes from the knowledge about

physical, psychologic, relationships/interpersonal, global, and transpersonal/spiritual domains.

In this healing system, there is no simple cause and effect, but there is the interrelationship of many factors. Healing cannot be the domain of allopathic curing, but must be a blend of human values and different practitioners when necessary.

The challenges are to integrate feminine values with masculine standards; to couple flexibility with decisiveness, perspective with focus, synthesis with analysis.

Nurses who have internalized the idea of healing can more easily help others through crisis and transition and facilitate the healing process in themselves and others. The continual process of healing the self is the first step in facilitating healing in others.

Eras of medicine

It is possible to delineate three different stages of medicine that are operational in the West (Table 1-4).[17,18] These stages can be referred to as *eras*. These eras are complementary; each has its strengths and weaknesses. A major nursing challenge is to blend the attributes of these eras within clinical practice.

Era I medicine began to take shape in the 1860s, at which time medicine began to become increasingly scientific. This approach is based on an understanding of health and illness that is completely physical in nature. It emphasizes a reductionistic, cause-and-effect approach to understanding the workings of the body, which is viewed largely as a machine. The emphasis in the Era I approach is on the use of *technology* in diagnosis, testing, and therapy.

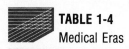

TABLE 1-4
Medical Eras

Era I	Era II	Era III
SPACE-TIME CHARACTERISTIC		
Local	Local	Nonlocal
SYNONYM		
Mechanical or "modern" medicine	Mind-body, complementary, or alternative medicine	Nonlocal medicine
DESCRIPTION		
Causal, deterministic, describable by classical concepts of space-time and matter-energy; mind not a factor; "mind" a result of brain mechanisms	Mind a major factor in healing within the single person; mind has causal power and, thus is not fully explainable by classical concepts in physics; includes but goes beyond Era I	Mind a factor in healing both within and between persons; mind not completely localized to points in space (brains or bodies) or time (present moment or single lifetimes); mind unbounded in space and time and thus ultimately unitary or One; healing at a distance is permitted; not describable by classical concepts of space-time or matter-energy
EXAMPLES		
Any form of therapy focusing solely on effects of things on the body, including acupuncture and homeopathy and the use of herbs. Includes almost all forms of "modern" medicine (e.g., drugs, surgery, irradiation, CPR)	Any therapy emphasizing the effects of consciousness solely within the individual body; psycho-neuroimmunology, counseling, hypnosis, biofeedback, relaxation therapies, and most types of imagery-based "alternative" therapies included	Any therapy in which effects of consciousness bridge between different persons; all forms of distant healing, intercessory prayer, "psychic" and shamanic healing, so-called "miracles," diagnosis at a distance, and noncontact therapeutic touch included; certain emotions—love, compassion, empathy—exerting nonlocal effects; when these emotions enter Era I and II therapies, these may take on Era III characteristics. Anytime a therapist is involved, this possibility holds.

For a detailed description of the three medical eras, see Dossey L: *Meaning and medicine: a doctor's tales of breakthrough and healing,* New York, 1991, Bantam Books.

All forms of treatment, including drugs, surgery, irradiation, diet, and exercise, as well as alternative measures such as acupuncture and homeopathy, are physical in nature. In Era I medicine, the mind or consciousness is regarded as a by-product of the chemical, anatomic, and physiologic aspects of the brain and is not felt to be a major factor in the origins of health or disease. The individual is considered to be "local" in nature; that is, he or she is localized to a specific location in space (the body itself) and in time (the present moment and a single lifetime).

In the 1950s, however, another era of medicine began to emerge, *Era II* medicine or "mind-body medicine." The hallmark of the Era II approach, originally called *psychosomatic medicine,* is the recognition that the actions of a person's mind or consciousness—thoughts, feelings, emotions, beliefs, meanings, and attitudes—exert important effects on the behavior of the physical body. This is a major departure from the Era I view. In the Era II approach, however, mind or consciousness continues to be seen as in Era I, as an individual phenomenon, localized to the brain and body of the person and thus fixed in space and time.

On the basis of emerging data, it is clear that another era of medicine is in the process of development, Era III or "nonlocal" medicine. The key feature of this perspective is the different way in which the mind is seen in relation to the brain and body. Firm evidence has accumulated, as a result of carefully controlled clinical studies, that there is some aspect of the human psyche that is not confined to points in space such as the brain or body or in time such as the present moment. There is evidence that this aspect of the mind, in addition to its ability to affect the body, can exert influences on distant bodies. Because of the evidence that the mind cannot be confined or localized to the brain or body of an individual and that it is not bound to the present moment, it can be called "nonlocal"—unbounded, unconfined, and not localized. Thus the experimental data have led to the hypothesis of a nonlocal form of medicine in which the mind of one person can influence the health of another, regardless of spatial separation.

Currently, the concept of nonlocality is generally unfamiliar to health care professionals. In modern physics, however, nonlocality has been established as an essential feature of how the world behaves in the subatomic realm. If it has proved essential to use nonlocal concepts in describing simple systems such as electrons, it is perhaps not surprising that it also is necessary to use this concept in describing the behavior of much more complex systems such as human beings. A challenge to health care professionals is to become familiar with the concept of nonlocality and to assess the ways in which it seems to manifest in our lives.

In addition to being important in health and illness, there are some surprising psychologic, religious, and spiritual implications of nonlocality. If there is indeed some aspect of the human psyche that is nonlocal—unbounded in space and time—this part of human consciousness begins to resemble the concept of the soul. Traditionally in the West, people have conceived of the soul as being infinite in time and space—eternal, immortal, and omnipresent. This is the definition of nonlocality. It can then be said that evidence for a nonlocal part of the mind is also indirect evidence for the existence of the human soul. The concept of nonlocality and the evidence for a nonlocal aspect of human consciousness are examined in Larry Dossey's *Recovering the Soul.**

These nonlocal and local states of consciousness are supported by Achterberg's concepts[1] of preverbal and transpersonal imagery. *Preverbal imagery* are images formed in the limbic system that act on persons' physical beings to change their physiologic activity (see p. 6). The second type of imagery is *transpersonal imagery,* in which the consciousness of one person can affect the physical substrate of another. These two types of imagery correspond to local versus nonlocal events. They also fall within, respectively, the Era II (local, mind-body) and Era III (nonlocal) healing methods (Table 1-4). Health and healing are indeed a collective affair.

Physical health, spirituality, and healing†

Healing is a process of bringing all parts of the self (the biologic, psychologic, sociologic, and spiritual) together to a deeper level of knowing. The feeling that results from deeper knowing and healing can be similar to the universal spiritual experience of oneness and unity. The result is a higher degree of integration, balance, and happiness in life while becoming aware of the importance and relationship of all of life's parts. To be healed, then, is to become whole, and the highest form of healing is to know and feel the wholeness and unity that has occurred.

---

*Larry Dossey: Recovering the soul, New York, 1989, Bantam Books.
†Adapted from Dossey B: Foreword: spirituality and healing, Holistic Nurs Prac 3(3):7, 1989.

Frequent misconceptions occur in contemporary thinking about the relationship between physical and spiritual health. For example, many people equate spiritual health with bodily health. It would seem that people who are highly evolved spiritually would be supremely healthy because healing and spirituality seem so closely related. Yet bodily health and spiritual attainment do not always correlate. Sometimes an inverse correlation seems to occur because some people experience a sense of wholeness with physical illness. When physical illness disappears as a person progresses on a spiritual path, it seems to be a gift. What is important is the inner life of the spirit, not the outer health of the body.

Equating spiritual and physical health is a practice that currently abounds in "holistic" health circles. It is heard that if a person is "really" spiritual enough, perfect bodily health follows. Cancer and heart disease will be cured, high blood pressure will decrease, and life will be long and healthy. This is not a holistic view because it excludes certain things from the whole. It places certain qualities such as suffering or illness apart from the ultimate and thus creates a dualism that is contrary to the principle of wholeness.

Another insidious problem occurs frequently when physical and spiritual health are considered the same. The problem takes place when a person tries to "be more spiritual" when thinking only of becoming healthier physically. Combining these two goals as if they are one frequently does not work. For example, if a person tries to meditate with an overt reason in mind, meditation simply does not work. This point can also be easily demonstrated in the biofeedback laboratory when a person *tries* to warm hands or relax muscles. As long as there is an intentional, active striving for a particular outcome, a person will fail. However, when a person puts personal agendas aside and learns to "let go" and not be attached to results, a real breakthrough occurs and the task is quickly learned. This "passive volition," this "doing by not doing," is the key to spiritual awareness and healing.

In some cases, "holistic" or "spiritual" therapies are acceptable, whereas orthodox drugs, surgery, and irradiation are not. This is an extreme attitude. It is common today for persons to believe that it is a sign of moral or spiritual ineptness to consent to surgery. This attitude can lead to an endless search for a magical cure that lies outside of traditional medicine.

The fact is that many therapies work, and as a result, persons should not categorically dismiss them. Although the natural, less invasive methods are preferred, the spiritual, psychologic, and physically oriented methodologies can work, and persons ought not consider themselves spiritual failures if they must resort to technologic therapies.

Physical and spiritual health are related in many ways. The *physical* and *spiritual* refer to two different domains. Spirit always includes the physical but cannot be explained by physical methods. In this way, physical and spiritual health can never be the same. Spiritual health will always be beyond physical health. It will always be transmaterial (beyond the body) and transmental (beyond the individual psyche and the ego).[18]

To assist others in tapping into their spirituality and healing, nurses must become aware of where they are on their own personal healing journey. As a person becomes aware of what can be achieved by inner recognition of spirit, a sense of healing awareness emerges. When nurses model healing awareness, consciously or unconsciously, they evoke the same awareness in others. Spirituality is timeless and infinite. It is the essence of wholeness. Thus, no one can attain it, but neither can a person escape it.

"Doing" and "being" therapies

Healing can be devised from any era approach, or a person can create a healing ritual that combines the eras. Moreover, healing can be categorized by a "doing" or a "being" approach (Figure 1-6).[18]

"Doing" therapies involve procedures, medications, surgery, and dietary manipulations. "Being" therapies do not use things but rather states of consciousness such as imagery, prayer, meditation, or quiet contemplation. Being therapies are therapeutic because of the ability of the mind to affect the body. They generally are used in either of two ways, *directed* or *nondirected*. When people use a directed mental strategy, they attach specific outcomes to the imagery, prayer, and meditation. For instance, someone might imagine heart disease decreasing and blood pressure normalizing, but when a nondirected approach is used, the person does not assign a specific outcome to the strategy. Rather, this person imagines that the best outcome for the particular situation will come about but does not try to steer the situation in any particular direction.

These therapies apply to nursing and medicine. The Era I approach involves doing therapies and is highly directed. Era II, on the other hand, is a classical bodymind approach that does not employ the use of things. For this reason it involves being therapies. However, it can be directed or nondirected, depending on the mental strategies that a person decides to use. Era III is similar in this regard. It involves being therapies and may be directed or nondirected.

However, the Era III approach also involves a nonlocal, transpersonal experience of being, in which an ordinary state of consciousness is raised above the strictly material level of the here-and-now. It involves honoring, not only the outer-directed, sensory experience, but also the inner experience. It involves a "not-doing" of releasing, emptying, trusting, and acknowledging that individuals have done their best, regardless of the outcome. As the understanding of the therapeutic potential of the mind is increased, it may be found that all therapies and all people take on a transcendent quality. There may be a sense of connecting with the consciousness of others—of experiencing a unity of consciousness—as they feel free to enter nonlocal forms of awareness. This felt oneness can aid persons to work with others to create healing rituals. This includes families and friends, colleagues, and other members of the health care team.

Rational and paradoxical healing

Approaches to healing can be arranged on a continuum of doing and being activities (Figure 1-7).[18]

Doing therapies fall into the *rational* category because they make sense to more linear, intellectual thought processes. These strategies are based on scientific data and often an algorithm or protocol, which dictates a step-by-

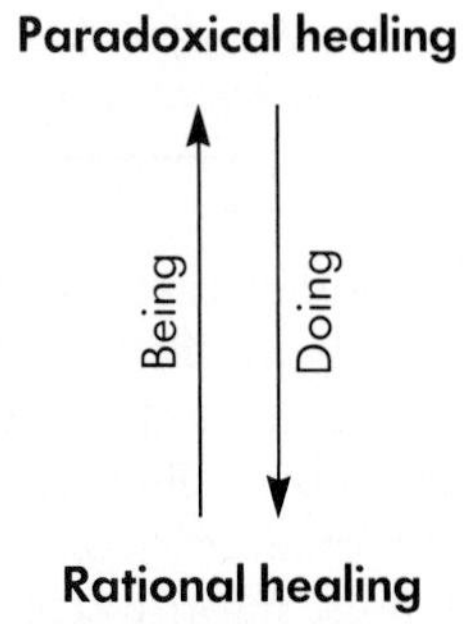

Paradoxical healing

Being ← → Doing

Rational healing

FIG. 1-6 "Being" and "doing" therapies.
From Dossey L: Meaning and medicine: a doctor's tales of breakthrough and healing, New York, 1991, Bantam Books.

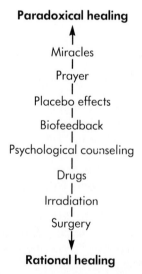

FIG. 1-7 Continuum of rational and paradoxical healing.
From Dossey L: Meaning and medicine: a doctor's tales of breakthrough and healing, New York, 1991, Bantam Books.

step approach on how to treat or advise the patient. Examples of rational healing include surgery, medications, exercise, and diet.

Being therapies are paradoxical because they frequently happen without a "scientific" explanation. A *paradox* is a statement or event that is seemingly absurd or contradictory but that is true.[18] An example, is psychologic counseling, in which a "breakthrough" for a patient is a paradox. Life assumes a new meaning for such a patient; however, there are no clearly delineated steps leading to the breakthrough. The progress is nonobjective, unmeasurable, and unpredictable, thus the term *paradox*.

The placebo is a paradoxical healing approach. If a patient has just a little discomfort, a placebo will not work very well. However, the more pain a patient has, the more dramatic the response to the placebo medication will be. Also patients respond best if they do not know that the medication is a placebo, an experience that is referred to as the "paradox of success through ignorance."[18]

Prayer and faith are paradoxical because there is no rational, scientific evidence for how they work. However, recent scientific studies are being reported, such as the prayer study done in a coronary care unit by Randolph Byrd,[9] a cardiologist. In this study, each patient in the experimental group of 201 patients was prayed for by five to seven Protestant and Catholic people each day across the United States. The control group of 192 patients was not the focus of prayer. This 10-month randomized, prospective, double-blind design study of patients with acute myocardial infarction demonstrated that there were significant decreases in the experimental group in the following events after acute myocardial infarction:

1. The experimental group was 5 times less likely than the control group to require antibiotics (3 compared with 16 patients).
2. The experimental group was 3 times less likely to develop pulmonary edema (6 compared with 18 patients).
3. None of the experimental group required endotracheal intubation (12 in the control group required mechanical ventilatory support).
4. Fewer patients in the experimental group died (although the difference was not significant).

This study, an example of a nonlocal phenomenon, is an Era III approach because it involves the intervention of people praying for others at a distance. Byrd[9] did not find that prayer groups in one city were any more effective than those in other cities, regardless of the patients' distance from the prayer group.

Religious faith may affect health. David Larson and others[25] recently reported on a link between the importance of religion and blood pressure. The researchers used questionnaires that investigated the significance of religion to individuals to determine the effect of religion on persons. About one fourth of the regular church goers revealed themselves as not especially religious. Overall, regular church goers who also portrayed their faith as very important had the lowest diastolic blood pressure. Nonchurch attendees who placed little significance on religion fared worst. The study also showed that religious smokers had much lower blood pressure than their nonreligious counterparts.

Every nurse has known, heard, or read about a patient who had an x-ray film showing evidence of metastatic cancer who created a "being approach" and later was diagnosed as well and cancer-free. These "miracle cures" are paradoxical because there is no scientific mechanism for them.[17] Some would say that such cases simply represent the natural course of the illness or that some die, whereas others live. The point is that there is a paradox in those who get well. We neither know nor can explain scientifically how these miracle cures occur. In the miracle cures reported at places such as Lourdes in France and Medjugorje in Yugoslavia, people who go to shrines and experience a miracle cure are said to be totally immersed in a being state. They do not try to make anything happen. When interviewed, they report experiencing a different sense of space and time. They get outside of the flow of time as past, present, and future and express an "eternal now." They reach a point of psychologic emptiness or enter into the void.[18] For many, there is mistrust of this state of emptiness or void; it is thought to be an "open door for the devil or evil to manifest itself."[18] However, others believe that it is necessary to go into this void or become empty to understand the meaning of illness and the eternal mystery involved in the complexities of life.

Clinical application of spirituality and healing

When technology, mind, and spirit are integrated into clinical practice, the demands of patient care responsibilities, documentation, and other constraints of the health care system are lessened because the model has changed from an allopathic approach to a holistic or a bio-psycho-social-spiritual model. Technology does not impede healing of the body-mind-spirit. It only becomes a problem when it obscures a patient's or nurse's wisdom or common sense.

This new model is a partnership versus an expert-novice relationship.[15] "Patient as partner" means that the patients are capable of making decisions about the course of treatment and about their own lives. This is often difficult when a patient chooses something other than what a physician or nurse recommends. The relationship is person centered rather than role centered.[13,15] This means that health care providers must come to terms with personal ego and the limitations of technology.

Communication with patients is open versus closed. Nurses must remember that there are usually many ways to reach health care goals and that more than one alternative is usually available to patients. Patients also are encouraged to focus on their strengths rather than on their limitations or the limitations imposed by technology. For example, Ornish[30] has demonstrated that even when technology is not able to help persons with severe coronary artery disease, patients can go beyond technologic constraints and use their strengths and potential for healing and changing their lifestyle and perceived meaning about heart disease; these patients can even reverse coronary artery disease.

Pioneering clinical programs

Three recognized pioneering programs at major medical centers use the bio-psycho-social-spiritual model and help patients form healing rituals for living. The first is the Behavioral Medicine Program at New England Deaconness Hospital in Boston.[36] Their Hypertension Group Program is a multiple cardiac risk reduction program that uses a nonpharmacologic approach to treating hypertension. The components of this program are seen in the box on pp. 21 and 22.

Another pioneering program, the Center for Human Caring is within the University of Colorado School of Nursing. The Center for Human Caring was established in 1986 by Dr. Jean Watson to support the continued development and utilization of the art and science of human caring as the foundation for a radically new Health Care System. The goal of the Center for Human Caring is to facilitate the emergence of a Health Care System that truly operationalizes the terms *health* and *care*. Such a system acknowledges that the healing of whole people may or may not include the curing of their diseases. Indeed, the vast majority of present-day diseases will never be cured but lived with for increasingly longer life-times. The drama of medical breakthroughs and seemingly miraculous cures is one that unfortunately will touch only a minute percentage of the population. For the rest, hospital discharge "sicker and sooner" and the phrase "there is nothing more we can do" become frightening realities for which most are ill-prepared to cope. When the goal is healing of the whole person and not curing of a disease, there is always something more that can be done. The art and science of human caring provides the foundation for that something more.

The Center for Human Caring believes that healing can be facilitated in a true Health Care System through creative utilization of existing knowledge about prevention, detection and treatment; through intervention strategies which capitalize on more complete understandings of the body-mind-spirit nature of person; through creative ontological designs of healing environments and educational programs which prepare healing professionals; and through public policy which is based on the moral ideal of caring as an end in itself. The goals of the Center of Human Caring are seen in the box, above.

CENTER FOR HUMAN CARING GOALS

The Center for Human Caring seeks to facilitate the re-visioning and re-creation of the existing Health Care System through projects derived from 4 major goals, consistent with the education, research, and service missions of the University of Colorado.

1. Facilitate the integration of knowledges from the humanities, the arts, cross-cultural spiritual disciplines, feminist theory, nursing, and emerging scientific disciplines such as psychoneuroimmunology and energy medicine into health care education, research and practice;
2. Develop and implement innovative approaches to the clinical practice of human caring and healing which balance and complement the traditional cure paradigm, and assist health care providers to utilize such approaches;
3. Provide a forum for interdisciplinary dialogue between scientists, scholars, artists, health care providers, government experts, and policymakers out of which may emerge new educational and clinical strategies for caring and healing;
4. Serve as an international resource and clearing house for information related to the theory and practice of human caring and healing.

From the Center of Human Caring, University of Colorado School of Nursing, 1990, Denver, Colo.

A third innovative program is at the University of Massachusetts Medical Center. The program, the Mindfulness Meditation Program, teaches patients a specific type of meditation called *mindfulness* and stress management strategies to reverse cardiovascular risk factors and stabilize heart disease while integrating healthy lifestyle changes.[23] It also addresses pain management; other illnesses are considered, as well.

Nurses can create the necessary steps to implement clinical programs that integrate a bio-psycho-social-spiritual model. It requires that nurses join other professionals to merge visions of such programs and create mission statements to guide them.

Mission statements

The mission statement of your hospital, clinic, or agency, as well as a nurse's personal mission statement, should reflect what that nurse values about healing work. A nurse should be empowered by these professional and personal mission statements. For healing to occur, personal and health care mission statements must reflect steps for healing.

HYPERTENSION GROUP PROGRAM SECTION ON BEHAVIORAL MEDICINE

PREPROGRAM SCREENING

Rule out secondary causes of hypertension and attain baseline physical examination. Establish motivation for attending and set mutual goals.

Session 1

Knowledge: Pathophysiology of hypertension
Skills: Instruction in diaphragmatic breathing

Session 2

Knowledge: Physiology of the relaxation response (RR)
Skills: Self-monitoring of blood pressure (BP)

Session 3

Knowledge: Instruction in low-sodium and weight-reducing diet
Skills: Self-monitoring of BP, daily elicitation of the RR, and 3-day food record to calculate sodium content and calories in diet

Session 4

Knowledge: Instruction in low-cholesterol diet
Skills: Daily: self-monitor BP, elicit RR, and follow 2-gram sodium diet and recommended calories
                Three-day food record to calculate cholesterol content in food and behaviors associated with eating

Session 5

Knowledge: Cardiovascular benefits of exercise
Skills: Daily: self-monitor BP; elicit RR; and follow recommended sodium, calorie, and cholesterol diet
                Identify a target heart rate and recommended rating of perceived exertion.

Session 6

Knowledge: Individual prescriptions for meditation practice, exercise, and diet, and a review of medical progress to date
Skills: Daily: self-monitor BP, elicit RR, and follow recommended sodium, calorie, and cholesterol diet
                Exercise within prescribed intensity 20 minutes 5 times per week

These skills are practiced daily and continue to be monitored for the remainder of the program. For the sake of brevity, they will not be repeated under skills for sessions 7 to 13.

Session 7

Knowledge: Behavior change theory
Skills: Identify past pattern of successful and unsuccessful behavior change
                Establish goals and make a plan to accomplish these goals

Attitudes

Throughout the 13 sessions the knowledge-based content and skills are designed to engender attitudes of mindfulness, openness, flexibility, positivity, and self-appreciation. Patients begin to view new experiences as a challenge versus a threat, with a sense of control versus helplessness and a feeling of commitment versus alienation.

Postprogram interview

Review progress in the program.
Set goals for maintaining progress and continued growth and health.

From Stuart E: Spirituality in health and healing: a clinical program, Holistic Nurs Pract 3(3):35, 1989.

Continued.

HYPERTENSION GROUP PROGRAM SECTION ON BEHAVIORAL MEDICINE—cont'd

Session 8

Knowledge: Stress pathophysiology and stress buffers

Skills: Identify physiological response to stress

Begin to *stop* and *take a breath* when encountering a stressor

Session 9

Knowledge: Benefits of Hatha Yoga in eliciting the RR

Skills: Practice in Hatha Yoga with emphasis on mindfulness of physical body and mental quieting

Recognize that emotions can influence the body and the effect of positive emotions on health

Practice positive affirmations each day

Session 10

Knowledge: Cognitive restructuring theory and automatic thoughts

Skills: Stop, take a breath, reflect on those automatic, unconscious, fleeting thoughts that influence behavior

Session 11

Knowledge: Cognitive restructuring theory

Beliefs, attitudes, and assumptions that cause difficulty

Skills: Stop, take a breath, reflect on the beliefs, attitudes, and assumptions that underlie automatic thoughts and response to stress

Session 12

Knowledge: Cognitive restructuring theory and alternative coping styles

Skills: Stop, take a breath, reflect on the beliefs, attitudes, and assumptions that underlie automatic thoughts and influence responses to stress, and choose how to respond (cope) (Stop, breathe, reflect, are you threatened, can you cope?)

Session 13

Knowledge: Creative thinking

Consider that the problems that we encounter cannot be solved by the level of thinking that created them

Skills: Stop, take a breath, reflect, choose how to respond based on a wide range of possibilities

CREATING THE TAPESTRY OF HEALING

Before you begin your "tapestry," choose a quiet, comfortable space. Consider the following: What will your room be like? Is there sunlight and fresh air? What kind of a chair will you sit in, or will you use a stool where your knees support your upper body as you work? Bring to your surroundings any special objects that will enliven your senses and make your work more productive, creative, and enjoyable. For example, you might play music or hang a favorite piece of art nearby. Flowers, incense, hot tea, or a warm or cold liquid to drink, or a light snack may also enhance your experience.

Begin by letting images appear that reveal the size your tapestry; now choose the size loom you will work on and the colors that appeal to the artist within you.

(Insert your name), as your mind becomes clearer and clearer, feel yourself becoming more and more alert. Somewhere deep inside of you, a light begins to glow. Sense this happening, the light growing brighter and more intense. This is your body-mind-spirit communication center. Breath into it; energize it with your breath. The light is powerful and penetrating, and a beam begins to grow out of it to guide you in creating your healing tapestry.

Sit for a while, with rhythmic breathing. Let the designs, colors, and movements of a spirit-filled tapestry begin to form. Let your rhythms of healing spirit begin to dance. You become at one with the work. Serve the work and the moment. Feel the energy of many high beings surrounding you, your soul expanding upward and outward, penetrating all of your energy systems, acknowledging the part of you in need of healing, honoring the challenges before you, asking for new understanding in this healing process, receiving the inner wisdom and new ways to connect with your higher self.

You are now beginning to create your warp of long vertical threads. You are joining each thread with your intrinsic rhythm. The tension on each thread is just right, like the violin strings on a finely tuned Stradivarius; the perfect tension is created and flows from you, the movement coming from your intrinsic beingness.

In front of you are exquisite threads of many colors and textures. Choose the threads to represent your healing, a beautiful thread to represent each of your healing potentials: your joy, peace, harmony, kindness, presence; your courage, truth, patience; your love, honor, trust; your fears, strengths, weaknesses; your light and shadow; your clarity, humor, abundance; your memories, magical places, compassion, forgiveness; your wisdom, purpose, meaning.

Select additional threads to represent releasing, opening, seeking, touching, caring, remembering, expressing, responding; more threads for affirming, changing, creating, intending; threads for sensing, planning, quieting, attuning; threads for softening, forgiving, clearing; threads for awakening, journeying, transcending, attending; threads for receiving, listening, doing; threads for being, enlivening, engaging; threads for letting go, entering the void.

Choose more threads to represent healing of family, friends, colleagues; for community, global nations, and relations; for all things living and nonliving; for healing moments, hurting moments. Spin your healing threads of light from your healing core, your healing source of beingness.

If it seems right, choose some healing objects to incorporate into your tapestry. As you choose these objects, let the sacredness of each object speak to you, such as stones, flowers, seashells, medallions, beads, grasses, representing you, people and things that are sacred, who may need to be remembered or healed.

Focus now on the patterns and designs, the squares, circles, mosaics, or others images, that will flow into your healing tapestry. Begin the next phase.

You feel the energy rising forth to begin the intermeshing, connecting, and coming together of the beautiful threads. Begin now to push and pull with the rhythm of creating, the in and out of the thread in your warp, woofing the threads with the beater, packing the threads, adding sacred objects, in and out, packing the thread, weaving in and out of your threads, in and out of the warp, breathing and feeling your intrinsic balance, journeying deep into your soul, tapping your inner wisdom, knowledge, and answers.

Now place the final threads into the tapestry; feel the energy, placing the final sacred objects in and on the tapestry. The work has reached a stopping point for now. Sit with your healing tapestry.

What patterns have emerged? What emotions do you feel? What kind of energy is present for you? What about you is still in need of healing? What can you do to bring about that healing? Do you feel a connection with your work? Do you feel open to the inner wisdom gained from this process? What are the notes and melody of your healing song? What truths resonates within you, coming from your always present, inner resonating healing core?

Take a few energizing breaths as you come back into full awareness of the healing space within you. As you sit in your healing room, know that whatever is right for you at this time is unfolding, just as it should, and that you have done your best, regardless of the outcome.

A hospital that is setting the prototype for a healing system is Riverside Methodist Hospitals in Columbus, Ohio.[41] Their mission statement is an example of what must occur for hospitals to move from a disease-management industry to a healing system. Riverside is a large medical complex where the best of Era 1 medicine is practiced. However, Riverside Methodist Hospitals is different from other hospitals because administrators, nursing directors, and managers are creating an environment for hospital employees to gain new knowledge and learn healing strategies for integrating technology, mind, and spirit in their personal and professional lives. Their Mission Statement is as follows:

We are committed to a partnership for healing and wholeness that integrates with the providence of God, the strengths of patients and their families, the care of the health care team and the service of employees.

The mission statement for their centennial year, which began in January, 1991, was as follows:

(We) will focus on the dynamic relationship between health and the healing process while challenging all employees to assume responsibility for enhancing or initiating new roles in delivering the healing process.

To actualize these statements, health care consultants and hospital educators are teaching new healing skills to employees. All employees are being challenged to communicate to upper management what is needed to enhance their healing work and evoke transpersonal human caring and caring transactions. For example, the idea of "renewal rooms" (see Chapter 2) are being discussed.

INCORPORATING HEALING CONCEPTS

A tapestry has always been a great symbol of the unfolding mystery, inner strengths, and harmonious interconnectedness about living and nonliving things. Throughout history, master weavers have always described the weaving of a tapestry as healing, as a calling, or as sacred work. For a few moments, allow yourself to imagine that you are a master weaver and you feel inspired to create a tapestry of healing. Take some time to read the box, p. 23, and allow your healing potential to emerge.

The healing tapestry of cardiovascular nursing blends the merging crossroads of technology, mind, and spirit. Participating in a holistic approach implies a deep sense of relatedness to patients and self. As nurses weave this tapestry, they must expand their framework of quality patient care and continue to explore the bio-psycho-social-spiritual model. They are co-learners and co-walkers with patients and their families, with colleagues, and with families and friends in this healing journey. They must be aware of the sharing, caring, and bonding that occurs at many different levels. This is the spirit of healing; however it arises and whatever it is, it is the human factor in the quest for meaning and unity.

KEY CONCEPT REVIEW

1. A bio-psycho-social-spiritual model:
   a. Combines spirituality with mind modulation of the autonomic nervous
   b. Differentiates between psychologic and spiritual elements
   c. Integrates and recognizes the interrelationship of biologic, psychologic, sociologic, and spiritual dimensions
   d. All of the above
2. Holism is:
   a. A theory that states that the functions of human beings are accounted for by behavior of the constituent parts of the body—atoms and electrons
   b. A theory that the universe and living nature are seen correctly in terms of interactional wholes that are more than the mere sum of their parts
   c. A theory of determinism
   d. A theory of molecular dysfunction
3. The new model of healing must:
   a. Integrate being and doing therapies
   b. Understand rational and paradoxical healing
   c. Evoke states of transpersonal human caring
   d. All of the above
4. According to Era III medicine consciousness is viewed as:
   a. Local in nature
   b. Nonlocal in nature
   c. A brain-bound mind state
   d. A body-bound mind state
5. Holistic nursing emphasizes:
   a. Fragmentation of the patient into physiologic and psychologic problems
   b. The organic or functional relationships between parts and wholes
   c. The nuisance of the placebo effect
   d. Limited evidence for the domain of spirituality

ANSWERS

1. d
2. b
3. d
4. b
5. b

REFERENCES

1. Achterberg J: Imagery in healing, Boston, 1985, Shambhala Publications, Inc.
2. Achterberg J: Woman as healer, Boston, 1990, Shambhala Publications, Inc.
3. Achterberg J, Dossey B, and Kolkmeier L: Rituals of healing, New York, 1992, Bantam Books.
4. Benner P and Wrubel J: The primacy of caring: stress and coping in health and illness, Menlo Park, Calif, 1989, Addison-Wesley Publishing Co, Inc.
5. Bevis EO: Accessing learning: determining worth or developing excellence—from a behaviorist toward an interpretive-criticism model. In Bevis EO and Watson J: Toward a caring curriculum: a new pedagogy for nursing, New York, 1990, National League for Nursing.
6. Borysenko J: Guilt is the teacher, love is the lesson, New York, 1990, Warner Books, Inc.
7. Brown M: The unfolding self, Los Angeles, California, 1983, Intermountain Associates for Psychosynthesis Press.
8. Burchardt M: Spirituality: an analysis of a concept, Holistic Nurs Pract 3(3):69, 1989.
9. Byrd R: Positive effects of intercessory prayer in a coronary care unit population, South Med J 81:826, 1988.
10. Derogatis LR: Psychological coping mechanisms and survival time in metastatic breast cancer, JAMA 242:1504, 1979.
11. Dossey B: Nurse as healer: toward the inward journey. In Dossey B and others: Holistic nursing: a handbook for practice, Gaithersburg, Md, 1988, Aspen Publishers, Inc.
12. Dossey B: The psychophysiology of bodymind healing. In Dossey B and others: Holistic nursing: a handbook for practice, Gaithersburg, Maryland, 1988, Aspen Publishers, Inc.
13. Dossey B: The transpersonal self and states of consciousness. In Dossey B and others: Holistic nursing: a handbook for practice, Gaithersburg, Md, 1988, Aspen Publishers, Inc.
14. Dossey B: Spirituality and healing, Holistic Nurs Pract 3(3):1, 1989.
15. Dossey B, Guzzetta C, and Kenner C: Body-mind-spirit. In Dossey B, Guzzetta C, and Kenner C: Critical care nursing: body-mind-spirit, Philadelphia, 1992, JB Lippincott Co.
16. Dossey L: Space, time, and medicine, Boston, 1982, Shambhala Publications, Inc.
17. Dossey L: Recovering the soul, New York, 1989, Bantam Books.
18. Dossey L: Meaning and medicine, New York, 1991, Bantam Books.
19. Engel G: A life setting conducive to illness: the giving-up—giving-in complex, Ann Intern Med 69:92, 1968.
20. Engel G: A need for a new model: a challenge for biomedicine, Science 196:129, 1977.
21. Freed CD and others: Blood pressure, heart rate, and heart rhythm changes in patients with heart disease during talking, Heart Lung 18:17, 1989.
22. Green WA, Goldstein S, and Moss A: Psychosocial aspects of sudden death, Arch Intern Med 129:725, 1972.
23. Kabat-Zinn J: Full catastrophe living, New York, 1990, Delacorte Press.
24. Kuhn C: A spiritual inventory of the medically ill patient, Psychiatr Med 6:87, 1988.
25. Larson D and others: The impact of religion on men's blood pressure, J Religion Health 28:265, 1989.
26. Lazlo E: The systems view of the world, New York, 1972, George Braziller, Inc.
27. Lipowski ZJ: Physical illness, the individual and the coping process, Psychiatr Med 1:90, 1970.
28. Lynch J: The language of the heart: the body's response to human dialogue, New York, 1985, Basic Books, Inc, Publishers.
29. Ornish D: Can lifestyle changes reverse coronary heart disease? Lancet 336:129, 1990.
30. Ornish D: Dr. Dean Ornish's program for reversing heart disease, New York, 1990, Random House, Inc.
31. Postlewaite LJ: Phenomenology of self: an experiential approach to the teaching and learning of caring. In Leininger M and Watson J, editors: The caring imperative in education, New York, 1990, National League for Nursing.
32. Rahe RH, Mahan JL, and Arthur RJ: Prediction of near-future health change from subject's preceding life changes, J Psychosom Res 14:401, 1970.
33. Riegel B and Dossey B: Acute myocardial infarction. In Dossey B, Guzzetta C, and Kenner C: Critical care nursing: body-mind-spirit, Philadelphia, 1992, JB Lippincott Co.
34. Rossi E: The psychobiology of mind-body healing, New York, 1986, WW Norton & Co, Inc.
35. Stein M: Influences of brain and behavior on the immune system, Science 191:435, 1976.
36. Stuart E: Spirituality in health and healing: a clinical program, Holistic Nurs Pract 3(3):35, 1989.
37. Thomas CB: Precursors of premature disease and death, Ann Intern Med 301:1249, 1976.
38. Thomas S: Spirituality: an essential dimension in the treatment of hypertension, Holistic Nurs Pract 3(3):47, 1989.
39. Vaillant GE: Natural history of male psychological health, N Engl J Med 301:1249, 1979.
40. von Bertalanffy L: General systems theory, New York, 1968, George Braziller, Inc.
41. Wimberely T: Riverside Methodist Hospital Mission Statement, Columbus, Ohio, 1991, personal communication.
42. Watson J: Nursing: human science and human care, East Norwalk, Conn, 1988, Appleton-Lange.
43. Whitman G and Guzzetta C: Cardiac surgery. In Dossey B, Guzzetta C, and Kenner C: Critical care nursing: body-mind-spirit, Philadelphia, 1992, JB Lippincott Co.
44. Wilbur K: Do we make ourselves sick? New Age Journal 6:50, 1988.

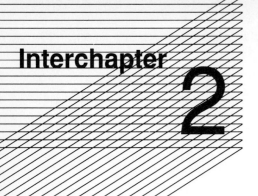

Interchapter 2

The Essence of Nursing

Throughout this book, the connections between body, mind, and spirit are explored and developed. To treat patients holistically, nurses must consider each of these aspects as integral to patient care. As early as 1929, Isabel Stewart reflected on the importance of addressing these aspects of care[8]:

The real essence of nursing, as of any fine art, lies not in the mechanical details of execution, not yet in the dexterity of the performer, but in the creative imagination, the sensitive spirit, and the intelligent understanding lying back of these techniques and skills. Without these, nursing may become a highly skilled trade, but it cannot be a profession or a fine art. All the rituals and ceremonials which our modern worship of efficiency may devise, and all our elaborate scientific equipment will not save us if the intellectual and spiritual elements in our art are subordinated to the mechanical, and if the means come to be regarded as more important than ends.

Spiritually, a vital human element, is a unique experience on the depth of life, vitality, energy and vision.[1,5,7] It is the cornerstone of holistic nursing practice.[6] How do you define spiritually for yourself? Can you identify what gives your life meaning? When you use the words "Guiding Force," "Higher Power," "God," or "Absolute," what do you experience?

The conscious decision to explore one's inner self in relation to the larger whole may be referred to as *spiritual journeying*.[4] This literal or figurative journey is an ongoing process of discovering the wisdom and strength of being human. The entry point of a spiritual journey may begin with a conscious awareness, or it may begin with an unexpected or disruptive event such as burnout, illness, death, or depression.[4]

Conscious awareness means that one recognizes the need for changes in behaviors, beliefs, and attitudes. This awareness creates a paradigm shift. The nurse must sort out old ways of thinking and being that create conflicts and decide what must be present to live what one values. Keegan refers to the sorting of the new information and experiences afforded the awakened individual as a *transformational process*.[2,4] *Trans* means "to move across, beyond, above, or through"; the root word *form* means "shape or structure." Thus *transform* means to move across or through structures or shapes.[2] Transformational change involves a fundamental shift in states of consciousness. There is a major difference in saying that we are human beings with occasional glimpses of spirituality and in recognizing that we are spiritual beings with human experiences.[3]

Each individual is the spiritual expert on his or her own life. The following list includes ways to incorporate the healing potential of spirituality in one's life[6]:

Connecting— connecting with self, others, Higher Power, universe; allows you to experience being grounded

Disconnecting— releasing to open yourself for new creative ways: relaxation, imagery, dance, and laughter

Skill development— challenging your mind to learn things other than nursing: exploring your inner wisdom; taking a class of a new interest; consulting a therapist if you feel stuck

Purifying— washing away, not necessarily with water: sitting quietly by a roaring fire or in the sunshine; being outdoors; taking a long bath or shower

Journeying— traveling in your imagination; reading a good book; walking or taking a leisurely drive; writing in a journal

Transforming— using raw materials to restore order and create something new: painting, weaving, needlepointing, or other craft; gardening or creative cooking

REFERENCES

1. Dossey B: The transpersonal self and states of consciousness. In Dossey B and others: Holistic nursing: a handbook for practice, Gaithersburg, Md, 1988, Aspen Publishers, Inc.
2. Hatcher M: Transformation and spiritual leadership, J Holistic Nurs 9(1):65, 1991.
3. Hover-Kramer D: Creating a context for self healing: the transpersonal perspective, Holistic Nurs Pract 3(3):27, 1989.
4. Keegan L: Spiritual journeying, J Holistic Nurs 9(1):3, 1991.
5. McGlone M: Healing the spirit, Holistic Nurs Pract 4(4):77, 1990.
6. Naigai-Jacobson M and Burkhardt M: Spirituality: cornerstone of holistic nursing practice, Holistic Nurs Pract 3(3):18, 1989.
7. Newman M: The spirit of nursing, Holistic Nurs Pract 3(3):1, 1990.
8. Stewart IM: The science and art of nursing (editorial), Nursing Education Bulletin 2:1, 1929.

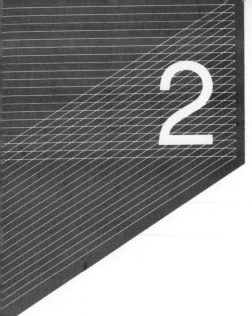

Nurses and Self-Assessment

Barbara Montgomery Dossey
Cathie E. Guzzetta

LEARNING OBJECTIVES

1. Investigate different qualities about healing that can enhance well-being.
2. Explore how perception shapes a person's response to stress.
3. Examine how personal goals lead to healing.
4. Analyze specific lifestyle changes that can be made to enhance healing.
5. Synthesize what occurs when nurses integrate healing modalities in daily life.

Many nurses understand the shift in health care from curing towards healing. Curing is predictable and objectively definable, and the curer is in control and usually inflexible. However, healing is unpredictable, objectively indefinable, and the healer is vulnerable and flexible.[21] Healing and working in a healing system involve the exploration about the nature, meaning, and purpose of being human. A healing system is made up of individuals who trust each other and recognize the invisible bond and forces of healing (see Chapter 1).[1] You should learn how to create a context for self-awareness and self-healing. As you integrate these basic principles in your life, you will become better facilitators in helping patients in their healing process.

THE "HEALING JOURNEY"

The conscious decision to explore the inner self is part of the "healing journey." This journey may begin with a conscious awareness of the need to change, or it may begin with burnout, depression, illness, a death of someone close to you, or another stressful life event.[14] With this conscious awareness, you will recognize the need for changes in behaviors, beliefs, and attitudes.[20] Many nurses do not recognize their own needs. This creates a vicious cycle in which the four characteristics of *codependency* occur. These are (1) caring for others and not caring for yourself, (2) perfectionism, (3) denial, and (4) poor communication.[10,15] This cycle is often due to feeling overworked and unloved, which leads to low self-esteem. The conscious awareness of the need to change creates a paradigm shift.

Part of the healing journey involves becoming aware of your perceptions of stress.[16,17] Every nurse has felt stress in his or her personal and professional life. Consider your perceptions of your stress. Think of a recent stressful event at home or work that involved you and someone else. Determine how you and the other person reacted. Ascertain whether you reacted differently to the same event. Stress is an individual matter. If you place two persons in a new situation, one may see it as a challenge, whereas the other may see it as a negative stressor. Take a few minutes to list the events of your day. Also include stressors that occurred yesterday. Determine your physiologic and mind-spirit states and the effective coping strategies or maladaptive strategies you used. Table 2-1 presents an example.

Because *perception* is an *intellectual* and *cognitive* process, you can pinpoint the stimuli that trigger negative defensive reactions, and you can develop effective coping strategies to use instead. Keep in mind the internal and external factors that govern stress. Internal factors are past experiences, behavior patterns that already exist, and heredity. Some external factors are environment, family, work, relationships, and drugs.

Participating in nursing is challenging and stressful. Identify your own perceptions and level of stress and determine whether this stress is chronic or episodic. Chronic stress is a state that is always present and can lead to disease. Episodic stress is of short duration and varies in intensity.

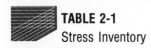

TABLE 2-1

Stress Inventory

My stressors	My physiologic states	My mind-spirit states	My coping strategies	My maladaptive strategies	Ways to change
I took care of patient in cardiogenic shock all day (arrested twice).	My pulse was around 100 beats per minute most of day. I had a headache. I felt tension in my neck and shoulders.	Tension Anxiety		I did not take a coffee or lunch break. I stayed tense all day.	Take breaks. Change pace. Ask for 5-minute breaks. Practice short relaxation skills at work.
I hate taking my son to soccer practice.	My headache continued from work.	Tension Anger		I got angry watching other parents put so much pressure on their kids for their performance to be near perfect.	Take some items from my low-priority list to do during son's soccer practice that do not require concentration. Take my needlepoint so that I can work on it.

Develop an awareness of stress and identify and experience body-mind-spirit changes that occur with stress. Recognize *eustress,* the positive stress that provides energy and helps you continue to entertain new ideas, gain insight, and reach your goals in a healthy manner.[22] Recognize when you fall into a *distress* zone, where negative stress can deplete your body-mind-spirit.

Creating a mission in life

An important part of your healing journey is creating and affirming your mission in life. Consider whether you have ever felt that time is just slipping by and you will never be able to do all those wonderful things you think about doing, such as cooking new recipes or taking a course in weaving, painting, or music. Determine whether you frequently say, "I don't have time to slow down" or "I don't have time to do anything for myself." Ask yourself whether you feel that you have primary control over your life or whether everybody else controls your life. Perhaps you should think about creating some new structure in which you are in control of your life. Reflect on your philosophy of life. Consider whether your life situation reflects your philosophy. To live more fully, you must have a *worthy personal mission.* Assess whether you ever think, "I always seem to make the same mistakes. I feel like I'm in a vicious circle, and I'm not surviving. I have no purpose, and I think I'll get out of nursing. It doesn't have anything to offer me."

If you do not have a worthy personal mission, you will make mistakes over and over again until you barely survive or do not survive the mistakes. Two big areas of personal mission are love and work. You have choices in both; they are not predetermined. You have a lot to say about where you work; and, although it may not seem like it, you even can decide whether you work.

A personal mission is a *survival technique.* Living in a society where there is so much freedom, people are very aware of themselves. This can create loneliness unless you know your mission and feel a sense of relatedness to your fellow humans, whether family, friends, or the people with whom you work. One of the only ways to survive, stay well, and feel whole on a continuous basis is to know who you are and what you care about and to spend effective time doing what it is you care about. You need to determine what the threads are that weave your life together— the special and important people, places, and pleasures. You need to concentrate on developing the best in you, not continually piecing the worst together. You are not *fixed* as a human who cannot change; you have *choices.*

Frequently, nurses act as though problems do not exist. When there is a problem, members of the staff can work together superficially, but underneath, real anger can mount. Because you may not correlate the problem with the facts, you may act inappropriately. Thus you should increase your skills with problem solving. This is another way to reduce stress and more clearly identify your personal mission.

Establishing goals

Another important part of the healing journey involves establishing goals that are used to achieve your personal mission in life. Scientific evidence clearly shows that mind, body, and emotions are one and act as such. The body is a complex machine that provides feedback during sickness and health. It is important to institute values that will allow you to dictate your own life and your own experience. Setting goals facilitates this because it serves as a reminder that you have the power to create new experiences in your life.

Simonton and Simonton[23] have found that determining goals serve the following purposes:

1. Determining goals is a declaration of your ability to create the experiences required to handle your emotional needs.
2. Goals direct energies in a positive direction, and they determine your expectations of life.
3. Goals are a confirmation of life.
4. Establishing goals reinforces meaning in life.
5. When you establish goals, you also are stating that you are in command and can make life work for you. You are acting on life rather than letting it act on you.
6. Setting goals and meeting them will allow you to start to build a positive image of yourself. It is a way of stating how important your needs are and what you are going to do to take care of them. By accepting your needs, you are saying that you are important to yourself.

Ideas for goal setting follow[23]:

1. Examine the *rewards* or *secondary gains* (e.g., getting attention) that you get from lack of health awareness or from being sick. Fix a goal that will allow you to get that same reward in a way that takes the form of health, not sickness.
2. Look at activities you always have wanted to do but have not because of lack of time, money, or whatever. Encouraging yourself to do these things can be a way to put more meaning in your life.

A plan for a positive life change follows[23]:

Goals that give my life meaning and purpose.	Steps I will take to accomplish this.	Dates I want to do this.
Goals that will put fun and play into my life.	Steps I will take to accomplish this.	Dates I want to do this.
Goals that are directed at increasing exercise in my life.	Steps I will take to accomplish this.	Dates I want to do this.
Goals that are directed at achieving nutritional balance.	Steps I will take to accomplish this.	Dates I want to do this.
Goals for relaxation and meditation.	Steps I will take to accomplish this.	Dates I want to do this.

Developing basic attributes

During the healing journey, you must develop and incorporate the following basic yet critical attributes: (1) a good self-image, (2) a positive attitude, (3) self-discipline, and (4) integration and balance of body-mind-spirit.[7,9] Each person develops and incorporates these factors differently in a way that works best for that individual.

Self-image means that people view themselves as good and healthy human beings. You must develop all your senses and see yourself as healthy in all respects—doing what you want to do with people, handling stressors with calmness and ease, and understanding your own feelings, as well as those of others. You must imagine yourself at your ideal body weight, doing exercises, being able to play, and practicing relaxation skills daily.

A *positive attitude* means that people like and respect themselves in all that they do. To thrive in this life, you have to learn to respect your body-mind-spirit.

You have to teach yourself *self-discipline*. This discipline is the idea of being calm and consistently following positive health patterns of relaxation, play, exercise, and nutrition.

Body-mind-spirit integration means that persons see themselves as a whole, not as separate from the rest of the community. You are a part of a whole universe, and you see this relationship in terms of interacting wholes that are more than the sum of the parts (see Chapter 1). You should feel a keen sense of balance and relatedness between who you are, where you are, and how you interact with everyone.

You continually need to do the following[4,6,8]:

1. Search for patterns and causes of stress and anxiety, as well as the patterns and causes of good feelings and emotions.
2. Emphasize your human values.
3. Assess pain and disease as valuable signals of internal conflict, not as being wholly negative.
4. Place emphasis on achieving maximal body-mind-spirit healing.
5. View your own body-mind-spirit as all coequal; one part is never more important than another.

Changing and taking risks

Identifying your mission, purpose, and goals in life involves *change* and *taking risks*. It does not imply that you are fragmenting your life and shirking responsibility. It is a natural process and a necessary step in the healing journey. You have to take responsibility for it; no one else can do it for you.

Think about whether you ever say, "I can't change. I try, and I never seem to get ahead." As a nurse, you do not allow your patients to preoccupy themselves with failure. You try all kinds of techniques to shift your patients' negative thinking to help them see how to live healthier and feel whole. You tell your patients constantly that there is a big difference between "I haven't changed" and "I can't change." You also need to apply positive affirmations to your own life. Thinking about failure can be detrimental when deciding a new plan of action for enhancing health. You have the capacity to change. For example, recently nurses have been sharing more ideas on how to be assertive rather than passive or aggressive. Learning these new concepts involves change.

Often when people try to change, they conclude they do not have the willpower. *Willpower* is a myth that researchers have disproved. Instead, you should think of *skillpower* rather than willpower. For high-level wellness and health, you must consciously and with commitment make a decision about your own survival-enhancement program. You will have to learn appropriate skills for managing your lifestyle that will keep you relatively serene and balanced in spite of daily stressors.

Change is a process of learning about your capacities through opening up to some new ways of being. Change implies that you can be flexible and that your lifestyle habits do not have to be permanent. Experiment. Try healthier ways of relating with friends, families, and colleagues and new ways of exercising, relaxing, eating, and playing. Try this easy exercise to help focus on change. Write down some specific ideas. Mark a piece of paper with a line down the center. Label one column *benefits for changing* and the other *cost for changing*. Write the best and worst reasons for changing. Writing it out on paper is an effective exercise to help recognize the things that need to be changed and ways to change them.

When you decide, for example, to start eating healthier or to begin an exercise program, first remember to stop berating yourself for poor eating habits or lack of exercise in the past. When you have relapses and eat junk food with 2000 calories instead of nutritionally sound food with calories, think of these as learning trials, and then *try again*. Think positively of the benefits of changing, and remember that you are making yourself healthier. Consider the consequences of changed behavior. Also, keep in mind that some people may not want you to be healthier and less stressed. Knowing that this can occur will make it easier to handle the situation if it does arise. Acting like the person you want to be will help in the change process. Also let your support people know that you are trying to change. Their encouragement is wonderful. Be proud of yourself. Be aware, however, that there are adjustment periods. When a new way of being does not seem quite right, give it a little time before jumping to conclusions.

Changing bad habits to healthier, happier patterns is essential for well-being. The more you do it, the better you get at it. Practice makes it easier and easier. As you make healthier changes in your life, you find that you more consistently select positive changes because your fear of changing is lessened.

Nine ways to begin to focus on healing follow:

1. Make body-mind-spirit connections. Assess daily attitudes, belief systems, and stressors, and evaluate physiologic, psychologic, and spiritual responses.
2. Achieve adequate sleep.
3. Eat three nutritious meals a day.
4. Participate in 30 minutes of aerobic exercise four or five times a week. Be certain to follow guidelines for exercises, as well as warm-up and cool-down exercises.
5. Practice some form of relaxation to achieve the relaxation response at least once a day (see Chapter 5).
6. Do specific body exercises and self-shiatzu to relieve accumulated tension (Fig. 2-1).
7. Include some form of play in your day.
8. Maintain an ideal weight.
9. Reduce or eliminate unhealthy lifestyle habits (e.g., excessive consumption of alcohol, drugs, caffeine, and smoking).
10. Know and seek support systems with family, friends, and others. Know where, with whom, and how to give and receive love and affection. Surround yourself with people who are not consistently saturated with the misery of human problems.[28]

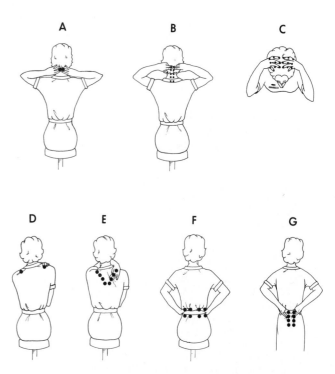

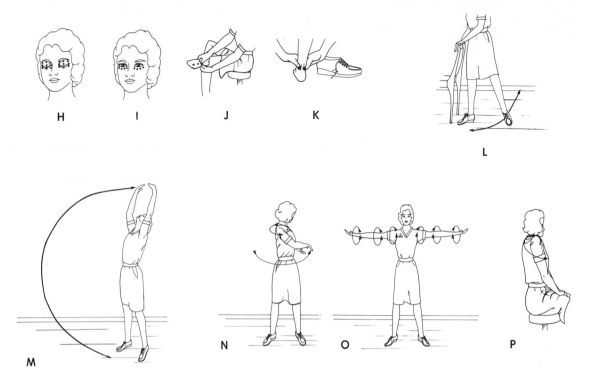

FIG. 2-1   Self-shiatzu is a gentle Oriental massage technique using light pressure (5 pounds), medium pressure (15 pounds), and deep pressure (20 pounds). To accurately know when you have this much pressure, push on a bedside scale with your thumbs or fingers to learn what different pressures feel like. **A,** Apply deep pressure below the base of the skull to release head and neck tension. Hold for 3 seconds, pause, repeat several times, and let go. **B,** To release tight neck muscles, again with deep pressure move down the muscle lines approximately two finger widths. Let your fingers feel the muscle bands. Hold for 3 or 4 seconds, pause, and move on down the neck. **C,** At the top of the head, use your index, middle, and third fingers of both hands. With moderate pressure, press at the three points shown for 3 or 4 seconds, pause, and move to the next two positions using the same technique. **D,** Relieve shoulder tension by placing your left hand on the back of your right shoulder. Locate what is called the *yipe point,* a key point where tension builds up. It is halfway between the base of the neck and edge of the shoulders. This point may be tender. Apply deep pressure for 3 or 4 seconds, pause, and repeat the sequence again on your opposite side. **E,** Stretch your left hand to your right shoulder to give yourself shiatzu to your upper back. Touch your index, middle, and third fingers to your spine. With deep pressure, find the pressure points as shown. Move two finger widths up on a line toward your shoulder, pressing in each position for 3 seconds; pause, and repeat the pressure at each point. **F,** To give self-shiatzu to your lower back, sit forward slightly in your chair. Place your fingertips above your hip bones, and extend your thumbs in toward your spine. Give deep pressure in each spot for 3 seconds, pause, and repeat. **G,** To give self-shiatzu to your spine, stand up, locate your coccyx. With your index and middle fingers, apply moderate pressure for 3 seconds; pause, and move up at two finger widths until you reach your waist. **H,** Apply self-shiatzu to your eyes. If you wear contact lenses, take them out first. The pressure points are on the inside edge of the eye sockets. With your index, middle, and third fingers of each hand, press on the points shown with light pressure for 3 seconds; pause, and repeat in the next two positions shown. **I,** To apply self-shiatzu to your cheeks, with your index and middle fingers side by side, apply moderate pressure at the outside of the bridge of the nose. Hold for 3 seconds, pause, and move one finger width across the cheeks. **J,** Apply self-shiatzu to your feet, one at a time. With deep pressure move down the line in the center of your foot using both of your thumbs side by side. Then move out to the point behind the ball of your foot, and apply pressure at each point for 3 seconds, pause, and move to the next position. **K,** Lean forward and rest your foot on the floor. Place a thumb on the outside of your ankle in the deepest recess between the rear of the anklebone and the Achilles tendon along the back of the heel. Apply moderate pressure for 3 seconds, pause, and repeat. **L to P,** You can stretch away tension in your entire body. While doing these tension-releasing exercises, remember to breathe in a rhythmic manner.

QUALITIES OF A NURSE-HEALER

Be aware that self-healing is a continual process.
Be familiar with the terrain of self-development.
Be open to self-discovery.
Continue to develop clarity about life's purposes to keep from acting mechanical and bored.
Be aware of present and future steps in personal growth.
Model self-care to help yourself and patients with the inward process.
Be aware that your presence is equally important as technical skills.
Respect and love patients regardless of who or how they are.
Offer patients methods for working on life issues.
Guide patients in discovering creative options.
Presume that the patients know the best life choices.
Listen actively.
Empower patients to recognize that they can cope with life processes.
Share insights without imposing personal values and beliefs.
Accept what patients say without judging.
See time with patients as being there for them to serve and share.

From Dossey B: Nurse as healer: toward the inward journey. In Dossey B and others, Holistic nursing: a handbook for practice, Gaithersburg, Md, 1988, Aspen Publishers, Inc.

Centering

An important step in the journey toward healing is exploring and acknowledging your inner wisdom.[18,19] True healing requires attention to your woundedness and the polarities, the purpose, and meaning in life. As you explore your inner dimension and recognize the innate wisdom that is present, your qualities of healing, as listed in the box, left, are more available to you.

Practicing and learning skills to quiet the mind create the necessary space for you to become centered and to recognize your intrinsic balance.[24] Time, solitude, practice, and conscious awareness will allow you to move to a place of centeredness more frequently. *Centering* is the state achieved when you move to an inner place of stability.[7] Centering allows you to devote time to inner silence to connect with your inner wisdom. When you are consciously aware of your involvement in life, you become more sensitive to your life patterns and processes.

As you recognize the aspects of your being that are in need of healing, you become able to live an authentic life. Think about how often you feel authentic. When you experience harmony in your actions, behaviors, thoughts, and feelings, you are participating from your authentic self. As you consciously participate from your spiritual nature and healing awareness, your actions have intention and purpose and are authentic.

Imagine having time at work to replenish your spirit. Consider a room on or near your unit that is designated

THE RENEWAL ROOM

Consider what it would take for you to be healed at work rather than physical and emotionally drained. As you read the following list of possibilities, stay open to the ideas. If you say they cannot happen, they will not. However, if you and your colleagues create your visions of healing and present them to the administration in the context of "This is what we need to facilitate healing in ourselves and our patients" and "This is how we see creating a Renewal Room," then it will become a reality. Here are a list of possibilities that can enhance your healing as the demands of cardiovascular nursing practice increase.

1. Is it possible for a room near the unit to be emptied and converted to a Renewal Room to nourish the staff?
2. Can you imagine signing up each day to go to the Renewal Room on or near the unit for 10 to 30 minutes to nourish yourself with relaxation and rest?
3. Is it possible to imagine that you have the support of your colleagues and administration to go to the Re-

newal Room? This rest period is valued and honored, and you are encouraged to nourish yourself.
4. Can you imagine the Renewal Room with comfortable pillows on a carpeted floor, beautiful pictures hanging on the wall, a few healing objects placed on several low tables for easy viewing, and an audio cassette library with a wide range of music, relaxation, and imagery tapes, headphones and tape recorders? There might also be a sign on the door that reads "This Renewal Room is for your relaxation and rest. Please enjoy." (For details of establishing an audio cassette relaxation, imagery, music library, see Chapter 5).

What were your experiences as you read the characteristics of the Renewal Room? What else would you add to your room? It is also important to create a similar kind of space for yourself where you live so that you allow time each day for inner reflection and healing to renew your body-mind-spirit.

From Dossey B, Guzzetta C, and Kenner C: Critical care nursing: body-mind-spirit, ed 3, Philadelphia, 1992, JB Lippincott Co.

as a renewal room for you and your colleagues to become nourished at least once each day. The box, lower left, discusses ways to create a renewal room at work. Remember if you think it can happen, you and your colleagues can develop the clarity, purpose and plans to create the steps to make it happen.

Affirmations of exceptional qualities

Affirmations are strong, positive statements that you select to affirm your intention and choices. Affirmations can help you develop clarity of goals that direct your actions and assist your self-evaluation. They help you increase responsibility for your actions, thoughts, beliefs, and values.

If your thoughts are hopeful and optimistic, your body responds with confidence, energy, and hope. On the other hand, if negative thoughts and emotions dominate, your body responds with tightness, uneasiness, and an increase in respirations, blood pressure, and heart rate, as well as other physiologic changes.

Affirmations can help you change your perceptions and beliefs. When you believe that an affirmation is true, your perceptions selectively reinforce a positive thought. Because your mind constantly engages in active thought processing, affirmations shape self-talk into positive thoughts. Because your self-dialogue continues into your dream states, make positive affirmations before falling asleep.

Consider how often you acknowledge the exceptional qualities that you bring to your workplace. All nurses can become exceptional.[13] Take a few minutes to reflect on the following affirmations of exceptional qualities. Read these affirmations, and let yourself experience them as if they already exist.
1. I am a critical thinker.
2. I take risks.
3. I manipulate time and resources wisely.
4. I am an advocate for nursing.
5. I am assertive.
6. I am caring.
7. I am future oriented.
8. I am self-aware.

Set aside time each day to use affirmations. Be aware of evoking your imagery process using all of your senses and inner experiences as you read the following affirmations:[9]
1. I operate from the perspective that life has meaning, direction, and value.
2. I am spirit filled.
3. I acknowledge a deeper understanding about my life that helps me solve or resolve old conflicts from a new perspective.
4. I am present and am aware of my worries, fears, hopes, faith, love, and compassion.
5. I feel a part of life and living.
6. I recognize that the different roles of my life are expressions of my true self.
7. I know a connection with some power higher than myself and feel a connection with the universe.

Laughter, humor, and joy

The healing journey includes laughter, humor, and joy. The stress in cardiovascular nursing can be lessened by laughter and humor because joy and sadness cannot occur simultaneously. These three lighter aspects of your human nature relieve tension, help manage pain, and act as distractors. Laughter and humor increase production of endorphins and are said to be the shortest distance between two people.[5] Moments of the lighter side of life can give you a sense of being in control, new hope, and alternatives to fear, anger, and grief.

Healing moments of being with yourself, patients, and others while talking, actively listening, and sharing times of life experienced together bring about humor and joy. Laughter and humor can come from telling stories or listening to others' stories. Reflecting on laughter shared can ease stress long after the story has been told. Laughing can often break the barriers for you or others to speak from your heart.

Moments of laughter and humor can be thought of as a "minirelaxation" strategy because they have a way of bringing a sense of balance, causing a person to be more objective and to release tension and unexpressed emotions.[5] Laughing at a situation allows you to contact your inner core of joy—to lighten the load of being human.

Building trust

You can help transform hospitals, clinics, and outpatient rehabilitation programs into healing environments. However, you cannot make changes in isolation. You must build trust among other nurses and share your visions and desires.

Nurses are notorious for not supporting each other with change. Try to turn this around and actively listen and support others in the change process. As you do this, your skills and awareness of love, respect, and trust between and among others will increase. When you negate and criticize another's wisdom, you create levels of fear within yourself that block your healing forces and trust. However, when you actively listen to new ways of participating, you build trust. These points are further developed in Table 2-2.[11]

Talking about healing work

Think about whether you have trouble talking about healing and what you do as a nurse to facilitate healing. Nurses can learn to be open and comfortable in talking about healing. Most nurses are very modest and take their skills and interactions for granted. Common comments by nurses are, "Well, that is what I do because I am a nurse" or "It is expected that I help patients." Frequently, nurses

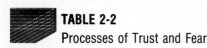

TABLE 2-2
Processes of Trust and Fear

Bodymind process	Effects	Bodymind process	Effects
TRUST LEVEL MOBILIZING LIFE FORCES		**FEAR LEVEL IMPAIRING LIFE FORCES**	
Motivation	Creates and mobilizes energy, increases strength and focus of motivation	Motivation	Often causes unfocused energy to be channeled into defense with reduced motivation
Consciousness	Unblocks energy flow, expands awareness, makes the unconscious more available	Consciousness	Reduces span of awareness, cuts off threatening areas of near-awareness and unconsciousness
Perception	Increases acuity of perceptions, improves vision and perspective	Perception	Decreases acuity of perceptions, impairs vision and perspective
Emotionality	Frees feelings and emotions to energize all processes of the bodymind	Emotionality	Disrupts feelings and emotions and is often defense oriented and dysfunctional
Cognition	Frees energy to allow focus on thinking and problem solving	Cognition	Possibly causes thinking and problem solving to be unfocused, displaced, defensive, ineffective
Action	Releases person for proactive and spontaneous behavior	Action	Causes reactive, congested, and inhibited behavior because of overconcern for consequences
Synergy	Frees total person for synergistic and holistic integration	Synergy	Causes processes and subsystems to be out of harmony, not synchronistic, and often segmented

From Hatcher M: Transformational and spiritual leadership, J Holistic Nurs 9(1):65, 1991.

do not give themselves credit for healing moments, and this leads to burnout and the expression, "Same old thing, day-in and day-out."

Critical patient incidents in which healing takes place are called *exemplars* by Benner.[2,3] Think about the last time that you created time within yourself to affirm the value of your actions and your presence with yourself or another. Ask whether you told yourself that you did a wonderful job. Remember whether you were inspired about your work and healing interactions.

The following are two examples of nurses at major medical centers who joined together to enhance their healing awareness. At Beth Israel Hospital in Boston, 21 nurses from 10 different subspecialties in the medical-nursing department exchanged healing moments every other Thursday at lunch.[27] To prepare for each meeting the group reviewed Benner's work and wrote exemplary moments that they had experienced. At each meeting, they would read two exemplars and discuss them.

Broad themes that surfaced in the discussions were patient-physician interactions, characteristics of novice and experienced nurses and physicians, the system's medical hierarchy, death and dying, advocacy, and patient-focused care. About 6 months into their series, Dr. Benner was invited to add her expertise. When these themes and concepts were grouped into a set of behaviors, they represented characteristics of the expert nurse's world that bring about exemplar moments of healing. These themes are summarized in Table 2-3.

At Maine Medical Center in Portland, Maine, a relaxation and imagery committee has been created.[26] A committee consisting of 12 nurses and a child-life specialist serve as a resource group for staff nurses interested in learning relaxation and stress-reduction techniques for use with their patients. This group also discusses healing moments with patients, families, and colleagues. A brochure has been developed and posted on each nursing unit with clearly stated objectives about the committee. Information is given in lectures and discussion and practice sessions about relaxation, imagery, and stress reduction. Other resources include a library of current audiovisual resource materials, as well as a resource library of printed information on these topics.

Joining your colleagues to do a critical analysis of patient interactions and identify the essential qualities of being a nurse-healer will inspire you. It can also bring together the minds of creative nurse thinkers who have the ability to institute healing practices within nursing.

TABLE 2-3
Practice Characteristics of Expert Nurses

Characteristics	Description
Mobilization of data	Has objective data to spur the medical hierarchy into action, has data to back up intuitive hunches about patient's changing condition
Persistence	Has confidence to keep trying until a patient's needs are met, regardless of being told to quit trying
Good listening skills	Hears what a patient says, is receptive and approachable, builds trust and mobilizes a patient's energy, even when faced with exhaustion, depression, or fear
Ability to create opportunity	Senses precise moment when to act and when to step back, creates space for open dialogue to discuss possible scenarios
Self-disclosure	Develops skills in sharing insight and experience with the patient, family, and colleagues
Incorporation of science into practice	Incorporates a wide range of knowledge into practice, knows the limits of science and when all data do not reflect what the intuitive bodymind feels, incorporates scientific and intuitive ways of knowing, advises novice nurses in incorporating science and intuition
Knowledge of how and when to relinquish control to the patient	Can step aside to reflect on various ways to help a patient reach a goal and recognizes that the patient's solution may be different, but lets it be if the patient needs control and if care and safety are not compromised
Knowledge of the patient	Uses instincts and intuition to help meet human needs while getting to know patient
Responsiveness	Is flexible, changes priorities according to patient's needs, listens to the patient and family to recognize their meanings of the situation
Avoidance of power struggles	Learns the system and how to use it; focuses on outcomes; consciously steers outcomes around the red-tape struggles to get what patients need; interprets, protects, and supports; maneuvers projects through the system and gets to the consumer what is needed—gets to the heart of advocacy

Adapted from Tofias L: Expert practice: trading examples over pizza; Am J Nurs 89(9):1193, 1989.

KEY CONCEPT REVIEW

1. Healing:
   a. Is an evolving process
   b. Involves self-responsibility
   c. Is a fluctuating state
   d. All the above
2. Perception is:
   a. A cognitive and intellectual process
   b. Always the same
   c. Goal setting
   d. A strategy
3. Setting personal goals helps nurses:
   a. Direct their energy in a positive direction
   b. Reinforce the meaning of life
   c. Build a positive image
   d. All the above
4. Changing lifestyle is:
   a. A learning process
   b. Associated with flexibility
   c. Dynamic
   d. All the above
5. Which of the following events is likely to take place when nurses model healing awareness?
   a. Nurses exhibit decreased tension.
   b. Nurses assess their own attitudes and beliefs.
   c. Nurses feel more creative.
   d. All the above

ANSWERS

1. d
2. a
3. d
4. d
5. d

REFERENCES

1. Achterberg J: Woman as healer, Boston, 1989, Shambhala Publication, Inc.
2. Benner P: From novice to expert: excellence and power in clinical nursing practice, Menlo Park, Calif, 1984, Addison-Wesley Publishing Co, Inc.
3. Benner P and Tanner C: Clinical judgement: how expert nurses use intuition, Am J Nurs 87(1):23, 1987.
4. Borysenko J: Guilt is the teacher, love is the lesson, New York, 1990, Warner Books, Inc.
5. Cohen M: Caring for ourselves can be funny business, Holistic Nurs Pract 4(4):1, 1990.
6. Diers D: Learning the art and craft of nursing, Am J Nurs 89(1):65, 1989.
7. Dossey B: Nurse as healer: toward the inward journey. In Dossey B and others: Holistic nursing: a handbook for practice, Gaithersberg, Md, 1988, Aspen Publishers, Inc.
8. Dossey B: The transpersonal self and states of consciousness. In Dossey B and others: Holistic nursing: a handbook for practice, Gaithersberg, Md, 1988, Aspen Publishers, Inc.
9. Dossey B and Keegan L: Holism and the circle of human potential. In Dossey B and others: Holistic nursing: a handbook for practice, Gaithersberg, Md, 1988, Aspen Publishers, Inc.
10. Hall S and Wray L: Codependency: nurses who give too much, Am J Nurs 89(11):1456, 1989.
11. Hatcher M: Transformation and spiritual leadership, J Holistic Nurs 9(1):65, 1991.
12. Hover-Kramer D: Creating a context for self healing: the transpersonal perspective, Holistic Nurs Pract 3(3):27, 1989.
13. Huston C: What makes the difference? attributes of the exceptional nurse, Nurs 90 90(5):170, 1990.
14. Keegan L: Spiritual journeying, J Holistic Nurs 9(1):3, 1991.
15. Krupnick S: Recognizing and avoiding negative addictions in your life, Holistic Nurs Pract 4(4):20, 1990.
16. Lakein A: How to get control of your life and time, New York, 1975, Signet.
17. McGlone M: Healing the spirit, Holistic Nurs Pract 4(4):77, 1990.
18. Naigai-Jacobson M and Burkhardt M: Spirituality: cornerstone of holistic nursing practice, Holistic Nurs Pract 3(3):18, 1989.
19. Newman M: The spirit of nursing, Holistic Nurs Pract 3(3):1, 1990.
20. Rew L: Intuition: nursing knowledge and the spiritual dimension of person, Holistic Nurs Pract 3(3):56, 1989.
21. Schunior C: Nursing and the comic mask, Holistic Nurs Pract 3(3):7, 1989.
22. Seyle H: Stress without distress, New York, 1975, Signet.
23. Simonton C and Simonton S: Getting well again, Los Angeles, 1978, Jeremy P Tarcher, Inc.
24. Stroebel C: Quieting response training, New York, 1980, BMA Audio Cassette Publication.
25. Taylor P and Ferszt G: Spiritual healing, Holistic Nurs Pract 4(4):32, 1990.
26. Thomas J: Relaxation/guided imagery committee, Portland, Maine, Maine Medical Center, personal communication, 1988.
27. Tofias L: Expert practice: trading examples over pizza, AM J Nurs 89(9):1193, 1989.
28. Vanore-Black N: Maintaining healthy relationships, Holistic Nurs Pract 4(4):39, 1990.

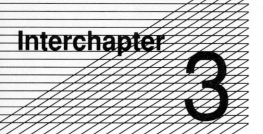

The Right and Left Brains

In 1836, Dax stated that the cerebral hemisphere opposite the preferred hand was dominant and mediated language.[4] The idea of cerebral dominance received much attention. The concept of split consciousness, however, was first developed by Al Wigans and published in 1844. After performing an autopsy on a man whom he had known well, Wigans found that the man had one cerebral hemisphere missing. His conclusion was that to be a person or have a mind, only one hemisphere is required. And if two hemispheres are present, one has two minds.

Today, modern brain research is referred to as "neowiganism." This means that each of us has two minds, the right brain and the left brain. The hemispheres are connected by the corpus callosum, a bundle of 200 million nerve fibers. Through the work of Sperry and colleagues[9-11] in the 1950s, it was determined that the corpus callosum provides hemispheric communication and transmission of learning and memory. Their continued research in the 1960s with neurosurgical patients allowed scientists to establish new information about the two hemispheres; that each hemisphere is different in goals, content, and modes of processing information. These researchers demonstrated that when the corpus callosum was disconnected, the two hemispheres continued to function independently (referred to as the split-brain studies).[2,3] Moreover, these researchers performed an elaborate series of tests that documented the separate functions of the right and left brain. For the first time, the right and left hemispheres were shown to perceive reality in special ways. It is for this exploration, clarification, and understanding of how the two hemispheres differ in function that Sperry was awarded the 1981 Nobel Prize for medicine.[1]

From Sperry's work, we know that the right and left hemispheres have highly specialized and different characteristics. The left hemisphere, for example, is logical, drawing conclusions based on the order of things; the right hemisphere is intuitive, using feeling, hunches, visual images, and patterns to draw conclusions. The left hemisphere is linear, keeping track of time; the right hemisphere is holistic, seeing parts and the relationship of the parts to form the whole. The left hemisphere functions sequentially, figuring things out in a step-by-step process with one part following another; the right brain functions integratively, having holographic perceptions. The left brain is verbal, using language, speech, naming, and reading; the right brain is nonverbal, using imagery and awareness of things. The left brain is concrete, selecting a small bit or part to represent the whole; the right brain is abstract, seeing the here and now in relation to whole. The left brain is rational, drawing conclusions based on reason and fact; the right brain is nonrational, not requiring facts or reasons to draw conclusions. The left brain involves convergent thinking seeing one meaning, one conclusion, and one alternative; the right brain involves divergent thinking, seeing many conclusions, many alternatives, and many meanings.[5]

This information has important applications in nursing. How can nurses use these two kinds of consciousness to effect healing, promote wellness, and facilitate a peaceful death for patients? If these modes of consciousness can alternate being in control, what kinds of modalities do nurses use and what guidelines can they develop to enhance hemispheric performance? Is it also possible, under certain conditions, that the hemispheres interfere with each other and prevent maximal hemispheric performance?[7,8]

There are probably times when the right and the left brain interfere with each other. It may be that patients who do not comply with diet, exercise, or medication regimens do so because of hemispheric conflict, that is, because of anger or lack of readiness to learn. It also may be possible that during crisis and stress, the right brain is in control, that is, the right brain predominates.[6] During such times, people may be processing information primarily from a right-brain mode. We have all seen patients and families, who under stressful illness conditions, say such things as "I don't know what to do! My brain is not working! I can't think!" These individuals are telling us that they cannot think from a rational and analytic left-brain mode.[6]

The problem should become apparent to any of us who have taught patients. Most of our traditional teaching is based on left brain functioning. For example, following an acute myocardial infarction, we focus teaching on an understanding of the pathophysiology and healing mechanisms of myocardial infarction and a therapeutic plan of care (e.g., reducing cholesterol, smoking cessation, exercise, and so forth). These activities involve left-brain teaching to stimulate the analytic, left hemisphere. Many of our patients, however, are in right-brain thinking. Hemispheric conflict results. Patients are unable to process the information. As a result, they do not understand or remember the information because learning has not taken place.[6]

An important nursing goal is to develop tools to help recognize what hemisphere is in control before patient teaching. When the right brain predominates, we need to initiate right-brain teaching. Self-regulation therapies such as relaxation, imagery, and music therapy provide patients with the intuitive experiences to stimulate the right brain and help them make bodymind connections. Patients who are in crisis or are experiencing stress tend to be receptive to these therapies because they are compatible with the way patients are processing information and are in harmony with their emotional needs.

Another important nursing goal is to develop patient teaching programs that incorporate both right- and left-brain learning modalities. To do so would permit *whole-brain learning* to take place. During the initial stress or crisis, for example, patients can be taught relaxation techniques such as deep breathing and muscle relaxation to help them cope with the immediate situation. When patients are in a more relaxed state, guided imagery techniques can be added progressively to help patients visualize and rehearse upcoming stressful procedures, tests, or surgery and to image positive short- and long-range healing outcomes (see Awakening the Inner Healer, p. 484 and Going Fishing During a Cardiac Catheterization, p. 542). Within or following such relaxed imagery sessions, left brain rational-analytic information can be introduced on heart functioning, risk factors, medication, diet, and exercise. Patients thereby are assisted in developing the skills to use the right and left brain in a complementary fashion to enhance hemispheric performance. Such whole-brain teaching programs can be developed for all traditional content taught by nurses. Patients then learn techniques to cope with the psychophysiologic response to the illness, as well as the necessary factual information about the illness.[6] The results of these whole brain programs might significantly impact on the learning outcomes of our patients by permitting hemispheric integration to occur. These outcomes, in turn, might revolutionize how and what we teach.[6]

REFERENCES

1. Bengelsdorf I: Medical news, JAMA 246:2316, 1981.
2. Bogen J: The other side of the brain, Bull La Neurol Soc 34:75, 1969.
3. Bogen JE: Some educational aspects of hemispheric specialization, UCLA Educ 17:24, 1975.
4. Crichley M: Dax's law, Int J Neurol 4:199, 1964.
5. Galin D: The two modes of consciousness and the two halves of the brain. In Goldman B, editor: Consciousness: brain states of awareness and mysticism, New York, 1979, Harper & Row.
6. Guzzetta CE: Infective endocarditis. In Dossey BM, Guzzetta CE, and Kenner CV: Critical care nursing: body-mind-spirit, ed 3, Philadelphia, 1992, JB Lippincott.
7. Levy J: Differential perceptual capacities in major and minor hemispheres, Proc Nat Acad Sci 61:1151, 1968.
8. Levy J: Psychobiological implications of bilateral asymmetry. In Diamond S, editor: Hemisphere function in the human brain, New York, 1974, John Wiley & Sons.
9. Sperry R: Hemispheric disconnection and unity in conscious awareness, Am Psychol 23:723, 1968.
10. Sperry R: Lateral specialization of cerebral function in the surgically separated hemispheres. In McGuigan F, editor: The psychophysiology of thinking, New York, 1973, Academic Press.
11. Sperry R and others: Interhemispheric relationships: the neocortical commissures; syndromes of hemisphere disconnection. In Vinken P, editor: Handbook of clinical neurology, Amsterdam, 1969, North Holland Publishing Co.

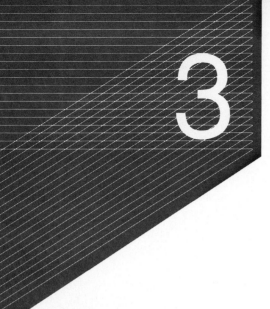

3 Cardiovascular Assessment

Cathie E. Guzzetta
Anita P. Sherer
Barbara Montgomery Dossey

LEARNING OBJECTIVES

1. Compare a holistic nursing assessment with a medical data base.
2. Identify the nine human response patterns and discuss the purpose of assessing each.
3. Explain the benefits of using a holistic cardiovascular assessment tool.
4. Assess a patient with cardiovascular disease using a holistic cardiovascular assessment tool.
5. Evaluate and revise the cardiovascular assessment tool based on the needs and requirements of your practice.

In the early 1970s, "assessment" was added to the expanded role of the nurse, although at the time, few nurses really knew what it meant. Soon it was discovered that it meant "physical" assessment. These new responsibilities were a logical extension of nursing practice, given the proliferation of critical care and step-down units across the country. In many cases, physicians first taught physical assessment to nurses. Later, as nurses became trained in physical assessment skills, they taught assessment courses at nursing schools and clinical institutions. As more nurses became proficient in physical assessment, assessment books written by nurses became available, nursing assessment articles were written, and seminars, conferences, and in-service classes were devoted to the topic. Through the identification and synthesis of the components of a nursing assessment, nurses have established their own unique role in identifying, diagnosing, preventing, and treating physical problems and have significantly enhanced the outcomes of patient care.

Although admission assessment forms are not standardized throughout the country, they nevertheless contain comparable data. Most include conventional information such as pertinent demographic data, past medical history, family history, a review of systems, and a physical examination (e.g., heart sounds, breath sounds, pupil checks, reflexes, and jugular venous pressure). Most also include some psychosocial questions (e.g., sleep patterns, exercise habits, hobbies, and level of anxiety) at the beginning or end of the tool.[22,23] The physical assessment skills performed by nurses and the way that the findings are recorded

and documented reflect the learning imparted by the physician-teachers who were guided by the biomedical model. As a result, the kind of assessment most nurses perform reflects this biomedical model orientation. Data are recorded on nursing assessment tools that are really nothing more than a medical data base with some psychosocial questions tacked on.[22,23]

Professional nursing has claimed to have moved away from the biomedical model and turned toward the more complete holistic model of health and illness.[12] As a result, nurses view the patient differently than physicians, and their assessment and corresponding data base must be structured and developed to reflect this difference. Nursing is concerned with the way the patient responds, physiologically and psychologically, to disease or illness. From a holistic nursing assessment, the individual is viewed as a bio-psycho-social-spiritual unit who is constantly exchanging and interacting with living and nonliving elements of the environment to create unique patterns and processes.[13] From this framework, the mind and body are seen as operating on a continuum. Disease is much more than a body process; it involves the whole person. The holistic model asserts that any explanation about the reasons that molecules malfunction and cause disease must include consciousness as a central factor. Thus the conscious mind is viewed as equally involved in all matters of health and illness.[13]

The nursing diagnosis movement[17] has in nearly two decades tried to identify, standardize, and research nursing diagnostic terminology. Further, advances in assessment areas that fall outside of the physiologic realm are of increasing importance to nursing practice. There is no doubt, for example, that astute cardiovascular nurses can identify a grade IV systolic heart murmur or recognize the signs and symptoms of congestive heart failure. There is some doubt, however, about whether all nurses have learned the additional assessment skills necessary to identify the signs and symptoms of powerlessness, body-image disturbance, or impaired social interaction. Moreover if the necessary data are not collected to assess these problems, it is impossible to identify many nursing diagnoses and for a holistic assessment to emerge. Thus major obstacles are incurred when using a medical data base because only part of the data necessary to assess all of the patient's bio-psy-cho-social-spiritual problems is collected.[23]

CONCEPTUAL MODELS OF NURSING

Over the last several decades, nursing leaders have recommended that conceptual models or frameworks of nursing be used to guide nursing practice.[8,12,19] Models provide the building blocks of clinical practice. They provide the big picture of nurses' responsibilities and actions. Nursing models also provide direction for the nursing process (i.e., assessment, nursing diagnosis, patient outcomes, planning, intervention, and evaluation). Within the first step of the nursing process, assessment, the model serves as the blueprint to determine the data to be collected when assessing patients. The model guides data collection and influences assessment findings and their interpretation. It also guides the development of assessment tool forms.

Traditional nursing models include Roy's adaptation model,[36] Chrisman and Fowler's systems-in-change model,[9] Rogers' unitary model,[35] Watson's human care model,[44] and Newman's health-as-expanding-consciousness model.[32] One holistic model, called the *Unitary Person Framework,* developed by the North American Nursing Diagnosis Association (NANDA),[40] focuses on the health

NINE HUMAN RESPONSE PATTERNS OF THE UNITARY PERSON FRAMEWORK

Exchanging: a human response pattern involving mutual giving and receiving
Communicating: a human response pattern involving sending messages
Relating: a human response pattern involving establishing bonds
Valuing: a human response pattern involving the assigning of relative worth
Choosing: a human response pattern involving the selection of alternatives
Moving: a human response pattern involving activity
Perceiving: a human response pattern involving the reception of information
Knowing: a human response pattern involving the meaning associated with information
Feeling: a human response pattern involving the subjective awareness of information

From the North American Nursing Diagnosis Association, St Louis, 1990.

TABLE 3-1
Taxonomy I Revised 1990*

Number	Nursing diagnosis	Number	Nursing diagnosis
PATTERN 1: EXCHANGING		**PATTERN 1: EXCHANGING, cont'd**	
1.1.2.1	Altered nutrition: more than body requirements	1.2.2.4	Ineffective thermoregulation
		1.2.3.1	Dysreflexia
1.1.2.2	Altered nutrition: less than body requirements	‡1.3.1.1	Constipation
		1.3.1.1.1	Perceived constipation
1.1.2.3	Altered nutrition: potential for more than body requirements	1.3.1.1.2	Colonic constipation
		‡1.3.1.2	Diarrhea
1.2.1.1	Potential for infection	‡1.3.1.3	Bowel incontinence
1.2.2.1	Potential altered body temperature	1.3.2	Altered urinary elimination
1.2.2.2	Hypothermia	1.3.2.1.1	Stress incontinence
1.2.2.3	Hyperthermia	1.3.2.1.2	Reflex incontinence

*This list represents the NANDA-approved nursing diagnoses for clinical use and testing (1990). NANDA-approved diagnoses currently designated as "potential for" will be changed to "high risk for" in 1992.
†New diagnostic categories approved 1990.
‡Categories with modified label terminology.
From the North American Nursing Diagnosis Association: St Louis, Mo, 1990, The Association.

Continued.

TABLE 3-1

Taxonomy I Revised 1990*—cont'd

Number	Nursing diagnosis
PATTERN 1: EXCHANGING, cont'd	
1.3.2.1.3	Urge incontinence
1.3.2.1.4	Functional incontinence
1.3.2.1.5	Total incontinence
1.3.2.2	Urinary retention
‡1.4.1.1	Altered (specify type) tissue perfusion (renal, cerebral, cardiopulmonary, gastrointestinal, peripheral)
1.4.1.2.1	Fluid volume excess
1.4.1.2.2.1	Fluid volume deficit
1.4.1.2.2.2	Potential fluid volume deficit
‡1.4.2.1	Decreased cardiac output
1.5.1.1	Impaired gas exchange
1.5.1.2	Ineffective airway clearance
1.5.1.3	Ineffective breathing pattern
1.6.1	Potential for injury
1.6.1.1	Potential for suffocation
1.6.1.2	Potential for poisoning
1.6.1.3	Potential for trauma
1.6.1.4	Potential for aspiration
1.6.1.5	Potential for disuse syndrome
†1.6.2	Altered protection
1.6.2.1	Impaired tissue integrity
‡1.6.2.1.1	Altered oral mucous membrane
1.6.2.1.2.1	Impaired skin integrity
1.6.2.1.2.2	Potential impaired skin integrity
PATTERN 2: COMMUNICATING	
2.1.1.1	Impaired verbal communication
PATTERN 3: RELATING	
3.1.1	Impaired social interaction
3.1.2	Social isolation
‡3.2.1	Altered role performance
3.2.1.1.1	Altered parenting
3.2.1.1.2	Potential altered parenting
3.2.1.2.1	Sexual dysfunction
3.2.2	Altered family processes
3.2.3.1	Parental role conflict
3.3	Altered sexuality patterns
PATTERN 4: VALUING	
4.1.1	Spiritual distress (distress of the human spirit)
PATTERN 5: CHOOSING	
5.1.1.1	Ineffective individual coping
5.1.1.1.1	Impaired adjustment
5.1.1.1.2	Defensive coping
5.1.1.1.3	Ineffective denial
5.1.2.1.1	Ineffective family coping: disabling
5.1.2.1.2	Ineffective family coping: compromised
5.1.2.2	Family coping: potential for growth
5.2.1.1	Noncompliance (specify)
5.3.1.1	Decisional conflict (specify)
5.4	Health-seeking behaviors (specify)

Number	Nursing diagnosis
PATTERN 6: MOVING	
6.1.1.1	Impaired physical mobility
6.1.1.2	Activity intolerance
6.1.1.2.1	Fatigue
6.1.1.3	Potential activity intolerance
6.2.1	Sleep pattern disturbance
6.3.1.1	Diversional activity deficit
6.4.1.1	Impaired home maintenance management
6.4.2	Altered health maintenance
‡6.5.1	Feeding self-care deficit
6.5.1.1	Impaired swallowing
6.5.1.2	Ineffective breastfeeding
†6.5.1.3	Effective breastfeeding
‡6.5.2	Bathing/hygiene self-care deficit
‡6.5.3	Dressing/grooming self-care deficit
‡6.5.4	Toileting self-care deficit
6.6	Altered growth and development
PATTERN 7: PERCEIVING	
‡7.1.1	Body-image disturbance
‡7.1.2	Self-esteem disturbance
7.1.2.1	Chronic low self-esteem
7.1.2.2	Situational low self-esteem
‡7.1.3	Personal identity disturbance
7.2	Sensory/perceptual alterations (specify) (visual, auditory, kinesthetic, gustatory, tactile, olfactory)
7.2.1.1	Unilateral neglect
7.3.1	Hopelessness
7.3.2	Powerlessness
PATTERN 8: KNOWING	
8.1.1	Knowledge deficit (specify)
8.3	Altered thought processes
PATTERN 9: FEELING	
‡9.1.1	Pain
9.1.1.1	Chronic pain
9.2.1.1	Dysfunctional grieving
9.2.1.2	Anticipatory grieving
9.2.2	Potential for violence: self-directed or directed at others
9.2.3	Post-trauma response
9.2.3.1	Rape-trauma syndrome
9.2.3.1.1	Rape-trauma syndrome: compound reaction
9.2.3.1.2	Rape-trauma syndrome: silent reaction
9.3.1	Anxiety
9.3.2	Fear

of the person, who is viewed as an open system interacting with the environment. Within this framework, each person has unique patterns of organization, which describes his or her state of health, as manifested by the nine human response patterns outlined in the box[7], p. 41. These patterns are believed to reflect all parts of the whole person.

The nine human response patterns also have been used to classify all NANDA-approved nursing diagnoses. In the past, NANDA-approved nursing diagnoses were organized alphabetically.[2,29,37] Currently, the alphabetical list has been replaced by *Taxonomy I*, which organizes nursing diagnoses according to the nine human response patterns (Table 3-1). (Also see Taxonomy I, p. 81.)

HOLISTIC CARDIOVASCULAR ASSESSMENT TOOL

Fig. 3-1 is an example of a holistic cardiovascular assessment tool.[22,23] This tool was developed so that all parts of the whole person could be assessed by evaluating each of the nine response patterns that compose the whole. When the tool was developed, the nine response patterns were rearranged and thus became the skeleton of the tool.[23] The *Standards of Cardiovascular Nursing*[1] and the *Standards for Nursing Care of the Critically Ill*[38] have been incorporated. Also, specific assessment parameters (signs and symptoms) related to most nursing diagnoses have been added to the appropriate nine human response patterns in the tool. NANDA's defining characteristics were used, as well.[7]

This assessment tool groups assessment parameters for a particular problem so that the nurse can determine whether a specific nursing diagnosis exists. Subjective data are followed by objective data within each major category of the tool. Summary assessment parameters (e.g., "willingness to comply with future health care regimen" under the Choosing Pattern) help the nurse to evaluate each nursing diagnosis. To clarify the data that are to be extracted from these summary assessment parameters, the questions and parameters on pp. 50 to 74 can be used.[18]

Although the original prototype tool was developed to assess the problems of the critically ill cardiovascular patient, it can be adapted for use with other patients (e.g., neurosurgical, neonatal, transplant, labor and delivery, psychiatric, and rehabilitation patients). Twenty-three assessment tools, all based on the Unitary Person Framework and Taxonomy I, have been developed for use with diverse patient populations.[23] The theory, process, structure, and outcome of these tools are the same, thereby offering a model for standardizing nursing data bases throughout nursing practice.[23]

USING THE HOLISTIC CARDIOVASCULAR ASSESSMENT TOOL

A nursing assessment is a logical, systematic, and ordered collection of data used to evaluate the health status of a patient to identify bio-psycho-social-spiritual problems.[21] A holistic assessment, however, involves more than just collecting appropriate data.[11] Nurses and patients are open systems; they exchange energy and information at many levels.[20,21] As in all human interactions, the quality and type of relationship between two persons influence the depth of information given and received. The nurse's sensitivity and perceptiveness greatly affect each nurse-patient encounter. Nurses function at their highest level when they are open to subtle cues, environmental changes, and intuitive feelings; each cue, change, or feeling can have an enormous impact on data collected and conclusions formulated during assessment. Nurses who are focused during assessment become aware of collecting data with purposeful intention. They become receptive to the encounter, thus allowing a free flow of information at many levels. They are able to use analytic and intuitive thinking when assessing a patient's nine human response patterns, which provide a rich data base by which to understand holistic patterns and processes.[30,34]

Moving from the more traditional organization of a medical data base, however, requires an effort on nurses' part. Nurses must cultivate a new way of collecting, synthesizing, and interrelating data so that the whole person can be understood. It requires the realization that problems in one human response pattern influence the other patterns.[30] The ability to identify signs and symptoms for each pattern is enhanced with practice.

Patients should be assessed within an appropriate time period, usually within 24 hours of admission. If the patient is in critical condition, priority sections are identified first; for example, rapid evaluation of the patient is done using the ABCs of basic life support in the Exchanging Pattern, disregarding the order of the variables in this section, and assessing only variables pertinent to the situation. After the patient has stabilized, the other response patterns can be assessed.[23]

When specific signs and symptoms that indicate a diagnosis are identified, the nurse circles the diagnosis in the right-hand column of the tool. A circled diagnosis does not confirm the diagnosis but simply alerts the nurse to a possible problem. If a particular problem is suspected, a complete evaluation is required to assess the critical defining characteristics of the diagnosis. The diagnoses are listed in the right-hand column as a learning technique to focus thinking, direct more detailed attention to a possible problem, and assist in identifying appropriate nursing diagnoses.[23]

Assessment variables are arranged with the diagnosis most likely to result from the data assessed. Some signs and symptoms, however, can indicate a number of diagnoses (e.g., tachycardia identified under the Exchanging Pattern may support the diagnosis of "anxiety" under the Feeling Pattern).[23] Therefore synthesis of all data is essential because data to support one diagnosis may be found

Text continued on p. 50.

HOLISTIC CARDIOVASCULAR ASSESSMENT TOOL*

Name _____ Age _____ Sex _____
Address _____ Telephone _____
Significant other _____ Telephone _____
Date of admission _____ Medical diagnosis _____
Allergies _____

COMMUNICATING ▪ A pattern involving sending messages   **Nursing Diagnosis**
Read, write, understand English (circle) _____   Impaired verbal
Other languages _____   communication
Intubated _____ Speech impaired _____
Alternate form of communication _____

KNOWING ▪ A pattern involving the meaning associated with information
Current health problems _____
_____
Previous illnesses/hospitalizations/surgeries _____
_____

History of the following problems: Knowledge deficit
    Heart _____
    Peripheral vascular _____
    Lung _____
    Liver _____ Kidney _____
    Cerebrovascular _____ Rheumatic fever _____
    Thyroid _____
    Other _____
Current medications _____
_____
_____

Risk factors   Present   Perceptions/Knowledge of
  1. Hypertension   _____ _____
  2. Hyperlipidemia   _____ _____
  3. Smoking   _____ _____
  4. Obesity   _____ _____
  5. Diabetes   _____ _____
  6. Sedentary living   _____ _____
  7. Stress   _____ _____
  8. Alcohol use   _____ _____
  9. Oral contraceptives _____ _____
 10. Family history   _____ _____

Perception/knowledge of illness/test/surgery _____
_____
Expectations of therapy _____
Misconceptions _____
Readiness to learn _____
    Requests information concerning _____
    Educational level _____
    Learning impeded by _____

*Adapted from: Guzzetta C et al: Clinical assessment tools for use with nursing diagnoses, St Louis, 1989, The CV Mosby Co.

FIG. 3-1 Holistic Cardiovascular Assessment Tool.

Orientation   Altered thought processes
    Level of alertness _____
    Orientation: Person _____ Place _____ Time _____
    Appropriate behavior/communication _____

Memory
    Memory intact: Yes _____ No _____ Recent _____ Remote _____

VALUING ▪ A pattern involving the assigning of relative worth
Spirituality or religious preference _____   Spiritual distress
Important spiritual or religious practices _____
Spiritual concerns _____
Cultural orientation _____
Cultural practices _____

RELATING ▪ A pattern involving establishing bonds
Role
    Marital status _____   Altered role performance
    Age & health of significant other _____   Parenting
                                                                  Sexual dysfunction
    Number of children _____ Ages _____   Work
    Role in home _____
    Financial support _____
    Occupation _____   Altered family processes
        Job satisfaction/concerns _____   Parental role conflict
        Physical/mental energy expenditures _____
    Sexual relationships (satisfactory/unsatisfactory) _____   Altered sexuality patterns
        Physical difficulties/effects of illness related to sex _____

Socialization   Altered socialization
    Quality of relationships with others: Impaired social interaction
        Patient's description _____
        Significant other's description _____
        Staff observations _____
        Verbalizes feelings of being alone _____   Social isolation
        Attributed to _____

FEELING ▪ A pattern involving the subjective awareness of information
Comfort
    Pain/discomfort: Yes _____ No _____
        Onset _____ Duration _____   Pain/chronic
        Location _____ Quality _____ Radiation _____   Pain/acute
        Associated factors _____
        Aggravating factors _____
        Alleviating factors _____
        Objective manifestations _____

Emotional Integrity/States
    Recent stressful life events _____

    Verbalizes feelings of _____   Anxiety
        Source _____   Fear
                                                             Grieving
    Physical manifestations _____   Dysfunctional
                                                                 Anticipatory

Continued.

MOVING ▪ A pattern involving activity
Self-care
Ability to perform self-care (specify level) _____

Specify deficits _____

Discharge planning needs _____

Self-care deficit
   (Level 0-4)
Feeding
   Impaired swallowing
Bathing/hygiene
Dressing/grooming
Toileting

Activity
Limitations of movement (specify level) _____

_____

Limitations in activities _____

_____

Verbal report of fatigue _____

Exercise habits _____

Impaired physical mobility
   (Level 0-4)
Activity intolerance
   Fatigue

Rest
Sleep/rest pattern _____
   Sleep aids (pillows, meds, food) _____
   Difficulty falling/remaining asleep _____

Sleep pattern disturbance

Recreation
Leisure activities _____
Social activities _____

Diversional activity deficit

Activities of Daily Living
Home maintenance management
   Size & arrangement of home (stairs, bathroom) _____
   _____ Safety needs _____
   Home responsibilities _____

_____

Impaired home maintenance
   management

Health maintenance
   Health insurance _____
Regular physical check-ups _____

Altered health maintenance

PERCEIVING ▪ A pattern involving the reception of information
Body image/Self-esteem
Perception of self and situation _____

_____

Description of body structure/functioning _____

_____

Self-esteem disturbance
   Chronic low
   Situational low
Body image disturbance

Meaningfulness
Verbalizes hopelessness _____
Verbalizes loss of control _____

Hopelessness
Powerlessness

Sensory/Perception
History of restricted environment _____
Vision impaired _____ Glasses _____
Auditory impaired _____ Hearing aid _____
Kinesthetics impaired _____
Gustatory impaired _____
Tactile impaired _____
Olfactory impaired _____

Altered sensory/perception
   Visual
   Auditory
   Kinesthetic
   Gustatory
   Tactile
   Olfactory

Reflexes: Biceps   R ____ L ____   Triceps R ____ L ____
           Brachioradialis R ____ L ____   Knee   R ____ L ____
           Ankle   R ____ L ____   Plantar R ____ L ____

EXCHANGING ▪ A pattern involving mutual giving and receiving
Circulation
  Cerebral   Altered cerebral tissue
    Neurologic changes/symptoms _____   perfusion
    Complaints of syncope _____
    Pupils   Eye Opening
      L 2 3 4 5 6 mm   None (1)
      R 2 3 4 5 6 mm   To pain (2)   Fluid volume
      Reaction: Brisk _____   To speech (3)   Deficit
      Sluggish _____ Nonreactive _____   Spontaneous (4)   Excess
      Retina _____
    Best Verbal   Best Motor
      Mute (1)   Flaccid (1)
      Incomprehensible sound (2)   Extensor response (2)   Decreased cardiac output
      Inappropriate words (3)   Flexor response (3)
      Confused conversation (4)   Semipurposeful (4)
      Oriented (5)   Localized to pain (5)
                           Obeys commands (6)
  Glasgow coma scale total _____   Altered cerebral tissue
                                                perfusion
  Peripheral   Altered peripheral tissue
                                              perfusion
    Arterial pulses: A = absent   B = bruits   D = Doppler
      +3 = bounding   +2 = palpable   +1 = faintly palpable
    Carotid   R _____ L _____   Popliteal   R _____ L _____
    Brachial   R _____ L _____   Posterior tibial   R _____ L _____   Fluid volume
    Radial   R _____ L _____   Dorsalis pedis   R _____ L _____   Deficit
    Femoral   R _____ L _____   Excess
    BP: Sitting   Lying   Standing
          R _____ L _____   R _____ L _____   R _____ L _____
          A-Line reading _____   CVP _____
    Venous pulse _____   Jugular venous distention R _____ L _____
    Peripheral veins _____
    Skin temp _____ Color _____ Cyanosis _____
    Capillary refill _____ Edema _____
    Clubbing _____
  Cardiovascular
    PMI _____ Pacemaker _____   Altered cardiopulmonary
    Apical rate & rhythm _____   tissue perfusion
    Heart sounds/murmurs _____
    Dysrhythmias _____
    Cardiac output _____ Cardiac index _____   Decreased cardiac output
    PAP _____ PAWP _____
    IV fluids _____
    IV medications _____   Dysreflexia
    _____
    Serum enzymes _____
Physical Integrity
  Tissue integrity _____   Impaired skin integrity
    Skin: Rash _____ Lesions _____   Impaired tissue integrity
    Petechiae _____ Bruises _____   Disuse syndrome
    Abrasions _____ Surgical incision _____   Infection
                                             Altered protection

Continued.

Oxygenation

Complaints of dyspnea _____ Precipitated by _____

Orthopnea _____

Rate _____ Rhythm _____ Depth _____   Ineffective breathing patterns

Labored/unlabored (circle)   Use of accessory muscles _____

Chest expansion _____ Splinting _____   Ineffective airway clearance

Cough: Productive/nonproductive _____

Sputum: Color _____ Amount _____ Consistency _____   Impaired gas exchange

Breath sounds _____   High risk for aspiration

Arterial blood gases _____

Oxygen percent and device _____

Ventilator _____

Physical Regulation

Immune   Infection

    Lymph nodes enlarged _____ Location _____   Hypothermia

    WBC count _____ Differential _____   Hyperthermia

    Temperature _____ Route _____   Altered body temperature

    Ineffective thermoregulation

    Altered protection

Nutrition

Eating patterns

    Number of meals per day _____   Altered nutrition

    Special diet _____   More than body

    Where eaten _____   requirements

    Food preferences/intolerances _____   Less than body

    Food allergies _____   requirements

    Caffeine intake (coffee, tea, soft drinks) _____

    _____

    Appetite changes _____

    Presence of nausea/vomiting _____

Condition of mouth/throat _____   Impaired oral mucous

_____   membranes

    Height _____ Weight _____ Ideal body weight _____   Altered nutrition

    More than body

Current therapy   requirements

    NPO _____ NG suction _____   Less than body

    Tube feeding _____   requirements

    TPN _____   High risk for aspiration

Labs

    Na _____ K _____ Cl _____ Glucose _____

    Cholesterol _____ Triglycerides _____ Fasting _____

    Hct _____ Hgb _____

    Other _____

Elimination

Gastrointestinal/Bowel   Altered bowel elimination

    Usual bowel habits _____   Constipation

    Use of laxatives, enemas, and/or suppositories _____   Perceived

    Alterations from norm _____   Colonic

    Abdominal physical exam _____   Diarrhea

    Incontinence

    Altered GI tissue perfusion

Renal/Urinary

    Usual urinary pattern _____   Altered urinary elimination

    Alteration from norm _____   Incontinence

    Bladder distention _____   Retention

    Color _____ Catheter _____   Altered renal tissue perfusion

    Urine output: 24 hour _____ Average hourly _____

    BUN _____ Creatinine _____ Specific gravity _____

    Urine studies _____

CHOOSING ▪ A pattern involving the selection of alternatives
Coping
    Patient's ability to cope _____   Ineffective individual coping
    _____   Defensive coping
    Family's ability to cope/give support _____   Ineffective denial
    _____   Impaired adjustment
    Patient's acceptance of illness _____
    _____   Ineffecitve family coping
    Patient's adjustment to illness _____   Disabled
    _____   Compromised

Judgment
    Decision making ability:
      Patient's perspective _____   Decisional conflict
      Other's perspective _____
    Ability to choose from alternatives _____

Participation
    Compliance with past/current health care regimen _____   Noncompliance
    _____
    Willingness to comply with future health care regimen _____

Health seeking
    Express desire to seek higher level of wellness _____   Health seeking behaviors
    _____

Prioritized nursing diagnoses/problem list:
1. _____
2. _____
3. _____
4. _____
5. _____
6. _____

Signature _____   Date _____

in other patterns. After data are synthesized, the nurse may discover that the data suggesting one diagnosis may indicate a more global nursing diagnosis. For example, data identified for "fear" and "social isolation" may support the diagnosis of "altered self-concept related to chronic illness." Therefore all diagnoses circled may not appear on the problem list at the end of the tool. Also the words "high risk for" are written next to the diagnosis if the patient is highly vulnerable to developing the problem.[23]

Because Taxonomy I is still being developed, many patient problems (nursing diagnoses) are missing from the list. Thus patients may exhibit signs and symptoms that support the existence of a new diagnosis not found in Taxonomy I. New diagnoses can be written in the right-hand column of the tool and circled.[23]

When the assessment is complete, the nurse reviews the circled problems, synthesizes the data, and formulates the appropriate list of nursing diagnoses and their probable etiologies. The diagnoses are then put in order of priority and are written on the problem list at the end of the tool. Patient outcomes and the plan for intervention (written in terms of nursing prescriptions) are identified for the most critical diagnoses. Less critical diagnoses are considered at a later date or are referred to other health care members as appropriate.[23]

There are many reasons for using a holistic cardiovascular assessment tool. The tool elicits data about holistic patterns from a nursing point of view. Because data measure human response patterns, the information is pertinent to nursing diagnoses. The tool provides the data necessary to validate and document the existence of nursing diagnoses. In fact, frequently the data are so rich that nursing diagnoses appear to "fall out" of the assessment.[23]

Nine human response patterns*

The following questions and parameters were developed to elicit meaningful data using the nine human response patterns. They follow the order of the tool in Fig. 3-1; however, the sequence in which the data are collected will depend on the type and condition of the patient.[23]

COMMUNICATING PATTERN

The purpose of this assessment is to determine whether the patient is able to communicate verbally and nonverbally with others. This pattern is evaluated first because the rest of the assessment depends on the patient's ability to communicate. If the patient is unable to communicate, the information may need to be obtained from family or a significant other.[3]

---

*Adapted from Guzzetta CE and others: Clinical assessment tools for use with nursing diagnosis, St Louis, 1989, The CV Mosby Co.

Language skills

Begin the assessment by evaluating the patient's written and oral language skills, including the ability to understand, speak, read, and write Engish. You can easily obtain this information by asking the patient about demographic data such as name, age, address, and telephone number. If any difficulty is identified, first determine whether there is a physiologic or psychologic cause (e.g., reduced blood pressure or brain circulation, stroke, brain tumor, oral anatomic defect, severe anxiety, or psychosis). Identify the primary language spoken in the home, as well as other languages spoken. Use an interpreter if the patient's primary language differs from yours and you find that communication is ineffective. Document whether the patient can use an alternate form of communication such as sign language, a sign board, writing, a typewriter, or a computer.[26]

Intubation and speech impairment

Determine whether the patient is able to speak and whether there are any barriers to communication. If the patient is unable to speak, document whether the patient is intubated or has a tracheostomy. Determine the reason and date that the intubation or tracheostomy was done. Also assess severe shortness of breath, facial paralysis, facial lacerations or burns, or a mandibular fracture as other possible reasons for an inability to speak. Evaluate whether the patient has slurred speech, stutters, is able to modulate speech, find words, name words, identify objects, and speaks in sentences.[6,15,26] Determine whether the patient has difficulty with phonation (i.e., ability to utter vocal sounds).

KNOWING PATTERN

The purpose of this assessment is to determine patient knowledge about the current and past health status and to evaluate readiness to learn, misconceptions, and level of orientation.

Current health problems

First seek information about the health problem that prompted the patient to seek health care assistance by simply asking, "What brought you to the hospital or clinic?" or "Why are you seeking medical attention?"[26] The problem should be succinctly and accurately stated. Elicit information about the severity and chronicity of the major concerns.

Assess current health problems by a chronologic overview of symptoms, including the circumstances around their onset and the changes and developments that followed.[26,43] This information provides a focus for collection of more specific data in the associated patterns of concern;

(e.g., for a patient who was admitted to a coronary care unit for syncope, a comprehensive assessment of the neurologic and cardiac categories under the Exchanging Pattern would be performed.)[21] Using communication and listening skills, assist the patient as much as possible during this phase of the assessment. In addition to objective complaints, recognize and note the patient's observations and perceptions of the complaints. As the patient expresses perceived physiologic or psychologic changes, reorganize the information according to the data base format to identify the patterns and processes underlying each sign and symptom.

Comprehensively describe individual symptoms. For each sign and symptom identified within a pattern, determine the time when and the circumstances under which the sign or symptom occurred. Explore the onset, duration, frequency, precipitating and alleviating factors, as well as the location, severity, and chronicity of the complaint.[43] Identify the absolute quantity (that is, the number of episodes per unit of time) and the severity of each episode. Make every effort to avoid inconclusive or general remarks, but remember that the relative quality of the symptom at present (compared with the past) may provide valuable information about the course of the illness.

In determining a clear symptomatology, record pertinent negative responses because the descriptions of some symptoms are so typical in many instances that the lack of an expected characteristic may be highly meaningful. For example, a patient who strongly verbalizes a perceived lack of control over the current situation (suggesting the diagnosis of "powerlessness") may be observed to be participating in self-care and decision making with a high degree of control.

Avoid the mistake of grouping or relating one complaint to another when the justification of such a grouping is unclear. Keep complaints separate unless you find a definite reason to support the grouping in the initial phases of the assessment.

Health history

Know that information on previous illnesses, hospitalizations, surgeries, and other problems may be extremely valuable in understanding the present complaints, as well as reactions to these problems. Be systematic in questioning so that areas requiring further evaluation are uncovered and important data are not obscured.

Understand that prior illnesses, hospitalizations, and surgeries are often identified most easily by the patient. Assess childhood illnesses, the patient's birth (especially birth weight and complications), a childhood history of rheumatic fever, and episodic cyanosis.

Determine whether the patient has been told of any previous cardiac disorders, such as a heart murmur, dysrhythmia, cardiac enlargement, angina pectoris, a possible myocardial infarction (MI), and heart failure, and whether any of these conditions were treated and the length of treatment.

Pay specific attention to a history of chest surgery or trauma and possible infections such as periodontal disease and other chronic bacterial infections that may predispose the individual to infective endocarditis. Determine whether there are metabolic disorders such as thyroid disease, glucose intolerance, or diabetes mellitus that may predispose the patient to premature atherosclerosis.

Look for signs or symptoms of peripheral vascular disease such as those related to intermittent claudication (e.g., calf cramping and fatigue when walking or exercising that is relieved by rest). Inquire about a history of lung disease such as tuberculosis, asthma, lung infections, or bronchitis. Identify frequent respiratory infections, which may indicate a possible intracardiac shunt.

Also identify the following: history of liver disease such as liver enlargement or hepatitis; kidney disease such as infections or stones; cerebrovascular problems such as dizziness, fainting, transient ischemic attacks, or strokes; gallbladder, gastrointestinal, or genitourinary problems; or hyperuricemia, or clinical gout.

Current medications

Investigate drug allergies. Identify previous life-threatening reactions to blood transfusions or contrast media (iodinated dyes) such as those used in angiographic and computed tomographic studies.

Identify medications that the patient is taking, including the name, dosage and frequency, length of therapy, and side effects. Also determine whether the patient is taking over-the-counter medications such as aspirin, acetaminophen, ibuprofen, laxatives, sleeping pills, or diet pills. Ask the patient to pick a typical day and describe all medications (physician- and self-prescribed) taken from morning until bedtime. In addition, specifically and accurately record current medications so that errors, incompatibilities, or inadvertent changes are not made in the a patient's pharmacologic regimen. Be particularly careful to obtain a medication history for the elderly patient, who may see more than one health care provider and consume several drugs that have synergistic or mutually inhibitory effects.[21]

Risk factors

Determine if patients have *coronary artery disease risk factors* and assess their perception and level of understanding[21,43] (see Chapter 8). Determine whether patients are aware of the way that the risk factors affect the heart and whether they consider the risk factor to be a significant threat to their health. Query patients about a history of *hypertension* and *hyperlipidemia,* especially hypercholesterolemia and hypertriglyceridemia. Ask about when the hypertension or hyperlipidemia was diagnosed (refer to "diet, current medications, and rest" for how it was treated). Identify a history of *smoking,* as well as the type of tobacco (e.g., cigarettes, cigars, pipe, or chewing tobacco), the age at which smoking began, the extent of daily use, and the age at which the smoking habit increased, decreased, or ceased. Inquire whether the patient has attempted to quit smoking in the past and whether there is an interest to stop.

Identify whether the patient has a history of *obesity* and determine the length of time that this condition has existed (refer to "ideal body weight" under "nutrition" in the Exchanging Pattern to determine the number of pounds/kilograms overweight; refer to "diet, exercise, and medications" for length of treatment). Investigate whether there is an interest in losing weight.

Identify whether the patient has a history of *diabetes mellitus* and the age at which it was diagnosed and whether treatment consists of diet, pills, or insulin injections (refer to "current medications and diet"). Explore the patient's lifestyle, especially with regard to activity levels and *sedentary living* (also refer to "exercise habits" under the Moving Pattern to determine the type and amount of daily exercise).

Explore high levels of *psychophysiologic stress,* especially stress related to work or family interactions (also refer to "recent stressful life events" under the Feeling Pattern), and assess behavior traits, especially type A personality. Document *substance abuse* such as alcohol or cocaine use, noting the type, amount, duration, and pattern of use.[45] Explore whether the substance abuse has interferred with the patient's job, marriage, or health and whether the patient has been hospitalized or is motivated to receive help regarding this problem. Identify the date and time the patient last used or ingested such substances. Also document the use of oral contraceptives, cessation of menses, or the beginning of menopause.

To better estimate the risk of cardiovascular disease for the patient, obtain a *family history,* which includes the history of blood relatives, especially parents and children. Identify age, sex, and health status of living family members, including parents, siblings, children, and spouse or significant other. Determine age, sex, and cause of death for deceased family members. Determine a family history of heart disease or premature atherosclerosis. Assess for certain familial diseases (e.g., assess for a family history of the coronary artery disease risk factors from the list outlined previously). Also determine a family history of cancer, other heart problems, peripheral vascular disease, cerebrovascular disease, hypertension, stroke, respiratory disease, diabetes mellitus, nervous or mental conditions, kidney disease, arthritic conditions, hematologic abnormalities, rheumatic fever, sickle cell anemia, or thyroid disease.

Perceptions and expectations

Investigate current knowledge and perceptions of the illness, tests, or surgery. Query patients about their perceptions of their biggest health problem. Ask them to discuss the problem and its cause. Also determine patient knowledge and understanding of upcoming tests, procedures, or surgery. Because patients can have assorted expectations about hospitalization and therapy, explore patient expectations of treatments and results.

Misconceptions

Identify misconceptions or lack of understanding regarding hospitalization, illness, tests, surgery, or therapy. When evaluating misconceptions, assess risk factors, perception and knowledge of the current situation, and expectations of therapy. Evaluate the answers given by the patient and the family. Determine whether the information is correct, whether the patient and family have a good understanding of the information, and whether the understanding is realistic for the situation.

Readiness to learn

Also assess readiness to learn because patients frequently request information that relates only to the immediate situation when they are critically ill. Evaluate the questions asked and the kind of information requested. For example, the patient might ask questions about the therapy, treatments, illness, or prognosis, or the patient might deny that a health problem exists.[19,21] (Integrate this data with the information associated with "coping" in the Choosing Pattern). Determine the patient's educational level so that teaching content and material can be selected appropriately. Also evaluate barriers to learning such as pain, environmental distractions, or other physical, emotional, or psychologic conditions.

Orientation and memory

Determine whether the patient is alert and oriented to person, place, and time. Evaluate the appropriateness of the patient's behavior and communication. Determine whether the patient is confused or lethargic.

Evaluate the patient's memory. Assess recent memory by asking where the patient lives or the current day, month, and year. Assess remote memory by asking whether the patient recalls the holidays that were celebrated in a particular month.

VALUING PATTERN

The purpose of this assessment is to determine patient spiritual and cultural values and the influence that such values have on illness, hospitalization, therapy, and recovery.

Spirituality

Assess the spiritual dimension related to the purpose and meaning of the patient's life; harmony with self, others, the environment, and a higher power; and a sense of awareness of inner strengths and unifying forces (see box on p. 9).

Identify the patient's religious preference and whether the patient practices the religion and attends church or synagogue. Explore the importance of religion in the patient's life and whether the patient would like to talk to a religious representative. Ask whether the patient considers any specific religious items important to have while in the hospital. Also investigate religious beliefs or practices that might affect treatment (for example, treatments prohibited by the religion). Explore spiritual concerns by determining whether the patient is absorbed with issues of life or death or is voicing distress about a relationship with a higher unifying force. Note when the patient questions the meaning of suffering and illness, creating inner conflicts about beliefs.

Cultural orientation and practices

Identify patients' cultural background or heritage. Identify strong ties to the customs and practices of the country of origin. Investigate the cultural definition of "illness" and the role of the family during times of illness. Ask patients to describe special customs during illness. Explore whether medical treatments are unacceptable because of cultural beliefs. Investigate how the nursing staff might aid in the continuation of family practices.

RELATING PATTERN

The purpose of this assessment is to determine ways that the patient relates to others in terms of home, work, and sexual and social roles.

Role in the home

Determine patients' marital status and the ages and health of significant others. Inquire about children, their ages, and whether they are living in the home. Investigate patients' roles in the home to determine whether they are responsible for running the household, making the major decisions, and providing care and discipline for the children. Explore whether this illness will alter the ability to carry out expected home and parenting responsibilities and the way that patients feel about such changes.

Financial support

Identify whether the patient is the major source of financial support and whether there are any financial concerns because illness often has a major impact on family finances.

Identify whether the patient verbalizes the need for financial assistance.

Occupation

Identify the patient's occupation, documenting hours worked per week, the physical workload and mental energy involved, and the amount of stress perceived. Determine whether the patient likes the job and whether there are any major concerns or problems. Investigate the patient's perceptions regarding the effects of the illness on the job. Also determine whether this illness will affect the patient's ability to return to work and the way that the patient feels about this situation.

Sexual relationships

Investigate difficulties, limitations, or changes in sexual interests, behaviors, or activities[16,26] because illness can have major repercussions on the patient's desire for sexual activity and the ability to perform sexually. Determine whether the patient has been at risk for contracting human immunodeficiency virus (HIV) infection. Ask whether the patient has received blood transfusions and the date and reason. Identify whether the patient has a history of homosexuality, prostitution, or intravenous drug abuse and whether the patient admits to multiple sexual partners or to sexual contact with a person who is HIV positive.

Socialization

To assess the quality of relationships with others, ask patients to describe how they get along with others and whether they feel a sense of belonging, caring, and interest when they are with family or friends. Determine whether patients feel comfortable in most social situations or whether they prefer to be alone most of the time. Do patients verbalize that they feel isolated, alone, or rejected by family and friends?[26] Validate patients' perceptions with family or significant others. Observe their interactions and relationships with family, friends, and staff to corroborate these perceptions.

FEELING PATTERN

The purpose of this assessment is to gather information that will reveal the physical and emotional feelings of the patient.

Pain and discomfort

Query the patient about *pain* or *discomfort*. Ask the patient to describe specifically any chest pain and to characterize the quality of the pain as crushing, squeezing, aching, heavy, tight, dull, burning, pleuritic, or associated with a feeling of indigestion (see Chapters 9 and 10). Have the patient rate the severity of the pain on a scale of 1 to 10. Ask the patient to identify the location of the pain by pointing to the body area involved.[20,43] Identify whether the pain radiates to other parts of the body and whether there are any associated, aggravating, or alleviating factors. For the pain of angina pectoris, identify any of the classic "4E" precipitating factors: exposure to extreme temperature, exertion, eating, and excitement. Determine whether the pain or discomfort is acute or chronic, whether it was sudden or gradual and intermittent or continuous, and whether the patient has ever had the pain before.[20,21] Ask about the time of onset and duration.

Explore whether patients have experienced *palpitations* that may be associated with changes in rate, rhythm (especially premature beats), or hemodynamic states. Know that patients may describe this unpleasant awareness of the heart beat by using such terms as *skipping, pounding, stopping,* and *turning over.* Ask them also to describe sensations of rate, rhythm, or forcefulness of the beat. Explore what they were doing at the onset of the symptoms because dysrhythmias can be caused by emotional or physiologic factors (e.g., psychologic stress, coughing, gagging, or vomiting). Query patients regarding associated chest pain, diaphoresis, dizziness, or syncope.

Explore a history of *dyspnea,* a symptom described by the patient as shortness of breath. Ask the patient to describe the time of onset, duration, and frequency. Determine whether the dyspnea is associated with any other symptoms (i.e., nausea, vomiting, diaphoresis, dizziness, or syncope). Identify factors that precipitate the dyspnea such as exertion or lying down and factors that alleviate it such as resting, walking, or sitting up.

Dyspnea accompanies chronic lung disease and a number of cardiac conditions. It is a manifestation of congestive heart failure. Commonly, this occurs with strain and may be affected by position. Dyspnea is categorized by type, degree, progression, and duration. The amount of exertion required to cause it and the amount of rest necessary to relieve it should be quantified carefully. It may be referred to as one of three types: dyspnea on exertion, orthopnea, or paroxysmal nocturnal dyspnea.

Exertional dyspnea is commonly associated with heart failure and lung disease. Frequently the patient describes that it is brought on by activities such as climbing a flight of stairs or a hill, having sexual intercourse, or exercising the upper extremities. You will need to know the amount of activity necessary to produce symptoms and whether the dyspnea has become more severe over time.

Another form of dyspnea is *orthopnea,* which is most often associated with congestive heart failure. Within a few minutes of lying flat in bed, the patient has difficulty with breathing. The orthopnea is relieved when the patient sits or stands. Often patients report that they require two or more pillows for sleep.

Paroxysmal nocturnal dyspnea is specific for left ventricular failure. It occurs at night, with the patient having little difficulty going to sleep. However, after 1 or 2 hours, the patient awakens with a terrifying sensation of suffocating. Although paroxysmal nocturnal dyspnea is not immediately relieved when the patient assumes an upright position, the distress is diminished after sitting up for a few minutes.

Objective manifestations

Observe for objective psychophysiologic manifestations of pain or discomfort. Identify guarding or protective behaviors such as self-focusing (e.g., altered time perception, withdrawal from social contact, or impaired thought processes), moaning, crying, restlessness, and grimacing. Examine the patient for altered muscle tone or autonomic nervous system response to pain (i.e., diaphoresis; blood pressure, pulse, and respiratory rates above normal; and pupillary changes). With chronic pain, query the patient about anorexia and weight or sleep pattern changes. Investigate fears of reinjury or physical and social withdrawal.

Emotional integrity

Evaluate emotional integrity to uncover recent (within the past 18 months) stressful life events such as family, financial, or work-related problems. Explore whether the patient has been particularly upset or worried recently. Investigate feelings of anxiety, fear, or grieving.[7,26]

To assess for *anxiety,* investigate whether patients believe they are jittery, distressed, scared, "rattled," or overexcited. Explore whether patients are experiencing a threat to self-concept, death, or change in health status, socioeconomic status, role functioning, environment, or interactional patterns. Note whether patients voice complaints of increased tension, apprehension, uncertainty, or inadequacy.

When assessing for *fear,* identify feelings of dread related to an identifiable source. Document physical manifestations of anxiety and fear such as increased heart rate; blood pressure and respiratory rates above normal; startle reflex to normal sounds; nonpurposeful activity such as picking at sheets, hair, or fingernails or constant leg motion; and darting eye movements.[7,15,26]

Evaluate signs and symptoms that indicate *grieving.* Explore personal or anticipated losses. Determine whether the patient is denying a loss or having difficulty expressing a loss. Also determine the impact of grieving on functional ability such as difficulty concentrating, eating, sleeping, or performing normal daily activities.[7]

MOVING PATTERN

The purpose of this assessment is to gather data to evaluate the effects of illness on the patient's ability to maintain self-care, move, and perform activities of daily living. Exercise, sleep, play, and the ability to sustain environmental and health maintenance are also investigated.

Self-care

To assess ability to perform self-care, identify whether patients are able to feed themselves independently, adequately swallow fluids and solids, bathe themselves, brush their own hair and teeth, use a toilet or commode, dress themselves, and maintain a satisfactory appearance. Document needs for self-care discharge planning.

The following code is used to define the patient's functional ability level. It is used to classify the nursing diagnoses listed under self-care deficits (i.e., "feeding; impaired swallowing; bathing/hygiene, dressing/grooming, and toileting self-care deficits") and the diagnosis of "impaired physical mobility" (see next section).[7]

0 = Completely independent
1 = Requires use of equipment or device
2 = Requires help from another person for assistance, supervision, or teaching
3 = Requires help from another person and equipment device
4 = Dependent, does not participate in activity

Activity

Limitation of movement and activities

Investigate a history of limitations in movement ("impaired physical mobility"), including moving, walking, and getting in and out of chairs and beds. Determine whether the patient has observed a decrease in muscle size, tone, strength, or control. Assess for perceptual, cognitive, neuromuscular, or musculoskeletal impairments. Observe for limitations of movement such as a reluctance to move, limited range of motion, or impaired coordination. Use the functional code previously outlined to classify functional level.

Also investigate "activity intolerance." Ask about pain or discomfort during activity. Ask whether there are any activities the patient can no longer perform. Query the patient about diminished strength or endurance. Observe the patient during daily activities and note symptoms associated or precipitated by such activity.

Verbalization of fatigue

Because fatigue, a subjective feeling, is frequently associated with cardiac illness, particularly congestive heart failure, and can have an enormous impact on a person's ability to carry out daily activities, query each patient about lack of energy, irritability, listlessness, or an inability to concentrate. Ask about constant feelings of weariness, weakness, or exhaustion. Determine whether the patient can maintain daily routines.

Exercise habits

Assess the patient's level of daily exercise. Ask whether the patient is involved in any type of exercise program. Determine the type of program, the number of times per week the exercise is performed, and the length of each exercise session. Explore the importance of exercise to psychophysiologic well-being. Query the patient also about the amount of exercise involved with job, home, sports, or outside activities.

Rest

Assess sleep-rest patterns by identifying the patient's bed time, number of hours slept per night, and rest periods routinely set aside for naps, relaxation, or meditation. Ask whether the patient usually feels rested after sleeping. If the patient verbalizes difficulty with sleeping, inquire about changes in behavior such as irritability, restlessness, lethargy, or listlessness. Observe whether the patient demonstrates signs of "sleep pattern disturbances" (e.g., mild fleeting nystagmus, light hand tremor, ptosis of eyelids, expressionless face, dark circles under eyes, frequent yawning, or changes in posture).[21]

Ask about use of sleep aids such as warm showers, music, food, alcohol, tranquilizers, or hypnotics. Determine also whether the patient has trouble falling asleep, remaining asleep, and returning to sleep once awakened.

Recreation

To assess leisure and social activities, explore hobbies and leisure time activities (e.g., sports, fishing, yardwork, sewing, painting, reading, and listening to music). Identify complaints of boredom. Assess whether the patient's home or hospital environment and condition would permit involvement in diversional activities, as well as activities the patient might be able to do while in the hospital.

Assess the patient's involvement in social activities (i.e., church groups, clubs, or organizations). Query the patient about the extent of the involvement and the importance of such activities.

Health and environmental maintenance

Assess the level of health maintenance. Determine whether the patient routinely sees a physician or a dentist for regular physical checkups or other physicians or nurses for any other reason. Identify whether the patient verbalizes an understanding of basic health practices and a responsibility for meeting basic health needs. Explore patient interest in improving health behaviors.[7,26,43]

To assess environmental maintenance, evaluate the size and lay out of the home. Identify obstacles such as steps at the entrance or within the home. Evaluate whether the kitchen, bedroom, and bathroom are accessible and whether safety rails are needed in the bathroom.

Determine whether the current illness might interfere with daily activities such as meal preparation, household chores, shopping, cleaning, or child care. (Also integrate this data with information under "role in home" in the Relating Pattern).

PERCEIVING PATTERN

The purpose of this assessment is to evaluate the patient's self-perception in terms of self-esteem and body image. Perceived hopelessness and powerlessness, as well as sensory perception, are also evaluated.[23]

Self-concept

To assess *self-esteem,* ask patients to describe the kind of person they are. Determine whether they are comfortable about the way they look, feel, and function. Ask patients to describe the meaning of illness/surgery to them and their families. Note whether patients express negative self-talk and whether such talk is *chronic* or is *situational* in response to the illness. Note patient comments about the ability to deal with the current situation. Identify whether patients project blame onto others.

When assessing for *body-image disturbances,* identify verbal or nonverbal patient statements reflecting actual or perceived changes in body structure or functioning.[6,26] Observe whether the patient refuses to discuss the illness, injury, or surgery. Identify negative expressions regarding the integrity of the body or uncertainty of heart functioning.[26] Observe whether the patient demonstrates responsibility for self-care.

Meaningfulness

Many cardiovascular problems can evoke feelings of hopelessness and powerlessness, which can have a heavy impact on patient illness and recovery. When assessing for *hopelessness,* ask patients to describe possible solutions to their problems. Ask about their future plans and their feelings about the future. Investigate signs and symptoms of hopelessness such as passivity, decreased verbalization, flat affect, lack of initiative, negative feelings, decreased appetite or response to stimuli, increased sleep, or lack of involvement in care.[7,20] (Synthesize this data with that found under "emotional integrity" states in the Feeling Pattern).

When assessing for *powerlessness,* notice whether the patient voices perceived loss of control regarding self-care and the outcomes of medical and nursing care. Notice patient dissatisfaction or frustration because of an inability to perform certain tasks or activities.[7,21,26] Identify whether the patient verbalizes ways to change, improve, or help the current situation or problem. Note participation in decision making.

Sensory perception

Assess sensory perception to determine whether the patient has experienced restricted environments, isolation, surgery, intensive care, prolonged bed rest, traction, or confining illness.[21,26]

Identify whether the patient has difficulty with seeing. Ascertain whether the patient has cataracts, a false eye, contact lenses, or glasses. Investigate the visual fields by direct confrontation because visual field deficits, or blind spots, commonly result from cerebrovascular accidents.

Evaluate whether the patient is able to hear normal conversation. Note whether the patient wears a hearing aid. If possible, assess the degree of demonstrated coordination while the patient walks or performs other activities (kinesthetics) and note the patient's sense of balance. Identify loss or impairment of taste (gustatory sensation). Note patient descriptions of metallic or unusual tastes. Question the patient regarding loss in the sense of touch (tactile impairment). Determine whether the patient can distinguish between dull, sharp, and light touch. Explore complaints of numbness, tingling, hypersensitivity, or decreased sensation. Investigate changes in the sense of smell.

Assess deep tendon reflexes (see the box, p. 57). Compare responses on corresponding sides, and grade the responses using the following code:[31,39]

0 = No response
1 = Sluggish or diminished
2 = Active or expected response
3 = More brisk than usual
4 = Brisk or hyperactive

EXCHANGING PATTERN

The purpose of this assessment is to evaluate the patient's physical condition. The assessment focuses on the cerebral, peripheral, cardiovascular, respiratory, nutritional, gastrointestinal, and renal variables, as well as laboratory values. Physical assessment, interviewing, communicating, listening, and intuitive skills are needed.[21]

Cerebral circulation

When assessing the cerebral circulation, evaluate for a history of neurologic changes or symptoms. Investigate difficulty with walking or complaints of dizziness, loss of balance, falls, weakness, numbness, or development of tremors. Explore whether the patient's family reports changes in personality.[19]

Determine whether the patient has experienced *syncope,* a temporary loss of consciousness resulting from inadequate oxygen supply to the brain. Know that syncope may be caused by heart block, cardiac asystole, severe sinus bradycardia or arrest, or ventricular tachydysrhythmias.

Assess the pupils for size, shape, and equality. Determine the pupillary reaction to light (e.g., brisk, sluggish, or nonreactive).[19] Evaluate the direct-light pupillary reflex (i.e., constriction of the lighted eye) and consensual pupillary reflex (i.e., constriction of the unlighted eye).

Perform a direct funduscopic examination of retinal color, arteriolar caliber and tortuosity, venous caliber, and arteriovenous nicking. Know that the normal retinal fundus reflects light well and that this light reflex is seen as an orange-red reflection through the pupil. First, observe the optic disc and emerging retinal vessels with respect to their caliber, areas of spasm, or collections of atheroma within their walls, which are normally invisible. Recognize that early atheroma collections give the arteriole a copper color, referred to as a *copper wire deformity,* and that severe atheroma collections obstruct transmission of light completely and are referred to as *silver wire deformities.*

Funduscopic examination may identify a patient as being diabetic by showing characteristic *microaneurysms,* which represent small dilations of arterial walls. Chronic hypertension also may be apparent from abnormalities present that are collectively referred to as *retinopathies.* The findings of various types of retinopathy delineate states of chronic vascular disease because the vessels represent end organs damaged by pathologic conditions, including diabetes mellitus, collagen vascular diseases (such as lupus erythematosus), and hypertension. Classifying findings into retinopathy grades such as the hypertensive retinopathy classification or arteriosclerotic changes provides a guide to the severity and chronicity of these two disease states. For arteriosclerosis, the changes range from an increased or bright-light reflex to increased arteriovenous nicking, copper wire deformities, and silver wire deformities in the most severe state. The changes in hypertension range from a slight reduction in arteriolar caliber to areas of focal constriction, areas of hemorrhage, and finally *papilledema.*

Assess the patient's level of consciousness using the Glasgow Coma Scale.[11] Score and total the three categories of this scale—eye opening, best verbal response, and best motor response.[19] The patient who is completely awake will score 15.

TESTING FOR DEEP TENDON REFLEXES

Biceps: The patient's arm is flexed at a 45-degree angle at the elbow. Palpate the biceps tendon in the antecubital fossa. Place your fingers over the biceps muscle and your thumb over the tendon. With the reflex hammer, strike your thumb. Flexion of the elbow should occur.

Brachioradialis: The patient's arm is flexed up to a 45-degree angle and rests on your arm with the hand slightly pronated. With the reflex hammer, directly strike the brachioradialis tendon. Observe for flexion and supination of the forearm.

Triceps: The patient's arm is flexed up to a 90-degree angle, with the patient's hand resting against the side of your body. Palpate the triceps tendon and strike it directly with the reflex hammer just above the elbow. Contraction of the triceps muscle causes extension of the elbow.

Knee: The patient's knee is flexed up to a 90-degree angle, with the lower leg loosely hung. Support the patient's upper leg with your hand without allowing it to rest against the side of the table. With the reflex hammer, strike the patellar tendon just below the patella. The lower leg will extend when the quadriceps muscles contract.

Ankle: With the patient sitting, flex the knee and dorsiflex the ankle up to a 90-degree angle holding the heel of the foot in your hands. Strike the Achilles tendon at the level of the ankle malleolus. Contraction of the gastrocnemius muscle causes plantar flexion of the foot at the ankle. Note also the speed of relaxation after muscular contraction.

Plantar: The patient's ankle is held in one hand while a sharp object is stroked from the lateral surface of the sole, starting at the heel of the foot and going to the base or the foot, curving medially across the ball and ending beneath the great toe. The normal response is flexion of all toes (negative Babinski's reflex). Extension or dorsiflexion of the great toe and fanning of the others represents a positive Babinski's reflex, which may reflect upper motor neuron disease.

From Guzzetta CE and others: Clinical assessment tools for use with nursing diagnosis, St Louis, 1989, The CV Mosby Co.

Peripheral circulation

Arterial pulses

Evaluate each set of peripheral pulses, including the brachial, radial, femoral, popliteal, posterior tibial, dorsalis pedis, and carotid. Palpate the arterial pulses for rate, rhythm, character, contour, amplitude, and bilateral equality. If the presence of a pulse is questionable, use a Doppler ultrasonic anemometer to determine its audible quality, symmetry, and the presence of a bruit.[3,41]

Palpate the radial pulse for 30 seconds when a regular rhythm is present and for 1 minute if an irregularity exists. If an irregularity is discovered, check the apical and radial pulses for a deficit (see later section). The *character* of the normal arterial wall, when palpated, will feel soft and pliable to the touch. With atherosclerosis, the wall will be resistant to compression and will feel like a hard rope.[21] The *contour* is evaluated by lightly compressing the artery. It is normally smooth and rounded with a sharp upstroke and a more gradual downstroke. Exercise or conditions such as hyperthyroidism, aortic regurgitation, hypertension, fear, or arteriosclerotic changes in the elderly will produce large, bounding pulses. In contrast, when stroke volume is reduced, such as with severe aortic stenosis, heart failure, or cardiogenic shock, small, weak pulses will be observed. Also assess the arterial pulses for bilateral *amplitude* using the following scale[24,33]:

    0 = Not palpable

    1+ = Faintly palpable (weak and thready)

    2+ = Palpable (normal)

    3+ = Bounding

Check the *carotid arterial pulse* for bilateral equality and quality of the pulsation, and visually inspect the head for movement. Unlike other arteries in the body, the carotid sinus at the bifurcation of the common carotid artery represents a risk to the patient during palpation. Excessive stimulation of this structure with vigorous palpation may result in significant bradycardia and occasionally symptoms of hypotension and cerebral insufficiency. Care must be taken when palpating the carotid arteries, especially in the elderly because this reflex may be excessively sensitive (Fig. 3-2). The index finger is pressed gently at the base of the neck, and carotid sinus massage is avoided at the carotid bifurcation just below the mandible. The rate, rhythm, and upstroke velocity of the carotid pulse are carefully noted. Furthermore palpation of the carotid arteries should be done one side at a time and gently to avoid possible reductions in cerebral blood flow.[40]

The contour of the carotid arterial pulse is valuable in determining the presence of a vascular obstruction. Obstructions at the aortic valve or within the innominate or common carotid arteries reduce the upstroke velocity, or normal tapping nature, of the carotid pulse. In this case, the carotid pulse rises slowly, and the transmission of the pulsation to the palpating finger is reduced.

An often neglected but important tool for determining vascular obstruction or tortuosity is auscultation of the vessels for *bruits*, which are blowing sounds produced by turbulent blood flow through these obstructions (Fig. 3-3). Although at times they are present without any significant obstruction to flow, vascular bruits of long duration, especially those that are nearly continuous, may represent important vascular obstructions. Evaluate the carotid, femoral, and abdominal aorta arteries for bruits. When arterial sounds are detected as bruits, the vibrations also can be palpated frequently as *thrills*.

Arterial pressure

Normal blood pressure in the aorta and large arteries ranges between 100 to 140 mm Hg systolic and between 60 to 90 mm Hg diastolic. Wide variations exist in the healthy adult outside this given range. Thus blood pressure trends rather than isolated readings are evaluated.

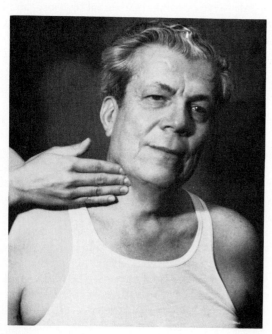

FIG. 3-2 The nurse palpates the carotid below and just medial to the angle of the jaw.

From Malasanos L, Barkauskas V, and Stoltenberg-Allen K: Health assessment, ed 4, St Louis, 1990, Mosby–Year Book, Inc.

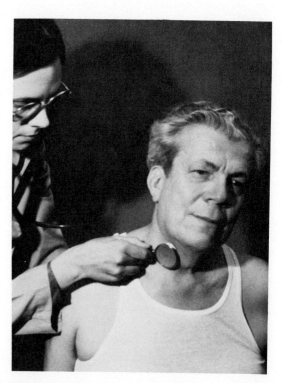

FIG. 3-3 The nurse listens with the bell of the stethoscope for bruits over the carotid artery.

From Malasanos L, Barkauskas V, and Stoltenberg-Allen K: Health assessment, ed 4, St Louis, 1990, Mosby–Year Book, Inc.

Determine arterial blood pressure by *indirect* (i.e., manual or automated devices) or *direct* methods (i.e., direct arterial cannulation). Indirectly determine arterial blood pressure by using a sphygmomanometer, whose proper usage and maintenance are important for reliability and continued accuracy. For ambulatory patients, take blood pressure measurements while the patient sits with the legs dangling and arm flexed slightly at the side or comfortably placed on an adjacent flat surface. Take measurements in both arms. There is a normal 5-to-10 mm Hg difference between the two arms. If the pressure changes with body positioning, take it with the patient lying, sitting, and standing.

Snugly apply the inflatable and appropriately sized cuff over the brachial artery with the lower cuff border approximately 2 to 3 cm above the antecubital crease and the length of the cuff bladder encircling half of the arm. Ensure that the width of the cuff is about 40% of the circumference of the arm. While palpating the radial pulse, inflate the cuff to approximately 30 mm Hg above the level at which the radial pulse is obliterated. Slowly reduce the cuff pressure about 3 mm Hg per heart beat as you auscultate the *Korotkoff* (or blood pressure) *sounds* with the diaphragm of the stethoscope placed over the brachial artery. Further reductions in cuff pressure are associated with changes in the pitch of the Korotkoff sounds.

Korotkoff sounds normally consist of five phases. *Phase 1* is characterized by the appearance of a faint, clear tapping sound that increases in intensity and represents the systolic pressure. The systolic pressure is the greatest pressure of blood against the vessel wall reached at the end of the rapid ventricular ejection phase. *Phase 2* is marked by the beginning of a murmur sound, presumably the result of the blood flow into a wider distal artery caused by the pressure of the cuff. *Phase 3* has a crisper, more intense tapping sound and is louder and higher pitched, with no discernible murmur. *Phase 4* represents a distinctive change in sound, which is muffled, less intense, and lowered pitched. It is the sound of diastolic pressure or the lowest pressure that occurs just before the next ventricular ejection. *Phase 5* is the point at which the sound disappears.[25] There is some conflict as to whether phase 5 or phase 4 is a more accurate indicator of the diastolic pressure.[24] Thus when documenting the arterial pressure, phase 1 (systolic pressure), phase 4 (diastolic pressure), and phase 5 (disappearance of the sound) should be recorded (e.g., 126/82/74 mm Hg). In aortic regurgitation, the diastolic sound can be heard until 0 mm Hg. In this situation, the systolic, muffled, and zero values are all recorded (e.g., 130/98/0 mm Hg).

Some patients who are hypertensive may have an auscultatory gap, which is a silent period between the systolic and diastolic pressures. Blood pressure measurements may be incorrectly recorded if the auscultatory gap is not recognized. The length of an auscultatory gap may range from 20 to 40 mm Hg. Such a gap occurs when auscultatory sounds are absent during phase 2. The complete blood pressure measurements and length of the auscultatory gap are recorded together (e.g., 190/100/90 mm Hg with an auscultatory gap from 170 to 140 mm Hg). The nurse also must be keenly aware of the potential for inaccuracies because of technical problems (e.g., a false-high or false-low blood pressure measurement because of obesity, misplacement of the cuff, or inadequate cuff size).

The average pressure that exists in the aorta during systole and diastole is called the *mean arterial pressure (MAP)*. The MAP can be calculated from the following equation:[4]

$$MAP = Pd + \frac{1}{3}(Ps - Pd)$$

where *Pd* is diastolic pressure and *Ps* is systolic pressure. For example, if a patient's blood pressure is 120/80, the MAP is 93 mm Hg.[10] The MAP is related to the mean blood volume in the arterial system and the peripheral vascular resistance, and it is influenced by the elastic properties of the arterial wall.[4]

The *arterial pulse pressure* is the difference between the systolic and the diastolic pressures. It represents the range of pressure in the arteries, normally from 30 to 40 mm Hg. (Causes of a widened and narrow pulse pressure are discussed under intraarterial monitoring in Chapter 7). It depends primarily on the stroke volume and arterial capacitance.[4]

In situations of very low arterial pressure such as shock, it may be difficult to hear Korotkoff sounds. In such cases after the cuff has been inflated, the radial pulse is palpated while the cuff pressure is reduced, and the systolic pressure is estimated by observing the pressure at which the pulse is felt first. (Because the diastolic pressure cannot be determined by palpation, the pressure would be recorded, for example, as 90/p). Use of an ultrasound (Doppler) device may provide more accurate systolic measurements. The Doppler technique is commonly used during low-flow hypotensive states to augment Korotkoff sounds when they cannot be heard by auscultation. Such devices use amplified reflected ultrasound to identify blood flow. As the blood pressure cuff is slowly deflated, the Doppler device is applied with conduction gel over the brachial artery to determine the systolic pressure.

Automated blood pressure monitors are used as another indirect method for measuring blood pressure. One type uses infrasound waves to detect arterial wall motion. Another type uses a double-air-bladder cuff that is applied in the same manner as a conventional cuff to detect arterial wall oscillations. The proximal bladder is inflated to occlude arterial blood flow in the arm and then is slowly deflated. The distal bladder then senses arterial wall oscillations and records the systolic, mean, and diastolic pressures.[24]

Direct blood pressure monitoring is accomplished by inserting a catheter or needle into an artery and attaching the catheter to a plastic tubing connected to a transducer. The transducer converts the mechanical energy that the blood exerts on the recording membrane into electrical voltage or current that can be calibrated in millimeters of mercury. The electrical signal is then transmitted to an electronic recorder and an oscilloscope, which continually record and display the pressure waves (see Chapter 7).

In some situations, major discrepancies exist between direct and indirect blood pressure measurements.[24] The discrepancies occur because the indirect blood pressure auscultation methods measure a different phenomena than do direct arterial methods. Auscultatory methods are blood-flow dependent, whereas arterial line pressures reflect the normal physiologic changes that occur when the pressure pulse travels to the periphery.[24] Thus in patients whose Korotkoff sounds might be diminished or absent because blood flow is markedly reduced, direct arterial measurements should be used. Such patients include those who are in shock, have high peripheral vascular resistance, or are hypothermic, obese, or edematous. In these low-blood-flow situations, discrepancies between direct and indirect pressure readings are likely to occur. Nurses are then often left to wonder which is the more accurate blood pressure measurement. Therefore when a high degree of accuracy is required, such as in patients in shock or when titrating intravenous drugs (especially those prescribed for hypertension or hypotension), direct arterial monitoring is recommended, and the routine of obtaining and comparing direct and indirect methods is discouraged. Arterial monitoring is also beneficial in providing continuous pressure monitoring and can be used for frequent arterial sampling to determine blood gas levels.[24]

Venous pulses

Examination of the neck veins is a valuable and accurate method of estimating right ventricular filling pressures and hence right ventricular function. It requires good lighting, patient cooperation, and comfortable positioning of you and the patient. Pulsations may be accentuated and their visualization enhanced by silhouette lighting and slight elevation and rotation of the patient's chest away from you. Attention should be directed to the base of the neck, and bilateral inspection is done. It is crucial to distinguish arterial pulsations from venous pulsations (see section on carotid arterial pulse).

Because neck veins normally are distended when the patient is supine (Fig. 3-4, *A*), jugular venous pulsations often are most apparent with the patient's head and chest elevated to approximately a 45-degree angle.[3] Pulsations of the large internal jugular veins, which connect to the central venous system and right atrium, reflect not only the absolute central venous pressure but also the cyclic changes in pressure within the right atrium, indicating the competence of right ventricular function. The ideal pulsation to observe is from the right internal jugular vein and not the variable array of external jugular veins. The external jugular veins are often slow to empty and transmit pressure changes poorly because of their course through the platysma muscle and the presence of intravascular valves. These problems do not affect the internal jugular veins. Because pressure in these veins normally is 0 to 5 mm Hg, unlike the arterial pulse, they normally are not palpable.

Evaluate jugular venous pulsations with respect to their contour (i.e., elevation and decline with time), as well as

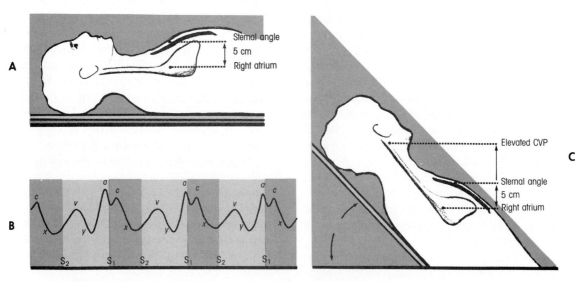

FIG. 3-4   Venous pressures and contour. **A,** Internal jugular vein normally is distended with patient supine. **B,** Jugular venous pulsations, illustrating the *a, c,* and *v* waves and the *x* and *y* descents. **C,** Determination of jugular venous pressure by measuring the vertical distance from the top of the internal jugular vein to the sternal angle.

their pressure. The contour of the jugular venous pulse reflects alterations in pressure secondary to changes in the cardiac cycle. The jugular venous pulse consists of the *a*, *c*, and *v* waves, although normally only the *a* and *v* waves are visible (Fig. 3-4, *B*). The *a* wave represents venous distention produced by right atrial contraction during diastole, which causes an increase in atrial pressure reflected in the central veins. It slightly precedes carotid pulsation. An amplified *a* wave indicates increased right atrial pressure. During atrial fibrillation, the *a* wave disappears. In atrial flutter, *a* waves occur at a fast rate, reflecting the mechanical consequences of rapid atrial depolarization. This may be the first clue that a dysrhythmia exists because the pulse rate that reflects ventricular contraction may be normal despite such atrial rhythm disturbances.

The *c* wave, not generally visible in the neck, occurs simultaneously with the carotid pulse and is caused by closure of the tricuspid valve, after which the atrium relaxes. The venous *c* wave is observed when the ventricles begin to contract during the rapid ejection phase of systole. The increase in ventricular pressure causes an increase in atrial and central venous pressures. As ventricular systole begins, the right atrial pressure declines, causing the height of the jugular venous blood column to decline also, thereby producing the *x* descent. The *v* wave is initiated by increased atrial pressure during the latter part of systole because of continued atrial filling when the tricuspid valve is closed. Its peak occurs during diastole. The upslope of the *v* wave is caused by the increase in pressure in the atria before the atrioventricular (AV) valves open, and the downslope of the wave occurs when the atrial pressure is suddenly reduced because the AV valves open.[14,25] An exaggerated *v* wave indicates right ventricular overload or tricuspid regurgitation. As right atrial pressure begins to fall again during diastole when the tricuspid valve opens to pour blood into the ventricle, the *y* descent is produced.

Venous pressure

Venous pressure is the pressure exerted by the blood within the venous system. It is highest in the venules of the extremities and lowest at the point where the vena cava enters the heart. Venous blood flow is continuous rather than pulsatory. In the inferior vena cava, venous pressure ranges from 6 to 8 cm H_2O.

Determine venous pressure by measuring the height of pulsation in the internal jugular vein.[25] Theoretically the venous pressure is calculated by measuring with a spinal fluid manometer the distance between the maximum height of one jugular venous pulsation and the right atrium. In practice, however, the level of the right atrium is difficult to determine, and thus the sternal angle, or angle of Louis, is used instead (located at the junction of the sternum with the second rib). The sternal angle lies approximately 5 cm above the right atrium for all positions between supine and 90 degrees upright. Thus the venous

pressure is determined by measuring the vertical distance from the top of the distended internal jugular vein to the sternal angle (Fig. 3-4, *C*). The upper normal limit for the jugular venous pressure is 3 cm H_2O above the sternal angle, which also represents a central venous pressure of 8 cm H_2O (because the sternal angle is 5 cm above the right atrium).

An increased jugular venous pressure is perhaps the most commonly recognized sign of right ventricular failure. However, jugular pressure also may be elevated by increased blood volume, obstructed central venous inflow to the right atrium (superior vena caval syndrome), increased pressure in the pericardium secondary to constriction by fibrotic tissue, or cardiac tamponade.

In critically ill patients, direct measurement of *central venous pressure (CVP)* is indicated. The CVP indicates right atrial pressure, which primarily reflects alterations in right ventricular pressure and only secondarily reflects changes in pulmonary venous pressure or the pressures in the left side of the heart. The CVP provides valuable information about blood volume, right ventricular function, and central venous return.

When a CVP is obtained, a vein is cannulated, and the catheter is threaded into the vena cava. The pressure can be measured in centimeters of water by a water manometer or in millimeters of mercury by a pressure transducer. The normal CVP ranges from 4 to 15 cm H_2O or 3 to 11 mm Hg.[20] (The value of centimeters of water can be converted to millimeters of mercury by dividing the former by 1.36 because 1 mm Hg equals 1.36 cm H_2O). A low CVP may indicate hypovolemia or peripheral blood pooling (e.g., as in septic shock). Elevated CVPs may signify right ventricular failure, pulmonary hypertension or embolism, or cardiac tamponade.

In situations in which the jugular venous pressure is not elevated but mild right ventricular failure is present, *hepatojugular reflux* is assessed by placing the hand over the liver and exerting mild pressure for 1 minute while the neck veins are observed. The patient should be lying comfortably and positioned at the point where the highest venous pulsation can be visualized in the middle of the neck. The patient is instructed to breath normally and special care is taken to avoid pain and prevent the patient from performing a Valsalva maneuver. An elevation in the jugular venous pressure of more than 1 cm during and immediately after compression suggests that right ventricular pressure is persistently elevated and implies that the right ventricle is unable to deal with an increased venous return. This is a sign of right ventricular failure, although occasionally it reflects an increased blood volume or a disorder associated with elevated levels of epinephrine and norepinephrine, which can reduce venous capacitance.

Auscultation of the neck veins may reveal a "roaring," continuous murmur that represents turbulence in the internal jugular vein. This phasic sound may be heard normally in patients under 30 years of age only when they are in an upright position. Unlike carotid arterial bruits, these *venous hums* diminish or disappear with jugular vein compression more distal to the stethoscope endpiece, a Valsalva maneuver, or the recumbent position.

Peripheral veins

The peripheral veins are a highly variable system that returns blood to the central circulation. Evaluation requires observation for abnormal distention, tortuosity, abnormal dilation, and associated edema. Evaluate peripheral veins with the patient in an upright position. A less optimal but adequate evaluation sometimes may be made as the patient sits with the legs dangling. Evaluate the lower extremities for tenderness, pain, warmth, and edema to help exclude thrombophlebitis. Performance of dorsiflexion of the foot may reveal pain in the calf (a positive *Homans's sign*) in the presence of thrombophlebitis.

Skin temperature and color

Assess skin temperature to determine whether it is normal, warm, hot, cool, clammy, or moist. Also evaluate skin color, noting whether it is pink, pale, or red and whether the patient exhibits pallor, jaundice, mottling, increased pigmentation, or blanching.

Cyanosis

The patient is assessed for cyanosis. Cyanosis in the mucous membranes (e.g., conjunctiva and inside the lips), the earlobes, the cheeks, and the extremities is termed *central cyanosis*. These areas are usually warm to the touch. Central cyanosis represents an excessive amount of unsaturated arterial hemoglobin (estimated to be at least 5 g/100 ml before it is appreciable). The arteriovenous oxygen difference is usually normal. It almost always reflects cardiopulmonary disease (e.g., congenital right-to-left shunts or pulmonary diseases such as pneumonia) and should be differentiated clearly from peripheral cyanosis.[21]

Peripheral cyanosis is more common than central cyanosis. It reflects reduced peripheral blood flow with increased extraction of oxygen by the peripheral tissues, resulting in reduced oxygen saturation in the venous blood. The arterial oxygen saturation may be normal. The arteriovenous oxygen difference is much greater than normal since the tissues use more oxygen because of blood stasis. Cyanosis is observed in the distal extremities, and the skin temperature of those areas is usually cold to the touch. Peripheral cyanosis is caused by exposure to cold, heart failure, and shock.[21,27]

Capillary refill and pulsation

Assess capillary refill by pressing the nailbed, earlobe, or forehead so that it blanches and release the pressure. Observe whether skin color returns to normal within 2 seconds.[27]

Capillary pulsation should also be assessed if the pulse pressure is elevated. Severe capillary pulsation can occur with bradycardia, an increased stroke volume (e.g., with an increased venous return or aortic regurgitation) and arteriolar dilation (causing decreased resistance). To assess for abnormal capillary pulsations, the anterior portion of the fingernail is pressed so that blood is forced out of the capillary nailbed. This produces blanching of the anterior nailbed, with the posterior part turning red because blood is trapped in the capillaries. Significant capillary pulsation can be demonstrated when the border between the red and white areas shifts back and forth with each pulsation. This is called *Quincke's sign* and is observed in patients with aortic regurgitation.[25]

Edema

Assess the patient for edema because fluid retention and edema are often characterized by a sudden weight gain and are frequently associated with cardiac failure. Because edema tends to accumulate in the dependent areas of the body, inspect the hands, feet, and ankles of the ambulatory patient and the sacrum, thighs, and abdomen of the bedridden patient.[43] Assess edema by firmly indenting the skin with the fingertips. Quantify and describe the degree of pitting by noting the depth of the finger indentation in the skin and the length of time necessary for it to disappear by using the following scale:[3,20]

> 0 = None present
> +1 = 0 to ¼ inch (trace); indentation disappears rapidly
> +2 = ¼ to ½ inch (moderate); indentation disappears in 10 to 15 seconds
> +3 = ½ to 1 inch (deep); indentation disappears in 1 to 2 minutes
> +4 = More than 1 inch (very deep); indentation present after 5 minutes

Clubbing

Clubbing of the nail beds should be observed.[20] With clubbing, the proximal nailbeds are convex and rise above the flat plane of the finger. The skin proximal to the nailbed feels spongy in clubbing, and in some cases the fingernails pulsate and flush. Clubbing is associated with certain pulmonary and cardiac diseases such as endocarditis[5,25] (see Fig. 13-3).

Cardiovascular circulation
Inspection, palpation, and percussion

Begin the cardiac assessment by inspecting and palpating the precordium. Cardiac location, chamber size and movement, movement of the great vessels, and amplitude and radiation of heart murmurs and sounds can be estimated through careful examination of the precordium.

Begin the precordial examination by actively observing

the thorax for abnormal configuration and movement. Examine the patient in the supine position with the chest exposed, especially from the foot of the bed, to facilitate the detection of certain asymmetric structures and pulsating chest movements.[43] Observe for an internal or external pacemaker. If internal, record the type and the way it functions. If external, record the type, settings, and how it functions.

Use tangential lighting that silhouettes movements or enhances shadows to enhance chest movements at eye level. Because shifting movements of underlying mediastinal structures may occur with lateral decubitus positioning, inspect the chest with the patient flat or sitting upright.

Refer to areas of the chest wall and precordium by certain descriptions that have become conventional. These topographic areas are defined as follows[20,21] (Fig. 3-5):

1. The aortic area is to the right of the sternal border at the second intercostal space (sometimes abbreviated 2ICS, RSB).
2. The pulmonary area is to the left of the sternal border at the second intercostal space (2ICS, LSB).
3. The tricuspid area is to the left of the lower sternal border at the fifth intercostal space (5ICS, LLSB); alternate terms are *septal* or *right ventricular area*.
4. The mitral area is at the midclavicular line overlying the fifth intercostal space (5ICS, MCL). Normally within the mitral area, the left ventricular apical beat

can be palpated; hence this area sometimes is called the *apical* or *left ventricular area*. The apical impulse is also known as the *point of maximal impulse* (PMI).

5. The secondary aortic area (or Erb's point) is to the left of the sternal border at the third intercostal space (3ICS, LSB).

These names may be a useful shorthand when documenting the results of the physical examination; however, they are not as helpful as simply describing locations on the chest using the vertical and horizontal coordinates. Imaginary vertical lines include the midsternal, midclavicular, anterior axillary, midaxillary, and posterior axillary lines. Usually the number of the intercostal spaces lying just below the identically numbered rib is a satisfactory horizontal coordinate.

Palpation follows inspection and should proceed in an orderly manner, from the primary aortic, pulmonic, secondary aortic, tricuspid, and mitral areas, as well as sternoclavicular and costochondral joints (Fig. 3-6). Palpation requires the recognition of vibratory sensations that most commonly represent transmitted sound energy from heart murmurs or vascular bruits, as well as larger areas of movement most often representative of cardiac chamber enlargement or pulsation of one of the great vessels. The term *thrill* is used to describe the palpable vibration produced by a loud heart murmur or vascular bruit.

Palpate the apical impulse or the PMI first. It is often identical in location with the midclavicular line and is palpable only over a small area, within one intercostal space. It is a tapping impulse with rapid retraction. Abnormalities of the apical impulse may indicate cardiac hypertrophy or enlargement. Evaluation of the apical impulse may be more valuable than the chest x-ray examination for detecting left ventricular hypertrophy. The location of the PMI helps in assessing heart size because, in situations of cardiac enlargement, the heart is displaced laterally from its midclavicular position. The contour of the apical beat is also important because ventricular hypertrophy (i.e., thickening of the heart muscle secondary to many disease states [e.g., hypertension, aortic valvular stenosis, or hypertrophic cardiomyopathy]) will increase the duration of the outward movement of the apical impulse; this is referred to as a *sustained apical impulse*. Other areas of the precordium are then systematically palpated during careful examination of sections where palpations are visible.

Percussing the heart for size and shape is largely a skill of yesteryear. Currently the incorporation of a chest x-ray examination into any complete cardiovascular assessment minimizes the value of cardiac percussion, which is difficult to master.

Cardiac auscultation

The patient's *apical heart rate* should be determined. It should be timed for a full minute and, when possible, be assessed with the patient supine, sitting, and standing to

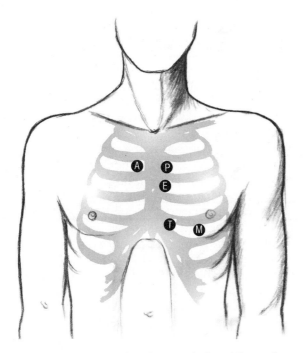

FIG. 3-5 Anatomic locations for auscultation of the cardiac sounds. *A*, Aortic area; *P*, pulmonary area; *E*, Erb's point; *T*, tricuspid area; *M*, mitral area.

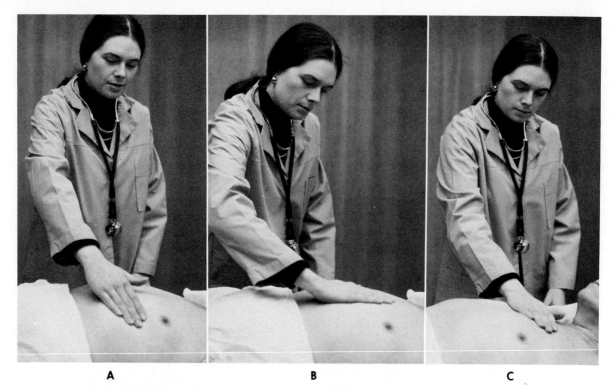

A   B   C

FIG. 3-6 The nurse palpates three areas of the precordium. **A,** Over the apex. **B,** Over the left sternal border. **C,** Over the base of the heart.

From Malasanos L, Barkauskas V, and Stoltenberg-Allen K: Health assessment, ed 4, St Louis, 1990, Mosby–Year Book, Inc.

determine whether orthostatic changes are excessive. *Orthostatic changes* are alterations in the heart rate and particularly blood pressure that result from changes in position with respect to gravity. A rise in pulse rate of greater than 15 beats per minute or a fall in blood pressure of greater than 20 mm Hg when the patient stands (compared with the values when the patient is supine) indicates excessive orthostatic changes. Such changes most often reflect an absolute or relatively reduced intravascular volume. This may result from bleeding, excessive diuretics, antihypertensive drugs, or anatomic dysfunction.

The regularity or irregularity of the resting pulse rate is assessed for the present evaluation and future reference. If the rhythm is irregular, it is assessed to determine whether it is regularly or irregularly irregular and whether a peripheral pulse deficit is present. An *apical-radial deficit* indicates that the apical heart rate (counted by auscultation) exceeds the radial pulse rate (counted by palpation). A deficit means that not every cardiac systole is forceful enough to produce a palpable radial pulse, which can occur with rhythm disturbances such as premature extrasystoles or atrial fibrillation. Because review of the patient's electrocardiogram (ECG) is an integral part of each cardiovascular assessment, the pulse rate observed and its regu-

larity are correlated with ECG tracings to detect discrepancies.

Also auscultate the heart to identify the normal first and second heart sounds and to determine whether there is a third or fourth heart sound or whether there are ejection sounds, midsystolic clicks, opening snaps, or heart murmurs.

Developing the skill of auscultation requires practice, a quiet environment, and a systematic approach. You must learn to focus on one sound at a time and proceed in an orderly fashion, identifying additional sounds and events. Make every effort to avoid being distracted by "interesting" or unusual auscultatory events.

Apply the diaphragm of the stethoscope to the LLSB and listen first for heart rate, rhythm, and regularity. Next proceed in a stepwise manner, focusing on the first, second, third (ventricular gallop), and fourth heart sounds (atrial gallop) and murmurs and miscellaneous sounds. Determine the location of maximum intensity, duration, quality, and radiation of each event. To recognize all available information, listen in each of the major precordial areas, including the aortic, pulmonary, tricuspid, and mitral areas (Fig. 3-5). Enhance auscultation by having the patient lie in the left lateral decubitus position with the hips and knees

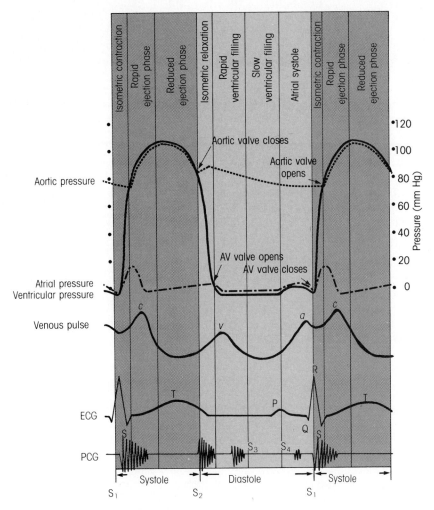

FIG. 3-7 Cardiac cycle, showing events of systole and diastole, venous pressure waves, ECG, and heart sounds.

flexed to bring more blood to the central circulation and thereby accentuate the sounds.[14,25] During auscultation, do not be concerned about the order of the areas; be sure to auscultate each area systematically.

During cardiac auscultation, use the stethoscope advantageously. Use the diaphragm to listen to high-pitched sounds such as the first and second heart sounds, to ascertain aortic or mitral insufficiency, and to listen for rubs or clicks. Press it firmly against the skin. Identify low-pitched sounds, such as the third and fourth heart sounds and the murmurs of aortic and mitral stenosis, with the bell of the stethoscope.[25] Place it lightly on the skin, with just enough pressure to seal the edge of the bell.

Never perform auscultation of the heart as an isolated event. Integrate the findings with the data collected in other categories of the Exchanging Pattern, such as the arterial pulse contour, venous pulse waves, and precordial movements to validate the judgments derived during this portion of the assessment.

Heart sounds

Several theories have been proposed to explain the generation of heart sounds. Heart sounds may be produced by the acceleration and deceleration of blood in the cardiac chambers; they may arise from energy sources within the heart, great vessels, or both. Cardiac sounds occur after closure of the heart valves, however, and the pressure gradients within the heart and great vessels are related to these sounds. The components of the cardiac cycle, venous pressure, ECG, and heart sounds are described in the box, p. 66, and are illustrated in Fig. 3-7.[4,5,16,25]

First heart sound. The first heart sound (S_1) is caused by the deceleration of blood associated with closure of the mitral and tricuspid valves (Fig. 3-8). This closure occurs when ventricular pressure is greater than atrial pressure. S_1 commonly has two high-frequency sounds designated M_1 (pronounced "M one") and T_1 for the mitral and tricuspid components. Because right-sided events follow left-sided events in the heart, the tricuspid valve closes slightly

CARDIAC CYCLE

Fig. 3-7 illustrates the cardiac cycle, the venous pressure waves, electrocardiogram (ECG), and heart sounds.

Ventricular systole

Ventricular systole can be divided into two phases: (1) the isometric contraction phase and (2) the ejection phase.*

Isometric contraction phase. The isometric (isovolumetric) contraction phase marks the onset of ventricular contraction (ventricular systole). It coincides with the peak of the R wave on the ECG and S_1. During this phase the AV valves have just closed, and the semilunar valves are not yet open. Ventricular pressure exceeds atrial pressure but is lower than aortic (and pulmonary) pressures. The ventricular pressure rapidly rises, increasing ventricular force or active tension to overcome the high aortic pressure (afterload). Because all the valves are closed, however, there is no ejection of blood and no external muscle fiber shortening. At this phase, the peak of force development is reached. When ventricular pressure exceeds aortic (and pulmonary) pressure, the ejection phase begins.

Ejection phase. The two ejection phases of the cardiac cycle, rapid ejection phase and reduced ejection phase, are marked by the opening of the semilunar valves and the onset of external muscle fiber shortening and ejection of blood to the aorta.

Rapid ejection phase. The rapid ejection phase is the rapid expulsion of blood from the ventricle to the aorta. It is a shorter phase than the reduced ejection phase and is characterized by a sharp rise in aortic pressure and an abrupt decrease in ventricular volume. During this phase the rate of cardiac output (Qi) exceeds the rate of peripheral runoff (Qo).

Reduced ejection phase. The reduced ejection phase is a slow expulsion of blood from the ventricle to the aorta. It is a longer phase than the rapid ejection phase. The cardiac output is less than peripheral runoff (Qi < Qo), so aortic pressure begins to decline. As ventricular pressure also declines and becomes lower than aortic pressure, the semilunar valves close, and ventricular diastole begins. The volume of blood remaining in the ventricles at the end of ejection is called the *residual volume.* Normally the residual volume is equal to the volume ejected during systole. With left ventricular failure the residual volume may be greatly increased. Increasing the inotropic state of the heart with drugs such as digitalis may reduce this residual volume and improve stroke volume.

Ventricular diastole

Ventricular diastole can be divided into four phases: (1) isometric relaxation, (2) rapid ventricular filling, (3) slow ventricular filling, and (4) atrial systole.*

Isometric relaxation phase. The time between closure of the semilunar valves and opening of the AV valves is the isometric (isovolumetric) relaxation phase and marks the beginning of diastole. This occurs when ventricular pressure becomes lower than aortic pressure, and there is a momentary backflow of blood from the aorta to the left ventricle. The pressure reversal and backflow of blood close the aortic valve, producing S_2 and causing an incisura on the pressure pulse wave. There is a rapid decline in ventricular pressure but no change in ventricular volume during isometric relaxation because both sets of valves are closed. Ventricular pressure is lower than aortic pressure but higher than atrial pressure.

Rapid ventricular filling phase. When ventricular pressure falls below atrial pressure, the AV valves open and blood rapidly rushes in from the atria to the ventricles, marking the onset of the rapid ventricular filling phase. During this phase the largest volume of blood is transferred into the ventricles because of the large pressure gradient between the atria and ventricles.

Slow ventricular filling phase. The slow ventricular filling phase, also called *diastasis,* is characterized by a slow transfer of blood from the atria to the ventricles. This phase contributes only a small additional volume of blood to the ventricles and is due primarily to the return of venous blood from the periphery and the lungs.

Atrial systole. During atrial systole, the last phase of ventricular diastole, the atria contract and are responsible for contributing 30% more of normal ventricular filling volume. Atrial systole begins with the peak of the P wave. The end of atrial contraction denotes a reduction in atrial pressure, the end of ventricular filling, and the end of ventricular diastole.

The ventricular filling that occurs during atrial contraction is not essential under most circumstances. For example, ventricular filling volumes are generally adequate in most patients with atrial fibrillation (when atrial contraction is not present). The atrial contribution for a patient with bradycardia also is not important. During bradycardia, ventricular filling almost stops at the end of the slow ventricular filling phase, and therefore atrial contraction contributes very little to ventricular filling volumes. In a patient with tachycardia, however, when the rapid and reduced ventricular filling phases are shortened, atrial contraction may contribute significantly to ventricular filling.

The importance of the atrial contribution to ventricular filling also depends on the characteristics of the AV valves. In mitral stenosis, for example, ventricular filling is impaired during the rapid and reduced filling phases of the cardiac cycle because the stenotic valve impedes blood flow. In such a situation the atrial contribution significantly contributes to ventricular filling.

*Data from Berne RM and Levy MN: Cardiovascular physiology, ed 6, St Louis, 1992, Mosby–Year Book, Inc; Guyton AC: Textbook of medical physiology, ed 8, Philadelphia, 1990, WB Saunders Co.

Heart sounds	Events	Cause	End-piece	Location	Pitch	Respirations	Position	Variables
First heart sound = S_1 (M_1T_1)		Closure of tricuspid and mitral valves	Diaphragm	Entire precordium (apex)	High	Softer on inspiration	Any position	Increased with excitement, exercise, amyl nitrate, epinephrine, and atropine
Second heart sound = S_2 (A_2P_2)		Closure of pulmonary and aortic valves	Diaphragm	A_2 at 2nd RICS; P_2 at 2nd LICS	High	Fusion of A_2P_2 on expiration; physiologic split on inspiration	Sitting or supine	Increased in thin chest walls and with exercise
Third heart sound = S_3 (ventricular gallop)		Rapid ventricular filling	Bell	Apex	Low	Increased on inspiration	Supine or left lateral	Increased with exercise, fast heart rate, elevation of legs, and increased venous return
Fourth heart sound = S_4 (atrial gallop)		Forceful atrial ejection into distended ventricle	Bell	Apex	Low	Increased on forced inspiration	Supine or left semilateral	Same as for S_3
Quadruple rhythm		S_1, S_2, S_3, and S_4 all heard separately	Bell	Apex	Low	Increased on inspiration	Supine or left lateral	Same as for S_3
Summation gallop = triple gallop		S_3 and S_4 fuse with fast heart rates	Bell	Apex	Low	Increased on inspiration	Supine or left lateral	Same as for S_3
Ejection sounds		Opening of deformed semilunar valves	Diaphragm	2nd RICS, 2nd LICS, or apex	High	Increases on expiration with pulmonary stenosis	Sitting or supine	Aortic ejection sound same as S_1 and S_2; pulmonary ejection sound increased on expiration
Systolic click		Prolapse of mitral valve leaflet	Diaphragm	Apex	High	Increased on expiration	Sitting or supine	Occurs later in systole with increased venous return (e.g.) with elevated legs or supine position
Opening snap		Abrupt recoil of stenotic mitral or tricuspid valve	Diaphragm	Apex	High	No effect	Any position	May be confused with S_3

FIG. 3-8 Heart sounds. *RICS*, Right intercostal space; *LICS*, left intercostal space.

after the mitral valve, and the pulmonic valve normally closes after the aortic valve. The higher pressures within the left heart chambers probably contribute to the amplitude of sounds, and hence M_1 is louder than T_1. The first heart sound corresponds with the onset of ventricular contraction and indicates the beginning of systole. It is heard shortly after the depolarization of ventricular muscle, which is marked by the inscription of the QRS complex on the ECG. Compared with the second sound, the first heart sound is lower in pitch, slightly longer in duration, and somewhat duller. Its intensity is determined by factors such as chest wall configuration, the PR interval (which determines position of the AV valve leaflets before closing), and the level of atrial pressure.

S_1 can be differentiated from other heart sounds because it closely corresponds to each carotid pulsation. Thus the nurse can correctly identify S_1, especially in patients with fast heart rates, by palpating a carotid artery during auscultation. S_1 is heard best with the diaphragm of the stethoscope over the entire precordium (although frequently it is loudest at the apex). During inspiration the sounds may become softer as the distance between the heart and chest wall increases with expansion of the lungs. Excitement and drugs such as amyl nitrate, epinephrine, or atropine sulfate, as well as exercise, may intensify S_1, probably as a result of increased myocardial contractility, heart rate, and rate of pressure development.

Although easily audible in children, the *split* of S_1, into M_1 and T_1 may be difficult to hear in adults. Abnormally wide splitting sometimes is heard in adults and results from mechanical or electrical problems that cause the ventricles to contract at different times. Right bundle branch block is an example of an electrical problem that can cause an abnormally wide split between M_1 and T_1, whereas mitral stenosis is a mechanical delay problem that can produce a reverse split of S_1 because the tricuspid valve closes before the mitral valve (T_1M_1).[25]

Second heart sound. The second heart sound (S_2) results from events associated with closure of the aortic and pulmonic valves, when pressure in the aorta and pulmonary arteries exceeds that within the right and left ventricles respectively (Fig. 3-8). S_2 corresponds with the onset of ventricular relaxation and marks the beginning of diastole. It is higher pitched and shorter in duration than S_1 and is heard best with the diaphragm of the stethoscope along the LSB. The designations A_2 and P_2 for the aortic and pulmonary components of the second heart sound indicate the normal sequence of these high-frequency sounds. The two components of S_2 are heard best with the diaphragm of the stethoscope in the pulmonary area, where P_2 usually is louder than A_2.

Varying degrees of splitting of A_2 and P_2 occur throughout the respiratory cycle. *Physiologic splitting* (i.e., normal splitting of A_2 and P_2) implies an increase in the separation of A_2 and P_2. This occurs with inspiration because of increased venous return to the right ventricle resulting from a more negative intrathoracic pressure. The extra volume of blood in the right ventricle increases the ejection time of the right ventricle and delays pulmonic valve closure. The delay of P_2 and a slight prematurity of A_2 as blood is withheld in the lungs, which transiently act as reservoirs, widen the separation of A_2 and P_2. The split commonly increases with exercise and often is heard easily in persons with thin chest walls.

The absence of physiologic splitting (i.e., the *fixed split* of S_2) is one of the most common findings used to identify an atrial septal defect (ASD). The balancing of blood volume between the right and left atria throughout the respiratory cycle produces this fixed split. This contrasts with the normal heart with an intact atrial septum, in which inspiration is associated with an increase in right atrial volume and a decrease in left atrial volume. An assessment of the splitting of S_2 should be part of every cardiovascular evaluation and is especially important in patients with a systolic or diastolic murmur that may be a result of an ASD. Also evaluated is the intensity of the components of S_2, which correlates with the pressure in the corresponding great vessels.

Paradoxical splitting, or reverse splitting, of S_2 occurs when left ventricular systole is delayed, causing aortic valve closure to follow pulmonic valve closure. Consequently, instead of the two components of the second heart sound fusing during expiration, the pulmonary sound occurs before the aortic sound during expiration (P_2A_2). Furthermore during inspiration the P_2 moves closer to the abnormally delayed aortic sound to produce a fusion of the two components and a reversal of the normal splitting pattern. Left bundle branch block, patent ductus arteriosus, aortic stenosis, uncontrolled hypertension, or severe left ventricular disease may be causal factors.

Gallop sounds. Gallop sounds are ventricular filling sounds. The third heart sound (S_3) occurs in early diastole, whereas the fourth heart sound (S_4) occurs in late diastole. They often are subtle, low in pitch, and easily overlooked. They may be heard best with the bell of the stethoscope and with the patient in the left lateral decubitus position and legs drawn up during auscultation.

Third heart sound. S_3, also called a *ventricular gallop, protodiastolic gallop,* or *early diastolic filling sound,* is common in children and young adults and in patients with hyperkinetic circulations. S_3 reflects early rapid ventricular filling (Fig. 3-8). It also may be an abnormal sound associated with high ventricular filling pressures such as those observed with heart failure or valvular regurgitation. S_3 is identified by its close association with S_2 and its occurrence in early diastole. S_3 increases with exercise, inspiration, elevation of the legs, or other factors that augment the return of blood flow to the heart. S_3 decreases by reducing the venous return, such as when standing or using venous tourniquets.

Fourth heart sound. S$_4$, also called an *atrial gallop* or *presystolic gallop,* is an abnormal finding in adults; there is increased intensity of the sound associated and synchronous with atrial contraction (Fig. 3-8). It is heard commonly in situations in which the ventricle has hypertrophied such as aortic stenosis, hypertension, and hypertrophic cardiomyopathy or situations in which the ventricle has been damaged with resultant scar tissue such as ischemic heart disease and specifically myocardial infarction. There also is a resultant loss of elasticity, or compliance, in these cases, which may further contribute to the audibility of this sound. S$_4$ is identified by its close proximity with S$_1$ in presystole. It is a low-pitched, soft, diastolic sound heard best at the apex and LLSB.

To differentiate gallop rhythms in the cardiac cycle, you may simulate the rhythm and patterns of the heart sounds with the cadence of two commonly used words. The pronunciation of these words resembles the sounds produced by gallop rhythms of S$_3$ and S$_4$:

Ken -tuc -ky

S$_1$ -S$_2$ -S$_3$

Ten -nes -see

S$_4$ -S$_1$ -S$_2$

Quadruple rhythms and summation gallops. Quadruple rhythms are the cadence of the normal S$_1$ and S$_2$ plus S$_3$ and S$_4$ (Fig. 3-8). When the heart rate is not abnormally fast, all four components may be heard separately and have been described as sounding like a cogwheel or a locomotive.

A summation gallop is a triple gallop produced by tachycardia or a delayed AV conduction time (Fig. 3-8). In such a condition, S$_3$ and S$_4$ may fuse in mid-diastole to form a single sound almost as loud as S$_1$ and S$_2$. A summation gallop has been compared to the sound of a horse cantering on a dirt track.

Miscellaneous sounds. Miscellaneous sounds of short duration include ejection sounds, systolic clicks, and opening snaps. *Ejection sounds* are brief, occur in early systole, and are associated with valvular or great vessel vibrations; they occur simultaneously with ejection of blood from the ventricles, hence their name (Fig. 3-8). They are identified most readily when heard in addition to the two components of the first heart sound; such a complex of sounds is called a *trill* (i.e., a trilogy of three sounds) when heard at the beginning of the cardiac cycle. The most common condition producing an ejection sound is aortic stenosis. Pulmonary ejection sounds typically occur with pulmonary hypertension. Ejection sounds also are caused by idiopathic great vessel dilation. Ejection sounds are high pitched and are heard immediately after S$_1$ with the diaphragm of the stethoscope and with the patient sitting or lying down.

Systolic clicks are brief, high-frequency sounds that occur most often in middle-to-late systole (Fig. 3-8). They may be followed by late systolic murmurs representing mitral regurgitation. They are heard best during forced expiration with the diaphragm of the stethoscope with the patient lying, sitting, or standing. Ejection clicks must be differentiated from ejection sounds, which usually occur much earlier in systole and are louder throughout the precordium.

Systolic clicks are best heard in the mitral area and are almost pathognomonic for mitral valve prolapse (also termed a *billowing mitral valve* or *Barlow's syndrome*). Systolic clicks occurring with mitral valve prolapse are caused by the ballooning of the leaflet tissue toward the left atrium in systole. A maneuver of great value is to listen for a systolic click with the patient standing. Because standing is associated with a reduced blood volume in the central circulation, prolapse of the mitral valve leaflets occurs earlier in systole than during sitting, causing the click to "move" earlier into systole.

The *opening snap* is an early diastolic sound occurring simultaneously with the opening of the mitral valve when it is thickened in mitral stenosis (Fig. 3-8). It is virtually diagnostic of rheumatic mitral valvular disease and, because of its timing in comparison with S$_2$, may indicate the severity of mitral stenosis. The closer in time these two sounds occur, the more severe the mitral stenosis. Opening snaps are high-pitched snaps heard with the diaphragm of the stethoscope over the mitral area.

Heart murmurs

Heart murmurs are vibratory sounds of increased duration that result from turbulent flow within the heart. Sounds of turbulence are referred to as *bruits* when they are generated from within a blood vessel and as murmurs when they emanate from passage of blood across a heart valve. Heart murmurs are characterized most importantly by their timing within the cardiac cycle (i.e., systolic or diastolic).[25] Other important descriptors of murmurs that should be assessed individually include configuration, intensity or loudness, location and radiation, pitch, and quality. Such descriptors also are used in differentiating pericardial friction rubs from murmurs (see Chapter 12).

Timing and configuration. It is useful to contrast systolic murmurs that are pansystolic (holosystolic) from those that are crescendo-decrescendo, or diamond-shaped, murmurs. Pansystolic murmurs are initiated with S$_1$ and terminated by S$_2$. They most often are plateau shaped and represent backward or regurgitant flow from the ventricle to the atrium (e.g., mitral or tricuspid regurgitation and ventricular septal defect [VSD]). The crescendo-decrescendo murmur, sometimes referred to as an *ejection murmur,* begins after S$_1$, increasing and then decreasing in intensity, and terminates before S$_2$. Most often this murmur reflects obstruction of right or left ventricular outflow. These murmurs may be generated below the valve, termed *subvalvular obstruction,* at the level of the valve as in pulmonary or aortic stenosis, or above the level of the valve, termed *supravalvular aortic* or *pulmonary stenosis.* Murmurs that are early, are soft crescendo-decrescendo, and often are heard best in the aortic or pulmonary areas are usually innocent, whereas murmurs that are loud, of long duration, especially pansystolic, and heard in the mitral or tricuspid areas usually indicate a pathologic condition.

Diastolic murmurs are almost always pathologic. Two common types of diastolic murmurs are those of aortic or pulmonary regurgitation. They are characterized by a decrescendo murmur with a high-pitched blowing quality. Another common diastolic murmur is the low-pitched rumbling murmur of a stenotic AV valve, most likely mitral stenosis because tricuspid stenosis is quite rare. Examination for aortic or pulmonary regurgitation is best accomplished by listening with the patient sitting upright, leaning forward, and holding in expiration. The diaphragm should be used at the LSB.

Intensity. Murmurs also may be divided according to the six categories or grades characterizing the intensity of sound. A grade 1 murmur is so faint that it can be recognized only after special effort on the part of the examiner. A grade 2 murmur is faint but can be heard easily. A grade 3 murmur is moderately loud. A grade 4 murmur is loud and usually associated with a thrill. A grade 5 murmur is very loud, and a grade 6 murmur is so loud that it can be heard with the stethoscope slightly removed from the chest wall.

Location and radiation. When murmurs are assessed, the area where the murmur is heard the loudest should be identified (i.e., mitral, tricuspid, aortic, or pulmonary areas). *Radiation* refers to the transmission of the sound to areas other than the anatomic location of the murmur. Radiation of a heart murmur in a specific direction may help in determining the site of origin. For instance, mitral murmurs appear to propagate, or radiate, to the axilla, whereas murmurs of left ventricular outflow project to the carotid arteries and base of the heart.

Pitch and quality. Murmurs may be classified as *high, medium,* or *low pitched.* A high- or medium-pitched murmur, such as that of aortic regurgitation, is heard best with the diaphragm of the stethoscope (Fig. 3-9); it sounds much like the forceful expiration of air through an open mouth. A low-pitched murmur, such as that found with mitral stenosis, makes a rumbling noise and is heard best with the bell. Murmurs may be further identified by their quality of sound; they may be described as *harsh, rumbling, blowing,* or *whooping.*

Types. The characteristics of timing, configuration, quality, pitch, location, and radiation are used to classify murmurs associated with abnormalities of the AV and semilunar valves (see Table 12-2).

Dysrhythmias

Evaluate the cardiac rhythm to determine the presence of dysrhythmias, including tachydysrhythmias, bradydysrhythmias; atrial, junctional or ventricular dysrhythmias;

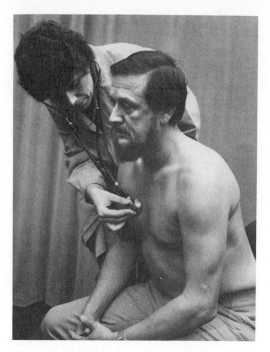

FIG. 3-9 Using the diaphragm of the stethoscope while the patient leans forward and holds the breath in full expiration, the nurse listens for high-pitched murmurs at the base of the heart. From Malasanos L, Barkauskas V, and Stoltenberg-Allen K: Health assessment, ed 4, St Louis, 1990, Mosby–Year Book, Inc.

first-, second-, or third-degree AV heart blocks; and premature atrial, junctional, or ventricular beats. Also document the rhythm and hemodynamic symptoms associated with the dysrhythmia such as hypotension, dizziness, syncope, confusion, or decreased cardiac or urinary output (see Appendix B).

Hemodynamic monitoring pressures

Assess hemodynamic monitoring variables, as indicated. (Normal cardiac output is 5 L/min[20,21] [see Chapter 7]). Also evaluate the cardiac index. (Normal cardiac index is 3.5 L/min/m^2 and ranges from 2.5 to 4.5 L/min/m^2.) Determine the cardiac index by dividing the cardiac output by the body surface area.[43] Evaluate pulmonary artery pressure (PAP) and pulmonary artery wedge pressure (PAWP). Normal PAP is less than 25 mm Hg systolic and 5 to 10 mm Hg diastolic, with a mean PAP of less than 13 mm Hg.[20,21] Normal PAWP ranges from 4 to 12 mm Hg (see Chapter 7).

Intravenous fluids, medications, and serum enzyme levels

Identify the type, amount, and rate of administration of all intravenous fluids that the patient is receiving. Record all intravenous medications, noting the name, dosage, and rate of administration. Evaluate the levels of serum cardiac enzymes, including creatine phosphokinase (CPK), CPK-MB isoenzyme, lactate dehydrogenase (LDH), LDH isoenzymes, and serum glutamic-oxaloacetic transaminase (SGOT)[20,42] (see Chapter 6). Refer to your institution's designated normal values.

Physical integrity

Explore whether the patient has corneal, mucous membrane, integumentary, or subcutaneous tissue damage such as a crushing injury or intravenous infiltration. Assess skin integrity in terms of hydration, vascularity, elasticity, texture, turgor, mobility, and thickness. Document skin rashes, lesions, bruises, abrasions, surgical incisions, or signs and symptoms of poor wound healing ("altered protection"). Also investigate other causes of disrupted skin surfaces such as invasive hemodynamic lines, stomas, or tubes.[31,39]

Assess the patient for *conjunctival petechiae* (associated with infective endocarditis) and for pale conjunctival tissue (associated with anemia). Assess for *xanthelasma*, or a yellow lipid plaque on the eyelids and elbows that is frequently associated with hyperlipidemia and a predisposition to atherosclerosis. Observe for arcus senilis, or a whitish opaque ring around the iris in the elderly patient. In younger patients, this finding is called *arcus cornealis* which is associated with hyperlipidemia and is abnormal.

Oxygenation
Dyspnea and orthopnea

The unique anatomic and functional interrelationship of the cardiac and respiratory systems requires a careful and complete evaluation of the chest, lungs, and respiratory system. Assess whether the patient is currently experiencing any dyspnea or orthopnea (integrate findings with Feeling Pattern).

Respiratory rate, rhythm, depth, and expansion

Assess the rate, rhythm, and depth of respirations; the adult breathes comfortably about 16 to 20 times per minute under normal conditions. Observe whether the depth of the breathing is shallow, moderate, or deep and whether the breathing is labored or unlabored. Observe whether the patient uses accessory muscles to breathe, whether the chest expands symmetrically, and whether the patient expends a great deal of energy to breathe. The entire rib cage should uniformly move laterally and upward with respiration. Evaluate abnormal breathing patterns such as asymmetric, obstructive, or restrictive breathing.

Cough and sputum

Identify whether the patient has a cough. If so, observe whether it is productive or nonproductive and whether the cough effort is effective. Determine the color, amount, odor, and consistency of sputum. Investigate hemoptysis that may be associated with pulmonary edema or a pulmonary embolus.

Breath sounds

The chest is palpated and auscultated during inspiration and expiration to assess for vibrations and breath sounds. *Fremitus* is a palpable vibration that may be associated with a friction rub (friction fremitus), loud rhonchi (rhonchal fremitus), or voice vibrations (vocal or tactile fremitus). The loudness, or intensity, of fremitus and that of breath sounds almost always are parallel. The grating quality, associated pain, localized area of abnormality, and presence of fremitus during inspiration and expiration help differentiate friction fremitus from rhonchal fremitus. *Rhonchal fremitus* is predominantly inspiratory, may clear with cough if it is produced by secretions obstructing a large airway, and generally is diffuse in location. The presence of *friction fremitus* may indicate pneumonia or another pulmonary process, especially one involving inflammation of the pleural surfaces because of its tendency to produce pleural friction rubs and fremitus.

Percussion of the chest is also used to determine the density of underlying structures. The sounds produced by structures such as bone are different in pitch and quality from those elicited from areas overlying normal lung, which are usually resonant, and those overlying fluid, which are characteristically dull. Percussion is most valuable for determining the presence of *pleural effusion* or changes in pulmonary consistency and density secondary to consolidation. Consolidation is intense inflammation with loss of aeration secondary to replacement of lung air spaces by liquid or solid material. It also is referred to as *atelectasis,* which describes collapse of lung spaces. The percussion note may reflect the absence of structural density such as with the presence of pneumothorax, air in the pleural space, or emphysema with its characteristic increase in aeration of the lung secondary to destruction of pulmonary structures.

After percussion, auscultation of the chest is performed to assess for breath sounds, bruits, pleural rubs, or any other adventitial or abnormal sounds. It is essential that the nurse be familiar with normal breath sounds to adequately assess the patient. Normal breath sounds may be bronchial (tracheal), brochovesicular, or vesicular according to the structure that characteristically produces them (Fig. 3-10, *A*).

Vesicular breath sounds originate in the alveolar air sacs. They are heard best during inspiration when air is moving into the terminal bronchioles and alveoli. Normally expiration is quiet or silent, and the inspiration/expiration ratio is 3:1. *Bronchial breath sounds* emanate from the bronchi and trachea. A combination of bronchial and vesicular breath sounds, or *bronchovesicular breath sounds,* normally are heard in the region below the trachea and peripheral

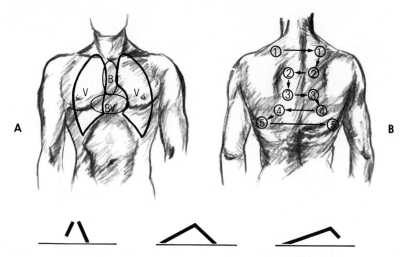

FIG. 3-10 A, Areas of the chest wall that overlie pulmonary regions associated with the three major types of breath sounds. *B,* Bronchial sounds; *BV,* bronchovesicular sounds; *V,* vesicular sounds. **B,** An approach to auscultation of the posterior aspects of the chest emphasizing the comparison of right and left pulmonary regions. Breath sounds are graphically represented at the bottom as bronchial *(left),* bronchovesicular *(middle),* and vesicular *(right).*

lung areas. Also, there are several types of abnormal breath sounds, termed *adventitious sounds*[21]:

1. Crackles: coarse or fine discontinuous, interrupted explosive sounds that emanate from fluid in the smallest airways, bronchioles, and alveoli (referred to in the past as *rales*)
2. Rhonchi: long, continuous, coarse sounds that emanate from turbulence in medium-sized airways or bronchi
3. Wheezes: whistling, hissing sounds produced by partial obstruction of large airways; possibly produced in small airways when turbulence is sufficient to produce audible noise
4. Pleural friction rubs: scratchy sound, which characteristically is heard only during inspiration and expiration and is silent during held respiration; produced by movement of inflammatory surfaces of pleurae over one another

Auscultate the patient's breath sounds on deep inspiration with the mouth open. Perform auscultation in an ordered sequence, beginning with the upper lung fields; auscultate one side and then the other, and compare both down to the level of the diaphragm. Firmly apply the diaphragm of the stethoscope to the chest wall to listen for the quality and amplitude of breath sounds (Fig. 3-10, *B*). Systematically auscultate all portions of the lung fields— posterior, anterior, and lateral. Concentrate first on normal breath sounds and then on abnormal sounds.

One maneuver that may help in evaluating the pulmonary system is auscultation of the chest during certain voice sounds. *Vocal resonance,* or the transmission of normal voice sounds, is increased in lung tissue with greater density or stiffness caused by pathologic processes. *Broncho-*

phony describes the increased intensity of vocal sounds, and *egophony* is a change in quality of the spoken word. Egophony is detected by having the patient speak the long "e" sound during auscultation of the chest. In areas of consolidation of the lung, the sound is heard as a long "a." In these areas the whispered speech of the patient is transmitted remarkably well through the stethoscope. This observation is termed *whispered pectoriloquy.* Examination of the chest is not complete until chest x-ray films are reviewed. The chest x-ray examination is indispensable; it gives information unavailable by physical examination.

Arterial blood gas and oxygen levels

Evaluate arterial blood gas levels. Describe any type of oxygen therapy and the percentage delivered. If the patient is on a mechanical ventilator, describe the type, settings, and the psychologic reaction to the ventilator.

Physical regulation

Determine the size, shape, mobility, tenderness, and enlargement of the lymph nodes. Assess lymph nodes in the head, neck, axillae, and inguinal and pelvic areas. Also assess the total white blood cell (WBC) count (leukocyte level) to determine elevations. The differential count is performed to determine the percentage of the types of leukocytes (i.e., neutrophils, lymphocytes, monocytes, eosinophils, and basophils) in the blood. Elevation of the neutrophil level indicates a bacterial infection. Elevation of the levels of lymphocytes and monocytes indicates a bacterial or viral infection.[39,42] Determine immune disorders or other abnormal blood disorders (e.g., leukopenia or thrombocytopenia) that might support the nursing diagnosis of "altered protection."

The patient's temperature is assessed. Temperature is measured on a Fahrenheit or centigrade scale. The formula for converting centigrade measurement to Fahrenheit and vice versa follows:

$$\text{Fahrenheit} = 1.8\,(^\circ\text{C}) + 32$$
$$\text{Centigrade} = \frac{^\circ\text{F} - 32}{1.8}$$

Rectal temperatures, which are the most accurate,[28] range from 36.1° C (97° F) to 37.0° C (99.6° F). In patients with acute myocardial infarction, measurement of rectal temperatures was usually avoided as a precaution against undue vagal stimulation. Recent studies suggest, however, that rectal temperatures are no longer contraindicated in these patients.[28]

Nutrition

When assessing nutritional status, determine the number of meals the patient eats each day. Ask patients to describe what they eat and drink in a typical day. Identify dietary needs or restrictions such as low-sodium, low-fat, low-calorie, low-protein, or low-sugar diets and whether there are any food allergies or foods not well tolerated by the patient. Identify types of foods the patient prefers and whether most of the meals are eaten at home or out. Determine the number of caffeinated beverages consumed each day (i.e., caffeinated coffee, teas, or soft drinks and amount of chocolate intake). Investigate changes in appetite such as eating or drinking more or less. Ask the patient whether there is an explanation for this change in eating pattern (e.g., nausea or vomiting).

Mouth and throat

Assess the condition and function of the mouth, lips, buccal mucosa, teeth, hard and soft palate, and throat. Ask whether the patient is able to bite, chew, taste, and swallow and whether there is oral pain or odor. Determine the condition and color of the gums and teeth, as well as the symmetry, color, mobility, and hydration of the tongue.

Height and weight

Assess height and weight and calculate the patient's ideal body weight. For men, 5 feet equals 106 pounds; for each additional inch, add 6 pounds. For a man 5 feet 8 inches tall, ideal body weight is 154 pounds. For women, 5 feet equals 100 pounds; for each additional inch, add 5 pounds. For a women 5 feet 5 inches, ideal body weight is 125 pounds.[21]

Current nutritional therapy and laboratory data

Document whether the patient is receiving nothing by mouth; nasogastric suctioning; tube feedings, including the type, amount, and frequency; or total parenteral nutrition (TPN), including the type, additives, and rate.

Assess laboratory data, which may include serum sodium, potassium, and chloride levels, glucose, cholesterol, and triglyceride levels (determine whether these were drawn under fasting conditions); and hematocrit and hemoglobin. Other laboratory data might include a blood coagulation profile ("altered protection") or drug toxicity screening.

Gastrointestinal and bowel pattern

Investigate usual bowel habits and whether the patient uses laxatives, enemas, suppositories, bran, or fruits to regulate bowel movements. Explore whether the patient has difficulty with constipation, hemorrhoids, bowel cramping, diarrhea, or bowel incontinence. Determine whether the patient has pain or bleeding with defecation. Document whether the patient has a colostomy or ileostomy and if so, the reason for it and the date of surgery.

Inspect the abdomen for rashes, scars, lesions, striae, or dilated veins. Assess for *ascites* or edema of the abdominal cavity. Observe the size, shape, and contour of the abdomen and auscultate the bowel sounds with the diaphragm of the stethoscope to determine their frequency, quality, and pitch. (Perform auscultation before palpation or percussion so that bowel sounds will not be altered). Use the following code for classifying bowel sounds:

0   = absent
1 + = hypoactive
2 + = normal
3 + = hyperactive

Percuss the abdomen to determine liver borders, gastric air bubbles (in left upper quadrant), splenic dullness, air, fluid, or masses. Palpate the abdomen to determine organ enlargement, muscle spasm or rigidity, masses, involuntary guarding, rebound tenderness, or pain.[19] Note the location, size, shape, mobility, tenderness, consistency, and pulsation of any masses.

Renal and urinary pattern

Determine the patient's usual urinary pattern. Explore whether the patient limits fluid during the day or night or whether excessive amounts of fluid are consumed. Investigate complaints of incontinence or retention of urine and ask the patient to describe frequency, burning, pain, dribbling, urgency, hematuria, nocturia, oliguria, or polyuria. Document whether the patient has a urostomy or is receiving dialysis (including type, frequency, and cause). Observe whether the bladder is distended. Examine the color, odor, and consistency of urine. Determine whether the patient has a urinary catheter (including type, duration, and problems). Measure the 24-hour urinary output or hourly output as indicated.

Document blood urea nitrogen (BUN) and creatinine levels. Evaluate additional urine studies such as urine culture and urine pH, acetone, glucose, blood, and protein levels.[19,27]

CHOOSING PATTERN

The purpose of this assessment is to determine whether the patient is successfully selecting alternatives consistent with medical, nursing, and health promotion recommendations. Coping abilities, judgment, participation, and wellness behaviors are evaluated.

Patient's ability to cope

To assess *individual coping* behaviors, explore whether patients believe they satisfactorily solve problems. Investigate who helps them to solve problems and whether it is easy or hard for them to accept needed help. Also ask patients how they deal with major problems (e.g., whether they become depressed, anxious, or nervous; eat food, drink alcohol, take drugs; ask someone for help, call the family, or try to solve the problem). Inquire about activities used to reduce stress such as listening to music, exercising, or using relaxation techniques. Verify the patient's perceptions by asking the family whether the patient is able to ask others for needed help.[7] Evaluate *defensive coping behaviors*. Identify whether the patient denies obvious problems or weaknesses, blames others for health or functioning, rationalizes failures, projects a falsely positive self-evaluation; or overreacts to slight criticism.[7]

Family's ability to cope and give support

To assess *disabling family coping,* observe whether family members are able to offer and give physical and emotional support to the patient. Determine whether they are able to make decisions and demonstrate behaviors supportive of the patient's psychophysiologic, social, or economic well-being.[7] Assess whether they appear to neglect the patient's basic needs, deny the patient's health problem and its extent and severity, or demonstrate rejection, intolerance, or abandonment.

When assessing for *compromised family coping,* determine whether the patient expresses concerns regarding the family members' response to the illness. Discover whether the family has inadequate knowledge of the patient's illness, treatment, or recovery that might interfere with their ability to support and assist the patient.[7]

Acceptance and adjustment to illness

To evaluate *denial,* observe whether patients fail to recognize the importance of symptoms and their danger, minimize symptoms, or displace the source of symptoms to other organs (e.g., chest pain dismissed as indigestion or gas). Delay in seeking health care assistance when symptoms appear is also characteristic of denial.[7]

To assess the level of *adjustment* to the illness, explore whether the patient accepts the change in health status brought about by the illness. Identify whether the patient exhibits a prolonged period of shock, disbelief, or anger regarding the current health status.[7] Evaluate the patient's movement toward independence as demonstrated by a willingness to become involved in problem solving or goal planning for the future.

Judgment

Assess *decision-making ability* by asking patients whether they believe they usually make good decisions. Identify the circumstances under which patients have difficulty making decisions. Observe whether patients verbalize uncertainty regarding the possible choices, vacillate between possible alternatives, or demonstrate unusual delay in making decisions regarding health care or treatment.[7] Also ask family members their opinion regarding the soundness and timeliness of patient's decisions.

Compliance

During discharge planning, take into consideration patients' past and current compliance with the health care regimen. Investigate whether patients have had difficulty in the past remembering to take their medication, following their diet, or adhering to a prescribed exercise program. Explore with patients the reasons they believe such difficulties occurred.[7]

Explore patients' motivation and willingness to comply with the future health care regimen. Investigate whether they foresee difficulty with following their new diet, exercise program, prescribed activities and treatments, or taking their medications. Ask patients whether they anticipate anything that is particularly difficult regarding the medical regimen instructions.[7,26] Determine whether the family understands the regimen and will support patients in complying with the recommendations.

Health-seeking behaviors

To assess the level of health-seeking behaviors, investigate whether patients are interested in finding ways to change or modify health habits and/or the environment to move toward a higher level of wellness (e.g., desire to stop smoking or overeating). Explore programs or resources that patients can use for health promotion.[7]

ADAPTING THE CARDIOVASCULAR ASSESSMENT TOOL

The tool in Fig. 3-1 was intended to be a working prototype demonstrating how human responses are assessed within the nine response patterns. As a working prototype, we encourage you to revise and adapt the tool to meet the needs of your practice. To further provide examples, we have included several case studies (see Chapter 17 and Appendix A) to demonstrate the ease at which nursing diagnoses can be identified using this type of assessment.

Because the needs and problems of cardiovascular patients differ based on the medical diagnosis and treatment plan, we have expanded this tool and developed several others. These include tools for assessing cardiac rehabilitation and transplant patients and a more abbreviated version for screening cardiovascular patients. These tools are presented in Appendix A with a case study and the data collected to demonstrate several approaches to a holistic patient assessment.

KEY CONCEPT REVIEW

1. The medical data base is inconsistent with current nursing practice because it:
   a. Is guided by the biomedical model
   b. Does not provide direction for how physiologic data should be interrelated to the psychologic realm
   c. Does not provide a complete holistic data base by which to assess all of the patient's body-mind-spirit problems
   d. All of the above
2. The choosing human response pattern involves:
   a. Selecting alternatives
   b. Sending messages
   c. The reception of information
   d. Establishing bonds
3. The benefits of using a holistic cardiovascular assessment tool include all of the following except:
   a. It provides the necessary data to support and document the existence of specific nursing diagnoses.
   b. It incorporates the tenets of the biomedical model.
   c. It demands a new way of synthesizing and interrelating data collected during assessment to determine holistic patterns.
   d. It offers a model for standardization of the nursing data base.
4. Data related to the current health problems and to coronary artery disease risk factors are collected and synthesized within the:
   a. Knowing Pattern
   b. Communicating Pattern
   c. Exchanging Pattern
   d. Choosing Pattern
5. Within the Valuing Pattern, the purpose of the assessment is to determine:
   a. Whether the patient is successfully selecting alternatives
   b. The patient's spiritual and cultural values as they relate to health and illness
   c. The patient's self-perception in terms of body image and self-esteem
   d. All of the above
6. Elevated jugular venous pressures may result from which of the following cardiac conditions?
   a. Tricuspid regurgitation
   b. Right ventricular failure
   c. Cardiac tamponade or constriction
   d. All the above

7. The mitral area on the precordium is located at the:
   a. Left sternal border, fourth intercostal space
   b. Right sternal border, second intercostal space
   c. Left sternal border, third intercostal space
   d. Midclavicular line, fifth intercostal space
8. All of the following are true with respect to the third heart sound except:
   a. It can be a normal sound in children and young adults.
   b. It may be the result of abnormally high ventricular filling pressures.
   c. It is identified by its close association with the second heart sound.
   d. It is associated with atrial contraction.
9. Match the following:
   a. First heart sound
   b. Second heart sound
   c. Third heart sound
   d. Fourth heart sound
   e. Ejection sound
   f. Systolic click
      1. Filling sound in early diastole
      2. Occurs simultaneously with ejection of blood from the ventricles
      3. Forceful ejection of blood during atrial contraction into a noncompliant ventricle
      4. Closure of the mitral and tricuspid valves
      5. Occurs in middle to late systole and represents mitral valve prolapse
      6. Closure of pulmonary and aortic valves
      7. Opening of the mitral and tricuspid valves
10. For an overview of the sounds of the cardiac cycle, stethoscope placement should be on the:
    a. Midclavicular border
    b. Right sternal border
    c. Left midaxillary border
    d. Left sternal border
11. Which of the following statements is true about central cyanosis?
    a. It is much more common than peripheral cyanosis.
    b. It reflects increased extraction of oxygen from peripheral tissues.
    c. It almost always reflects cardiopulmonary disease.
    d. It may be seen in mild degrees in normal individuals exposed to cold temperatures.

12. Sleep rest patterns and health maintenance management are assessed and synthesized in the:
    a. Exchanging Pattern
    b. Moving Pattern
    c. Perceiving Pattern
    d. Knowing Pattern

ANSWERS

1. d		9. a 4	
2. a		b 6	
3. b		c 1	
4. a		d 3	
5. b		e 2	
6. d		f 5	
7. d		10. d	
8. d		11. c	
		12. b	

REFERENCES

1. American Nurses' Association Division of Medical-Surgical Nursing Practice and American Heart Association Council of Cardiovascular Nursing: Standards of cardiovascular nursing practice, Kansas City, Mo, 1981, The Association.
2. Aydelotte MK and Peterson KH: Keynote address: nursing taxonomics: state of the art. In McLane AM, editor: Classification of nursing diagnoses: proceedings of the seventh conference, St Louis, 1987, The CV Mosby Co.
3. Bates B: A guide to physical examination, ed 3, Philadelphia, 1983, JB Lippincott Co.
4. Berne RM and Levy MN: Cardiovascular physiology, ed 6, St Louis, 1992, Mosby–Year Book Inc.
5. Braunwald E: Heart disease: a textbook of cardiovascular medicine, ed 3, Philadelphia, 1988, WB Saunders Co.
6. Carpenito LJ: Nursing diagnoses: application to clinical practice, ed 3, Philadelphia, 1989, JB Lippincott Co.
7. Carroll-Johnson RM, editor: Classification of nursing diagnoses: proceedings of the eighth conference, Philadelphia, 1989, JB Lippincott Co.
8. Chinn P: Advances in nursing theory, Rockville, Md, 1983, Aspen Publishers, Inc.
9. Chrisman MD and Fowler MD: The systems-in-change model for nursing practice. In Riehl J and Roy C, editors: Conceptual models for nursing practice, ed 2, New York, 1981, Appleton-Century-Crofts.
10. Daily EK and Schroeder JS: Techniques in bedside hemodynamic monitoring, ed 4, St Louis, 1989, The CV Mosby Co.
11. Dossey GM, Guzzetta CE, and Kenner CV: Essentials of critical care nursing: body-mind-spirit, Philadelphia, 1990, JB Lippincott Co.
12. Dossey BM and others: Holistic nursing: a handbook for practice, Gaithersburg, Md, 1988, Aspen Publishers, Inc.
13. Dossey L: Space, time, and medicine, Boston, 1982, Shambhala Publications, Inc.
14. Goldberger E: Textbook of clinical cardiology, St Louis, 1981, The CV Mosby Co.
15. Gordon M: Manual of nursing diagnosis, St Louis, 1989, The CV Mosby Co.
16. Guyton AC: Textbook of medical physiology, ed 8, Philadelphia, 1990, WB Saunders, Co.
17. Guzzetta CE: Nursing diagnoses: effect on the profession, Heart Lung, 16:629, 1987.
18. Guzzetta CE: General focus question and parameters for eliciting appropriate data. In Guzzetta CE and others: Clinical assessment tools for use with nursing diagnoses, St Louis, 1989, The CV Mosby Co.
19. Guzzetta CE: Nursing assessment: In Dossey BM, Guzzetta CE, and Kenner CV: Critical care nursing: body-mind-spirit, ed 3, Philadelphia, 1992, JB Lippincott Co.
20. Guzzetta CE and Casey P: Cardiovascular assessment. In Dossey BM, Guzzetta CE, and Kenner CV: Critical care nursing: body-mind-spirit, ed 3, Philadelphia, 1992, JB Lippincott Co.
21. Guzzetta CE and Seifert PC: Cardiovascular assessment. In Kinney MR and others, editors: Comprehensive cardiac care, ed 7, St Louis, 1991, Mosby–Year Book Inc.
22. Guzzetta CE and others: Unitary person assessment tool: easing problems with nursing diagnoses, Focus Crit Care 15:12, 1988.
23. Guzzetta CE and others: Clinical assessment tools for use with nursing diagnoses, St Louis, 1989, The CV Mosby Co.
24. Henneman EA and Henneman PL: Intricacies of blood pressure measurement: reexamining the rituals, Heart Lung, 18:263, 1989.
25. Hurst JW and others, editors: The heart, ed 7, New York, 1990, McGraw-Hill, Inc.
26. Kim MJ, McFarland GK, and McLane AM: Pocket guide to nursing diagnoses, ed 3, St Louis, 1989, The CV Mosby Co.
27. Kinney MK, Packa DR, and Dunbar SB, editors: AACN's clinical reference for critical care nursing, ed 2, St Louis, 1988, The CV Mosby Co.
28. Kirchhoff KT: An examination of the physiologic basis for "coronary precautions," Heart Lung 10:874, 1981.
29. Kritek PB: Development of a taxonomic structure for nursing diagnoses: a review and update. In Hurley M, editor: Classification of nursing diagnoses: proceedings of the sixth conference, St Louis, 1986, The CV Mosby Co.
30. Macrae JA: Listening: an essay on the nature of holistic assessment. In Krieger D, editor: Foundations for holistic health nursing practices: the renaissance nurse, Philadelphia, 1981, JB Lippincott Co.
31. Malasanos L and others: Health assessment, ed 4, St Louis, 1990, The CV Mosby Co.
32. Newman MA: Health as expanding consciousness, St Louis, 1986, The CV Mosby Co.
33. Quinless F: Assessing the client with acute cardiovascular dysfunction, Top Clin Nurs 8:45, 1986.
34. Quinn JF: Client care and nurse involvement in a holistic framework. In Krieger D, editor: Foundations for holistic health nursing practices: the renaissance nurse, Philadelphia, 1981, JB Lippincott Co.
35. Rogers M: Introduction to the theoretical basis of nursing, New York, 1969, FA Davis Co.
36. Roy C: Introduction to nursing: an adaptation model, Englewood Cliffs, NJ, 1976, Prentice-Hall.

37. Roy C: Framework for classification systems development: progress and issues. In Kim MJ, McFarland GK, and McLane AM, editors: Classification of nursing diagnoses: proceedings of the fifth conference, St Louis, 1984, The CV Mosby Co.
38. Sanford SJ and Disch JA: American Association of Critical-Care Nurses standards for nursing care of the critically ill, ed 2, East Norwalk, Conn, 1989, Appleton-Lange.
39. Seidel HM and others: Mosby's guide to physical examination, St Louis, 1987, The CV Mosby Co.
40. Strobeck JE: Approach to the patient with cardiac disease: the physical examination, Cardiovasc Rev Rep 1:760, 1980.
41. Swartz MH: Physical diagnosis: history and examination, Philadelphia, 1989, WB Saunders Co.
42. Thompson J and others: Clinical nursing, St Louis, ed 2, 1989, The CV Mosby Co.
43. Underhill SL and others: Cardiac nursing, Philadelphia, 1989, JB Lippincott Co.
44. Watson J: Nursing: human science and human care, Norwalk, Conn, 1985, Appleton-Century-Crofts.
45. Yacone LA: Cardiac assessment: what to do, how to do it, RN p. 43, May 1987.

Interchapter 4

The Critical Link Between Body and Mind

What is the critical link between body and mind? How do the body and mind communicate? Each of us has experienced the physiologic increases in heart rate and respirations when we become angry, fearful, or scared. We also have experienced the physiologic responses of relaxation when we are balanced, calm, and at peace. How then can our emotions change our physiology? It is just an autonomic system event? Or does it entail more?

Our understanding of how the body and mind communicate has been revolutionized by the discovery of the *neuropeptide system*. Neuropeptides, which come directly from the body's DNA, are amino acids that can open the lock to receptor sites to facilitate or block a specific cellular response. Endorphins (meaning the morphine within) were the first neuropeptides discovered.[2] Candace Pert, former Chief of Brain Chemistry of the Clinical Neuroscience Branch of the National Institute of Mental Health, was the codiscoverer of the endorphins with Solomon Snyder, who was awarded the Nobel Prize for his work.[4] Endorphins were called neuropeptides because they were first identified in the brain and consist of peptides.[2,7]

Since the discovery of endorphins, 50 to 60 other neuropeptides have been identified.[3] It is now known that brain function can be regulated by these various neuropeptides, which can alter behavior, mode states, and cellular function.[8] It also has been discovered that neuropeptides are located not only in the brain but also in the brain stem, spinal cord, and gastrointestinal system and are capable of circulating throughout the body.[5] Moreover, the autonomic, immune, and endocrine systems are integrated by the neuropeptides, which are responsible for connecting the body and emotions.[9]

The body and mind are an interrelated network of informational systems.[9] The brain, immune, endocrine, and autonomic nervous systems, however, have their own set of rules or codes. To transmit information between these systems, some type of transducer is necessary to allow the code of one system (e.g., the immune system) to be translated to the code of another (e.g., the endocrine system).[1] Transduction refers to the conversion of energy (or information) from one form to another[9] (e.g., in arterial pressure monitoring the transducer converts the mechanical energy that the blood exerts on its recording membrane into electrical voltage that can be calibrated in millimeters of mercury and electrically displayed as a pressure wave on an oscilloscope).

We know that the limbic-hypothalamic system is the primary mindbody transducer of information.[9] The limbic-hypothalamic system mediates and biochemically modifies emotions, moods, and feelings.[7] Our understanding of how emotions are transduced by the limbic-hypothalamic system has been enhanced, however, when researchers analyzed the distribution of neuropeptide receptors throughout the body. The limbic-hypothalamic region was found to have an abundance of neuropeptide receptors suggesting that an "informational center" exists in these areas.[9]

The brainstem and spinal cord also have multiple neuropeptide receptors. For this reason, it has been proposed that limbic system boundaries be extended to include the sensory information obtained from these areas.[9] The dorsal horn of the spinal cord transmits information from peripheral organs, skin, and glands to the central nervous system. The grey region of the brainstem and the dorsal horn of the spinal cord also are important centers for the transmission of pain. They are enriched with receptors for substance P, a chemical that enhances the transmission of pain. They also are enriched with receptors for endorphins that block the transmission of pain by inhibiting the release of substance P.[2,7]

The enteric system also has a rich supply of neuropeptides receptors. When it was discovered that the entire lining of the gastrointestinal tract contained receptor sites for endorphins and the ability to manufacture these mind-altering chemicals,[4] Pert stated, "It seems entirely possible to me that the richness of the receptors may be why a lot of people feel their emotions in their gut—why they have 'gut feelings'."[7]

The neuropeptides of the immune system are the immunotransmitters (e.g., thymosins, lymphokines, endorphins, adrenocorticotrophic hormone, thyroid-stimulating hormone, and so forth) and the neuropeptides of the endocrine systems are the endocrine hormones (e.g., adrenocorticotrophic hormone, vasopressin, endorphins, oxytocin, and so forth). Although it has been known that the endocrine system can control immune function, it also is becoming clear that the immune system can control endocrine function. Because both the immune and endocrine systems are able to produce the same molecules (hormones) and both systems have common receptors for these molecules, they are able to transmit information to one another.[10]

Neuropeptides and their receptors explain how emotions are experienced throughout the body. Neuropeptides are called *messenger molecules*. Because the autonomic, endocrine, and immune systems all make and use messenger molecules, they are able to "talk" within themselves and with each other.[4] These messenger molecules travel

78

throughout the body in various and diverse ways capable of translating the code of one system to the code of another to enable widespread and versatile communication patterns.[9] When the neuropeptide receptors are activated by the appropriate neuropeptide messenger molecules, the internal activities of the cell are triggered. Thus the endocrine hormones, the autonomic nervous system neurotransmitters, and the immunotransmitters of the immune system all act as messenger molecules that can open the receptor lock on the cell surface. These messenger molecules are communication channels between the receptor and the cell, which allow the mind to activate internal cellular functions.[9] The term *information substrate* is used to describe the neuropeptide system that has bridged our understanding of previously divided fields such as psychology, neurology, endocrinology, immunology, and biochemistry.[8] Neuropeptides and their receptors integrate the central and autonomic nervous systems, glands, and immune system to explain the biochemistry of emotions and the communication link between mind and body.

How then does the mind transduce emotions such as fear or peacefulness to the body? First, emotions, attitudes, and feeling are transmitted to the limbic-hypothalamic system as neural signals or messages. The limbic-hypothalamic system then acts as a transducer to convert the neural messages it receives into messenger molecules. These messenger molecules, in turn, activate the receptors on the cell's surface to produce physiologic changes. Fear, for example, triggers the limbic-hypothalamic system, which transduces the neural messages into the neurotransmitters of the autonomic nervous system (e.g., norepinephrine), the immunotransmitters of the immune system, and the hormones of the endocrine system to alter nervous system, endocrine, and immune function.

We now have the information to explain the critical link between the mind and body. The neuropeptide system is responsible for this communication. The hypothalamus is the central information center of neuropeptide activity and the bridge between the mind and body.[9] We also know that positive emotions have specific chemical correlates that produce specific desired physiologic effects on the body.[6] Since the functions of the endocrine, immune, and the autonomic system are mediated by the limbic-hypothalamic system, they are accessible to mind therapies that can change negative emotions into positive ones.[9] Mental suggestion, beliefs, and self-regulation therapies such as relaxation, guided imagery, and music therapy can activate the limbic-hypothalamic system to transduce positive feelings, emotions, thoughts, words, and images into the desired messenger molecules causing physiologic healing at the cellular level.[9]

From the work of Sperry and colleagues on the hemispheric function of the brain (p. 38), it appears that the ability of the brain to transduce emotions, images, and feelings to the limbic-hypothalamic system is enhanced when the right brain is permitted to process the information without any interference from the left hemisphere. Thus in a state of relaxation or guided imagery, any intruding signals of doubt from the critical, analytic, left brain are suppressed.[11] It is as if interhemispheric communication between the right and the left brain are blocked during states of relaxation and other forms of self-regulation allowing the right brain to work, uninhibited by the left.

What are the implications for nursing? First, we must realize that, as nurses, we are able to facilitate the process of this communication in a more intentional and deliberate way.[9] If positive emotions and thoughts are best transduced by the right brain, then our role is to assist patients in shifting their cerebral hemispheric dominance to the right hemisphere. This can be accomplished when we implement mind therapies such as relaxation and guided imagery into our daily plan of care. In doing so, we help patients not only to cope with the anxiety and stress of the illness but also to transform their negative emotions into desired thoughts and feelings to activate inner psychophysiologic healing.[4]

REFERENCES

1. Bowers K: Hypnosis: an informational approach, Ann New York Acad Sci, 296:222, 1977.
2. Davis J: Endorphins, New York, 1984, Dial Press.
3. Dossey BM, Keegan L, Guzzetta CE, and Kolkmeier L: Holistic nursing: a handbook for practice, Gaithersburg, Md, 1988, Aspen Publishing Co.
4. Dossey L: Recovering the soul, New York, 1989, Bantam Books.
5. Margules D: Beta-endorphins and endoloxone: hormones of the autonomic nervous system for conservation or expenditure of bodily resources and energy for anticipation of famine or feast, Neuroscience and Behavioral Review 3:155, 1979.
6. Melnechuk T: Neuroimmunology: crossroads between behavior and disease. Report on selected conferences and workshops, Advances 2:54, 1985.
7. Pert C: The wisdom of the receptors: Neuropeptides, the emotions, and bodymind, Advances 3:3, 1986.
8. Pert C, Ruff M, Weber R, and Herkenham ML: Neuropeptides and their receptors: a psychosomatic network, J Immunology 135:820, 1985.
9. Rossi EL: The psychobiology of mind-body healing: new concepts of therapeutic hypnosis, New York, 1986, WW Norton.
10. Smith E, Harbour-McMenamin D, and Black J: Lymphocyte production of endorphins and endorphin-mediated immunoregulatory activity, J Immunology 135:779s, 1985.
11. Wickramasekera I: A conditioned response model of the placebo effect: predictions from the model. In White L, Tursky B, and Schwartz G, editors: Placebo: theory, research, and mechanisms, New York 1985, Guilford Press.

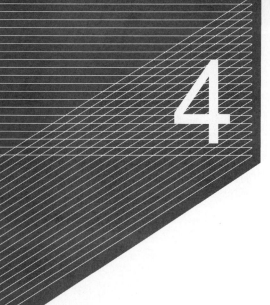

4

Nursing Diagnoses

Cathie E. Guzzetta
Barbara Montgomery Dossey

LEARNING OBJECTIVES

1. Examine the status of the nursing diagnosis movement.

2. Compare and contrast the definitions for a nursing diagnosis versus a medical diagnosis.

3. Examine the steps involved in the nursing diagnostic process.

4. Compare the parts included in the nursing diagnostic statement for actual, high-risk, and wellness nursing diagnoses.

5. Explore four different ways to write a diagnostic statement.

6. Formulate a diagnostic statement for an actual, a high-risk, and a wellness nursing diagnosis.

7. Analyze the academic and clinical impact of the nursing diagnosis movement.

8. Evaluate some of the issues confronting the nursing diagnosis movement.

Before the nursing diagnosis movement, which began in 1973, problem identification was the weak link in the nursing process. Within the past decade, the nursing diagnostic process has been accepted in academic and clinical settings as a means of delineating the remaining steps in the nursing process. Thus problem identification has been judged to be a clear and distinct phase (the second phase) of the nursing process. Because of the nursing diagnosis movement, problem identification is no longer the weak link. From a clinical, academic, and legal viewpoint, it appears that the nursing diagnosis movement will continue to gain momentum because of its major contribution in guiding nursing practice.

DEFINITION

The term *nursing diagnosis* has been defined in many ways in the literature. Recently the North American Nursing Diagnosis Association (NANDA) has revised and accepted the following definition:[44]

A nursing diagnosis is a clinical judgment about individual, family, or community responses to actual or potential health problems/life processes. Nursing diagnoses provide the basis for selection of nursing interventions to achieve outcomes for which the nurse is accountable.

The term *nursing diagnosis* has engendered strong criticism by some medical and nursing groups. Physicians have claimed, for example, that only they can diagnose. To avoid such criticism, other terms, such as *problems* or *needs,* have been used. In 1965, Levine[38] coined the term *trophicognosis* to replace the words *problems, needs,* and *diagnosis,* but her terminology was not accepted by the nursing community. Although the term *nursing diagnosis* continued to appear in the nursing literature, it was not until the nursing diagnosis movement that it gained acceptance and recognition. However, some nursing and medical groups continue to react negatively to the term.

By definition, *diagnosis* means the act of gathering or seeking information about what is causing some difficulty, what is interfering with normal function, or what is in need of correction.[7] From this definition, it is clear that nurses can diagnose as effectively as physicians.

Nursing versus medical diagnosis

To thoroughly understand the concept of nursing diagnosis, it is important to distinguish between a nursing and medical diagnosis. At times, this distinction has been confusing, especially in critical care.

The difference between a medical and a nursing diagnosis lies in its purpose. Medicine traditionally has been guided by a biomedical model based on the belief that all disease is caused by a malfunction of specific molecules or organs.[14] As a result, medicine is involved with the pathologic characteristics, diagnosis, and cure of disease. The purpose of a medical diagnosis is to identify the cause of the disease, and the treatment is directed by its cause.[16]

Nursing, however, is guided by a holistic model that reflects the interconnections of the mind and body. It conveys the oneness and unity of the individual; thus any change in the mental state always is accompanied by a change in the physiologic state and vice versa.[12,13,22] Nurses who use holistic models realize that human interaction is translated into physiologic responses and changes in consciousness. These psychophysiologic changes occur during all nurse-patient interactions because the nurse and patient are open systems and the omnidirectional information flow between them is continuous (see Chapters 1 and 2).

Because of the holistic model, a nursing data base, as opposed to a medical data base, is mandatory to the assessment of the whole patient.[26-28] Use of a nursing data base such as the Holistic Cardiovascular Assessment Tool (see Fig. 3-1) permits the nurse to collect and evaluate the necessary data about human responses so that judgments can be made about actual or high-risk health problems or life processes. Data obtained in the nursing data base are analyzed, conclusions are drawn, and nursing diagnoses are made.

The purpose of a nursing diagnosis then is to identify human responses to stressors or other factors that adversely affect the attainment of optimal health. Treatment is directed toward the cause of the response or factors influencing it. Thus nursing diagnoses are used to guide the steps of the nursing process. They are used to select nursing interventions that will successfully achieve desired patient outcomes for which the nurse is accountable.[13]

NANDA

Nurses always have identified patient problems, and writing a nursing diagnosis is not really a different activity. The difference is that NANDA (formerly called the National Group for Classification of Nursing Diagnoses) has been involved over the past two decades in developing, refining, and promoting a taxonomy of nursing diagnostic terminology.[9,44] This group has standardized labels or terms for patient problems that nurses encounter. Such work has lead to testing and research so that specific patient outcomes and nursing interventions can be developed for each diagnosis. This entire process is being used to identify activities unique to nursing.[25]

TAXONOMY I

For many years, the NANDA-accepted list of nursing diagnosis was organized alphabetically. However, the alphabetic list has been replaced by Taxonomy I, which uses the nine human response patterns of the Unitary Person Framework[44] (i.e., communicating, knowing, valuing, relating, feeling, moving, perceiving, exchanging, and choosing [see box on p. 41]).

The taxonomy was developed to systematically order the diagnoses into categories with relevant characteristics. It offers a major advantage to the alphabetic system because the taxonomy can be used to identify relationships and conceptual gaps among the diagnoses. It also facilitates communication of the diagnoses, information retrieval, and computer access.[44]

All NANDA-approved nursing diagnoses have been placed within the relevant response patterns at various category levels of Taxonomy I, according to their degree of abstractness (see Table 3-1). Abstract concepts are theoretic, frequently are not directly measurable, and may not be clinically useful in planning nursing care. Concrete concepts, on the other hand, are observable and measurable, and are generally useful in directing nursing care.[44] Within Taxonomy I, first-level categories, which are the most abstract, are used to define the response pattern of interest (for example, Exchanging Pattern). Second-level categories include the diagnostic qualifiers such as *altered* (for example, "altered circulation"). Third-level categories define the specific area of concern (for example, vascular). Fourth- and fifth-level categories are more specific and concrete in defining the particular problem and in directing the plan of care. A fourth-level category is "altered vascular fluid volume," and a fifth-level category is "fluid volume excess." The numbering system represents the way the diagnoses are related to one another and does not reflect any purposeful attempt to put the diagnoses or the patterns in order of priority[44] (e.g., 1.6.2 in Taxonomy I is "altered protection," and 1.6.2.1 is "impaired tissue integrity").

The nursing diagnoses listed in Taxonomy I have been approved by NANDA for clinical testing and continuing development.[44] These diagnoses are still under evaluation. It has not been determined whether each label actually exists in clinical practice or that it is useful in describing patient problems. As research is conducted to validate each label, its related factors, and its defining characteristics, the accepted list of nursing diagnoses will be modified, expanded, and supported.[20,21,34,35,41]

TYPES OF NURSING DIAGNOSES

In addition to arranging the diagnoses by Taxonomy I, NANDA also has divided nursing diagnoses into three categories: actual, high-risk, and wellness.[44]

Actual nursing diagnoses

Actual nursing diagnoses describe the patient's actual health problem. The diagnostic *label,* or the name for the diagnosis, is identified from Taxonomy I (see Table 3-1). The diagnostic label is a "concise phrase or term which represents a pattern of related cues" that defines the diagnosis in practice.[44] The diagnostic qualifiers outlined in Table 4-1 are used with the diagnostic label. Other qualifiers not listed can be used, as well.

Related factors are identified as "conditions or circumstances that can cause or contribute to the development of the diagnosis."[44] Related factors can be antecedent to, related to, associated with, contributing to, or abetting the problem.[44] They help identify situations maintaining the problem and preventing improvement. Related factors are used to guide the plan of care because they convey circumstances the nurse and the patient must change so that the patient can achieve a state of health.[10]

For actual problems, the diagnosis and related factors are connected by the phrase *related to*, thereby forming the *two-part diagnostic statement*; an example follows:

"Knowledge deficit about acute myocardial infarction (AMI) related to newly diagnosed health problem"

The phrase *related to* is legally recommended rather than *caused by* or *due to* because cause and effect have not been established yet for most nursing diagnoses.[43] The diagnostic statement should be specific to guide the remaining steps of the nursing process.

When making a judgment about whether the patient actually exhibits a specific nursing diagnoses, the nurse assesses the defining characteristics of the diagnosis. *De-fining characteristics* refer to behaviors or signs and symptoms that cluster to represent the diagnosis.[44] They are necessary to identify the diagnostic entity and to differentiate between nursing diagnoses. The defining characteristics should be measurable and are divided into major and minor categories.

Major defining characteristics are the *critical indicators* of the diagnosis occurring in 80% to 100% of patients experiencing the diagnosis. *Minor* defining characteristics are *supporting indicators* occurring in 50% to 79% of patients. They are not always present, but they complete the clinical picture in describing the diagnosis.[44]

The actual nursing diagnosis can be written in a two-part diagnostic statement (as described previously) or in a *three-part diagnostic statement* if signs and symptoms are included. Including the signs and symptoms in the diagnostic statement provides on-the-spot documentation to validate that the patient exhibits the defining characteristics. This format is recommended when teaching students or when initially implementing nursing diagnoses in the clinical setting. The appropriate signs and symptoms can be documented in or after the diagnostic statement; an example follows:[24]

"Knowledge deficit about AMI related to newly diagnosed health problem manifested by inability to describe meaning and signs and symptoms of an AMI"

OR

"Knowledge deficit about AMI related to newly diagnosed health problem:
1. Patient asked, "What is a heart attack?"
2. Patient was unable to list early warning signs of AMI.
3. Patient was unable to describe CAD risk factors."

Partial lists of defining characteristics have been published to assist the nurse in verifying a particular nursing diagnosis.[18,32,44] After assessing the patient's condition and formulating possible nursing diagnoses, the nurse should refer to the list of defining characteristics to determine whether the critical indicators actually were observed. If they were, the nursing diagnosis is made. The complete list of defining characteristics for many nursing diagnoses, however, is still being developed. For some diagnoses, the defining characteristics have not been identified and in most cases, they have not yet been validated by research. In the clinical setting, this lack of information can be perplexing. Therefore if the defining characteristics for a particular diagnosis are incomplete or missing, nurses must use their knowledge, education, and experience to determine whether the signs and symptoms observed during the nursing assessment are sufficient to confirm the existence of the actual health problem. If the nurse judges that they are, the nursing diagnosis is made.

The introduction of defining characteristics brings with it an important advancement to nursing assessment. It is no longer adequate to say, "I think the patient is de-

TABLE 4-1

Diagnostic Qualifiers for Actual and High-Risk Nursing Diagnoses

Qualifier	Definition
Altered	A change from baseline
Impaired	Made worse, weakened; damaged, reduced; deteriorated
Depleted	Emptied wholly or partially; exhausted of
Deficient	Inadequate in amount, quality, or degree; defective; not sufficient; incomplete
Excessive	Characterized by an amount or quantity that is greater than is necessary, desirable, or useful
Dysfunctional	Abnormal; incomplete functioning
Disturbed	Agitated; interrupted, interfered with
Ineffective	Not producing the desired effect
Decreased	Lessened; lesser in size, amount or degree
Increased	Greater in size, amount, or degree
Acute	Severe but of short duration
Chronic	Lasting a long time; recurring; habitual; constant
Intermittent	Stopping and starting again at intervals; periodic; cyclic

From North American Nursing Diagnosis Association: Taxonomy I: revised 1990, St Louis, 1990, The Association.

pressed." Defining characteristics eliminate guesses and hypotheses. Before a nursing diagnosis is made, it must be supported by actual data obtained from the nursing assessment.

High-risk nursing diagnoses

Diagnostic labels also consist of high-risk nursing diagnoses. As of 1992, all NANDA-approved diagnoses designated as *potential for* were changed to *high risk for*.[44] A high-risk nursing diagnosis is[44]:

a clinical judgment that an individual, family, or community is more vulnerable to develop the problem than others in the same or similar situation. High-risk nursing diagnoses are supported by risk factors that guide nursing interventions to reduce or prevent the occurrence of the problem.

The qualifiers listed in Table 4-1 also are used with the high-risk nursing diagnosis.

Within this category, risk factors associated with the diagnosis are identified. *Risk factors* are "behaviors, conditions, or circumstances that make an individual, family, or community more vulnerable to a particular problem than others in the same or similar situation."[44] Signs and symptoms are not identified for high-risk diagnoses. The diagnosis and the risk factors are connected by the phrase *related to* and written as a two-part statement; an example follows:

"High risk for altered nutrition: less than body requirements related to fatigue, activity intolerance, and progressive cardiac failure"

Changing the terminology of *potential* problems to *high risk for* is another major advance in the nursing diagnosis movement. All critically ill patients, for example, may have the "potential" for infection. Specifically stating which patients are at "high-risk" for such infection, however (e.g., those who are immunosuppressed or those with invasive lines), is essential to providing quality nursing care to prevent or reduce this problem in susceptible patients. Moreover, nurses will be better able to demonstrate and document their contribution to achieving desired patient out-

 ALTERED HEALTH MAINTENANCE

DEFINITION

Inability to identify, manage, and/or seek out help to maintain health

DEFINING CHARACTERISTICS

Demonstrated lack of knowledge regarding basic health practices
Demonstrated lack of adaptive behaviors to internal/external environmental changes
Reported or observed inability to take responsibility for meeting basic health practices in any or all functional pattern areas
History of lack of health seeking behavior
Expressed interest in improving health behaviors
Reported or observed lack of equipment, financial, and/or other resources
Reported or observed impairment of personal support systems

RELATED FACTORS

Lack of, or significant alteration in, communication skills (written, verbal, and/or gestural)
Lack of ability to make deliberate and thoughtful judgments
Perceptual/cognitive impairment (complete/partial lack of gross and/or fine motor skills)
Ineffective individual coping
Dysfunctional grieving
Unachieved developmental tasks
Ineffective family coping
Disabling spiritual distress
Lack of material resources

From North American Nursing Diagnosis Association: Taxonomy I: revised 1990, St Louis, 1990, The Association.

 HEALTH-SEEKING BEHAVIORS (SPECIFY)

DEFINITION

A state in which an individual in stable health is actively seeking ways to alter personal health habits and/or the environment in order to move toward a higher level of health*

DEFINING CHARACTERISTICS
Major

Expressed or observed desire to seek a higher level of wellness

Minor

Expressed or observed desire for increased control of health practice
Expression of concern about current environmental conditions on health status
Stated or observed unfamiliarity with wellness community resources
Demonstrated or observed lack of knowledge in health promotion behaviors

From North American Nursing Diagnosis Association: Taxonomy I: revised 1990, St Louis, 1990, The Association.
* Stable health status is defined as age-appropriate illness-prevention measures achieved, client reports good or excellent health, and signs and symptoms of disease, if present, are controlled.

comes when, for example, infection is found not to occur in this high-risk patient because of the quality of nursing care administered. In addition, the high-risk category will be beneficial in justifying allocation of resources and personnel and in the reimbursement for third-party payment.

Wellness nursing diagnoses

Wellness nursing diagnoses also have been addressed by NANDA. A wellness nursing diagnosis is a "clinical judgment about an individual, family, or community in transition from a specific level of wellness to a higher level of wellness."[44] The diagnoses listed in Taxonomy I are now used with the phrase *potential for enhanced* (in which *enhanced* means to "make greater or more desired or to increase in quality") to formulate wellness nursing diagnoses. Such diagnoses are written as one-part statements; an example follows:

"Potential for enhanced adjustment to illness"

The inclusion of wellness diagnoses is a major milestone of the nursing diagnosis movement. In the past, nursing diagnoses were criticized for excluding behaviors that maintained and promoted wellness. Wellness and health promotion are national priorities. Wellness nursing diagnoses broadens the perspective from an illness-dominated framework, which focuses primarily on unhealthy responses, to one that incorporates a positive wellness orientation.

A distinction must be made between the concepts of illness prevention (or risk reduction), health maintenance, and health promotion. *Illness prevention* or *risk reduction* involves behaviors aimed at actively protecting against or reducing the chances of encountering disease, illness, or accidents.[1,45] High-risk nursing diagnoses are directed at prevention. Nursing interventions are actively selected to reduce or prevent the particular problem.[6]

Health maintenance implies sustaining a neutral state of health. Patients unable to identify, manage, or seek help to maintain health would be diagnosed as having "altered health maintenance."[51] Nursing interventions would be aimed at activities to prevent and to protect health (e.g., following a balanced diet, stopping smoking, obtaining regular medical examinations, and sleeping 6 to 8 hours per night).[16] The definition, defining characteristics, and related factors for altered health maintenance are outlined in the box on p. 83.

Health promotion, however, goes beyond health prevention or maintenance. It involves a personal responsibility for health. It places the individual in an active role. Thus individuals strive actively to improve their lifestyle to achieve high-level wellness.[51] The diagnosis of "health-seeking behaviors" (i.e., health-promoting behaviors) is consistent with the concept of health promotion. Health-seeking behaviors might include activities such as requesting additional information and recipes to enhance a low-cholesterol, low-fat, low-salt, low-sugar, and high-fiber diet; practicing daily relaxation techniques; and participating in aerobic exercises 3 to 5 times per week. The definition and defining characteristics of health-seeking behaviors are outlined in the box on p. 83. The new category of wellness nursing diagnoses using Taxonomy I with the qualifier of *potential for enhanced* also addresses health promotion activities and allows the nurse to focus on wellness, facilitate responsibility for self-care, and promote healthy behaviors.

WRITING DIAGNOSTIC STATEMENTS

Different approaches to writing nursing diagnoses have been identified by several authors.* Use of one or more of these variations may help, depending on the problems observed and the expertise of the nurse. The following examples illustrate some possible variations. Because the nursing diagnosis movement is growing and developing, there are many correct ways to implement the process in clinical practice.

One-part statements

The cause (related factor) of an actual problem may initially be undefinable, and further assessment and observation may be necessary before it can be written in the diagnostic statement. When this occurs, the diagnostic statement consists only of the first main clause. The cause or related factors are written later, after they have been established. However, this variation does not happen frequently, and it should not be used as an excuse for omitting the related factor in the diagnostic statement. When it is omitted, the nurses neither know the elements maintaining the unhealthy state nor the conditions needing to be changed to achieve a state of health.

For example, the diagnosis, "altered sensory perception," may be formulated for a patient demonstrating disorientation to time, place, and person; restlessness; and altered communication patterns. The cause might be an acute pathologic condition caused by drug toxicity, high fever, or electrolyte imbalance; a chronic pathologic condition caused by generalized atherosclerotic disease; or sensory deprivation or overload caused by interrupted sleep patterns, constant pain, or loss of hearing or vision. It may not be possible to establish the cause (or related factor) for this problem until further diagnostic testing and observations are completed.

Two or more related health problems

Occasionally two or more health problems may be so closely related that their cause, plan, and intervention are the same. When this occurs, related problems are written together in the first main clause; an example follows:

---

*References 7, 16, 18, 25, 32, and 37.

"Depression and anxiety related to impending open-heart surgery"

Unrelated problems, however, should not be written in the first main clause, even though the cause of the problems may be the same. Problems may be seen as unrelated when the nursing plan requires separate interventions for each problem; an example follows:[24]

Wrong: "Anxiety and decreased activity level related to frequent episodes of chest pain"

Right: "Anxiety related to frequent episodes of chest pain"

Right: "Decreased activity level related to frequent episodes of chest pain."

Two or more related factors

In contrast, two or more related factors may be associated with the same problem. If this information would help in developing the care plan, then both related factors should be listed in the diagnostic statement; and example follows:[26]

"Impaired skin integrity related to immobility and altered circulation"

Levels of diagnoses

Nursing diagnoses sometimes are organized into levels to enhance descriptiveness, specificity, and conciseness.[7] The central diagnosis is written as a broad diagnostic statement followed by related subdiagnoses, which are sufficiently specific to direct nursing intervention. Thus the nurse can organize the plan of care around related problems that characterize the patient's total response pattern (central diagnosis) by formulating specific nursing diagnoses (subdiagnoses), which are more concrete and narrower in focus. Patient outcomes and nursing orders then are developed for each subdiagnosis. This variation is more complex than many of the others and is recommended for the clinician with more advanced diagnostic skills; an example follows:[24]

"High level of psychophysiologic stress related to unexpected cardiac illness

1. Extreme anxiety related to fear of death
2. High risk for decreased cardiac output due to dysrhythmias related to sympathetic nervous system overactivity and myocardial irritability
3. Sleep pattern disturbance related to the intensive care unit (ICU) routine and invasive monitoring equipment"

Avoiding errors

Several errors also may be encountered in writing the diagnostic statement,[7,10,43,46] which can reduce the specificity, descriptiveness, and usefulness of the diagnosis. The nursing diagnosis should be written as a nursing diagnosis rather than a medical diagnosis. Nurses should ask what they are treating related to the medical diagnosis; an example follows:[24]

Wrong: "Congestive heart failure"

Right: "Decreased cardiac output related to mechanical factors (preload, afterload, or inotropic state of the heart)" (see Chapter 10)

The nursing diagnosis should be written in terms of a problem, not a patient need. All patients have a hierarchy of needs, but after a need is identified as being unmet, it becomes a patient problem; an example follows:[24]

Wrong: "Need for maintenance of nutritional intake"

Right: "Altered nutrition: less than body requirements related to nausea and vomiting"

A common error in writing the diagnostic statement is making it too general so that it does not give sufficient direction for the nursing interventions; an example follows:

Wrong: "High risk for complications related to prolonged intravenous (IV) therapy"

Right: "High risk for infective or phlebotic vascular complications related to prolonged IV therapy"

Occasionally the nursing diagnosis is written in terms of a nursing problem or a nursing goal. Rather, it should be stated in terms of a patient problem; an example follows:

Wrong: "Teach patient about the hazards of valvular reinfection"

Right: "High risk for valvular reinfection related to an insufficient knowledge about infective endocarditis"

The nurse should be careful when writing the diagnostic statement so that the problem and related factors do not say the same thing; an example follows:[24]

Wrong: "Feeding self-care deficit related to inability to feed self"

Right: "Feeding self-care deficit related to weakness, fatigue, and dyspnea"

The nurse should not write a diagnostic statement that might have serious legal ramifications; an example follows:[24]

Wrong: "High risk for physical injury related to lack of safety precautions"

Right: "High risk for physical injury related to mental confusion"

The first main clause should reflect an actual or high-risk problem and not an environmental problem. Environmental factors are stated in the second main clause; an example follows:[24]

Wrong: "Excessive environmental stimuli related to monitoring equipment"

Right: "Altered sensory perception (auditory and visual) related to excessive environmental stimuli"

The nurse should not formulate a nursing diagnosis that should not or cannot be corrected[7]; an example follows:

Wrong: "Denial related to recent acute illness (AMI)"

Patients frequently are in a state of denial after an AMI, a situation that may be helpful in the early stages of coping. In the acute stage, denial is not a problem unless it extends into the recovery period and the patient denies the illness, symptoms, and need to comply with the medical regimen. The diagnosis of "ineffective denial" would then be appropriate.

The nurse should be careful not to write the diagnosis in judgmental terms. Judgmental terms label the patient and are derived from a subjective interpretation of behavior; an example follows:

Wrong: "Noncompliance with daily antihypertensive medication related to lack of cooperation and irresponsibility"

Right: "Noncompliance with daily antihypertensive medication therapy related to perceived side effects of medication (i.e., sexual dysfunction)"

When writing the diagnostic statement, abbreviations and specialized jargon should be avoided. These may be confusing to other health team members and may defeat the purposes of the diagnostic process.

USING NURSING DIAGNOSES

Using a nursing diagnosis does not take time from the nurse's usual busy day. It helps the nurse determine the priority of patient problems and directs the plan of care, and it provides purpose and direction to the nursing process. Standardization, clarification, and communication about the patient's health problems to all members of the health team are facilitated. It increases the nurse's accountability and helps convey holistic and humane nursing care.

The nurse who wants to begin using nursing diagnoses should consider the following suggestions.[10,24,46] They should carry Taxonomy I, the list of NANDA accepted nursing diagnoses, and should not be afraid to use it. Taxonomy I is worded in a new way to establish a standardized terminology for patient problems to enhance efficiency and communication. Thus it is imperative to be thoroughly familiar with the terminology and to use it correctly.

Early in the day, nurses should establish the habit of doing a holistic nursing assessment, using a standardized nursing data base such as the one described in Chapter 3, being certain to include a review of the nurses' notes from the previous 24 to 48 hours, as well as progress notes, laboratory results, and medical orders.

After establishing a baseline assessment of the patient, nursing diagnoses are put in order of priority and are written on the patient's care plan. The nurse should never wait until the end of the shift. The accepted list of nursing diagnoses outlined in Taxonomy I does not consist of all possible problems observed by nurses. Undoubtedly many important clinical health problems remain to be identified and added to the accepted list. Because the list is incomplete, sometimes the nurse will identify a problem that is not on the list. If the patient exhibits observable signs and symptoms that support a new diagnosis, the nurse words the problem concisely, identifies the related factors, and writes the diagnostic statement on the problem list. Moreover, if the new diagnosis is useful in defining a patient problem, the nurse should consider obtaining the detailed criteria for submitting a new nursing diagnosis to NANDA to be considered for inclusion in Taxonomy I (see the box).

Next the patient outcomes for the nursing diagnoses are identified, the nursing prescriptions (plan) are developed, the nursing actions are implemented, and patient

 PROCEDURE FOR SUBMITTING NEW NURSING DIAGNOSES TO NANDA

If a new diagnosis, not found on the list, is identified as a useful label, nurses are encouraged to submit it to NANDA's Diagnosis Review Committee. They can write to NANDA—the address can be found at the end of this chapter—to obtain the criteria for submission. The submission must comply with NANDA's guidelines and include the following:

1. The label or the name of the diagnosis
2. A definition of the diagnosis that is defined clearly and precisely so that its meaning can be understood and differentiated from other related diagnoses
3. For actual nursing diagnoses, the related factors that can cause or contribute to the development of the problem; for high-risk diagnoses, the risk factors that make a patient more susceptible than others to develop a particular problem
4. For actual nursing diagnoses, the major and minor defining characteristics of the diagnosis
5. A literature review that supports the diagnostic label, the defining characteristic, the related factors, the associated risk factors, and when possible, the results of scientific investigation
6. The diagnosis (i.e., the three-part statement for actual nursing diagnoses, the two-part statement for high-risk diagnoses, and the one-part statement for wellness diagnoses), with the associated outcome criteria and nurse-prescribed interventions

After submission the new diagnosis is reviewed by the Chairperson of NANDA's Diagnosis Review Committee and the Expert Advisory Panel of this committee. If it is accepted, the new diagnosis is forwarded to NANDA's Board of Directors for approval. The last step involves presentation of the new diagnoses at the NANDA Conference and then mailing the diagnosis to the membership for a vote. If approved at each step, the new diagnosis is then added to the taxonomy.

Data from North American Nursing Diagnosis Association: Taxonomy I: Revised 1990, St Louis, 1990, The Association.

outcomes for each nursing diagnosis are evaluated.[39] Throughout the day, the nurse should be cognizant of the nursing diagnoses generated and the patient outcomes that have developed. The expected patient outcomes are compared and documented with the ones actually observed. Because the nursing process is dynamic and continuous, reassessment and reevaluation are essential.[10]

Each nursing diagnosis should be referred to when giving nursing care, having health team conferences, charting patient responses, giving change of shift reports, retrieving patient data, and carrying out health care follow-up procedures. Nursing diagnoses also can provide a focal point for updating education and knowledge, and they provide an important area for research on the quality of patient care.[10]

NURSING DIAGNOSES AND STANDARDS OF CARE

The American Nurses' Association Division on Medical-Surgical Nursing Practice and the American Heart Association Council on Cardiovascular Nursing[5] have developed the *Standards of Cardiovascular Nursing Practice.* These standards, outlined in the box, pp. 88-93, were developed from the steps of the nursing process and include assessment, nursing diagnosis, goals, plan, implementation, and evaluation. Also the American Association of Critical-Care Nurses[48] have developed and revised their structure, process, and outcome standards for care of the critically ill. The process standards likewise were developed from the nursing process and include collecting data, identifying problems and needs, formulating the plan of care, implementing the plan, and evaluating care. Units III & IV of this text incorporate both the standards for cardiovascular nursing and the process standards for care of the critically ill.

These standards of practice provide model statements that direct the nurse in delivering care during each step of the nursing process. They also are used as the basis for evaluating the effectiveness and quality of care. These standards should be used when caring for all patients with cardiovascular dysfunctions. Because standards of practice are written in general terms, it is usually necessary to use them with more specific standards of care tailored to the patient's illness and modified according to hospital policy, as well as state nurse practice acts.[30]

In most clinical settings, standards of nursing care are written for many nursing and medical diagnoses. When standards are available for a specific diagnosis, the nurse should list the diagnosis on the care plan and write in a notation to refer to standards of care. This eliminates the need to recopy the standard and allows the nurse to direct attention to problems that are unique to the individual. To effectively use the standards, the nurse must have ready access to them (via computer or by multiple copies typed on index cards that can be attached to the care plan); also, the nurse must know and understand the standards.

Cardiovascular patients may be at high risk for developing certain problems more frequently than others.[33] The nursing diagnoses formulated in Units III & IV of this book represent the more common human responses associated with each cardiovascular dysfunction. However, the nurse must be warned against applying these problems to all patients with a similar illness and thereby labeling the patient without sufficient data. Thus the diagnostic statement should not be written in terms of the nurse's expectations.[7] For example, not all patients experience depression after an AMI, and therefore the nurse should not assume that all AMI patients are depressed. All patients must be assessed individually.

The nursing plan also should not be written in terms of nursing goals that do not conform to patient goals. Nurses should not assume, for example, that all patients want a preoperative visit to the ICU or cardiac catheterization laboratory or that all cardiac surgical patients desire comprehensive preoperative teaching.

IMPACT OF THE NURSING DIAGNOSIS MOVEMENT

The nursing diagnosis movement has had a greater impact on the nursing profession than anyone could have imagined when it first began back in 1973.[23] The progressive acceptance of nursing diagnosis by educators in baccalaureate and higher-degree nursing programs was recently confirmed by McLane and Kim[42] in a survey of 496 nursing programs accredited by the National League for Nursing. About 99% of generic programs, 97% of masters programs, and 92% of doctoral programs in nursing have integrated nursing diagnostic concepts into their curricula. These statistics have rapidly increased over the past several years[40] and suggest that the nursing diagnosis movement has rapidly grown within our academic institutions.[23]

The nursing diagnosis movement also has had an impact on our professional organizations. In a publication by the American Nurses' Association (ANA) Congress for Nursing Practice,[4] nursing was defined as "the diagnosis and treatment of human responses to actual or potential health problems." This statement is exciting, not only because a definition of nursing was agreed on and accepted by the ANA, but also because it validates the importance of nursing diagnosis within the profession. Furthermore the five divisions of nursing practice of the ANA have accepted nursing diagnosis as an integral part of the nursing process.[4] Many states have revised or are revising their nurse practice acts to include nursing diagnosis as a responsibility of the nurse.

The American Heart Association[5] and the American Association of Critical-Care Nurses[48] have included problem identification (nursing diagnosis) in their standards of care. The American Association of Colleges of Nursing has cited identification of nursing diagnoses as an essential component of provider care.[2] Likewise, the Joint Commission for Accreditation of Healthcare Organizations has

Text continued on p. 93.

STANDARDS OF CARDIOVASCULAR NURSING PRACTICE

STANDARD 1

The collection of data about the health status of the individual is systematic and continuous. These data are recorded, retrievable, and communicated to appropriate persons.

Interpretive statement

Data are obtained by observation, interview, physical examination, review of records and reports, and consultation. Priority of data collection is determined by the immediate health care problems of the individual.

Criteria

1. Health data include, but are not limited to, the following:
   a. History regarding the following:
      1) Information about perceptions, expectations, and adherence with past prescribed and/or self-initiated dietary, medication, and activity programs
      2) Symptoms identified by the individual, including description of onset, duration, quality, location, radiation, associated symptoms, precipitating factors, relieving factors of each symptom
      3) Cardiovascular risk factor profile, including the following:
         Family history of heart disease or vascular disease
         Hypercholesterolemia/hypertriglyceridemia—serum lipid levels
         Smoking
         Hypertension
         Obesity
         Sedentary living
         Diabetes
         Psychosocial factors
         Alcohol intake
         Oral contraceptives
      4) Previous health state, including the following:
         Hospitalizations
         Operations
         Injuries
         Infectious diseases
      5) Personal and social factors, including the following:
         Habits
            Coffee, tea, soft drink intake
         Meals
            Usual number taken daily
            Where eaten
            Description of self as "slow" or "fast" eater
         Sleep
            Sleeps well/restless/poorly
            Dreams/nightmares
            Sleeps flat/upright
            Number of pillows
            Number of hours of sleep, including individual's perception of adequacy
            Use of sleeping pills
         Occupation
            Job description
            Physical energy expenditure
            Mental energy expenditure
            Working hours
            Shift changes
            Length of time at this work
            Job satisfaction/employer/associates
            Energy expenditure in traveling to and from work
            Chemical/physical hazards
         Activities
            Hobbies
            Sports
            House/yard work
            Organizations and clubs
         Living arrangements
            Marital status
            Ages and health of spouse and children
            Number of persons in the home
            Domestic harmony/problems
         Environment
            Size and arrangement of home
            Neighborhood: terrain, transportation, safety
            Pollutants
            Pets
         Economic situation
            Health insurance
            Financial resources/obligations
         Psychosocial readjustments
            Recent stressful life events
            Changes in role relationships
         Cultural orientation, values, and beliefs
            Spiritual belief
         Education
            Ability to read and understand preferred major language
            Number of years of school completed
      6) Systems review
         Skin
            Diaphoresis
            Bruising
            Petechiae

From American Nurses' Association Division on Medical-Surgical Nursing Practice and American Heart Association Council on Cardiovascular Nursing: Standards of cardiovascular nursing practice, Kansas City, Mo, 1981, The Association.

STANDARDS OF CARDIOVASCULAR NURSING PRACTICE—cont'd

Head, eyes, ears, nose, and throat
  Headaches
  Visual problems
  Nasal stuffiness
  Allergies
  Thyroid
Respiratory
  Cough
    Dry/productive
    Time of day/coughing at night
    Position/dependent
    Hemoptysis/secretions
  Wheezing respirations
  Dyspnea or shortness of breath
    Exertional—amount of activity that pre-
      cipitates it
    Orthopnea
    Paroxysmal nocturnal dyspnea
Cardiovascular
  Discomfort or pain in chest, arms, shoul-
    ders, back, neck, jaw
  Degree and duration of pain
  Aggravating and alleviating factors for
    pain
  Fatigue—change in activity tolerance
  Edema
  Claudication
  Heart consciousness
    Aware of normal heart action
    Aware of irregular beating
    Aware of pounding or palpitations
  Rheumatic fever
  Scarlet fever
  Frequent tonsillitis as a child
  "Growing pains"
  Murmur
Gastrointestinal
  Food preferences
  Appetite change
  Food intolerance
    How manifested
    Use of antacids
  Heartburn
  Difficulty with swallowing
  Hematemesis
  Stools
    Color change
    Diarrhea/constipation
Genitourinary
  Change in urinary pattern
  Nocturia
  Hematuria
  Change in sexual desire/function

Metabolic
  Weight changes and what does individual
    attribute it to
Neuropsychiatric
  Dizziness
  Vertigo
  Fainting spells
    Sudden without warning
    Precipitating factors
    Fade out/gray out
  Convulsions
  Tremors
  Incoordination
  Gait changes—staggering
  Memory changes, confusion
  Changes in comprehension, understand-
    ing
  Speech changes, slurring
  Numbness, tingling
  Paralysis
  Fatigue
    When noticed
    Build up during the day versus waking
      up tired
  Emotional changes
    Recent mood changes
    Irritable/depressed/tense/nervous/anx-
      ious/insomnia
  b. Current medical diagnosis and therapy
  c. Information about previous use of and access to
     health services
  d. Individual's psychosocial behavior and response
     to illness or predicted illness/individual's expres-
     sion of fears, patterns of coping/adaptation
     1) individual's understanding of previous health
        problems
     2) individual's interest in learning about health
        problems
  e. Clinical assessment of cardiovascular functions
     and status in the following areas:
     1) Cardiac
        Chest wall, size, configuration, and move-
          ments
        Point of maximal intensity, thrills, heaves,
          pulsations
        Heart sounds and murmurs
        Pericardial friction rub
        Apical/radial pulses; rate, quality, and
          rhythm
        Korotkoff sounds
     2) Pulmonary
        Respiratory rate, quality, and pattern
        Chest expansion
        Intercostal retractions/bulging
        Position of trachea

Continued.

STANDARDS OF CARDIOVASCULAR NURSING PRACTICE—cont'd

Diaphragm excursion
Tactile fremitus
Breath sounds
Rales, rhonchi, wheezes, pleural friction rub
"E" to "A" changes, whispered pectoriloquy,
   brochophony
Clubbing

3) Vascular
   Skin, color, moisture, temperature
   Petechiae
   Nailbed, mucous membrane color
   Peripheral pulses
   Homan's sign
   Blood pressure
   Pulsus alternans
   Pulsus paradoxus
   Bruits, carotid, renal artery
   Eye grounds

4) Circulatory
   Jugular venous distention
   Jugular venous pulsations
   Hepatojugular reflux
   Kussmaul's sign
   Edema
   Ascites
   Liver engorgement and enlargement
   Skin turgor

5) Effects on the neurologic system
   Visual acuity
   Level of consciousness
   Restlessness
   Confusion
   Syncope
   Pupil response

6) Related responses
   Body temperature
   Xanthaloma
   Arcus senilis

7) Laboratory results
   Electrocardiogram
   Chest x-ray examination
   Exercise testing
   Complete blood count
   Serum electrolyte level
   Fasting blood sugar
   Uric acid level
   Blood coagulation studies
   Serum creatinine and blood urea nitrogen
     levels
   Serum lipid level
   Serum enzyme level
   Arterial blood gases
   Urine studies

2. Health data are collected by appropriate methods.

3. Health data collection is ongoing.
4. Health data includes historical summary of health problems.

STANDARD II

Nursing diagnosis is derived from health status data.

Interpretive statement

The nursing diagnosis is a statement of the individual's actual or potential health problems and limitations that nurses are able to identify and treat.

Criteria

1. The nursing diagnosis identifies the individual's presenting problems and limitations.
2. Nursing diagnosis may be developed for individuals in any one of the following phases of illness:
   a. *Acute:* occurring in response to stimuli in the immediate environment (internal and/or external) but not enduring for any length beyond the removal of those stimuli
   b. *Chronic:* continuously present for an extended period of time
   c. *Intermittent:* recurring regularly at short intervals with absence of symptoms in the interim
   d. *Potential:* likely to occur given the combination of this person, place, and time
3. Nursing diagnosis is derived from the following:
   a. Clinical manifestations (characteristics) of or human responses to cardiovascular problems
   b. Hygiene, mobility, comfort, safety, sleep/rest, ventilation, circulation, nutrition, elimination, sexuality, skin integrity, prevention, and education.
   c. The recognition of the individual's unique response to each situation (e.g. diagnostic procedures, the medical therapeutic regimen, a change in lifestyle, or the use of specialized equipment)
   d. Analysis of human and community resources
4. The nursing diagnosis provides the basis for nursing orders and should include the etiology or probable cause to ensure an appropriate treatment plan.

Examples of nursing diagnoses	*Possible etiologies*
Alteration in cardiac output	Congestive heart failure, dysrhythmias, ischemic heart disease, or shock
Mobility impairment	Physiologic or physical limitations within the environment (e.g. being on a respirator, intraaortic balloon pump insertion, or being on bed rest)

STANDARDS OF CARDIOVASCULAR NURSING PRACTICE—cont'd

Skin integrity impairment	Mobility impairment, dehydration, invasive diagnostic tests, intravenous therapy, or self-care deficit
Fluid volume deficit	Decreased oral intake, prolonged vomiting, diarrhea, excessive diuretic therapy, or hemorrhage
Fluid volume overload	Decreased cardiac output, congestive heart failure, renal failure, excessive intravenous fluids, or electrolyte imbalance
Alterations in electrolyte balance	Potassium deficit and excess digitalis, fluid overload, or alteration in nutrition
Sensory/perceptual alteration	Excessive, insufficient, or inappropriate environmental stimuli, clinical alterations (either exogenous [e.g. drug ingestion] or endogenous [e.g. electrolyte imbalance]) or psychologic stressors
Self-care deficit (in any or all areas of activities of daily living)	Intolerance to activity, pain, perceptual cognitive impairment, neuromuscular impairment, musculoskeletal impairment, impaired transfer ability or depression/severe anxiety
Knowledge deficit	Lack of exposure, lack of recall, nonuse of information, information misinterpreted, cognitive limitations, disinterest, or lack of familiarity with available resources
Nonadherence	Knowledge deficit, lack of motivation, cultural/spiritual factors, fear, organic brain dysfunction, or lack of financial resources
Alteration in comfort	Ischemic chest pain, myocardial infarction, trauma, infection, or tension/anxiety
Sleep pattern disturbance	Ischemic chest pain, fear, anxiety, environmental surroundings, or depression
Ineffective coping	Situational crises, personal loss, death, illness, social changes, lack of resources, or ego fragility
Infection	Invasive procedures, mobility impairment, skin integrity impairment

STANDARD III

The plan of nursing care includes goals.

Interpretive statement

A goal is the end state toward which nursing action is directed.

Criteria

1. Goals are derived from nursing diagnosis.
2. Goals are assigned appropriate priorities.
3. Goals are stated in terms of observable outcomes.
4. Goals are formulated by the individual, family, significant others, and health personnel.
5. Goals are congruent with the individual's present and potential physical capabilities and behavioral patterns.
6. Goals are attainable through available human and community resources.
7. Goals are achievable within an identifiable period of time.

Examples of goals of nursing care

The goals of cardiovascular nursing for an individual with a known or predicted cardiovascular alteration are prevention of complications; restoration, maintenance, and promotion of optimum cardiac function; and acceptable quality of life. The following outcomes are specific to individuals with known or predicted cardiovascular alterations but may also be applicable to any individual with any physiologic alterations. Identification of outcomes depends on the known health status of the individual.

1. The individual is free from preventable adverse effects that may be directly related to nursing practice.
   Criteria—the individual will:
   a. Maintain cardiovascular status without further deterioration due to specific condition
   b. Be free of complications (e.g. thrombophlebitis, skin impairment, respiratory problems) due to decrease in physical activity and/or temporary maintenance of bed rest
   c. Maintain good body alignment while on bed rest to promote rest and relaxation and to decrease the workload of the heart
   d. Maintain electrolyte balance with appropriate electrolyte supplements as indicated by laboratory data to prevent cardiac complications
   e. Be free of infection at the site of insertion of invasive devices
   f. Maintain urinary output as measured every _____ hours
   g. Be free of cardiac dysrhythmias due to electrical hazards
2. The individual maintains a pharmacologic regimen that is compatible with therapeutic and personal goals.
   Criteria—the individual will:
   a. Explain the rationale for the specific drug regimen prescribed
   b. State the specific action and side effects of prescribed medications
   c. Assist in determining the schedule for taking medications in the hospital or elsewhere

Continued.

STANDARDS OF CARDIOVASCULAR NURSING PRACTICE—cont'd

   d. Plan an appropriate method to assist with drug compliance in the home

3. The individual maintains an activity pattern that is compatible with therapeutic and personal goals.
   Criteria—the individual will:
   a. Explain the rationale for the specific activities prescribed
   b. State the rationale for activities to be avoided due to specific condition
   c. Develop a schedule for increasing activity and/or return to as normal a lifestyle as appropriate
   d. Evaluate tolerance to new activities based on prescribed guidelines

4. The individual maintains a dietary intake that is compatible with therapeutic and personal goals.
   Criteria—the individual will:
   a. Explain the rationale for the specific dietary regimen prescribed
   b. Maintain adequate intake of fluids as allowed
   c. Maintain weight records as prescribed

5. The individual demonstrates a knowledge level that will enable modification of lifestyle.
   Criteria—the individual will:
   a. Explain the rationale for the specific therapeutic regimen prescribed
   b. Identify those factors that will promote or impede compliance
   c. Demonstrate correctly how to take radial pulse
   d. Identify symptoms due to specific disease process or therapeutic intervention that indicate the need for medical assistance
   e. Know how to obtain medical assistance
   f. Know how to obtain and use community resources

6. The individual participates in planning the modification of lifestyle and accepts the modification.
   Criteria–the individual will:
   a. State potential risk factors and relate these to own lifestyle and environment
   b. Develop a plan for modifying own risk factors within a specific period of time

7. The individual demonstrates effective coping mechanisms to adapt to altered lifestyle.
   Criteria—the individual will:
   a. Identify coping mechanisms previously used
   b. Maintain therapeutic regimen as prescribed by the physician or nurse
   c. State the rationale for activities to be avoided due to specific condition
   d. Develop a schedule for increasing activity and/or return to as normal a lifestyle as appropriate
   e. Evaluate tolerance to new activities based on prescribed guidelines

   f. Express feelings about specific condition and therapeutic regimen

STANDARD IV

The plan for nursing care prescribes actions to achieve the goals.

Interpretive statement

The determination of the results to be achieved is an essential part of planning care.

Criteria

1. The plan for nursing care is part of the multidisciplinary plan of care.
2. The plan for nursing care describes a systematic method to meet the goals.
3. The plan for nursing care is initiated after nursing diagnosis and the formulation of goals.
4. The plan for nursing care is based on current scientific knowledge of pathophysiologic and psychosocial components.
5. The plan for nursing care incorporates available and appropriate material resources and environmental controls, including the following:
   a. Proper functioning of equipment
   b. Safety from electrical hazards
   c. Physical safety
   d. Noise control
   e. Humidity, temperature, and light
   f. Control of excess traffic in the clinical setting
   g. Potential and actual contaminants
6. The plan for nursing care reflects the considerations of the "Patient's Bill of Rights."*
7. The plan for nursing care specifies the following:
   a. What actions are to be performed
   b. How the actions are to be performed
   c. When the actions are to be performed
   d. Who is to perform the actions
   e. Anticipated outcomes
8. The plan for nursing care is developed with and communicated to individual, family, significant others, and health personnel as appropriate.
9. The plan for nursing care is realistic and achievable.
10. The plan for nursing care is documented in the individual's permanent record.

STANDARD V

The plan for nursing care is implemented.

* American Hospital Association, 1972.

STANDARDS OF CARDIOVASCULAR NURSING PRACTICE—cont'd

Interpretive statement

The plan is implemented to achieve the goals and is documented to enhance communication among health professionals to promote continuity of care.

Criteria

1. The nurse does one or more of the following:
   a. Provides direct care
   b. Delegates tasks and supervises the work of others
   c. Refers the individual to other professionals for specialized services
   d. Coordinates the efforts of health team members
2. Nursing actions must:
   a. Be documented by written records
   b. Reflect the plan of care including, for example, physical ministrations, counseling, and teaching
   c. Be performed with safety, skill, and efficiency
   d. Reflect consideration of the individual's and family's dignity, beliefs, values, and desires

STANDARD VI

The plan for nursing care is evaluated.

Interpretive statement

The evaluation of nursing care is an appraisal of progress toward meeting the goals of care.

Criteria

1. The individual's response to nursing action is compared with the outcomes stated in the goals.
2. Information is gathered by all health care personnel involved. Examples of such information include the following:
   a. Physiologic signs, such as heart rate and rhythm, body fluid pressures, temperature, urinary output, weight, skin condition, laboratory data, and presence or absence of complications
   b. The individual's demonstrated ability to verbalize information or to perform tasks in a self-care regimen, such as drug information and self-administration, diet, activity, treatment, and a medical follow-up routine
   c. The individual's expressed ability to cope with imposed alterations in lifestyle
   d. The individual's perceived achievement of mutually identified goals
   e. The contribution of the family and significant others to the achievement of the goals of care, including their willingness and ability to participate in and adjust to the altered lifestyle
   f. The availability and effectiveness of human, community, and material resources utilized, including timely discharge planning and access to appropriate services.

STANDARD VII

Reassessment of the individual, reconsideration of nursing diagnosis, setting of new goals, and revision of the plan for nursing care are a continuous process.

Interpretive statement

The steps of the nursing process are taken concurrently and recurrently.

Criteria

1. Revision of the nursing diagnosis is based on the results of the evaluation.
2. New goals formulated are consistent with the evaluation of the individual's progress and with the revised plan of care.

---

mandated that each patient's nursing care be based on identified nursing diagnoses or patient care needs.[31]

Recently the ANA has become involved in a major project to develop a uniform classification system for describing all of nursing practice.[36] The ANA will direct its efforts toward classifying the areas of assessment, outcomes, and intervention, whereas NANDA will continue its work with nursing diagnoses.[3] ANA and NANDA also have been working together to develop a coding translation of Taxonomy I that has been submitted to the World Health Organization for possible inclusion in the next International Classification of Diseases (ICD-10).[15,36,44] Acceptance of the taxonomy would augment the international use of nursing diagnoses.

CRITICAL ISSUES IN NURSING DIAGNOSES

As the impact of the nursing diagnosis movement continues to be evaluated, nurses will be forced to face some of its critical issues. A major issues involves the understanding that a nursing diagnosis reflects only the independent role of the nurse.[13,17,19,26,50] This problem is realized on any day when caring for an acutely ill patient (e.g., when only 10% of the nurse's responsibilities might include independent activities). If most of the day therefore involves interdependent functioning, then it is clear that the nursing diagnoses in Taxonomy I do not capture the essence of nursing practice.[13,49]

Much of this discussion appears to focus on the problems of physiologic nursing diagnoses; some nurses be-

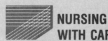

NURSING DIAGNOSES ASSOCIATED WITH CARDIOVASCULAR PATIENTS

EXCHANGING PATTERN

Vascular instability
High risk for tissue destruction
High risk for organ failure
Altered electrolyte regulation
Altered coagulation
High risk for bleeding
High risk for infective/phlebotic vascular complications
High risk for transmitting infection
Psychophysiologic stress

COMMUNICATING PATTERN

Altered nonverbal communication

RELATING PATTERN

Role incapacities
Impaired work functioning
Social withdrawal

VALUING PATTERN

Despair

CHOOSING PATTERN

Nonadherence
Inadequate self-monitoring
Inadequate self-protection
Reduced use of health services
Ineffective stress management
Dysfunctional adaptation to change
Exposure to hazards

MOVING PATTERN

Ineffective rest-activity pattern
Altered psychomotor activity
Altered health maintenance: ineffective prevention or reversal of coronary artery disease (CAD) risk factors

PERCEIVING PATTERN

Dependence and independence conflict

KNOWING PATTERN

Altered level of consciousness
Memory deficit
Confusion

FEELING PATTERN

Depression
Anger
Guilt

lieving that certain physiologic problems, such as "decreased cardiac output" and "impaired gas exchange," should not be called *nursing diagnoses*.[52,53] These nurses believe that such diagnoses should be deleted from the accepted list because most of the interventions related to these diagnoses cannot be implemented independently by nurses. To deal with this issue, Carpenito[8] has recommended use of collaborative problems that she defines as "physiologic complications for which nurses use monitoring skills to detect onset or status so that nurses can collaborate with medicine to provide definitive therapy." Because collaborative problems require medical and nursing intervention, Carpenito believes that it is not appropriate to develop outcome criteria for such problems.[8] Even if collaborative problems are used with nursing diagnoses, the list of nursing diagnoses will still reflect only part of what nursing does.[12]

Physiologic problems, however, are not diagnosed and treated solely by physicians. Nurses have and will always identify and treat the physiologic problems of their patients. A holistic approach to patient care involves caring for the whole patient—their bio-psycho-social-spiritual problems. If the dependent and interdependent roles of the nurse are reflected in the medical diagnoses or in collaborative problems, the nursing diagnosis movement will never be able to develop labels and research nursing interventions for all of nursing practice.

Thus it is time that nurses begin to question why nursing diagnoses should only reflect the independent role of the nurse and only part of what nurses do.[13] It is time to challenge traditional thinking. Nurses should develop an accepted list of nursing diagnoses that enables them to document their role in preventing the catastrophic complications of injury and disease.[49] They should develop labels (nursing diagnoses) that reflect all problems encountered and dealt with by nurses.

To address this issue, the independent and dependent roles of the nurse need to be reevaluated. Although these roles theoretically can be defined, the lines that separate them in practice are not as clear.[13] For example, consider the "dependent role" of the nurse when administering digoxin to a patient on order of the physician. Before administering the drug the nurse assesses the patient, determines that first-degree atrioventricular heart block is present, evaluates the patient's hemodynamic status, withholds the drug, and notifies the physician. If dependent means "determined by another,"[54] then these actions are not really dependent. Rather, these actions are interdependent and reflect the coparticipation of the nurse in assisting the patient and physician in treating the illness. In this light, no nursing action is totally dependent.[12,24] Conversely, if *independence* means "not affiliated with a larger unit" or "not subject to control by others," no nursing actions are totally independent. Moreover, the amount of current nursing practice that is 100% independent is highly questionable in terms of being independent of what or whom.[33]

Perhaps the nurse's dependent and independent roles cannot be clearly defined because, in practice, these roles do not exist. Perhaps the nurse's role is one of *interdependence* and coparticipation with the patient, family, physician, and other members of the health team. This viewpoint is grounded in the holistic model, which considers the interrelatedness of all individuals. It establishes a new kind of perception that goes beyond "either/or" issues of role definitions and establishes the process and relational aspects of the roles.[12]

If nursing diagnoses are to reflect things that nurses do, they must include labels for all problems encountered by nurses. A comprehensive taxonomy is needed that includes all the patient's actual or high-risk body-mind-spirit problems and wellness, health-promotion, and health-maintenance behaviors that are identified and dealt with by nurses. Such a taxonomy would reflect the interdependent role of the nurse and all of what nursing does.[12]

The reasons for developing this comprehensive system are compelling.[12] A comprehensive taxonomy is needed to direct nursing therapies so that holistic care can be delivered. Nurses will be recognized consistently for the care administered and reimbursed for services rendered only when they can label and document their responsibilities and actions clearly and concisely. Comprehensive labels will provide additional support for justifying staffing patterns and prospective payment for nursing care and will direct third-party payments. They will permit information to be easily retrievable from computers for quality assurance programs and for research. Labels that incompletely identify problems nurses encounter or labels that reflect medical diagnoses, however, will be counterproductive to nursing research and advancing the practice of nursing.[12] A comprehensive taxonomy, therefore, is essential for documentation of the complex responsibilities and skills needed in caring for patients with complicated psychophysiologic problems.[49] They will provide the focus to test and validate a scientific body of knowledge for predicting and controlling the outcomes of our nursing care.[12]

The box, left, offers a list of new nursing diagnoses that have not been approved by NANDA. This list reflects problems that nurses encounter with cardiovascular patients.[2,11] Use of these new diagnoses may assist nurses to better demonstrate and document their role in helping cardiovascular patients to achieve desired outcomes. Many of these diagnoses could be added to Taxonomy I to achieve a more comprehensive system that represents nursing practice (see the box).[13,25,33,37,49]

There is no evidence to support "one right way" to use nursing diagnoses. All approaches have value, and one approach may be more appropriate, depending on the nurse's beliefs, values, and frame of reference. Because there are a number of ways to formulate nursing diagnoses and the plan of care, several approaches have been used in Units III & IV of this text to provide a broad and flexible view of the process. Many of the diagnoses in Units III & IV represent health problems interdependently treated by the nurse. For example, the nursing diagnosis, "decreased cardiac output related to disturbances in electrical, mechanical, or structural factors," is a nursing diagnostic label that describes the specific physiologic problems and complications that an AMI patient (or other patients) may develop and that nurses identify and treat. These approaches are presented here so that nurses can confront the issues as they exist in clinical practice and decide which approach to use. Reevaluation also will be necessary to confirm the efficacy of the choice in practice.

Nurses in the nursing diagnosis movement should remain open minded and carefully consider the controversial issues and problems that exist. Controversy can be beneficial when it is directed toward examining and expanding the issues involved. As we confront the problems, we will also move toward developing solutions.

LEARNING ABOUT NURSING DIAGNOSES

There are many ways the nurse can learn about nursing diagnoses,[10,47] including the following:

1. Attend a local, state, or regional nursing diagnosis conference.
2. Ask the head nurse, supervisor, clinical nurse specialist, in-service educator, or invite an outside consultant to give a workshop on nursing diagnosis.
3. Read recent literature on the topic, including the proceedings from the national NANDA conferences that are held every 2 years.
4. Join NANDA.* Membership includes information about conferences, literature, recent changes, and new developments in nursing diagnoses related to practice, education, and research. Membership also includes a subscription to *Nursing Diagnosis,* the official journal of NANDA.
5. Begin using nursing diagnoses.

---

*Clearinghouse, North American Nursing Diagnosis Association, St. Louis University, Department of Nursing, 3525 Caroline St., St. Louis, MO 63104; telephone: (314) 577-8954.

KEY CONCEPT REVIEW

1. The term *nursing diagnosis* refers to all the following except:
   a. Patient needs
   b. Patient problems
   c. High-risk health problems
   d. Response to life processes
2. Within the framework of the nursing process, formulating nursing diagnoses:
   a. Assists the nurse in evaluating whether nursing orders have been carried out
   b. Can be identified easily by using a comprehensive medical data base
   c. Is viewed as the second step in the nursing process
   d. Is viewed along with assessment as the first step in the nursing process
3. All the following are parts of the nursing diagnostic process except:
   a. Outcome criteria
   b. Related factors
   c. Signs and symptoms
   d. Problems
4. Which of the following is a correctly written nursing diagnostic statement that describes an actual nursing diagnosis?
   a. "Alterations in sleep and rest patterns"
   b. "Knowledge deficit about AMI related to newly diagnosed health problem"
   c. "Anxiety and decreased activity levels related to frequent episodes of chest pain."
   d. "Need for maintenance of nutritional intake"
5. Wellness nursing diagnoses are:
   a. Written as one-part diagnostic statements
   b. Written as two-part diagnostic statements
   c. Written as three-part diagnostic statements
   d. Not considered nursing diagnoses
6. All the following are acceptable variations of the diagnostic statement except:
   a. Writing two or more closely related problems in the first main clause
   b. Writing nursing diagnoses that are organized into levels
   c. Writing the patient's signs and symptoms in the diagnostic statement
   d. Placing environmental factors in the first main clause
7. The following is/are/ true about the impact of the nursing diagnosis movement:
   a. About 99% of the generic programs in nursing have integrated nursing diagnosis concepts into their curricula.
   b. About 25% of the master's programs in nursing have integrated advanced nursing diagnoses concepts into their curricula.
   c. The Joint Commission for Accreditation of Healthcare Organizations has not yet addressed the issue of using nursing diagnoses in their standards.
   d. All of the above are true.
8. The need to develop a comprehensive taxonomy of nursing diagnoses that includes all problems encountered and dealt with by nurses is necessary for all of the following reasons except:
   a. It would provide support for justifying staffing patterns.
   b. It would demonstrate the nursing contribution to affecting desired patient outcomes.
   c. It would prevent physiologic nursing diagnoses from being added to the accepted list.
   d. It would allow nurses to research and advance all of nursing practice.

ANSWERS

1. a	3. a	5. a	7. a
2. c	4. b	6. d	8. c

REFERENCES

1. Allen CJ: Incorporating a wellness perspective for nursing diagnosis in practice. In Carroll-Johnson RM, editor: Classification of nursing diagnoses: proceedings of the eight conference, Philadelphia, 1989, JB Lippincott Co.
2. American Association of Colleges of Nursing: Essentials of college and university education for professional nursing: final report, Washington, DC, 1986, The Association.
3. American Nurses' Association: Classification systems for describing nursing practice, Kansas City, Mo, 1989, The Association.
4. American Nurses' Association Congress for Nursing Practice: Nursing: a social policy statement, Kansas City, Mo, 1980, The Association.
5. American Nurses' Association Division on Medical-Surgical Nursing Practice and American Heart Association Council on Cardiovascular Nursing: Standards of cardiovascular nursing practice, Kansas City, Mo, 1981, The Association.
6. Bulechek GM and McCloskey JC: Nursing interventions: treatments for potential nursing diagnoses. In Carroll-Johnson RM, editor: Classification of nursing diagnoses. proceedings of the eighth conference, Philadelphia, 1989, JB Lippincott Co.
7. Carlson J, Craft C, and McGuire A: Nursing diagnoses, Philadelphia, 1982, WB Saunders Co.
8. Carpenito LJ: Nursing diagnoses in critical care: Impact on practice and outcomes, Heart Lung 16:595, 1987.
9. Carroll-Johnson RM, editor: Classification of nursing diagnoses: proceedings of the eighth conference. Philadelphia, 1989, JB Lippincott Co.
10. Dossey BM and Guzzetta CE: Nursing diagnosis, Nurs 81 11:34, 1981.
11. Dossey BM and Tucker D: The use of nursing diagnoses in a critical care setting, Nurs Diag Newsletter 8:82, 1981.
12. Dossey BM, Guzzetta CE, and Kenner CV: Essentials of critical care nursing: body-mind-spirit, Philadelphia, 1990, JB Lippincott Co.
13. Dossey BM, Guzzetta CE, and Kenner CV: Critical care nursing: body-mind-spirit, ed 3, Philadelphia, 1992, JB Lippincott Co.
14. Dossey L: Space, time, and medicine, Boston, 1982, Shambhala Publications, Inc.
15. Fitzpatrick JJ and others: Translating nursing diagnosis into ICD code, Am J Nurs 89:493, 1989.
16. Gleit CJ and Tatro S: Nursing diagnoses for healthy individuals, Nurs Health Care 11:456, 1981.
17. Gordon M: Nursing diagnosis and diagnostic process, Am J Nurs 76:1298, 1976.

18. Gordon M: Manual of nursing diagnosis, New York, 1987, McGraw-Hill, Inc.

19. Gordon M: Nursing diagnosis: process and application, New York, 1987, McGraw-Hill, Inc.

20. Grant JS, Kinney M, and Guzzetta CE: A methodology for validating nursing diagnoses, Ad Nurs Sci 12:65, 1990.

21. Grant JS, Kinney M, and Guzzetta CE: Using magnitude estimation scaling to examine the validity of nursing diagnoses, Nurs Diag 1:64, 1990.

22. Green E and Green A: Beyond biofeedback, New York, 1977, Delta Books.

23. Guzzetta CE: Nursing diagnoses: Effect on the profession, Heart Lung 16:629, 1987.

24. Guzzetta CE and Dossey BM: Nursing diagnosis: framework-process-problems, Heart Lung 12:281, 1983.

25. Guzzetta CE and Forsyth GL: Nursing diagnostic pilot study: psychophysiologic stress, Adv Nurs Sci 2:27, 1979.

26. Guzzetta CE and Kinney MR: Mastering the transition from medical to nursing diagnosis, Prog Cardiovasc Nurs 1:41, 1986.

27. Guzzetta CE and others: Unitary person assessment tool: easing problems with nursing diagnoses, Focus Crit Care 15:12, 1988.

28. Guzzetta CE and others: Clinical assessment tools for use with nursing diagnoses, St Louis, 1989, The CV Mosby Co.

29. Jenny J: Classifying nursing diagnoses: a self-care approach, Nurs Health Care 10:83, 1989.

30. Johanson BC and others: Standards for critical care, St Louis, 1988, The CV Mosby Co.

31. Joint Commission for Accreditation of Healthcare Organizations: AMH: Accreditation Manual for Hospitals: The 1991 Joint Commission. I. Standards for nursing care, Oakbrook Terrace, Ill, 1991, JCAHO.

32. Kim MJ, McFarland GK, and McLane AM: Pocket guide to nursing diagnoses, ed 2, St Louis, 1989, The CV Mosby Co.

33. Kim MJ and others: Clinical use of nursing diagnosis in cardiovascular nursing. In Kim MK and Moritz DA, editors: Classification of nursing diagnosis: proceedings of the third and fourth national conferences, New York, 1982, McGraw-Hill, Inc.

34. Kinney ME and Guzzetta CE: Identifying critical defining characteristics of nursing diagnosis using magnitude estimation scaling, Res Nurs Health 12:373, 1989.

35. Kinney ME and Guzzetta CE: Testing a measurement technique to study nursing diagnosis. In Carroll-Johnson RM, editor: Classification of nursing diagnoses: proceedings of the eighth conference, Philadelphia, 1989, JB Lippincott Co.

36. Lang NM and Gebbie K: Nursing taxonomy: NANDA and ANA joint venture toward ICD-10CM. In Carroll-Johnson RM, editor: Classification of nursing diagnoses: proceedings of the eighth conference, Philadelphia, 1989, JB Lippincott Co.

37. Lengel NL: Handbook of nursing diagnosis, Bowie, Md, 1982, Robert J Brady Co.

38. Levine M: Trophicognosis: an alternative to nursing diagnosis: exploring progress in medical-surgical nursing, American Nurses' Association Regional Clinic Conference 2:55, 1965.

39. McFarland GK and McFarlane EA: Nursing diagnoses and intervention: Planning for care, St Louis, 1989, The CV Mosby Co.

40. McLane AM: Nursing diagnosis in baccalaureate and graduate education. In Kim MJ and Moritz DA, editors: Classification of nursing diagnoses: proceedings of the third and fourth national conferences, New York, 1982, McGraw-Hill, Inc.

41. McLane AM: Measurement and validation of diagnostic concepts: a decade of progress, Heart Lung 16:616, 1987.

42. McLane AM and Kim MJ: Integration of nursing diagnosis in curricula of baccalaureate and graduate programs of nursing: a survey. In Carroll-Johnson RM, editor: Classification of nursing diagnoses: proceedings of the eighth conference. Philadelphia, 1989, JB Lippincott Co.

43. Mundinger MD and Jauron G: Developing a nursing diagnosis, Nurs Outlook 23:94, 1975.

44. North American Nursing Diagnosis Association: Taxonomy I: revised 1990, St Louis, 1990, The Association.

45. Pender NJ: Languaging a health perspective for NANDA taxonomy on research and theory. In Carroll-Johnson RM, editor: Classification of nursing diagnoses: proceedings of the eighth conference, Philadelphia, 1989, JB Lippincott Co.

46. Price MR. Nursing diagnosis: making a concept come alive, Am J Nurs 80:668, 1980.

47. Rossi L: Guidelines for planning programs on nursing diagnosis. In Kim MJ and Moritz DA, editors: Classification of nursing diagnosis: proceedings of the third and fourth national conferences, New York, 1982, McGraw-Hill, Inc.

48. Sanford SJ and Disch JM: American Association of Critical-Care Nurses: Standards for nursing care of the critically ill, ed 2, Norwalk, Conn, 1989, Appleton & Lange.

49. Steele D and Whalen JA: A proposal for two new nursing diagnoses: potential for organ failure and potential for tissue destruction, Heart Lung 14:426, 1985.

50. Tanner CA: Symposium on nursing diagnoses in critical care: overview, Heart Lung 14:423, 1985.

51. Tripp S and Stachowiak B: Nursing diagnosis: health seeking behaviors (specify). In Carroll-Johnson RM, editor: Classification of nursing diagnoses: proceedings of the eighth conference. Philadelphia, 1989, JB Lippincott Co.

52. Wake M: Special interest groups report: nursing diagnosis in critical care. In Kim MJ, McFarland GK, and McLane AM, editors: Classification of nursing diagnoses: proceeding from the fifth national conference, St Louis, 1984, The CV Mosby Co.

53. Wake M: Symposium: nursing diagnosis in critical care: overview, Heart Lung 16:593, 1987.

54. Webster's New Universal Unabridged Dictionary, ed 2, New York, 1983, New World Dictionaries/Simon & Schuster.

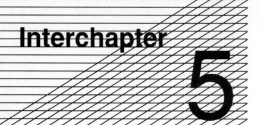

Interchapter 5

Heart Disease and Self-Regulation Therapies

What we think and feel can change our physiology. Our thoughts and emotions are transduced into neural messages that are converted in the brain to neurohormonal messenger molecules that move through the body to communicate directly with the autonomic, endocrine, immune, and neuropeptide systems. Patients who participate in self-regulation or mind therapies are capable of changing negative imagery, thoughts, and feelings into positive and healthy neural messages. Positive emotions have distinct biochemical correlates that have specific effects on tissues and diseases.[13] Thus researchers are beginning to understand the biochemical steps by which the mind can regulate molecules at the cellular and genetic levels.

The evidence supporting the link between negative emotions and illness is discussed in Interchapters 4 and 11. Evidence also is accumulating rapidly to support the link between positive emotions and healing. Consider the results, for example, of several investigations evaluating the effects of music on cardiovascular patients. These studies document that acute cardiac patients who participate in music sessions report significant psychologic benefits,[4,6] reduced anxiety,[3,5,15] reduced depression,[15] lowered heart rates, increased peripheral temperatures, reduced cardiovascular complications,[6] lowered systolic blood pressures,[5,15] and lowered mean arterial pressures.[15]

Self-regulation therapies such as progressive relaxation and Benson's relaxation technique also have been studied in patients undergoing cardiac rehabilitation; the results were significant effects on diastolic blood pressure[8] and lowered levels of anxiety and depression.[2] Likewise, the use of progressive relaxation with patients undergoing coronary revascularization surgery

significantly lowered values related to length of time that the patient was under anesthesia, the length of time that the patient was on cardiopulmonary bypass, the number of units of blood used, and the degree of postoperative hypothermia.[1] In a study by Patel and others,[11] 192 men and women with major coronary artery disease risk factors were randomly assigned to a control or treatment group consisting of deep-breathing exercises, relaxation, meditation, and stress management. At 8 weeks and 8 months, the experimental group had lower diastolic and systolic blood pressures and serum cholesterol levels and had smoked fewer cigarettes than the control group. After 4 years of follow-up study for this same group,[12] the differences in blood pressure were maintained. The control group reported more episodes of angina and treatment for hypertension and its complications. The incidence of ischemic heart disease and fatal myocardial infarction and the electrocardiographic evidence of myocardial ischemia also was greater in the control group at 4 years.[12]

Ornish and others[9] studied the effects of stress management training that included meditation and dietary changes for patients with ischemic heart disease. Patients in the experimental group demonstrated an increase in the duration of exercise, total work performed, left ventricular regional wall motion during peak exercise, and left ventricular ejection fraction. Also a 21% decrease in plasma cholesterol levels and a 91% reduction in anginal episodes occurred.

Synder[14] reviewed 13 studies testing the outcomes of relaxation therapy with a variety of patients. Although significant differences were not found between all test measurements before and after therapy, 12 of the 13 studies demonstrated positive documented outcomes. Likewise, Hyman and

others[7] analyzed 48 research studies of nonmechanically assisted relaxation techniques and found that all therapies except Benson's relaxation technique demonstrated evidence of effectiveness, particularly for nonsurgical patients with problems such as hypertension, headache, and insomnia.

Medical science has focused on the anatomic, physiologic, cellular, genetic, and pharmacologic methods of accessing healing. This focus has concentrated solely on the body side of the bodymind equation.[13] Data are now available to help health care workers understand the way that the mind and body are connected and the way that they communicate. We now know that mind therapies also can be used to access healing. This knowledge may provide the missing link between bodymind communication. It also may provide the missing link in treating patients. After all of these centuries, the body approach to treating illness may have missed its mark because it has not taken into account the profound, devastating effects nor the enormous healing effects of the mind. Treating body ailments with body-oriented therapies may be only half of the answer. There might be amazing outcomes if both sides of the bodymind equation were addressed.

The outcomes of bodymind therapies are dramatically exemplified in the recent study conducted by Ornish and others[10] (see Chapter 1). Experimental subjects who ate low-fat food, exercised, stopped smoking, and participated in stress-management techniques and group support had a regression of coronary artery lesions when compared to a control group. Bodymind therapies were used in this study and achieved what has never been done before—the ability to reverse coronary artery disease.

The role of nurses is clear. They must

learn to incorporate mind-oriented therapies at the bedside to treat the psychologic sequelae inherent to all illness. In addition, however, nurses must learn to supplement the best of traditional medical therapy with the best of mind therapies as a means of activating inner healing and augmenting the effects of drugs, surgery, and technologic therapies. The results could revolutionize the way care is delivered and might significantly improve morbidity and mortality rates and the quality of life. Then the essence of real healing might be unveiled.

REFERENCES

1. Aiken LH and Henrichs TF: Systematic relaxation as a nursing intervention technique with open heart surgery patients, Nurs Res 20:212, 1971.
2. Bohachick P: Progressive relaxation training in cardiac rehabilitation: effects on psychologic variables, Nurs Res 33:283, 1984.
3. Bolwerk CA: Effects of relaxing music on state anxiety in myocardial infarction patients, Crit Care Nurs 13:63, 1990.
4. Davis C and Cunningham SG: The physiologic responses of patients in the coronary care unit to selected music, Heart Lung 14:291, 1985.
5. Guzzetta CE: Effects of relaxation and music therapy on coronary care units patients admitted with presumptive acute myocardial infarction, Department of Health and Human Services Division of Nursing, Grant NU 00824, Aug 1987.
6. Guzzetta CE: Effects of relaxation and music therapy on coronary care unit patients with presumptive acute myocardial infarction, Heart Lung 18:609, 1989.
7. Hyman RB and others: The effects of relaxation training on clinical symptoms: a meta-analysis, Nurs Res 38:216, 1989.
8. Munro BH and others: Effect of relaxation therapy on post-myocardial infarction patients' rehabilitation, Nurs Res 37:231, 1988.
9. Ornish D and others: Effects of stress management training and dietary change in treating ischemic heart disease, JAMA 249:54, 1983.
10. Ornish D and others: Can lifestyle changes reverse coronary heart disease: the lifestyle heart trial, Lancet 336:129, 1990.
11. Patel C, Marmot MG, and Terry DJ: Controlled trial of biofeedback-aided behavioral methods in reducing mild hypertension, Br Med J 282:2005, 1981.
12. Patel C and others: Trial of relaxation in reducing coronary risk: four year follow up, Br Med J 290:1103, 1985.
13. Rossi EL: The psychobiology of mind-body healing: new concepts of therapeutic hypnosis, New York, 1986, WW Norton & Co, Inc.
14. Synder M: Progressive relaxation as a nursing intervention: an analysis, ANS 6:47, 1984.
15. Updike P: Music therapy results for ICU patients, Dimens Crit Care Nurs 9:39, 1990.

5 Biobehavioral Interventions

Barbara Montgomery Dossey
Cathie E. Guzzetta

LEARNING OBJECTIVES

1. Examine three characteristics of psychophysiologic self-regulation.
2. Evaluate the relaxation response in the cardiovascular patient.
3. Synthesize the types of imagery.
4. Analyze how music alters perception of time.
5. Explore potential outcomes when the nurse uses a body-mind-spirit framework.

Biobehavioral interventions are strategies that help evoke simultaneous, positive, body-mind-spirit experiences to enhance well-being. These interventions assist the nurse in practicing and integrating philosophic and scientific frameworks. Research has demonstrated that psychophysiologic stress associated with the physiologic events of bodily illness produce corresponding psychologic events. Thus nurses can reduce the effects of cardiovascular illness by teaching patients to use biobehavioral interventions. The positive changes that occur are links to the patient's deeper understanding about the meaning of and emotions involved in the cardiovascular illness.

PSYCHOPHYSIOLOGIC SELF-REGULATION

Psychophysiologic self-regulation is a process of learning conscious control of the autonomic nervous system and bringing involuntary body responses (i.e., heart rate, blood pressure, respirations, and muscle tension) under voluntary control.[2] Biobehavioral interventions are used to teach cardiovascular patients psychophysiologic self-regulation skills. Self-regulation skills are easily incorporated as nursing interventions for all nine human responses patterns (see Chapter 3) and should be incorporated early in teaching. As self-regulation is learned, patients may reverse the negative effects of cardiovascular disease and are better able to select bodymind responses to manage stressors. Cardiovascular patients who learn, practice, and integrate biobehavioral interventions are most successful at decreasing anxiety and fear, thus preventing, decreasing, and reversing symptoms, and stabilizing their cardiovascular disease (see

Chapter 1).[17] Biobehavioral interventions also help patients develop positive lifestyle patterns, increase self-awareness and creativity, improve learning, clarify personal values, and cope more effectively with cardiovascular dysfunctions. The three steps in psychophysiologic self-regulation follow:[2]

1. Assess for negative bodymind responses to stress.
2. Learn biobehavioral skills (relaxation, imagery, and music) to evoke inner peace and calmness.
3. Use biobehavioral skills daily to make effective choices.

RELAXATION

Relaxation is a psychophysiologic state characterized by parasympathetic dominance involving many visceral and somatic responses. It is the absence of physical, mental, and emotional tension. This response may be achieved in many ways, including breathing exercises, relaxation techniques, biofeedback, prayer, and certain forms of meditation. Two other strategies for evoking states of relaxation are imagery and music. A degree of discipline is required to evoke this response, which results in mental and physical well-being. Table 5-1 guides the nurse in use of relaxation as a nursing intervention.

Relaxation skills allow a person to do the following:[14]

1. Focus inward, which may be goal-directed
2. Evoke inner calmness
3. Alter perceptions of linear time—past, present, and future—to the present moment
4. To control awareness

TABLE 5-1
Nursing Intervention: Relaxation

Patient outcomes	Nursing prescriptions	Evaluation
Patient will demonstrate decreased anxiety, tension, and other manifestations of the stress response as a result of the relaxation intervention.	Guide patient in relaxation exercise. Evaluate for decrease in anxiety, tension, and other manifestations of the stress response as evidenced by heart rate within normal limits, decreased respiratory rate, return of blood pressure toward normal, resolution of anxious behaviors such as anxious facial expressions and mannerisms, repetitious talking or behavior, inability to sleep or restlessness.	Patient exhibited decreased anxiety, tension, and other manifestations of the stress response as evidenced by normal vital signs; a slow, deep breathing pattern; and decreased anxious behaviors.
Patient will demonstrate a stabilization or decrease in pain as a result of the relaxation intervention.	Evaluate for decrease in pain as evidenced by reduction or elimination of pain control medication and increase in activities or mobility.	Patient intake of pain medication stabilized and then decreased with relaxation skills practice. Patient began to participate in activities previously limited by pain.
Patient will link breathing awareness to a commonly occurring cue and use this combination to reduce tension.	Teach awareness of breathing patterns and habitual linking of relaxing breathing to a cue in the environment.	Patient used turning in bed as a cue to take a slow, deep breath and relax jaw muscles.

From Dossey B and others: Holistic nursing: a handbook for practice, Gaithersburg, Md, 1988, Aspen Publishers, Inc.

Strategies for teaching relaxation

There are many ways to teach relaxation. The box (right) includes guidelines on visual cues to relaxation. The box, p. 102, provides guidelines for relaxation and imagery.

Breathing exercises

One of the most effective strategies for achieving relaxation is the power of the breath. The patient pays attention to the breath, counts one on each exhalation, or counts the breaths sequentially up to four and then starts over with one. After these methods are learned by the patient, imagery exercises are combined with them. Some simple breath imagery suggestions follow:

1. Imagining the body as hollow and allowing each breath to fill the hollow body slowly with relaxation
2. In the mind's eye, seeing the breath as a soft color and breathing that color into all parts of the body
3. Breathing the relaxation up one side of the body and down the other
4. Breathing the relaxation up the front of the body and down the back
5. Breathing the relaxation up through the soles of the feet and relaxing the inside of the body
6. Breathing the relaxation down from the top of the head, over the skin, and back into the feet

VISUAL CUES TO RELAXATION

A change in breathing pattern: slower, deeper breaths progressing to slow, somewhat shallower breathing as relaxation deepens
More audible breathing
Fluttering of eyelids
Blanching of the skin around the nose and mouth
Easing of jaw tightness, sometimes to the extent that the lips part and jaw drops slightly
If patient is supine, toes pointing outward, rather than straight up
Complete lack of muscle holding (Ask permission to lift arm gently by the wrist: you should feel no resistance, and arm should move as easily as any other object of similar weight.)

From Dossey B and others: Holistic nursing: a handbook for practice, Gaithersburg, Md, 1988, Aspen Publishers, Inc.

GUIDELINES FOR PRACTICING RELAXATION AND IMAGERY

Never listen to a relaxation tape while driving. However, you can use music to help you relax while you are driving.
Arrange for uninterrupted time for practice.
Provide yourself with at least one 20-minute practice period a day, preferably twice a day.
Control room temperature for comfort; have a light blanket available if needed.
Get in the most comfortable position possible for a relaxed state.
If you choose to work with your eyes closed, give yourself the suggestion that your "eyes are open behind your closed eyelids and that you are wide awake." This will help you stay awake during states of deep relaxation.
Try not to practice after eating because you will most likely go to sleep. Sleep and relaxation are two different things.
Use audiotapes of relaxation and imagery that you purchase or tapes made during guided imagery sessions by the guide. Graduate to using imagery tapes created by you.
Use headsets if necessary.
Practice early in the day when your mind is clear or before falling asleep so that you take positive thoughts and healing resources into sleep.
Learn ways of using positive imagery throughout the day.
Establish an audiotape library (see box on p. 109).

Autogenics

The nurse can also teach the patient to use the repetition of different autogenic phrases. By using these direct positive inner phrases or dialogues, a patient can change physiologic conditions from within. Autogenic phrases are a way of altering the normal homeostatic mechanisms of the autonomic nervous system. Combined with other techniques that use inner dialogue, these phrases are extremely effective when the nurse uses cognitive processes or strategies to enable the patient to utilize intellectual and intuitive processes to relax (see pp. 116-121).

The nurse can repeat autogenic phrases to patients, or patients can repeat them to themselves; examples are, "My right arm is warm and heavy," "My right leg is warm and heavy," and "Heaviness and warmth are flowing through my body."

Relaxation response

Benson[4] describes the *relaxation response* as a hypometabolic state of decreased sympathetic nervous system arousal. This strategy involves passive concentration on the slow repetition of a neutral word such as *one* or *relax*. This word is repeated during each exhalation for 15 to 20 minutes to produce deep relaxation. The technique works best when used in a quiet environment.

Progressive muscle relaxation

Progressive muscle relaxation (PMR) is consciously tensing and relaxing muscle groups to become more aware of subtle degrees of tension. This conscious decision to tense and then relax teaches the patient a new way of being in control when stress occurs. Because the body responds to stressful events and thoughts with muscle tension, a patient can learn to deliberately increase tension in certain muscle groups and slowly release the tension and discomfort and evoke calmness and relaxation.

Body scanning

Body scanning is the conscious focusing of awareness on various parts of the body to detect areas of accumulated tension. For example, a patient scans the body and finds that there is accumulated tightness in the back and upper shoulders. With this awareness the patient then might use breathing, relaxation, and imagery strategies to focus on the tense area to reverse or decrease the tension. It is useful for a patient to learn to create a system for scanning; an example includes a head-to-toe scan. The patient starts at the top of the head and goes down the body to the feet. A systematic scan helps the patient learn deeper levels of body and inner awareness.

Biofeedback

Biofeedback is the use of instrumentation to mirror psychophysiologic processes of which a patient is usually unaware. As a patient learns to recognize different body areas of tension, temperature, and brain wave states and then learns relaxation skills, involuntary body responses can be brought under voluntary control.

Biofeedback research and clinical application for specific cardiovascular dysfunction have been done in the areas of migraine headaches, hypertension, Raynaud's phenomenon, paroxysmal atrial tachycardia, atrial fibrillation, premature ventricular contractions, angina, acute myocardial infarction (AMI) and recovery from open heart surgery, and peripheral vascular disease.

Prayer

When patients have deeply held philosophical or personal religious beliefs, prayer may elicit the relaxation response. With prayer, patients can connect to their religious and spiritual roots. Prayer may be directed or nondirected or said silently or aloud as a focusing device. Benson[5] has referred to this as the "faith factor." He suggests repeating the following words from various spiritual traditions:

Roman Catholics and Christians from related traditions may wish to use the following:
1. A variation on the prayer: "Lord Jesus Christ, have mercy on me"
2. A line from the Our Father or the Lord's Prayer: "Our Father, who art in heaven," or "Hallowed be Thy name"
3. A line from the Hail Mary: "Hail Mary, full of grace"

Protestants may wish to use the previous phrases that seem appropriate to their personal beliefs or any of the following:
1. Words from Psalm 23: "The Lord is my shepherd"
2. Words from Psalm 100: "Make a joyful noise unto the Lord"

Jewish people of any tradition (and many Christians, as well) may be comfortable with focus words and phrases such as these:
1. The Hebrew word for *peace:* Shalom
2. The Hebrew word for *one:* Enchod
3. The Hebrew words for *Hear Oh Israel:* Shema Yisroel

Moslems might want to repeat words such as the following:
1. The word for *God:* Allah
2. The word of the first Moslem who called the "faithful" to prayer: Ahadum

Those from the Eastern traditions might use meditative techniques of those faiths:
1. The Bhagavad-Gita, the Hindu Scriptures, that say: "Joy is inward"
2. Mahatma Gandhi, who said: "Turn the spotlight inward"
3. Buddhist literature containing phrases like these: "Life is a journey" and "I surrender indifferently"
4. Ham Sah: "I am that"
5. Om Namah Shivava: "I honor my inner self"

If the patient does not affirm a traditional religious faith, the relaxation response can still be an important part of therapy by choosing a neutral word or phrase of the patient's choice, such as *one, love, peace,* and so forth.*

Meditation

Meditation is another way of quieting the mind, but it differs from relaxation. Meditation takes much more discipline and practice. Meditation is the inward focusing of attention to reach deeper levels of inner awareness. Patients may repeat a chosen word or phrase (mantra), silently or aloud, as a means of achieving this inward focus. During meditation, the ordinary state of awareness moves above a lower, material level, and a person becomes aware of what is true in inner and outer experience.

IMAGERY

Imagery is the information a person gains through sensory modes—visual, auditory, olfactory, gustatory, and tactile. A sixth sense is an inner-felt sensation of knowing, referred to as a *felt sense.* An example is when persons state that they just know something because they feel as if they have received a message of knowing, often located in their abdomen or chest. Because imagery involves all of the senses, it can give remarkable messages to persons about their body-mind-spirit throughout each day. Images are connected to physiologic states and are the bridge between the conscious processing of information and physiologic change.[1] Images may precede or follow physiologic changes and can be induced by conscious, deliberate behaviors, and by subconscious acts (e.g., reverie or dreaming).

Imagery is an important nursing intervention; guidelines for its use are in Table 5-2. The nurse must assess patients to determine the degree to which they can understand the imagery process. The major variables that affect the successful use of imagery are varying levels of consciousness resulting from physiologic or traumatic alterations, anxiety, fear, pain medication, education levels, cultural symbols, and belief systems.

To achieve the most effective results, imagery should be preceded with general relaxation interventions such as head-to-toe relaxation (see pp. 414-415) or general relaxed breathing exercises. Music can also assist the patient with the imagery process.

Types of imagery

Imagery assists patients in gaining access to the imagination. Patients can consciously create healing images of their disease or disability and of the reversal or stabilization of

---

*From Benson H: Beyond the relaxation response, New York, 1984, Times Books/Random House.

TABLE 5-2

Nursing Intervention: Imagery

Patient outcomes	Nursing prescriptions	Evaluation
Patient will demonstrate skills in imagery.	Guide the patient in an imagery exercise.	Patient practiced imagery and reported learning basic skills.
	After the imagery process experience, assess anxiety and fear, individual coping, power over daily events, ability to move toward an effective lifestyle, ability to change image of self-defeating lifestyle habits, recognition of images created by self-talk, and creation of end-state images of desired health, habits, feelings, wants, and needs for daily living.	Patient reported a decrease in anxiety and fear, demonstrated increased effective individual coping, demonstrated increased personal power over daily events, imaged strengths that moved toward an effective lifestyle, changed images of self-defeating lifestyle behavior, recognized images that were created by self-talk, and created end-state images of desired habits, feelings, wants, and needs for daily living.
Patient will participate in drawing (if appropriate)	Encourage patient to participate in drawing of symptoms and free drawing as appropriate.	Patient participated in drawing of symptoms and free drawing as appropriate.
Patient will demonstrate an understanding of drawing as a communication process.	Instruct patient that drawing is a form of communication with the self and symptoms, that choosing colors has personal meaning, that imagery drawings have special meaning, and that drawing should be done in a nonjudgmental manner.	Patient demonstrated an understanding of drawing as a form of communicating with the self and symptoms, chose colors that had personal meaning, expressed images that had special meaning, allowed drawing to be done in a nonjudgmental manner.

From Dossey B and others: Holistic nursing: a handbook for practice, Gaithersburg, Md, 1988, Aspen Publishers, Inc.

their cardiovascular dysfunctions. When nurses learn the different types of imagery in Table 5-3, they find that guiding patients in the imagery process is much more effective because they more easily recognize the patients' unique imagery patterns. Nurses can also assess patients' imagery processes to avoid flooding them with too many suggestions. Nurses are also more aware of when patients are ready to engage in more in-depth imagery.

The patients should be encouraged to use imagery skills for 20 minutes 2 to 3 times a day. Although the following steps may seem easy, they require focused concentration to effect health or recovery or facilitate peaceful dying[2]:
1. Identify the problem, disease, or goal of imagery.
2. Begin with several minutes of relaxation by paying attention to rhythmic breathing or using a general relaxation exercise.
3. Develop images of the following:
   a. The problem or disease
   b. Inner healing resources, including beliefs and attitudes
   c. External healing resources, including treatments, procedures, medications, and surgery

4. End with images of the final, desired state of well-being.

Receptive versus active imagery

Receptive imagery involves images that appear in conscious thought and seem to just "bubble up." They are received without effort. Receptive images are common when daydreaming and falling asleep.

To experience receptive imagery, persons let imagery experiences just "bubble up" as they focus on where their body accumulates tension, such as the back of the neck or shoulders. They mentally record the sights and sensations. Common imagery expressions are tightness, tingling, warmth, or knots.

Active imagery occurs as persons focus on the conscious formation of images. They pay attention to the images that come from the area of the neck or shoulders. Common images are popping or grinding of muscles or knots in muscles. It is possible to "speak" to a body part by imagining seeing, feeling, hearing or touching smooth muscles or feeling the release of tension. The box on p. 105 provides information on relaxation and imagery for the hypertensive patient.

RELAXATION AND IMAGERY INFORMATION FOR THE HYPERTENSIVE PATIENT

Think of the number of patients you have discharged with a diagnosis of essential hypertension and prescriptions for several antihypertensive medications. Did you let patients hear their own blood pressure readings when elevated, as well as when they were in normal ranges? Patients with high blood pressure become accustomed to physiologic changes and pressure elevation without knowing it. Try incorporating the following suggestions in your patient teaching methods:

1. Record the baseline pressure and teach patients to check their own blood pressures.
2. Have the patients check their blood pressure *several times a day or more often* to learn to identify the sounds and feelings of varying levels of blood pressure. Have patients keep diaries of physical manifestations associated with blood pressure elevations, including head pounding and neck tension. This is a very effective strategy for outpatients.
3. Teach relaxation and imagery techniques.
4. Get patients to focus on increasing hand and foot temperatures, which increase with relaxation.
5. Have patients focus on positive images such as relaxed blood vessels.
6. Suggest that patients purchase personal blood pressure cuffs and check for accuracy their measurements with those from a cuff in the physician's office or clinic.

You may disagree with this approach for the following reasons. It will be counterproductive; you might get patients who are so anxious that their blood pressures will be difficult to control or patients might develop a compulsive fixation on their illness. In addition, recording how the body feels serves little purpose, because hypertension is usually asymptomatic.

However, after using these strategies in the treatment of hundreds of hypertensive patients in an outpatient clinic and biofeedback department, we have found that patients are more compliant and enjoy participating in their care. Patients, if taught to be aware of their bodies, can associate specific feelings with increased blood pressure. By using relaxation, imagery, music, biofeedback skills, and effective dialogue with proper use of the voice and breath, patients can learn to keep their blood pressures in a normotensive range. Some patients are even able to reduce medications or stop taking them altogether. If this is done, the patients also are taught that, if they again assume a frantic lifestyle and stop using relaxation and imagery techniques, medication may once again be needed.

Case Study. A 45-year-old man with hypertension was referred for stress management and blood pressure control. He began to learn such strategies, including drawing. His first drawing (Fig. 5-1, *A*) shows the way he saw his blood pressure in his mind before therapy. He said, "They (the vessels) are very tense and irregular." At this time, his systolic pressure was 160 mm Hg, and his diastolic pressure was 90 mm Hg. After a 20-minute relaxation and imagery session his blood pressure was 124/70 mm Hg. He felt an internal shift toward relaxation, and he attributed this feeling to his imagery change from blood vessels as "tight as a spring and very tense with high pressure" to "blood vessels without tension having easy blood flow." He said, "I feel all smoothed out. You're right. I know that feeling of tension means that my blood pressure is up. For the first time, I know that I can learn to keep my blood pressure in a normal range. I feel a new lease on life" (Fig. 5-1, *B*).

Concrete versus symbolic imagery

Concrete images are images that are physiologically and anatomically correct. It is important to help patients use correct biologic images because inaccurate images often block inner resources. Because people communicate with the body by images, emphasis on correct biologic imagery and use of natural imagery must be emphasized. Images and their associated thoughts get converted via state-dependent memory (see Chapter 1) to the body through the neurotransmitters of body systems. Some creative and helpful

TABLE 5-3
Types of Imagery

Subtype	Characteristics
Receptive journey	"Bubbling up": unexpected reception of images
Active	Inward journey: attention to bodymind
	Conscious formation of image
	Direct image regarding body area or activity that requires attention
Concrete	Real life: under the microscope
	Biologic correctness
Symbolic	Metamorphosis: personal energy of a person
	Images that cannot be forced
Process	Step-by-step goal to be achieved
	Mechanics of biologic correct images
End state	Imagination of final healed state
General healing	Event, healing light, forgiveness, inner guide or advisor
Packaged	Commercial tapes that have general images
Customized	Images that become personalized

From Achterberg J, Dossey B, and Kolkmeier L: Rituals of healing, New York, 1992, Bantam Books.

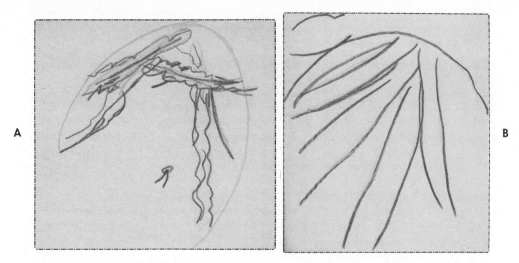

FIG. 5-1   Imagery with hypertension. **A,** Patient's first drawing showing hypertension. **B,** Second patient drawing after relaxation and imagery techniques were practiced showing normotensive state.

images for teaching biologic correctness can be found in drug advertisements and anatomy coloring books. Other sources are education information pamplets from professional organizations that focus on specific diseases or health problems, such as the American Heart Association or American Lung Association.

Symbolic imagery is a metamorphosing process for each patient; it cannot be forced. As patients enter into and deepen relaxation, their innate inner wisdom releases symbolic images. These images come from attitudes, belief systems, cultural experiences, and the unconscious and may have healing qualities. Thus the nurse must assess with patients the images that emerge. If patients develop negative images, the nurse can help facilitate exploration of the images and guide patients in developing positive images.

An example of symbolic imagery is from an individual with supraventricular tachycardia who formed images of a huge computer that symbolized his bodymind communications center. It contained files with many programs to help him change his aggressive, competitive nature. He had an elaborate sinoatrial (SA) control panel, and in his mind he could push a button to start his SA program that sent the impulses correctly down his normal conduction pathways. He chose another program that instructed him in recognizing and altering his perception of time when he felt himself getting angry.

Concrete and symbolic images are important and helpful, but symbolic images are more powerful because patients are more involved in the process, thus more symbolism and healing occurs.

Case study. Sam, a 58-year-old man, 4 days after coronary artery bypass surgery, was having extreme anxiety and pain. When asked about the location of his pain, he responded while breathing in a shallow manner, "It's all over—in my legs, my arms, my chest. The worst pain is in my chest. It's like a tight, constricting band of pain squeezing the very life out of me." As Sam described his pain, he was using his hand to form a band of pain. The nurse suggested to Sam that he would have great success at reducing his pain because his images and description were so clear to him. The nurse began to help Sam work with his pain by teaching him rhythmic breathing. As he inhaled, she had him image his lungs filling from the bottom upward, just like water poured in a glass fills from the bottom up. Within a few breaths, Sam's breathing was relaxed, deep, and regular.

The nurse had several crayons in her jacket pocket. She gave them to Sam with a piece of paper and asked him to draw his pain (Fig. 5-2, *A*). As he finished drawing the tight constricting band of pain, the nurse suggested that, in his mind, he could take the end of the band of pain and uncoil it in the opposite direction when pain occurred. The nurse demonstrated this motion with her hands and then had Sam do it. He started at his belly and upcoiled the black band until he could no longer see it around his abdomen and chest.

As he did this, he was amazed at how his pain diminished, and he even had moments of no pain. The nurse discussed how pain and anxiety were connected and the positive effect of relaxed breathing and images on the management of pain. Sam required only oral pain medication at bedtime.

Why did this simple technique work? It was effective because the nurse helped the patient use his own consciousness in his own behalf. Instead of being anxious and out of control, Sam learned to evoke his own inner healing resources and to shift negative images to positive images in conjunction with abdominal breathing.

Sam continued to practice relaxation and imagery techniques in cardiac rehabilitation. He developed strong images of his new jump grafts as open with blood flowing in a regular fashion (Fig. 5-2, *B*). He said that these strong images were important reminders that were extremely helpful in learning new lifestyle patterns to keep his new vessels open. (See Interchapter 10.)

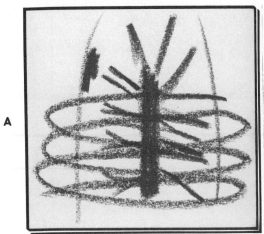
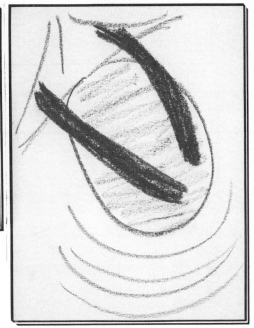

FIG. 5-2 Imagery after CABG surgery. **A,** Sam's first drawing showing chest pain. **B,** Drawing by Sam after he practiced relaxation and imagery techniques showing jump grafts as open.

Case study. This interaction took place with J.D. and his wife in the CCU 3 days after J.D.'s massive AMI. J.D. had symptomatic heart failure and pericarditis secondary to his AMI, and he was discouraged. After an assessment, the nurse concluded that J.D. and his wife were ready to learn some new ideas. A relaxation and imagery session were suggested. This session worked for the following reasons: (1) the patient had a readiness to learn; (2) the patient and wife agreed to participate; (3) the nurse knew techniques to help the patient and wife make positive bodymind connections and use their inner healing resources; and (4) a trusting, caring relationship was present. Before the 10-minute relaxation induction, the nurse asked J.D. to assess his imagery. J.D. described his heart as a big bag of water that wasn't pumping very good (his congestive heart failure). He said that it had another awful, inflamed bag around it that still caused him a lot of pain when he moved certain ways or took deep breaths (his pericarditis). He said, "I don't see anything good, and I don't see me getting better. I'm depressed about the whole damn thing."

The nurse decided to help J.D. begin to create positive images about his healing process and show him how to use his inner healing resources so that he could focus on his recovery with less stress. The nurse started with a short relaxation exercise with J.D. and his wife. While they were still quietly relaxing, the nurse asked them to continue focusing on the breath with each inhalation and each exhalation. She left the room to obtain crayons and paper from her locker. The nurse returned to the room and then concluded the relaxation exercise, returning J.D. and his wife to a wakeful, alert state. The nurse asked J.D. to choose a few crayons and pick colors that had meaning to him. He was asked to draw a few images of his heart.

J.D. talked as he drew: "I'll start with the purple and draw a circle for my heart (Fig. 5-3, *A*). Well, blood tries to get into my heart like it always does, but it gets blocked. A part of my heart has died. I'll use black around this area since it's dead. My heart doesn't pump very good, so that's why it's such an irregular shape. Blood is still

going in and out of my heart, but not in this area. Now this outside area is that sac around my heart. It's big and swollen and hot and painful. All these little marks out here are the pain it caused me [color chosen was orange]. The figure in the center is a dancing and singing girl who used to be in my heart; she has a black muzzle on her mouth now because she is not singing anymore."

The nurse asked J.D. how he felt. He answered, "Really sad, really. I feel angry that I had this heart attack now. I'm too young to have a heart attack. I hope I can recover and get strong again."

The nurse realized that clarification was needed to help J.D. understand more about the normal-healing process and how to focus on his inner strengths. His drawings had shown misunderstanding about coronary artery blood flow. J.D. thought that his coronaries were on the inside of his heart. To instruct him, the nurse used prominent veins on the back of J.D.'s hand to represent his coronary arteries, which followed a left anterior descending, circumflex, and right coronary line. She used his hand in a slight fist position to represent his heart. The nurse also used a plastic heart model that can be opened to show the inside of the heart to explain normal blood flow, congestive heart failure, pericarditis, collateral circulation, scar tissue formation, and the cardiac medications and their therapeutic action.

Based on the nurse's explanations, J.D. began to form another image in his mind. He began to see himself forming a very strong scar where the heart damage was. He said, "All this solid red is new blood supply; it is a lattice network. All the rest of the red is blood flow throughout my heart. These other lines are channels of normal blood flow in and out of my heart." (Fig. 5-3, *B*) The nurse began to investigate the meaning of the dancing girl J.D. had drawn; she asked how he saw himself involved in his healing process. J.D. stated that he felt as if he was not doing much. The nurse shared some ways that he could participate more in his healing. He was told "Every time you swallow a pill, feel it entering your mouth and going to your

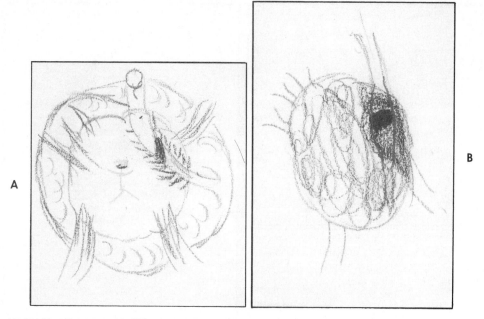

FIG. 5-3 Imagery after AMI. **A,** J.D.'s first drawing showing CHF, pericarditis, and infarction. **B,** Drawing by J.D. after he learned relaxation and imagery techniques showing heart healing with strong scar and new collateral circulation.

stomach. Acknowledge to yourself that it is being absorbed and is in your blood stream and working. Instead of resenting the fact that you are taking medication 4 times a day, focus on the purpose of why you are taking these medications. The purpose of taking the pills on schedule is to obtain a therapeutic blood level."

The nurse also encouraged J.D. to focus on positive powerful images to help him have a therapeutic level of positive emotions. He was told to recognize negative self-talk about how slowly recovery was going and to create a positive image to help manage discomfort. He was instructed to see his heart healing in his mind moment by moment, to believe he was making steady progress, to feel that his chest pain and irregular heart beats were gone. Then he was asked to imagine the dancing girl under these conditions. J.D. said that she was swimming very fast and that his recovery would go faster. He stated, "I can't believe how shifting my thoughts helps."

Process, end-state, and general healing images

Process imagery is a strategy of guiding a patient in a step-by-step biologic healing process in the imagination. For example, when teaching a patient about heart healing after an AMI, the nurse includes the normal evolution from damage to buildup of collateral blood flow to healthy scar formation. (Fig. 5-3, *B*). Information should also be included on medication, rest, and other specific aspects of cardiac rehabilitation.

Process imagery also involves helping a patient decrease emotions such as fear or anxiety before tests or surgery. Negative emotions can be decreased or eliminated with process imagery rehearsal. Patients should be encouraged to do a step-by-step rehearsal of procedures, treatments or surgery before the event (e.g., before cardiac catheterization, percutaneous transluminal coronary angioplasty, and cardiac surgery). With relaxation and imagery skills, a patient can also increase self-esteem, independence, and commitment to healthy living.

End-state imagery occurs when the patient rehearses being in a final, healed state. An end-state image for an AMI patient would be a healed heart and a return to exercise, work, and healthy sexual activity.

General healing images are events rather than a process. The best general images have personal healing significance. An example might be patients being bathed with relaxation and the warmth of the sun. Another example might be patients experiencing a sound or color penetrating the core of their being. General healing images also come in the form of a felt sense of unity, universal power, spirit, or God. They frequently appear as an inner spiritual guide such as an animal or a totem or rhythmic images such as a wise old person.

Packaged versus customized imagery

Packaged imagery involves using another person's images such as those purchased with tapes on self-hypnosis, relaxation, and imagery or the scripts at the end of this chapter. Commercial tapes or tapes prepared by the nurse using the scripts at the end of this chapter can be therapeutic and serve as general guides. They can facilitate healing and learning of skills when a nurse cannot be present.

ESTABLISHING AN AUDIOTAPE LIBRARY

TAPES AND RECORDERS

Have several tape recorders with comfortable headsets.

Place all equipment in a safe and convenient location.

Have a variety of music tapes available. Commercial tapes are relatively inexpensive and readily available. A complete tape library will include music, relaxation, imagery, stress-management tapes, and specific tapes for smoking cessation, presurgery and postsurgery, weight reduction, pain management, insomnia, self-esteem, and subliminal learning. Consider different types of music, such as easy listening, light and heavy classical, popular, jazz, hymns, choral, and nontraditional selections.

Ask staff members to donate one favorite tape to the library.

Write the different tape companies listed in the resource box on p. 114, and request their tape selections and descriptions.

Encourage nurses to develop tapes for specific patient problems that can help with procedures, tests, and treatments (see box on p. 115). The tapes may or may not have soothing background music.

Have brochures and catalogues of recording companies available on request for the patient.

Encourage use of different tapes for further relaxation, imagery, and stress-management training.

TAPE, RECORDER, HEADSET CHECK-OUT PROCEDURE

If tapes are checked out by the patient's family, have the person make a deposit for it. It is suggested that the deposit cover the cost of the tape in case it is not returned.

Establish who will have authority to check out the tapes and recorders. If in the hospital, a volunteer could assist in checking out the equipment for the patient after the nurse has assessed the patient's needs and selected the appropriate tape.

Prepare a sign-out log that records the patient's name, room, date, and check-out time.

Instruct the patient in the use of the recorder and specific tapes if required.

Allow 20 to 30 minutes of listening without interruption twice a day. Place a sign on the patient's door stating, "Session in Progress—Do Not Disturb."

After the listening session, evaluate the patient's response to the tape and answer questions.

Chart the patient's specific response to tapes. For example, were the desired outcomes achieved (e.g., lowered respiratory rate, decreased heart rate and blood pressure, decreased muscle tension and anxiety)? Identify the patient's subjective evaluation, (e.g., found the experience relaxing, helped with sleep, assisted in coping with pain, assisted with painful procedure).

Return the tape, recorder, and headset to the library, and record the check-in information in the log.

From Dossey B and others: Holistic nursing: a handbook for practice, Gaithersburg, Md, 1988, Aspen Publishers, Inc.

Customized imagery are images that "bubble up" in unique ways after the patient listens to packaged imagery. An example of customized images is from a patient who used a commercial tape before open heart surgery. After surgery, he customized his images and saw his new jump grafts as golden strong pipes through which blood flowed without tension. As he continued to alter his aggressive nature, he also learned to concentrate on the golden light that would then fill his whole body. He said, "This lets me get in touch with a new skill. I have learned about my softer nature, which is part of my total healing. It is the sharing of emotions first with myself and then with others."

Integrating imagery in practice

The box above gives guidelines for establishing an audiotape library within a hospital or outpatient clinic. To maintain a tape library, each nursing unit must have a system for lending cassette tapes, master tapes, recorders, and headsets, as well as a check-out and return procedure. If this system is not established, the best library can disappear in a matter of weeks because people forget to return equipment, master tapes are lost, given out and forgotten, or equipment disappears.

Some degree of imagery is always present in the way that patients imagine their body functioning. Imagery associated with illness or symptoms is almost always negative, particularly when a patient has a known illness. As patients who have conditions that are undiagnosed wait for tests results, it is common for them to create many scenarios of what is wrong and often the images are untrue. As soon as possible, patients should be taught the use of imagery skills to decrease anxiety and to develop a clear picture of what the physician has told them. Patients who leave the physician's office with confusion may create negative images that take their toll on the patient and family. Encourage patients to ask for clarification. Patients also have the right to get answers that can help them in healing and recovery. Edu-

IMAGERY RITUAL

First, mesh all your senses into your physical problem:
  See, hear, taste, feel, smell the problem.
  Sense the problem clearly without *judgment* or criticism.
Second, mesh your senses into the internal and external healing resources:
  See, hear, taste, feel, smell the internal healing resources.
  See, hear, taste, feel, smell the external healing resources.
Third, mesh your senses into the total healing:
  See, hear, taste, feel, and smell yourself totally, completely and successfully functioning as you want to do.
  See, hear, taste, feel, smell yourself accepting that whatever is right for you at this point in time is unfolding just as it should and that you have done your best, regardless of the outcome. Do this last part for 1 to 2 minutes.

From Achterberg J, Dossey B, and Kolkmeier L: Rituals of healing, New York, 1992, Bantam Books.

cation about correct biologic images of specific problems is important because it can assist the healing process.

Patients should also be taught to assess their belief systems and to identify two types of solutions for working with problems—internal healing resources (beliefs and attitudes) and external healing resources (treatments, procedures, medications, and surgery), as well as ways to use correct biologic images of a physical problem.

Use of internal and external healing resources is effective. As patients work with physical problems, they can learn the skill of meshing their senses into the physical problem, then into the solution, and then into total healing. This part of the imagery ritual should take about 10 minutes. Steps for instructing a patient in a basic imagery ritual are listed in the box above.

Healing force of imagery

When assessing and facilitating patients in exploring feelings and perception about their cardiovascular illness, hospitalization, and rehabilitation, the nurse should become aware of the images and patterns occuring as patients tell their story, personal myths, and symbols. The constant inner dialogue of these stories creates patients' unique images. Patients are also the best interpreters of their own images. Frequently the turning point for mobilizing patients' innate healing ability is when they recognize the negative imagery invading their lives.

The nurse must assess when patients' images of disease are more powerful than internal and external healing resources. Even when patients do not return to health and move toward death, the same imagery process is used. Images evoke profound inner strength by assisting patients or family members in the release of life at the appropriate time. Patients then can begin to move toward peaceful dying.

Drawing images

Drawing allows a patient access to internal mental and emotional images, symbols, and felt sense shifts.[2,8] When a patient draws images, emotions are externalized, and they often reveal another level of rich inner wisdom. The most important thing in facilitating a patient with drawing is to know that it has nothing to do with skills of drawing. It is merely a reflective expression to help the patient better communicate with inner healing resources.

When patients are drawing, a constant inner dialogue (self-talk) occurs on many levels. Patients are instructed to imagine the dialogues as internal advisors with special messages. If patients learn to listen without judging when drawing, messages from their wise selves will continue to come forth. Thus drawing often breaks down the resistance to discovering the inner spirit or soul. This unique drawing experience allows quiet time and the space for emergence of insights toward solving problems, meeting challenges, and taking new life directions.

Drawing guidelines and drawing interpretation

Drawing guidelines and drawing interpretations that are in the box, p. 111, are written as if a nurse is instructing a patient with drawing. Each nurse should add a personal style to these guidelines. To be an effective facilitator with drawing, it is *essential* that the nurse experience the drawing process.

MUSIC

Different types of music can evoke therapeutic changes in physiologic conditions, emotions, attitudes, and behavior.[11] Music, like relaxation and imagery techniques, is used with traditional therapy. This provides patients with integrated experiences that encourage them to be active participants in health care. Table 5-4 guides the nurse in the use of music as a nursing intervention.

Music has measurable psychophysiologic effects on cardiovascular patients. One study has demonstrated the effectiveness of music and relaxation interventions in reducing the stress in patients in a coronary care unit who were admitted with presumptive diagnoses of AMI.[12] Patients' stress was evaluated by apical heart rates, peripheral temperatures, cardiac complications, and qualitative patient evaluation data. The relaxation and music group partici-

GUIDELINES FOR DRAWING IMAGES

PATIENT INSTRUCTIONS

Gather your drawing supplies. You might draw at a desk or spread your supplies on the floor, particularly if you are using a large piece of paper. In a few minutes, I will be turning on music that will help you with your creativity. If you wish to continue this process at home, place your tape recorder and several music selections nearby so that you can choose music to match your mood or choose selections to let your images flow.

After you have created your space for drawing, choose your favorite breathing or general imagery exercise to help you focus. Turn on the music that you have chosen and sit calmly and quietly telling yourself that there is no place where you have to be or anything that needs to be done; there is just the present moment.

Listen to your constant self-talk. Do not judge your drawing or images; just allow your body, mind, and spirit to connect as you begin to be with the paper, crayons, and other drawing supplies.

Become aware of the energy that seems to "bubble up." Be receptive to your images. Your body will begin to develop its own creative rhythm. You can't predict what will happen, which is the exciting part of this experience.

Let your body energy resonate with your imagery and inner body vibration. If one seems to get ahead of the other, just notice and let the energies slowly begin to resonate together or in a parallel fashion. Let go of trying to control your energy. Your inner quality of knowing your inner experience happens as you become immersed in your images and inner wisdom.

Notice images that come forth. Remember that images involve all of the senses—hearing, seeing, feeling, tasting, smelling, and any inner-felt sensations. These imagery expressions represent your current feelings and thoughts.

Now let yourself draw some of your images on your paper. Choose colors that appeal to you. If you start working with a color and wish to change, feel free to do so. There is no one best way to draw. Drawing can be realistic or symbolic. When you feel stuck in your insight or overwhelmed with emotions, let the music in and continue drawing the feelings.

Stay with the drawing as long as you need to do so. You will know when you are done.

After you draw, you might want to write down some details of your images or list words that represent patterns of your thoughts. Sometimes you may hear or feel more of your experiences rather than seeing images. It also adds to your reflective experience if you keep your drawings and place a date on them. Over time, your images will change, creating new patterns of insight.

PATIENT INSTRUCTIONS FOR DRAWING INTERPRETATION

You are the best interpreter of your drawing process. What you draw reflects your personal journey at this time. Many emotions may come forward—laughter, anger, excitement, or tears. There is no such thing as a good or bad emotion. Emotions surface because they are ready to be expressed.

If you feel stuck in the experience, invite the music in to your conscious awareness. It will help you release the block in your creative process.

All images that come forth are part of your healing. Images and symbols that you draw have both positive (light) and negative (dark) aspects that have meaning for your life. You cannot know one without knowing the other. For example, you can identify health because at some time you have experienced sickness. When you acknowledge light and shadow as part of life's journey, you create the time that is essential for self-awareness and self-healing.

---

pated in three sessions over a 2-day period. Patients in the relaxation and music group had decreased apical heart rates, increased peripheral skin temperatures, and fewer cardiac complications compared with the control group. This study indicated that the use of relaxation and music are effective in reducing psychophysiologic stress in patients in coronary care units.

At the Institute for Music, Health, and Education (IMHE), clinical research has been done with patients using relaxation, imagery, and music as complementary healing interventions. To further develop the use of these interventions in clinical practice, the following four areas were researched:

1. Music to alter time and space relationships
2. Music to modify environment
3. Music to evoke integration and grounding
4. Music to facilitate the imagery process

Time and space are influenced and modified by the vertical and horizontal position of a patient's ears.[7] Blood flow to the ear's vestibular system is affected by position, and it is different when a patient's body is in a standing, sitting, or lying position. Thus the message to the brain is also changed. In the relaxed, reclining position, slow music can facilitate more images and associations than when the patient is in other positions because the body is not constantly working to determine its exact position and actions. This more relaxed position allows the bodymind to slow the internal clock, which also slows the "sense of time." Music also alters a sense of time and space because it changes physiologic states as a result of vibrational resonance.

Rapid and intense music selections are also important

TABLE 5-4
Nursing Invervention: Music

Patient outcome	Nursing prescriptions	Evaluation
Patient will demonstrate skills in music therapy. Patient will demonstrate positive physical and psychologic effects of response to music.	Guide the patient in a music therapy session. Provide patient with opportunity to select music of choice for listening.	Patient used music 1 to 2 times a day to facilitate healing. Patient chose music of choice for listening.
	Evaluate patient's positive physical and psychologic effects to music: *Physical effects:* Decreased respiratory and heart rates, blood pressure, muscle tension, and fatigue	Patient demonstrated positive physical and psychologic effects: *Physical effects:* Decreased respiratory rate from 28 to 18/minute, heart rate from 120 to 90 beats/minute, blood pressure from 160/100 to 130/70, muscle tension, and fatigue
	Psychologic effects: Positive emotions; decreased restlessness, agitation, anxiety, depression, isolation; and increased motivation; nonverbal expression of feelings; and positive images	*Psychologic effects:* Positive emotions; decreased restlessness, agitation, anxiety, depression, isolation; and increased motivation; nonverbal expression of feelings; and positive imagery

From Dossey B and others: Holistic nursing: a handbook for practice, Gaithersburg, Md, 1988, Aspen Publishers, Inc.

 GUIDELINES FOR LISTENING TO MUSIC

Begin with a general relaxation session
Listen to the music for 15 to 20 minutes.
Tell yourself that you would like to go wherever the music takes you.
Let the music suggest to you what to think and feel. Let the feelings arise from your inner knowing.
Do not analyze the music, its composition, or structure.
Imagine that the music is bathing away tension, worries, or fear.
Let the music suggest different sounds, colors, and textures.
If listening to soft music let it suggest softness, openness, and gentleness.
Listen to music that matches your mood; if you are discouraged or depressed, choose music to lift your spirits.
Create your own music. Allow an audible groan such as "ohhh" or "ahhh" to escape. Let the groan go as deep as possible without forcing it. Notice the vibration within your bodymind and the releasing and emptying of tension.
Ask yourself whether the music stirred unpleasant memories. If it did, once again let the images come, and allow a dialogue between them. Keep in mind that the only reason you can identify negative images (shadows) is that you know the opposite—the positive images (light). Look for the messages that light and shadow have for you.

in the imagery process. With music selections with faster rhythms, the notes come closer together, and a patient does not have time to relax or come to resolution between the notes. The images are intensified, and the types of images and breakthroughs experienced are different than when using slow music.

Music evokes a change in the environment by the vibrations of the musical tones.[7] It can alter space in many ways. The choice of music can create peace, calmness, safety, or spaciousness, or it can manifest a tension, clutter, or heaviness. Music should be carefully chosen for hallways, waiting rooms, and nursing units.

To achieve optimal patient outcomes with music, the patient, not the nurse, should choose the music. No "best" type of music exists. Music that one patient considers relaxing might make another patient tense. Patients should be encouraged to experiment with solo instruments such as the harp, piano, flute; nature sounds such as ocean waves, rain, and wind or different musical arrangements such as classical, jazz, contemporary, and choral. The music will also evoke different feelings and images depending on the length of time that a patient listens to a selection and the extent to which the patient releases the need to analyze the musical arrangement and instruments. The box, left, provides guidelines for listening to music, and the box on p. 113 is a guide for evaluating the patient's subjective experience with music.

Personal experience allows the nurse to guide patients in more effective use of music selections. As the nurse masters relaxation and imagery skills, a deeper level of healing, integration, and grounding is gained. *Integration* im-

EVALUATION OF THE PATIENT'S SUBJECTIVE EXPERIENCE WITH MUSIC

Was this a new kind of music listening experience for you? Can you describe it?

Did you have any visual experiences? Of people, places, or objects? Can you describe them?

Did you see any colors while listening? Did the color change as the music changed?

Were you less aware of your surroundings? Were you able to concentrate on the music?

Did you like the music?

Did the music produce feelings or emotions?

Did you notice textures, smells, movements, or tastes while experiencing the music?

Was the experience pleasant?

Did you feel relaxed and refreshed after the experience?

Would you like to try this again?

What would be helpful to make this a better experience for you?

From Dossey B and others: Holistic nursing: a handbook for practice, Gaithersburg, Md, 1988, Aspen Publishers, Inc.

plies a sense of inner peace, a place of inner being and quietude. A person feels truly unified and focused. *Grounding* is the state achieved when a person moves within oneself to an inner reference of stability.

The nurse must experiment with different types of music to find music selections that can enhance integration and grounding for the self and to understand the depth to which music selections can evoke psychophysiologic experiences that can heal. Different music selections can be suggested to the patient before, during, and after relaxation and guided imagery sessions. Practice is required to skillfully change and use different music selections and not interfere with the therapeutic guiding process. Nurses must experiment with and learn to choose music to begin relaxation, music to evoke the integration of the imagery process, and music to ground the relaxation and imagery process.

Music to facilitate the relaxation and imagery process

Music not only facilitates deep relaxation but also evokes different types of imagery.[2,7] When the imagery process is first used, it is common for images to be concrete. Frequently patients get stuck in concrete images without using other types of imagery (Table 5-3). A variety of music selections have been tested at the IMHE to help patients evoke certain experiences. These different experiences and music selections are listed in the box on p. 114, top. The

box on p. 114, bottom, provides a resource list for relaxation, imagery, and music tapes.

Music should be chosen based on the *iso-principle* (i.e., matching music to the mood of the patient and then slowly changing it to the mood that a patient wants to evoke).[11,15] When a patient is not feeling good, has acute or chronic pain, or is grieving, moods vary from mild discouragement to depression. If the goal of the music is to reduce depression, the patient might start out listening to a musical selection that helps to relax for several minutes and then change to music that evokes a lighter, yet related response. Music selections made by the patient depend on the kinds of feelings and experiences the patient wishes to achieve. Certain kinds of music evoke calmness and peace; other types can help a patient work through grief, depression, or death imagery. Music selections stimulate images that assist one in connecting with emotions.

Music also can unblock tension, worry, and fear, which prevent a patient from achieving a deep level of healing. During a relaxation and imagery session, patients should be encouraged to experiment with slow and fast music, depending on current life events. Pleasant and unpleasant images emerge with music. If unpleasant images occur, nurses can suggest ways that a patient may work with these images or stop them. To stop or change the images, the patient takes a deep breath, deepens the relaxation, and lets the images once again emerge; then the patient sees how the images change.

The use of music to facilitate imagery and healing has received attention by many researchers since the 1970s. One influential healing modality, known as Guided Imagery and Music (GIM) was developed by Bonny and Savary.[6] This method is a one-to-one process in which a "guide" facilitates a patient in exploring life's journey using selected classical music. It is a dynamic inner experience that can bring about physical, emotional, and spiritual wholeness. After the assessment, music is selected to help a patient evoke different states of emotional awareness and experiences. In this specific imagery process, the guide encourages the patient to verbalize without analyzing the images associated with the music during the session. After a session the patient is brought back slowly to a wakeful state. The guide then assists the patient in integrating the experience through drawing images, journaling, or using dialogue.

NURSING PROCESS AND BIOBEHAVIORAL INTERVENTIONS

The nursing process must be used with biobehavioral interventions. Assess the patient's present state and willingness to participate in interventions. Based on the assessment, identify information that needs to be taught; then choose the appropriate interventions. After assessing the patient and formulating nursing diagnoses, use these in-

CHOOSING MUSIC FOR USE IN IMAGERY AND HEALING

The following music has been selected after experimentation at the IMHE. It is important to remember, when choosing music to create a specific environment, that habituation can occur. For example, 2 minutes of listening to music to evoke images may be enough to trigger activation; 15 minutes may negate the effects. About 20 to 30 minutes of listening to baroque music to enhance concentration is effective; listening longer has less value.

MUSIC SELECTIONS THAT HELP ACTIVATE IMAGERY

J. S. Bach, *The Well Tempered Klavier*
Cambridge Buskers, *Not Live from New York*
Don Campbell, *Dances for a Sleep Walker*
Scott Joplin, soundtrack from *The Sting*
Eugene Ormandy, *Fireworks*
Sousa marches
Mannheim Steamroller, *Saving the Wildlife*
Tomita, *Snowflakes are Dancing, Cosmos*
Paul Winter, *Earthbeat*

MUSIC SELECTIONS THAT HELP CONCENTRATION

Don Campbell, *Angels* (side 2), *Cosmic Classics, Crystal Mediations*
Eugene Friesen, *New Friends*
Gregorian *Chants*
Mozart, *C Major Piano Concerto* (Elvira Madigan)
Ranier, *Songs of the Indian Flute*
Relax with the Classics, Andante (Lind Institute)
Paul Winter, *Sunsinger*

MUSIC SELECTIONS THAT HELP TO RELAX

Don Campbell, *Angels* (side 1), *Birthing, Crystal Rainbows, Runes* (deep relaxation)
Eno, *Music for Airports, The Pearl*
Key Gardner, *The Rainbow Path*
Jonathan Goldman, *Dolphin Dreams*
Relax with the Classics, Adagio and Largo

MUSIC SELECTIONS IN CONCERT WITH ACTIVE IMAGERY

Beethoven, *Piano Concerto no. 5 in E Flat Major*
Brahms, *Violin Concerto in D Major*
Handel, *Royal Fireworks Suite*
Haydn, *Symphony no. 94 in G Major*
Mozart, *Symphonies in C Major, G Minor; Violin Concerto no. 5 in A Major*
Relax with the Classics, Allegro
Tchaikovsky, *Piano Concerto no. 1 in B Minor*

MUSIC SELECTIONS IN CONCERT WITH PASSIVE IMAGERY

Don Campbell, *Dances for a Sleepwalker, Lightning on the Moon*
Corelli, *Concerto Grossi no. 4, no. 10, no. 11, no. 12*
David Hykes, *The Harmonic Choir*
Handel, *Water Music Suite*
Kitaro, *Silk Road*
Mascagni, *Intermezzo from Cavalleria Rusticana*
Satie, *Gymnopedies*
Vivaldi, *Flute concertos*

From Campbell D: Music, physician for times to come, Wheaton, Ill, 1991, Theosophical Publishing House. For information on where to get tapes that are hard to find, write Institute for Music, Health, and Education, PO Box 1244, Boulder, CO 80306, (303)443-8484.

RESOURCES FOR RELAXATION, IMAGERY, AND MUSIC TAPES

Awakening Productions, 4132 Tuller Avenue, Culver, CA 90230.
Bodymind Systems, 910 Dakota Drive, Temple, TX 76504, (817)773-2337.
Health Horizons, 3919 N. Twin Oaks Road, San Marcos, CA 92069, (619)471-9349.
Institute for Music, Health, and Education, P.O. Box 1244, Boulder, Co 80306, (303)443-8484.
Mind/Body Health Sciences, 22 Lawson Terrace, Scituate, MA 02066, (617)545-6890.

New Era Media, 425 Alabama Street, San Francisco, CA 94110 (415)863-3555
Narada Distributing, 207 East Buffalo, Milwaukee, WI 53202.
Windham Hill Productions, P.O. Box 9388, Stanford, CA 94305
Sources Cassette, Department 99, P.O. Box W, Stanford, CA 94305, (415)328-7171.

**MAKING YOUR OWN RELAXATION
AND IMAGERY TAPES**

Use the scripts in this book (see pp. 118 to 121) to make tapes for your unit or clinic. Start first with a relaxation script of your choice. Change, add, or delete any part of the script to create your own unique tape to fit specific protocols of your practice area.

Reinforce exactly what you want patients to hear to help them engage their inner healing resources.

Review ways to empower patients' senses and inner dialogue. Modulate your voice to increase the power of your words.

If you are preparing patients for a procedure or surgery, use imagery information for the senses such as smells, sounds, and textures that the patient will encounter. Reinforce that patients are to rehearse in their mind a successful procedure from start to finish, including a rapid recovery.

As you record your script, you might have two tape recorders, one recorder playing music and the other recording your voice accompanied by music.

NURSE AS FACILITATOR

To be the best possible facilitator with guided relaxation, imagery, or music interventions, nurses should have personal experience and a knowledge of the interventions. They must learn to use these interventions as healing rituals rather than as step-by-step techniques. Nurses who learn such skills gain balance and increase their energy and joy. It is only through personal experience that nurses can facilitate and integrate these interventions so that nurse-patient interactions becomes a transforming experience.[9,25]

Often patients ask about the next step of recovery. The nurse can explain external resources such as drugs or procedures. However, patients really may be searching for meaning and the answers to questions about life. A nurse can never know the answers for another but can help patients find their own answers.

Biobehavioral interventions can be used to evoke self-reflection and states of inner calmness and peace for patients, families, and significant others. Patients must learn to access their inner healer and wisdom. These moments are unpredictable, and there is no formula for how a person does this. The real healing in such sessions cannot be predicted.

Before the session, establish the degree of the patient's readiness and willingness to learn. Assess the patient's understanding about the nature of the problem and concerns. For example, determine what the patient understands about the medical diagnosis, the prognosis, medical treatment, and side effects. Assess the positive or negative aspects of the patient's imagery in regard to the problem or disease. Note areas that are not understood. As a guide, you may need to speak with the patient's physician, particularly when medical or surgical therapy is complex. This will give you more information to help the patient with the imagery process.

Before the session, assess the patient's general concerns, including health, stressors, and relationships. Assess anxiety and tension levels to determine the types of relaxation techniques that will be the most effective. Ask the patient about symptoms and the way that they are interpreted. Inquire about how the patient is handling the problem or situation. Assess body and verbal language as events in the patients life are being described. Determine the length of time the problem has existed and the reason the patient is seeking help. Also assess the patient's perception about significant others, family members, and friends.

Assess for behaviors that a patient would like to possess, or help the patient identify a more desirable situation. Determine the patient's dominant senses so that you can give suggestions such as, "See yourself. . . " or "Hear yourself saying. . ." during each session. Relate imagery in scripts to the wants, needs, desires, or recurrent and dominant themes in the patient's life. Determine the patient's internal and external healing resources, and use this infor-

terventions for decreasing, eliminating, or stabilizing alterations in all nine human responses patterns (see Tables 5-1, 5-2, and 5-4). Incorporate interventions into a bedside session, a private counseling session, or a group cardiac rehabilitation class.* The box above provides guidelines for making relaxation and imagery tapes for cardiovascular patients.

When using these interventions in the acute care setting such as the coronary or critical care unit, prepare the patient's room for quiet, comfort, and no interruptions. Place a sign on the patient's door that states, "Relaxation session in progress. Please do not enter." Assist the patient to get comfortable as needed, for example, have the patient empty the bladder and place a light blanket nearby for warmth because a person is more sensitive to subtle changes in air temperature when relaxed. Set aside 15 to 20 minutes for the patient to experience relaxation, imagery, or music. To assist patients in incorporating biobehavioral interventions on a long-term basis, use the three phases of a *ritual*.[2] The first phase is *separation,* which involves locating a special quiet place for creating a healing state of consciousness. The second phase is *transition,* which involves becoming aware of being changed through the healing process. The third phase is *reincorporation,* which involves re-entering life's activities with a sense of being renewed and changed.

*References 3, 5, 10, 13, 16-18, 20, 22-24.

mation during guided imagery sessions to help the patient develop personal symbols and rituals. If a patient is returning for a session or if you are returning to the patient's bedside for the next session, elicit questions, successes or problems with relaxation and imagery that have occurred since the last session. Stimulate discussion about the insight that the patient has gained. As the patient shares relaxation and imagery experiences, listen for recurrent patterns that were recognized from previous sessions or diary or journal entries.

During the session, assist the patient in creating personal images by using relaxation, imagery, and music scripts with music for integration and grounding. Continue to reassess the patient's state of relaxation throughout the session by observing body position, change in skin tone, and eyelid movement as listed in the box on p. 101. Watch for clues in shifts of emotions during the session, including those indicated by body language and facial expression such as smiles, frowns, or tears. Assess involvement in the relaxation and imagery process. Ask the patient to raise a finger to indicate *yes* to determine whether the relaxation and imagery process is satisfactory, whether the pace needs to be slower, whether the patient is awake or whether a position change would increase comfort.

Pace the relaxation script and images given to the patient. Avoid flooding the patient with information and images because this blocks the creative process. When guiding the patient with the scripts, use techniques to affect the patient's senses and inner dialogue.

Assist the patient to stay with the flow of images without talking. Interpreting specific images is an intellectual process. When the patient talks during the session, the free flow of spontaneous images, feelings, and emotions is interrupted. However, during certain types of guided imagery that work with music (i.e., GIM), the patient should verbalize to the guide the images as they occur in relationship to the music. The guide assesses and facilitates the patient to continue work on specific phases of images during deep relaxation. This requires specific training that can be obtained from workshops on imagery training.[6]

Advance to different relaxation and imagery exercises when the patient's health status changes, treatment changes, boredom occurs, new information is received about the problem or healing resources, or the current exercises are no longer effective. Make a tape of the session so that the patient can practice, or let a patient check out a tape from the audiotape library as outlined in the box on p. 109.

In closing the session, help the patient interpret the relaxation and imagery experiences by weaving questions into the conversation. Ask the patient reflective questions for further introspection such as:

1. How does your bodymind register that you are tense?

2. What are the special messages that you can give yourself that will convey reassurance, openness, calmness, and trust?

3. As you work with your imagination, what are the questions that you still have about interpreting your images?

4. Do you notice any sensations (kinesthetic or felt sense) when you let go of tension or worries? What other sensory experiences do you have?

Offer the patient paper and crayons to express states of relaxation and their images and feelings with drawing or journaling. Refer to drawing previously discussed. Make notes on the patient's record to add more detail in future sessions if the patient desires more complexity or if the patient is ready to move to another area of healing or problem solving, (i.e., changing coronary artery disease risk factors or reducing stress at work or in relationships). Give the patient feedback and also ask about which imagery scripts worked best. Suggest referral to other sources or therapists if necessary. Offer the patient guidelines on how to practice relaxation and imagery and evaluate with the patient techniques that have and have not worked during sessions.

APPLICATION OF BIOBEHAVIORAL SCRIPTS*

All of the following script excerpts and complete biobehavioral scripts include intellectual and intuitive thought processes. The bodymind responds in a healthy manner when suggestions of relaxation and healing images are given, particularly when different phrases and voice inflections are integrated into those suggestions.

The following strategies combine tonal inflection, different phrases, and special use of words so that patient's intellectual and intuitive processes work together at a higher level.[8,19,21] Packaged relaxation and imagery tapes include some of these voice inflections, but when the nurse makes a tape or when patients are encouraged to make their own tapes, special healing cues can be included. In the examples that follow a series of dots and dashes such as . . . . and . . . . will appear. These dots mean to pause and change your tonal inflection when reading or recording a script.

Truism

The patient's intellectual mind likes facts that are organized. As a result, when a patient hears a statement and can *believe* or *accept it as accurate or as truth*, the intuitive mind is free to accept a relaxed experience or a healing statement. The script excerpt that follows connects true

---

*Source: Adapted from Peterson G and Mehl L: Pregnancy as healing: a holistic philosophy for prenatal care, Berkeley, Calif, 1984, Mindbody Press.

statements that may precede a suggestion and be connected to another true statement. When this occurs, a patient's intellectual thought process is satisfied that the facts are logical. A person does not need to examine the facts, and it leaves the intuitive mind free to accept the suggestion.

An example follows of how connecting true biologic statements in relaxation and imagery scripts works for a patient with hypertension:

As you take your next breath in, become aware of the fact that you are breathing air into your lungs (truism) and the oxygen from that breath moves from your lungs into your bloodstream (truism) . . . you can let yourself imagine that your blood vessels are very relaxed (suggestion) . . . free of excess tension (suggestion). . . . and at this time you can continue this deep state of relaxation (suggestion).

The suggestion "to let yourself imagine" is preceded by two true statements: (1) that you are breathing air into your lungs and (2) that the oxygen moves from your lungs into your bloodstream. The true statements are followed by suggestions of desired biologic changes (relaxed blood vessels) while the patient maintains a deep state of relaxation. The patient's intellectual thought process is occupied with the true statements and leaves the intuitive process free to go with the suggestion of deep relaxation and to feel the sensations associated with relaxed blood vessels.

Embedded commands

In the guiding process, the nurse should use embedded commands by changing the intonation of the voice, such as pitch, volume, or speed of the spoken words. Embedded commands are *short phrases* that *stand out* because of pauses in the sentence. Unusual grammatical structure appears in the following script excerpt to occupy the patient's logical thought process; thus the phrases stand out. If the patient's name is inserted while reading or recording the script, the patient's intuitive process may comprehend the short message more easily. An example would be: "You can, . . . (insert patient's name), relax more deeply (embedded command) . . . if you want to." When using changes in the quality of the voice, pauses, and calling a patient by name, the suggestion, "relax," is more easily heard by the patient.

The nurse can make the volume or tone of voice more dramatic by increasing the power of specific words or phrases. An example might be, "(insert patient's name), . . . allow yourself to . . . relax into the pain with the next breath . . . feel . . . as you breathe into that pain now." The words to change with voice inflection would be "relax into the pain" and "feel . . . breathe into that pain now."

Linkage

Intellectual thoughts can be diverted by connecting certain *statements, behaviors,* and *actions* with *suggestions,* which serve as a diversion to satisfy a patient's logical thought process. An example would be rehearsing relaxation while preparing for cardiac catheterization. The nurse would say:

"(Insert patient's name), relax into the surface under your body. Before the physician begins . . . once more . . . relax more deeply and really sink into the mattress on the table where you are . . . feeling yourself being supported by this surface . . . and let it be a reminder to take a deep breath and relax more deeply."

Reframing

Reframing helps a patient contact the part of a behavior that may be preventing or prohibiting healthier thoughts or behaviors. It helps a patient reflect on old or current belief systems about an existing problem or experience so that new actions and beliefs can be created to lead a healthier state. For example, if an AMI patient repeats that his or her heart is big, overstretched, and ineffective, these words create negative imagery that further interferes with psychophysiologic recovery. A reframe would be, "My heart is healing, moment by moment and is a strong effective pump (see Fig. 5-3, *B*). Another example is a patient who is scheduled for a second cardiac catheterization who reports to the nurse memories of pain and discomfort during the previous procedure. This patient is reinforcing the anticipated fear and pain and is also more likely to have these symptoms or complications. The nurse can instruct the patient correctly about the procedure and then encourage the patient to change the negative self-talk of "I dread it, because it is going to hurt" to a *reframe* of "I am relaxed and the procedure is going smoothly." The patient would practice this reframe and "rehearse" a successful procedure until the experience of positive sensations that are associated with the suggestions are felt.

Metaphors

Metaphors are *figures of speech* or *implied comparisons* in which a word or phrase ordinarily and primarily used for one thing is applied to another. When metaphors are used in relaxation and imagery tapes, healing is enhanced because the intuitive self can deepen the experience of the words as they are heard. For example, "(Patient's name), . . . imagine the relaxation flowing from the top of your head to your toes . . . like a warm waterfall." The metaphor here of relaxation is implied to be a gentle, warm waterfall. Other metaphors might be relaxation as gentle as snow flakes falling or as gentle and cool as a spring breeze.

Therapeutic double-bind

A patient's bodymind will relax more quickly when intellectual thought processes are *occupied* and *involved* in making several different choices. This will lead the patient to participate in the given suggestion. An example follows:

the dome-shaped accumulation of sticky cholesterol that has collected over an old injury to the blood vessel wall. . . . In your mind's eye, see yourself gently peeling off the layers of fatty material and handing them over to special cells that stream by. . . . Like little garbage trucks, these cells cart the cholesterol to the intestine where it joins other unneeded materials and eventually leaves the body. . . . You may continue with this process until you feel you have accomplished enough. . . .

As you continue on your journey, you notice the small globes of cholesterol are also free-floating in the clear liquid portion of the blood stream. . . . On closer inspection it is apparent that there are two types of cholesterol, one is a bit darker and heavier, almost jewel-like; this is your high-density lipoprotein, or HDL. The other form is lighter and opaque; it is the low-density lipoprotein or LDL. . . . As you continue to relax and learn more about your internal world, you see the HDL move toward the LDL and surround it. . . . The LDL is herded toward the garbage trucks and is taken away, some of the HDL riding along as guards. . . . After a period of time, you notice that there is far less cholesterol floating by, and what is there is predominantly the HDL. . . .

You may now choose to travel on the beam of light to the upper right quadrant of your abdomen, to that marvelous internal factory that is your liver. . . . The liver performs many different functions, one of which is to manufacture cholesterol. You speak with the supervisor of the cholesterol division and suggest that perhaps the workers have been under too much stress. . . . They have been turning out more cholesterol than is needed and they deserve some time off. . . . It is agreed that they will begin to work at partial speed, and that their output will be maintained at a lower, healthier level. . . .

As you come toward the end of this journey, you feel confident that you will continue to make subtle adjustments in your lifestyle, adding pleasurable forms of exercise into your routine and eating tasty, healthy foods. . . . You can feel the warmth and peace that comes with taking time out to relax, even if it is just for a few minutes each day. . . .

Dysrhythmias and mitral valve prolapse

As you prepare to focus on a calm, regular heart beat . . . gently place your thumbs and first fingers together and allow the air to breathe in and out of you all by itself. . . . You can begin to feel the pulse of your heartbeat in your fingertips. . . . Is it possible for you to imagine that you are resting on a beautiful, warm, sandy beach? . . . Can you feel the ocean breeze on your face, and the warmth of the morning sun on your skin? . . . As you relax on the beach, you begin to notice the waves breaking softly on the sand and a line of foam washing up the damp sand to your feet . . . and then the foam bubbles sink into the sand and the waves move back to the edge of the water. . . . As you continue to watch the waves, you notice that they are

moving up the beach as you breathe in . . . and back down the beach as you breathe out . . . in . . . and out . . . in . . . and out . . . continue to focus on smooth, even, body rhythms . . .

Occasionally you may feel a variation in your heartbeat as you sense it through your fingertips or even as you become aware of a change in rate or regularity in your chest. . . . Allow a picture to come into your mind of a healthy young animal like a horse. . . . Imagine watching that strong young horse running playfully across a field. Hear the hoofbeats, and see the horse running in slow motion. . . . Once in a while, as an expression of the pure joy of living, that horse simply kicks its hind feet up into the air and keeps on running, getting stronger and more beautiful every day. . . . It is sturdy, vibrant and full of life. . . . Visualize your heart . . . sturdy . . . vibrant . . . full of life . . .

(For mitral valve prolapse, continue with the following script.)

In your imagination, allow yourself to become very tiny and powerful, perhaps seeing yourself as a mighty magician or even something mechanical like a computer chip . . . tiny, but with great powers. . . . Travel on a beam of light to the interior of your heart where you can see, hear, and touch the wonderful structures that regulate blood flow . . . valves, chambers, sparkles of electrical energy. . . . As you make your way through your heart, you can reach out and stroke the muscular walls. . . . You can tighten up any loose cords or valve leaflets. . . . You can make any changes that you know will increase the efficiency of your heart. . . . Take all the time you need to do this . . .

Angina

(If a patient has known angina, practice of this ritual should be encouraged before an attack. This script is to be used with the nitroglycerin therapy. Then when an attack occurs, the patient will have more success at aborting it with general relaxation, hand-warming, and breathing exercises. With an acute angina attack, this script is used as the nitroglycerin is placed under the patient's tongue. Breathing and hand-warming scripts are incorporated with this imagery script.)

As you place the powerful nitroglycerin under your tongue . . . it immediately dissolves in the saliva in your mouth. . . . Right now, the medicine is in your blood stream and working. . . .

For a few moments . . . travel on a beam of light . . . to your heart and just observe your coronary arteries . . . on the surface of your heart. With the medicine and your relaxed breathing . . . your whole body relaxes. . . . Your coronary vessels are opening more . . . relaxing . . . delivering more nourishing blood to your heart muscle. . . . Your pain is leaving.

Just continue to watch in your mind's eye as your coronary arteries respond to your relaxed breathing. Notice your hands warming. . . . As your hands warm . . . your coronary arteries open more . . . allowing blood to flow and nourish your heart muscle. Imagine the muscle tissue in the coronary arteries relaxing . . . relaxing even more . . . becoming more open and larger . . . allowing more blood to flow through them. . . . Sense this experience of opening and softening . . . feeling comfortable. . . . Know that with your relaxed breathing . . . and your relaxed body . . . your coronary vessels also are relaxed and sending more blood to your heart muscle.

MI and open heart surgery

Travel on a mental journey to your heart . . . just observe it for a while. As you watch your heart, see vividly all of its parts that make it such a wonderful part of your body. Observe your heart functioning . . . like a magnificent pump, the finest and most efficient that you can imagine. . . . Listen to how regular your heartbeats are and how strong your heart muscle is. In your mind, go to the area where you had your (jump grafts) (MI). Feel (the jump grafts) (your MI scar) becoming stronger and stronger every day. . . . Think about blood flowing (through your jump grafts) (to the healthy muscle around your scar), nourishing that area, as well as sending oxygen and nourishment to the rest of your whole heart. Just think about how (big and strong your jump grafts are now since surgery) (normal blood flows through your heart muscle). . . .

In your mind now . . . begin to go through all aspects of the cardiac rehabilitation process. See yourself participating in every phase to help stabilize your heart disease and improve all aspects of your life. . . .

If you are taking medications, take a few moments now to think about them. Imagine yourself taking each pill, or if the medication is in ointment form, applying it to your body as a very natural process. Remember to relax all your muscles as you take your medications so that they may have the best possible effect on your heart . . . body. Go over those medications in your mind now and see if you understand the dosage of each drug, the specific schedule for taking each one, and the action of each. Feel relaxation as you do this. . . .

Scan your mind now about your current diet. As you eat, be aware of not being tense or anxious. . . . Pay attention to what you are eating. . . . Notice the texture, taste, smell, and temperature of your food as you eat it. . . . Notice the sensation of the food against your teeth and gums. Chew your food slowly and carefully. Adjust your rate of eating so you feel relaxed and comfortable. Whether you are eating alone or with other people, feel yourself relaxed and at ease. . . .

If you get hungry before mealtime, think about what you have a taste for and how you can eat healthy foods. . . . If you are buying food, allow yourself to spend some time reading labels to know the content of the food. If you are eating out, choose places that will have the right kinds of food for you. If you are preparing your food, smell the food, feel it, see yourself preparing fresh fruits and vegetables, fish, chicken, or meat in a relaxed manner. . . .

In your mind now visualize yourself getting ready to exercise. Feel yourself preparing your body for conditioning as you do your warm-up exercises. . . . Feel each muscle as you stretch very slowly. Just let go of tension in those muscles. . . . Now move through your exercise routine on the treadmill, walking or riding the bicycle, seeing yourself doing very well. . . . And now you are at the end of your exercising doing your cool-down exercises. Feel your body energized and free of tension.

In your mind . . . see yourself taking 15 to 20 minutes twice a day to do your relaxation exercises. . . . As you inhale now, feel yourself breathing in energy and balance. . . . As you exhale feel yourself letting go of doubts, fears, anger, sadness, illness, and imbalance. . . .

Identify in your mind now the people who are important to you. . . . Feel yourself giving and receiving comfort . . . support and being receptive with these people. Allow your relationships with these people to become more meaningful. . . . Continue to see yourself with these people . . . allow yourself to tell them things that you want them to know but have not told them. . . .

In your mind . . . see yourself beginning to feel a sense of play on a daily basis . . . a time when you allow yourself to play spontaneously . . . laughing out loud . . . and having fun with your friends. Feel the experience now of what it is like to laugh inside and outside. . . . Let your eyes dance and your face smile. Permit yourself to experience play without guilt, even when there is more work to be done. . . .

Again, let's go over the events that you are participating in . . . all areas of cardiac rehabilitation (medications, diet, exercise, and relaxation). Think of positive thoughts about healing and that your body will be healing itself in a wonderful and remarkable way. Feel yourself working with your body and mind to heal. Feel your heart continuing to get stronger and stronger day by day, stabilizing your disease process, and balancing your life.

KEY CONCEPT REVIEW

1. The three characteristics of psychophysiologic self-regulation can best be described as:
   a. Truisms, embedded commands, and synesthesia
   b. Correct biologic images, rituals, and music
   c. Body inner awareness, self-regulation skills, and effective choices
   d. Dominant right hemispheric function, self-awareness, and correct biologic images
2. The relaxation response is:
   a. Increased sympathetic nervous system arousal

b. Decreased sympathetic nervous system arousal
c. Relaxation techniques
d. Imagery techniques
3. Which of the following statements is true about imagery:
a. Imagery provides a focus for organizing psychophysiologic energy.
b. Strong positive imagery helps the patient activate the inner healer.
c. Imagery processes created by the patient translate into measurable psychophysiologic change.
d. All of the above are true.
4. Music helps the patient:
a. Maintain awareness of clock time
b. Focus on pain
c. Increase stimuli
d. Alter perception of clock time

5. When the nurse uses a body-mind-spirit framework this can:
a. Serve as a unifying guide for gaining insight about the patient's self-concept
b. Help organize patient problems
c. Help establish multiple nursing interventions
d. All of the above

ANSWERS

1. c
2. b
3. d
4. d
5. d

REFERENCES

1. Achterberg J: Imagery in healing, Boston, 1985, Shambhala Publications, Inc.
2. Achterberg J, Dossey B, and Kolkmeier L: Rituals of healing, New York, 1992, Bantam Books.
3. Acosta F: Biofeedback and progressive relaxation in weaning the anxious patient from the ventilator: a brief report, Heart Lung 19(2):299, 1988.
4. Benson H: The relaxation response, New York, 1975, William Morrow & Co, Inc.
5. Benson H: Beyond the relaxation response, New York, 1984, Times Books.
6. Bonny H and Savary L: Music and your mind , New York, 1978, Harper & Row, Publishers, Inc.
7. Campbell D: Music, physician for times to come, Wheaton, Ill, 1991, Theosophical Publishing House.
8. Dossey B: Imagery: awakening the inner healer. In Dossey B and others: Holistic nursing: a handbook for practice, Gaithersburg, Md. 1988, Aspen Publishers, Inc.
9. Dossey B: Relationships: learning the patterns and processes. In Dossey B and others: Holistic nursing: a handbook for practice, Gaithersburg, Md, 1988, Aspen Publishers, Inc.
10. Frenn M, Fehring R, and Kartes S: Reducing the stress of cardiac catheterization by teaching relaxation, DCCN 5(2):108, 1986.
11. Guzzetta C: Music therapy: hearing the melody of the soul. In Dossey B and others: Holistic nursing: a handbook for practice, Gaithersburg, Md, 1988, Aspen Publishers, Inc.
12. Guzzetta C: Effects of relaxation and music therapy on patients in a coronary care unit with the presumptive diagnosis of acute myocardial infarction, Heart Lung 18(6):609, 1989.
13. Horowitz B, Fitzpatrick J, and Flaherty G: Relaxation techniques for pain relief after open heart surgery, DCCN 3(3):364, 1984.
14. Kolkmeier L: Relaxation: opening the door to change. In Dossey B and others: Holistic nursing: a handbook for practice, Gaithersburg, Md, 1988, Aspen Publishers, Inc.
15. McClellan R: Music and altered states, Dromenon 2(winter):7, 1979.
16. Miller K and Perry P: Relaxation technique and postoperative pain in patients undergoing cardiac surgery, Heart Lung 19(1):136, 1990.
17. Ornish D: Can lifestyle changes reverse coronary heart disease, Lancet 336:129, 1990.
18. Pender N: Effects of progressive muscle relaxation training on anxiety and locus of control among hypertensive adults, Res Nurs Health 8(1):67, 1985.
19. Peterson G and Mehl L: Pregnancy as healing: a holistic philosophy for prenatal care, Berkeley, Calif, 1984, Mindbody Press.
20. Puntillo K: The phenomenon of pain and critical care nursing, Heart Lung 17(2):262, 1988.
21. Sheikh A: Techniques to enhance imaging ability. In Sheikh A: Anthology of imagery techniques, Milwaukee, Wisc, 1986, American Imagery Institute.
22. Stuart E: Non-pharmacologic treatment of hypertension: a multiple-risk-factor-approach, Cardio Vasc Nurs 1(1):1, 1987.
23. Stuart E, Decko J, and Mandle C: Spirituality in health and healing: a clinical program, Holistic Nurs Pract 3(3):35, 1989.
24. Thomas S: Spirituality: an essential dimension in the treatment of hypertension, Holistic Nurs Pract 3(3):47, 1989.
25. Vaughan F: The inward arc, Boston, 1986, Shambhala Publications, Inc.

UNIT II

SELECTED CARDIOVASCULAR TESTING AND MONITORING TECHNIQUES

Cholesterol: Another Side to the Story

What do you think of when you consider the causes of hypercholesterolemia? Do you think the cause is genetic or that it's primarily a result of a high fat diet, obesity, or lack of exercise? These reasons are, of course, ones we hear about the most. All these causes are overwhelmingly physical in nature. They are rooted in our body chemistry, our cells, our genes, or they are related to what we eat. But there is another side to high cholesterol we never hear about. It is a nonphysical side, and it has to do with feelings and emotions. Studies suggest that these factors can be just as important as the physical ones.

Schottstaedt and co-workers[5] examined the fluctuations of certain hormones in the blood of patients who were hospitalized on a metabolic ward. They found that several vitally important hormones fluctuated when the patients underwent "interpersonal difficulties" that caused psychologic stress. The problems usually centered on the patients' most significant relationships.

Wolf and others[6] used the metabolic ward to study changes in cholesterol levels in patients who had coronary artery disease. In this situation, it was possible to keep factors such as diet and exercise rigidly controlled. They found that reassuring and supportive types of relationships could significantly lower cholesterol levels, while stressful human interactions could significantly elevate it. They found that within the hospital setting, the blood cholesterol went up or down, depending on the closeness of the relationships experienced by the patients. One patient was a 49-year-old man who had experienced several myocardial infarctions and had a history of disrupted human relationships. During his hospital stay, here is what they observed:

. . . the patient seemed happy and reasonably relaxed, although very eager to please during the first few days of the study while receiving daily visits from his new woman friend. When she left town for a few days without telling him, however, he became anxious. Serum cholesterol concentration rose somewhat until she returned, revisited, and reassured him. While out of town, however, she had met another man whom she preferred. Her daily visits to the patient fell off and . . . she [eventually] told him she had abandoned the plan to marry him and would not see him again. He became intensely depressed. Again the serum cholesterol rose and the following day he had a recurrent AMI. Four days later he died.

In a dramatic study at Ohio State School of Medicine, a group of rabbits was fed a diet that was high in cholesterol and triglycerides. At the end of the study period the rabbits were autopsied and their coronary arteries were examined for evidence of coronary artery disease. All the rabbits were riddled with typical coronary artery disease except for a particular subgroup who, however, had eaten the same diet. The only uncontrolled variable in this study seemed to be that this particular subgroup of rabbits was cared for by a female graduate student who removed them from their cages daily and held, touched, petted, and talked to them—and then placed them back in their cages and fed them their atrocious diet. But how could this possibly protect the rabbits from the effects of their high cholesterol diet? Skeptical about the effects of touching and petting, the researchers repeated the study (three times in all) with identical findings: the touched and petted rabbits were largely spared the effects of coronary artery disease, which devastated the other rabbits who were not held, touched, nor petted.[3]

But what do touched and petted rabbits have to do with human beings? Similar events also seem to occur in human beings. In a study of 10,000 males with coronary artery disease, researchers found that the incidence of angina was reduced by 50% if the man had a loving, supportive wife.[2]

Can emotions be used purposefully to lower the cholesterol level, or are we simply the helpless victims of our emotional life and our interpersonal stresses? In a landmark study, Cooper and Aygen[1] studied a group of men who had marked elevations of cholesterol levels. They taught them to do something that men in our society seldom do—sit silently in a chair twice a day for 15 minutes and simply clear their minds. If a thought intruded, they were asked to let it pass by without dwelling on it. As they did this, keeping their diet, body weight, and exercise levels constant, their cholesterol levels fell by up to one third.

So what do we make of the cholesterol story? There is no doubt that the physical factors are vitally important: genetics, diet, weight, and exercise. We ought to do everything in our power to attend to these factors, and if the cholesterol levels do not fall, drugs may be necessary. Yet the story does not end here. As the precious studies clearly show, our mental life is clearly involved—our emotions, attitudes, feelings, and relationships. (see Chapter 5 and Chapter 19 for further information.)

But if these issues are so important, why is it that physicians often do not include them with discussions of the physical factors? For the most part, physicians may view "disturbed relationships and interpersonal stress" as too complex to deal with. Thus physicians tend to address the physical factors of diet, weight, exercise, and medication. In addition, many people would rather "take a pill" than expend the hard work needed to repair their family relationships, job stress, or improve their quality of life. However, as people realize that they can affect their physiology by learning relaxation, imagery, and biofeedback skills, the emphasis of a positive change about our mental life will continue to change.

There continues to be a growing awareness in nursing, medicine, and our culture that human illness is vastly more complex than we imagined a few years ago. Ornish's[4] landmark study, which clearly demonstrated that people with devastating coronary artery disease (see Chapter 1) can reverse supposedly fixed coronary lesions, supports the importance of emotions and attitudes in health and illness. Nurses must learn biobehavioral skills and integrate these in their own lives and in their clinical to be effective facilitators for patients.

REFERENCES

1. Cooper M and Aygen M: Effect of meditation on blood cholesterol and blood pressure. J Israel Medical Assn. 95:1, 1978.
2. Medalie JH and Goldhourt U: Angina pectoris among 10,000 men. II. Psychosocial and other risk factors, Am J Med 60:910, 1976.
3. Neren RM and others: Social environment as a factor in diet-induced atherosclerosis, Science 208:1475, 1980.
4. Ornish D: Dr. Dean Ornish's program for reversing heart disease, New York, 1990, Random House.
5. Schottstaedt WW and others: Sociologic and metabolic observations on patients in the community of a metabolic ward, Am J Med 25:248, 1958.
6. Wolf S and others: Changes in serum lipids om relation to emotional stress during rigid control of diet and exercise, Circulation 26:379, 1962.

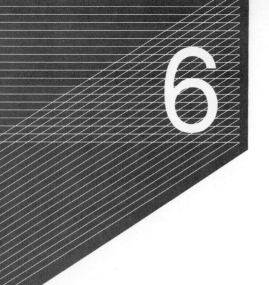

6

Diagnostic Testing

Linda A. Prinkey

LEARNING OBJECTIVES

1. Synthesize the basic principles used to formulate a care plan for all patients undergoing cardiovascular diagnostic testing.
2. Explain the rationale for serial cardiac enzyme testing for patients with suspected myocardial infarction.
3. Discuss the role of sodium, potassium, and calcium in the four phases of the cardiac action potential.
4. Describe three diagnostic testing procedures that involve recording the transmission of electrical impulses through the heart.
5. List two indications for echocardiography.
6. State the purpose of technetium-99m pyrophosphate nuclear scans.
7. Compare and contrast the two forms of thallium-201 scanning.
8. Describe the possible applications of magnetic resonance imaging, positron emission tomography, and computerized tomography in the diagnosis of cardiac disorders.
9. Describe the sensations a patient is likely to experience during cardiac catheterization.
10. Discuss two indications for electrophysiologic studies.

Modern technology offers many new testing methods for determining and quantifying cardiovascular disorders. However, these tests are only adjunctive methods for data collection. A careful bio-psycho-social-spiritual assessment provides the foundation for directing further inquiry and for confirming the diagnosis of cardiovascular disease.

NURSING PROCESS

Assessment

Nursing assessment for all diagnostic testing focuses on determining the knowledge base that the patient and family possess regarding the disease process, the purpose of the test, the procedure itself, and finally the possible findings and their implications. Therefore Knowing is the critical response pattern to assess for all patients undergoing diagnostic testing (see Chapter 3).

The most helpful assessment technique for the Knowing Pattern is the use of open-ended questions that allow the patient and family to summarize their understanding of the information that they have received from many sources. Some helpful assessment questions follow:

1. Can you tell me why you are here today?
2. Why you are having this test?
3. Did the doctor say what the problem might be?
4. Can you tell me what you think the problem might be?
5. What do you know about the test?
6. What are the most important things you would like to know about your test?
7. What do you expect to find out from this test? What might these results mean to you?

Not only is it important to assess the patient's and family's knowledge, it is also essential to determine their readiness to learn and any barriers that might impede the learning process. People who are ready to learn often ask questions. They may also express a desire to learn. Interested individuals maintain eye contact and appear to listen. Barriers that can impede learning include the language spoken, educational level, reading ability, level of consciousness, sedation, and distractions such as noise, pain, fear, and anxiety. All factors should be considered before formulating a nursing diagnosis and a plan of care for a patient undergoing diagnostic testing.

Nursing diagnosis

The nursing diagnosis common to almost every patient and family is knowledge deficit of diagnostic testing related to lack of exposure to pertinent information. Lack of knowledge can lead to fear and anxiety, which increase stress that patients and families experience related to diagnostic procedures.

Planning

Because lack of knowledge and resultant fear and anxiety are common among patients and families involved in test-

ing, information should decrease their fear and anxiety. Further, minimizing the patient's anxiety may reduce the possibility of detrimental effects during the procedure.[41]

Although each procedure requires that some test-specific information be given to patients and families, there are some common elements in patient teaching for diagnostic testing. The following plan of care can be used as a teaching framework for all cardiovascular diagnostic procedures. Test-specific patient education information is included with the discussion of each procedure or group of related procedures in this chapter.

NURSING DIAGNOSIS	Knowledge deficit of diagnostic procedures related to lack of exposure to pertinent information (knowing pattern)	

PATIENT OUTCOMES	NURSING PRESCRIPTIONS	EVALUATION
The patient will describe normal cardiovascular function relevant to the test being performed	Teach normal cardiovascular function relevant to the test being performed.	Described normal function of the portion of the cardiovascular system being investigated
The patient will describe the suspected pathophysiologic condition in patient's own words	Teach the suspected pathophysiologic condition in layperson's terms.	Verbalized the suspected pathophysiologic condition in patient's own words
The patient will explain the purpose of the test	Explain the purpose of the test.	Explained the purpose of the test
The patient will list possible test results	Teach possible test results.	Listed the possible results of the test
The patient will describe the procedure in the patient's own words	Describe the procedure in layperson's terms.	Described the procedure in patient's own words
The patient will describe possible sights, sounds, and sensations associated with the test	Describe possible sights, sounds, and sensations associated with the test.	Described possible sights, sounds, and sensations associated with the test
The patient will list complications that might occur	Ask patient about complications the physician said might occur. Correct misconceptions or refer questions or misconceptions to the physician.	Listed complications that might occur
The patient will describe the expected postprocedure care in patient's own words	Describe expected postprocedure care.	Described the expected postprocedure care in patient's own words

Intervention

Patient education related to diagnostic testing should address the suspected or known disease process, the purpose of the test, a description of the procedure, possible findings, and care before and after the procedure. When possible, the patient and family must know what to expect before the test takes place. Several studies[5,41,42,44] have shown that patients are more interested in what they will see, hear, and feel than in lengthy descriptions of the procedure and technique. For the nurse to provide accurate information regarding the sights, sounds, and sensations

associated with a particular test, the nurse should have observed one or more of these procedures. Also, audiovisual aids appropriate to patient learning needs and abilities should be provided. The nurse should use these aids only to enhance patient learning. Audiovisual materials should never be the only source of information used. Regardless of the teaching methods used, the nurse should be available to answer questions and provide other information such as relaxation techniques. In this way, the nurse can provide holistic care in meeting the needs of the body-mind-spirit.

For invasive procedures such as cardiac catheterization and electrophysiologic studies, a *written informed consent* is required. Informed consent is permission given by an individual for a specific test or procedure. The person is not considered to be informed until all available options, as well as the risks and benefits of the procedure, have been fully explained. Therefore adequate and appropriate patient teaching is an essential prerequisite for obtaining valid informed consent.

BLOOD TESTING
Lipid studies
Background information

Lipids are a normal component of plasma. The types of lipids normally found in the blood include triglycerides, cholesterol, and phospholipids. Laboratory tests for plasma lipids and lipoproteins include total serum cholesterol, total serum triglyceride, high-density lipoprotein (HDL), and low-density lipoprotein (LDL) levels; cholesterol/HDL ratio; and lipoprotein phenotyping. The significance of tests and normal values are discussed in Chapter 8.

Indications

Quantification of various serum lipid forms helps in determining an individual's risk for heart disease (see Chapter 8). They are also used in monitoring the effectiveness of dietary and drug interventions to reduce the risk of coronary artery disease associated with hypercholesterolemia.

Procedure

The test to determine serum cholesterol levels is often performed for preliminary screening. This test can be performed by a fingerstick or by venipuncture. The remaining lipid studies are performed via venipuncture.

Patient teaching

Explain the purpose of the tests. Advise the patient to fast for 12 hours and to abstain from drinking alcohol for 24 hours before the test. If possible, encourage the patient to continue his or her regular diet for 7 days before testing. Also ask the patient to refrain from taking medications, such as estrogen, oral contraceptives, and salicylates before the test because these drugs may alter results.[21]

Cardiac enzyme studies
Background information

Enzymes are substances that assist in cellular chemical reactions. They exist in all living tissues. Normally, enzymes are inside the cell walls. However, when cells die, their membranes leak, allowing enzymes to escape into the circulation. Because some cells are always dying and being replaced by others, there are always small amounts of enzymes in the blood. Large serum concentrations of en-

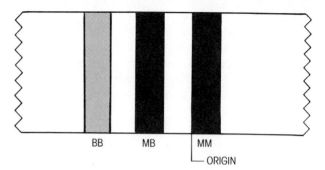

FIG. 6-1 CPK isoenzyme electrophoresis. At a pH of 8.0, CPK-MM is essentially neutral and remains at the origin. CPK-MB and CPK-BB are negatively charged and move toward the positive electrode.

Adapted from Roberts R: Diagnostic assessment of myocardial infarction based on lactate dehydrogenase and creatine kinase isoenzymes, Heart Lung 10:488, 1981.

zymes suggest an abnormal amount of cellular destruction (for example, an acute myocardial infarction [AMI]).

Creatine phosphokinase levels. *Creatine phosphokinase* (CPK or CK) is an enzyme found in the myocardium, skeletal muscle, kidneys, and brain. It exists in three forms, called *isoenzymes,* which can be separated through *electrophoresis* (Fig. 6-1). Cells of the kidneys and the brain contain mostly CPK-BB. CPK-MM is found mainly in skeletal muscle. CPK-MB exists primarily in cardiac muscle tissue. Because CPK-MB is found almost exclusively in cardiac muscle, the concentration of this isoenzyme correlates closely with myocardial infarct size.[26]

The normal serum concentration of CPK is 5 to 75 milliunits (mU)/ml. This level begins to rise within 4 to 8 hours after cellular insult and peaks in 12 to 24 hours. Total CPK values usually return to normal within 48 to 72 hours.[37] Reperfusion interventions such as percutaneous transluminal coronary angioplasty (PTCA), and administration of thrombolytic agents may cause an early and exaggerated rise in CPK levels.[11] CPK values in these settings may not correlate closely with infarct size.

Like all tests, CPK is not a perfect indicator because other conditions can cause elevations in this enzyme. Intramuscular injections, surgery, trauma, strenuous exercise, and some disease states can raise CPK levels. However, CPK-MB values greater than 10% to 15% of the total serum CPK indicate AMI.[55]

Lactate dehydrogenase levels. *Lactate dehydrogenase* (LDH) is another enzyme used to determine myocardial damage. Like CPK, LDH is found in many tissues and has several isoenzymes. Normal total serum LDH is 200 to 400 Wroblewski units/ml or 100 to 225 mU/ml.[37] LDH_2 concentrations normally are higher than those of LDH_1, the LDH isoenzyme found primarily in cardiac cells. In AMI, total LDH levels increase 5 to 6 times the normal in the first 48 hours. They remain elevated for 6 to 14 days.[37] In addition, LDH_1 levels become disproportionally elevated and exceed LDH$_2$ concentrations. This pattern is referred to as a *flip*.

Indications

Cardiac enzyme (CPK and LDH) levels are obtained to determine the presence or absence of AMI. Cardiac enzymes in the concentrations and patterns described, with data from the patient history and other diagnostic tests, can distinguish between AMI and angina pectoris. In angina pectoris, the myocardium is ischemic, not necrotic; therefore cardiac enzyme values should be normal.

Procedure

Blood samples are usually obtained by peripheral venipuncture. When thrombolytic agents are administered, a heparin lock should be inserted before starting the medication so that samples can be drawn without increasing the risk of bleeding from repeated venipunctures. Heparin locks can also be helpful for patients lacking good venipuncture sites and in reducing patient discomfort.

Total CPK and CPK-MB samples should be drawn on admission and then 12 and 24 hours later. If chest pain recurs, samples should be drawn during the episode, at 12 hours, and again at 24 hours. Total LDH levels should be ordered if an AMI is suspected to have occurred more than 24 hours before admission. LDH isoenzymes should only be ordered if the total LDH is elevated.[35]

Patient teaching

Explain the need for repeated blood samples and their anticipated timing. Explain that the substances being tested are released when part of the heart muscle dies. Also tell the patient that certain levels of these substances in the blood indicate that an AMI or heart attack has occurred. Discuss the rationale for additional testing such as electrocardiograms. Allow the patient and family to verbalize questions or concerns. Further patient teaching concerning risk factors, angina pectoris, and AMI may be appropriate (see Chapters 8, 9, and 10).

Coagulation studies
Background information

Coagulation is an essential protective mechanism. Its primary purpose is maintenance of an adequate circulating blood volume. The process of clot formation is complex and involves many enzymes and other proteins referred to as *clotting factors* (Fig. 6-2). There are two ways to activate the final common clotting pathway, which begins with factor X. These are called the *intrinsic* and *extrinsic pathways*. The intrinsic pathway consists of clotting factors that normally circulate in the blood. The pathway is activated when factor XII contacts an abnormal surface. In contrast, activation of the extrinsic pathway requires the release of factor III (tissue thromboplastin) from endothelial or other tissue cells when they become damaged.

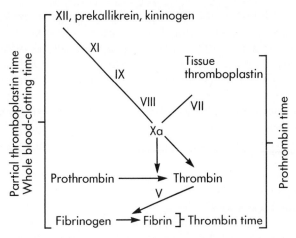

FIG. 6-2   Clotting cascade and coagulation tests. PTT and APTT measure global clotting function and provide information about the intrinsic pathway. The PT measures clotting that occurs via the extrinsic pathway (which begins with tissue thromboplastin).

From Nossel HL: Bleeding. In Isselbacher I et al, editors: Harrison's principles of internal medicine, ed 9, New York, 1980, McGraw-Hill, Inc.

Normally, prompt coagulation is desirable. However, for many cardiovascular disorders, prolongation of the clotting process is recommended to reduce the risk of thromboembolism. Anticoagulants lengthen clotting times by acting on specific factors. Therefore the effects of anticoagulants can be measured by tests that examine the functioning of certain portions of the clotting cascade.

Partial thromboplastin time and activated partial thromboplastin time. Partial thromboplastin time (PTT) and *activated partial thromboplastin time* (APTT) are one-stage clotting tests. These tests measure the same functions and are essentially the same. However, the APTT is a more sensitive test.[21] PTT and APTT detect factor deficiencies and drug interactions in the intrinsic pathway. PTT and APTT are also considered global tests for coagulation because proper functioning of the final common clotting pathway is necessary to achieve clot formation.[30]

Heparin, a commonly used anticoagulant, affects clotting by enhancing the ability of naturally occurring antithrombin III to inactivate thrombin, activated factor IX (IXa), and activated factor X (Xa). The most widely used test for monitoring heparin therapy is the APTT.[51]

Normal values for PTT and APTT depend on the phospholipid and activator reagents used. Thus laboratories usually report a control value with the patient's results. Typically, the PTT is 60 to 85 seconds, and the APTT is 20 to 35 seconds.[37] The recommended APTT for therapeutic anticoagulation is at least 1.5 times the control.[51]

Prothrombin time. Prothombin time (PT) measures the clotting ability of five factors: prothrombin, fibrinogen, and factors V, VII, and X. Because it measures factor VII, the PT can be used to assess the function of the extrinsic pathway. The PT also assesses common pathway function.

Laboratory normals vary, depending on the type of thromboplastin used. Therefore laboratories usually report their normal values with the patient's results. Some laboratories may use a more standardized reporting system adopted by the World Health Organization (WHO) in 1982. This system converts the local PT ratio observed (patient value ÷ laboratory control = local PT ratio) to an International Normalized Ratio (INR) that reflects the result that would have been obtained if the WHO reference thromboplastin had been used to perform the test.[29] Use of this system allows physicians to prescribe anticoagulant therapy consistent with current national and international recommendations.

Coumarin derivatives are commonly used oral anticoagulants. The primary agent used in North America is warfarin sodium.[30] Warfarin and other coumarin derivatives inhibit hepatic synthesis of four vitamin K–dependent clotting factors: II (prothrombin), VII, IX, and X. The PT test uses tissue thromboplastin (factor III) and calcium to activate the extrinsic pathway to produce a clot. Therefore prolongation of the PT may indicate deficiencies of factor VII (extrinsic) and the common pathway factors (prothrombin and factor X) caused by warfarin therapy or other pathway abnormalities such as factor deficiencies related to liver disease. Of course, when pretherapy PT values are normal, subsequent prolongation during warfarin administration usually can be attributed to drug effect.

A normal PT is usually 9.5 to 12 seconds.[37] The Committee on Antithrombotic Therapy of the American College of Chest Physicians (ACCP) and the National Heart, Lung, and Blood Institute (NHLBI) have recommended two levels of oral anticoagulant therapy based on PT results expressed as INR values. The less-intense therapeutic range recommends warfarin administration to achieve an INR of 2.0 to 3.0. This value translates roughly into a PT value of 1.3 to 1.5 times the control value for tests using thromboplastins generally available in North America. The more-intense therapeutic range suggests warfarin dosing to obtain an INR of 3.0 to 4.5, which corresponds approximately with a PT value of 1.5 to 2.0 times the control for tests using North American thromboplastins.[29]

Indications

Coagulation studies (PTT or APTT and PT) are often performed as screening tests before surgery. These tests are also necessary to establish a baseline for anticoagulant therapy. The appropriate tests for adjusting heparin and warfarin administration were discussed previously.

Continuous intravenous heparin administration is used primarily as the initial agent to accomplish anticoagulation in patients requiring oral anticoagulant therapy. Because warfarin and other oral anticoagulants affect coagulation by interfering with clotting factor synthesis, their action is delayed until the factors already present in the plasma are cleared (24 to 48 hours). In contrast, heparin affects co-agulation immediately and directly by enhancing the action of antithrombin III. Therefore patients receive an initial dose of intravenous heparin, followed by a continuous infusion for 5 to 7 days. Oral anticoagulant therapy is started on day 1 or 2.[30]

Continuous intravenous heparin, followed by 3 months of less-intense oral anticoagulant therapy, is indicated for treatment of deep venous thrombosis and pulmonary embolism.[30,69] It is also recommended as a preventative therapy for AMI patients with an increased risk of systemic embolism related to (1) an anterior transmural myocardial infarction (MI), (2) atrial fibrillation, (3) a history of previous systemic emboli or pulmonary embolism, (4) poor left ventricular function, or (5) chronic congestive heart failure (CHF).[54] This type of therapy is also used with thrombolytic agents such as streptokinase and tissue plasminogen activator (tPA). However, the ACCP/NHLBI committee has no recommendation regarding this practice.[15]

Less-intense therapeutic oral anticoagulation without previous heparin administration is indicated for (1) prevention of venous thromboembolism in patients undergoing neurosurgery, major knee surgery, and elective or fractured hip surgery;[30] (2) atrial fibrillation in patients who have experienced a systemic embolism, have mitral valve disease, or have thyrotoxicosis;[20] (3) atrial fibrillation in patients expected to undergo elective cardioversion;[20] (4) rheumatic heart disease and normal sinus rhythm when the left atrial diameter is greater than 5.5 cm;[36] and (5) the first 3 months after tissue valve replacement.[63] More-intense therapeutic oral anticoagulation is recommended only for patients with mechanical prosthetic heart valves or recurrent systemic embolism.[30]

Procedure

PTT, APTT, and PT are usually obtained by peripherial venipuncture using a syringe containing sodium citrate or a blue-top Vacutainer tube, which already contains an appropriate anticoagulant. If a heparin lock, arterial line, or heparinized central intravenous line are used to obtain the sample, a volume of blood equal to the volume contained in the device or tubing distal to the sampling port must be drawn and discarded before obtaining the laboratory sample.

When intravenous heparin therapy is initiated, the PTT or APTT is checked 6 hours after starting the constant infusion and is repeated until the result is consistently 1.5 to 2 times the control value. After the first few days of heparin therapy, the APTT can be obtained daily.[30]

For oral anticoagulant monitoring, PT samples are drawn daily until the desired therapeutic effect is achieved. When overlapping heparin therapy is used, the first PT is drawn 4 hours after the heparin is stopped. After a maintenance dose is determined, the frequency of monitoring depends on physician preference and patient compliance with medication and diet instructions.

Patient teaching

Explain the purpose and expected frequency of the test to the patient and describe heparin and oral anticoagulants as medications that slow the blood's ability to clot. Caution the patient to report bruises and bleeding to the nurse or physician immediately. Explain the importance of adhering to medication instructions and dietary restrictions because many medications and foods can affect the action of oral anticoagulants.

ELECTROCARDIOGRAPHIC STUDIES
Common principles

The electrocardiogram (ECG) was one of the first tests used to diagnose cardiac disorders. Today the ECG remains a major diagnostic tool. The ECG records the electrical activity of the heart as impulses travel through the myocardium. Each impulse causes the cardiac muscle to change its electrical charge through processes known as *depolarization* and *repolarization*.

Resting membrane potential

Electrically charged particles called *ions* exist intracellularly and extracellularly throughout the body in varying concentrations. These variations are created, in part, by the semipermeable nature of cell membranes, which allow certain ions to move freely across them but prevent or slow the movement of others. Thus the cell membrane participates in creating *electrical* and *concentration* gradients for potential ion movement. When conditions permit, ions travel down their concentration gradient (that is, from an area of higher concentration to an area of lower concentration).

In quiescent cardiac cells, differences in membrane permeability and the concentration gradients of sodium ions (Na^+) and potassium ions (K^+) combine to make the inside of the cell more negative than its external environment. This condition is referred to as the *resting membrane potential (RMP)*. Normally the RMP is -90 millivolts (mV). In this state, the K^+ concentration is higher intracellularly, and the concentration of Na^+ is higher extracellularly. Be-

cause the membrane is very permeable to K^+, these ions readily diffuse outward. However, the membrane is less permeable to Na^+. As a result, more K^+ leave the cell than are replaced by Na^+ moving inward. The relatively lower concentration of intracellular cations creates a transmembrane electrical gradient of -80 mV. The remaining -10 mV of the RMP is generated by the sodium-potassium pump. This pump uses adenosine triphosphate (ATP) to actively transport three Na^+ out of the cell while it allows only two K^+ to enter. By actively transporting Na^+ outward, the sodium-potassium pump helps maintain the RMP, creates a Na^+ gradient across the cell membrane, and rids the cell of Na^+ after rapid depolarization.[17]

Action potentials

The rapid changes that occur in the transmembrane potential of cells in response to a stimulus are collectively referred to as an *action potential*. Each action potential can be divided into five phases (Fig. 6-3).

Phase 0: depolarization. According to the *gate theory*, cardiac cell membranes have channels that control the inward flow of ions. These channels are regulated by gating particles known as G proteins.[13] When cardiac cells are stimulated, the *fast sodium channels* open, allowing Na^+ to rapidly diffuse into the cells. This rapid influx of positive ions reduces the negativity of the membrane potential and produces the upstroke of the action potential waveform known as *depolarization*. Optimal opening of the fast sodium channels occurs when the stimulus causes the cell to reach the *threshold potential* (-70 mV). While the fast channels are open, the cell also reaches the threshold for the *slow calcium channels* (-30 to -40 mV), and calcium ions (Ca^{++}) begin to move intracellularly.

As Na^+ and Ca^{++} rush into the cell, the transmembrane electrical potential reaches zero. However, because a Na^+ concentration gradient still exists, this ion continues to enter the cell until all the Na^+ channels have been depleted or inactivated ($+20$ mV). At this point, depolarization ends.

Phase 1: rapid repolarization. The abrupt closure of the fast sodium channels, combined with outward move-

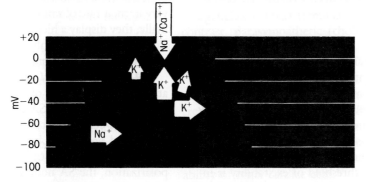

FIG. 6-3 Cardiac action potential. The flow of ions during phases 0 to 4.

permeable to potassium. This results in a rapid efflux of potassium from the cells, causing their membrane potentials to be more negative than normal. Because of this increased negativity, the cells are less excitable. This state is referred to as *hyperpolarization.* Hyperpolarization of SA node cells decreases their rate of discharge and therefore decreases the heart rate. PNS stimulation also slows the rate of impulse conduction from the atria to the ventricles.[43]

Recording conduction

The ECG and other related tests record the differences in electrical potentials between segments of cardiac muscle. Because the measuring probes, called *electrodes,* are not attached directly to the cardiac cells, the wave form recorded differs in appearance from the action potential tracing from an individual cell. The electrocardiographic wave form is the summation of the electrical events occurring throughout the heart.

When cardiac tissue is in a resting state, there is no difference in electrical potential from one segment to another. This period corresponds to the flat baseline, or *isoelectric,* portion of an ECG recording. Depolarization and repolarization of regions of cardiac tissue cause negative or positive deflections on the ECG, depending on the spatial relationship between the recording electrode and the direction of the tissue's electrical transmission. In general, a wave of depolarization advancing toward a positive electrode is recorded as a positive deflection. As a wave of depolarization moves away from a positive electrode, a negative deflection is recorded. In addition, the amount of tissue involved influences the magnitude of the wave form, whereas the rate of conduction influences the width.

ECG waveform

Depolarization of the atria by the SA node impulse produces a small, rounded deflection called the *P wave.* It is normally positive in leads I, II, aV_F, aV_L, V_3, to V_6, but it may be diphasic or inverted in the remaining leads. The P wave usually is not longer than 0.1 second in duration or greater than 3 mm in amplitude. (For information concerning ECG paper time and amplitude measurements, see Appendix B). Widening and notching of the P wave usually are associated with *left atrial enlargement.* Right atrial enlargement, most often secondary to cor pulmonale, tricuspid stenosis, or congenital cardiac disease, produces a characteristic tentlike increase in the P wave amplitude. Inverted P waves most commonly are seen with ectopic atrial or junctional beats.

The time between atrial depolarization and repolarization is electrically quiet, and no deflection is observed. An *isoelectric,* or straight, line is recorded by the ECG. Simultaneous with the end of atrial depolarization and before atrial repolarization, the electrical wave is carried through the AV junction to the ventricles. The speed of interventricular conduction contributes to the concurrent timing of atrial repolarization and ventricular depolarization. The larger forces associated with ventricular activity overshadow the forces of atrial repolarization, and thus only ventricular depolarization is recorded. The time from the beginning of atrial depolarization to the beginning of ventricular depolarization is called the *PR interval.* From the beginning of the P wave to the beginning of the ventricular complex, the total duration of the PR interval ranges from 0.12 to 0.2 second.

Ventricular depolarization inscribes a triphasic deflection on the ECG: the QRS complex (Fig. 6-6). The initial negative deflection, the *Q wave,* is related to the reversal of cardiac force from the predominantly right-to-left orientation as interventricular activation begins on the left side of the septum and spreads from left to right. The diagnosis of a transmural MI is based on the presence of *significant Q waves,* that is, a Q wave amplitude that is a fourth or greater than the height of the R wave or a QS

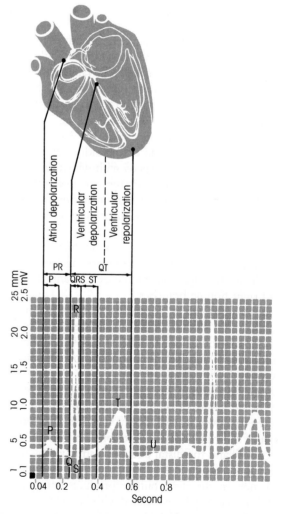

FIG. 6-6 Electrical impulse conduction as recorded by ECG.
From Gary LC and Guzzetta CE: Cardiac monitoring and dysrhymias. In Dossey BM, Guzzetta CE, and Kenner CV, editors: critical care nursing: body-mind-spirit, ed 3, Philadelphia, 1992, JB Lippincott & Co.

configuration. Because Q waves may be found routinely in many leads, a final decision about their significance is impossible unless it is correlated with the patient's clinical history and physical examination.

Septal depolarization is followed by activation of the large free left ventricular wall, and cardiac forces again are directed toward the left, producing a large positive deflection on the ECG, the *R wave*. The last portion of the ventricle to be depolarized is the base, which lies superiorly and to the right. Forces again are directed to the right, producing the second negative deflection, the *S wave*. Regardless of whether the ventricular complex is composed of two or three waves, *QRS* is a generic term used to describe a wide range of ventricular patterns. In describing the morphology of a particular QRS complex, lowercase letters denote small waves, and capital letters indicate large waves. If more than one positive wave is present, the second wave is labeled *R or r prime (R′ or r′)*. Some possible QRS descriptions are qRs, QS, or RSr′.

The QRS duration is measured from the end of the PR interval to the beginning of the ST segment and ranges from 0.06 to 0.10 second. The amplitude and morphology of the QRS complex corresponds with the particular lead being examined and the patient's age and clinical conditions, particularly those that increase the distance of the electrode from the heart, such as emphysema or obesity. A QRS amplitude of less than 5 mm in the bipolar limb leads is abnormal. In the precordial leads the amplitude of the R waves becomes progressively larger from V_1 to V_6. A total QRS amplitude (obtained by subtracting the value of any negative deflection from that of the positive deflection) of greater than 25 mm in the precordial leads indicates *ventricular hypertrophy*.

There is a period of electrical quiet, similar to that observed in the atria, between ventricular depolarization and repolarization. The isoelectric line associated with that stage is the *ST segment*. The point at which the ST segment takes off from the ventricular complex is the *J point*. Myocardial ischemia displaces the ST segment. ST segment depression greater than 0.5 mm or ST elevation greater than 1 mm indicates myocardial ischemia.

Ventricular repolarization produces the *T wave*, a rounded deflection slightly larger than the P wave. The pattern of repolarization causes the T wave to be upright in most leads. T waves usually are not taller than 5 mm in the standard limb leads or 10 mm in the precordial leads. Abnormally tall (hyperacute) T waves are associated with AMI and hyperkalemia.

The *U wave* is a small, rounded deflection that directly follows the T wave and is thought to represent an after-depolarization of a papillary muscle. The U wave's polarity is the same as that of the T wave, and the normal amplitude of the U wave usually is not greater than a fourth that of the T wave. U waves are more prominent at slower heart rates and become more apparent when hypokalemia is present.

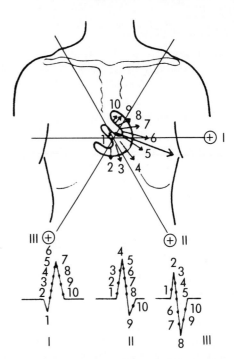

FIG. 6-7   Relationship of QRS configuration to ECG lead. Initial depolarization of the ventricular septum *(1)* moves away from the positive electrode of lead I, resulting in a negative deflection, and toward the positive electrode of lead III, resulting in a positive deflection. The sequence of ventricular depolarization and its relationship to the QRS in leads I, II, and III are also shown.

Adapted from Conover MB: Understanding electrocardiography: arrhythmias and the 12-lead ECG, ed 5, St Louis, 1988, The CV Mosby Co.

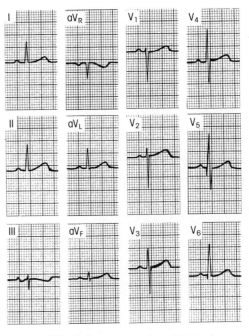

FIG. 6-8   Normal 12-lead ECG.

Twelve-lead ECG

Background Information

A standard ECG consists of three bipolar limb leads (leads I, II, and III), three unipolar limb leads (aV$_R$, aV$_L$, and aV$_F$), and six unipolar chest (precordial) leads (V$_1$ to V$_6$). Limb leads record electrical potential from the frontal plane and precordial leads from the horizontal plane.

The morphologic characteristics of the ECG complex in each lead are directly related to the orientation of each lead to the wave of depolarization as it courses through the cardiac chambers (Fig. 6-7). Based on an understanding of the normalcy of each lead, evaluation of all 12 leads allows the nurse to assess the individual's cardiac status more precisely (Fig. 6-8).

Bipolar leads (standard limb leads). The bipolar leads—leads I, II, and III—record the potential between two points on the body. Lead I connects the right shoulder and the left shoulder; lead II connects the right shoulder and left leg; and lead III connects the left shoulder and left leg. Because of the right-to-left cephalocaudal orientation of the wave of depolarization, the QRS complexes are upright in the bipolar limb leads, except for the presence of a nonsignificant q wave recording initial left-to-right depolarization of the interventricular septum. Because lead II parallels the wave of depolarization, complexes are taller than those of the other leads (Fig. 6-9, *A* and *B*).

Unipolar limb leads. The unipolar, or *augmented*, limb leads, aV$_R$, aV$_L$, and aV$_F$, record the potential in only one direction, toward the lead. By having all connections except the recording electrode grounded into a central terminal,

only one pole of the lead axis is recorded. Because of their low amplitude, the ECG recorder augments the deflections 1.5 times, as denoted by the prefix a in the lead names. The QRS complex is negative in aV$_R$ because the wave of depolarization travels away from that lead (Fig. 6-9, *C*). Generally, biphasic deflections may be seen in aV$_L$, and aV$_F$ records positive deflections as the wave of depolarization advances toward the positive pole. A small q wave showing left-to-right depolarization of the interventricular septum is normal in aV$_F$.

Precordial leads. The precordial leads are six unipolar chest leads placed in these locations on the chest wall:

V$_1$ Fourth intercostal space, right sternal border
V$_2$ Fourth intercostal space, left sternal border
V$_3$ Halfway between V$_2$ and V$_4$
V$_4$ Fifth intercostal space, midclavicular line
V$_5$, V$_6$ Fifth intercostal space in the anterior and midaxillary lines, respectively

Precordial leads record electrical potential in the horizontal plane (Fig. 6-10). V$_1$ and V$_2$ usually reflect a small r wave of initial left-to-right ventricular activation, but because the bulk of the depolarizing forces are directed

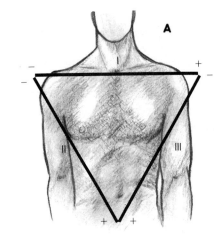

FIG. 6-9 Hexaxial reference system. Constructing the hexaxial reference system. **A,** The bipolar limb leads I, II, and III form Einthoven's triangle. **B,** The triaxial system is formed by intersecting leads I, II, and III at their midpoints. **C,** The orientation of the unipolar limb leads aV$_R$, aV$_L$, and aV$_F$. **D,** The hexaxial reference system with the polarity and electrical value of each lead axis indicated.

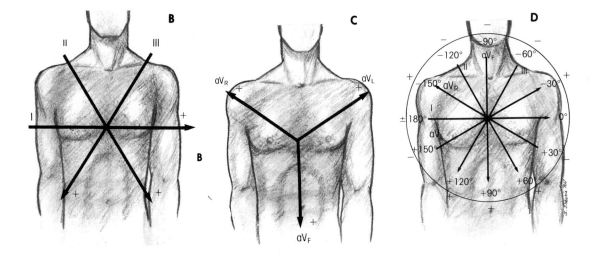

away from these leads, toward the left ventricle, a deep S wave follows (Fig. 6-8). The height and depth of the R and S waves in V_3 and V_4 are equal, with no q wave present. Initial left-to-right ventricular activation is recorded in V_5 and V_6 as a small q wave, followed by a tall R wave representing the large forces directed toward the left ventricle. Terminal depolarization of the basal portions of the ventricles shifts the depolarization forces to the right and inscribes a small s wave after the R wave.

Electrical axis. A *vector* is a force that has magnitude and direction.[16] The wave of depolarization produces many electrical forces of varying magnitude and direction; each one is an instantaneous vector. The *mean instantaneous vector* is the overall direction of the wave of depolarization, and its direction can be determined by calculating the electrical axis.

Hexaxial reference system. The hexaxial reference system is used to calculate the electrical axis. It is constructed by intersecting the midpoints of the axes of leads I, II, and III and then superimposing the axes of the unipolar leads aV_R, aV_L, and aV_F.

Each pole of any lead has a value of 30 degrees; all poles above lead I are negative in value, and all poles below lead I are positive (Fig. 6-9, *D*). A *normal axis* lies between 0 and +90 degrees; *left axis deviation* (LAD) lies in the 0 to −90 degree range, and *right axis deviation* (RAD) is in the +90 to ±180 degree range. An indeterminate or extreme right axis deviation (ERAD) is −90 to ±180 degrees.

Calculating axis. Because the four quadrants of the hexaxial reference system are found by the intersection of leads I and aV_F, an immediate determination of the general orientation of the axis can be made by examining the ECG complexes in only those two leads. With this simplified method of determining the electrical axis, the axis is normal when the QRS complexes are positive in leads I and aV_F. A positive complex in lead I and a negative complex in aV_F indicate a LAD (Fig. 6-11). A *negative* complex in lead I and a *negative* complex in aV_F indicate a ERAD, and a *positive* complex in aV_F and *negative* complex in lead I indicate a RAD in the +90 to ±180 degree range (Fig. 6-12). Although this approach provides a simple method for determining the general orientation of the electrical axis, a more precise calculation involves some additional steps.

To calculate axis to within 30 degrees:[43]

1. Determine the appropriate quadrant of the hexaxial reference system by looking at leads I and aV_F. Examine the QRS wave forms in both leads. For each lead, choose one QRS complex that best represents the majority of QRS complexes recorded in that lead. Subtract the number of small blocks on the ECG paper below the isoelectric line from the number of small blocks above this line.

   a. Lead I. A positive result (that is a predominantly positive QRS) indicates that the vector is to the left. A negative result or negative QRS indicates that the vector is to the right.

   b. aV_F. A positive result or a positive QRS complex indicates that the vector is inferior. A negative result or a negative QRS complex indicates that the vector is superior.

   c. Combine the information from leads I and aV_F to identify the proper quadrant.

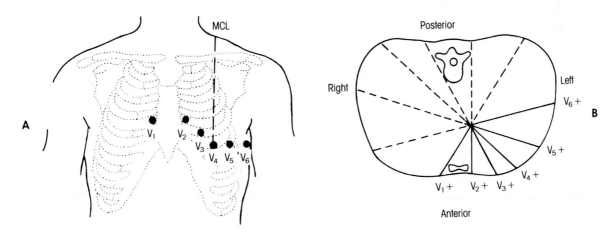

FIG. 6-10 Electrode positions of the chest (precordial) leads. **A**, V_1—fourth intercostal space to the right of the sternum; V_2—fourth intercostal space at the left sternal border; V_3— halfway between V_2 and V_4; V_4—fifth intercostal space at the midclavicular line; V_5—anterior midaxillary line directly lateral to V_4; V_6—midaxillary line directly lateral to V_5. **B**, Precordial reference figure—V_1 and V_2 are right-sided precordial leads; V_3 and V_4 are midprecordial leads; and V_5 and V_6 are left-sided precordial leads.

Adapted from Andreoli KG and others: Comprehensive cardiac care: a textbook for nurses, physicians and other health practitioners, ed 5, St Louis, 1987, The CV Mosby Co.

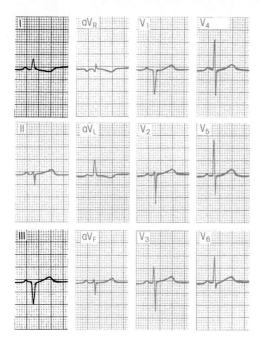

FIG. 6-11   Left axis deviation.

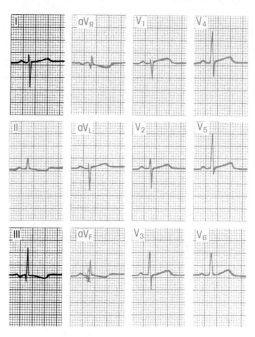

FIG. 6-12   Right axis deviation.

2. Identify the most equiphasic or isoelectric QRS from leads I through aV$_F$. (Hint: It is the lead with the result closest to zero using the subtraction method described in Step 1.)

3. Select the lead that is perpendicular to the lead identified in Step 2. (Hint: Lead I is perpendicular to lead aV$_F$, lead II is perpendicular to lead aV$_L$, and lead III is perpendicular to lead aV$_R$). This lead should have the tallest QRS complex (net height − positive or negative). If not, double check Steps 1 to 3. If the tallest QRS is still not the lead perpendicular to the most isoelectric lead, the true mean QRS axis lies between the perpendicular lead and the lead with the largest QRS complex.

4. Note the degrees of axis for the portion of the lead selected in Step 3 that corresponds with the quadrant identified in Step 1.

For example:
1. *Figure 6-8:*
   a. Step 1a = positive, left. Step 1b = positive, inferior. Step 1c = left inferior quadrant, normal axis.
   b. Step 2 = aV$_F$.
   c. Step 3 = lead I is perpendicular to aV$_F$, but lead II is taller, therefore the true mean QRS axis lies between leads I and II.
   d. Step 4 = +30 degrees is between leads I and II in the left inferior quadrant (normal axis).
2. *Figure 6-11.*
   a. Step 1a = positive, left. Step 1b = negative, superior. Step 1c = left superior quadrant, left axis deviation.

   b. Step 2 = aV$_R$.
   c. Step 3 = lead III is perpendicular to aV$_R$; it also has the tallest (largest-amplitude) QRS complex.
   d. Step 4 = −60 degrees is in the left superior quadrant (LAD).
3. *Figure 6-12.*
   a. Step 1a = negative, right. Step 1b = positive, inferior. Step 1c = right inferior quadrant, right axis deviation.
   b. Step 2 = aV$_R$.
   c. Step 3 = lead III is perpendicular to aV$_R$; it also has the tallest QRS complex.
   d. Step 4 = +120 degrees is in the right inferior quadrant (RAD).

The most frequently calculated axis is the mean QRS vector. However, the electrical axis of P and T waves can also be determined using the same general steps by substituting the wave form of interest for the QRS as it appears in the instructions.

Both structural and electrical conduction disturbances can cause changes in axis. Because axis is the mean vector of depolarization, changes in the size and thickness of cardiac structures, such as atrial enlargement and ventricular hypertrophy, can affect the electrical axis. An MI alters the QRS axis because the necrotic area no longer conducts electrical impulses. This allows the instantaneous vectors of the remaining electrically active tissue to exert a greater-than-normal influence on the mean vector. Displacement of the entire heart by tumors, fat, fluid, an elevated diaphragm, and other mechanisms can change the electrical axis. In these instances, conduction through cardiac tissue may be normal, but the position of the heart in relation to the standard 12-lead ECG electrodes is abnormal. Abnormal ventricular conduction is another, more common cause of axis deviation.

Intraventricular conduction defects. *Intraventricular conduction defects* are disorders of the bundle of His and its branches. They frequently are associated with AMI and in these instances may be temporary or permanent. Many cardiac drugs affect the refractoriness of the conduction system in general and the intraventricular system in particular. Other factors that contribute to bundle branch blocks and hemiblocks include valvular disease, congenital anomalies, ventricular hypertrophy, primary myocardial disease, infective cardiac disease, and atherosclerotic disease of the conduction system.

Loss of any segment of the intraventricular conduction system is associated with decreased conduction velocity as the wave of depolarization spreads through slower conducting muscle in the area normally supplied by the blocked bundle. Some prolongation of the QRS complex is expected. *Complete bundle branch block* of either bundle branch is confirmed when the QRS duration is greater than 0.12 second. When the QRS is between 0.1 and 0.12 second, *incomplete bundle branch block* is present.

In addition to a wider total QRS complex, a late *intrinsicoid deflection* is inscribed. A late intrinsicoid deflection is a reflection of the time taken for the activation wave to reach the epicardial surface under the recording electrode. It is measured from the beginning of the ventricular complex to the peak of the R wave.[17] Right bundle branch blocks and left bundle branch blocks are associated with secondary ST and T wave changes; that is, the ST segment and T wave are directed opposite to the direction of the QRS complex. Intraventricular conduction defects usually are accompanied by a RAD or LAD as terminal forces activate the area of myocardium normally supplied by the blocked conduction segment.

RIGHT BUNDLE BRANCH BLOCK. Right bundle branch block (RBBB) does not interfere with the initial left-to-right direction of the depolarizing force in the ventricles. Because left ventricular activation time remains normal, the *intrinsicoid deflection* in the left precordial leads (V_5 and V_6) occurs on time. Late activation of the right ventricle, as depolarizing forces spread from the left ventricle through the septum, produces a *late intrinsicoid deflection* in the right precordial leads (V_1 and V_2) and, in most cases, a RAD. Asynchronous activation of the ventricles results in a secondary component to the ventricular complex in the right precordial leads. Called an R′ wave, the ventricular complexes in RBBB may take a variety of shapes, including rsr′, rSR′, rR′, or the M-shaped pattern usually cited in describing RBBB in V_1 and V_2 (Fig. 6-13).

In the left precordial leads, V_5 and V_6, the initial q wave is preserved, the intrinsicoid deflection is normal, but the S wave is widened because of the delayed right ventricular activation. Lead I also shows a wide S wave.

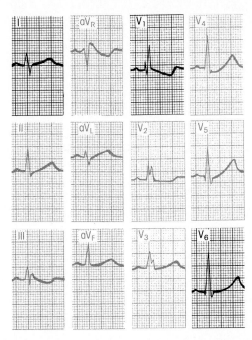

FIG. 6-13 Right bundle branch block. The right precordial leads demonstrate the characteristic M-shaped pattern. The duration of the QRS complex is less than 0.12 seconds, indicating the block is incomplete.

A RBBB commonly is seen in normal and diseased hearts and, because of the extensive conducting tissue remaining, generally is accorded little significance.

LEFT BUNDLE BRANCH BLOCK. Block of the main left bundle (LBBB) disrupts the normal left-to-right activation pattern of the ventricles. The depolarizing force instead travels down the right bundle and follows a right-to-left direction as it spreads through the interventicular septum to the left ventricle. In lead V_1, this altered activation pattern causes loss or reduction of the r wave and a wide, predominately negative ventricular complex. The most common QRS morphologic characteristic in lead V_1 is QS. In the left precordial leads, V_5 and V_6, the initial q waves are absent, and the main QRS deflection is wide and notched with a late intrinsicoid deflection. Q waves are also absent in lead I and aV$_L$, with a broad, notched R wave (Fig. 6-14). Because the terminal ventricular forces are directed to the left, LAD is usually present.

The distinctive QS complex in lead V_1 and the wide, notched R waves in leads I and V_6 are the hallmarks of LBBB. Therefore leads I, V_1, and V_6 can be examined to differentiate between LBBB and RBBB.

An LBBB can easily mask the ECG signs of an anterior infarction. The presence of q waves in V_5 and V_6 with a concomitant LBBB strongly suggests an underlying acute myocardial process.

HEMIBLOCKS. A block occurring in either fascicle of the left bundle is known as a *hemiblock*. Involvement of the anterosuperior fascicle is called a *left anterior hemiblock (LAH),* and block of the posteroinferior fascicle is called a *left posterior hemiblock (LPH)*. Left ventricular activation

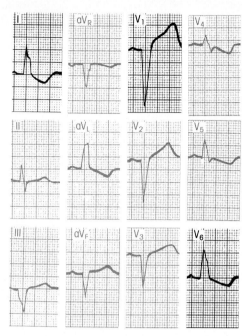

FIG. 6-14 Left bundle branch block. The wide QRS complexes are obvious in the left precordial leads. There is a QS complex in V_1, and an absence of normal q waves in V_5 and V_6.

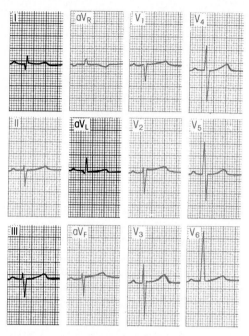

FIG. 6-15 Left anterior hemiblock. There is a small q wave in lead I and a small r in lead III. The duration of the QRS complex is normal. The axis is shifted to the left.

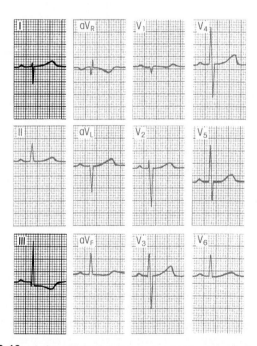

FIG. 6-16 Left posterior hemiblock. Lead I shows a small r and deep S wave. Lead III shows a small q and tall R wave. The axis is shifted to the right.

is a product of simultaneous depolarization of both fascicles. Block of either division of the left bundle shifts the terminal QRS forces in the direction of the division blocked, resulting in an axis deviation.

Because the anterosuperior fascicle is believed to be contiguous with the bifurcating bundle, an LAH frequently is associated with a RBBB. The anterosuperior fascicle lies in the left ventricular outflow tract, is less diffuse than the posteroinferior fascicle, and receives its blood supply from only the LAD coronary artery; all three factors contribute to its friable nature. On the ECG an LAH is diagnosed by a small *q* wave in lead I and an rS pattern in lead III (Fig 6-15). The axis is shifted to the left, usually at least −60 degrees. The QRS may be normal in duration.

When the anterosuperior division is blocked, initial activation forces are directed to the right through the posteroinferior division, but terminal forces move toward the left because the area normally depolarized by the anterosuperior fascicle is stimulated by the propagated wave front. The *q* waves in the anterior leads produced by an LAH can mimic the pattern of an anterior infarction. An LAH most often is associated with an anterior infarction and by itself is not significant because of the extensive conduction tissue remaining.

The posteroinferior fascicle receives a dual blood supply from the right coronary and the left circumflex coronary arteries and is a much more diffuse system than the anterosuperior fascicle. Although these factors probably contribute to the lower incidence of posteroinferior block, its occurrence should be accorded more significance. Because intraventricular conduction is supported only by the un-

certain anterosuperior division, a combination of new RBBB and LPH requires constant vigilance.

When conduction through the posteroinferior fascicle is blocked, initial forces are directed leftward, through the anterosuperior division, inscribing a small *r* in lead I and a small *q* in lead III (Fig. 6-16). Subsequently the activation wave spreads rightward to the area normally supplied by the posterior fascicle. Lead I shows a deep S wave, and lead III shows a tall R wave. The rightward spread of terminal forces is associated with a RAD, usually about +120 degrees. The pattern of LPH may be misdiagnosed as an anterior infarction. By itself, an LPH does not require supportive therapy. When RBBB and LPH are present, the patient must be monitored closely for signs of antero-superior involvement (e.g., development of a concomitant, first-degree AV heart block) or complete involvement indicating third-degree AV heart block.

Indications

A patient admitted with a known or suspected cardiac problem routinely has at least one ECG. Any episode of suspicious chest pain or other indications of angina pectoris or MI necessitates an ECG during and after the episode (see Chapters 9 and 10). Certain ECG changes, such as symmetric and deeply inverted T waves and negative T waves in V_2 and V_3, are sensitive indicators of left main coronary artery disease.[48] Most people admitted to hospitals or clinics for surgery have an ECG to screen for conditions that could cause problems during or after surgery. Other common indications for an ECG are cardiac drug therapy, rhythm and conduction disturbances, electrolyte imbalances and therapy, hemodialysis or peritoneal dialysis, trauma patient evaluation, and workups before and after cardiac surgery.[47,59]

Procedure

If possible, the patient should lie supine on a bed or examination table. The chest should be exposed, and very hairy areas should be shaved to reduce the resistance to current flow into the electrode. The skin should be dry and clean. Skin areas where the electrodes will be placed are cleaned with alcohol sponges and sometimes lightly rubbed with fine sandpaper or gauze to improve conduction by removing surface skin cell debris. Furthermore, if serial ECGs are required, the chest should be marked so that the same site is consistently used for chest leads. ECG changes that occur between recordings can then be correctly attributed to the heart and not to a change in lead position.

The patient should be comfortable, and shivering should be stopped before the ECG because muscle tremors produce their own electrical current, which make the ECG difficult to interpret. The correct electrodes must be placed on their respective limbs because misplacement causes incorrect interpretations. If the patient has an amputated limb the electrode should be placed on the stump.

After the leads are in place, the recording can begin. The ECG normally takes about 5 minutes and can be performed by physicians, nurses, or technicians. The date, time, patient name, and room should be recorded on the ECG itself. Any other valuable information that the phy-

sician may find useful in interpreting the ECG, such as chest pain, palpitations perceived by the patient, special medication, or treatments during the ECG,[47] should also be recorded.

Patient teaching

Tell the patient that the electrical recordings will not cause discomfort and that there is no danger of electrocution. Encourage the patient to ask questions before recording begins, because talking increases the heart rate and may also cause artifacts on the recording.

Ambulatory electrocardiography
Background information

The term *ambulatory electrocardiogram* (ambulatory ECG) refers to a wide variety of continuous and intermittent ECG recording procedures. All ambulatory ECG methods record time intervals longer than those of the standard 12-lead ECG and are intended to record cardiac electrical activity as patients participate in normal daily routines. Unlike the standard 12-lead ECG, ambulatory devices usually only record one or two leads.

Continuous recorders. Continuous ambulatory ECG monitors use tape or semiconductor computer-chip memory to record cardiac electrical events. The tape recorder monitors use magnetic tape cassettes or reels and record at very slow speeds. Timing accuracy depends on the precision of the motor drive and the recording of time signals with the ECG.[33] Digital recording monitors store digitalized and encoded ECG information on semiconductor computer chips. These devices are more compact, have no moving parts, and require less energy to run.

Tape-system, 24-hour recordings can be scanned in 15 to 30 minutes for heart rate, QRS configuration, and dysrhythmias. Reports include heart rate graphs and frequency distributions of dysrhythmias. Segments of particular interest, such as dysrhythmias, can be printed on ECG graph paper for further analysis. Some systems also provide "full disclosure," which is a compressed printout of every QRS complex that occurred during the recording period. This type of report allows evaluation of isolated premature ventricular complexes (PVCs), sequences of PVCs, and ventricular tachycardia, as well as the initiation and termination of other dysrhythmias.

Intermittent recorders. Intermittent ambulatory ECG monitors record short segments of data. They are activated by the patient at the onset of the symptoms being investigated. The most important type of intermittent recorders are those with transtelephonic capability. Transtelephonic monitors can transmit the patient's recorded ECG over standard telephone lines to a physician's office, hospital, or other interpretation facility. This type of device is especially useful when the events being studied occur infrequently.

Indications

One of the primary and most widely accepted purposes of ambulatory ECG monitoring is evaluation of symptoms such as palpitations, dizziness, and syncope, which may be related to dysrhythmias or cardiovascular dysfunction.[33] Ambulatory ECGs also allow examination of beat-to-beat changes in heart rate (R-R intervals) and therefore aid in the diagnosis of certain conditions such as sleep apnea.[25]

The 24-hour recordings also help in evaluating pacemaker function. Monitors that record the pacing stimulus artifact on a separate channel from the ECG facilitate this type of analysis. Ambulatory ECGs are a widely accepted method of investigating pacemaker-mediated tachycardia, evaluating the effectiveness of antitachycardia pacing, and analyzing the function of rate-responsive physiologic pacing.[33]

Ambulatory ECGs can also be used to assess the risk of future cardiac dysrhythmias in symptomatic and asymptomatic patients. Patients with known coronary artery disease (CAD) and ventricular dysfunction who have frequent PVCs or complex ventricular dysrhythmias are at higher risk for future cardiac events.[58] Patients who have had a myocardial infarction and patients who have idiopathic hypertrophic cardiomyopathy with ventricular ectopy are also at increased risk for future dysrhythmias and can benefit from early identification.[38,57]

Ambulatory ECGs are also ordered for less common indications such as evaluation of antidysrhythmic or antianginal medication efficacy, Wolff-Parkinson-White syndrome, and prolonged QT syndrome. Although 24-hour ECG recordings generally are indicated for patients suspected to have Prinzmetal's angina, the use of ambulatory monitoring to evaluate angina pectoris is somewhat controversial. Because ST segment morphologic characteristics can be altered by many physiologic events other than ischemia, including postural changes, tachycardia, and hyperventilation, the specificity of ambulatory ECG changes in the ST segment in diagnosing or evaluating angina pectoris is still under investigation.[33]

Procedure

An ambulatory ECG can be an inpatient or outpatient procedure. The patient's chest is prepared as for other ECG-related studies, and three to five electrodes are attached and secured with tape. The electrodes are connected via a cable to the recorder, which is slightly larger than a transister radio. Usually, the recorder is carried on a shoulder strap or belt loop. The patient is given a diary card and is instructed to record important activities and symptoms. The patient should also be instructed to denote symptoms by pushing the marker button on the monitor and noting this action in the diary. If the recorder has a visible clock, the patient should use this clock for timing diary entries. Important activities to note include shaving, sexual activity, exercise, and defecation.

The monitor records one or two leads simultaneously. Usually V_5 and either V_1 or lead II are used.[59] When the monitoring period is completed, the patient returns the device for analysis of the recordings.

Patient teaching

Emphasize that the patient should continue all normal daily activities, including work, household chores, and exercise, while wearing or using the monitor. Because monitors are not waterproof, include swimming and tub bathing or showering as exceptions. Stress the importance of completing the diary and using the marker button to indicate symptoms. If the patient is unable to record the necessary data, explain that a hospital staff member or a significant other will need to perform these tasks.

Exercise electrocardiography (stress testing)
Background information

Exercise ECGs, also referred to as *graded exercise tests* (GXTs) or *stress testing*, have been a valuable and proven diagnostic tool in detecting and evaluating CAD and the individual's functional capacity to work or exercise. The principle of GXTs is to assess the ability of the coronary arteries to supply adequate blood flow to the heart during periods of increased myocardial oxygen demand generated by increased physical activity. This test also directly evaluates the ability of the heart to increase the rate (chronotropism) appropriately and indirectly evaluates its ability to appropriately increase the intramyocardial oxygen tension, the force of contraction, and stroke volume of the left ventricle.[59] (Also see Figure 9-3.)

The test has some risks; however, if it is done properly with appropriately trained personnel, the incidence of AMI or serious dysrhythmias during or immediately after the test is 2.4 in 10,000 tests. The mortality rate is 1 in 10,000 tests.[59,68]

As with most tests GXT is not perfect, especially in regard to detecting CAD in persons with no symptoms of CAD; the percentage of false test results is as high as 65% in one study.[12] Women are as much as 4.5 times more likely to have a false-positive result than men, and men were reported to be only 2.8 times as likely to have a false-negative.[12] (*False positive* means that the GXT test was positive for CAD, although angiography was negative for CAD. *False negative* means that the GXT did not indicate CAD, whereas the angiogram proved the presence of CAD.) Thus GXT is more accurate for men (88% of true-positive tests) than for women (46% of true-positive tests).[59] The reason for this is not known. Because of this variance, physicians may order a combined GXT and a nuclear scan if the GXT is positive or questionably negative. Combined testing is the preferred procedure for evaluating women suspected of having CAD.

Testing protocols. The GXT may consist of a single

exercise level or multiple stages. Single-stage tests, such as the *Master's two-step exercise test,* do not always elicit meaningful data because maximal effort may not be achieved. Multiple-stage tests gradually increase the cardiovascular work load through the use of predetermined protocols. For example, the *Bruce protocol* increases the exertion level every 3 minutes. Like other multiple-stage tests, it also includes warm-up and cool-down periods, intended to reduce the risk of complications such as ventricular tachycardia or fibrillation.

GXT tests are also classified as *maximal* or *submaximal.* Maximal tests are terminated by the onset of symptoms or exhaustion. Submaximal tests end when the patient reaches the target heart rate, usually calculated as 85% of the maximum predicted heart rate for the patient's age and sex.

Exercise modes appropriate for GXT testing include steps, treadmills, and bicycle ergometers. The unit of measurement for work load is METs (1 MET equals the amount of effort required to use 3.5 ml O_2/kg/minute). Most untrained adults who do not have CAD can perform activities requiring 10 or more METs.

Indications

Two of the primary uses of the GXT are detection and confirmation of CAD. Other applications include determination of the prognosis of patients with CAD, evaluation of antianginal therapy and dysrhythmias, analysis of the function of rate-responsive pacemakers, assessment of effort-related symptoms, and determination of the functional level of patients with congestive heart failure or noncoronary cardiovascular disease. One study of 3600 men found that positive GXT results were a stronger predictor of cardiovascular death than abnormal serum lipid levels, a history of smoking, or hypertension.[23] Contraindications for GXT are AMI, unstable angina, acute myocarditis or pericarditis, congestive heart failure, left main coronary artery stenosis, rapid atrial and ventricular dysrhythmias, severe aortic stenosis, uncontrolled hypertension, and advanced AV block.[52]

Procedure

The patient lies on an examining table, and 10 or more electrodes are placed on the chest. Skin preparation is similar to that used for 12-lead ECGs. The electrodes and their cables are taped securely to the body to reduce motion artifact. Sometimes a mesh vest is worn to hold the electrodes in place. Baseline 12-lead ECG and blood pressure measurements are obtained supine, standing, and after 30 to 45 seconds of hyperventilation. A 12-lead ECG taken after hyperventilation is necessary to distinguish T-wave abnormalities caused by this activity and those resulting from ischemia.[17]

The patient then begins the prescribed activity. Continuous recording of at least one lead is performed throughout the test. Periodically, according to the selected protocol, one, three, or more leads are recorded, and blood pressure measurements are obtained. If a multiple-stage protocol is used, the work load is increased after each set of measurements. The patient continues to exercise until the desired end point is reached or one of the following occurs:

1. The patient experiences excessive fatigue, leg pain, dyspnea, dizziness, or exhaustion.
2. There is evidence of progressive ischemia such as chest pain, ST-segment changes, decreased heart rate or blood pressure, or widening of the QRS.
3. Dysrhythmias such as sustained supraventricular tachycardia, frequent PVCs, or ventricular tachycardia occur unless the purpose of the GXT was dysrhythmia evaluation.[52]

After the test has ended, the patient cools down by walking or pedaling slowly. The patient's heart rate, blood pressure, and ECG measurements are monitored until they return to baseline.

Patient teaching

Instruct the patient to have a light meal about 2 hours before the test. Stress the importance of fasting after this time because food in the stomach decreases the blood supply available to the heart and can precipitate nausea and vomiting. Also request that the patient refrain from smoking for at least 2 hours before the test. Depending on the purpose of the test, inform the patient that regularly scheduled medications may need to be omitted. Tell the patient that cardiac medications are frequently omitted when the purpose of the test is to determine the extent of CAD and that medications are not omitted if the GXT is done to assess functional capacity. Drugs that may effect GTX results include digitalis preparations, procainamide, quinidine, nitroglycerin, nifedipine, beta-blockers, and atropine.[52] Also instruct the patient to wear clothes and shoes that will be comfortable during exercise.

Before the test, ask the patient to sign an informed consent form. Instruct the patient to report the development of angina pectoris, leg discomfort, or dyspnea during the test. Finally, emphasize that the patient can stop the test at any time.

AMBULATORY BLOOD PRESSURE MONITORING
Background information

Ambulatory blood pressure monitoring (ABPM) is similar in concept to ambulatory ECG monitoring. As with continuous ambulatory ECG monitoring, a recording of data for up to 24 hours can be obtained. Blood pressure (BP) readings can be measured invasively, via a fine intraarterial catheter inserted in the radial or brachial artery, or noninvasively. The invasive technique records information about beat-to-beat variations in BP. The noninvasive method stores readings at preset intervals during the monitoring period. For example, readings might be obtained every 30 minutes. ABPM differs from ambulatory ECG monitoring in that there are no definitive abnormalities in ABPM. Whereas ambulatory ECG readings can quantify dysrhythmias, ABPM provides frequency distributions of systolic and diastolic pressures or average pressures over time. Pressure data must then be interpreted by the physician to determine its significance.

Noninvasive pressure measurements are obtained via Korotkoff sounds or by oscillometry. Devices using the aucultatory method can be affected by movement artifact picked up by the microphone in the BP cuff. Combining ECG R-wave gating (see p. 149) with pressure monitoring helps eliminate this problem. Machines using the oscillometric approach detect fluctuations in the brachial artery and compute the systolic and diastolic pressures from an algorithm.

BP measurements obtained by invasive or noninvasive ABPM are accurate and reliable.[24,67] Further, average pressures obtained by ABPM are more prognostic of target organ involvement and cardiovascular complications of hypertension than so-called casual readings taken in a physician's office.[19,34] As many as 20% of patients diagnosed as hypertensive on the basis of casual readings have been found to be normotensive outside the physician's office.[50] This phenomenon, referred to as *white-coat hypertension,* results in unnecessary antihypertensive treatment of affected individuals. ABPM may help in discriminating between this phenomenon and hypertension requiring intervention.[19]

Indications

The primary indication for ABPM is diagnosis of hypertension. However, not all patients being evaluated for hypertension require ABPM. Patients who already demonstrate hypertensive effects such as left ventricular hypertrophy, abnormal renal function, or ocular fundal changes do not require ABPM for diagnostic confirmation. ABPM is recommended as a screening tool for individuals diagnosed in the office as having mild-to-moderate hypertension. These patients should also have a negative history of heart disease and no secondary hypertensive changes.[67] ABPM may also help in monitoring the effects of antihypertensive therapy. However, further research is needed in this area.

Procedure

Noninvasive devices are used most commonly in outpatient settings. For noninvasive ABPM, a BP cuff containing a small microphone or sensor is placed around the patient's arm using standard technique. Taping the tubing to the patient's arm just below the cuff, may help in maintaining the proper cuff position. The tubing for inflating and deflating the cuff is attached to the device. Monitors using Korotkoff sounds may also require placement of several

chest ECG electrodes that are connected to the recorder by a cable. The recording device may be carried using a shoulder strap. The patient also receives a diary to record activities and other information during the monitoring period.

Patient teaching

As with ambulatory ECG monitoring, emphasize that the patient should continue all normal daily activities, including work, household chores, and exercise, although strenuous exercise should be avoided because of the motion artifact it may generate. Because the devices are not waterproof, inform the patient that swimming, tub bathing, and showering are contraindicated. Stress completion of the diary by the patient because it gives the physician helpful information for interpreting the test results. If the patient cannot write in the diary, request that a family member assist in this task.

ECHOCARDIOGRAPHY
Background information

Echocardiography is used extensively to diagnose cardiac disorders. It provides a safe, painless, and noninvasive method to obtain valuable information about cardiac cavity dimensions, chamber wall and interventricular septum thicknesses, and motion of valve leaflets and individual segments of the left ventricle during systole and diastole. Systolic, diastolic, and stroke volumes can also be estimated. This information is graphically recorded using time, distance, and ECG references. Echocardiograms frequently are used serially to evaluate therapy or follow disease progression.

A transducer, containing a piezoelectrode crystal, is placed on the chest. The crystal generates a high-frequency sound beam, that can be directed at structures, somewhat like shining a flashlight beam into a dark room. The transducer converts mechanical energy to electrical energy, and vice versa, and can send and receive the sound waves. Sound waves are sent for a brief period, and then the transducer converts to a listening mode to record the sound "echoes" that return when reflected off thoracic structures. This is similar to sonar techniques used to detect ship movements and distances at sea.

Echoes are graphically recorded on paper with a simultaneous ECG lead (usually lead II) for reference to the cardiac cycle. Structures can be viewed from different angles by simply changing the position of the transducer. Cavities filled with fluid do not reflect the waves and usually are represented on the graphic record as empty areas (Fig. 6-17).[59] It is possible to view very specific structures such as the posterior leaflet of the mitral valve in systole or diastole. The pulsed sound waves also can be varied to achieve different objective data such as the flow rates of regurgitant jets.[59]

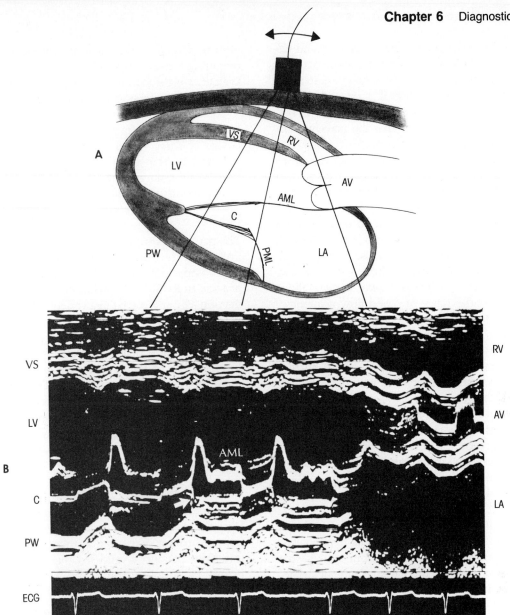

FIG. 6-17 M-mode echocardiography. **A,** Echo transducer on the chest. **B,** The graphic recording. *Arrow* indicates the posterior leaflet of mitral valve. *RV,* Right ventricle; *VS,* ventricular septum; *LV,* left ventricular cavity; *AV,* aortic valve; *AML,* anterior leaflet of mitral valve; *PML,* posterior leaflet of mitral valve; *C,* chordae; *LA,* left atrium; *PW,* left ventricular posterior wall.
From Nanda NC and Gramiak R: Clinical echocardiography, St Louis, 1978, The CV Mosby Co.

Modes. Unidimensional and *two-dimensional* techniques are available.

Unidimensional. The M-mode (motion) portrays the echoes as dots on a vertical axis relative to the distance between it and the transducer; a horizontal axis represents time. The M-mode provides this information on an oscilloscope, and it may be printed on paper. M-mode echocardiograms allow the physician to assess the motion of cardiac structures as they change shape and positions relative to the transducer position during the cardiac cycle.[59,60] However, the M-mode does not depict structures as a whole. M-mode recordings view one very thin cross section over time.

Two-dimensional. Two-dimensional imaging (2D mode) is the foundation of current echocardiographic examination. The image is produced by rapidly sweeping ultrasound signals through an arc and then reconstituting the acquired signals at very high speeds so that all data slices appear as a fan-shaped single image.[60] This mode provides better information concerning the spatial orientation of cardiac structures. Five techniques are used to obtain 2D mode images: the *short-* and *long-axis tomograms, four-chamber cardiac apical image,* and *suprasternal* and *subcostal images.* The subcostal technique is one of the most useful because the lateral orientation allows simultaneous viewing of both mitral valve leaflets.[40]

DOPPLER ECHOCARDIOGRAPHY. Doppler echocardiography is based on the principle that the perceived frequency of a sound varies as the source moves toward or away from the receiver. Because sound waves can be reflected by the cellular elements of the blood, the velocity and direction of blood flow can be determined by the shift in echo frequencies. The *pulsed Doppler mode* allows calculation of blood velocity from an electronically created sample volume. The pulsed Doppler mode provides only intermittent sampling, which limits its use to the quantification of high-velocity jets such as those associated with stenotic valvular lesions. *Continuous-wave Doppler* allows assessment of a broader range of blood flow velocities.[22] *Color Doppler flow mapping* assigns colors to pulsed Doppler–derived flow velocities and superimposes them on a 2D image of the area being investigated. Thus blood flow through the cardiac structures can be observed. Further, color Doppler flow data correlate well with data obtained during cardiac catheterization.[4]

TRANSESOPHAGEAL ECHOCARDIOGRAPHY. Transesophageal echocardiography uses the 2D and color Doppler flow mapping modes to examine cardiac structures, particularly the aortic and mitral valves or their protheses. This approach is especially helpful in evaluating prosthetic valve malfunction in patients with obesity, emphysema, or chest deformities.[45]

The transesophageal transducer is mounted at the tip of an adult gastroscope. After the patient's hypopharynx is topically anesthetized with lidocaine spray, the gastroscopic tube is inserted with the patient lying in the left lateral position. The transducer is oriented anteriorly and positioned in the esophagus against the left atrium. Because the ultrasound waves are not impeded by lung or fat tissue, signal quality is improved. This position also prevents wave attenuation caused by AV valve prostheses.[45] Transesophageal determinations of regurgitation correlate very well with those obtained via cardiac catheterization.[4,45]

Indications

Echocardiography has several advantages. It does not use radiation or create any known biologic hazard. It can also be performed at the bedside and repeated as necessary. In addition, with the exception of the transesophageal approach, echocardiography is painless and noninvasive.

Echocardiograms are used to evaluate disorders of the valves, chambers, and other cardiac structures. They are frequently used to assess valvular function and size. In fact, direct or transesophageal procedures can be used intraoperatively to evaluate mitral valve function.[4] Echocardiograms are also useful in detecting atrial and ventricular masses and thrombi, as well as chamber dilation or hy-

pertrophy. Left ventricular wall motion and aneurysm formation can also be studied. Pericardial disease can also be evaluated via echocardiograms, which are the procedure of choice for assessing pericardial effusions.

Qualitative assessments of cardiac output, stroke volume, and ejection fraction can be made. Although calculations of these values can be performed, they are based on diameters that may not truly reflect global cardiac function. More accurate data for these hemodynamic parameters are obtained from nuclear studies.

Procedure

The patient lies supine in bed or on an examination table. Frequently the head is elevated 30 to 45 degrees. The chest is exposed, and two or three electrodes are attached to provide an ECG. The transducer probe is coated with conduction jelly and placed in a variety of angles and positions as the technician or physician views the echos on a screen. The patient may be asked to change positions or lie on the left side to enable better visualization of certain structures. Key portions of the examination are printed on long or snapshot-size photographic paper. The entire test can also be videotaped for later, detailed examination or comparison. The lights may be dimmed during the procedure to facilitate viewing. Drugs such as amyl nitrite may be given to increase contractility and provide additional data on valve function.

Patient teaching

Know that little preparation is required for this procedure. With the exception of transesophageal studies, patients do not need to fast. Explain that there is little if any discomfort. Give patients a mild sedative and a local anesthetic before transesophageal procedures, if they are ordered.

Instruct all patients to lie still and refrain from talking during the study. Also inform the patients that multiple position changes and transducer probing are routine.

NUCLEAR CARDIOVASCULAR TESTING
Common principles

Nuclear scanning provides several noninvasive methods for assessing cardiovascular disorders. By combining computer programs with scanning techniques, very accurate determinations of cardiac function can be made. In general, these tests involve injecting small amounts radioactive substances via a peripheral venipuncture and then scanning at predetermined time intervals.

Patient teaching

Remember that certain patient teaching information is common to all nuclear cardiovascular tests. First, describe the equipment that patients will see, including the camera scanners. Then emphasize that the tests are not painful. Explain that an intravenous infusion, heparin lock, or single venipuncture may be used to inject the radioactive material. Emphasize that the radiation dose is very small and is usually eliminated from the body within 24 hours. Finally, inform patients that they may need to change positions several times during the test.

Myocardial imaging
Background information

Myocardial imaging detects recent MIs and delineates the extent of tissue involvement. The radionuclide, technetium-99m pyrophosphate, is used in this study because it is taken up by calcium. Cellular necrosis causes high levels of intracellular calcium. Pyrophosphate is therefore taken up by these cells and appears as a *hot spot* when scanning is performed. Normal cardiac tissue does not take up pyrophosphate and does not appear in the scanned image.

There are four degrees of uptake graded from + to + + + +. Subendocardial infarction demonstrates diffuse uptake, + or + +. Transmural infarction causes the myocardium to take up more pyrophosphate than surrounding bone and results in a grading of + + + or + + + +.[59] (See Figure 10-7.)

Several factors influence the sensitivity of test results. The location of the infarction can affect the accuracy of the test. Anterior infarctions are much more easily located than inferior infarctions.[59] Time also can affect the degree of uptake. The scan will be negative if done within 12 hours of the infarction. Uptake peaks 36 hours after the infarction and returns to normal in about 7 to 10 days.[2] Patients whose scans remain positive for 2 to 6 months after the infarction usually have a poor prognosis, probably because of the large amount of infarcted tissue and poor healing. Sometimes old areas of infarction can appear as a hot spot, falsely indicating a new infarction. Infarction size also can affect whether it is detected by this test. An infarct of less than 3 g usually is not detected, and sometimes subendocardial infarctions will not appear.[59]

Indications

This test is indicated when it is difficult to determine by standard enzyme analyses and ECGs whether there has been an AMI. A patient with complete LBBB, equivocal enzyme determination, or a permanent pacemaker or who has just undergone surgery is a typical candidate for this procedure. It also helps in diagnosing a right ventricular infarction, locating a true posterior infarction, assessing cardiac trauma after an injury to the chest, estimating the size of an infarction, especially if the enzymes continue to rise several days after the event, and determining whether an infarction has occurred after cardiac resuscitation.[59] The test is contraindicated in pregnant patients to spare the fetus from exposure to even minute amounts of radiation.[47]

Procedure

The patient receives an injection of about 15 millicuries (mCi) of technetium-99m pyrophosphate in a peripheral vein.[59] After 1½ to 2 hours the patient is taken to the nuclear medicine department where the scan is performed. The patient lies on a hard x-ray table, and a standard scintigraphic camera and scanner measure the uptake in the bone and tissue. The camera is placed close to the chest, and the results are recorded on an instant camera. The areas that take up the substance appear as hot spots on the film, indicating the infarcted tissue, its location, and its size. The left anterior oblique (LAO), left lateral, and anterior positions are usually photographed.[2,59]

If the patient is very ill, some centers do this test at the bedside in the coronary care unit (CCU). For safety, personnel who are pregnant should not participate in this test or care for a patient who has had the test done within the last 24 hours, while minute amounts of radiation are given off by the patient. There is not thought to be any hazard to persons who are not pregnant.[14]

The test is almost 100% accurate for diagnosing transmural infarctions if done 12 hours to 7 days after the infarction. For subendocardial infarction, it is less accurate, at 40% to 90%, depending on the investigator.[2,59]

Patient teaching is the same as for perfusion imaging and blood pool imaging and is covered later.

Perfusion imaging (thallium scanning)
Background information

Thallium-201 is the usual radionuclide substance used to determine perfusion in the myocardium. Methoxy-isobutyl-isonitrile (MIBI), an isonitrile with higher energy and better image resolution properties, may also be used.[53] Evaluation of coronary artery and ventricular function is the most common reason for performing this type of test.

Thallium is in the same group of ions as potassium on the periodic chart and behaves physiologically like potassium in the body. It is actively transported into the healthy myocardial cells through the cell membrane at a rate proportional to regional blood flow.[46] (All muscle cells will take in thallium if there is adequate perfusion, but this discussion only considers the process in healthy myocardial muscle cells.) As thallium enters the body, it begins to give off tiny amounts of radiation from the nucleus. By tracking and measuring this radioactivity, it is possible to pinpoint areas of poor uptake of the isotope, usually signifying poor or no circulation to the area. Myocardial fibrosis, caused by an old MI, also would have a poor uptake of the isotope. Areas that do not take up the thallium well or at all appear as dark spots, or *cold spots,* on the computer composite image. The test also may be performed in conjunction with an exercise test to measure the myocardial perfusion pattern and cell function under stress or maximal performance.[1]

The computer composite shows a doughnut-shaped myocardium. The center of the doughnut is the ventricular cavity, which does not show up well because it is filled with fluid.[59]

Indications

Thallium scanning almost always is used to diagnose or evaluate CAD. It especially helps in the following diagnostic situations[6,10,47,59]:

1. Detecting the presence of early infarction, before enzyme levels rise
2. Evaluating the viability of cardiac tissue adjacent to the infarction
3. Evaluating the functional significance of borderline lesions found during coronary angiography (e.g., if a 50% to 60% obstruction is located, it is used to determine whether the patient should have PTCA or myocardial revascularization or whether there would be no benefit to the remaining cells or the cells in the area supplied by that coronary arterial branch)
4. Evaluating the person with symptoms of angina pectoris and a normal angiogram to assist with evaluation for coronary artery spasm
5. Evaluating the person with symptoms of angina pectoris and an abnormal ECG
6. Evaluating the person's functional capacity after PTCA or myocardial revascularization
7. Evaluating the person who has no symptoms and has a positive GXT
8. Evaluating the extent of CAD, its impact on the coronary circulation, and patient survival
9. Localizing and defining MI

Procedure

If the procedure is to be done on a resting basis, the patient is taken to the nuclear medicine department and given 2 mCi of thallium-201 into an indwelling intravenous line.[59] The γ-scintillation camera is positioned over the patient's chest, and imaging begins within 10 minutes.[10] Thallium is extracted by the cells in large measure during the initial passes through the circulation.[8]

The usual views are anterior and 45- and 70-degree LAO. Some laboratories use the supine, as well.[40,59,72] Computer-assisted scanning allows the myocardium to be recorded "in motion," and documentation of akinesia, dyskinesia, and hypokinesia of localized myocardium can be done, based on the amount of thallium-poor areas, which signal infarction or ischemia (Fig. 6-18). The results are recorded on film or videotape.

If the test is done in conjunction with exercise, the patient is prepared in the usual manner. An intravenous infusion is started, and the patient exercises according to one of the protocols (usually the Bruce) or pedals a modified bicycle while lying on the x-ray table.[7] After the patient reaches exhaustion or develops angina pectoris, the injection of thallium-201 is given through the intravenous line. Exercise is continued, if possible, for another 30 to 60 seconds to allow the circulation to distribute the thallium-201. The patient then is taken off the treadmill or bicycle, and imaging begins no later than 10 minutes after the exercise has ceased.

If a cold spot, signifying a defect in perfusion, is seen, another scan must be done to determine whether the defect represents a scar or ischemic tissue.[72] This process is called *redistribution analysis*. Although 85% to 90% of thallium is extracted by the myocardium on the first pass, the radionuclide does not remain fixed to the cells. After the initial pass, thallium is continuously exchanged between normally perfused myocadial cells and the pool of thallium circulating in the bloodstream. Areas that are ischemic during exercise but receive adequate bloodflow at rest will take up the radionuclide, depending on the bloodflow they receive. If a cold spot or defect resolves when the patient

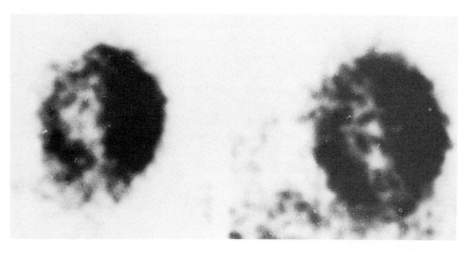

FIG. 6-18 Exercise (stress) thallium scanning. The left image taken soon after exercise shows a large *cold spot* indicating a perfusion defect. The right image, obtained 4 hours later, shows that the defect has resolved, indicating reversible ischemia.

Adapted from Sanderson R and Kurth C: The cardiac patient: a comprehensive approach, ed 2, Philadelphia, 1983, WB Saunders Co.

receives the second scan 2½ to 4 hours after initial testing, the area is considered to have undergone redistribution (Fig. 6-18). Thus redistribution identifies regions of myocardium supplied by narrowed arteries, whereas unresolved defects indicate scar tissue from an MI. Depending on the study, this test is 80% to 95% accurate for documenting CAD and cardiac function.

If patients are unable to exercise because of claudication or other physical disabilities, thallium can be administered during the peak vasodilatory effect of an intravenous injection of dipyridamole. Scanning is performed approximately 10 minutes later. In this case, thallium is redistributed to viable but normally underperfused tissue. The sensitivity and specificity of this method is comparable to thallium exercise scintigraphy.[6]

Blood pool imaging (radionuclide angiography)

Background information

Blood pool imaging differs from myocardial and perfusion imaging in that the isotope stays in the bloodstream and is not picked up by myocardial tissue. Determinations can be made of blood volumes by a computer-assisted γ-camera. Technetium pertechnetate commonly is used for this test because it attaches to the red blood cell and remains in the circulation for several hours. Other substances that may be used are technetium-tagged albumin or red blood cells. Both versions of the procedure—the *first pass* and the *multiple-gated acquisition (MUGA) scan*—are used to determine ejection fractions and ventricular functional ability. The test is quite accurate and involves little risk to the patient.

Indications

The test is used to determine cardiac function in patients with CAD, valvular disease, or MI. Blood pool imaging can be used to predict survival of MI patients based on ejection fraction determinations. Sequential studies can assist in determining the optimal time for valve replacement.[22] It also can be used to measure the effect of medications that increase the pumping ability of the myocardium.

Procedure

First pass scan. The patient is intravenously infused with a bolus of the radionuclide substance into a peripheral vein over a calculated period. Radioactivity counts are recorded rapidly by the γ-camera as the substance passes through the right side of the heart, pulmonary artery and veins, left atrium and ventricle, and out of the aorta. Each chamber can be identified by the computer and scanner.

The ejection fraction is calculated from the counts for systole and diastole. Higher counts are obtained in diastole because there is more blood and hence more isotopes in the ventricular chamber during this part of the cardiac cycle. When the blood is ejected during systole, the counts fall. With the data of 3 to 5 cardiac cycles a *representative cycle* is constructed by the computer. The fraction of the isotope ejected with each beat can be determined and hence the ejection fraction (the fraction of blood ejected compared with the volume present in the ventricle at the beginning of diastole). This method is very accurate and compares favorably with the ejection fraction obtained by the cardiac catheterization method. It may even be more accurate because ventricular geometric shape is measured.[59,72]

The function of the ventricular walls is analyzed by having the computer draw systolic and diastolic rings and superimpose them; then the degree of motion of various ventricular areas can be analyzed. Most patients with CAD have asymmetric myocardial blood distribution, and segmental ventricular wall motion abnormalities are seen. By contrast, patients with other types of cardiac muscle disease have uniformly global dysfunction. The computer also can calculate the time required for blood to move through each chamber and the cardiac output for the ventricles.

Sometimes areas of the myocardium adjacent to infarcted tissue are still alive but function poorly because of ischemia. Drugs, such as nitroglycerin, may be given during the scan to determine whether drug therapy will cause a significant area to become functional again. This technique also may be used to determine whether a bypass graft will help in that area. An akinetic scarred area will not respond to drug therapy. Thus surgery of the area would be useless.

Multiple-gated acquisition scan. The MUGA scan can be done immediately after first-pass scanning or as a separate test. Both methods involve the administration of only one dose of technetium. For the MUGA scan, an ECG monitor and cable are connected to a computer, which measures the R-R interval and divides it into 14 to 28 segments called *gates*. Images are recorded for each segment. The computer then analyzes these sequential images to determine regional wall motion, ventricular volumes, and ejection fraction.

An exercise MUGA is performed with the patient riding a conventional stationary bicycle or lying on a bicycle table. As for other exercise tests, the patient is subjected to gradually increasing workloads. The γ-camera is usually placed in the LAO position. Rest images are taken before beginning the exercise. These are later compared to images taken during exercise to determine changes in ejection fraction and wall motion. Generally, with ischemia, the ejection fraction decreases. However, for women, a decreased or unchanged ejection fraction during exercise is not a reliable indicator of ischemia.[27] Regional wall motion abnormalities during exercise indicate discrete coronary lesions, whereas global dysfunction suggests severe triple vessel disease, cardiomyopathy, or valvular disease.[31]

Positron emission tomography
Background information

Positron emission tomography (PET) is a noninvasive test that can be used to assess myocardial perfusion and metabolism. Research indicates that this study can be useful in determining ischemic but salvagable myocardial tissue.[32,64] This information can be invaluable in determining potential bypass graft and PTCA sites and in evaluating the results of such interventions.

Positrons are positively charged nuclear particles. Positron-emitting radionuclides release positrons that interact with electrons. This reaction creates two photons that are emitted at a 180-degree angle. These photons are high-energy particles that can be counted by a pair of scintillation detection devices positioned 180 degrees apart. Usually a ring of paired detectors is used to collect particle activity data from many angles. Computer assisted tomographic, or multiple "thin-slice" images, are then constructed from this data. Because accurate data acquisition requires the imaged object to remain stationary, gating like that used in MUGA scanning is used for cardiac imaging.

Many radioactive substances are used for this test. In general, they are radioactive forms of elements such as oxygen, nitrogen, and carbon or are metabolic substrates tagged with positron-emitting isotopes (e.g., fluorine-18 deoxyglucose [FDG] and carbon-11–labeled palmitate [¹¹C-palmitate]). Often, two radioactive tracers are used, one to assess perfusion and one to assess metabolism. Myocardial perfusion is measured by the uptake of tracers like oxygen-15–labeled water, nitrogen-13–labeled ammonia, and rubidium-82 by cardiac cells. As in thallium scanning, defects or cold spots indicate poor or no perfusion.

Metabolic activity of the myocardium is measured by the uptake of ¹¹C-palmitate or FDG. The normal energy substrate used by the heart is fatty acids. ¹¹C-palmitate is a tracer-labeled fatty acid. Decreased uptake indicates a derangement in myocardial fatty acid metabolism and is associated with ischemia. No uptake indicates necrosis.

When fatty acids are unavailable as an energy source, the heart uses a variety of other substrates, including glucose. In the absence of oxygen, myocardial cells switch to anaerobic metabolism and metabolize glucose exclusively. FDG, a tagged form of glucose, is used to evaluate this activity. FDG uptake is increased in underperfused myocardium, indicating ischemic but viable tissue.[39]

Images obtained using a perfusion tracer are compared with those taken after injection of a metabolic tracer. When FDG is used as the metabolic tracer, areas of increased uptake that correspond to perfusion tracer cold spots indicate ischemic but metabolically active myocardium.

Indications

PET can be used to evaluate patients with CAD for a variety of reasons. It can be used to determine areas of ischemic yet viable tissue that may benefit from interventions such as myocardial revascularization or PTCA. The study can also evaluate the results of thrombolytic therapy, myocardial revascularization, or PTCA. Finally, PET can distinguish ischemic from nonischemic heart failure.[9]

Procedure

The patient lies on a narrow x-ray table that will pass through the PET machine. ECG electrodes are attached for gating. The patient receives an intravenous injection of the perfusion or metabolic tracer and then is positioned inside the PET machine. Images are obtained and reviewed. The procedure is repeated with the other tracer when adequate tracer clearance time has elapsed. Because of the short half-life of most tracers, repeated imaging can occur in a very short period.

For cardiac glucose metabolism studies, 50 grams of glucose is given by mouth 60 to 90 minutes before FDG tracer administration. This ensures adequate tracer uptake. Images are then obtained 45 to 60 minutes later.

Magnetic resonance imaging
Background information

Magnetic resonance imaging (MRI), also known as nuclear magnetic resonance (NMR), is a noninvasive test that provides high-resolution tomographic images like those produced by PET and computed tomography (CT) scans. Unlike PET and CT scans, no radioactive tracers, x-rays, or contrast media are used making it comparatively safer.

MRI or NMR studies the behavior of hydrogen ions as they respond to magnetic and radiofrequency forces around them. When a magnetic force is applied to the hydrogen ions, they align in the direction of that force. The application of specific radiofrequency waves (resonant frequency) causes hydrogen nuclei to rotate away from their magnetic field alignment. When the radiofrequency pulse stops, the hydrogen nuclei realign with the magnetic field. As the nuclei realign, they emit energy at the same frequency as the radiofrequency pulse (resonant frequency). This energy is detected by a radiofrequency coil.

Resonance frequency and therefore the emission frequency of nuclei at a specific site are influenced by the local magnetic field. If a magnetic gradient exists in one or more planes, specific emission frequencies will pinpoint nuclei location. Applying a radiofrequency pulse corresponding to the resonant frequency of a plane will cause only the nuclei in that plane to resonate. This enables precise image plane or "slice" analysis of structures in that plane.

Another unique characteristic of MRI is that blood, which is moving through the image plane, causes a loss of signal intensity. This loss of intensity appears as dark areas and provides a natural contrast for visualizing the walls of blood vessels and heart chambers (Fig. 6-19).[28] Although this property is useful for some cardiovascular studies, it can cause blurred images of cardiac structures. Gating techniques like those used for MUGA scans provide sharper resolution for studies involving the heart.[49]

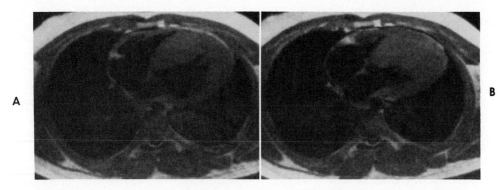

FIG. 6-19 Magnetic resonance imaging scan. Idiopathic hypertrophic subaortic stenosis (IHSS). **A,** A transverse image obtained near end-diastole. The septum is markedly thickened compared to the posterior ventricular wall. Involvement of the anterior left ventricular wall in the hypertrophic process is also present. **B,** Same level during systole. The left ventricular outflow tract is seen to be narrowed.

From Peshock RM: Heart and great vessels. In Stark DD and Bradley WG Jr, editors: Magnetic resonance imaging, ed 2, St Louis, 1992, Mosby–Year Book, Inc.

Indications

The potential uses for MRI scanning in the diagnosis of cardiovascular disease have not been fully explored. Some indications include evaluation of (1) congenital abnormalities of the aorta, pulmonary arteries, and superior vena cava; (2) gross patency of myocardial revascularization conduits; and (3) pericardial disease. In addition, AMIs can be visualized using a technique that analyzes tissue relaxation times. However, changes in tissue relaxation times are not specific to AMI.[49]

Procedure

Because MRIs generate strong magnetic fields, the patient must remove all metal jewelry and appliances before scanning. Very small amounts of metal such as surgical hemoclips are not adversely affected. Larger, permanent metal appliances or devices, such as pacemakers and prosthetic valves, are contraindications for MRI. However, evaluation of the response of specific devices to MRI conditions can be performed.[49]

For gated MRI studies, electrodes are applied. Unlike other nuclear studies, no radioactive tracers are injected. Therefore an intravenous line is not required. The patient lies on a narrow table that moves into the center of the scanner. During scanning the patient must remain very still because talking or movement may distort the images.

Patient teaching

Ask the patient about metal implants and other contraindicated devices. Instruct the patient to remove all jewelry and other metal objects. Explain that the procedure is not painful or dangerous. Also tell the patient that the machine may be very noisy but that this is normal. Most importantly, request that the patient lie very still during the scan.

RADIOGRAPHIC STUDIES
Common principles

Radiographic procedures use x-rays, a form of electromagnetic radiation, to diagnose disorders. X-rays penetrate substances to varying degrees. The degree of penetration, for the most part, is related to the density of the material. X-rays that pass through an object expose photographic plates positioned behind the subject or cause phosphor in a receiver tube to emit visible light (fluoroscopy). Because the heart and great vessels are filled with blood, they absorb most of the x-rays and appear as white or opaque areas on film. In contrast, the lungs, which are filled with air, allow most of the x-rays to pass through them to the film and appear as dark, almost completely black areas.

Chest x-ray studies
Background information

Chest x-ray studies, like ECGs, are commonly performed as part of the diagnostic profile for patients with cardiovascular disorders. They provide valuable information about the location and size of the heart and its chambers, as well as the position of invasive catheters and other devices. X-ray films also show the size of the great vessels, the presence of calcium in the heart and surrounding vessels, and pulmonary changes that may occur secondary to heart disease, such as pulmonary congestion resulting from congestive heart failure.

Indications

Chest x-ray examinations are part of the standard diagnostic testing regimen for all patients with heart disease. Patients with AMI or congestive heart failure frequently have chest x-ray examinations performed daily during hospitalization to determine the existence and extent of pulmonary involvement. Patients with transvenous pacemakers, pulmonary artery catheters, central venous catheters, or endotracheal tubes often have chest x-ray tests taken to evaluate catheter or tube placement.

Procedure

For routine chest x-ray studies, patients usually go to the radiology department. There, patients sit or stand erect with their chests against the x-ray plates. In general, all chest films are taken during deep inspiration. A *cardiac series* includes a posteroanterior film, as well as lateral, RAO, and LAO views. The anteroposterior view is used for portable chest x-ray tests.

Patient teaching

Recall that chest x-ray examinations require little patient preparation and instruction. Ask patients to remove all clothes above the waist and dress in a fabric or paper gown with ties or nonmetal snaps. Inform patients that they may be requested to sit or stand in specific positions and to hold their breath. Emphasize that they must not move until instructed to do so.

Computed tomography
Background information

Computed tomography (CT) scanning uses thin, fan-shaped x-ray beams that pass through the patient and are then registered by a 180-degree arc of detectors. The number of x-rays deleted from a beam as it passes through the patient is directly proportional to the density of tissue in its path. The computer uses this information to reconstruct images that are then transferred to x-ray film. These images can also be viewed on a screen.

Standard CT image acquisition is slow. Therefore movement of the heart would normally distort cardiac images. ECG gating or high-speed (fast CT) scanning overcomes this problem. Exposure times for fast (cine CT) scanning are only 50 milliseconds (msec), and imaging occurs at a rate of 17 scans/second. Intravenous iodinated contrast medium is administered for almost all cardiac CT scans.

Indications

CT scanning can be used to evaluate myocardial function by determining the dynamics of wall thickening, left ventricular volume, stroke volume, and ejection fraction. Areas of infarction can be detected by CT scanning with contrast media because the distribution of the iodinated contrast varies between normal and infarcted tissue. Contrast media–enhanced CT can also be used to assess gross myocardial revascularization patency. The pericardium is easily visualized by CT scanning; therefore this test is useful in assessing pericardial fluid and diagnosing constrictive pericarditis. Cardiac masses and abnormalities of the great vessels can also be studied.[28]

Procedure

The patient lies on a narrow x-ray table that moves into the center of the CT scanner. If a contrast medium is used, an intravenous line must be present or started before the procedure. If gating is used, ECG electrodes are attached to the patient. ECG electrodes should not be placed in areas that might interfere with imaging. The patient and x-ray table are positioned in the center of the CT scanner, and scanning begins. Periodically the table moves slightly forward or backward to obtain different cross-sectional images. A contrast medium is sometimes administered after initial images are scanned; otherwise, it is administered just before imaging as an intravenous bolus or a rapid infusion.

Patient teaching

Ask patients about allergies to iodine or shellfish. If patients are allergic, notify the physican and the CT technician. Instruct patients to lie completely still during the study because movement distorts the images. Explain to patients that they will lie on their backs and move through a round hole in the center of the CT scanner, which is just large enough for the narrow x-ray table to pass through. Patients may be asked to place their arms over their heads throughout the study to facilitate the acquisition of certain images.

Fluoroscopy
Background information

Images produced during fluoroscopy differ from those of standard x-ray studies. The heart, great vessels, and bones appear dark because they absorb x-rays as they penetrate the body. The rays that pass through less dense matter, such as the lungs, cause the receiving phosphor tube to convert the x-rays to visible light, resulting in light areas on the television viewing screen. The major advantage of this technique is that images can be viewed as they are produced (real time).

Indications

Fluoroscopy is frequently used during the insertion of pulmonary artery or transvenous pacing catheters. This technique is also used during cardiac catheterization, coronary arteriography, and electrophysiology studies to correctly position catheters.

Procedure

The patient lies supine on an x-ray table. Antiseptic scrubs and sterile drapes appropriate for the procedure are applied. The fluoroscopic camera is positioned over the patient's chest and is often operated by foot pedals. Personnel assisting in the procedure wear lead aprons and sterile caps, gowns, and masks. Lead gonadal shields should be provided for the patient. The fluoroscopic camera is operated intermittently rather than continuously during the procedure to check catheter location. This reduces patient and personnel radiation exposure.

Patient teaching

When possible, explain the procedure to the patient. Often the patient's condition may preclude lengthy explanations. Provide information to significant others as time permits. Also explain that fluoroscopy is a special type of x-ray examination. Instruct the patient to lie very still during the procedure.

Cardiac catheterization and coronary arteriography

Background information

Cardiac catheterization involves passing a radiopaque catheter via an artery or vein into the chambers of the heart. The purpose of the study is to obtain chamber pressures and oxygen saturation values. Ventricular function and wall motion can also be evaluated.

Pressures inside the cardiac chambers help in diagnosing and measuring abnormalities and the degree of hemodynamic compromise. The shape of the pressure wave recording can be used to distinguish valvular stenosis from insufficiency. The presence or absence of pressure differences or *gradients* on either side of a valve can also indicate the type of pathologic condition present. Elevations in peak ventricular pressures can signify the obstruction of outlet valves (aortic and pulmonic), decreased ventricular compliance caused by hypertrophy or constrictive pericarditis, or myocardial muscle weakness caused by cardiomyopathy or congestive heart failure.[59]

Oxygen saturation levels obtained in the heart chambers and vessels can indicate the presence of shunts. Shunting can be caused by congenital septal defects (usually atrial) or septal defects resulting from infarction or mechanical perforation. A *left-to-right shunt* occurs when blood from the left side of the heart, which is under more pressure, flows into a chamber on the right side. This results in higher-than-normal oxygen saturation values in the affected right chamber. The normal oxygen saturation values for the heart and its surrounding vessels follow:[59]

Superior vena cava	70%
Inferior vena cava	80%
Coronary sinus	20%*
Right chambers	75%
Pulmonary artery	75%
Left chambers	95%

Coronary arteriography (angiography) examines abnormalities in coronary artery blood flow via injection of contrast medium directly into vessels. Coronary arteriography is considered the best modality for evaluating CAD.[56]

---

*Due to high oxygen extraction of the myocardium.

Indications

The indications for cardiac catheterization depend on the side of the heart being studied. Right heart catheterization is performed to evaluate valvular disease, congenital heart disease, and pericardial tamponade or constriction. It can also be done as part of electrophysiologic studies, endocardial biopsies, and some studies of the left side of the heart.[65] Catheterization of the left side of the heart allows evaluation of aortic and mitral valvular disease and left ventricular function. Coronary arteriography is often performed with left heart catheterization. Some indications for coronary arteriography include high risk of sudden death as indicated by noninvasive testing, new onset or unstable angina pectoris, Prinzmetal's angina, atypical chest pain, and evaluation of CAD in patients who have had heart transplant. Coronary arteriography is also performed during the first hours of AMI to initiate intracoronary thrombolytic therapy or PTCA, although this indication is controversial.[56,65]

Procedure

Cardiac catheterization and coronary arteriography are performed under sterile conditions in a specially equipped x-ray room or catheterization laboratory. The patient is frequently given a mild sedative and usually is not permitted to eat or drink for 6 hours before the procedure. Most medications are continued up to the time of the procedure. After the patient arrives in the procedure room, the area where the catheter is to be inserted is shaved if necessary, and the area is scrubbed with an antiseptic solution. Sterile drapes are then applied. A local anesthetic is administered at the site of catheter insertion. A child under the age of 12 may be given a general anesthetic. After the procedure, patients usually remain in the hospital overnight. However, the studies can be performed on an outpatient basis.

Right heart catheterization. This procedure is performed by puncturing a peripheral vein such as the femoral or antecubital vein. The catheter is guided through the vein under fluoroscopy until it reaches the right atrium. After the catheter is in the right atrium, blood samples and pressure measurements are taken. The catheter is then moved across the tricuspid valve and into the right ventricle, where more blood samples and pressures are obtained. Frequently, right ventriculography is performed by injecting contrast media into the right ventricle during fluoroscopy to examine the right ventricular outflow tract, as well as pulmonic and tricuspid valve function. The catheter is then advanced across the pulmonic valve and into the pulmonary artery, and more samples of blood and pressure readings are collected. Finally the catheter is guided through the pulmonary artery into a wedge position where pressure measurements indirectly reflect the pressures in the pulmonary veins and left atrium. After all the information is obtained, the catheter is withdrawn and

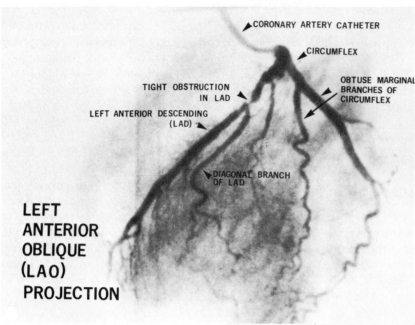

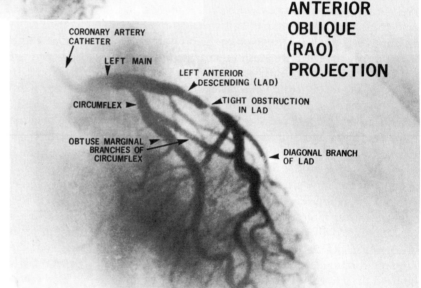

FIG. 6-20 Left coronary arteriogram. Note the coronary catheter (Judkins) in the left coronary orifice, the different branches of the coronary artery system, and the tight obstruction in the left anterior descending artery.

Adapted from Sanderson R and Kurth C: The cardiac patient: a comprehensive approach, ed 2, Philadelphia, 1983, WB Saunders Co.

pressure is applied to the puncture site. When the bleeding is stopped, the site is covered with a pressure dressing, and the patient is returned to the nursing unit or to a recovery area (outpatient) for further observation.

Left heart catheterization and coronary arteriography. For this procedure, an introducer is inserted into the femoral or brachial artery. Catheters with special shapes so that they can be guided easily into various areas are inserted via the introducer during the test. Only one catheter is used at a time. Under fluoroscopy, catheters are guided retrograde to the blood flow toward the aortic root.

If only left heart pressures are desired, a catheter is passed across the aortic valve, and pressures are obtained on either side of the valve. Then the catheter is advanced into the left ventricle, where oxygen saturation samples

and pressures readings are obtained. The catheter and introducer are then withdrawn, and pressure is applied at the site for at least 15 to 30 minutes.

If coronary arteriography is performed, a preformed catheter is manipulated from the aortic root into the left coronary ostium. The catheter's position is verified by injection of a small amount of contrast media under fluoroscopy. After the catheter is properly positioned, several injections of contrast media are made while motion pictures called *cines* are taken from several different angles. The most common views used are RAO, LAO, and cephalic (Fig. 6-20). When these pictures are completed, this catheter or another specially formed catheter is positioned in the right coronary ostium, and the procedure is repeated.

Because the contrast material fills the coronary artery

completely during injection, oxygenation of the myocardium may be compromised, causing angina. Nitroglycerin can be administered sublingually, intravenously, or via the catheter just before the constrast media injection to dilate the artery and decrease ventricular workload through a reduction in preload (see Chapter 7).

After the coronary arteriography is completed, left ventriculography is often performed by injecting contrast media into the left ventricular cavity. Usually a catheter that curls into a loop at the tip, called a *pigtail,* is used to reduce the risk of ventricular dysrhythmias caused by mechanical irritation.[65] Left ventriculography is done to evaluate left ventricular performance and mitral valve competency. Left ventricular wall motion is assessed, and aneurysms are identified. Stroke volume and ejection fraction are also determined. Mitral valve competency is evaluated by the amount of contrast media reflux (regurgitation) into the left atrium. The extent of regurgitation is graded from I to IV, with I being the smallest amount of reflux.

After the ventriculogram is completed, the catheter and introducer are withdrawn. Pressure is held over the puncture site for 15 to 30 minutes. Then a pressure dressing is applied, and patients are returned to their rooms or a recovery area (outpatient).

Patient teaching

Explain the risks and complications of cardiac catheterization and coronary arteriography to patients and their families. Obtain written informed consent when patients are able to verbalize an understanding of the procedure and its risks.

Explain common complications of cardiac catheterization and coronary arteriography, which include allergic reaction to the contrast media, dysrhythmias, bleeding from puncture sites, and back pain. Ask patients whether they have allergies to iodine or seafood. Report such allergies to the physician because often the physician will attempt to suppress the allergic response by administering steroids and diphenhydramine hydrochloride. Dysrhythmias that can occur include PVCs, ventricular tachycardia, ventricular fibrillation, premature atrial contractions, supraventricular tachycardia, and atrial fibrillation. Remember that these dysrhythmias are usually caused by irritation of the endocardium by the catheter tip. Explain that palpitations or dizziness may be experienced. Tell patients about the importance of coughing when requested to do so by the physician or other personnel. Remember that coughing increases the intrathoracic pressure in a manner similar to external chest compressions and can provide cerebral and coronary perfusion during ventricular tachycardia or fibrillation.[18]

To prevent bleeding from puncture sites, patients remain on bed rest for 4 to 6 hours after the procedure. When femoral punctures are made, the head of bed can only be elevated to 30 degrees, and a sandbag is placed over the puncture site. Brachial access sites should be immobilized on an arm board. If a left heart catheterization was performed, arterial occlusion can also occur. Explain that a nurse will check the puncture site and pulses in the affected extremity every 15 minutes during the first hour after the procedure, then every 30 minutes for 2 hours, and then every hour for 4 more hours. Instruct patients to immediately report numbness or warm, wet sensations.

Tell patients that back pain is usually caused by prolonged supine positioning on the x-ray table and in bed. Instruct patients to request analgesics for this discomfort. They also can ask to be log-rolled toward the affected side to receive back rubs or be propped in a side-lying position.

Also explain other risks and complications when coronary arteriography is performed. Remember that physicians should inform patients of the mortality rate associated with this procedure (0.1%, or 1 in 1000) and should also explain the risks of myocardial infarction (0.2%) and stroke (0.1%).[65]

Explain other important aspects of the procedure. Describe the sights, sounds, and sensations that patients will experience in the procedure room, especially the flushing sensation often produced by the injection of contrast media. Instruct patients to report chest discomfort immediately during and after the procedure. (Also see the relaxation script for cardiac catheterization, Interchapter 17.)

ELECTROPHYSIOLOGIC STUDIES

Electrophysiologic studies permit detailed analysis of cardiac electrical events. The use of intracardiac catheters or epicardial electrodes permits a more intimate and precise view of local and regional myocardial conduction than a 12-lead ECG. In general, these studies are invasive because they require the insertion of catheters like those used in cardiac catheterization or exposure of the heart during surgery.

Endocardial electrophysiologic studies
Background information

The test most commonly referred to as an *electrophysiologic study (EPS)* involves the percutaneous insertion of catheters under fluoroscopy. These catheters are electrodes that sense local electrical activity. Some catheters also have pacing capability. Simultaneous multichannel ECG recordings are taken from the electrode catheters and body surface electrodes so that the timing and location of impulse initiation can be identified (Fig. 6-21). EPS studies are performed in the cardiac catheterization laboratory or a specially designed EPS laboratory equipped with fluoroscopy.

Indications

The most common indications for EPS are cardiac arrest not related to myocardial infarction or electrolyte imbal-

FIG. 6-21 EPS recording. This baseline recording was performed on photographic paper at 100 mm/sec. The first three tracings are surface leads I, II, and III; the next four represent intracardiac electrograms—the high right atrial *(HRA)* electrogram demonstrates a discrete atrial *(A)* potential; the coronary sinus *(CS)* electrogram demonstrates both atrial and ventricular *(V)* potentials; and the distal and proximal His electrograms demonstrate atrial, His bundle, and ventricular potentials.

From Wiener I: Electrophysiologic studies. In Tilkian AG and Daily EK, editors: Cardiovascular procedures: diagnostic techniques and therapeutic procedures, St Louis, 1986, The CV Mosby Co.

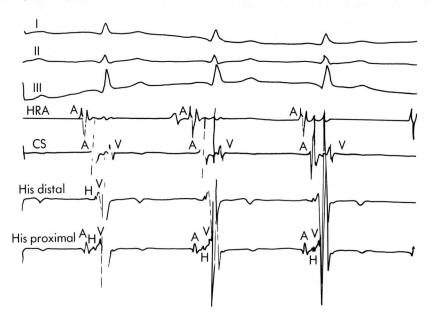

ance, recurrent sustained ventricular tachycardia, and suspected Wolff-Parkinson-White syndrome. Other indications include unexplained recurrent syncope, symptomatic supraventricular tachycardia, and conduction delays not clearly delineated by noninvasive testing.[70]

Procedure

The procedure is similar to that used in cardiac catheterization. Usually catheters are inserted percutaneously into the femoral vein and advanced through the inferior vena cava into the heart. To obtain a recording from the bundle of His, a multipolar catheter is advanced across the tricuspid valve and into the right ventricle. It is then withdrawn slowly until a His bundle tracing is seen on the recorder. Often, three other catheters are also inserted. A quadripolar high right atrial catheter records sinus node activity. Another catheter, placed in the coronary sinus records left atrial impulse formation and conduction. A fourth catheter, positioned in the right ventricle records activity there. If left ventricular stimulation is necessary, a quadripolar catheter is usually inserted in the femoral artery and advanced retrograde through the aorta to the left ventricle.

Two basic types of stimulation, incremental pacing and premature stimulation, are used. Incremental pacing is synchronized to the native QRS complex. Commonly used pacing intervals are 600, 500, 400, 350, 300, and 250 msec. This type of pacing is used to evaluate sinus node function and AV conduction. It can also be used to induce and terminate supraventricular and ventricular dysrhythmias.[71]

Premature stimulation involves the introduction of a precisely timed premature stimulus or multiple stimuli during sinus rhythm, paced rhythm, or tachycardias. It is used to measure refractory periods and to stimulate or terminate tachycardias.

After tachycardias are stimulated, drugs can be tested to determine their effectiveness in controlling or preventing the dysrhythmia. The drugs tested are chosen, based on the nature of the dysrhythmia. Sometimes drug testing can require repeated EPS procedures.

Mapping

Mapping refers to tracing the reentrant pathways of supraventricular tachycardias or the origin of ventricular tachycardias. Mapping can be performed with intracardiac catheters during laboratory EPS procedures or with epicardial electrodes attached to the heart during cardiac surgery.

Simultaneous electrode recordings reveal the earliest site of dysrhythmia activation. Locating pathways and ventricular ectopic foci are important for the success of surgical ablative or cryoablative techniques. These techniques are used to interrupt the pathway or destroy the irritable focus.

Other methods of conducting electrophysiologic studies

Some newer, less invasive methods of performing limited electrophysiologic studies include atrial electrocardiograms from transvenous or epicardial pacing wires and ECGs from esophageal electrodes. In addition, some newer permanent pacemakers can be instructed to give programmed stimulation via the pacing catheter.[61]

Patient teaching

Know that these tests can be extremely frightening to a patient because they often involve the induction of ventricular tachycardia, which a patient may recognize as a life-threatening dysrhythmia. Allow patients to verbalize their concerns.

KEY CONCEPT REVIEW

1. For patients undergoing diagnostic testing, which human response pattern is the most critical to assess?
   a. Feeling
   b. Perceiving
   c. Knowing
   d. Exchanging
2. Patient education related to diagnostic testing should include which of the following?
   a. An explanation of the suspected disease process
   b. A description of the procedure
   c. A list of possible findings
   d. All of the above
3. Total serum CPK and serum CPK-MB samples should be drawn on admission and then 12 and 24 hours later because:
   a. CPK values peak in 6 to 8 hours.
   b. Total serum CPK only rises when an AMI has occurred.
   c. CPK values return to normal in 12 hours.
   d. CPK values peak 12 to 24 hours after an AMI.
4. Serum LDH levels should be obtained when an AMI is suspected to have occurred more than 24 hours before admission because:
   a. LDH levels remain elevated for 6 to 14 days.
   b. LDH levels do not begin to rise until the third day after an AMI.
   c. LDH is an enzyme found only in myocardial cells.
   d. None of the above.
5. The resting membrane potential (-90 mV) of most cardiac cells is maintained by all of the following *except:*
   a. Passive diffusion of K^+ out of the cells
   b. Active transport of Na^+ out of the cells
   c. Active transport of Cl^- into the cells
   d. An imbalance in Na^+ and K^+ movement
6. During phase 0 (depolarization) of an action potential:
   a. Fast sodium channels open.
   b. K^+ rushes into the cell.
   c. Ca^{++} is actively transported out of the cell.
   d. All of the above.
7. The 12-lead electrocardiogram:
   a. Consists of six limb-lead and six chest-lead recordings
   b. Records the heart's electrical activity from 12 different views
   c. Is indicated for patients experiencing chest pain
   d. All of the above
8. Exercise electrocardiography (stress testing):
   a. Involves the recording of an ECG over a 24-hour period while the patient performs normal daily activities
   b. Never yields false negative or positive results
   c. Is primarily used to detect or confirm CAD
   d. Is more sensitive than thallium-201 exercise testing
9. Echocardiography is used to assess:
   a. Valvular function

Explain the risks and complications of the procedure. The complications are basically the same as those for cardiac catheterization. In addition, tell the patient that the mortality rate from these procedures is also the same as that for cardiac catheterization.[70] Obtain an informed consent when the patient has verbalized understanding of the procedure, its complications, and its risks.

   b. The presence of atrial and ventricular masses and thrombi
   c. Cardiac output, stroke volume, and ejection fraction
   d. All of the above
10. Two-dimensional echocardiography (2D mode)
    a. Produces images by rapidly sweeping ultrasound signals through an arc
    b. Is an invasive procedure requiring the insertion of catheters
    c. Provides less information about the spatial orientation of cardiac structures than M-mode echocardiography
    d. Uses pulsed sound waves to calculate blood velocity
11. Hot spots seen during technetium-99m pyrophosphate scanning indicate:
    a. Ischemia
    b. Necrosis
    c. Ectopic foci for ventricular dysrhythmias
    d. Adequately perfused myocardium
12. Technetium-99m pyrophosphate scanning is most accurate when performed:
    a. Less than 12 hours from the onset of chest discomfort
    b. During chest discomfort
    c. About 36 hours after the onset of chest discomfort
    d. About 6 months after an AMI
13. Cold spots seen during rest thallium-201 scanning indicate:
    a. Myocardial fibrosis from an old infarction
    b. Areas of ischemia
    c. Areas of new infarction
    d. All of the above
14. An exercise thallium-201 scan can pinpoint areas of ischemia when cold spots:
    a. Disappear on a second scan performed 1 to 4 hours later
    b. Disappear with exercise
    c. Are not seen
    d. Remain unchanged on a second scan performed 2 to 4 hours later
15. PET scanning uses radioactive tracers to assess:
    a. Ventricular wall motion
    b. Myocardial perfusion and metabolism
    c. Myocardial perfusion
    d. Myocardial metabolism
16. MRI imaging:
    a. Requires injection of radioactive isotopes
    b. Uses the natural properties of hydrogen ions
    c. Involves the use of x-rays
    d. Is a highly invasive and dangerous procedure
17. All of the following are sensations a patient may experience during coronary arteriography *except:*
    a. Chest discomfort
    b. Palpitations caused by PVCs
    c. Flushing
    d. Abdominal cramping

18. All of the following are complications of coronary arteriography *except:*
    a. Allergic reaction to contrast media
    b. Ventricular fibrillation
    c. Hepatic failure
    d. Stroke
19. One indication for electrophysiology studies is:
    a. Murmurs
    b. Atypical chest pain
    c. Recurrent sustained ventricular tachycardia
    d. History of previous MI
20. Testing methods used for electrophysiology studies include all of the following *except:*
    a. Injection of contrast media into the left ventricle
    b. Multichannel ECG monitoring
    c. Pacing stimulation
    d. Administration of antidysrhythmic drugs

ANSWERS

1. c	5. d	9. d	13. d	17. d
2. d	6. a	10. a	14. a	18. c
3. d	7. d	11. b	15. b	19. c
4. a	8. c	12. c	16. b	20. a

REFERENCES

1. Adam WE and others: Assessment of left ventricular function during exercise by radionuclide ventriculography, CVP 2:47, 1981.
2. Allen H: Radionuclide studies in coronary artery disease, CVP 2:21, 1981.
3. Allessie MA and Bonke FIM: Atrial arrhythmias: basic concepts. In Wandel WJ, editor: Cardiac arrhythmias: their mechanisms, diagnosis, and management, Philadelphia, 1980, JB Lippincott Co.
4. Assey ME, Usher BW, and Hendrix GH: Valvular heart disease: use of invasive and noninvasive techniques in clinical decision-making. II. Mitral valve disease, Mod Concepts CV Dis 58(11):61, 1989.
5. Barret N and Schwartz M: What patients really want to know, Am J Nurs 81:1642, 1981.
6. Beller GA: Noninvasive assessment of myocardial ischemia, Baylor Cardiol Series 12(1):5, 1989.
7. Bentley LJ: Radionuclide imaging techniques in the diagnosis and treatment of coronary heart disease, Focus Crit Care 14(6):27, 1987.
8. Berger H and Zaret B: Nuclear cardiology. II. N Engl J Med 305:855, 1981.
9. Bergmann S and others: Positron emission tomography of the heart, Prog Cardiovasc Dis 28(3):165, 1985.
10. Berman D: Thallium-201 imaging and exercise testing. In Hamilton G and Pohost G, editors: Diagnostic visualization of the ischemic myocardium, New York, 1978, Proclinics for New England Nuclear.
11. Blanke H and others: Patterns of creatine kinase release during acute myocardial infarction after nonsurgical reperfusion: comparison with conventional treatment and correlation with infarct size, J Am Coll Cardiol 3:675, 1984.
12. Borchat J and others: Treadmill exercise testing and coronary cineangiography following first myocardial infarction, J Cardiac Rehabil 1:206, 1981.
13. Brown, AM and Birnbaum L: Ion channels and G proteins, Hosp Pract 24(7):189, 1989.
14. Burks, J and others: Radiation exposure to nursing personnel from patients receiving diagnostic radionuclides, Heart Lung 11:217, 1982.
15. Cairns JA and others: Coronary thrombolysis, Chest 95(2) Suppl:73S, 1989.
16. Castellanos A and others: Didactic vectorcardiography: general concepts, Heart Lung 4:699, 1975.
17. Conover MB: Understanding electrocardiography: arrhythmias and the 12-lead ECG, ed 5, St Louis, 1988, The CV Mosby Co.
18. Criley JM, Blaufuss AH, and Kissel GL: Cough-induced cardiac compression: self-administered form of cardiopulmonary resuscitation, JAMA 236:1246, 1976.
19. Devereux RB and Pickering TG: Relationship between ambulatory and exercise pressure and cardiac structure, Am Heart J 116(4):1124, 1988.
20. Dunn M and others: Antithrombotic therapy in atrial fibrillation, Chest 95(2)Suppl:118S, 1989.
21. Fischbach FT: A manual of laboratory diagnostic tests, ed 3, Philadelphia, 1988, JB Lippincott Co.
22. Gawlinski A: New diagnostic techniques. In Kern L, editor: Cardiac critical care nursing, Gaithersburg, Md, 1988, Aspen Publishers, Inc.
23. Gordon DJ and others: Predictive value of the exercise tolerance test for mortality in North American men: the Lipid Research Clinics' Mortality Follow-Up Study, Circulation 74:252, 1986.
24. Graettinger WF and others: Validation of portable noninvasive blood pressure monitoring devices: comparison with intra-arterial and sphygmomanometer measurements, Am Heart J 116(4):1155, 1988.
25. Guilleminault C and others: Cyclical variation of the heart rate in sleep apnea syndrome: mechanisms and usefulness of 24 hr. electrocardiography as a screening technique, Lancet 1:126, 1984.
26. Hackel DB and others: Comparison of enzymatic and anatomic estimates of myocardial infarct size in man, Circulation 70:824, 1984.
27. Higginbothom MB and others: Sex-related differences in normal cardiac response to upright exercise, Circulation 70(3):357, 1984.
28. Higgins CB: Newer cardiac imaging techniques: Digital subtraction angiography; computed tomography; magnetic resonance imaging. In Braunwald E, editor: Heart disease: a textbook of cardiovascular medicine, ed 3, Philadelphia, 1988, WB Saunders Co.
29. Hirsh J and others: Optimal therapeutic range for oral anticoagulants, Chest 95(2)Suppl:5S, 1989.
30. Hyers TM, Hull RD, and Weg JG: Antithrombotic therapy for venous thromboembolic disease, Chest 95(2)Suppl:37S, 1989.
31. Kline LW and Helfart RH: Value of noninvasive techniques following acute myocardial infarction. In Kotler MN and Syeiner, editors: Cardiac imaging: New technologies and clinical applications, Philadelphia, 1986, FA Davis Co.
32. Knabb RM and others: The temporal pattern of recovery of myocardial perfusion and metabolism delineated by positron emission tomography after coronary thrombolysis, J Nucl Med 28:1563, 1987.
33. Knoebel SB and others: Guidelines for ambulatory electrocardiography: a report of the American College of Cardiol-

ogy/American Heart Association Task Force on Assessment of Diagnostic and Therapeutic Cardiovascular Procedures, J Am Coll Cardiol 13(1):249, 1989.

34. Lavie CJ, Schmieder RE, and Messerli FH: Ambulatory blood pressure monitoring: practical considerations, Am Heart J 116(4):1146, 1988.

35. Lee T and Goldman L: Serum enzyme assays in the diagnosis of acute myocardial infarction: recommendations based on quantitative analysis, Ann Intern Med 102:221, 1986.

36. Levine HJ, Pauker SG, and Salzman EW: Antithrombotic therapy in valvular heart disease, Chest 95(2)Suppl:98S, 1989.

37. Malasanos L, Barkauskas V, and Stoltenber-Allen K: Health assessment, ed 4, St Louis, 1990, Mosby–Year Book, Inc. Co.

38. Maron BJ and others: Prognostic significance of 24 hour ambulatory electrocardiography monitoring in patients with hypertrophic cardiomyopathy: a prospective study, Am J Cardiol 48:252, 1981.

39. Marshall M and others: Identification and differentiation of resting myocardial ischemia in man with positron computed tomography, ^{18}F-labeled fluorodeoxyglucose and N-13 ammonia, Circulation 67:766, 1983.

40. Mason D, Demaria A, and Berman D: Principles of noninvasive cardiac imaging echocardiography and nuclear cardiology, New York, 1980, Le Jacq Publishing, Inc.

41. McHugh N, Christman N, and Johnson J: Preparatory information: what helps and why, Am J Nurs 82:780, 1982.

42. Michigan Nurses' Association's Conduct and Utilization of Research in Nursing Project: Sensory information can reduce children's fears of threatening procedures, Nurs 82, p 24, May 1982.

43. Miers LJ: Cardiac electrical activity. In Kinney MR, Packa DR, and Dunbar SB: AACN's clinical reference for critical care nursing, ed 2, New York, 1988, McGraw-Hill, Inc.

44. Murray R and Zertner J: Guidelines for more effective health teaching, Nurs 76, p 44, Feb 1976.

45. Nellessen U and others: Transesophageal two-dimensional echocardiography and color Doppler flow velocity mapping in evaluation of cardiac valve prostheses, Circulation 78(4):848, 1988.

46. Nielson AT and others: Linear relationship between distribution of thallium-201 and blood flow in ischemic and nonischemic myocardium during exercise, Circulation 61:797, 1980.

47. Pagana KD and Pagana TJ: Diagnostic testing and nursing implications, St Louis, 1982, The CV Mosby Co.

48. Paul SC and Johnson P: Early recognition of critical stenosis high in the left anterior descending coronary artery, Heart Lung 19(1):27, 1990.

49. Peshock RM: Heart and great vessels. In Stark DD and Bradley WG Jr, editors: Magnetic resonance imaging, ed 2, St Louis, 1992, Mosby–Year Book, Inc.

50. Pickering TG and others: How common is white coat hypertension? JAMA 259:225, 1988.

51. Poller L, Tomson JM, and Yee KF: Heparin and partial thromboplastin time: an international survey, Br J Haematol 44:161, 1980.

52. Rabbani LE and Antman EM: Exercise testing and ambulatory monitoring. I. Exercise testing methods and applications, Cardio Rev Reports 10(9):46, 1989.

53. Ratner S: Myocardial perfusion imaging: is MIBI better than thallium? Cardiol Trends Prod News 10(2):14, 1990.

54. Resnekov L and others: Antithrombotic agents in coronary artery disease, Chest 95(2)Suppl:52S, 1989.

55. Roberts R: Enzymatic diagnosis of acute myocardial infarction, Chest 93(1 suppl):3S, 1988.

56. Ross J and others: Guidelines for coronary angiography: a report of the American College of Cardiology/American Heart Association Task Force on Assessment of Diagnostic and Therapeutic Cardiovascular Procedures, J Am Coll Cardiol 10(4):935, 1987.

57. Ruberman W and others: Ventricular premature beats and mortality after myocardial infarction, N Engl J Med 297:750, 1977.

58. Ruberman W and others: Ventricular premature complexes in prognosis of angina, Circulation 61:1172, 1980.

59. Sanderson R: Diagnostic techniques. In Sanderson R and Kurth C, editors: The cardiac patient: a comprehensive approach, ed 2, Philadelphia, 1983, WB Saunders Co.

60. Sanfilippo AJ and Weyman AE: The role of echocardiography in managing critically ill patients. I. Currently available techniques and obtainable measurements, J Crit Illness 3(4):30, 1988.

61. Schneller SJ: Noninvasive electrophysiology studies using permanent cardiac pacemakers, Cardiol Trends Prod News 10(2):1, 1990.

62. Spear JF and Moore EN: Supernormal excitability and conduction. In Wellens HJ, Lie KI, and Janse MJ, editors: The conduction system of the heart: structure, function, and clinical implications, Philadelphia, 1976, Lea & Febiger.

63. Stein PD and Kantrowitz A: Antithrombotic therapy in mechanical and biological prosthetic heart valves and saphenous vein bypass grafts, Chest 95(2)Suppl:107S, 1989.

64. Tamaki N and others: Positron emission tomography using fluorine-18 deoxyglucose in evaluation of coronary artery bypass grafting, Am J Cardiol 64:860, 1989.

65. Tilkian AG and Daily EK: Cardiac catheterization and coronary arteriography. In Tilkian AG and Daily EK, editors: Cardiovascular procedures: diagnostic techniques and therapeutic procedures, St Louis, 1986, The CV Mosby Co.

66. Touloukian JE: Calcium channel blocking agents: physiologic basis of nursing intervention, Heart Lung 14(4):342, 1985.

67. Weber MA: Evaluating the diagnosis and prognosis of hypertension by automated blood pressure monitoring: outline of a symposium, Am Heart J 116(4):1118, 1988.

68. Weiner D: Exercise testing for the diagnosis and severity of coronary artery disease, J Cardiac Rehabil 1:433, 1981.

69. Wheeler AP, Jaquiss RD, and Newman JH: Physician practices in the treatment of pulmonary embolism and deep venous thrombosis, Arch Intern Med 148:1321, 1988.

70. Wiener I: Electrophysiologic studies. In Tilkian AG and Daily EK, editors: Cardiovascular procedures: diagnostic techniques and therapeutic procedures, St Louis, 1986, The CV Mosby Co.

71. Wit AL: Cellular electrophysiologic mechanisms of cardiac arrhythmias, Ann NY Acad Sci 432:1, 1986.

72. Zeluff G, Cashion W, and Jackson D: Evaluation of coronary arteries and the myocardium by radionuclide imaging, Heart Lung 9:344, 1980.

Interchapter 7

Stress and Ventricular Fibrillation

The relationship between psychologic stress and the occurrence of malignant ventricular dysrhythmias is well documented in the research literature. For example, Wellens and co-workers[6] documented the recurrent onset of ventricular fibrillation in a young girl whenever she was awakened by an alarm clock. The initial episode of fibrillation occurred after she was awakened by a thunderclap. In another study, Reich and colleagues[5] found that of 117 patients referred to a major medical center for management of ventricular dysrhythmias, 26 patients were experiencing emotional disturbances during the 24 hours before onset. Although the predominant emotion accounting for the disturbance was anger, other common affective states such as depression and grief were identified. Interestingly, these 26 patients were distinguished from the rest of the study group by having *less* severe coronary artery disease.

Lown and associates[4] have described the case of a 39-year-old man who experienced two episodes of ventricular fibrillation. The initial episode occurred when he was rough-housing with his sexually mature daughters. This event was interrupted by a neighbor ringing the doorbell, at which time the man looked up, said "I'm sorry," and had a cardiac arrest that was documented to be due to ventricular fibrillation. He was resuscitated and later underwent coronary angiography without any findings of structural heart disease. He was defensive and covertly hostile and denied being depressed or angry. His lifestyle was one of controlled aggression. Although outwardly calm and controlled, during psychiatric interviews he would develop increases in the frequency and grade of ventricular premature beats. A second cardiac arrest occurred during the REM stage of sleep documented by his EEG.

When his dysrhythmia could not be controlled with a variety of pharmacologic agents, he was taught to meditate, using a noncultic technique. While meditating he could control his dysrhythmias successfully. Only through the combined use of medication and psychologic methods, including meditation, could his ventricular ectopy be controlled.

Anxiety, anger, depression, and grief are not simply the ways in which patients respond to being hospitalized; these emotions are frequently the precipitating events that trigger the need for hospitalization in the first place. Clearly those at higher risk for emotionally induced ventricular dysrhythmias are patients with underlying cardiac disease. Lethal ventricular dysrhythmias also can be triggered by psychologic factors, however, in patients who have no structural cardiac disease.[3]

Although it has been documented that a single emotional event can trigger ventricular dysrhythmias such as in the Lown case study, more frequently it has been reported that for several weeks before the major stressful event, patients experience feelings of hopelessness, emotional vulnerability, grief, and depression[2] that culminate in a *giving-up/given-in* response.[1] Thus it is critical to assess patients for reports of recent stressful life events (i.e., loss of a loved one, loss of a job, severe disappointments) and newly identified anxiety producing situations and to evaluate them for new signs and symptoms of fatigue and depression. Patients can be taught to record stressors during the day to become aware of which incidents are triggering emotional responses. They can be instructed to avoid stressful settings, people, and situations whenever possible.[3] They can be taught ways to change their perception of emotionally stressful situations and exert conscious control over their emotional responses (e.g., "Is this worth dying for?").[3] They also can be guided to learn a variety of strategies to reduce the impact of their emotional responses (e.g., deep breathing, muscle relaxation, imagery, music therapy).

Cases such as these suggest that the traditional way of regarding the heart as a mere object of therapy is short-sighted and incomplete. It is necessary to transcend our habitual ways of envisioning the heart as a malfunctioning end-organ that can invariably be treated with mere surgical or pharmacologic approaches. No matter how much we wish to objectify our approaches to cardiac disorders, research reports such as these remind us, perhaps uncomfortably, that disorders of the cardiac rate and rhythm are not always as objective as we might wish to make them. Sometimes the most surprising variables creep in, variables that truly may be disconcerting—such as alarm clocks and thunderclaps.

REFERENCES

1. Engel G: A life setting conducive to illness: the giving-up-given-in complex, Ann Int Med 69:293, 1968.
2. Green WA, Goldstein S, and Moss AJ: Psychosocial aspects of sudden death: a preliminary report, Arch Intern Med 129:725, 1972.
3. Hackett RP, Rosenbaum JFM, and Resar GE: Emotion, psychiatric disorders, and the heart. In Braunwald E, editor: Heart disease, ed 3, Philadelphia, 1988, WB Saunders.
4. Lown B, Temte JV, Teich P, and others: Basis for recurring ventricular fibrillation in the absence of coronary artery disease and its management, N Engl J Med 294:623, 1976.
5. Reich P and others: Acute psychological disturbances preceding life-threatening ventricular arrhythmias, JAMA 246:233, 1981.
6. Wellens HJJ, Vermeulen A, and Durrer D: Ventricular fibrillation upon arousal from sleep by auditory stimuli, Circulation 46:661, 1972.

7

Hemodynamic Monitoring

Elaine Kiess Daily

LEARNING OBJECTIVES

1. Evaluate the four factors that regulate the heart as a pump.
2. List the disease states for which hemodynamic monitoring is used.
3. Compare and contrast the normal values with the meaning of the abnormal values obtained through hemodynamic monitoring.
4. Describe nursing care of a hemodynamically monitored patient.
5. List the complications and treatment of hemodynamic monitoring problems.
6. Synthesize the steps that should be used to troubleshoot monitoring equipment.

Since the development of the balloon-tipped flotation catheter by Doctors Swan and Ganz in 1970, its use for bedside hemodynamic monitoring has become an integral component in the care of critically ill, hemodynamically unstable patients. Although controversy exists regarding the risks versus benefits of its use, it continues to play an important role in the current care and management of critically ill patients.[20,40,47]

The purpose of bedside hemodynamic monitoring is to survey and optimize the determinants of oxygen delivery by measurement of intracardiac and intravascular pressures and calculation of hemodynamic parameters.

The safe and effective use of hemodynamic monitoring in the care of critically ill patients requires a clear understanding of cardiovascular physiologic conditions and knowledge of the associated technical aspects.

CARDIAC PUMP

The primary function of the cardiopulmonary system is to transport sufficient oxygen to tissues for maintaining aerobic metabolism and tissue viability and removing metabolic waste products. The accomplishment of this goal requires optimal performance of the lungs for gas exchange and the heart to pump blood to the lungs and into the systemic circulation.

Cardiac ultrastructure

The basic unit of the ventricular myocardium is the myocardial cell or fiber. Each myocardial muscle fiber (myocardial cell) (Fig. 7-1) is covered by a membrane called the *sarcolemma* and is separated by a modified cell membrane called an intercalated disk. This disk holds the myocardial muscle fiber together, permits molecule exchange between cells, and probably provides a low-resistance pathway for conduction between cells, which results in a functional syncytium.

Within each myocardial muscle fiber are hundreds of *myofibrils*. Each myofibril is composed of *sarcomeres* that contain *myosin* and *actin* filaments, which are the contractile elements of the heart. The myosin filaments are called the *thick filaments,* and the actin filaments are called the *thin filaments;* they interdigitate and form the *dark* and *light bands* (Fig. 7-1).

The light bands or the I bands, consist only of the thin actin filaments. The dark bands, or A bands, contain the thick filaments and represent areas where the actin overlaps with the myosin. Small projections on each side of the myosin filaments are called *cross-bridges*. The center of the myosin filament contains no cross-bridges. Each actin filament is attached to a Z membrane *(Z line)*. A sarcomere extends from one Z line to another.

The myofibrils lie suspended inside the sarcoplasm (a cellular matrix) (Fig. 7-1), which consists of fluid and many mitochondria, which supply energy to the myocardium. The sarcoplasmic reticulum lies in the sarcoplasm and consists of longitudinal tubules that are parallel to the myofibrils. Cisternae and junctional feet (bulbous structures) are found at the end of each of the longitudinal tubules.

The sarcolemma forms deep invaginations into the cell called the transverse tubules, or T tubules, which lie per-

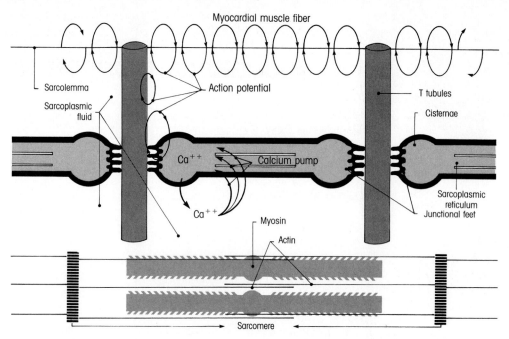

FIG. 7-1   Structure of a myocardial muscle fiber, also showing excitation of the muscle that produces the release of calcium from the sarcoplasmic reticulum and the uptake of calcium by the calcium pump. Myocardial muscle fiber structures also include the sarcolemma (cell membrane), T tubles that contain extracellular fluid and transmit the action potential, sarcoplasmic fluid (cellular matrix containing the myofibrils), sarcoplasmic reticulum (longitudinal tubules), and junctional feet (that abut on the T tubules and transmit the action potential to the sarcoplasmic reticulum).

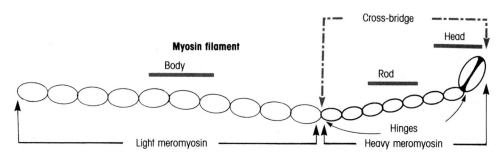

FIG. 7-2   Myosin filament, showing the body, rod, and head.
Redrawn from Guyton AC: Textbook of medical physiology, ed 6, Philadelphia, 1981, WB Saunders Co.

pendicular to the myofibrils. The T tubules contain extracellular fluid and extend through the muscle fiber and open to the exterior of the cell. Each muscle fiber has T tubules that lie between the ends of the longitudinal tubules and abut on the cisternae (Fig. 7-1).

T tubules are located on both sides of the sarcomere at the point where the actin and myosin overlap. Myocardial contraction is activated because of the changes that occur in the longitudinal and T tubules.[22]

The myosin filaments can be divided into two parts: (1) *light meromyosin,* or the *body,* which consists of two peptide strands wound around each other to form a helix;

and (2) *heavy meromyosin,* which possesses adenosine triphosphatase activity and is composed of the *rod,* which is a double-helix, and the *head,* which is two globular protein masses attached to the rod.[2,22] The heads and rods make up the cross-bridges of the myosin filament. There is a flexible hinge between the body and the rod and another between the rod and the head (Fig. 7-2).

Each actin filament is composed of an actin double helix, troponin, and tropomyosin. Each strand of the helix is attached to one molecule of adenosine diphosphate, which is believed to be the active site that interacts with the myosin cross-bridges to produce myocardial contrac-

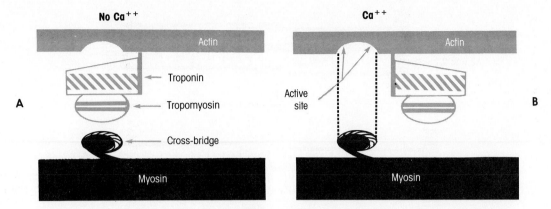

FIG. 7-3 Actin filament. **A,** Inhibitory effect of the troponin-tropomyosin complex without calcium. **B,** Inhibitory effect of the troponin-tropomyosin complex removed with calcium to produce muscle contraction.

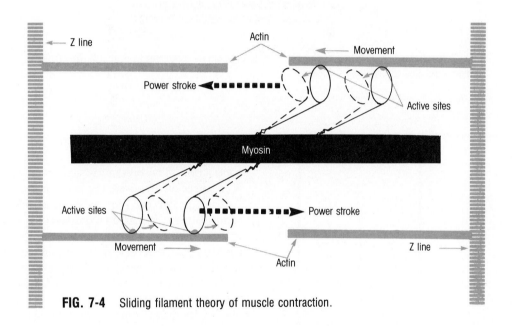

FIG. 7-4 Sliding filament theory of muscle contraction.

tion. The actin helix also contains troponin and tropomyosin.

The troponin, with the tropomyosin attached to it, lies in the groove formed by the actin helix. When the troponin and tropomyosin are bound together, the active sites on the actin filament are covered, the muscle is relaxed, and interaction between the myosin cross-bridges and actin filament is inhibited (no contraction) (Fig. 7-3, A).[2]

Myocardial contraction can occur when the active sites on the actin filament are uncovered. This is accomplished by the presence of calcium. Because troponin has high-affinity calcium binding sites, it is believed that, when present, calcium combines with troponin. This combination allows troponin to undergo a structural change such that it pulls the tropomyosin deep into the groove of the actin

strand, thereby uncovering the active sites on the actin (Fig. 7-3, B).[3] The heads of the myosin filaments are attracted to the active sites to trigger muscle contraction.

Myocardial contraction is believed to occur because of a sliding filament (ratchet) theory of contraction. When the sarcomere is activated electrically, the filaments slide by each other, shortening the sarcomere and allowing the myosin head to attach to the active sites on the actin filament. This hinge between the head and the rod allows the head to tilt forward toward the center of the myosin filament. As the head tilts forward, it pulls the actin filament with it and moves the actin toward the center of the myosin. Each *head tilt* is called a *power stroke* (Fig. 7-4).[2,22]

After each head tilt, the head breaks away from the active site and rises again to combine with a new active

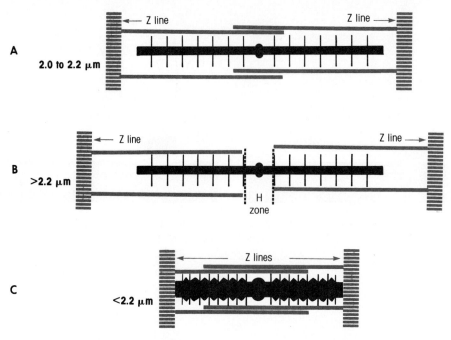

FIG. 7-5   **A,** Sarcomere stretched to 2.2 μm. **B,** Sarcomere stretched to over 2.2 μm. **C,** Sarcomere stretched to less than 2.2 μm.

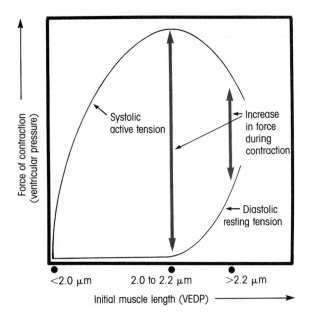

FIG. 7-6   Relationship between muscle length and force of contraction. The increase in developed tension is large when the muscle is stretched to 2.2 μm; the increase in developed tension is small when the muscle is stretched beyond normal limits (more than 2.2 μm).

site farther down the actin filament. A series of head tilts creates a sliding or ratcheting effect and causes muscle contraction. The breakaway activity of actin and myosin is an effect of adenosine triphosphatase.

The greater the number of cross-bridges pulling the actin filament, the greater the force of contraction. Peak myocardial contraction occurs when there is maximal overlap between the actin and the myosin cross-bridges. At the sarcomere's normal stretched length of 2.0 to 2.2 microns (μm), the actin overlaps with the myosin and begins to overlap with other actin[2,5,22] (Fig. 7-5, *A*). Stretched to this length, the sarcomere produces the maximal contractile force.

When the resting muscle is stretched, a *resting tension* or *resting pressure* (preload) develops. This occurs during diastole, when the ventricle is filled with blood, before contraction takes place. The increase in tension that occurs during contraction (systole) is called *active tension* or *active pressure.*[2]

Fig. 7-6 illustrates the relationship of initial muscle length (*ventricular end-diastolic volume* [VEDV]) and force of contraction (or ventricular pressure). The upper curve represents the pressure developed during systole, and the lower curve represents the pressure developed during diastole. Peak systolic pressures are achieved by a ventricular end-diastolic pressure (VEDP) of approximately 12 mm Hg. At this pressure the sarcomere is stretched to 2.0 to 2.2 μm. Note also that the diastolic pressure curve is initially flat, indicating that large diastolic volumes can be accommodated by the normal ventricle with only small increases in the diastolic resting tension.[2]

If the sarcomere is stretched at rest to greater than 2.2 μm, the number of myosin cross-bridges overlapping with the actin is reduced. The ends of the actin begin to pull apart, creating a light area in the center of the A band called the *H zone* (Fig. 7-5, *B*). Note also in Fig. 7-6 that, when the sarcomere is stretched greater than 2.2 μm, the resting tension rapidly increases while the active tension and the force of contraction are reduced.[5]

If the sarcomere is stretched to less than 2.0 μm (Fig. 7-5, *C*), the two Z membranes abut on the ends of the myosin. The myosin filaments begin to crumple, and the active tension and the force of contraction are reduced.[5,22]

ELECTRICAL AND CHEMICAL EVENTS OF MUSCLE CONTRACTION

Action potential is the electrical activity that initiates or causes muscle contraction (see Chapter 6). The action potential travels along the sarcolemma and into the T tubules, which spread the action potential deep within and throughout the muscle fiber.

As it travels, the action potential produces a flow of current in the junctional feet of the cisternae of the sarcoplasmic reticulum. This current flow causes calcium to be released from the sarcoplasmic reticulum into the sarcoplasmic fluid.[2,22,26] The calcium then diffuses to the myofibrils, where it combines with troponin to uncover the active sites on the actin and produce muscle contraction. The released calcium is almost immediately returned by a calcium pump in the sarcoplasmic reticulum, which induces relaxation after contraction. The calcium concentration is generally low in the sarcoplasm except during the action potential.[3,14,22]

DETERMINANTS OF MYOCARDIAL FUNCTION

The velocity of muscle fiber shortening (velocity of contraction) and the force of contraction are related to the presence of intracellular calcium and the presence of a volume load.

Preload

As the VEDV rises, the cardiac muscle fiber is stretched to its initial muscle fiber length, thereby raising the VEDP. The VEDV, or preload, determines the length of muscle fiber at the onset of contraction. The length of the muscle fiber in turn determines the force of contraction and the velocity of muscle fiber shortening.

The ability of the peripheral vessels to return blood to the heart can alter the preload and hence cardiac output. Factors that reduce peripheral vascular resistance—augmenting venous return and VEDV—include pregnancy,

fever, and anemia. Preload is also increased by factors that cause venoconstriction, such as exercise, anxiety, and sympathomimetic drugs. Decreasing intrathoracic pressure (i.e., making it more negative) increases thoracic blood volume and cardiac filling. The normally negative intrathoracic pressure becomes more negative during inspiration, thereby increasing venous return and stroke volume.

Frank-Starling phenomenon

The Frank-Starling phenomenon is based on a length–active tension relationship concerning the ability of the ventricle to change the force of contraction from heartbeat to heartbeat because of its initial end-diastolic size.[2,5,26] The Frank-Starling curve illustrates that the stroke volume is increased as the preload is increased (Fig. 7-7).[2,5,22,26] The optimal left ventricular end-diastolic pressure (LVEDP) is 12 mm Hg. When it is increased to 15 to 20 mm Hg (in the normal heart), no appreciable increases in stroke volume are seen (plateau of the curve). When filling pressures are greater than 20 mm Hg, stroke volume may begin to fall because there is not an optimal relationship between the actin and myosin filaments.

If the preload is increased to within physiologic limits (as defined by the Frank-Starling law), the rate and extent of muscle fiber shortening, and the work of the heart are increased. Also, as the preload is increased, the isometric force is increased and the ventricle is able to contract optimally against progressively larger afterloads. The LVEDP can be raised by increasing the blood volume, preload, or

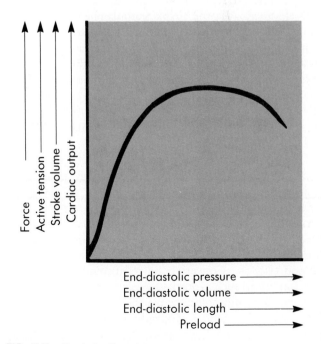

FIG. 7-7   Frank-Starling phenomenon.

by decreasing the inotropic state of the heart (i.e., decreasing contractility).

Preload is reduced when venous return is reduced due to hemorrhage, a sudden change to an upright position, or increased intrathoracic pressure associated with positive pressure ventilation. Venodilatation caused by drugs such as nitroglycerin produces venous pooling and reduced venous return and preload. When the pericardial pressure is increased, such as during pericardial effusion or tamponade, cardiac filling and end-diastolic volume are reduced. Because preload also can be augmented by atrial contraction, the loss of atrial contraction during atrial fibrillation may reduce end-diastolic volumes.

Afterload

Afterload refers to impedance that the ventricle must overcome during ejection. Afterload does not affect the myocardial muscle fibers until after the onset of contraction.[2,5,26] Impedance is determined by arterial pressure, ventricular radius and wall thickness, and blood viscosity. External shortening of the muscle fibers during contraction does not occur until the active tension developed in the ventricle is equal to the afterload (i.e., after the semilunar valves open and blood is ejected into the aorta).[5,26]

Stroke volume is inversely related to afterload. When afterload is increased beyond physiologic limits, such as during peripheral vasoconstriction, the arterial blood pressure increases and thereby reduces the rate and extent of muscle fiber shortening and therefore stroke volume. Under normal circumstances, however, when the stroke volume is reduced, the LVEDV or preload, is increased, which in turn stretches the resting length of the myocardial muscle fibers. Via the Frank-Starling phenomenon, this increased stretch produces an increase in stroke volume. This regulatory mechanism not only increases the stroke volume against a greater afterload but also the work of the heart (where *work* equals the mean arterial pressure [MAP] multiplied by the stroke volume), which can be detrimental to a patient with an ischemic myocardium (increasing the work increases the myocardial oxygen demand [MVo_2], which cannot be met).

Impedance to left ventricular (LV) ejection can be altered by valvular heart disease. In mitral regurgitation, for example, impedance to blood flow is lowered during LV ejection because blood flows forward through the open aortic valve while simultaneously flowing back through the regurgitant or incompetent mitral valve. Afterload can also be reduced by arteriolar dilation, vasodilators, and lowered blood viscosity. Conversely, impedance may be increased by conditions such as aortic stenosis, arterial and arteriolar constriction, and polycythemia.[5,26]

When the afterload is greatly increased from normal, the *onset* of muscle fiber shortening is delayed.[2,3] This occurs because there is a longer isometric contraction time

because of the increased afterload. Thus a greater ventricular active tension must develop before it is equal to the increased afterload so that external muscle fiber shortening can occur. With an increased afterload, there is also a reduction in the rate and extent of muscle fiber shortening.[2,5,26]

Inotropic state of the heart

The inotropic state of the heart, or myocardial contractility, determines the force developed during systole, the velocity of muscle fiber shortening, and the extent of the muscle fiber shortening. These factors in turn depend on the interaction of calcium, actin, and myosin.[5,26]

The inotropic state of the heart can be increased, shifting the Frank-Starling curve to the left, by factors such as central nervous system stimulation, circulating epinephrine and norepinephrine, cardiac glycosides, β_1-adrenergic receptors, calcium, glucagon, and caffeine. Myocardial contractility may be depressed, shifting the Frank-Starling curve to the right, by factors such as ischemia, heart failure, anoxia, acidosis, hypoxia, local and general anesthetics, and barbiturates.[4,34,41,46] Although these factors may influence myocardial contractility, they may or may not be responsible for producing changes in cardiac output.

PHYSIOLOGIC BASIS OF HEMODYNAMIC MONITORING

The physiologic function of the circulatory system depends on a series of complex interactions. The heart serves as a pump. The vascular system serves as a reservoir and a conduit. The kidneys control blood volume through a complex balancing system.

Adequate oxygen delivery is determined by cardiac output, the oxygen saturation of arterial blood (SaO_2), and the concentration of hemoglobin. This relationship is depicted in Figure 7-8. Bedside monitoring is used to assess the determinants of cardiac output (and hence oxygen delivery) through measurement of the hemodynamic parameters reflecting preload, afterload, and contractility.

Preload

Preload, the volume of blood in the ventricle before contraction, depends on the capacity of the venous system. The clinical measurement of preload of the right side of the heart is the pressure during filling of the right ventricle (RV) at end-diastole (end-diastolic pressure [EDP]). Except with tricuspid stenosis, the pressure in the right atrium (RA) is the preload or filling pressure of the RV. Thus the RA pressure (RAP) or the central venous pressure (CVP) is clinically used to assess preload of the right side of the heart.[4,5,17,26]

The clinical measurement of preload of the left side of

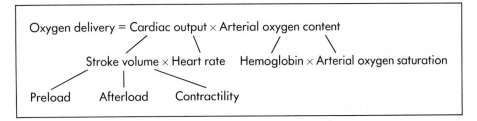

FIG. 7-8 Oxygen delivery (ml/min) is a product of the cardiac output and the oxygen content of arterial blood. In turn, cardiac output is a product of stroke volume and heart rate. The stroke volume is subsequently determined by preload, afterload, and contractility. The arterial oxygen content is a product of the hemoglobin and oxygen saturation of arterial blood (Sao_2). Alterations in oxygen delivery can be achieved by manipulation of any of these parameters.
Redrawn from Daily EK and Schroeder JS: Techniques in bedside hemodynamic monitoring, St Louis, 1989, The CV Mosby Co.

the heart is the diastolic filling pressure of the LV reflected by the left atrial pressure (LAP). This pressure can be measured indirectly by wedging the pulmonary artery (PA) catheter in a small branch of the PA, occluding blood flow in that segment of the vessel. This technique permits backward reflection of the LAP to the catheter tip and is termed a *pulmonary artery wedge pressure* (PAWP) and is used clinically to reflect left-sided heart preload.

Afterload

Afterload is the tension developed by the myocardium during contraction and is inversely related to cardiac output. Afterload of the left side of the heart can be estimated by calculating the systemic vascular resistance according to the formula in Table 7-1.* Normal systemic vascular resistance is 900 to 1400 dyne-seconds-cm^{-5}. To index this parameter to the individual body size, the denominator of the formula should be the patient's cardiac index in place of the cardiac output. The normal values of *systemic vascular resistance index* are between 1700 and 2500 dyne-seconds-cm^{-5}/m^2.

Afterload of the right side of the heart is estimated by calculation of the pulmonary vascular resistance, also listed in Table 7-1. Normally, the resistance to flow through the pulmonary circuit is substantially lower than the corresponding systemic circulation with values of less than 200 dyne-seconds-cm^{-5}. The normal pulmonary vascular resistance index is 200 to 450 dyne-seconds-cm^{-5}/m^2.

Optimal resistance, or afterload, results in production of the least tension in the heart during maintenance of adequate coronary and systemic blood flow.[4]

Contractility

Contractility is the inotropic state of the myocardium. Although contractility cannot be measured directly or even

approximated in the clinical setting, an index of ventricular work *(stroke work index)* is used to assess changes in contractility. The stroke work indices of either ventricle can be calculated according to the formulas listed in Table 7-1. Studies by Shoemaker and others[44] have shown that maintenance of a LV stroke work index greater than 55 $g \cdot m/m^2$/beat is associated with improved survival in shock patients.

Heart rate

Heart rate is a major determinant of cardiac output, coronary blood flow, and myocardial oxygen use. It is measured in the number of beats per minute. Within limits, increases in heart rate can increase cardiac output. However, heart rates greater than 120 to 125 beats per minute may be associated with reductions in stroke volume and hence cardiac output because of the decreased duration of diastole and ventricular filling. Fast heart rates with shortened diastolic duration also decrease left coronary perfusion time and increase myocardial oxygen consumption (MVo_2), causing an imbalance between myocardial oxygen supply and demand.

Cardiac output

Cardiac output is the amount of blood ejected by the ventricles per minute. It is the product of heart rate and stroke volume (cardiac output = heart rate × stroke volume). Normal cardiac output is between 4 to 8 L/min. A more individualized measurement of flow is the cardiac index, which can be calculated according to the formula in Table 7-1. The normal resting cardiac index is 2.5 to 4.0 L/min/m^2.

Numerous and varied pathologic conditions can result in a low cardiac output and hence reduce oxygen delivery resulting from inadequate LV filling, or inadequate LV ejection. The box on p. 169, top left, lists some of the pathologic conditions responsible for these inadequacies.

---

*References 10,12, 21, 29, 34, 38, and 52.

TABLE 7-1

Normal Values and Equations for Hemodynamic Monitoring

Normal resting range	Equation

CENTRAL VENOUS PRESSURE (CVP)

4-15 cm H_2O or 3-11 mm Hg

LEFT VENTRICULAR END-DIASTOLIC PRESSURE (LVEDP)

8 ± 4 mm Hg

PULMONARY ARTERY PRESSURE (PAP)

Systole: 20 ± 5 mm Hg
Diastole: 12 ± 3 mm Hg
Mean: 15 ± 5 mm Hg

PULMONARY ARTERY WEDGE PRESSURE (PAWP)

4-12 mm Hg

RIGHT ATRIAL PRESSURE (RAP)

4 ± 2 mm Hg

CARDIAC OUTPUT (CO)

4-8 L/min   CO = Stroke volume × Heart rate

STROKE VOLUME (SV)

60-130 ml/beat $SV = \dfrac{CO}{\text{Heart rate}}$

CARDIAC INDEX (CI)

2.5-4.0 L/min/m² $CI = \dfrac{CO}{\text{Body surface area}}$

STROKE INDEX (SI)

46 ± 8 ml/beat/m² $SI = \dfrac{SV}{\text{Body surface area}}$

MEAN ARTERIAL PRESSURE (MAP)

80-95 mm Hg $MAP = \text{Diastolic pressure} + \dfrac{\text{Systolic} - \text{Diastolic}}{3}$

SYSTEMIC VASCULAR RESISTANCE (SVR)

900-1400 dyne-seconds-cm^{-5} $SVR = \dfrac{MAP - \text{Mean venous pressure (MVP)}}{CO} \times 80$

PULMONARY VASCULAR RESISTANCE (PVR)

<200 dyne-seconds-cm^{-5} $PVR = \dfrac{MPAP - \text{Mean PAWP}}{CO} \times 80$
  (normally ⅙ of SVR or less)

LEFT VENTRICULAR STROKE WORK INDEX (LVSWI)

40-75 g·m/m²/beat   LVSWI = SI × (MAP − Mean PAWP) × 0.0136

RIGHT VENTRICULAR STROKE WORK INDEX (RVSWI)

4-8 g·m/m²/beat   RVSWI = SI × (MPAP − Mean RAP) × 0.0136

FACTORS CAUSING LOW CARDIAC OUTPUT

INADEQUATE LV FILLING

Tachycardia
Rhythm disturbance
Hypovolemia
Mitral or tricuspid stenosis
Pulmonic stenosis
Constrictive pericarditis or tamponade
Restrictive cardiomyopathy

INADEQUATE LV EJECTION

LV ischemia or infarction
Myocardial disease
Increased afterload
   Aortic stenosis
   Hypertension
Mitral regurgitation
Metabolic disorders
Drugs with negative inotropic effects

Modified from Daily EK and Schroeder JS: Techniques in bedside hemodynamic monitoring ed 4, St Louis, 1989, The CV Mosby Co.

 INDICATIONS FOR HEMODYNAMIC MONITORING

Complicated acute myocardial infarction
   Evidence of hypoperfusion
   Significant pulmonary congestion
   Unexplained dyspnea
   Refractory dysrhythmias
   Persistent myocardial ischemia
   RV infarction
Suspected anatomic lesions
   Ventricular septal rupture
   Papillary muscle rupture
   Pulmonary embolism
   Pericardial tamponade
Shock states
   Cardiogenic
   Hypovolemic
   Septic
High-risk patients undergoing surgery

The procedure for bedside monitoring of thermodilution cardiac output is discussed in a later section.

Cardiac function

Cardiac function or ventricular performance is best expressed or depicted by a ventricular function curve (see Fig. 7-7). This curve compares changes in the preload, or distending pressure of the ventricle, with cardiac output and indicates that the stretch of the myocardial muscle is directly related to the force generated by the myocardium.[1,21,54] Increases in preload result in increases in cardiac output or stroke volume, within physiologic limits. The upper limit of left ventricular filling pressure is the oncotic pressure that will result in pulmonary venous hypertension, causing movement of fluid out of the vascular space resulting in overt pulmonary edema. Measurement of the PAWP permits assessment and regulation of an optimal left ventricular filling pressure to maintain a maximal cardiac output while preventing pulmonary edema.

CLINICAL APPLICATIONS

In the critically ill, hemodynamically unstable patient, hemodynamic monitoring is used to obtain a more accurate and detailed assessment of cardiovascular function, to prevent complications, and to titrate therapy. When combined with careful assessment of the patient, hemodynamic monitoring provides detailed information regarding cardiovascular status and thus expands the scope of cardiovascular evaluation. It does not, of course, take the place of careful patient assessment and observation but rather is an adjunct to meticulous assessment.

In certain pathologic conditions, hemodynamic monitoring is extremely useful to determine the specific hemodynamic derangements and to guide therapeutic interventions appropriately. In general, hemodynamic monitoring is indicated in patients with complicated acute myocardial infarction, anatomic cardiac lesions, shock states, and in high-risk patients undergoing surgical procedures (see the box, above).

Complicated acute myocardial infarction

Patients who suffer acute myocardial infarction can be classified according to clinical parameters that relate to the prognosis and reflect LV function. The most common prognostic index is the *Killip classification*. Killip Class I patients have no evidence of heart failure, and a 6% to 12% mortality rate exists. The evaluation of hemodynamic function should indicate that systemic arterial pressure, cardiac output, peripheral resistance, and left ventricular filling pressure are within normal limits.[28,38,41]

Killip Class II patients have evidence of heart failure, as indicated by basilar crackles, an S_3 gallop, and evidence of venous hypertension on an x-ray film. The mortality rate is 17% to 21%. Systemic arterial pressure and cardiac output are usually normal. Peripheral vascular resistance may be normal but occasionally is slightly increased, and left ventricular filling pressure is elevated.

Patients in Killip Class III have severe heart failure as evidenced by frank pulmonary edema. There is an associated mortality rate of 30% to 40%. Hemodynamically, these patients are seen first with normal or decreased systemic arterial pressure, reduced cardiac output, and significantly increased peripheral vascular resistance and PAWP.

Patients in Killip Class IV have cardiogenic shock, as indicated by hypotension, with a systolic blood pressure of less than 90 mm Hg. The associated mortality rate with this classification is 90% to 95%. Hemodynamic measurements indicate significant reductions in systemic arterial pressure and cardiac output, with increases in peripheral vascular resistance. A subgroup of patients who have apparent cardiogenic shock also are classified in Killip Class IV, but they have a low or normal PAWP. The hemodynamic abnormalities found in this subgroup can be corrected with volume replacement, and the associated mortality rate is only 10% to 15%.[38,41]

Suspected anatomic cardiac lesions

Hemodynamic monitoring also permits rapid identification of complications of myocardial infarction, including ventricular septal rupture, papillary muscle rutpure, and cardiac tamponade. Patients with ventricular septal rupture can be identified by measuring oxygen saturations from the RA and the PA. An increase in oxygen saturation of greater than 5% between the RA and the PA confirms the presence of a left-to-right intracardiac shunt.

Papillary muscle rupture resulting in acute mitral regurgitation is identified by the presence of a large, early *v* wave in the pulmonary artery wedge (PAW) waveform. Cardiac tamponade may occur secondary to myocardial rupture and can be recognized by an elevation of all right-sided pressures with equalization of mean right atrial pressure (MRAP), right VEDP, PA diastolic pressure (PADP), and PAWP.[42] Pulsus paradoxus with a greater than 10 mm Hg decline in arterial systolic pressure during spontaneous inspiration also is usually evident in patients with cardiac tamponade. Pulmonary embolism is hemodynamically evidenced by pulmonary hypertension accompanied by a normal or even low PAWP.

Shock states

Shock is a common indication for hemodynamic monitoring. Shock may be divided into four categories: hypovolemic shock, cardiogenic shock, septic shock, and shock associated with obstruction to blood flow.

Hypovolemic shock

Patients who suffer shock from hypovolemia may have a readily identifiable cause such as acute blood loss, dehydration, or vomiting. Adequate replacement of volume usually can be monitored via a central venous catheter. The exception is with cardiac or pulmonary disease, in which the CVP often is not an accurate reflection of left ventricular filling pressure. Under these conditions monitoring the PAWP is necessary to determine whether adequate volume has been replaced to maintain LV function.[51]

Cardiogenic shock

Cardiogenic shock requires measurement of both right and left ventricular filling pressures. An acute myocardial infarction may selectively alter RV or LV function, and both chambers need to be monitored to determine ideal filling pressures for maintenance of optimal cardiac output or to guide therapy.[16]

Hemodynamic evidence of cardiogenic shock secondary to LV failure includes an elevated PAWP (greater than 18 to 22 mm Hg) accompanied by hypoperfusion with a cardiac index of less than 2.2 L/min/m². Cardiogenic shock associated with RV failure is hemodynamically manifested by an elevated RAP to values greater than the PAWP with accompanying hypoperfusion. Table 7-2 lists specific hemodynamic alterations associated with shock states.[8]

Septic shock

In septic shock, there is a sequestration of volume in the venous system and therefore a reduction of venous return.[5] The problem is not one of absolute hypovolemia but rather of faulty blood distribution within the peripheral blood channels resulting in relative hypovolemia. Vasodilation associated with sepsis produces reduced systemic vascular resistance (usually in association with high cardiac outputs) and low filling pressures (RA and PAW). Hemodynamic monitoring is done for evaluation of intravascular volume and systemic perfusion and for determination of proper filling pressures and fluid requirements.

Pulmonary disease

Hemodynamic monitoring is helpful in differentiating pulmonary disease from acute LV failure as a cause of dyspnea and hypoxia. Patients with pulmonary infiltrates, who have elevated mean pulmonary artery pressure (MPAP) and normal left ventricular filling pressure have pulmonary disease. In patients with known heart disease who are undergoing extensive surgical procedures, continuous evaluation of left ventricular filling pressure is important to prevent cardiogenic shock and pulmonary edema.[34,42]

CENTRAL VENOUS CATHETERIZATION
CVP

The CVP is a fairly simple measurement of the body's blood volume and vascular tone. However, it is a poor indication of left-sided heart failure. CVP is a direct measurement of RAP and an indirect measurement of right ventricular diastolic pressure (RVDP).

CVP can be measured in centimeters of water by a

TABLE 7-2
Differentiating Hemodynamic Features Associated with Cardiogenic Shock States

Pathophysiology	RAP	PAP	PAWP	Differentiating features
Acute LV failure	Normal or high	High	High	Increased *v* wave secondary to functional mitral regurgitation
RV infarction	High	High or low	Normal or low	RA pressure greater than PAWP Increased *a* wave in RAP Prominent *y* descent in RAP Kussmaul's sign
Acute mitral regurgitation	Normal or high	High	High	Large, early *v* wave (at or shortly after QRS) (*v* wave may exceed PA systolic)
Acute ventricular septal defect	High	High	High	Oxygen saturation step-up between RA and PA Possible increased *v* wave in PAWP, occurring later in systole (well after QRS) High thermodilution cardiac output values
Acute cardiac tamponade	High	High	High	Prominent *x* descent with brief or absent *y* descent in RAP Normal respiratory response in RAP Diastolic equalization (RA approximately equal to PAEDP approximately equal to PAW) Pulsus paradoxus in arterial pressure
Acute massive pulmonary embolism	High	High	Normal or low	PAEDP greater than PAW Pulsus paradoxus in arterial pressure

From Daily EK: Use of hemodynamics to differentiate pathophysiologic causes of cardiogenic shock, Crit Care Nurs Clin North Am 1:589, 1989.

water manometer or in millimeters of mercury by a pressure transducer. The normal CVP ranges from 4 to 15 cm H_2O or 3 to 11 mm Hg. It is important to understand the conversion factor between the two values. Mercury is 1.36 times heavier than water. Thus to convert millimeters of mercury to centimeters of water, it is multiplied by the conversion factor of 1.36; for example[33]:

$$10 \text{ mm Hg} \times 1.36 = 13.6 \text{ cm } H_2O$$

Conversely, to convert centimeters of water to millimeters of mercury, the manometrically obtained value (in cm H_2O) is divided by 1.36.

As blood volume decreases, the CVP decreases correspondingly. A CVP of less than 4 cm H_2O indicates a hypovolemic state in which fluid volume can be given safely without overloading the heart. Conversely, a CVP higher than normal may indicate a hypervolemic state, and the patient may need to be treated with diuretics, inotropic agents, vasodilators, or rotating tourniquets.[15,29] Decreased compliance of the RV alters the pressure-volume relationship, however, resulting in elevated CVP or RAP that does not accurately reflect the volume status of the right side of the heart.

Central venous catheters

There are many types of central venous catheters. Their selection usually depends on the insertion site to be used and the diameter of the catheter and its length. An ante-

cubital site requires a longer catheter than a subclavian site. The diameter sizes for adults range from a 24-gauge introducer needle to a 17-gauge needle and finally a 14-gauge introducer needle. Each introducer needle comes with a smaller intracatheter, which remains in the vein.[18]

Procedure

The procedure for insertion of a central venous catheter involves selecting an appropriate insertion site. The antecubital area, subclavian area, or jugular vein may be chosen. Although arm vein cannulation for insertion of central venous catheters is associated with the lowest complication rate, the catastrophic complication of acute cardiac tamponade is more likely to occur when this insertion site is used.[7] Movement of the arm can cause forward migration of the catheter tip, resulting in perforation of the RA wall.

Before beginning the procedure, the catheter length required for proper positioning of the catheter tip in the superior vena cava, just above the RA junction is estimated. This can be done by laying the packaged catheter over the patient from the proposed insertion site to the sternal notch and determining the corresponding catheter length.

The patient is placed in a supine position, or in Trendelenburg's position if a central vein is cannulated, and the area is prepared with an antibacterial solution. With sterile technique the needle and intracatheter are inserted until the tip of the intracatheter rests in the superior vena cava according to the previously determined catheter length.

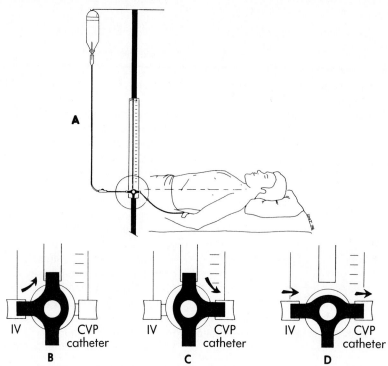

FIG. 7-9 Procedure for measuring CVP with manometer. **A,** Manometer and intravenous tubing in place. **B,** Turn the stopcock so that the manometer fills with fluid above the level of the expected pressure. **C,** Turn the stopcock so that the intravenous line is off and the manometer flows to the patient. Obtain a reading after the fluid level stabilizes. **D,** Turn the stopcock to resume the intravenous line flow to the patient.

From Daily EK and Schroeder JS: Techniques in bedside hemodynamic monitoring, St Louis, 1989, The CV Mosby Co.

The catheter is then connected to a transducer or a water manometer via a stopcock and fluid-filled tubing. (The setup and procedure for measurement of CVP via a water manometer are depicted in Figure 7-9.) When the initial CVP reading is satisfactory, the intracatheter is sutured to the skin at the insertion site. An occlusive dressing is applied over the site. After insertion, a chest x-ray film is taken to rule out a pneumothorax caused by insertion.

The CVP setup has five basic parts: an intravenous fluid bottle, fluid-administration set, three-way stopcock, fluid adjuster attached to the intravenous extension tubing, and manometer, usually scaled from 0 to 30 cm H_2O.

To obtain a CVP reading with a manometer, the zero-level of the manometer is aligned at the approximate level of the RA, commonly considered to be at the midchest level measured at the fourth intercostal space. (To ensure continuity of zero-leveling, an X is marked on the patient's chest at this position.)

The nurse then turns the stopcock to fill the manometer with fluid from the intravenous bottle to the 25-cm mark. The stopcock is then turned to open the manometer to the patient. The CVP measurement is obtained at the end of expiration, when the fluid level in the manometer stabilizes. The fluid fluctuates with each deep respiration; this is not to be confused with a stabilizing fluid level. Ventilator-assisted respirations produces a falsely high CVP reading. If the patient is unable to tolerate a supine position, the elevation of the head of the bed should be recorded on the patient's chart, and all further readings should be taken at that angle.

PA CATHETERIZATION

The development of the flow-directed, balloon-tipped PA catheter has provided the opportunity to indirectly acquire important diagnostic and therapeutic information regarding LV function. As the major pumping chamber of the heart, the LV's performance correlates closely with overall cardiac function and indicates the severity of cardiac dysfunction. The LVEDP or preload is one of the primary determinants of LV performance because it affects the myocardial fiber stretch during diastole when the LV passively fills. In the patient with normal lungs and a normal mitral valve, the PA end-diastolic pressure (PAEDP)

…

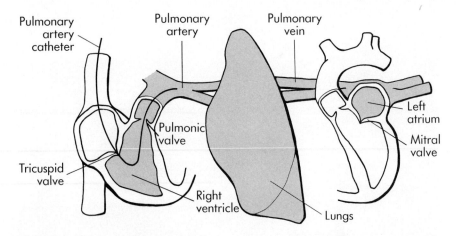

FIG. 7-10 Measurement of PAP. PA systolic pressure equilibrates with the RV systolic pressure, whereas the PAEDP equilibrates with the LVEDP, in the absence of pulmonary or mitral valve disease.

Adapted From: Dossey BM, Guzzetta CE, and Kenner CV: Critical care nursing: body-mind-spirit, ed 3, Philadelphia, 1992, JB Lippincott Co.

closely reflects the LVEDP and can be used as an index of LV function or dysfunction. At the end of diastole, just before the next systole, the mitral valve is still open, and the LV is filled with blood. During this period, there is an equilibration of pressures between the pulmonary veins, the pulmonary capillaries, and the PA at end-diastole (Fig. 7-10). At this point, the pressure in the PA is equal to the LVEDP.

Inflation of the balloon at the tip of the PA catheter occludes the vessel and causes a cessation of forward blood flow in that branch of the PA. The tip of the catheter, which extends beyond the balloon, "sees" only the pressure ahead in the pulmonary venous system, which is retrogradely transmitted to the catheter tip. This is actually the LAP, which is the filling pressure of the LV. Thus the PAWP is used as a reflection of left-sided heart preload or LVEDP.

PA catheters

Balloon flotation PA catheters are available to meet virtually every need in hemodynamic monitoring. In addition to thermistors, which allow measurement of cardiac output by the thermodilution technique, these catheters come equipped with pacing wires and an additional RA port for the infusion of fluids or drugs or measurement of RV ejection, as well as a sensor to continuously measure venous oxygen saturation.

Procedure

Before pressure measurements are obtained, the reference port of the transducer must be set level with the patient's phlebostatic axis or midchest height, approximately the

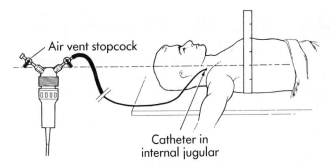

FIG. 7-11 Illustration showing measurement of the patient's chest to determine the midchest position and placement of the transducer reference port at this level. In this way the two open "ends" (the air vent stopcock and the catheter tip) are at the same level and negate the effects of hydrostatic pressure.

From Daily EK and Schroeder JS: Techniques in bedside hemodynamic monitoring, St Louis, 1989, The CV Mosby Co.

level of the RA (Fig. 7-11). The transducer is then connected to the monitor. With the reference stopcock open to air, the zero dial on the monitor is set, and the calibration is checked.

Before catheter insertion and under sterile conditions, the catheter is flushed with sterile solution, and the integrity of the balloon is assessed by inflating it with the maximum amount of air and immersing it in water to check for air bubbles (Fig. 7-12). If a thermodilution catheter is used, the integrity of the thermistor wires should be assessed by connecting the catheter to the cardiac output computer with the appropriate computer cable.

The catheter is connected to the transducer by short, stiff extension tubing and stopcocks (Fig. 7-13). The connecting tubing should be just long enough to connect the

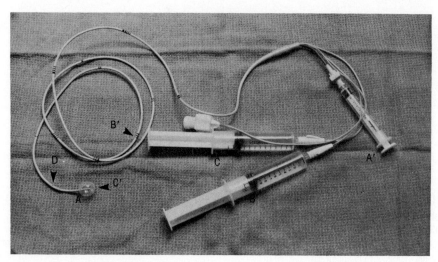

FIG. 7-12   The PA flow-directed thermodilution catheter. Before insertion, the catheter is inspected for defects and surface is lubricated with a sterile solution. *A,* Care should be taken not to damage the latex balloon during catheter preparation. Note the maximal balloon inflation capacity printed on the catheter shaft. *A',* The balloon integrity is checked by inflating the balloon to capacity while it is immersed in a sterile solution (filtered carbon dioxide is the manufacturer's recommended inflation medium). *B,* The monitoring RA (proximal) lumen is filled with sterile fluid to minimize the chance of introducing air into the circulatory system. *B',* Note the patency of the atrial port *(arrow). C,* The monitoring PA (distal) lumen is filled with sterile fluid as in *B. C',* Note the patency of the PA port *(arrow). D,* Thermistor site.

Courtesy American Edwards Laboratories.

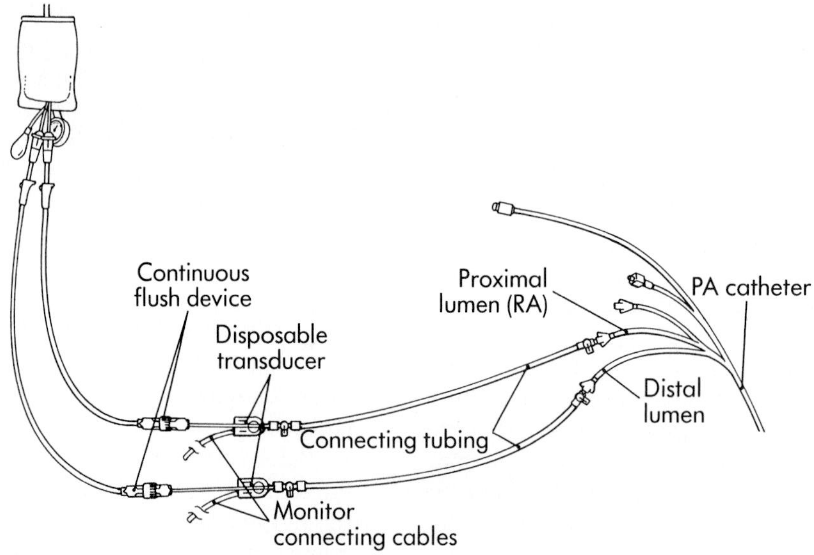

FIG. 7-13   An appropriate setup for monitoring of PAP and RAP using disposable transducers and one intravenous solution bag.

From Daily EK and Schroeder JS: Techniques in bedside hemodynamic monitoring, St Louis, 1989, The CV Mosby Co.

catheter to the transducer. Excessive tubing lengths cause distortion of pressure waveforms. Ideally, the transducer should be connected directly to the catheter via a stopcock. The connector tubing must be flushed with an intravenous fluid before it is connected to the catheter. To prevent thrombus formation at the tip of the catheter, 1 unit of heparin per milliliter of intravenous fluid is added and a continuous flush device is used. Pressure waveforms are continuously monitored during insertion to ensure proper location of the catheter tip.

Patient preparation

Give the patient and family information relating to the necessity of the procedure, risks involved, techniques used, and sensations that may be felt. Make these explanations relatively short and simple, depending on the needs of the patient and the acuteness of the situation. Reduce or totally eliminate stress because it can inhibit the teaching-learning process. Frequently ascertain the patient's stress by listening to the questions asked.

"Am I going to die? Will it hurt? What will it feel like? How long will it take? Can I see my spouse? What if my heart stops during the procedure? Have you talked this over with my spouse?" These are questions frequently asked by patients before a catheter insertion. Answer them in lay terms to increase the patient's understanding. Use assurance to relieve stress and enhance the teaching-learning process. Obtain informed consent before the procedure.

Insertion

The antecubital, femoral, internal jugular, or subclavian vein can be used as an insertion site (Fig. 7-14). The latter two are preferred because they permit the patient full freedom of the arms and because there is less pulling and tugging of the catheter. A higher risk of venous thrombosis accompanies the use of the femoral vein, and pneumothorax or arterial puncture can occur in the subclavian approach.

Preparation of the insertion site is performed in the same manner as for central venous catheterization. After topical anesthesia is injected, the vein is identified by venipuncture with a needle and syringe to withdraw blood. The guide wire then is passed into the vein through the needle; the needle is removed and a dilator and sheath are inserted as a unit over the guide wire. The dilator and wire are removed, leaving the sheath in place. The catheter is inserted through the sheath and advanced to the level of the superior vena cava, which is approximately 50 cm from the antecubital fossa and 25 cm from the entrance to the internal jugular and subclavian veins.[17] The distal lumen of the catheter then is attached to the fluid-filled monitoring system and transducer, and the catheter is positioned

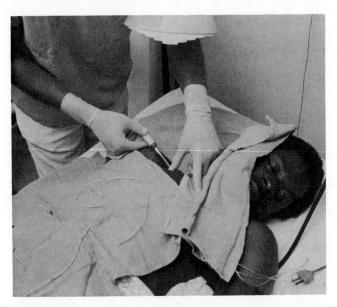

FIG. 7-14 The subclavian approach with the introducer needle. The needle, inserted under the midclavicle, is aimed at the top of the posterior aspect of the sternal manubrium. (Note the fingertip in the suprasternal notch.) Because this lies parallel with the frontal plane of the patient, the needle will enter the anterior wall of the subclavian vein.

to record the RAP (Fig. 7-15). The balloon is inflated with air according to the manufacturer's directions: 0.8 cc for a 5 French (Fr) catheter and a 1.5 cc for a 7 Fr catheter. Then with the use of pressure monitoring, the catheter is advanced, and the RVP (Fig. 7-16), and then the PAP are recorded. After it is in the PA, the balloon is deflated and the catheter advanced approximately 5 cm. The catheter is in a good position when a clear PAP is recorded with the balloon deflated and PAWP is recorded with the balloon inflated (Fig. 7-17).

If the balloon does not advance easily and appropriate RAP, RVP, and PAP are not recorded, the balloon is deflated, and the catheter is withdrawn to the superior vena cava. The balloon is again inflated, and another attempt at passage is made. When possible, the patient is placed in a fluoroscopic bed so that bedside fluoroscopy can be used for assistance if there is difficulty in advancing or positioning the catheter. When fluoroscopy is not available, a regular portable chest x-ray machine is used.

After insertion, the catheter is tied to the skin with sutures and looped, with the suture being used to secure a thumb loop. This ensures that any tension on the catheter will not be placed directly on the insertion site. A similar technique is used at other insertion sites so that tension placed on the catheter will not withdraw it inadvertently from the PA. The area is cleaned, antibiotic ointment is applied, and a sterile dressing is put in place. The catheter

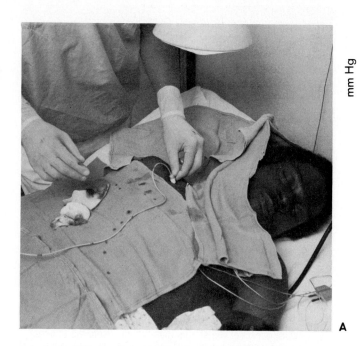

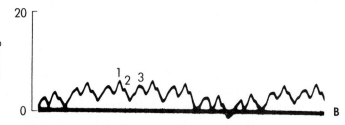

FIG. 7-15   A, PA catheter is advanced through the sheath. **B,** Right atrial waveform as the catheter tip reaches the atrium. *1, a* wave; *2, c* wave; *3, v* wave.

B From Daily EK and Schroeder JS: Techniques in bedside hemodynamic monitoring, St Louis, 1989, The CV Mosby Co.

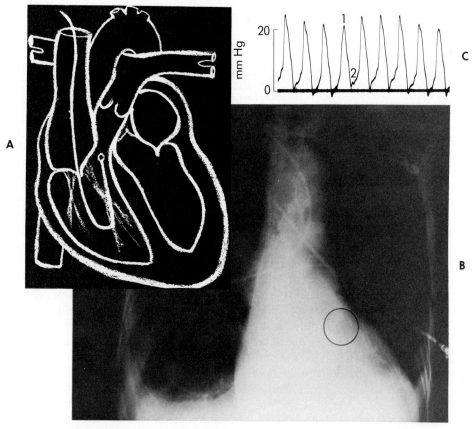

FIG. 7-16   A, Catheter with balloon partially inflated in the RV. **B,** X-ray film of catheter tip in the RV. **C,** Strip of RV waveform. *1,* Systole; *2,* diastole.

C From Daily EK and Schroeder JS: Techniques in bedside hemodynamic monitoring, St Louis, 1989, The CV Mosby Co.

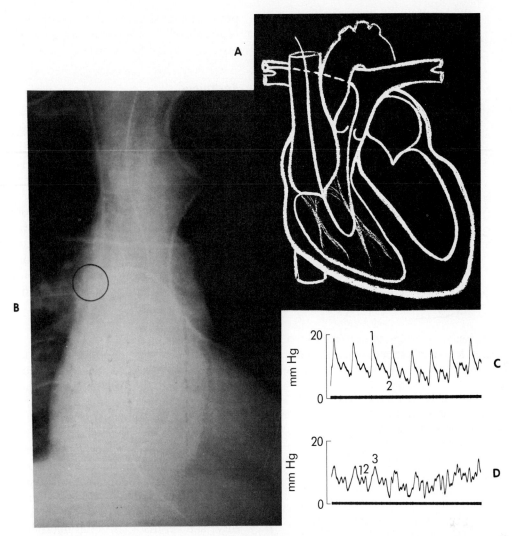

FIG. 7-17   **A,** Catheter with balloon partially inflated in the PA. **B,** X-ray film of catheter tip in the PA. **C,** Strip of PAP waveform with balloon deflated. *1,* Systole; *2,* diastole. **D,** Strip of PAWP waveform with balloon inflated. *1, a* wave; *2, c* wave; *3, v* wave.
D From Daily EK and Schroeder JS: Techniques in bedside hemodynamic monitoring, St Louis, 1989, The CV Mosby Co.

is taped down firmly to the skin so that it will not catch on the bed or dislodge accidentally.

After the catheter is in position, it is important to continuously monitor the PAP to ensure that the catheter is not lodged in a wedge position, a complication that could cause pulmonary infarction or injury to the PA.

THERMODILUTION CARDIAC OUTPUT DETERMINATION

The thermodilution method of cardiac output measurement was first described by Fegler in 1954.[35] This method is an adaptation of the indicator-dilution method using a known temperature as the indicator. The change in blood temperature downstream (from the RA to the PA) is re-

corded by a thermistor near the tip of the PA catheter. The resultant change in temperature over time produces a curve that is inversely proportional to blood flow. A special cardiac output computer analyzes the temperature/time curve and applies appropriate constants to determine the rate of blood flow according to the Stewart-Hamilton indicator-dilution equation.

Initially, chilled injectates with temperatures near zero were used to maximize the difference between the injectate and the blood in the PA. However, studies have demonstrated that cardiac output determinations obtained with iced injectate and room-temperature injectate correlate closely with each other, as well as with other methods of cardiac output determination.[9,50] The ease of operation and other considerations regarding infection and cost have

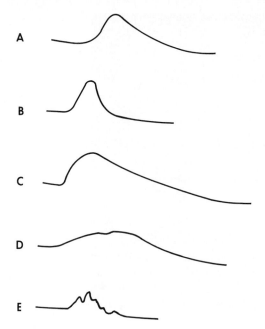

FIG. 7-18 Schematic representation of various thermodilution cardiac output curves. **A,** Normal cardiac output curve showing smooth upstroke. **B,** Small area beneath the curve as seen in patients with high cardiac outputs. **C,** Large area beneath the curve as seen in patients with low cardiac outputs. **D,** Uneven injection indicated by uneven upstroke on curve. **E,** Artifact in both upstroke and decline of curve resulting in erroneous cardiac output measurement.

From Tilkian A and Daily EK: Cardiovascular procedures, St Louis 1986, The CV Mosby Co.

made the use of room-temperature injectate a more popular practice. However, it may be necessary, at times, to use iced injectates to increase the sensitivity of the computer and obtain more reproducible data. This may be the case in patients who are markedly hypothermic or who are on mechanical ventilation causing extreme variation in baseline PA temperature or if reduced injectate volumes are required (such as 5 or 3 ml).

Because thermodilution cardiac-output determinations measure flow over only a few seconds of time, numerous (three to five) determinations are made, and the mean of these values are used to reflect the average flow rate.

All cardiac output curves should be visually inspected for accuracy. The upstroke of the curve should be smooth and even (Fig. 7-18).[49] Bumps or steps apparent on the upstroke indicate an uneven injection, and the measurement should be disregarded. The downslope of the curve determines the total area beneath the curve, which is inversely proportional to cardiac output. A rapid downstroke is seen in patients with a high cardiac output, whereas a slow, gradual downslope is seen in patients with low stroke volumes. The numerical value displayed by the cardiac out-

put computer should correlate with the visual appearance of the curve. If an apparent disparity exists, troubleshooting steps should be carried out (see later section).

Technique
Preparation

The injectate solution and closed system are assembled according to the manufacturer's directions. The injectate syringe is attached to the port of the stopcock of the injectate system. The thermistor hub of the PA catheter is then connected to the cardiac output computer via the appropriate connecting cable. The correct computation constant is dialed on the cardiac output computer, according to the volume and temperature of the injectate and the size and type of PA catheter. The computer is activated and a "ready" signal occurs. The PA waveform from the distal lumen of the catheter is checked to verify that the tip is in the PA position.

Procedure

The stopcock near the proximal port is turned off to the transducer, and *exactly* 10 ml (or 5 ml) of injectate is slowly withdrawn into the injectate syringe via the closed system. The "start" button on the cardiac output computer is pressed, and the contents of the syringe are injected immediately into the proximal lumen. The injection must be done smoothly and rapidly (within less than 4 seconds). The nurse notes the patient's heart rate and rhythm during the cardiac output determination. This is particularly important if there is considerable variation between readings. Then the nurse observes the corresponding cardiac output curve and verifies a fast, even injection with an apparent area that correlates with the displayed numerical value. Cardiac output measurements are repeated until three have been completed. If cardiac output values vary markedly, it may be necessary to perform and average 5 or 6 successive determinations.

Although greater reproducibility of cardiac output values can be achieved by injecting the solution at a specific point in the respiratory cycle, these values may not represent the patient's average flow rate. For this reason, it is better to perform cardiac output determinations randomly during the respiratory cycle.[10]

Evidence from several studies indicates some statistically significant differences in cardiac output values obtained while the patient is in a lateral position instead of a supine position.[11,53] The actual differences, however, are small and clinically insignificant.

CONTINUOUS MONITORING OF VENOUS OXYGEN SATURATION

PA catheters that contain fiberoptics provide continuous monitoring of the oxygen saturation of mixed venous (PA) blood (SvO_2) in addition to the usual hemodynamic parameters. Optical fibers transmit and receive reflected light from blood. The reflected light signal is converted to an electrical signal and transmitted to a remote data processor, which displays the signal on a screen or on a slow-speed paper recorder. A corresponding digital value is also displayed continuously and updated every 1 to 2 seconds.

Oxygen is taken up in the lungs and delivered to the tissues by hemoglobin molecules in blood. The rate at which oxygen is delivered depends on the flow rate of blood, or the cardiac output. The relationship of these determinants to overall oxygen delivery can be expressed as:

$$\text{Oxygen delivery} = \text{cardiac output} \times \text{Hemoglobin} \times 1.34 \times \text{SaO}_2 \times 10$$

where 1.34 is the number of milliliters of oxygen carried by each gram of hemoglobin and 10 is the conversion factor.

Any decline in cardiac output, hemoglobin, or arterial oxygen saturation (SaO_2) can reduce oxygen delivery to the tissues. When this occurs or when tissue oxygen demands are increased, the tissues must increase the amount of oxygen extracted from the blood to maintain aerobic metabolism. This increase in oxygen extraction results in a reduction in the SvO_2 of blood returning to the heart. Thus SvO_2 is a reflection of the adequacy of oxygen delivery. Normally, the SvO_2 is between 65% to 77%. SvO_2 levels below 60% reflect an imbalance between oxygen

supply and oxygen demands. If the SvO_2 begins to decline (no matter what the value), immediate assessment of the components of oxygen delivery and oxygen consumption (demands) should be performed. Increases in oxygen demands are usually clinically apparent (Table 7-3).

If increases in oxygen demands are not apparent, assessment of the determinants of oxygen delivery must be performed. Marked reductions in hemoglobin, as a result of significant bleeding, usually occur slowly, and are seldom responsible for sudden decreases in SvO_2. Hypoxemia, with low SaO_2 values, can be assessed immediately via pulse oximetry. SaO_2 reductions greater than 10% are uncommon in most clinical situations.[19]

Hypoperfusion, the most common cause of declining SvO_2 values, is evaluated by thermodilution cardiac output determinations when SvO_2 values decline 10% or more over a 3 to 5 minute period. Brief, minor changes in SvO_2 are clinically insignificant and are likely caused by some type of interference rather than changes in cardiac output.[24]

Technique
Preparation

Fiberoptic PA catheters are available in 4, 7.5, and 8 Fr sizes. The 7.5 and 8 Fr catheters contain cardiac output thermistor wires, which should be checked before catheter insertion. The catheters should be handled gently, avoiding

TABLE 7-3
Various Causes of Alterations in SvO_2

SvO_2 reading	Physiologic alteration	Clinical causes
HIGH 80%-95%	Decreased oxygen consumption	Hypothermia Anesthesia Induced muscular paralysis Sepsis
	Increased oxygen delivery Mechanical interference	Hyperoxia Catheter wedging Left-to-right shunt
NORMAL 60%-80%	Oxygen supply equal to oxygen demand	Adequate perfusion
LOW <60%	Increased oxygen consumption	Shivering Pain Seizures Activity or exercise Hyperthermia Anxiety
	Decreased oxygen delivery	Hypoperfusion (decreased cardiac output) Anemia Hypoxemia

From Daily EK and Schroeder JS: Techniques in bedside hemodynamic monitoring, St Louis, 1989, The CV Mosby Co.

sharp bending to prevent damage to the optical fibers within them.

Calibration of the oximeter must be performed at the onset of individual use. This requires obtaining laboratory analysis of a sample of venous blood for entry of the known oxygen saturation. This calibration procedure should be carried out on a daily basis or when there are doubts regarding the displayed SvO_2 readings.

COMPLICATIONS OF PA MONITORING

Although the relative ease of catheter insertion and the information obtained make PA monitoring a valuable diagnostic tool, it has risk. Reported overall complications rates for PA catheters are as high as 75%.[13,43] However, this high rate relates to the frequent occurrence of transient

and clinically benign dysrhythmias. The majority of complications that occur with PA catheterization are minor, although fatalities may be associated with major complications. A brief overview of the complications, their causes, and the nursing intervention associated with PA catheters is listed in Table 7-4.

Dysrhythmias

The major complication encountered with PA catheter insertion is the occurrence of dysrhythmias, including premature atrial contractions, premature junctional contractions, transient premature ventricular contractions, or potentially life-threatening ventricular tachycardia. As the catheter advances through the RA, tricuspid valve, and RV, its tip frequently irritates the endocardium. This

TABLE 7-4
PA Catheter Complications

Causes	Nursing care	Causes	Nursing care
DYSRHYTHMIAS		**PULMONARY INFARCTION OR HEMORRHAGE**	
Irritation of endocardium	Monitor electrocardiogram continually.	Prolonged wedging	Passively deflate balloon immediately after PAWP readings.
	Have emergency cart, antidysrhythmic drugs, and defibrillator available.	Frequent wedging	Follow balloon inflation and deflation guidelines.
		Catheter migration	
		Thrombus formation	Obtain a chest x-ray film to verify catheter position.
INFECTIONS			
Local		**PNEUMOTHORAX**	
Breakdown in sterile technique	Wet catheter before insertion.	Accidental intake of air into pleural space	Instruct patient to lie as still as possible during catheterization.
Irritation of skin	Use sterile technique for daily dressing and tubing changes.		Obtain chest x-ray film after insertion.
Endocardial			
Breakdown in sterile technique	Maintain sterile technique.	**AIR EMBOLISM**	
Irritation of endocardium	Recognize signs of endocarditis.	Air intake via the insertion needle, loose connections, open stopcocks, or inadvertant injection	Tighten all connecting sites every 4 hours; check them frequently.
PA PERFORATIONS			Place dead-ender caps on all stopcock ports.
Arterial wall overdistension	Follow guidelines for balloon inflation.		Keep all connections or possible openings into the vascular system below the level of the heart.
Eccentric balloon inflation	Check balloon inflation before insertion.		
Catheter migration	Ensure that there is no fluid in balloon.		Instruct patient to hum or suspend respirations when the vascular system is open and near or above heart level.
	Watch for evidence of PAWP waveform.		
BALLOON RUPTURE			
Loss of balloon elasticity or integrity	Follow guidelines for balloon inflation and deflation.		
	Stop inflating if no resistance is felt or PAWP is not obtained.		
	Use carbon dioxide for balloon inflation in patients with suspected intracardiac shunt.		

added stimulation to tissue already coping with a physiologically diseased state can change the balance from a basically harmless premature ventricular contraction to ventricular tachycardia or fibrillation.[12,18,52]

Transient premature ventricular contractions and nonsustained ventricular tachycardia usually subside with completion of catheter passage out to the PA. If sustained ventricular tachycardia occurs despite catheter withdrawal back to the RA, prompt cardioversion is necessary. Rarely, ventricular fibrillation may occur, requiring immediate defibrillation. Ventricular dysrhythmias occur more commonly with shock, acute myocardial ischemia or infarction, hypokalemia, hypocalcemia, hypoxemia, acidosis, and prolonged catheter insertion times. The prophylactic use of lidocaine to control cardiac dysrhythmias has been reported,[48] but it is not routinely used.

Dysrhythmias also may be caused by a knotting of the catheter in the RA or RV. This rare occurrence needs immediate attention. If an RV waveform is not evident after inserting 50 cm of catheter from the right antecubital approach or 30 cm from the subclavian or jugular approach, the catheter tip probably is coiling in the RA.[37]

Successful removal of a knotted catheter can be accomplished with millimeter-by-millimeter maneuvering using fluoroscopic guidance. Dysrhythmias frequently are provoked with this procedure. The defibrillator and emergency cart should be nearby and ready for use at all times. The nurse should make certain that the patient is attached to the cardiac monitor, and the leads should be placed to provide a good baseline and QRS complex. The monitoring electrodes should not be placed near the insertion site.

The patient should already have an intravenous or an intermittent therapy (Heparin Lock) needle to facilitate the immediate injection of antidysrhythmic drugs if necessary. Prefilled syringes of lidocaine (or bretylium) should be immediately available. With a little forethought the complications of dysrhythmias, although not entirely preventable, can be reduced to minor occurrences.

Bundle branch block

Right bundle branch block may occur during manipulation of the catheter in the RV. This is generally not a problem unless the patient has preexisting left bundle branch block resulting in complete atrioventricular block. Patients with left bundle branch block undergoing PA catheterization should have transvenous or transcutaneous pacing equipment readily available to prevent ventricular asystole.

Infection

Infection secondary to catheterization can range from contamination to colonization. Obviously, a breakdown in sterile technique is the major cause.

Infective endocarditis is a major but rare complication of PA catheterization that may occur as a result of catheter irritation of the endocardium in association with bacterial growth. The symptoms of endocarditis include reactions to infection, cardiac manifestations, and the hypersensitive reactions produced by the immunologic derangements (see Chapter 13).[5,23,39]

Prevention of infection includes meticulous aseptic technique during catheter insertion, daily observation and care of the insertion site (including cleansing with a bactericidal agent and application of iodophor ointment and a new sterile dressing), and an abbreviated time of catheter placement. Catheters left in place longer than 4 days have a higher incidence of infection.[25,32] To reduce the incidence of infection, the Centers for Disease Control recommends changing the intravenous solution, tubing, stopcocks, and transducer every 48 hours, using nonglucose intravenous solutions, and removing and replacing the catheter, if necessary, after 4 days. Advancement of PA catheters after initial placement should only be done if the proximal portion of the catheter has been maintained sterile inside a protective sleeve. All intravascular catheters should immediately be removed if infection or sepsis develops, and appropriate antibiotic therapy should be instituted.

PA perforation

PA perforation is a dramatic and usually fatal complication that occurs infrequently with the use of PA catheters. Predisposing conditions to PA rupture include pulmonary hypertension, advanced age (over 60 years), anticoagulation, and cardiopulmonary bypass surgery. High PAP from any cause drives the catheter tip distally into smaller vessels, thereby increasing the risk of perforation. Vascular changes that occur in elderly patients also result in lower rupturing pressures. The use of hypothermia, as well as manipulation of the catheter during cardiac surgery, also increase the risk of PA rupture. This complication is avoided if care and attention are given to hemodynamic monitoring techniques. The PA waveform should be continuously displayed and changes in its configuration observed while the balloon is inflated slowly. As soon as the wedge pattern appears, the nurse should stop inflating the balloon and quickly obtain a reading.

Although the recommended balloon capacity of the 7 Fr catheter is 1.5 cc of air, an inflation volume of 0.8 to 1.0 cc is often sufficient, depending on the size of the vessel in which the catheter tip lies. If a PAW waveform is obtained with balloon inflation volumes of less than 0.8 cc of air, the catheter tip has migrated distally into a small branch of the PA and should be withdrawn slightly. At no time should any fluid be injected into the balloon port of the catheter.

A small perforation of the PA, evidenced by the sudden appearance of a small amount of hemoptysis, may be managed by placing the patient in a lateral recumbent position with the affected side down and closely monitoring and observing the patient. Any anticoagulation therapy should be stopped and reversed. A small amount of hemoptysis (15 to 30 ml) should prompt consideration of a "wedge" angiographic study to determine the size and location of the perforation. Massive hemoptysis can be controlled with insertion of a double-lumen endotracheal tube to prevent bleeding into the unaffected lung and to aid ventilation until surgical repair can be performed.

Balloon rupture and air embolism

Rupture of the latex balloon of the PA catheter is usually a minor complication that can occur as a result of very frequent or improper wedging techniques. Although faulty manufacturing may be responsible for the incidence of balloon rupture, assessment of the balloon's integrity is always made before insertion. Evidence of air leakage when the fully inflated balloon is immersed in water indicates an incompetent balloon, which should be replaced with another catheter.

Rupture of the balloon is indicated by a lack of resistance during inflation with no change in the waveform configuration. The appearance of blood in the balloon lumen also indicates balloon rupture. If balloon rupture is suspected, no further inflations should be attempted, and the balloon lumen should be sealed tightly.

Venous air embolism is a rare but catastrophic complication of central venous catheterization. Although large amounts of air (200 to 300 cc) can cause patient fatality, even small amounts of air (as little as 20 cc) may cause harm to a critically ill patient.[2] Air can enter the venous system through any opening in the catheter, tubing, or infusion sites; through the needle or sheath during catheterization; or along the formed track of a removed catheter that has been in place for a prolonged period. This complication is more likely to occur when the patient is in an upright position, takes a deep breath, or is in a state of hypovolemia with a low CVP.

Prevention of venous air embolism requires meticulous nursing attention to the assessment and maintenance of the patency of monitoring lines. The security of all connecting sites should be checked frequently, and the sites should be kept positioned below the RA. If venous air embolism is clinically suspected, the patient should be immediately placed in a left lateral Trendelenburg position to prevent RV outflow obstruction. Oxygen should be administered with ventilatory support, if necessary. The central venous or PA catheter should be aspirated to attempt to remove the air within the system.

Pulmonary infarction or hemorrhage

Pulmonary infarction or hemorrhage may occur as a result of frequent and prolonged wedging of the catheter. Forward migration of the catheter occurs primarily during the first 24 hours as the catheter loop tightens with repeated RV contractions. Frequent wedge readings may damage the PA walls and predispose the patient to thrombus formation in and around the catheter.

To help prevent this problem, the manufacturer recommends that the balloon never be inflated over 1.5 cc while in the patient.[36,37] After the PAWP is obtained, the balloon should be passively deflated immediately. If there is a damped waveform, the nurse should not forcefully flush the catheter but try to aspirate the clot.[54] The catheter should not be flushed while in the wedge position; if there is an indication that the catheter tip is situated in a small artery (continual wedge pattern), a chest x-ray film is taken and the physician notified immediately. The physician probably will have the nurse pull the catheter back until a PA pattern is obtained.

Pneumothorax

A pneumothorax may occur during catheter insertion into the internal jugular or subclavian vein with inadvertent puncture of the pleural space. Instructing and helping the patient to remain still during cannulation are important ways of preventing this complication. The treatment depends on the size of the pneumothorax, the patient's symptoms, and the results of arterial blood gas analysis.

INTRAARTERIAL MONITORING

Intraarterial pressure can be measured directly via a small catheter placed in a peripheral artery. Directly measured arterial pressure is not only more accurate, but the ability to assess the arterial pulse waveform visually can often provide important diagnostic information.

The arterial system can be cannulated percutaneously or via an arterial cutdown at various sites, including the femoral, axillary, brachial, and radial arteries. Femoral and brachial arteries traditionally have been cannulated primarily in the cardiac catheterization laboratory on a short-term basis for pressure measurements and angiography, whereas the radial artery is commonly used for bedside, continuous intraarterial monitoring.

Physiologic review

The arterial blood pressure is generated by ejection of blood into the arterial vasculature from the LV. The amount of pressure generated is determined by the volume of blood ejected, as well as the resistance to ejection within the arterial vascular system. This is best expressed as:

$$Pressure = Flow \times Resistance$$

During LV ejection, the aorta is distended with blood. This distention is transmitted peripherally along adjacent segments of the aorta, producing a *pressure wave* that is transmitted through the arterial circulation and produces a palpable pulse peripherally.

The velocity of the pressure wave is slow in the aorta (3 to 5 m/sec) and gradually increases in the smaller arteries (15 to 35 m/sec). The rate at which the pressure wave travels down the aorta is determined by the *compliance* or distensibility of the arterial system. Decreases in vascular compliance (as seen in elderly patients with arteriosclerosis) result in a rapid transmission of the pressure wave.

Components of the pressure wave

The pressure wave in the aorta (Fig. 7-19, *A*) is characterized by a rapid rise in pressure during systole, followed by a slower rise in pressure, until the peak systolic pressure is achieved. The pressure curve then begins to fall and is interrupted by the *incisura*. The incisura occurs just after the aortic valve closes.

During systole, aortic pressure is raised. When the ventricles begin to relax, ventricular pressure rapidly decreases, causing a sudden transient backflow of blood from the high-pressure aorta to the ventricle. This backflow causes a small drop in aortic pressure, thus producing a small drop in the curve (the incisura). The backflow of blood also causes the aortic valve to close, and so extra blood fills the aortic root, thereby increasing aortic pressure slightly and causing a small rise in the pressure curve.[5] (On the peripheral pressure wave this is referred to as the *dicrotic notch*.)

After the incisura the pressure in the aorta rapidly decreases during early diastole and then continues to decrease more slowly during the end of diastole as peripheral runoff continues. As the pressure wave travels from the aorta to the periphery, the wave becomes distorted and is characterized by the following:

1. There is an initial delay in the onset of the pressure rise (Fig. 7-19, *B*, point *1*).
2. The upstroke of the curve is steeper (Fig. 7-19, *B*, point *2*).
3. The systolic curve is narrow and peaked and reaches higher levels (Fig. 7-19, *B*, point *3*).
4. The incisura is replaced by a dicrotic notch, which occurs later and lower in the diastolic curve than the incisura[5,26] (Fig. 7-19, *B*, point *4*).

As it is transmitted from the aorta to the periphery, the pressure wave increases, and the shape of the curve changes because of reflection, tapering, resonance, and damping. *Reflection* of the pressure wave occurs when vessels branch and when they diminish in size. As the wave distends the smaller vessels, some of the waves travel backward along the same vessel. When the retrograde wave coincides with an oncoming wave, the two waves summate and produce a larger wave. Thus the pressure wave reflects the summation of the retrograde and antegrade waves. As much as 80% of the waves are reflected back, causing a higher pulse pressure (20% to 30% higher in peripheral arteries than in the aorta) and distortion and peaking of the wave in the periphery. When the peripheral vessels are constricted and narrowed, a larger percentage of waves is

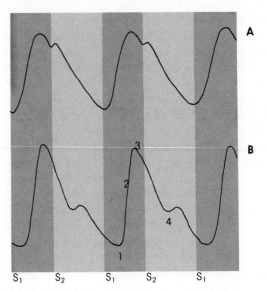

FIG. 7-19 Pressure waves. **A,** Carotid pressure wave. **B,** Radial pressure wave.

reflected back. Conversely, when the peripheral vessels are dilated, the percentage of waves recycled back is reduced.

The pressure wave is amplified as it travels down tapered vessels. *Tapering* produces peaking of the curve.

The shape of the pressure wave is also affected by resonance. The arterial pressure wave is a complex wave composed of a series of sine waves of differing frequencies and amplitudes. There is one fundamental frequency and a number of harmonics that usually have a smaller amplitude than the fundamental frequency. The arterial vessels resonate at certain frequencies, thereby intensifying some waves, whereas others are damped and disappear. This phenomenon is called *resonance*.

Damping is produced by resistance to blood flow. Because the resistance of the smaller arteries and arterioles is higher, blood flow is greatly reduced and the transmission of the pressure is lessened. Thus the pressure wave becomes smaller and smaller in the arterioles until it is almost absent in the capillaries.

Damping is also produced because the distensibility of the smaller arteries and arterioles is decreased. The small amount of blood that flows with each wave causes a smaller pressure rise, resulting in smaller and smaller waves in the more distant vessels.

Pulse pressure

The arterial pulse pressure is the difference between the systolic and diastolic pressures and normally ranges from 30 to 40 mm Hg. It depends primarily on the stroke volume and arterial compliance.

Factors that increase the pulse pressure. Increasing the stroke volume can affect pulse pressure. With an *increase in stroke volume,* a larger volume of blood must be accommodated in the arterial system with each heartbeat, thereby increasing the pressure rise during systole and increasing the pressure fall during diastole (increased recoil). In sinus bradycardia, for example, the reduced heart rate produces large ventricular filling pressures, resulting in a larger stroke volume to increase the pulse pressure. Likewise, in hypervolemia, filling pressures are increased, augmenting stroke volume and raising pulse pressure.[26]

A second factor responsible for increasing pulse pressure is a change in the systolic ejection velocity of the ventricle. This factor is closely related to increasing stroke volume. When the *ejection velocity* of the ventricle is increased during the rapid ejection phase of systole, the sudden ejection of blood causes aortic pressure to rise rapidly before blood can run off to the peripheral vessels, causing the pulse pressure to increase. This is observed in patients receiving β_1-adrenergic receptor drugs such as isoproterenol, dobutamine, and moderate doses of dopamine.[26]

A third factor that increases the pulse pressure is *reduction of the peripheral vascular resistance*. When resistance is lowered, it permits a rapid flow of blood from the arteries to the veins, thereby increasing venous return, increasing ventricular filling pressures, and thus increasing stroke volume. Furthermore, when resistance or afterload is reduced, it is easier for the heart to eject a given stroke volume. Resistance is lowered with a resultant increase in pulse pressure during circumstances such as exercise, hot weather, anemia, fever, and hyperthyroidism.

A fourth factor responsible for increasing the pulse pressure is *decreased arterial compliance*. Arterial compliance is reduced when the arterial blood pressure is increased to a high (or decreased to a low) range. The less compliant the arterial tree, the greater the rise in pressure for a given stroke volume. In a patient with hypertension, for example, there is reduced compliance because less blood can be accommodated in the arterial system for a given stroke volume when the arterial pressure is high. Thus pulse pressure rises even in the presence of a normal stroke volume. During aging the arterial walls lose their elasticity and become fibrotic and calcified. The rigid vessels cannot stretch, thereby reducing compliance. The loss of compliance causes the arterial pressure to rise higher than normal during systole and to fall lower than normal during diastole (decreased recoil), thereby increasing the pulse pressure. For the same reasons a rise in pulse pressure is also observed in arteriosclerotic disease.[5,26]

Factors that reduce the pulse pressure. The same factors that increase pulse pressure can reduce it. When the *stroke volume* is reduced, a smaller amount of blood is accommodated by the arterial tree with each heartbeat. This causes a decrease in the pressure rise during systole and reduces the pressure fall during diastole. Clinical conditions that reduce stroke volume and pulse pressure include hypovolemia, heart failure, and shock.[26]

A second factor responsible for reducing the pulse pressure is prolonging the period of *systolic ejection*. This occurs in aortic stenosis, when the time required to eject a given stroke volume is increased due to the stenotic aortic valve. A large part of the ejected stroke volume has time to run off to the peripheral vessels during systole, thereby reducing the pulse pressure.

A third factor, *increasing peripheral vascular resistance*, is closely related to the first two factors in reducing pulse pressure. When resistance or afterload is increased, less stroke volume is ejected with each heartbeat than at lower or normal levels of resistance. Resistance is increased with a resultant decrease in pulse pressure during conditions such as severe cold, shock, exogenous or endogenous increases in catecholamines (norepinephrine), and metabolic acidosis.[26]

Arterial catheterization

The radial artery is the most commonly used arterial catheterization site because the hand receives good collateral circulation from the ulnar artery. Before cannulation of the radial artery, the adequacy of collateral blood flow to the hand should be assessed by performing the *Allen's test*.[10,23,30] With the patient's arm elevated well above heart level, the nurse presses a thumb on the radial artery and the other thumb on the ulnar artery while the patient makes a tight fist, squeezing the blood from the palm and fingers. The ulnar artery is then released while radial compression is maintained. If the blood returns rapidly (3 to 5 seconds) to the palm and fingers when the patient opens the hand, ulnar patency is present. If patency of the radial artery needs to be tested, the test can be repeated with release of the radial artery.

Before the insertion the nurse must assess the color, pulses, and temperature of the selected extremity. The condition of the extremity should be checked during the insertion, if possible, and immediately after, and the nurse should report changes immediately to the physician. The limb used for the arterial line insertion should remain uncovered or accessible for viewing. The pulses distal to the catheter should be checked every 2 hours for signs of thrombosis or total occlusion.

Arterial catheter insertion

As with venous catheterization, the area is carefully scrubbed with an iodine solution, and a sterile drape is positioned before catheter insertion. One percent lidocaine hydrochloride is used to anesthetize the area, and the needle with the catheter sheath is inserted percutaneously into the artery. After the needle is withdrawn, the catheter usually is positioned 4 to 6 cm within the artery, and a heparinized intravenous solution and stopcock are attached. Care should be taken to secure the catheter with sutures, and a sterile dressing is applied. The monitoring setup for intraarterial pressure monitoring is the same as that used for PAP monitoring (Fig. 7-20). (See Chapter 3.)

syrine should be heparinized if an arterial blood gas sample is needed.)

4. Withdraw the amount of blood needed using one syringe. To prevent infection, use the exact size syringe for total volume needed in multiple laboratory tests. This eliminates unnecessary opening and handling of the site.
5. Turn the stopcock off to the port site and on between the flush system and the patient and briefly "fast flush" the line with the use of the continuous flush device.
6. Remove the syringe, immediately remove air bubbles from the blood sample, and cap the syringe. (If blood is drawn for blood gas analysis, immediately immerse the arterial blood sample in an ice bath.)
7. Turn the stopcock off to the patient and open between the flush system and the port site. Flush the open port site onto some sterile gauze without contaminating the port site.
8. Put a sterile cap on the port site.
9. Turn the stopcock so that the system is on a continual flush to the patient at 3 to 5 ml/hour.

Complications

The risks and complications associated with intraarterial monitoring include hemorrhage, infection, and arterial thrombosis.[25,33]

Extensive blood loss through arterial line disconnection is the greatest risk of intraarterial pressure monitoring. It is of primary importance to use Luer-Lok connections that screw together. Also, the cannulated site must be left uncovered to permit observation for bleeding caused by loose connections. Activating the high-low pressure alarms on the monitor will alert the nurse to a disconnection because of the associated immediate drop in pressure. Disconnections could result in hemorrhage rapidly because of the pressure in the arterial system.

Infection of arterial lines is usually due to contamination of stopcocks connected to the system. An increased incidence of infection is associated with prolonged duration of catheter placement. For this reason, arterial catheters should be removed after 72 to 96 hours. In addition, all components of the fluid-filled system, including the intravenous fluid bag, stopcocks, transducer, and tubing should be changed every 24 to 48 hours.[6] The backup of blood, encrusted blood on the port site, and leaks in the pressure system may lead to bacteremia. Nonocclusive dressings and poor taping techniques over the sutured insertion site also increase this risk. An occlusive dressing is recommended. Sterile dead-ender caps should be used to occlude all open stopcock ports. The use of syringes to occlude a stopcock port or leaving the port open to air increases the risk of infection. Iodinized preparations, sterile daily dressing changes, and frequent inspection of the

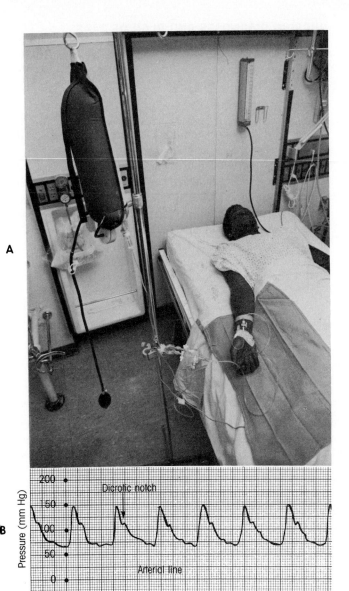

FIG. 7-20 **A,** A pressurized arterial line setup is attached to a radial artery catheter. **B,** Recording of an arterial waveform with calibration.

Blood sampling

An indwelling arterial catheter frequently is used to obtain blood samples for laboratory tests, including arterial blood gas analysis. The following steps outline the procedure for obtaining blood samples from an arterial line:

1. Make certain the line is patent by checking the pressure and waveform readings.
2. Turn the stopcock off to the intravenous solution and open the capped port site. Remove the cap, attach a 10-ml syringe in the port site, and withdraw and discard 5 ml of blood.
3. Place a new sterile syringe in the port site. (The

site are other measures of prevention. The line should be removed immediately if inflammation is present. The line is maintained only with a heparinized flush; no other fluid should be infused through the system.[23,30,39,45]

The heparinized normal saline, continuously infused through a pressurized flush valve, also helps control thrombus formation. This flush system valve allows the fluid to flow under pressure at a rate of 3 to 5 ml/hour, depending on the valve used.[5,30] To prevent flushing of thrombus material, the catheter should always be aspirated before flushing, and the blood, which could contain a clot from the catheter tip, should be discarded. This should be followed by gentle, manual flushing of a small volume (2 to 4 ml) of solution. If the continuous flush device is activated, the flush valve should be opened for only a few seconds because vigorous flushing with as little as 7 ml of fluid into a radial artery catheter could reach the aortic arch and possibly result in cerebral embolization.[31]

NURSING DIAGNOSES AND PLAN OF CARE

Table 7-5 outlines the nursing diagnoses and plan of care for patients undergoing hemodynamic monitoring.

TROUBLESHOOTING

The use and benefits of hemodynamic monitoring are predicated on the accuracy of the data obtained. It is the critical care nurse's responsibility to obtain hemodynamic data accurately. Careful standards and procedures as outlined by the institution should be followed and logical troubleshooting steps undertaken when a problem exists. In this way, accuracy of the data can be optimized and potential complications minimized or avoided. Table 7-6 lists problems and associated troubleshooting interventions associated with hemodynamic monitoring.

TABLE 7-5

Nursing Diagnoses and Plan of Care for Patients Undergoing Hemodynamic Monitoring

Patient outcomes	Nursing prescriptions	Rationale
DECREASED CARDIAC OUTPUT RELATED TO MYOCARDIAL DYSFUNCTION		
Optimal hemodynamic function as evidenced by: Cardiac index (CI): 2.5-4 L/min/m² PAEDP/mean PAWP or mean LA 15-20 mm Hg Mean RAP 4-8 mm Hg MAP: 70-80 mm Hg Heart rate (HR): 50-100 beats per minute without ectopic occurrence	Monitor preload (RA and PAEDP, PAW or mean LAP) and administer appropriate medications and fluids as ordered. Measure cardiac output (CO) and CI and calculate SVR and/or PVR. Administer appropriate medications as ordered. Plot ventricular function curves.	Preload is optimized to increase systolic ejection according to Starling's law.
Systemic vascular resistance (SVR): <1400 dyne-seconds-cm⁻⁵ Pulmonary vascular resistance (PVR): <250 dyne-seconds-cm⁻⁵	Calculate LV stroke work index (LVSWI) and/or RV stroke work index (RVSWI). Administer appropriate medications as ordered.	High LVSWI or RVSWI increases heart work and oxygen needs (MVO₂).
Normal arterial blood gas levels Normal hemoglobin level Urinary output: ≥40 ml/hr SvO₂: 60%-77% Oxygen delivery to tissues: ≥900 ml/min	Monitor electrocardiogram for rate, rhythm, and ectopic occurrence, and determine hemodynamic response to changes in rate or rhythm. Treat according to protocol. Implement emergency measures as necessary.	Very fast heart rates may decrease stroke volume by decreasing LV filling. Very slow heart rates (<50) may produce inadequate CO (CO = HR × SV). Dysrhythmias reduce CO.
	Physically assess patient (vital signs, heart and lung sounds, skin color and temperature, fluid balance, mentation, and jugular vein distention) and report significant changes.	Baseline heart and lung sounds are necessary to determine the onset of new sounds associated with cardiac pathology; decreased mentation or increased restlessness may be an early indication of decreased CO.

Adapted from: Daily EK and Schroeder JS: Techniques in bedside hemodynamic monitoring, ed 4, St. Louis, 1989, The CV Mosby Co.

TABLE 7-5

Nursing Diagnoses and Plan of Care for Patients Undergoing Hemodynamic Monitoring—cont'd

Patient outcomes	Nursing prescriptions	Rationale
	Measure arterial blood gas and hemoglobin levels and report significant changes. Administer appropriate therapy as ordered.	Oxygen delivery is optimized by maintaining CO, SaO_2 and hemoglobin at normal levels.
	Measure hourly urine output and report if <30 ml/hr.	Measurement used to determine renal perfusion and function and prevent dysfunction resulting from ischemia.
	Measure SvO_2 and report reductions of 10% for 2-3 min or if <60%.	Decrease in SvO_2 indicates inadequate tissue perfusion. SvO_2 <60% is associated with poor prognosis.
	Reduce patient's activity and stress.	Reduced activity and stress will decrease oxygen demands.

ALTERED PERIPHERAL PERFUSION RELATED TO COMPROMISED CIRCULATION ASSOCIATED WITH INVASIVE MONITORING

Optimal skin integrity Normal skin color and temperature Equal arterial pulses in all extremities	Assess catheter insertion site daily; cleanse site, apply iodophor ointment and new sterile dressing.	Inflammation at catheter insertion site is associated with infection and/or thrombophlebitis.
	Assess skin color, temperature and sensitivity in area around insertion site. Report significant changes.	Alteration in tissue perfusion may result in an increase in skin temperature below catheter site. An increase in skin temperature with pain or tenderness is associated with thrombosis or thrombophlebitis.
	Palpate and compare pulses in each extremity. Report changes.	A decrease or loss in arterial pulsations distal to catheter insertion site is associated with arterial insufficiency secondary to thrombus formation.
	Assess catheterized extremity for edema by measuring the other extremity at the same anatomic location.	Edema is a characteristic manifestation of decreased tissue perfusion caused by venous interference.

HIGH RISK FOR INFECTION RELATED TO INVASIVE MONITORING

Lack of infection as demonstrated by: Normal temperature Normal WBC Negative cultures of blood or catheter tip	Check patient's temperature every 4 hours and as needed, and report any significant changes.	Increase in temperature is associated with infectious process.
	Change catheter and catheter site every 4 days.	Risk of infection increases with duration of catheter placement more than 5 days.
	Change intravenous fluid, tubing, stopcocks and disposable transducer every 48-72 hours.	Static fluid is a potential source for bacterial growth.
	Inspect and cleanse catheter insertion site every day; apply iodophor ointment and clean sterile dressing.	Skin and old blood are potential sources for infection. Iodophor ointment reduces bacterial growth.
	Do not use intravenous solution containing glucose.	Glucose solutions promote growth of bacteria.
	Place sterile dead-ender caps on all stopcocks.	Open stopcock port allows bacteria to enter.
	Use aseptic technique when withdrawing from or flushing the catheter.	Aseptic techniques prevent contamination of open system.

Continued.

TABLE 7-5

Nursing Diagnoses and Plan of Care for Patients Undergoing Hemodynamic Monitoring—cont'd

Patient outcomes	Nursing prescriptions	Rationale
	If reusable transducers are used, sterilize transducer before patient use.	Minute flaws in disposable transducer domes allow contact between infusing fluid and transducer contaminating intravenous fluid.
	Carefully remove all traces of blood from stopcock ports after obtaining blood sample from catheter.	Old blood promotes growth of bacteria.
	Use sterile plastic catheter sleeve over PA catheter.	Method keeps external portion of catheter sterile to permit catheter advancement, if necessary.

HIGH RISK FOR INJURY RELATED TO HEMORRHAGE

Lack of hemorrhage	Keep all catheter connecting sites visible and observe them frequently for possible hemorrhage.	Major blood loss can occur without notice from stopcocks or loose connections hidden beneath dressings or bed linens.
	Tighten all catheter connecting sites and stopcocks every 4 hours and as needed.	Plastic connections become loose over time, and leakage can occur.
	Restrain patient, if necessary.	A restless or confused patient may pull catheter out or connecting tubing apart.
	After removal of arterial catheter, apply firm pressure to insertion site for 10 minutes before checking and applying pressure dressing.	Method allows clot to form at insertion site to seal vessel opening.
	Discontinue systemic heparinization several hours before catheter or sheath removal.	

HIGH RISK FOR INJURY RELATED TO THROMBOEMBOLI

Lack of thrombus as evidenced by: Patent catheter Unimpeded infusion or flush Undamped waveform	Use heparinized intravenous solutions with continuous flush device to continuously infuse all catheter ports and sideport of sheath, if used.	Continuous forward flow and use of heparin is associated with a decrease in thrombus formation at catheter tip or around catheter in sheath.
	Always aspirate and discard before gently flushing catheter. If unable to aspirate, do not flush catheter. Periodically aspirate and manually flush catheter or activate flush device (every 4-6 hours).	Technique removes fibrin or clot from within or at tip of catheter to prevent injection of clot material. Forward movement of heparinized fluid prevents clot formation.
	Do not fast-flush arterial catheter longer than 2 seconds; manually flush arterial catheter by gently tapping plunger of flush syringe with no more than 2-4 ml of fluid.	Vigorous flushing of arterial catheter with large amounts of fluid can result in cerebral embolization.
	Maintain 300 mm Hg pressure on intravenous cuff.	About 300 mm Hg pressure is required to maintain a forward flow of heparinized solution via the flush device.

TABLE 7-5

Nursing Diagnoses and Plan of Care for Patients Undergoing Hemodynamic Monitoring—cont'd

Patient outcomes	Nursing prescriptions	Rationale
	Remove all traces of blood from catheter, tubing, and stopcocks after withdrawing blood; flush completely.	Residual blood in catheter, tubing, or stopcock can form small clots that can occlude catheter or be injected into patient.

HIGH RISK FOR INJURY RELATED TO VENOUS AIR EMBOLISM

Patient outcomes	Nursing prescriptions	Rationale
Lack of venous air embolism	Tighten all catheter connecting sites and stopcocks every 4 hours and as needed; check frequently.	Plastic connections become loose over time, permitting intake of air into system.
	Place dead-ender caps on all stop cock ports.	Open or vented ports permit intake of air.
	Keep all connections or possible openings into vascular system below level of the heart.	Air intake is more likely to occur through loose connection or open port when the patient is in an upright position and takes a deep breath.
	Remove all air from intravenous solution bag.	Air in the bag and solution can enter tubing and catheter.
	Have patient hum or suspend respirations when vascular system is open and near or above heart level.	Air intake through the open port occurs during inspiration.
	After removal of venous catheter which was in place for a long time, apply petrolatum jelly and occlusive dressing to insertion site.	Air intake can occur through the open tract formed by catheter that was in place for a long time, especially in a thin person with minimal subcutaneous tissue.

HIGH RISK FOR INJURY RELATED TO PULMONARY INFARCTION OR HEMORRHAGE

Patient outcomes	Nursing prescriptions	Rationale
Lack of pulmonary infarction or hemorrhage as evidenced by: Normal respirations Lack of hemoptysis Normal arterial blood gas level	Continuously monitor PA waveform at distal tip of PA catheter.	Forward migration of catheter into a wedged position will be evidenced by PAW waveform.
	Inflate balloon to wedge catheter briefly (<20 seconds).	Step minimizes cessation in blood flow to reduce risk of pulmonary ischemia or infarction.
	Leave balloon of catheter deflated with stopcock open and syringe removed.	Open stopcock with syringe off permits passive deflation in case air remains in the balloon.
	Monitor PAEDP instead of PAWP (if close relationship).	Monitoring PAEDP reduces risks caused by inflation of the balloon and cessation of blood flow in branch of the PA.
	Check location of catheter tip after insertion and as needed via chest x-ray film.	Catheter tip migrates forward with blood flow into a wedge position (particularly during first 24 hours).
	Continuously observe waveform during *slow* balloon inflation; stop inflation at first appearance of PAW waveform. Do not inflate 7 Fr catheter with more than 1.5 cc air.	Overinflation of balloon can cause rupture of vessel.

Continued.

TABLE 7-5

Nursing Diagnoses and Plan of Care for Patients Undergoing Hemodynamic Monitoring—cont'd

Patient outcomes	Nursing prescriptions	Rationale
	Do not inflate balloon with air if resistance is met.	Catheter may be in a small branch of the PA and already mechanically wedged, or balloon may already be inflated.

HIGH RISK FOR INJURY RELATED TO CARDIAC DYSRHYTHMIAS OR CONDUCTION DISTURBANCES

Lack of life-threatening dysrhythmias or conduction disturbances	Continuously monitor waveform from distal port of catheter.	Appearance of RV waveform indicates that catheter tip has fallen into RV and could cause ventricular dysrhythmias.
	Monitor daily x-ray chest film.	Check for coiling of catheter in RV or RA, which could cause dysrhythmias.
	If RV waveform appears, quickly inflate balloon of catheter.	Catheter tip in RV can produce ventricular dysrhythmias; with balloon inflation, catheter should float to PA.
	To remove catheter, deflate balloon actively and completely with syringe and quickly remove catheter.	Rapid removal of catheter with fully deflated balloon should result in few, if any, dysrhythmias.
	Follow emergency protocols for life-threatening dysrhythmias.	

ANXIETY RELATED TO FEAR OF TECHNOLOGIC EQUIPMENT AND PROCEDURES ASSOCIATED WITH HEMODYNAMIC MONITORING

Verbalization of feelings Relaxed manner Verbalization of familiarity with hemodynamic monitoring procedures and equipment	Initiate interventions to reduce anxiety (see Chapter 5).	Readiness to learn facilitates meaningful learning and retention of knowledge.
	Based on readiness to learn, explain reasons for hemodynamic monitoring, function and purpose of hemodynamic monitoring equipment, and procedures related to hemodynamic monitoring.	Knowing rationale and purpose of hemodynamic monitoring reduces anxiety.
	Instruct patient in biobehavioral interventions (see Chapter 5)	Use of energy-release techniques helps reduce anxiety.
	Listen attentively, encourage verbalization, and provide a caring touch.	Personal attention reassures patient.

SLEEP PATTERN DISTURBANCE RELATED TO INVASIVE MONITORING PROCEDURES

Undisturbed sleep	Do not awaken or reposition patient to obtain hemodynamic parameters.	Hemodynamic measurements may be obtained with patient in supine, right or left lateral positions, or 45-degree semi-Fowler's position as long as air-reference stopcock is adjusted to mid-RA level and transducer is rezeroed.
	Instruct patient in relaxation techniques (see Chapter 5).	Energy release techniques help patient to relax and aid in sleep.
	Provide quiet, dimly lit environment.	A quiet, dark environment is more conducive to sleep.

TABLE 7-6
Troubleshooting Inaccurate Pressure Measurements

Problem	Prevention	Intervention
Damped waveform or abnormally high pressure		
Catheter tip against vessel wall	Usually cannot be avoided.	Pull back or reposition catheter while observing waveform.
Partial occlusion of tip by clot	Use continuous drip with occasional hand flushing. Flush well after blood sampling. Use heparin-bonded catheters.	Aspirate catheter; flush with heparinized fluid.
Pressure trapped by improper sequence of stopcock operation	Turn stopcocks in proper sequence when two pressures are measured on one transducer.	Thoroughly flush transducers with intravenous solution; turn to zero, and turn stopcocks in proper sequence.
Stopcock partially turned	Turn stopcock completely.	Check stopcock handle; turn completely.
Kinked catheter	Check catheter at entry site during insertion; keep catheter straight or with large, loose coils to prevent pulling or bending.	Check catheter at entry site; straighten catheter and tape it in correct position.
Air bubbles in fluid line or transducer	Carefully remove all air bubbles during setup; check every 4 hrs and as necessary.	Check fluid system and transducer; fast-flush system.
Straight or drifting line		
Overwedged catheter	Carefully observe PA waveform during balloon inflation; stop inflation as soon as PAW waveform is obtained.	Deflate balloon; inflate while observing PA waveform. Stop inflation as soon as PAW waveform is obtained; if less than 0.8 cc of air is required, withdraw catheter slightly.
Eccentric balloon inflation	Check balloon inflation before catheter insertion.	Rotate and reposition catheter; monitor PAEDP pressure only.
Catheter in Zone I or II location with tip reading high alveolar pressure	Obtain lateral chest x-ray film after catheter insertion; reposition catheter if it is below the level of LA.	Place patient in lateral position with catheter tip down. Reduce positive end-expiratory pressure to less than 15 cm H_2O. Maintain LA pressure at less than or equal to 15 mm Hg.
Pressure trapped by improper sequence of stopcock operation	Turn stopcocks in proper sequence when two pressures are measured on one transducer.	Thoroughly flush transducers with intravenous solution; turn to zero, and turn stopcocks in proper sequence.
Stopcock partially turned	Turn stopcock completely open.	Check stopcock handle; turn completely.
Negative or inappropriately low pressure		
Transducer air reference port level higher than midchest	Mark midchest level and maintain air reference level at that level.	Recheck air reference position; adjust if necessary.
Loose connection	User Luer-Lok stopcocks; check connections periodically.	Check connections; retighten.

Modified from Daily EK and Schroeder JS: Techniques in bedside hemodynamic monitoring, ed 4, St Louis, 1989, The CV Mosby Co.

Continued.

TABLE 7-6
Troubleshooting Inaccurate Pressure Measurements—cont'd

Problem	Prevention	Intervention
Inappropriate pressure waveform		
Altered location of catheter tip (forward to PAW or back to RV or RA)	Establish optimal catheter position during insertion.	Identify waveform on scope. Reposition catheter. Obtain chest x-ray film.
	Suture catheter at insertion site and tape to skin.	
	Continuously monitor pressure from distal lumen of catheter	
	Mixed pressures (PA/PAW or PA/RV pressures) usually precede change.	
	If less than 0.8 cc of air is required to obtain a PAW waveform, withdraw the catheter slightly.	
	Obtain chest x-ray film daily and as necessary.	
No pressure		
Transducer turned off to patient	Follow routine, systematic steps for pressure measurement.	Check system and stopcocks.
Amplifier on "CAL," "zero," or "off"		

KEY CONCEPT REVIEW

1. Preload is measured in terms of end-diastolic volume or pressure and represents the volume in the:
   a. RA
   b. Lungs as tidal volume
   c. Ventricle before contraction
   d. Ventricle during systole
2. Afterload is the tension developed by the myocardium during:
   a. Infarction
   b. Contraction
   c. Diastole
   d. Hypotension
3. What are the four factors regulating the heart as a pump?
   a. Preload, afterload, heart rate, and automaticity
   b. Preload, afterload, heart rate, and contractility
   c. Preload, afterload, blood pressure, and automaticity
   d. Preload, afterload, contractility, and automaticity
4. What is a common indication for hemodynamic monitoring?
   a. Shock
   b. Uncomplicated myocardial infarction
   c. Unstable angina
   d. Chronic obstructive pulmonary disease
5. What is the normal mean pulmonary artery pressure?
   a. Less than 5 mm Hg
   b. Less than 13 mm Hg
   c. Between 12 and 25 mm Hg
   d. Greater than 25 mm Hg
6. Exaggerated PAW v waves are commonly seen in the following condition:
   a. Mitral stenosis
   b. Mitral regurgitation
   c. Cardiac tamponade
   d. Pulmonary embolus
7. Elevated PAWPs are commonly seen in:
   a. RV failure
   b. Hypovolemia
   c. LV failure
   d. Pulmonary disease
8. What does the CVP primarily measure?
   a. RV volume
   b. Pulmonary filling pressure
   c. The body's blood pressure
   d. The body's blood volume
9. What is the ratio of centimeters of water to millimeters of mercury?
   a. 1.36 cm $H_2O = 1$ mm Hg
   b. 13.6 cm $H_2O = 1$ mm Hg
   c. 1 cm $H_2O = 1.36$ mm Hg
   d. 1 cm $H_2O = 13.6$ mm Hg

10. What part does hemodynamic monitoring play in total patient care?
    a. It provides vital life-saving measures.
    b. It relieves the patient's symptoms.
    c. It gives the patient needed security.
    d. It permits trend monitoring, allows assessment of therapy, and, at times may be a diagnostic tool.
11. Monitoring mixed venous oxygen saturation is used as an indicator of:
    a. Oxygen delivery
    b. Oxygen demands
    c. Cardiac output
    d. All of the above
12. Evidence of improper thermodilution cardiac output injection technique includes:
    a. A small cardiac output curve
    b. A large cardiac output curve
    c. An uneven downslope of the cardiac output curve
    d. An uneven upslope of the cardiac output curve
13. What is the greatest risk of intraarterial monitoring?
    a. Discomfort to the patient
    b. Exsanguination
    c. Thrombus formation
    d. Infection
14. What is the major complication encountered during a PA catheter insertion?
    a. Dysrhythmias
    b. Catheter contamination
    c. PA perforation
    d. Balloon rupture
15. How can the incidence of PA balloon rupture be decreased?
    a. Never overinflate.
    b. Inflate the balloon slowly and gradually.
    c. Use the catheters well within their shelf life.
    d. All the above are correct.
16. What complication occurs from the frequent and prolonged wedging of the PA catheter?
    a. Pulmonary infarction
    b. Dysrhythmias
    c. Infection
    d. All the above
17. What is the first action the nurse takes when the PA waveform becomes severely dampened?
    a. Check the stopcocks.
    b. Assess the patient.
    c. See if the digital display matches the waveform.
    d. Check for backup of blood in the line.
18. What is the cause of an unobtainable wedge pattern?
    a. Catheter introducer site infection
    b. Catheter slipping out of position
    c. Dysrhythmias
    d. All the above

ANSWERS

1. c	5. b	9. a	13. b	16. a
2. b	6. b	10. d	14. a	17. b
3. b	7. c	11. d	15. d	18. b
4. a	8. d	12. d		

REFERENCES

1. Alpert JS: Hemodynamic monitoring: the basics, Primary Cardiol 5:113, 1981.
2. Berne RM and Levy MN: Cardiovascular physiology, ed. 6, St Louis, 1992, Mosby–Year Book, Inc.
3. Braunwald E: Regulation of the circulation, N Engl J Med 290:1124, 1974.
4. Braunwald E: Determinants and assessment of cardiac function, N Engl J Med 296:87, 1977.
5. Braunwald E, editor: Heart disease: a textbook of cardiovascular medicine, ed 3, Philadelphia, 1988, WB Saunders Co.
6. Centers for Disease Control: Guidelines for prevention of infections related to intra-vascular pressure-monitoring systems, Infect Control 3:68, 1982.
7. Collier PE, Ryan JJ, and Diamond DL: Cardiac tamponade from central venous catheters: reports of a case and review of the English literature, Angiology 35:595, 1984.
8. Daily EK: Use of hemodynamics to differentiate pathophysiologic causes of cardiogenic shock, Crit Care Nurs Clin North Am 1:589, 1989.
9. Daily EK and Mersch J: Comparison of Fick method of cardiac output with thermodilution method using two indicators, Heart Lung 16:294, 1987.
10. Daily EK and Schroeder JS: Techniques in bedside hemodynamic monitoring, ed. 4, St Louis, 1989, The CV Mosby Co.
11. Doering L and Dracup K: Comparisons of cardiac output in supine and lateral positions, Nurs Res 37:114, 1988.
12. Dossey BM, Guzzetta CE, and Kenner CV: Critical care nursing: body-mind-spirit, ed. 3, Philadelphia, 1992, JB Lippincott Co.
13. Duncan JW and Powner DJ: Complications associated with the use of pulmonary artery catheters, Ariz Med 39:433, 1982.
14. Fabiato A and Fabiato F: Calcium and cardiac excitation-contraction coupling, Annu Rev Physiol 41:473, 1979.
15. Fischer RE: Measuring central venous pressure, Nurs 79 9:74, 1979.
16. Forrester JS and others: Filling pressures in the right and left sides of the heart in acute myocardial infarction: a reappraisal of central venous monitoring, N Engl J Med 285:190, 1971.
17. Ganz W and others: A new technique of measurement of cardiac output by thermodilution in man, Am J Cardiol 27:392, 1971.
18. Gernert CF and Schwartz S: Pulmonary artery catheterization, Am J Nurs 73:1182, 1973.
19. Gore JM and others: Handbook of hemodynamic monitoring, Boston, 1985, Little, Brown & Co.
20. Gore JM and others: A community-wide assessment of the use of pulmonary artery catheters in patients with acute myocardial infarction, Chest 92:721, 1987.
21. Gorlin R: Practical cardiac hemodynamics, N Engl J Med 296:203, 1977.
22. Guyton A: Textbook of medical physiology, Philadelphia, 1991, WB Saunders Co.
23. Horowitz JH and Luterman A: Postoperative monitoring following critical trauma, Heart Lung 4:269, 1975.

24. Hoyt JW and others: Continuous SvO_2 as a predictor of changes in cardiac output: clinical observations. In Schweiss JF, editor: Continuous measurement of blood oxygen saturation in the high risk patient, vol 1, San Diego, 1983, Beach International, Inc.

25. Hudson-Civetta JA and others: Risk and deletion of pulmonary artery catheter-related infection in septic surgical patients, Crit Care Med 15:29, 1987.

26. Hurst JW: The heart: arteries and veins, ed. 6, New York, 1986, McGraw-Hill, Inc.

27. Kashuk JL and Penn I: Air embolism after central venous catheterization, Surg Gynecol Obstet 159:249, 1984.

28. Killip T and Kimball JT: A survey of the coronary care unit: concept and results, Prog Cardiovasc Dis 11:45, 1968.

29. Lalli SM: The complete Swan-Ganz, RN 9:65, 1978.

30. Lamb J: Intra-arterial monitoring: rescinding the risks, Nurs 77 7:65, 1977.

31. Lowenstein E, Little JW, and Lo HH: Prevention of cerebral embolization from flushing radial artery cannulas, N Engl J Med 285:1414, 1971.

32. Michel L, March HM, and McMichan JC: Infection of pulmonary artery catheters in critically ill patients, JAMA 245:1032, 1981.

33. Mitchell PH and Mauss N: Intracranial pressure: fact and fancy, Nurs 76 6:53, 1976.

34. Norris DL and Klein LA: What all those pressure readings mean and why, RN 10:35, 1981.

35. Pearl RG and others: Effect of injectate volume and temperature on thermodilution cardiac output determination, Anesthesiology 64:798, 1986.

36. Procedures for insertion of Swan-Ganz catheters, Swan-Ganz monitoring systems, Irvine, Calif, 1980, American Edwards Laboratories.

37. Product bulletin, Swan-Ganz monitoring systems, Irvine, Calif, 1980, American Edwards Laboratories.

38. Rackley CE and Russell RO Jr: Measurements in heart failure in patients with cardiac infarction: hemodynamic monitoring in a coronary intensive care unit, Mt Kisco, NY, 1974, Futura Publishing Co, Inc.

39. Rhoades C, Adcock M, and Javanovich J: Prevention of nosocomial infection in critical care units, Nurs Clin North Am 15:803, 1980.

40. Robin E: The cult of the Swan-Ganz catheter: Overuse and abuse of pulmonary flow catheters, Ann Intern Med 103:445, 1985.

41. Ross J: Hemodynamic changes in acute myocardial infarction, Hosp Pract 7:125, 1972.

42. Russell RO Jr and others: Current status of hemodynamic monitoring: indications, diagnosis complications, Cardiovasc Clin 11(3):1, 1981.

43. Shah KB and others: A review of pulmonary artery catheterization in 6,245 patients, Anesthesiology 61:271, 1984.

44. Shoemaker WC and others: Clinical trial of survivors' cardiorespiratory patterns as therapeutic goals in critically ill postoperative patients, Crit Care Med 10:398, 1982.

45. Smith RN: Invasive pressure monitoring, Am J Nurs 78:1514, 1978.

46. Sonnenblick EH and Strobeck JE: Derived indexes of ventricular and myocardial function, N Engl J Med 296:978, 1977.

47. Spodick DH: Physiologic and prognostic implications of invasive monitoring: undetermined risk/benefit ratios in patients with heart disease, Am J Cardiol 46:173, 1980.

48. Sprung CK and others: Prophylactic use of lidocaine to prevent advanced ventricular arrhythmias during pulmonary artery catheterization, Am J Med 75:906, 1983.

49. Tilkian A and Daily EK: Cardiovascular procedures, St Louis, 1987, The CV Mosby Co.

50. Vennix CV, Nelson DH, and Pierpont GL: Thermodilution cardiac output in critically ill patients: comparison of room temperature and iced injectate, Heart Lung 13:574, 1984.

51. Weil MH: Evaluation and treatment of the patient with cardiovascular collapse, Emerg Med 13:93, 1981.

52. Weisil RD, Berger RL, and Hechtman HB: Measurement of cardiac output by thermodilution, N Engl J Med 292:682, 1975.

53. Whitman G, Howaniak D, and Verga T: Comparison of cardiac output measurements in 20° supine and 20° right and left lateral recumbent positions, Proceedings of the Ninth Annual National Teaching Institute of the American Association of Critical Care Nurses, Irvine, Calif, 1982, The Association.

54. Woods SL: Monitoring pulmonary artery pressures, Am J Nurs 76:1765, 1976.

THE PERSON WITH CARDIOVASCULAR DYSFUNCTION

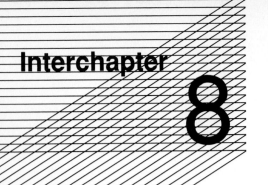

Interchapter 8

Risk Factors and Coronary Artery Disease

The link between arteriosclerotic heart disease and the major coronary artery disease (CAD) risk factors (i.e., cigarette smoking, hypercholesterolemia, and hypertension) is well known. These risk factors significantly increase the chance of developing heart disease. This association is so well established that these factors are thought to predominate in large groups of patients with CAD.

This is not the case. In fact, most persons who are first seen clinically with CAD have not one or two risk factors but *none*.[1] This is almost an embarrassment, considering the present state of knowledge about what really determines the development of the leading cause of death in American society and the world.[3]

Perhaps the origins of this illness lie elsewhere. In 1973 a special task force in Massachusetts reported to the Secretary of the Department of Health, Education, and Welfare their findings on the likelihood of surviving CAD.[4] They found that the most reliable factor in determining survival was not smoking, high blood pressure, or hypercholesterolemia, but job satisfaction. The second most reliable predictor was what the task force termed *overall happiness*.

Little attention usually is given to the satisfaction and happiness of patients with CAD, perhaps because it seems hopeless to deal with such broad subjective areas of persons' lives. Most want to focus on something about which they can do something, such as the serum cholesterol level or smoking, even if most new patients with CAD have none of these factors. However, nurses should not retreat from issues simply because they are difficult. No one else on the health care team spends as much time at a patient's bedside and interacts so regularly with family members. No one else has a better vantage point from which to evaluate patients' fears, anger, contentment, unhappiness, strengths and weaknesses, and coping skills.

It is not the nurse's role to reshape patients' entire personalities during the hospital experience. Nevertheless they can begin to move patients in the appropriate direction when encouraging them to openly examine their own lifestyles and behavior. They can guide the direction by assuring patients that it is acceptable to doubt, question, and reassess negative behavior patterns. They can reinforce the need for patients to accept more responsibility for their own health, to make sound choices that promote health, and to pursue healthy behaviors. They can inform patients about health-promoting activities known to prevent or reverse disease and can refer patients to the appropriate people and centers for help.[2] They also can motivate patients by giving them the permission to change.

When patients ask whether there could be a possible link between anxiety, worries, or unhappiness and CAD, we can say "yes." By doing this, we are being consistent with current scientific data.

REFERENCES

1. Jenkins CD: Psychological and social precursors of coronary disease, N Engl J Med 284:244, 1971.
2. Leaf A and Ryan TJ: Prevention of coronary artery disease, N Engl J Med 323:1416, 1990.
3. Okie S: Mortality: heart disease is world's worst scourge, Washington Post, April 30, 1990, p A2.
4. Work in America: Report of a special task force to the Secretary of the Department of Health, Education, and Welfare, Cambridge, Mass, 1973, The MIT Press.

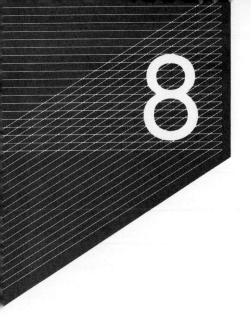

8

The Person with Coronary Artery Disease Risk Factors

Carolyn L. Murdaugh

LEARNING OBJECTIVES

1. Compare and contrast the major theories for the development of atherosclerosis.

2. Analyze the major modifiable and nonmodifiable risk factors for the development of atherosclerosis and coronary artery disease.

3. Explore the major nursing diagnoses based on the assessment of persons at risk for coronary artery disease.

4. Appraise the medical and nursing interventions for persons with identifiable risk factors for coronary artery disease.

The Framingham Heart Study began the investigation of coronary artery disease (CAD) over 40 years ago in Framingham, Massachusetts, a small town north of Boston. The study was one of the first to develop the concept known as *risk factors*. Because every man and woman in the town of Framingham were examined every 2 years, those who developed CAD could be compared with those who did not. Anything that was associated with a higher rate of heart attack or stroke became a risk factor. The identification of risk factors in Framingham formed an important base for many intervention studies that have since been conducted to establish a causal connection between risk factors and CAD. The three major risk factors that were identified and have been substantiated in other large studies are blood cholesterol level, hypertension, and cigarette smoking. Other major risk factors identified include obesity, diabetes mellitus, sedentary activity, and stress. In addition, nonmodifiable risk factors, including gender, family history, and age, have also been described as risk factors, beginning with the Framingham study.

Over the past 30 years, age-adjusted mortality for all cardiovascular diseases has decreased by 40% in the United States.[55] Goldman and Cook[24] estimated that 45% of the decline in death rate was related to changes in lifestyle such as cessation of cigarette smoking and that 40% could be attributed to medical interventions. An examination of the Framingham Heart Study also provides evidence for the role of risk factor reduction in the decrease in mortality from cardiovascular disease. However, evidence suggests that secondary rather than primary prevention may have been most effective because prevalence rates have increased, whereas the incidence rates remain constant.[70] Thus the Framingham study continues to contribute to the study of CAD and patient care.

ATHEROSCLEROSIS

Atherosclerosis is an extremely complex process that was recognized in humans even in the fifteenth century, when lesions were identified in Egyptian mummies. The development of atherosclerosis in humans depends on several factors, including age, genetic makeup, and physiologic status, as well as the number and extent of risk factors present. The lesions of atherosclerosis occur principally in the innermost layer of the artery wall, called the *intima*. These lesions have been called the *fatty streak,* the *fibrous plaque,* and the *complicated lesions*. Changes have also been observed in the media or middle layer underlying the lesion, principally in association with advanced lesions.

The *fatty streak* is a grossly flat, lipid-rich lesion consisting of macrophages and some smooth muscle. Fatty streaks are found in the aorta shortly after birth and in most children over 1 year of age in all populations. They increase in number between the ages of 8 and 18. Fatty streaks appear in the coronary arteries around age 15 and increase in these vessels through the third decade.[59] Fatty streaks are yellowish in appearance due to extensive lipid deposits. They cause little or no obstruction and do not cause any clinical problems. By themselves, fatty streaks are considered benign. It has not been resolved whether fatty streaks are the precursors for fibrous plaque and atherosclerosis.

More advanced lesions, called *fibrous plaques,* begin to develop in the coronary arteries after 20 years of age in countries with a high incidence of atherosclerosis. The fibrous plaque is grossly white in appearance and becomes elevated so that it may protrude into the lumen of the artery. Development of the lesion is due to an increased proliferation of intimal smooth muscle cells. The smooth muscle cells form a fibrous cap resulting from the accumulation of intracellular and extracellular lipids and deposition of connective tissue. Beneath the fibrous cap, the lesions consist of smooth muscle and macrophages, which contain lipid droplets surrounded by connective tissue. Be-

neath these cells, there may be an area of necrotic debris, cholesterol crystals, and calcification. Smooth muscle rich fibrous plaques are often found at the same anatomic sites in coronary and extracranial cerebral arteries where fatty streaks were found early in life.[68] This finding suggests that fibrous plaques may be derived from fatty streaks in which cell proliferation, lipid accumulation, and connective tissue formation have continued. However, fatty streaks can also occur in anatomic sites that differ from those in which fibrous plaques occur.

Advanced or *complicated lesions* occur in patients over the age of 30, when fibrous plaques undergo complex changes and increase in frequency. Fibrous plaques become vascularized, and the necrotic lipid-rich core increases in size and often becomes calcified. The intimal surface of the lesion may disintegrate and ulcerate, allowing thrombi to form on the surface of the plaque. The thrombi may further increase the size of the plaque and reduce the lumen of the artery, resulting in reduced blood flow (ischemia) or arterial occlusion (necrosis) (Fig. 8-1). Clinical symptoms occur as a result of the ischemia or necrosis and are manifested as myocardial infarction, stroke, aortic aneurysm, and gangrene of the extremities. Thus although clinical symptoms may occur suddenly, the atherosclerotic process began at an early age.

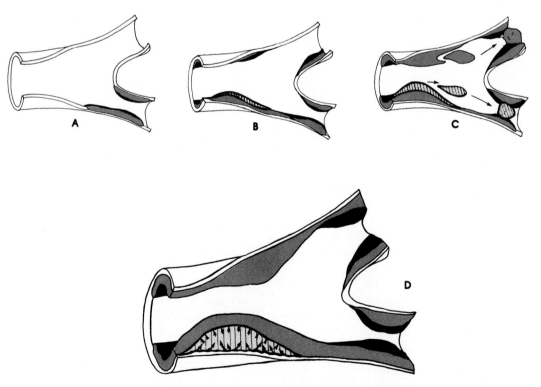

FIG. 8-1 **A,** Obstruction of coronary arteries from plaque formation (atheromas). **B,** Clot formation around plaques. **C,** Thrombi (plaque thrombus above and blood thrombus below). **D,** Vessel hemorrhage.

PATHOGENESIS

The key elements in the development of the atherosclerotic lesions are smooth muscle proliferation, connective tissue formation, and lipid accumulation. Recognition of these key components has led to the development of several theories to describe the cause and development of atherosclerosis. Theories receiving the most attention are the response-to-injury hypothesis, the lipoprotein hypothesis, and monoclonal hypothesis.[59,60]

Response-to-injury hypothesis

With the response-to-injury hypothesis, some form of injury occurs to the endothelium, resulting in structural or functional changes in the endothelial cells. Injury may result from factors such as chronic hypercholesterolemia, increased shear stress from blood flow at bifurcations in arteries, hypertension, and chemical toxins found in cigarette smoke that change the nature of the permeability barrier of the endothelial cells.

Endothelial cells, functionally active components of the intima, perform two vital functions. The cells normally are a permeability barrier to control the passage of molecules from the plasma to the underlying artery wall. The endothelium also forms a thromboresistant surface that promotes the continuous flow of blood by producing a heparinlike surface, proteoglycan, and synthesizing prostacyclin (PGI_2). *Prostacyclin*, the most potent vasodilator isolated to date, is also a potent inhibitor of platelet aggregation.

An immediate platelet response results when the endothelium is injured. Platelets begin to adhere to the subendothelial layer at the site of injury. The platelets aggregate and release their granule contents, which contain several mitogens, including *platelet-derived growth factor* (PDGF). PDGF binds to connective tissue at endothelial injury sites to attract smooth muscle cells from the media into the intima. Within 3 to 5 days after platelets release their contents, smooth muscle cells migrate from the media into the intima of the artery and proliferate. If the injury and the tissue response is limited and the integrity of the endothelium is restored, the lesion may be able to regress. Evidence of such regression is available from human and animal studies. For example, endothelial injury occurs when a balloon catheter is placed in an artery. However, when the catheter is removed, endothelial cells regenerate slowly. In young monkeys, complete regeneration of the endothelium can take as long as 9 months.[59] If the injury is long or chronically repeated, the lesions may continue to progress to advanced plaques with clinical consequences. One cause of long-standing injury is chronically elevated low-density lipoproteins, also called *chronic hypercholesterolemia*.

Fagiotto, Ross, and Harker[16,17] have conducted extensive research on the response-to-injury hypothesis. They studied the effects of inducing chronic hypercholesterolemia lasting from 12 days to 13 months in 40 pigtail monkeys. Levels of hypercholesterolemia between 300 to 1000 mg/dl were obtained within 12 days, and monocytes were observed attached to the endothelial surface throughout the arterial tree. These monocytes seemed to be migrating between endothelial cells into the intima. Within 1 month, many monocytes had begun to accumulate lipid and take on the appearance of foam cells.

Within 3 months the lesions began to resemble fatty streaks consisting of 2 to 3 layers of foam cells. After 4 months of hypercholesterolemia, breaks occurred between the endothelial cells separating the fatty streaks. Retraction of the endothelium resulted from the breaks, providing opportunity for platelet adherence, aggregation, and release of PDGF. Smooth muscle proliferation lesions of atherosclerosis then appeared over the next 2 months. Fagiotto and Ross' observations[16,17] support other studies that reported that smooth muscle proliferation lesions of atherosclerosis are preceded by endothelial injury in the form of breaks in the endothelium, exposure of macrophages, and platelet interactions.

Lipoprotein hypothesis

With the lipoprotein hypothesis, there are marked elevations of plasma low-density lipoproteins (LDL). *Low-density lipoprotein*, the major cholesterol-transporting lipoprotein, is the major carrier of cholesterol into tissues. Elevated levels of LDL may cause injury to the endothelial lining of the artery by infiltrating the intima from the blood.

Brown and Goldstein[7] contributed knowledge on the interaction of LDL with cells. They demonstrated that human cells possess specific receptors on their surface membranes that bind with high affinity to LDL. The "LDL pathway" is part of a complex biochemical pathway that regulates the uptake, storage, and synthesis of cholesterol by the cell. The number of receptors is adjusted to provide the cell with enough cholesterol to meet its needs. Thus the cholesterol needs of the cell determine LDL receptor synthesis, or the number of LDL receptors available for binding LDL. If LDL receptors are abnormally decreased or missing, the cell cannot adequately gain access to LDL, resulting in high plasma LDL concentrations. This is the case in familial hypercholesterolemia when LDL receptors are reduced or lacking.

Regardless of whether LDL levels are elevated due to a defect in the LDL receptor or other genetic or environmental factors, cholesterol esters are ultimately deposited in the arterial wall because of endothelial injury. Injury occurs from exposure of the endothelium to the high LDL levels. Smooth muscle cells fill with excess LDL and become foam cells. Thus LDL by itself may promote proliferation of smooth muscle cells and connective tissue components.

Monoclonal hypothesis

The monoclonal hypothesis suggests that each atherosclerotic lesion is derived from a single smooth cell that is the generator of all proliferating cells within the lesion. The hypothesis is based on the Lyon or inactive X chromosome hypothesis. The Lyon hypothesis states that only one of the two X chromosomes present in every adult female somatic cell is active. The progeny of each cell expresses the same inactive X chromosomes as its parent cell. Benign tumors exhibit similar phenomena, in that all tumor cells originate from a single cell, therefore being monoclonal. However, recent evidence indicates that the lesions of atherosclerosis are not derived from a single cell but rather a population of cells of identical phenotype or some combination. The lesions are more likely hyperplastic rather than neoplastic in nature, which provides rationale for the development of interventions to promote regression.

Regression of atherosclerosis

Animal models have commonly been used to study regression of atherosclerosis because of the inability, until recently, to conduct such research with humans. Rabbits, pigeons, swine, dogs, and nonhuman primates have served as subjects. Nonhuman primates, particularly the rhesus and macaque monkeys, are preferred because they develop lesions that clearly mimic lesions in humans such as xanthomata, myocardial infarction, cerebral ischemia, and stroke. Dietary cholesterol has been the major mechanism for the induction of atherosclerosis. Drug administration and mechanical injury of the endothelium have also been used. After treatment, some animals were occasionally sacrificed, and the arteries were examined at autopsy for pathologic conditions. Alternatively, serial laparotomies were performed to avoid the "one-time look" problem. Exercise and drug treatment for hypercholesterolemia were shown to decrease the severity of the atherosclerotic lesions. Documented regressive changes were related to a decrease in the size of the lesion. Changes included regeneration of the endothelium, decreased cell proliferation, decreased lipid accumulation and the development of foam cells, and decreased necrosis of plaque. Although more research is needed, evidence indicates that a reduction in risk factors can lead to a regression of lesions (see Ornish, p. 5).

Risk factors for CAD

Elevated blood cholesterol, hypertension, and cigarette smoking have been positively correlated with atherosclerotic lesions; these risk factors are referred to as *atherogenic traits*.[2] Diabetes mellitus, obesity, physical inactivity, and stress also contribute to the atherosclerotic process.

Elevated blood cholesterol

Dietary lipids are primarily responsible for the high incidence of atherosclerotic disease in the industrially developed world. The ingestion of cholesterol and elevated plasma cholesterol levels are associated with CAD within all population groups. Results from the Lipid Research Clinics Program[42] demonstrated a causal relationship between the plasma lipoprotein profile, cholesterol levels, and morbidity and mortality rates from coronary atherosclerosis.

Longitudinal studies such as the Framingham Study[32] and the Seven Country Study[46] clearly demonstrate that persons with symptomatic CAD have higher levels of cholesterol than individuals without clinical symptoms. Prospective studies have shown that serum cholesterol levels predict the occurrence of CAD disease and deaths. For persons with cholesterol values below 175 mg/dl, the risk of death is half as much as the risk of persons with cholesterol values of 250 mg/dl or higher. Persons with cholesterol levels of 240 mg/dl or above have double the risk of CAD of persons with a level of 200 mg/dl.

A high serum cholesterol level is a primary risk factor in patients age 65 and older.[25] For each 1% increase in total cholesterol, the risk of CAD increases by 2% to 3%, similar to risks in younger persons. However, a high total cholesterol level alone does not predict cardiovascular diseases in older persons; fractionation into LDL cholesterol and high-density lipoprotein (HDL) cholesterol is necessary. A high LDL cholesterol level is a risk factor for CAD in persons older than 50 years.[8] In Framingham women over age 50, but not in men, triglyceride rather than LDL cholesterol levels were slightly better predictors of CAD. The HDL cholesterol level, which has an inverse relation to CAD, remains significant in men to age 79 and women to age 69.[8] Because the rates of coronary artery disease increase significantly after menopause, elevated cholesterol levels are also an important risk factor in women.

Classification of lipoproteins. Cholesterol is a naturally occurring lipid component of cell membranes and a precursor of bile acids and steroid hormones. Cholesterol is also the predominant lipid component of the atherosclerotic lesion. Cholesterol travels in the circulation in spherical particles that contain lipids and proteins called *lipoproteins*.

Three major classes of lipoproteins can be measured in the serum of a fasting individual: LDLs, HDLs, and very-low-density lipoproteins (VLDLs). LDL, the primary atherogenic lipoprotein, contains approximately 60% of the total cholesterol and is positively correlated with risk for CAD. VLDL, which is largely composed of triglycerides, contains 10% to 15% of the total serum cholesterol.

VLDLs transport the majority of endogenous triglycerides and may be related to CAD incidence by an association with reduced HDL, diabetes, and obesity.

Because most of the cholesterol in the serum is found in LDL, the concentration of total cholesterol is closely correlated with the concentration of LDL cholesterol. The LDL cholesterol offers more precision in determining individual risk and is preferred for clinical decisions about interventions to lower blood cholesterol levels. However, total cholesterol levels can be used in initial serum lipid evaluation. Serum HDL levels reflect the process of cholesterol removal from the peripheral tissues to the liver for degradation. Higher levels of HDL facilitate cholesterol removal from the body. Thus the ratio of HDL to total cholesterol is significant in assessing cardiovascular risk.

Classification of patients. The National Heart, Lung, and Blood Institute (NHLBI) recommends measurement of serum total cholesterol levels in all adults 20 years of age and over at least once every 5 years.[48] Tests to determine total cholesterol levels are appropriate in initial evaluation because they are cost effective and can be measured accurately without fasting. Cholesterol testing, however, is only one component of a comprehensive risk factor evaluation. Optimal serum cholesterol values for American adults are 200 mg/dl or less. Patients with an optimal blood cholesterol level should be provided with educational materials designed to assist them in maintaining blood cholesterol levels below 200 mg/dl and reducing associated risk factors. These patients are advised to have serum cholesterol tests within 5 years or with their annual physical examinations. Serum cholesterol levels of 200 to 239 mg/dl are classified as "borderline high blood cholesterol." These patients are educated about dietary and associated risk factor modification and are rechecked annually. Individuals who have been diagnosed with CAD or two associated nonlipid risk factors are referred for measurement of serum LDL cholesterol levels. Cholesterol levels of 240 mg/dl and above are classified as "high blood cholesterol." Patients with high blood cholesterol levels need to be referred for testing for the serum level of LDL cholesterol.

The level of LDL cholesterol, as well as the total blood cholesterol level, serves as a key index for clinical decision making regarding therapy designed to lower cholesterol levels. Desirable LDL cholesterol levels are 130 mg/dl and below. Levels of LDL cholesterol of 160 mg/dl or greater are classified as "high-risk LDL cholesterol." High-risk patients need dietary therapy and frequent monitoring. Levels of 130 to 159 mg/dl are classified as "borderline high-risk LDL cholesterol." Borderline high-risk patients are advised to follow a fat-modified diet and are reevaluated annually. Persons with levels of 190 mg/dl or higher need an adequate dietary trial immediately because they are at very high risk. Pharmacologic therapy often is necessary in this group.

Lowering cholesterol levels reduces the incidence of CAD.[48,70,72] Clinical trial results indicate that dietary intervention is as effective in preventing recurrent myocardial infarction and death in patients with diagnosed CAD as it is in primary prevention. Although direct evidence is strongest in middle-age men with high initial cholesterol levels, epidemiologic observations and animal experiments also indicate that reduction of total and LDL cholesterol levels reduces the incidence of CAD in younger and older men, in women, and in individuals with more moderate cholesterol levels.

Dietary treatment. The goal of treatment is to lower LDL and total cholesterol levels and to reduce excess body fat. If normal plasma cholesterol levels are not achieved with dietary management, pharmacologic therapy is instituted. However, continued dietary management can reduce the drug dosage, lessening the occurrence of side effects.

A two-step program[47] may be used to progressively reduce the intake of dietary saturated fatty acids and cholesterol and eliminate excess total calories. The Step-One diet provides an intake of total fat less than 30% of calories, saturated fatty acids less than 10% of calories, and cholesterol less than 300 mg/day. Serum cholesterol levels need to be measured at 4 to 6 weeks and at 3 months after starting the Step-One diet. If the goals of therapy are not achieved on the Step-One diet by 3 months, the Step-Two diet is implemented. The Step-Two diet further reduces the intake of saturated fatty acid to less than 7% of calories and cholesterol intake to less than 200 mg/day.

The degree of reduction that can be achieved by dietary therapy depends on the dietary habits of the patient before starting the diet and adherence with dietary modifications. Changing a typical American diet to the Step-One diet can reduce cholesterol levels on the average by 30 to 40 mg/dl. Advancing to the Step-Two diet can further reduce levels by approximately 15 mg/dl. Most of this decrease occurs in the LDL cholesterol fraction.

Cholesterol reduction can be achieved by dietary therapy alone for many high-risk patients. Persons who do not have high LDL cholesterol levels or severe lipid abnormalities need to continue dietary therapy for at least 6 months before considering drug therapy. Associated risk factors such as obesity, sedentary lifestyle, and smoking need to be modified as part of cholesterol-lowering therapy. If the goals of LDL cholesterol reduction are met by diet modification, long-term monitoring is indicated. If reduction of LDL cholesterol is not achieved, lipid-lowering drugs are considered in conjunction with continued dietary intervention.

Pharmacologic treatment. Patients with high LDL cholesterol levels after dietary therapy are candidates for drug treatment. Most interventions require 4 to 6 weeks before an effect is seen. Therefore a minimum of 3 months of dietary therapy is required to provide a baseline before evaluating the efficacy of pharmacologic therapy. According to the National Cholesterol Education Program Expert Panel,[47] drug therapy is considered when LDL cholesterol levels are 190 mg/dl or higher in patients without diagnosed CAD or when the patient has at least two associated CAD risk factors; it is also considered when LDL levels are 160 mg/dl or greater in patients with diagnosed CAD or with two associated CAD risk factors.

Treatment goals for pharmacologic therapy are the same as for dietary therapy. For patients without a diagnosis of CAD or with two associated CAD risk factors both treatments attempt to reduce LDL cholesterol levels to less than 160 mg/dl. For patients with diagnosed CAD or two associated CAD risk factors, the treatments attempt to reduce LDL cholesterol levels to less than 130 mg/dl.

Most lipid-lowering drugs have side effects, so they are generally used only when nonpharmacologic management has been unsuccessful. Guidelines established by the National Cholesterol Education Program Expert Panel[47] recommend the sequence of drugs. Bile acid sequestrants, (cholestyramine [Questran, Cholybar]) and nicotinic acid (Nicobid, Nicolar, Nia-Bid) are the initial drugs of choice for treatment of elevated levels of LDL. Both drugs are effective in lowering LDL cholesterol and CAD risk. Both are also generally safe for long-term use. Bile acid sequestrants are nonabsorbable anionic exchange resins that prevent the reabsorption of cholesterol in the gastrointestinal tract, causing it to be excreted in the feces. Nicotinic acid is the drug of choice when triglyceride levels are greater than 250 mg/dl because it lowers LDL cholesterol without exacerbating the hypertriglyceridemia. Nicotinic acid lowers cholesterol by decreasing the synthesis of VLDL, the precursor of LDL in the liver. Administration of bile acid sequestrants may increase hepatic VLDL production and increase the plasma concentration of triglycerides. Bile acid sequestrants are thus contraindicated as single-drug therapy in patients with hypertriglyceridemia (see Appendix C).

Gemfibrozil (Lopid) and clofibrate (Atromid-S) are fibric acid derivatives. These drugs increase lipoprotein lipase activity, resulting in an increase in VLDL triglyceride clearance. Fibric acids reduce plasma triglyceride levels and VLDL levels of cholesterol. Although gemfibrozil has been approved for treatment of hypertriglyceridemia, results of the Helsinki Heart Study[19] indicate that the drug is also effecive for the treatment of hypercholesterolemia. These two drugs reduce the total cholesterol/HDL cholesterol ratio without the side effects caused by bile acid sequestrants or nicotinic acid.

Lovastatin (Mevacor), a 3-hydroxy-3-methylglutanyl coenzyme A (HMG CoA) reductase inhibitor, is frequently successful when other pharmacologic agents have not been effective in lowering LDL levels. These drugs act by decreasing liver cholesterol synthesis, resulting in increased LDL receptor activity, increased clearance of LDL from plasma, and a reduced LDL plasma level. However, the

long-term safety (longer than 5 years) and effect on CAD risk have not been established.

The lipid-lowering effect of *fish oils* have also been investigated. The low incidence of CAD in Eskimos in Greenland may be related to their consumption of seal, whale, and fish, which contain eicosapentaenoic acid, a polyunsaturated fatty acid of the omega-3 series. Eicosapentaenoic acid may inhibit the metabolism of arachidonic acid, a potent inducer of platelet aggregation when converted to thromboxane A_2. Thus metabolism of arachidonic acid and platelet aggregation are inhibited.

Current dietary recommendations include the consumption of fish 2 to 3 times a week. However, no evidence to date warrants the use of omega-3 capsules as a dietary supplement. There is a potential for vitamin A and D toxicity because the capsules are available without a prescription.

Hypertension

Hypertension is one of the most potent risk factors for cardiovascular disease and death. Elevated blood pressure is the major factor contributing to strokes, and it is a major factor for heart attacks and death. The risk of cardiovascular complications intensifies with increasing systolic and diastolic blood pressures. Hypertension is a systolic blood pressure of 140 mm Hg and above or a diastolic blood pressure of 90 mm Hg and above. Of the 60 million Americans with hypertension, 75% have mild hypertension, or diastolic blood pressures between 90 and 105 mm Hg. The term *mild* refers only to the degree of elevation and must not be thought to be unimportant because persons with mild hypertension are at considerable excess risk of disease and death.[49] Persons with elevated blood pressure are twice as likely to develop peripheral vascular disease, sudden death, coronary heart disease and myocardial infarction, congestive heart failure, and kidney failure, and are four times more likely to have a stroke as those with normal blood pressure.[34]

The clinical complications of hypertension result from either a direct pathologic effect of the vasculature or promotion of the atherogenic process. Renin and other agents may cause cellular changes, or the increased shear stress of the flow of blood may be a factor. The findings of animal, human population, and postmortem studies suggest that hypertension is a stimulus for the development of atheromas in arterial endothelium.[41]

Hypertension is common among the elderly; a prevalence rate of 50% in the aging population has been reported.[74] In adults, diastolic blood pressure generally rises until age 55 to 60 and then levels off. Systolic blood pressure also rises with age.[20] Older people were once thought to tolerate high blood pressure better than younger patients. However, a direct link between systolic blood pressure and the incidence of stroke and CAD has been established for patients over the age of 40. The Framingham study demonstrated that the older the person, the greater the detrimental effects of high blood pressure.[8] In the elderly, hypertension is a major risk factor for CAD, congestive heart failure, stroke, renal failure, and intermittent claudication.

Hypertension is more common in blacks than in whites. Blacks have an average systolic blood pressure of about 6 mm Hg higher and a diastolic blood pressure of 5 mm Hg higher than whites.[73] The results of the Hypertension Detection and Follow-up Program[65] revealed that hypertension was 1½ to 2 times more common among black Americans than among white; severe hypertension (diastolic blood pressure greater than 115 mm Hg) was 5 times more common among black men than among white men and 7 times more common among black women than among white women. Death rates remain 2½ times greater for blacks.

Pathophysiology. The cause of essential hypertension remains unknown. Most hypotheses consider hypertension a "disuse of regulation" because abnormalities in the control systems fail to bring blood pressure back to normal when it becomes elevated. The basic hemodynamic fault proposed is a failure to control systematic vascular resistance, whatever the cause.[14] Hemodynamic characteristics (cardiac output and total peripheral resistance), neural and volume factors, and the renin-angiotension system have also been explored as potential causes. Findings vary, depending on the severity and type of hypertension. Stress is also considered a major factor by some investigators. Heredity has also been found to be a major contributor.

Detection of hypertension. The control of hypertension begins with detection. Accurate detection is based on proper measurement of blood pressure, but hypertension cannot be diagnosed on the basis of a single measurement. If elevated blood pressure is detected at an initial visit, two subsequent visits with elevated readings of 140/90 mm Hg or above are needed to make the diagnosis.

Blood pressure should initially be measured in both arms, with subsequent measurements taken in the arm with the highest reading. If blood pressure is measured in the sitting or standing position, the arm must be positioned at heart level. Measurement should not begin until the patient has rested quietly for 5 minutes. Smoking or caffeine ingestion should not have occurred for at least 30 minutes. The appropriate cuff size is necessary to ensure accurate measurement. The rubber bladder needs to encircle at least two thirds of the arm (see Chapter 3). Two or more readings should be averaged.

Guidelines for confirmation and follow-up have been outlined by the Joint National Committee on Detection, Evaluation, and Treatment of High Blood Pressure.[31] Follow-up depends on the blood pressure obtained. Normal blood pressure measurements (less than 140/85 mm Hg) should be rechecked within 2 years. A diastolic pressure of 85 to 89 mm Hg should be rechecked within 1 year. A diastolic pressure of 90 to 104 mm Hg should be rechecked within 2 months. A diastolic pressure of 105 to 114 mm Hg and a systolic pressure of 140 to 200 mm Hg requires further referral and evaluation within 2 weeks. A diastolic pressure greater than 115 mm Hg requires immediate referral and drug therapy. Twenty-four-hour ambulatory blood pressure devices are available to monitor persons with marked variability in blood pressure. However, these devices are not recommended for routine use because the technique is costly (see Chapter 6).

Treatment. The primary objective of the treatment of hypertension is to reduce and maintain blood pressure below 140/90 mm Hg. Nonpharmacologic and pharmacologic approaches to therapy are available. Nonpharmacologic therapy, which includes weight reduction, salt restriction, and moderation of alcohol consumption, lowers blood pressure and improves the efficacy of pharmacologic agents. The decision to implement pharmacologic therapy is based on the severity of blood pressure elevation and the presence of other complications.

Nonpharmacologic treatment. Nonpharmacologic therapies are instituted when the diastolic pressure is between 90 and 94 mm Hg in patients under age 50 without other cardiovascular risk factors or evidence of target organ damage. They are also used as an adjunct to pharmacologic therapy and should be considered in all antihypertension therapy.

DIETARY SALT RESTRICTION. Some persons are considered "salt sensitive" in that they tend to retain sodium, gain weight, and develop an elevated blood pressure on a high-salt diet. In contrast, "salt-resistant" persons do not have a change in blood pressure or weight on a high-or a low-salt diet. This variability helps explain why blood pressure is lowered in some but not all patients after sodium restriction. Moderate sodium restriction of 2000 mg per day (5 grams of sodium chloride or 88 millimoles [mmol] of sodium) is recommended to lower blood pressure. Sodium restriction can be accomplished by avoiding heavily salted food and omitting salt in cooking. Because there is no easy way to tell which patients may benefit, the restriction is not severe, and there are usually no serious consequences even if the patient's blood pressure does not respond to the restriction. All hypertensive patients should be counseled about reducing sodium intake.

WEIGHT REDUCTION. Obesity and blood pressure are closely related. Weight reduction has been associated with a decrease in blood pressure. Because of the clear relationship, all obese hypertensive adults need to be placed on weight-reducing diets. The patient should be within 15% of the desired body weight.[49] Each kilogram of weight loss usually is accompanied by a 1 to 2 mm Hg decrease in blood pressure.

RESTRICTION OF ALCOHOL INTAKE. Moderate alcohol consumption is recommended. More than 2 ounces of alcohol per day may produce hypertension because ethanol, even in small amounts, produces a pressor effect.[36] Therefore daily intake should be restricted to 2 ounces of whiskey, 8 ounces of wine, or 24 ounces of beer.

Pharmacologic therapy. Even when nonpharmacologic therapy is used, many persons with hypertension still need drug therapy, particularly to reduce the mortality rate in patients with diastolic pressures greater than 104 mm Hg.[36] Patients with mild hypertension or a diastolic blood pressure of 90 to 104 mm Hg also benefit from antihypertensive therapy, which decreases stroke, congestive heart failure, and the number of deaths. All persons with persistently elevated diastolic pressures greater than 94 mm Hg and those with other major risk factors or evidence of target organ damage should be treated with pharmacologic agents.

An individualized approach is necessary in choosing drug therapy. Until recently, diuretics were the initial drug of choice. However, diuretics may induce hypokalemia, glucose intolerance, and hypercholesterolemia without providing the extent of protection against CAD that was previously thought.[36] Diuretics may be safely used if biochemical aberrations are corrected and patients are followed closely. However, other drugs can be used initially in the absence of a diuretic; specifically beta blockers, angiotensin-converting enzyme (ACE) inhibitors, and calcium channel blockers can be used. Central and peripherally acting adrenergic inhibitors may be added to the first set of agents used.

DIURETICS. Hydrochlorothiazide remains the diuretic of choice for most patients. If patients need more potent diuretics, loop diuretics, such as furosemide, are prescribed. Attention must be given to the potential rise in the serum cholesterol level, fall in the potassium level, and worsening of glucose intolerance. In addition, much smaller doses than initially thought can be used in the elderly. Hypokalemia can be prevented by using smaller doses or prescribing potassium-sparing diuretics (see Appendix C).

BETA BLOCKERS. Beta blockers are often prescribed as initial therapy in younger, white patients. Many beta blockers are available today and differ in three major ways: (1) beta selectivity, (2) intrinsic sympathomimetic activity, and (3) lipid solubility. The major side effects are related to a magnification of their beta receptor blockade. For example, congestive heart failure may develop from decreased cardiac output (see Appendix C).

CALCIUM CHANNEL BLOCKERS. These vasodilator drugs may be used as a first, second, or third drug and have been found to be effective in elderly persons with hypertension.

ACE INHIBITORS. ACE inhibitors inhibit the enzyme that converts angiotensin I to the vasoconstrictor, angiotension II. Although these drugs are not any more effective than other antihypertensive agents, the absence of central nervous system and cardiac-mediated side effects provide an advantage for some patients. However, other side effects, such as loss of taste, chronic cough, rash, bone marrow depression, and proteinuria, have been reported.

OTHER AGENTS. Other agents may be used as a second drug with the previous agents. Vasodilators, such as hydralazine and minoxidil, are usually added as third drugs. Peripheral adrenergic inhibitors, reserpine and guanethidine, are expensive and produce unpleasant side effects.

Cigarette smoking

Cigarette smoking, the most important modifiable risk factor for CAD, causes 3 times more CAD deaths than deaths from lung cancer.[33] In almost all studies, death rates increase with the number of cigarettes smoked. Lower death rates are reported in persons who quit smoking than in persons who continue to smoke. Cigarette smoking also acts synergistically with other risk factors to greatly increase the risk for CAD. For example, smoking and the concurrent use of oral contraceptives greatly increase the risk of CAD in women compared to the risk in persons who neither smoke nor use oral contraceptives.

Cigarette smoking is less of a risk factor for CAD among the elderly than it is among younger persons. In people older than 65, the relationship between cigarette smoking and CAD disappears.[37] However, cigarette smoking remains a significant risk factor for intermittent claudication and stroke for older men and women.[35]

Cigarette smoking presents the same risk for CAD in blacks as in whites.[51] Smoking doubles the risk of CAD in persons with hypertension. Black and white men who smoke the same number of cigarettes have similar CAD mortality rates; however, for black women who smoke the same number of cigarettes as white women, black women have slightly lower mortality rates. The National Health Interview Survey and the National Health Examination Survey found that more black than white men smoked (44.9% versus 37.1%)[11,22] However, smoking among black and white women was the same (30%).[22] Recent analysis of national trends indicate that education has replaced gender as the major sociodemographic predictor of smoking status.[23] Smoking has declined 5 times faster among higher-educated persons; 34.2% of persons with less than a high school diploma smoke as compared with 18.4% of persons with 4 or more years of college.

Over 4000 substances have been identified in cigarette smoke; some are toxic, mutagenic, carcinogenic, and pharmacologically active.[28] Nicotine and carbon monoxide have been singled out as having significant roles in the development of atherosclerosis. The addictive properties of nicotine are responsible in the failure to quit smoking. Because nicotine crosses the blood-brain barrier and is distributed throughout the brain, its effects on the central nervous system are due to direct actions on brain receptors.[9] Nicotine excites nicotinic receptors in the spinal cord, autonomic ganglia, and adrenal medulla.

The link between cigarette smoking and atherosclerosis is thought to be mediated through the response-to-injury hypothesis. Carbon monoxide may produce hypoxia of the intima and increase endothelial permeability. In addition, nicotine may exert a toxic effect on the endothelium. In animal studies, repeated endothelial injury has resulted from hypoxia and the nicotine effects of cigarette smoking.[76]

Smoking a cigarette activates the central nervous system. Transient cardiovascular responses in healthy people include an increased heart rate and blood pressure, cardiac stroke volume and output, and coronary blood flow. In addition, peripheral cutaneous vasoconstriction and increased muscle blood flow occurs as a result of the release of vasopressin. Concentrations of free fatty acids, glycerol, and lactate are increased.

Carbon monoxide from cigarette smoke also produces cardiovascular effects. Carbon monoxide binds to hemoproteins such as hemoglobin. Cigarette smokers have 5 times greater carboxyhemoglobin levels than nonsmokers.[28] Thus the oxygen-carrying capacity of the blood is reduced.

Cigarette smoking has effects that facilitate the development of thrombosis. Increased platelet aggregation, increased platelet adhesiveness, shortened platelet survival, decreased clotting times, and an increased hematocrit have been recorded in smokers. Tobacco smoke may reduce the production of PGI_2 the potent inhibitor of platelet aggregation. Nicotine may be the agent responsible.[76] In animal studies, cardiac automaticity is increased, and the threshold for ventricular fibrillation is lowered. These effects may account for the increased risk for sudden death in cigarette smokers.

The adverse effects of "involuntary" or "second-hand" smoking on health in adults and children is being addressed. Second-hand smoking occurs when nonsmokers are exposed to cigarette smoke in an enclosed environment. This smoke has high concentrations of carbon monoxide and many toxic and carcinogenic substances.[18] In 15 studies of involuntary smoking, 10 found an increased risk of lung cancer in nonsmokers married to smokers. However, many of the studies were flawed. Four recent studies have addressed some of the earlier design problems and found the same results; involuntary smoking is associated with an increase risk for lung cancer in nonsmokers. Although additional studies are needed, accumulating evidence supports the carcinogenic effects of passive or second-hand smoke on nonsmokers. In addition, high mortality rates from cardiovascular disease have been observed in persons who lived with smokers.[18] No causal relationship, however, has been determined.

Nicotine-substitution therapy. Nicotine is the dependence-producing substance in tobacco. It easily crosses the blood-brain barrier to affect mood and cognitive function. Benowitz[3] provides considerable evidence to substantiate nicotine dependence in humans. For this reason, nicotine substitution therapy, using nicotine gum, has been a successful pharmacologic approach to smoking cessation.

Each piece of gum contains 2 mg of nicotine, equal to about half of a cigarette, without the other damaging components of cigarette smoke. When the nicotine gum is used regularly throughout the day, the levels of nicotine average one third to two thirds of the levels observed with smoking. Gum containing 4 mg of nicotine is available in Europe. Studies indicate that the higher level is more effective in highly dependent smokers.

Nicotine gum is most effective when used as one component of a comprehensive smoking-cessation program. The gum reduces nicotine withdrawal symptoms and provides a substitute oral activity. After the patient decides to quit smoking, the gum should be made available. The patient is instructed to chew the gum for 20 to 30 minutes when the urge to smoke arises. Up to 30 pieces of gum per day may be chewed; most persons chew 10 to 15 pieces per day. They should be told to chew slowly until a taste of tingling is experienced. The effects of nicotine will not occur as rapidly as cigarette smoking, but chewing will reduce withdrawal effects. The amount of gum chewed is decreased as the patient adapts to lower levels of nicotine.

Side effects of nicotine gum include a sore throat, tired jaws, hiccups, palpitations, nausea, and other gastrointestinal symptoms. Patients should be encouraged to chew more slowly if side effects are reported. No studies report on the safety of the gum for persons with diagnosed CAD or hypertension.

Diabetes mellitus

Diabetes mellitus is one of the leading causes of disability in persons over 45.[61] CAD is the major cause of death in more than half of diabetic patients; it tends to occur at an earlier age and with greater severity in diabetic than in nondiabetic persons.[50]

Diabetes mellitus contributes to cardiovascular risk, particularly in older women.[32] Older patients with diabetes have twice the risk for myocardial infarction. Elderly people with diabetes and hyperlipidemia have about a 15 times the risk, as do patients with hypertension and hyperlipidemia. In diabetic patients, the major lipid problem is "mixed hyperlipidemia" associated with low HDL cholesterol.[2]

Diabetes mellitus also represents a primary risk factor for CAD in Hispanic Americans. A prevalence of non-insulin-dependent diabetes mellitus is substantially greater in Hispanics than in non-Hispanics.[21] Hispanics also have a higher incidence of non-insulin-dependent diabetes mellitus than American whites.[64] An increased prevalence of diabetes has been observed among Hispanic Americans of lower sociocultural status.[27] The prevalence of non-insulin-dependent diabetes mellitus decreases with increasing socioeconomic status.

Accelerated atherosclerosis is a major complication of diabetes mellitus. This condition may be related to factors such as hyperglycemia, hyperinsulinemia, and plasma lipid abnormalities, all of which are common in diabetic persons.[67] Hyperglycemia is an independent risk factor in the development of CAD in persons with diabetes. Increased blood glucose is associated with increased plasma lipid levels,[32] elevated mean systolic and diastolic blood pressures, and a higher mean body mass. Accelerated atherosclerosis in patients with diabetes mellitus indicates an alteration in lipid and lipoprotein metabolism.[39] Comparisons of lipid values for diabetic and nondiabetic individuals have shown elevated cholesterol levels in diabetic persons. Increased fasting blood glucose levels among diabetic people are associated with significant increases in all lipid components except for HDL cholesterol.[52]

Control of hyperglycemia and plasma cholesterol and triglyceride levels may alter the predicted risk of CAD in non-insulin-dependent diabetics.[61,75] Although non-insulin-dependent diabetic patients have lower HDL cholesterol levels compared with nondiabetic controls, the relative decrease is greater for women.[39] One explanation for the loss of premenopausal protection from microvascular disease in women is the differing effect of diabetes on HDL cholesterol levels in the two sexes. Improved control of hyperglycemia may influence the course of CAD directly by diminishing risk factors such as hypercholesterolemia, increased LDL cholesterol levels, decreased HDL cholesterol levels, and increased plasma triglyceride levels.[61]

Another potential risk factor for CAD in the diabetic person is the level of circulating insulin. Hyperinsulinemia promotes ischemic vascular disease and is a risk factor independent of blood glucose level, plasma cholesterol levels, and blood pressure.[61] Because precursor stages of type II diabetes mellitus are characterized by hyperinsulinemia, subjects may be exposed to increased circulating insulin levels over time. Hyperinsulinemia is prevalent in type II diabetics secondary to insulin resistance related to obesity.

The primary factor in reduction of cardiovascular risk is dietary control. In diabetic individuals, caloric restriction and intake alteration can significantly decrease plasma insulin, triglyceride, total cholesterol, and VLDL cholesterol levels; decrease elevated blood pressure; increase HDL cholesterol levels; and aid in the control of serum glucose levels.[61] Current American Diabetes Association guidelines for dietary modification urge reduction in saturated fat and cholesterol intake and an increase in dietary fiber and complex carbohydrates. These recommendations parallel those of the American Heart Association for prevention of CAD in the general population.

In addition, education and intervention for the diabetic patient must include a reduction of caloric intake to reduce the risk of CAD resulting from obesity. The increased risk for CAD in obese individuals may result from association with atherogenic factors such as hypertension, hypercholesterolemia, hypertriglyceridemia, and hyperinsulinemia. Patients with type II diabetes have a higher incidence of obesity than nondiabetic patients from the same popula-

tion. Because atherogenic vascular disease is more prevalent in diabetic persons who have gained weight in adult life, the reversal or prevention of obesity by caloric restriction may reduce the incidence of many atherogenic risk factors.

Obesity

Obesity is the most prevalent, potentially controllable, and most neglected health problem in the United States. Obesity is an excess of relative body fat content, or a body-mass index (weight/height) greater than 20% above ideal. Obesity, in terms of body-mass index, is an independent risk factor for CAD.[29] Weight reduction favorably affects other risk factors such as hypertension, hyperlipidemia, and diabetes. In addition to total body weight, the distribution of fat is sometimes assessed by measurement of waist (abdominal) to hip (gluteal) circumference. An increased abdominal/gluteal ratio is generally associated with greater risk for cardiovascular disease. Generally an abdominal/gluteal ratio above 0.90 in women and above 1.0 in men puts an individual in the high-risk category.[6]

The degree of obesity may be an independent risk factor, especially in women.[43] The effects of increased weight include increased serum lipid levels and blood pressure, increased blood volume and resting cardiac output, elevated left ventricular filling pressure at rest and during exercise, diminished left ventricular chamber compliance, and increased pulmonary and systemic vascular resistance. Obesity also adversely affects the cardiovascular risk profile and increases atherogenesis through impaired glucose tolerance, increased plasma uric acid levels, elevated LDL cholesterol levels, decreased HDL cholesterol levels, and elevated serum triglyceride levels.[72]

Treatment. Obesity should be controlled because it adversely affects the major CAD risk factors, including blood pressure, LDL cholesterol and blood glucose levels, and physical inactivity. There is a high correlation between the body-mass index and serum cholesterol levels. Weight reduction lessens cardiac work and thereby decreases angina pectoris. Also, weight reduction improves exercise tolerance, exerts a favorable effect on blood pressure, glucose intolerance, and plasma uric acid levels and improves the HDL/total cholesterol ratio.

Weight loss reduces plasma cholesterol and serum triglyceride levels. Reduction in cholesterol and triglyceride levels is partly due to dietary modifications involving decreased intake of total fat and saturated fat, as well as a physiologic response to weight reduction. Weight reduction by low-saturated-fat, low-cholesterol diets lowers the risk of CAD. Dietary management of obesity is recommended because weight reduction is beneficial as a component of multifactorial risk reduction and lifestyle change.

Persons who are not obese but do have increased upper body fat and borderline or elevated serum cholesterol levels are called *metabolically obese.* A 10- to 20-pound weight loss in these people will result in dramatic reduction in cholesterol levels. Thus weight loss in the obese individual is part of the initial management of hyperlipidemia.

Dietary restrictions are the first treatment of choice for obesity. However, inadequate weight loss may necessitate other types of treatment.[5] Although controversial, appetite-suppressing drugs remain a treatment option. Major problems in drug therapy are related to central nervous system stimulation and abuse. Surgery is another option when massive obesity is a major health threat. Gastric bypasses are done more frequently than intestinal bypasses because of fewer complications and side effects. Mandibular fixation or jaw wiring is another radical option for patients when rapid weight loss is needed. However, the risk of aspiration also places the patient at high risk.

Physical inactivity

Despite the continuing debate, most persons believe that habitual physical activity reduces mortality rates from atherosclerotic CAD. Framingham data show reduced cardiovascular and CAD mortality rates with increased physical activity at all ages, including the elderly. Similarly, a higher level of physical fitness has been associated with decreased cholesterol and increased HDL levels, lower blood pressure, and reduction in cigarette smoking.[4]

Physiologic benefits of regular physical activity are related to its effects on several factors, including hyperlipidemia, hypertension, tobacco use, and diabetes mellitus. HDL cholesterol levels usually increase directly with the frequency and intensity of exercise, and LDL cholesterol and serum triglyceride levels decrease. These changes are observed only after several months, and they disappear if exercise is discontinued. Improvements in exercise capacity usually results in a lowering of systolic, diastolic, and mean arterial pressures.

Regular exercise has beneficial effects on other risk factors. Exercise programs increase motivation for smoking cessation. Weight reduction also occurs when exercise is initiated in previously sedentary, obese persons. Exercise also alters several blood coagulation factors. In diabetic persons, improved glucose tolerance and lower plasma insulin levels have been observed. Last, regular exercise is associated with decreased stress and depression.

Exercise recommendations. A complete history and physical examination is necessary in all persons before beginning an exercise program to identify all risk factors and symptoms of CAD. Guidelines have been established for graded exercise testing.[1] The exercise prescription includes instructions on the components of the conditioning session, including the warm-up period; the endurance phase prescribed in terms of intensity, duration, and frequency; and the cool-down period; as well as the type of exercise.

Warm-up phase. In the warm-up phase, low-level calisthenics or stretching exercises are performed to loosen muscles and joints and to gradually increase respiratory, metabolic, and cardiovascular rate. Warm-up exercises should include musculoskeletal and cardiopulmonary activity. Cardiopulmonary exercises involve total body movement and permit gradual elevation of the heart rate to an appropriate training level. This phase lasts from 5 to 15 minutes and ends with brisk walking or easy jogging.

Endurance phase. The endurance or conditioning phase produces the training effect. It directly stimulates the oxygen transport system. The three critical elements—intensity, duration, and frequency—are individually adjusted to achieve an effective, yet safe exercise program.

INTENSITY. The intensity of the exercise must be sufficient to attain the prescribed target heart rate. The target heart rate is the training heart rate selected for the patient. In general, a target heart rate range between 70% and 75% is recommended for unsupervised home exercise, and a range between 80% and 85% is recommended for supervised programs.

When the maximal heart rate has not been determined by an exercise test, the target rate is calculated from the age-predicted maximal heart rate. However, this method has disadvantages for patients with heart disease. The age-predicted heart rate may be unrealistically high because the maximal attainable rate may be reduced by the patient's disease or the appearance of signs and symptoms that prevent the patient from exercising at the predicted level. Therefore although the predicted maximal heart rate method is safe for healthy persons, it should not be used in patients with known heart disease.

DURATION. Exercise must be sustained long enough to achieve the desired cardiovascular effects. The duration necessary to produce a significant training response varies inversely with the intensity of exercise. The lower the intensity, the longer the duration. If the patient is able to exercise at 70% to 85% of maximal heart rate, 15 to 20 minutes produces substantial cardiovascular conditioning. Extending the duration beyond 45 minutes increases the risk of orthopedic complications.

FREQUENCY. Three or four exercise sessions per week on nonconsecutive days appear to be the most effective regimen. However, daily sessions may be necessary initially for patients to incorporate the exercise program into their daily routine. The risk of orthopedic injury increases with frequency of exercise. If the patient is not in proper condition, several short walks a day may be appropriate initially. Less fatigue and soreness results. Also, if a walk is missed, the patient has not "gone off the program" and is more likely to continue exercising.

Cool-down phase. The cool-down phase occurs immediately after exercise and lasts 5 to 10 minutes. A postexercise cool-down period prevents venous pooling and reduces leg soreness and stiffness. Cool-down activities permit appropriate circulatory readjustment and return of heart rate and blood pressure to near-preexercise levels.

Types of exercise. The type of exercise prescribed involves the rhythmic, repetitive movements of the large muscle groups and is aerobic in nature. *Aerobic* means "with oxygen." Thus, aerobic exercises are those that demand oxygen without producing an intolerable oxygen debt, so they can be continued for long periods. Walking, jogging, bicycling, swimming, rope jumping, cross-country skiing, and running games such as basketball, tennis, and racquet ball are considered aerobic exercises.

Age and gender

Age is a powerful predictor of CAD; risk increases as age increases. When adults enter their 40s, CAD becomes clinically evident. The incidence increases substantially beyond age 45 in men and 55 in women.[33] During childbearing years, women have about one fourth the risk of men for developing CAD. In women the rate of CAD is relatively slow before menopause. However, after menopause the rate of increase rises rapidly. Women lag behind men by 10 years or more in the occurrence of CAD, but the gap narrows with advancing age. Men have a higher incidence of CAD at all ages. However CAD is second to cancer as the major cause of death under age 40 and is the number one cause of death after age 60.

The exact role of the aging process in the development of CAD is unknown.[38] Earlier research suggested that cardiac atrophy occurred with aging. More recent research suggests that heart size does not change in normal, healthy elderly persons. However, a slight increase in the thickness of the left ventricular wall tends to occur with normal aging. Cardiac output also does not decline in healthy elderly persons. However, it is maintained by a different mechanism than in younger persons. Younger persons rely on an increase in heart rate and a decrease in end-systolic volume. Healthy elderly persons use the Frank-Starling mechanism, or an increase in end-diastolic volume, to increase stroke volume.[66] Decreased responsiveness to beta-adrenergic stimulation is theorized to mediate the shift in the mechanisms.

Family history

The Framingham study found that persons whose parents died from CAD had a 30% increase in risk for CAD occurring before age 60.[10] Genes and environment place family members at risk for CAD. For example, a person's smoking status, cholesterol level, and dietary sodium intake are determined to a large degree by the shared family environment. In other words, health habits are often similar in families.

The role of genetic factors in atherosclerosis is difficult to evaluate because of the clustering of other risk factors. However, certain inherited disorders predispose a person to premature CAD. In homozygous familial hypercholesterolemia, myocardial infarction often appears as early as age 20.[26] Three quarters of heterozygous parents die from CAD by age 60.

The genetic contribution of CAD has been shown in

hyperlipidemia, diabetes mellitus, and obesity. Hyperlipidemia and diabetes mellitus need aggressive correction in families with known histories of CAD before age 55. In such families, the family history needs to be evaluated and all relatives screened. Interventions can be used for those identified to be at high risk for CAD.

Oral contraceptives

Oral contraceptive use is associated with an increased incidence of cardiovascular disease. The risk of myocardial infarction in users of oral contraceptives with no predisposing medical conditions is related to age and the presence of other risk factors. Use of oral contraceptives in women over age 40 is associated with an increased risk of myocardial infarction, particularly in women with long-term use and other risk factors. For example, women younger than 40 who suffer a myocardial infarction have almost always been cigarette smokers.[57,63] The incidence of stroke or thromboembolism is increased with oral contraceptive use at all ages when compared to nonusers.

Oral contraceptives have an effect on lipid metabolism and blood pressure. Total serum cholesterol, triglyceride, and LDL cholesterol values are increased, and HDL cholesterol levels are decreased.[56,62] The magnitude of the changes depend on the estrogen and progestogen content of the oral contraceptive, as well as age, weight, and smoking history.[45] Systolic and diastolic blood pressure levels also increase slightly in oral contraceptive users.[69] The risk for hypertension may be 3 to 6 times greater, depending on the oral contraceptive formulation. Glucose tolerance is also decreased, especially in women with a family history of diabetes. In users of oral contraceptives, cigarette smoking increases the risk of myocardial infarction in premenopausal women. In studies of women smokers age 35 years or older who used oral contraceptives, the relative risk for myocardial infarction has been estimated to be 4 to 20 times that of nonusers who have never smoked.

Since the mid-1970s, estrogen and progestogen dosages in oral contraceptives have been decreased based on the relationship of these two hormones with CAD risks in oral contraceptive users. However, many young users of oral contraceptives are still at increased risk for development of CAD.[62] Young women who take oral contraceptives must be screened to detect risk factors. In addition, interventions are needed to reduce or eliminate major risk factors for CAD in women of childbearing age.

Menopause and noncontraceptive estrogen replacement

Estrogen replacement in postmenopausal women has been advocated because of the increased incidence of CAD after menopause. Controversy about the association between noncontraceptive estrogen treatment and risk of CAD still exists. However, most experts agree that the use of noncontraceptive estrogens by postmenopausal women is not associated with an increased risk for myocardial infarction and may possibly provide a protective effect.[40]

Estrogen replacement therapy is thought to produce a protective effect through its actions on lipids. In women who are taking estrogen, HDL cholesterol levels increase, and LDL cholesterol levels decrease. The side effects seen in oral contraceptive users are not a problem because the dosage of estrogen is much lower than that used in oral contraceptives. Currently progestins are prescribed with estrogen replacement medications because of the otherwise increased risk of endometrial cancer. The effects of progestins may counter the protective effects of estrogens because they have been associated with increased levels of LDL cholesterol and decreased levels of HDL cholesterol. Clinical trials are underway to establish the maximum therapeutic dosages of progestins.

Stress: type A behavior pattern

The type A behavior pattern (TABP), another major independent risk factor for CAD, is considered the occupational disease of high achievers.[44] The TABP is most prevalent among upwardly mobile, achievement-oriented managers and professionals, ranging from 50% to 75% in employed middle-class samples. The pattern is characterized by a chronic sense of time urgency, intense ambition, hostility, aggression, and excessive competition.[58] The characteristics form a behavior pattern that is seen in individuals reacting to stressful or challenging situations.

Persons who exhibit TABP are more likely to participate in challenging and demanding situations that further type A behavior. Many studies report that persons with TABP also exhibit exaggerated cardiovascular and neuroendocrine reactivity to stressors during the normal waking hours, which may be the basis for the behavior pattern as a cardiovascular risk factor.[71] Frequent activation of the sympathetic adrenal medullary system may be involved in the development of atherosclerosis.

In recent years, the expression of hostility and anger has been a more sensitive predictor of the development of CAD in men. Studies show significant relationships between TABP hostility scores and the severity of disease evidenced by coronary angiography.[44] However, the evidence is limited, and longitudinal studies that incorporate more accurate measures of TABP are needed before final conclusions can be made about biobehavioral mechanisms.

Strategies for altering TABP. Only one primary prevention trial, the Montreal Type A Intervention Project, and one secondary prevention intervention study, the Recurrent Coronary Prevention Project, for altering type A behavior have been reported in the literature.[58,71] In both reports, interventions were successful in altering TABP. Stress management, biofeedback, meditation, progressive relaxation, cognitive behavioral therapy, and aerobic exercise were used successfully in altering the hard-driven, competition-driven, speed and impatient behavior of the type-A person. Cognitive behavior modification has been successful in altering negative beliefs about the self and others.

In therapy, small groups have been more effective than large, impersonal groups. Interventions are also more likely to succeed when patients are taught to identify overt type-A behaviors and characteristics that need to be modified. Patients must be prepared for complex, long-term treatment that requires a commitment to change.

Pharmacologic treatment. Pharmacologic approaches for altering TABP have also been tried on the basis of the increased sympathetic reactivity that may cause this behavior pattern.[44] Patients who have been placed on beta-adrenergic blocker therapy have shown more of a decrease in intensity of behaviors than controls have. Thus although evidence is limited, the role of drugs in altering TABP is promising.

Nursing Process

Case study. Ms. B.T., a 48 year old Mexican American bank executive, was admitted to the Intermediate Care Unit with a 2-hour history of chest pain. Her electrocardiogram (ECG) taken in the emergency room was normal. However, her blood pressure was 170/90 mm Hg. She was given two nitroglycerin tablets 5 minutes apart, which relieved the pain. After admission, she was given 5 mg of diazepam (Valium). All cardiac enzyme levels and ECGs were normal over the next 3 days. Her total serum cholesterol level was 310 mg/dl. The physical examination revealed normal results.

Ms. B.T. stated she had been under extreme pressure in her work. She lives with her husband, a blue-collar worker, and has two children, ages 20 and 23, who are enrolled in the local university. She admitted to mild chest pain for the past 2 months, which was associated with her work and arguments with her husband over the children's college grades. She admitted to smoking 1 to 1½ packs of cigarettes a day. Her weight was 20 pounds above her ideal weight, which she attributed to work and home commitments interfering with her ability to maintain a regular exercise program and to a large intake of fast foods. Her blood pressure remained elevated throughout hospitalization.

Assessment
Exchanging pattern

Because Ms. B.T. did not suffer a myocardial infarction and her physical examination was normal, the assessment will focus only on the cardiovascular risk factors identified. The information under each major risk discusses signs and symptoms and pertinent findings for diagnosing each risk factor. In addition Chapters 9 and 10 provide an assessment of the patient with angina and myocardial infarction.

Communication pattern

In the Communicating Pattern, assess the ability of the patient to articulate responses that will enable you to validate the presence of CAD risk factors and their potential causes. Assess verbal and nonverbal communication because behaviors associated with nonverbal communication will assist you in diagnosing TABP.

For example, Ms. B.T. was a bilingual, articulate, educated Mexican American woman. Her speech was rapid, and her nonverbal communication indicated that she was impatient with the examiner and somewhat hostile in her comments.

Relating pattern

Remember that the Relating Pattern is a crucial part of the assessment of the patient with CAD risk factors because family and occupational roles exacerbate many risk factors and long-term, successful lifestyle changes depend on social support from others. Thus determine the type and quality of roles occupied by the patient. Assess the family structure, including child care responsibilities, and the financial and occupational status of all members of the household. If the patient is single, ask about social networks and social support needs. For single and married persons, explore the quality of the network and support within the family, social network, and occupation. In addition, assess the patient's ethnic origin because it often determines dietary preferences, family and role orientations, and attitudes toward change.

Ms. B.T.'s cultural practices were related to her heritage. The traditional Mexican diet is high in fat and sodium. She and her husband preferred Mexican food over American food. Moreover, the traditional Mexican female role is that of homemaker. Although the role has changed in recent years, the "macho image" is still predominant among many individual Mexican Americans.

Ms. B.T., a bank executive, was married to a blue-collar worker and admitted that she was embarrassed in some social situations because of her husband's lack of formal education. She also admitted feeling guilty for making a higher salary. She found it difficult to discuss her work pressures with him, thinking he did not understand. Their two children were in college, and the differences between her and her husband seemed to be exaggerated now that they were alone together, because her husband still maintained many of the traditional cultural practices.

Knowing pattern

In the Knowing Pattern, assess patient knowledge of cardiovascular risk factors, including knowledge of family history of risk factors, understanding of the identified risk factors, and the significance of the cause of atherosclerosis and CAD. In addition, determine the patient's level of readiness to learn how to eliminate or modify risk factors present.

The risk factors that were identified in Ms. B.T. were hypertension, cigarette smoking, elevated blood cholesterol, stress, mild obesity, and sedentary lifestyle. Although she knew that cigarette smoking caused lung cancer, she did not understand the role of cigarettes as a risk factor for CAD. In addition, although she had never been told that her blood pressure was elevated, she knew that being overweight was a contributing factor. She was very interested in discussing risk factors and wanted to learn to modify them and stated that it was time to start paying attention to her health.

Feeling pattern

When assessing the Feeling Pattern, evaluate the patients' emotional responses to the illness, as well as their understanding of the illness. Obtain information about recent life stressors that may have influenced the current episode of illness, including the family and work environment. Also identify healthy and unhealthy coping strategies used by the patient. For example, determine how the patient copes with stressful life events. Use statements such as "Tell me how you usually handle stressful situations" or "Tell me what is happening to you," to obtain an accurate picture of the patient's emotional status.

Ms. B.T. stated that her major coping strategies were cigarette smoking and eating. She confessed that she did not have a close relationship with her husband, and her major source of emotional support was her sister. She also stated that the increased responsibilities with a job promotion had added additional stress to her life because she was working extra hours and taking work home to complete at night, which irritated her husband. She was annoyed that her illness had taken her away from her work but understood that the stress of her work was a major factor in her illness. She also realized she was using unhealthy coping strategies and expressed a desire to change her behavior.

Moving pattern

In the Moving Pattern, assess the patient's participation in aerobic and social activities. Also ascertain exercise likes and dislikes. Explore the patient's leisure time to determine the amount of time spent in diversional activities and social networks.

Ms. B.T. indicated that very little time was spent on leisure activities. On Sundays, she attended mass with her family, and her family ate Sunday dinner with her parents. Before her promotion, she attended an aerobic dance class 3 times a week. She did not like to jog but enjoyed walking and lived in a neighborhood in which this exercise was feasible. Because her husband only enjoyed spectator sports, they did not do any exercise activities together. However, she thought he might also like to walk in the neighborhood.

Perceiving pattern

In the Perceiving Pattern, try to obtain an understanding of patients' self-concept and self-esteem because such judgments provide valuable information about whether patients feel that a change in lifestyle will be successful. Assess body image and sense of control. Determine whether patients feel that change is possible. Ask whether patients feel that they have the control to make the necessary changes to modify risk factors or whether they feel powerless or helpless. Obtain this information by observing patients' body language and direct and indirect cues in response to questions; these assessment parameters also are noted during evaluation of the other patterns.

Ms. B.T. believed she had control over events in her life but had let them slide out of control. However, she did not feel helpless or depressed about the situation. Her self-esteem remained high, and she was positive about her desire and ability to make the changes needed to eliminate the identified risk factors.

Choosing pattern

Determine whether the patient and family have the coping and problem-solving strategies to change unhealthy behavior. Also identify the support offered by family members and friends. Ask who the patient turns to for help. Identify whether the patient is satisfied with the amount of support available within or outside the family. Evaluate whether the patient has a realistic assessment of the situation and whether the patient can make realistic decisions about change based on the above information provided.

Ms. B.T. had advanced from a bank teller to an executive with a lot of responsibilities. She had reached this position by attending school in the evenings and working during the day. In addition she had raised two sons who were in college. She stated that she and her husband had drifted apart because her involvement with her career left little time or interest for anything else. However, the family had been close at one time, and she saw the potential to re-establish a more positive relationship with her husband,

especially since the children would soon be on their own. She saw how her work had taken over her life and began to talk about stepping down to a less-stressful position so that she could have more leisure time. She felt she had reached her career goals, and she expressed a desire to spend more time on her personal and family goals. Ms. B.T.'s appraisal of the situation was realistic because the hospitalization seemed to be a pivotal point, providing her with insight into what was happening in her life.

Nursing diagnoses

The presence of one major cardiovascular risk factor is cause for developing interventions to eliminate or reduce the patient's risk for CAD. When more than one risk factor is identified, the patient, physician, and nurse work together to set the behaviors needed for lifestyle change in order of priority. Change is first directed toward the risk factor most detrimental to the patient.

Common human responses that are anticipated for patients with CAD risk factors are indicated by the following nursing diagnoses:
1. Knowledge deficit related to CAD risk factors
2. Altered nutrition: more than body requirements related to poor nutritional habits, lack of exercise, and stress
3. High risk for nonadherence related to CAD risk factor reduction
4. Powerlessness related to lifestyle change
5. Inadequate social support related to lifestyle change

For each of these diagnoses, the patient outcomes, nursing prescriptions, and evaluation criteria are outlined with a discussion of the factual information that supports the plan and implementation of care.

NURSING DIAGNOSIS 1 **Knowledge deficit related to CAD risk factors (knowing pattern)**

PATIENT OUTCOMES	NURSING PRESCRIPTIONS	EVALUATION
Patient will verbalize the major modifiable and nonmodifiable cardiovascular risk factors present.	Teach major modifiable and nonmodifiable risk factors.	Patient verbalized the major modifiable and nonmodifiable cardiovascular risk factors present.
Patient will identify strategies to eliminate or reduce major modifiable risk factors.	Discuss strategies to eliminate or reduce major modifiable risk factors with the patient.	Patient identified strategies to eliminate or reduce major modifiable risk factors.
Patient will set in order of priority the strategies for risk factor reduction.	Inform patients about risk factors that are the most important to eliminate initially.	Patient set in order of priority strategies for risk factor reduction.

Plan and intervention for knowledge deficit

Knowledge deficit indicates a deficiency in cognitive information or psychomotor skills to the extent that the deficiency interferes with risk factor modification. The diagnosis is based on initial assessment of the patient's baseline knowledge. The nurses should determine what the patients know about risk factors and their modification. This information is used to identify factors that may interfere with patients' learning the necessary data about risk factor modification. Patients also need to perform self-assessment so that they are aware of their needs and desires to learn. A member of the social network should be involved, if possible.

Objectives are then formulated based on the knowledge assessment. Patients should know that the stated objectives are what is expected and what needs to be done to reach desired goals. Content to be taught can then be formulated. It must provide an adequate knowledge base. Content is chosen according to the patient's educational level, reading level, prior experiences with the health care system, age, and occupation. The nurse must be certain that the information is current and relevant.

Teaching to decrease knowledge deficit may be implemented in a group or individually. Group teaching is economical, and patients learn from each other. Audiovisual aids should be used when appropriate because multiple stimuli facilitate the learning process.

The effectiveness of the teaching program needs to be evaluated. Indications of success include increased knowledge, an attitude change, or a behavior change. Direct observations, written tests, or patient or family reports of knowledge gain are also used to measure success. Further teaching is based on the results of evaluation.

Evidence suggests that an increase in knowledge does not necessarily mean that a change in behavior will occur. Other factors, such as social support, stress reduction, and feelings of control, have an important role in successful lifestyle changes, as well. However, knowledge is the initial step and an essential one in the teaching-learning process.

NURSING DIAGNOSIS 2 **Altered nutrition: more than body requirements related to poor nutritional habits, lack of exercise, and stress (exchanging pattern)**

PATIENT OUTCOMES	NURSING PRESCRIPTIONS	EVALUATION
Patient will identify eating strategies for successful weight loss.	Discuss the ABCs of eating.	Patient identified three strategies to control negative eating behaviors.
Patient will verbalize the importance of low-calorie, low-cholesterol, low-fat foods.	Discuss low-calorie, low-cholesterol, low-fat foods.	Patient identified foods high in calories, cholesterol, and fat.
Patient will initiate a low-calorie, low-cholesterol, low-fat diet.	Evaluate the patient's acceptance of the new diet and encourage the use of a food diary.	Patient maintained a low-calorie, low-cholesterol, low-fat diet.
Patient will initiate an exercise program to facilitate weight loss.	Formulate an exercise program based on patient's needs and preferences.	Patient initiated and complied with a regular exercise program.
Patient will comply with pharmacologic therapy to reduce cholesterol (if ordered).	Discuss the purpose, dosage, and side effects of cholesterol-lowering medications.	Patient complied with pharmacologic therapy to reduce cholesterol levels.

Plan and intervention for altered nutrition

Altered nutrition: more than body requirements refers to body weight greater than desirable, according to life insurance tables. This diagnosis may be made for several risk factors, including elevated serum cholesterol levels, hypertension, physical inactivity, and obesity. First, nursing management for the patient with the diagnosis for the risk factor, obesity, with or without other risk factors, is discussed. Nursing management of the patient with the risk factor of an elevated cholesterol level is then discussed because weight loss is often the cornerstone of the management of an elevated serum cholesterol level and other risk factors.

Obesity

Nursing interventions are based on a thorough assessment. A detailed obesity history is obtained initially. The physical examination includes height, weight, and skinfold measures. Any other risk factors need to be identified and evaluated. Caloric requirements need to be assessed so that an appropriate caloric intake can be planned with a reasonable caloric deficit. Evaluation and management of obesity is important because of its relationship to other CAD risk factors.

The patient must make the commitment to changing eating behavior before it can be modified. Behavior modification, group therapy, and self-directed change techniques may be used in learning to maintain ideal weight. A program of weight reduction begins with education related to cardiovascular risk associated with excess body weight and strategies available to reduce weight. Health teaching includes nutrition, exercise, and stress-management techniques. The nurse assesses the patient's level of knowledge, available support systems, and level of motivation. The goal of appropriate body weight is more easily attained if the patient establishes a diet by using a food diary to identify mutually agreeable areas for behavior modification. After habits are identified, short- and long-term goals for weight reduction can be set. The family needs to be involved in planning to provide support. In addition, nonfood rewards can be established.

Throughout the weight-loss process, positive reinforcement is provided, and self-reinforcement is encouraged. Reinforcement of positive behavior enhances self-esteem and increases the likelihood of permanent behavior change.

The ABCs of eating incorporates behavioral strategies for change. First the antecedents (A), or triggers, in the environment that promote eating are identified. The eating behavior (B) is then assessed. Behavior includes places where one eats and the rate and frequency at which one eats. The consequences (C) of eating reflect the feeling that the patient has about eating. Patients learn to monitor the ABCs so that identified patterns and rewards can be modified.

Elevated blood cholesterol level

The management of hyperlipidemia must incorporate dietary modification, weight loss, exercise, and possibly drug therapy. The overall objective in cholesterol level reduction is implementation of an individualized program leading to permanent lifestyle change with self-management as the central focus. Dietary management requires long-term behavioral changes. Adherence to lifestyle changes may be increased through education and behavior modification strategies.

Initially, the patient must understand the rationale for recommended changes. The nurse needs to assess the patient's current level of knowledge, awareness of need for change, available support systems, perceived barriers to lifestyle change, and level of motivation.

The patient is then helped to identify and set in order of priority the problem areas related to dietary modification and associated risk factor reduction. Diet histories need to include previous dietary change attempts, habits of eating out, and grocery shopping habits. Physical activity also is assessed if obesity is a problem. Changes are implemented over time, with easier adjustments introduced first to increase feelings of success. Each problem area should be assigned a priority by the patient. The nurse and patient monitor progress and make change as needed. Long-term follow-up is necessary because dietary changes require life-long changes.

The institution of pharmacologic therapy must include patient education about the goals of drug treatment and the expected side effects of the medication. Side effects may occur with all cholesterol-lowering drugs; they should be monitored and reported to the nurse or physician. The need for a long-term commitment to pharmacologic therapy is emphasized. Dietary modification must be maintained, even after drug therapy is implemented. Patients must not be led to believe that the medication will enable them to forego dietary restrictions.

NURSING
DIAGNOSIS 3 **High risk for nonadherence related to CAD risk factor reduction (choosing pattern)**

PATIENT OUTCOMES	NURSING PRESCRIPTIONS	EVALUATION
Patient will verbalize actual and perceived barriers to adherence.	Explore actual and perceived barriers to adherence.	Patient identified three barriers to adherence in lifestyle change.
Patient will identify strategies to facilitate adherence to lifestyle change.	Identify strategies to facilitate adherence.	Patient identified three strategies to facilitate adherence to lifestyle change.
Patient will participate in developing and will sign a written contract for lifestyle changes.	Assist the patient in developing a written contract for lifestyle changes.	Patient helped develop and signed a written contract for lifestyle changes.

Plan and intervention for nonadherence

The goal of primary prevention is to develop the best possible therapeutic regimen to modify risk factors associated with cardiovascular disease and enhance adherence with the regimen after it has been established. Programs of change are successful only if individuals adhere to their regimen as a component of ongoing lifestyle change. Therefore major efforts are needed to understand the factors involved in adherence behavior, and plans need to be made to incorporate motivational interventions when possible. Because nonadherence is a major nursing diagnosis in cardiovascular risk reduction, a general discussion of interventions is followed by specific interventions for hypertension, smoking, and physical inactivity.

Nursing interventions begin with an assessment of the likelihood of early nonadherence in patients. Data on physical and psychologic status, as well as present lifestyle habits and available support systems, may provide an indication of potential adherence. The patient's value on health, perception of control, and perceived barriers to initiating change are needed to provide an individually tailored program. A detailed psychosocial assessment also helps in identifying motivational level and areas that will require special attention. Intervention strategies that meet the needs of the individual are more likely to be successful in helping the patient to adhere to the recommended lifestyle changes.

Because the initiation and maintenance of behavior change are essential to risk factor reduction, internal and external motivational interventions need to be planned. Interventions must break down barriers and motivate the individual by reinforcing new behaviors.

Extrinsic motivational strategies include reducing perceived barriers to lifestyle change through education about cardiovascular risk reduction techniques that can be controlled by the individual; increased involvement of supportive others in the change process; and collaborative decision making related to goal setting.

Intrinsic motivational strategies provide the base for long-term lifestyle change because adherence to new behaviors must be regulated by the person undergoing change. Intrinsically oriented interventions enable the patient to set health-related goals to be achieved and be involved in decision making and development of specific actions to achieve the goals; they also emphasize individual responsibility and self-directedness in risk reducing behaviors.

Adherence begins when the patient agrees that a problem exists. After the problem is acknowledged, viable solutions can be proposed, and an acceptable plan can be designed. Written contracts are often negotiated at this time. Continuous personal contact is necessary to provide feedback on progress. The personal contact also enables the patient to get all questions and concerns addressed. Involvement of the patient's social network, as well as a

maintenance of change behavior, needs to be encouraged during the early phases.

Ongoing monitoring of the patient's progress enables early diagnosis of relapse so that new strategies can be planned and implemented. The patient is encouraged to verbalize adherence problems. The actual and perceived barriers and facilitating factors are reassessed and monitored through the program.

Hypertension

Many drugs are available for the treatment of hypertension. However, all agents produce unpleasant side effects, making adherence to therapy a main problem in reducing hypertension. Patients diagnosed with hypertension usually have other risk factors, so a long-term lifestyle change program must be instituted to help eliminate smoking; reduce calories; decrease sodium, saturated fat, and alcohol consumption; and increase daily exercise. The patient should be guided to set in order of priority the risk factors for change and assist in selecting the one to alter first. The patient must also be given information about hypertension and the importance of controlling blood pressure. The mechanisms and potential side effects of medications also are discussed with the patient and family members. The partner also needs to be included in educational sessions related to diet (e.g., sodium restriction, grocery shopping, and reading labels). Home blood pressure measurements may help the patient understand how activities and emotions influence blood pressure. Patients must also learn that hypertension is not curable and life-long follow-up and attention will be needed (see boxes on pp. 21-22 and 105).

The elderly present special problems related to treatment adherence. Difficulties associated with decreased vision and hearing must be kept in mind when teaching these patients. Living alone may increase transportation problems. Dietary habits may lead to hypokalemia. Fixed incomes may limit their ability to have prescriptions filled or keep appointments. These issues need consideration when assisting patients over age 60 in making lifestyle changes and adhering to a medication regimen.

Smoking

Despite knowledge of the health consequences of smoking, one third of the adults in the United States continue to smoke. This percentage is increasing in young women between ages 15 and 24. Thus school, hospital and community-based interventions need to begin education about this risk factor by making smokers aware of the consequences of smoking. Motivation to stop must be increased by providing incentives to stop. Smokers should be taught strategies for stopping. During smoking cessation programs, role models and emotional support must be provided. In addition, long-term support is necessary to help maintain behavior change.

Smoking cessation counseling begins with assessment

of smoking habits, including the amount the patient smokes, date of start, and attempts to quit. In addition, psychosocial factors, such as the desire to quit, social support, perceived barriers and benefits to quitting, and perceived stress that may be interfering with quitting, are assessed. The assessment will enable the nurse to understand the role of smoking for patients, ascertain their knowledge level of smoking risks, and establish rapport before implementing interventions.

Next, the patient agrees on a quit date. Before the agreement, the benefits of quitting, as well as the consequences of smoking, are discussed. Also, all patient concerns about quitting should be addressed.

Patients may decide to quit on their own or request assistance in a smoking cessation program. Regardless of the option, the patient's progress is monitored. Support and positive reinforcement are provided during each visit. If patients are unable to quit completely, they should be encouraged to decrease the amount smoked by using various strategies. For example, implementing environmental restrictions, such as not smoking in the office, car, or certain rooms in the house, may be an initial step in cutting down on the amount smoked. In addition, self-help books, kits, and cassettes should be made available. Other tips for helping the patient quit are listed in the box.

Almost all smokers are able to quit initially; however, the majority resume smoking within a few months. Therefore attention to maintenance strategies is extremely important. The major factor for successful maintenance is social support. If patients do not identify supportive partners or friends, a group that can help sustain the motivation and decrease the stress of quitting needs to be made available. Partner support is extremely helpful in successful maintenance. Patients should also be taught self-control skills to manage the discomfort of withdrawal and loss of pleasure from smoking. They can learn to recognize and modify cues that previously triggered smoking and to develop substitute responses to replace smoking. Finally, cognitive restructuring approaches can be undertaken to facilitate maintenance. These approaches assume that some change first occurs in patients' attitudes toward smoking or their perception of their ability to maintain smoking cessation. In other words, patients are able to resist smoking because of a personal conviction that they can successfully maintain smoking cessation.

Physical inactivity

On the average, half of the patients who start an exercise program never finish. Dropout rates range from 20% to 60%, with the lowest attrition occurring during the first 3 months of a program and the highest after 40 months.[53] About 50% of exercise dropouts occurs between 6 and 12

 TIPS FOR QUITTING SMOKING

Write down reasons for desiring to stop smoking.
Use oral substitutes for cigarettes (e.g., toothpicks, sugarless gum, sugarless candy).
Leave the table immediately after a meal.
Initially avoid drinking beverages such as alcohol or coffee that are associated with smoking.
Wear a rubberband on one wrist and stretch and release it for a zap whenever there is a desire to smoke.
Inform family members and friends of the decision to quit.
If possible, quit with a friend.
Record all positive effects related to quitting.
Avoid smokers and places where smokers congregate.
Find behaviors to substitute when an urge to smoke surfaces.

months in supervised and unsupervised exercise programs.

The most frequently reported characteristic associated with dropout is smoking. Smoking patterns are indicative of an individual's general adherence with a healthy lifestyle. Blue-collar occupations are another frequently cited contributor to nonadherence with regular exercise. Blue-collar workers may have less knowledge of their disease process and use health care services in general less frequently.[54] Patients who are inactive in their leisure time also tend to have a higher dropout rate. Overweight participants and those with angina[13] also have lower adherence rates. A major factor that predicts nonadherence is lack of support from a significant other. Encouragement and ongoing support of others is needed to motivate persons to initiate and maintain a regular exercise program.

Nursing interventions begin with assessment of the existing level of physical activity, knowledge level, perceived barriers to exercise, available support systems, and level of motivation. The nurse must identify factors that will inhibit success and then help persons eliminate or modify such barriers. A mutually agreeable plan of exercise includes short- and long-term exercise goals. Small, flexible goals may increase feelings of success and achievement. Emphasis is placed on time rather than distance-oriented goals. Rewards are planned in advance as a reinforcement for goals achieved. Because adherence, not initiation of an exercise program, is the major problem, the nurse needs to focus on strategies that promote adherence.

NURSING
DIAGNOSIS 4 **Powerlessness related to lifestyle change (perceiving pattern)**

PATIENT OUTCOMES	NURSING PRESCRIPTIONS	EVALUATION
Patient will participate in decision making relating to lifestyle change.	Provide opportunities for the patient to participate in decisions.	Patient made decisions related to setting risk factor interventions in order of priority.
Patient will participate in designing risk factor reducing program.	Encourage the patient to actively participate in designing a creative, yet realistic risk factor reduction program.	Patient assisted in choosing realistic strategies to initiate a lifestyle change program.
Patient will verbalize feelings of control to initiate lifestyle changes.	Assess the patient's level of control regarding the ability to initiate lifestyle changes.	Patient verbalized feelings of control to initiate lifestyle changes.

Plan and intervention for powerlessness

Powerlessness describes a subjective state in which persons perceive a lack of personal control over their lives. Powerlessness inhibits motivation to initiate lifestyle change. Patients who feel they have no control do not participate in self-care to reduce their risk for cardiovascular disease. Therefore nurses must stress that the patient is a partner in decisions and has control over making successful lifestyle changes. Perceived control plays a significant role in lifestyle change behaviors. Patients who believe they have control over their lives and have the ability to make change are more likely to initiate and sustain programs of change.

After the nursing diagnosis of powerlessness is made, interventions are implemented to enable patients to increase control of their lives. If knowledge deficit contributes to the problem, teaching is implemented. Attention must be focused on identifying realistic, attainable goals, providing choices, and providing continuous positive feedback to change the patient's perception of powerlessness. The degree of participation in planned interventions is a measure of success in gaining or regaining control.

NURSING
DIAGNOSIS 5 **Inadequate social support related to lifestyle change (relating pattern)**

PATIENT OUTCOMES	NURSING PRESCRIPTIONS	EVALUATION
Patient will identify supportive persons in the social network.	Assist the patient to identify persons who will support lifestyle changes.	Patient stated at least one person or group who provides support.
Patient will verbalize the kind and quality of support in the social network.	Help the patient to identify the kind (i.e., informational, financial, emotional) and quality of the support that the person is able to give to facilitate desired lifestyle changes.	Patient described the kind and quality of social support from at least one person or group.

Plan and intervention for inadequate social support

Social support refers to the emotional and material resources available to the patient through relationships with others. Social support includes the provision of information, money, and emotional support. Positive social support is associated with adherence to lifestyle change in risk factor– reducing programs. Inadequate support has been identified by persons who have dropped out of lifestyle change programs. Spousal support has also been consistently linked to adherence in patients with cardiovascular disease.

Support may be beneficial in two ways. It may directly influence the motivation to change behavior, or it may indirectly modify or buffer other factors that influence behaviors. For example, a supportive person may provide a relaxing environment to reduce hassles and stress. Much controversy exists about the exact role of support in enhancing lifestyle change. Despite the unanswered questions, social support has consistently been found to be a positive factor. Therefore the nursing assessment needs to identify supportive persons in the patient's social network, the type of support provided, satisfaction with the support, and the actual quality of the support provided. After a detailed assessment, interventions can be tailored to ensure adequate provision of support. Family members of supportive friends need to participate fully in goal setting and program planning. Such support is fostered by the nurse and health care team. If the patient does not have an adequate social network, appropriate support groups or programs should be identified. The adequacy of the support is monitored through the lifestyle change program. New strategies are implemented as necessary to provide the necessary support for successful change.

KEY CONCEPT REVIEW

1. All of the following are well known theories describing the development of atherosclerosis *except:*
   a. Response-to-injury hypothesis
   b. Smoking hypothesis
   c. Lipoprotein hypothesis
   d. Monoclonal hypothesis

2. Which of the following structures is the site of injury and subsequent site for the development of atherosclerosis?
   a. Collagen cells
   b. Epithelial cells
   c. Myocardial cells
   d. Endothelial cells

3. All of the following risk factors are potentially modifiable *except:*
   a. Hyperlipidemia
   b. Cigarette smoking
   c. Family history
   d. Diabetes mellitus

4. All of the following are not modifiable risk factors *except:*
   a. Gender
   b. Family history
   c. Menopause
   d. Hypertension

5. Noncontraceptive estrogen replacement may provide a protective effect by *increasing:*
   a. LDL cholesterol levels
   b. HDL cholesterol levels
   c. Triglyceride levels
   d. VLDL cholesterol levels

6. The primary nursing diagnosis for persons who have major modifiable risk factors is:
   a. Impaired physical mobility
   b. Altered tissue perfusion
   c. Nonadherence
   d. Impaired verbal communication

7. Interventions for high blood cholesterol levels include all of the following *except:*
   a. Weight reduction
   b. Low-fat, low-cholesterol diet
   c. Low-sodium diet
   d. Regular exercise program

8. Risk factor reduction is set in order of priority according to:
   a. The nurse's judgment
   b. The patient's judgment
   c. The severity of the risks present
   d. All of the above

ANSWERS

1. b	3. c	5. b	7. c
2. d	4. d	6. c	8. d

REFERENCES

1. American College of Sports Medicine: Guidelines for exercise testing and prescriptions, Philadelphia, 1986, Lea & Febinger.
2. Assmann G and Schulte H: Diabetes mellitus and hypertension in the elderly: concomitant hyperlipidemia and coronary heart disease, Am J Cardiol 63:33H, 1989.
3. Benowitz NL: Pharmacologic aspects of cigarette smoking and nicotine addiction, N Engl J Med 319(20):1318, 1988.
4. Blackburn H and Jacobs DR: Physical activity and the risk of coronary heart disease, N Engl J Med 319(18):1217, 1988.
5. Bray GA: Complications of obesity. II. Health implications of obesity, Ann Intern Med 103:(6 suppl):1052, 1985.
6. Bray GA: Obesity and the heart, Mod Concepts Cardiovasc Dis 56(12):67, 1987.
7. Brown MS and Goldstein JL: How LDL receptors influence cholesterol and atherosclerosis, Sci Am 251(5):58, 1984.
8. Castelli WP and others: Cardiovascular risk factors in the elderly, Am J Cardiol 63:12H, 1989.
9. Clark PB: Nicotine and smoking: a perspective from animal studies, Psychopharmacology (Berl) 92:135, 1987.
10. Conroy RM, Mulcahy R, and Hickey N: Is a family history of CHD an independent coronary risk factor? Br Heart J 53:378, 1985.
11. Cooper R and Simmons BE: Cigarette smoking and ill health among black Americans, NY State Med J 85(7):344, 1985.
12. Criqui MH: Epidemiology of atherosclerosis: an updated overview, Am J Cardiol 57:18C, 1986.

13. Dishman R: Motivation and exercise adherence. In Silva JM and Weinberg RS, editors: Psychological foundations of sport, Champaign, Ill, 1984, Human Kinetics Publishers, Inc.

14. Dustin HP: Pathophysiology of hypertension. In Hurst JW, editor: The heart, ed 6, New York, 1985, McGraw-Hill, Inc.

15. Eder HA: Lipoproteins as risk factors for coronary heart disease, Heart 1(1):31, 1990.

16. Fagiotto A and Ross R: Studies of hypercholesteremia in the nonhuman primate. II. Fatty streak conversion to fibrous plaque, Arteriosclerosis 4:341, 1984.

17. Fagiotto A, Ross R, and Harker L: Studies of hypercholesteremia in the nonhuman primate. I. Changes that lead to fatty streak formation, Arteriosclerosis 4:323, 1984.

18. Fielding JE and Phenow KJ: Health effects of involuntary smoking, N Engl J Med 319(22):1452, 1988.

19. Frick M and others: Helinski Heart Study: primary prevention trial with gemfibrozil in middle-aged men with dyslipidemia, N Engl J Med 317:1237, 1987.

20. Frohlich ED: Hypertension in the elderly, Curr Probl Cardiol 13(5):319, 1988.

21. Gardner LI, Stern MP, and Haffner SM: Prevalence of diabetes in Mexican Americans: relationship to percent of gene pool derived from Native American sources, Diabetes 33:86, 1984.

22. Garfinkel L: Cigarette smoking and coronary heart disease in blacks: comparison to whites in a prospective study, Am Heart J 108:802, 1984.

23. Geizerova H and Masironi R: Cigarette smoking among children and adolescents: world view, J Int Soc Fed Cardiol 1:10, 1989.

24. Goldman L and Cook EF: The decline in ischemic heart disease mortality rates: an analysis of the comparative effects of medical interventions and changes in lifestyle, Ann Intern Med 101:825, 1984.

25. Gottlieb SO and Gerstenblith G: Silent myocardial ischemia in the elderly: current concepts, Geriatrics 43(4):29, 1988.

26. Hamly RI: Hereditary aspects of coronary artery disease, Am Heart J 101:639, 1981.

27. Hazuda HP and others: Effects of acculturation and socioeconomic status on obesity and diabetes in Mexican Americans, Am J Epidemiol 1:289, 1988.

28. Holbrook JH and others: Cigarette smoking and heart disease, Circulation 70(6):1114A, 1984.

29. Hubert HB and others: Obesity as an independent risk factor for cardiovascular disease: a 25-year follow-up of participants in the Framingham Heart Study, Circulation 67:968, 1983.

30. Hunter S and others: Social status and cardiovascular risk factors in children: the Bogalusa Heart Study, J Chronic Dis 32:441, 1979.

31. Joint National Committee on Detection, Evaluation, and Treatment of High Blood Pressure: the 1988 report, Archives Intern Med 148:1023, 1988.

32. Kannel WB: Lipids, diabetes, and coronary heart disease: insights from the Framingham study, Am Heart J 110:1100, 1985.

33. Kannel WB and Abbott RD: Incidence and prognosis of unrecognized myocardial infarction: an update on the Framingham study, N Engl J Med 311:1144, 1984.

34. Kannel WB, Dannenberg AL, and Abbott RD: Unrecognized myocardial infarction and hypertension, Am Heart J 109:581, 1985.

35. Kannel WB and others: Prevention of cardiovascular disease in the elderly, J Am Coll Cardiol 10(2):25A, 1987.

36. Kaplan NM: Arterial hypertension. In Stein JH, editor: Internal medicine, ed 3, Boston, Little, Brown, & Co.

37. Kashyap ML: Cardiovascular disease in the elderly: current considerations, Am J Cardiol 63:3H, 1989.

38. Kreisberg R and Kasim S: Cholesterol metabolism and aging, Am J Med 82(suppl 1B):54, 1987.

39. Laakso M and others: Lipids and lipoprotein abnormalities associated with CHD in patients with insulin dependent diabetes mellitus, Arteriosclerosis 6:679, 1986.

40. LaRosa JC: Effect of estrogen replacement therapy on lipids: implications for cardiovascular risks, J Reprod Med 30(suppl 10):811, 1985.

41. Leitshuk M and Chobanian A: Vascular changes in hypertension, Med Clin North Am 71(5):827, 1987.

42. Lipid Research Clinics Program: The Lipid Research Clinics Coronary Primary Prevention Trial Results. I. Reduction in incidence of coronary heart disease, JAMA 251:351, 1984.

43. Manson JE and others: A prospective study of obesity and risk of coronary heart disease in women, N Engl J Med 322:822, 1990.

44. Matthews KA and Haynes SG: Type A behavior pattern and coronary disease risk: update and critical evaluation, Am J Epidemiol 123:923, 1986.

45. Meade TW: Effects of progestogens on the cardiovascular system, Am J Obstet Gynecol 142:776, 1982.

46. Menotti A and others: Seven countries study: first 20 year mortality data in 12 cohorts in six countries, Ann Med 21(3):270, 1989.

47. National Cholesterol Education Program Expert Panel: Report of the National Cholesterol Education Program Expert Panel on Detection, Evaluation, and Treatment of High Blood Cholesterol in Adults, Arch Intern Med 148:36, 1988.

48. National Heart, Lung, and Blood Institute: High blood cholesterol in adults, National Cholesterol Education Program, Bethesda, Md, 1987, NHLBI.

49. National Heart, Lung, and Blood Institute: The 1988 report of the Joint National Committee on Detection, Evaluation, and Treatment of High Blood Pressure, NIH Publication No. 88-1088, USDHHS, PHS, NIH, 1988.

50. Nesto RW and Kowalchuk GJ: The ischemic cascade: temporal sequence of hemodynamic, electrocardiographic and symptomatic expressions of ischemia, Am J Cardiol 57:23C, 1987.

51. Office on Smoking and Health, Center for Health Promotion and Education: Cigarette smoking among blacks and other minority populations, MMWR 36:404, 1987.

52. Ohlson L and others: Fasting blood glucose and risk of coronary heart disease, stroke, and all cause mortality: a 17-year follow-up study of men born in 1913, Diabetic Med 3:33, 1986.

53. Oldridge NB: Compliance and drop-out in cardiac rehabilitation, J Cardiac Rehabil 7:166, 1984.
54. Oldridge NB: Cardiac rehabilitation, self-responsibility and quality of life, J Cardiopul Rehabil 6:153, 1986.
55. Pell S and Fayerweather WE: Trends in the incidence of myocardial infarction and in associated mortality and morbidity in a large employed population: 1957-83, N Engl J Med 312:1005, 1985.
56. Powell MG and others: Effects of oral contraceptives on lipoprotein lipids: prospective study, Obstet Gynecol 63:764, 1984.
57. Rosenberg M and others: Myocardial infarction in women under 50 years of age, JAMA 250:2801, 1983.
58. Roskies E and others: The Montreal Type A Project: major findings, Health Psychol 5:45, 1986.
59. Ross R: The pathogenesis of atherosclerosis: an update, N Engl J Med 314(8):488, 1986.
60. Ross R and others: The role of endothelial injury and platelet and macrophage interactions in atherosclerosis, Circulation 70(suppl 3):III-77, 1984.
61. Ruderman NB and Haudenschild C: Diabetes as an atherogenic factor, Prog Cardiovasc Dis 26:373, 1984.
62. Russel-Briefel R and others: Cardiovascular risk status and oral contraceptive use: United States, 1976-80, Prev Med 15:352, 1982.
63. Salonen JL: Oral contraceptives, smoking, and risk of MI in young women: a longitudinal population study in Eastern Finland, Acta Med Scand 212:141, 1982.
64. Samet JA and others: Diabetes, gallbladder disease, obesity, and hypertension among Hispanics in New Mexico, Am J Epidemiol 128(1):302, 1988.
65. Saunders E: Hypertension in blacks, Med Clin North Am 71(1):1013, 1987.
66. Schulman SP and Gerstenblith G: Cardiovascular changes with aging: the response to exercise, J Cardiopul Rehabil 9(1):12, 1989.
67. Sosenko JM, Breslow JL, Miettinen OS: Hyperglycemia and plasma lipid levels: a prospective study of young insulin-dependent diabetic patients, N Engl J Med 302:650, 1980.
68. Stacy HL: Evolution of atherosclerotic plaques in the coronary arteries of young adults, Arteriosclerosis 3:471a, abstract, 1983.
69. Stampfer MJ and others: A prospective study of past use of oral contraceptive agents and risk of cardiovascular disease, N Engl J Med 319:1313, 1988.
70. Sytkowski PA, Kannel WB, and D'Agostino RB: Changes in risk factors and the decline in mortality from cardiovascular disease: The Framingham Heart Study, N Engl J Med 322:1635, 1990.
71. Thoreson C: Altering type A behavior pattern in postinfarction patients, J Cardiopul Rehabil 5:258, 1985.
72. Tyroler HA, editor: Epidemiology of plasma high-density lipoprotein cholesterol levels. II. The Lipid Research Clinics Program Prevalence Study, Circulation 62(suppl 4):1, 1980.
73. Wallin JD: Hypertension in black patients: epidemiologic and pathophysiologic considerations, J Clinical Hypertension 1:7, 1986.
74. Wenger NK, Gersh BJ, and O'Rourke RO: Cardiovascular disease in the elderly, J Am Coll Cardiol 10(2):80A, 1987.
75. West KM and others: The role of circulating glucose and triglyceride concentrations and their interactions with other 'risk factors' as determinants of arterial disease in nine diabetic population samples from the WHO multinational study, Diabetes Care 6:361, 1983.
76. Zimmerman M and McGeachie J: The effect of nicotine on aortic endothelium, Atherosclerosis 63:33, 1987.

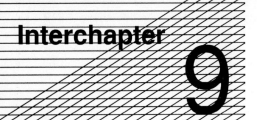

Interchapter

9

Killer Mondays

Sudden death is one of the most feared outcomes of myocardial disease. Variations in such deaths were studied by the University of Manitoba; 3983 male patients were observed from 1948 to 1980.[5] In men with no previous clinical evidence of ischemic heart disease, an increase in sudden cardiac deaths occurred on Mondays.

Acute myocardial infarctions (AMIs) occur more frequently on a particular day of the week and hour of that day—the so-called Black Monday Syndrome: Monday morning, 8 to 9 AM. No other species on earth dies more frequently on a particular day.[2]

Research suggests that the way people feel about their jobs may underly Black Monday Syndrome. In a Department of Health, Education, and Welfare survey, the best predictor of a first AMI is job satisfaction, a better predictor than cholesterol levels, blood pressure, cigarette smoking, or obesity.[6]

Psychologic stress has been associated with sudden cardiac death and AMI (see p. 300). Returning to work on Mondays poses an increase in emotional stress. Internal biologic variations also play a role, making people more susceptible to the underlying ischemic process.[3] Reintroduction to occupational stress, activity, or pollutants after a weekend may precipitate dysrhythmias or myocardial ischemia.[1]

Regardless of the mechanisms, we can educate our patients to decrease one variable that is controllable: psychophysiologic stress. This teaching is important for patients and nurses. Here are four significant steps that can be used to take charge of one's life[4]:

Who's running your life?

We should never cease to explore our level of job satisfaction at work. Is there meaning and fulfillment? Does our job stimulate and inspire us? Do we approach Mondays with enthusiasm or dread? Do we want to go to work? If not, the stage is set for adverse health events in our lives.

How do you start each morning? Early morning sets the mood for the day. If you wake up angry or discouraged, you set a negative mood for the day. Generating positive thoughts each morning can result in an improvement in the service, quality, rewards, and effectiveness of your job. Each morning think of your mind as a canvas on which you can paint events that affect you. When you empower yourself, it impacts you and colleagues, physicians, patients, family, and friends.

Do you choose positive or negative news?

Do you read the newspaper or listen to the news before going to work? The news is usually depressing and upsetting.

Start your day with as much peace and tranquility as possible. Eliminate the negative news, particularly first thing in the morning. Keep abreast of current news, particularly news that we can do something about such as community events. Have a selection of books of short inspirational thoughts or an audiocassette tape of positive affirmations.

Do you actively maintain a healthy lifestyle?

Do you have a healthy lifestyle? Do you ever say after a weekend, "I'll start eating healthier and exercising tomorrow?" Then before you realize it, another month goes by with sloppy eating habits and no exercise, resulting in a 5-pound weight gain and becoming spirit-drained.

We have heard the comparison of the body to a car. We can be unaware of our car—feeding it cheap fuel, getting low on oil, skipping maintenance. Then it starts breaking down. What steps do you take to avoid junk fuel and to exercise (20 to 30 minutes) and play (15 to 30 minutes) each day? As we create a healthy rhythm of nu-

tritious eating and exercising, we eliminate the toxins in overprocessed food, strengthen our cardiovascular system and body, and stimulate our endorphin system that increases our well-being. It's pay now or later in the form of acute or chronic illness.

Are you failing to plan?

Do you ever think that you don't have time to plan? When we fail to plan, we feel out of control and depressed, and we procrastinate and overreact. Planning allows us to be more spontaneous and in control and gains us more free time.

How do you plan your day? Do you have a habit of prioritizing and making a "to-do" list? Planning creates a positive step for each day. Unanticipated events occur, but by planning we are in control and can take steps for incorporating these events without being overwhelmed.

How many choices do you have?

These steps and choices may seem obvious. They involve good common sense but often are not practiced. To make consistent, successful changes, self-awareness skills and daily *practice* are required. These steps should be included in preventive cardiac education and rehabilitation.

REFERENCES

1. Lown B: Sudden cardiac death: the major challenge controling contemporary cardiology, Am J Cardiol 43:313, 1979.
2. Muller JE: Circadian rhythms in the frequency of sudden death, Circulation 75:131, 1987.
3. Pavedis T and Pinsker HM: Oscillator theory and neurophysiology, Fed Proc 36:2033, 1977.
4. Powers D: Powers Newlletter (spring issue), 1991, The Powers Group.
5. Rabkin SW, Matthewson FA, and Tate RT: Chronobiology of cardiac sudden death in men, JAMA 244:1357, 1980.
6. Work in America: report of a special task force to the Secretary of the Department of Health, Education, and Welfare, Cambridge, 1973, MIT Press.

9

The Person with Angina Pectoris

Sandra W. Haak
Sue E. Huether

LEARNING OBJECTIVES

1. Discuss the signs and symptoms of angina pectoris.
2. Describe the pathophysiologic basis for the clinical manifestations of angina pectoris.
3. Differentiate anginal symptoms from chest discomfort or pain unrelated to cardiac problems.

4. Analyze the importance of the patient history in assessing the person with angina pectoris.
5. Discuss diagnostic procedures used in evaluating the patient with angina pectoris.

6. Discuss patient outcomes, nursing prescriptions, and evaluation criteria for each nursing diagnosis for the patient with angina pectoris.
7. Describe the procedure, patient selection, and nursing care of a patient undergoing percutaneous transluminal coronary angioplasty.

Angina pectoris is a cardiovascular syndrome associated with myocardial ischemia and disturbance of myocardial function but without development of myocardial necrosis.[112] *Angina* is the Latin word for spasmodic, choking, suffocating pain, whereas *pectoris* means chest.[36] Thus *angina pectoris* is literally translated to "strangling chest."[112] The typical clinical manifestation is pain or discomfort, which is described as crushing, pressing, or constricting; is located in the substernal area of the chest; begins during exertion; is relieved by rest; lasts 3 to 5 minutes; and radiates to the neck, jaw, or left arm.[73,112] The symptoms are caused by disparity between myocardial oxygen demand and myocardial oxygen delivery.* Patients who have unpredictable episodes are considered unstable, and those with poor left ventricular function and poor exercise tolerance experience the complications of myocardial infarction (MI) or sudden death at a rate of 16% to 19% per year.[49] In contrast, stable patients with good left ventricular function and good exercise tolerance experience these complications at a rate of 1% to 2% per year.[49] The major goals of therapy are to improve myocardial perfusion, relieve symptoms during attacks, and prevent or delay the development of MI and sudden death.[72,112,119]

---

*References 70, 78, 86, 112, 119, 139, and 142.

INCIDENCE

The precise incidence rate of angina pectoris is unknown. Estimates based on the Framingham Heart Study are that 2.5 million people in the United States suffer from angina and about 300,000 new cases of angina are identified each year.[4] Although it is caused by underlying ischemic heart disease, angina rarely causes death in itself. Death from ischemic heart disease is usually attributed to MI.[4] Healthier lifestyles and advances in medical treatment are reflected in the 28.7% decline in the age-adjusted death rate from MI from 1977 to 1987.[4] Despite the declining mortality rate, heart disease was still the leading cause of death in 1987, with ischemic heart disease accounting for 24% of all deaths.[95] In 1989, 5 million Americans had a history of angina pectoris or MI. The American Heart Association predicted that in 1990, 1.5 million Americans would experience an MI and that more than 500,000 of these individuals would die.[4]

CORONARY BLOOD FLOW

Arterial blood to the heart is supplied by three major arteries, the left anterior descending (LAD) and circumflex (LCX) branches of the left coronary artery (LCA), as well as the right coronary artery (RCA) (Figure 9-1). The RCA and LCA arise directly from the aorta behind the right and

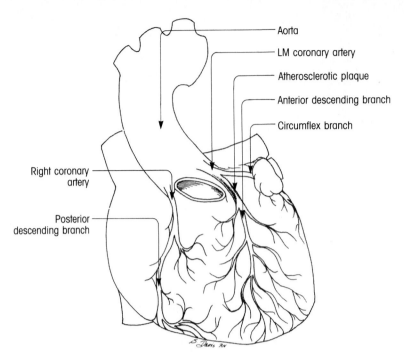

FIG. 9-1   Coronary circulation. The coronary arteries arise from the aortic arch and supply oxygen-rich blood to the myocardium. Note the atherosclerotic obstruction in the proximal portion of the left anterior descending coronary artery. *LM,* Left main coronary artery.

left cusps of the aortic valve. The LAD branch supplies blood to the anterior wall of the left ventricle, the anterior two thirds of the interventricular septum, and some of the inferior wall near the apex. The LCX branch extends laterally, in the atrioventricular (AV) groove, to supply blood to the lateral aspect of the left ventricle. The RCA runs in the right AV groove to supply the AV node. It then turns and becomes the posterior descending artery, which supplies the posterior third of the interventricular septum. A posterior left ventricular branch supplies the diaphragmatic wall of the left ventricle. The major vessels lie on the surface of the heart. Usually a rich system of branches ensures an adequate blood supply to the myocardium at all times by penetrating from the epicardium to the endocardium.[9]

The walls of normal coronary arteries are compliant and have three layers: the intima, the media, and the adventitia. The intima, the innermost layer, consists of a continuous layer of endothelial cells that provide a smooth internal surface. The middle layer, the media, makes up the bulk of the arterial wall and consists of smooth muscle cells separated from the intima and adventitia by sheets of elastic fiber, the internal and external elastic lamina. The outermost layer, the adventitia, consists of connective tissue, elastic fibers, and fibroblasts.[9]

Coronary perfusion is consistent with the pulsatile flow pattern of aortic pressure. Coronary blood flow is lowest during systole when the branches that penetrate the myocardium are compressed by the contracted muscle. During systole, left ventricular wall pressure is greatest near the endocardium and lowest near the epicardium. Coronary blood flow reaches a peak when the ventricles have relaxed during early diastole and compression of the vessels is nearly absent. Normally, increased blood flow to the endocardium during diastole compensates for greater blood flow to the epicardium during systole. Ischemia and consequent damage is greatest in the inner wall of the ventricle during abnormal conditions such as atherosclerosis, left ventricular hypertrophy associated with hypertension, or aortic stenosis because blood flow to the endocardial regions is more severely reduced than flow to the epicardial regions.[9]

Under normal resting conditions, the heart extracts about 75% of the oxygen from the coronary blood, leaving little reserve oxygen for use when there is increased myocardial work. Therefore increased oxygen demands are normally met by an increase in blood flow. *Autoregulation* (local, nonneural control) of coronary blood flow permits variation in coronary vessel resistance consistent with changes in aortic perfusion pressure and cardiac work. A local decrease in oxygen concentration releases adenosine or other substances such as carbon dioxide, hydrogen ions, bradykinin, and prostaglandins, which dilate arterioles. Nervous regulation of coronary blood flow can be direct or indirect. Sympathetic stimulation of coronary vessels provides the most direct influence with α_1-receptors mediating vasoconstriction and the more abundant β_2-receptors mediating vasodilation. α_2-receptors inhibit release of norepinephrine and promote vasodilation.[9]

ETIOLOGY AND PRECIPITATING FACTORS

Anginal episodes represent myocardial ischemia precipitated by factors or events that result in an imbalance between myocardial oxygen demand and supply. The underlying cause is usually coronary artery disease or coronary artery spasm, although cardiovascular disease or systemic illness that limit the heart's ability to increase coronary blood flow (oxygen supply) relative to increased myocardial work (oxygen demand) may also cause angina.

Myocardial oxygen supply can be reduced by (1) vascular factors such as increased resistance in coronary vessels due to vasospasm or atherosclerotic plaque; (2) cardiac factors such as decreased cardiac output resulting from cardiac dysrhythmias, dilated cardiomyopathy, or valvular stenosis or incompetence; (3) hematologic factors such as anemia, hypoxemia, or other decreases in the content or availability of oxygen in the blood; or (4) systemic disorders that reduce blood flow such as advanced pulmonary or systemic hypertension.[45,112] Factors and events that increase myocardial oxygen demand include (1) increased heart rate associated with exercise, stress, cardiac dysrhythmias, hypoxemia, anemia, fever, hyperthyroidism, or other excessive metabolic demands; (2) increased myocardial wall tension associated with elevated systolic pressure, increased ventricular volume, or ventricular hypertrophy;

and (3) increased myocardial contractility associated with release of catecholamines or sympathetic stimulation.[43,86,133,139] In the majority of cases, the underlying cause of angina pectoris is atherosclerotic plaque, which occludes 70% to 75% or more of the lumen of one or more coronary arteries. Coronary artery spasm can occur in normal or significantly stenosed coronary arteries as the only cause of obstruction or as a critical compounding factor.[72,86,112]

LESIONS OF ATHEROSCLEROSIS

In the process of *atherosclerosis*, arteries thicken and lose elasticity because of lipids and fibrin deposited in their walls. The lesions of atherosclerosis can be classified as fatty streaks, fibrous plaques, and complicated plaques (see Table 9-1 and Fig. 9-2). *Fatty streaks* may be the earliest lesion of atherosclerosis. They are composed primarily of cholesterol ester (oleic acid) and are present in the aorta by 10 years of age and in the coronary arteries by 15 years of age.[81] Fatty streaks do not inevitably progress to the more advanced lesions of atherosclerosis.[111]

Fibrous (pearly) *plaques* are characteristic of advancing atherosclerosis; they are elevated lesions of the intima that consist of lipid-filled smooth muscle cells and macrophages in a fibrous matrix. The lipid-filled macrophages have a foamlike appearance under the microscope and thus are described as *foam cells*. The plaques appear in men before women and in the aorta before the coronary arteries. Like

TABLE 9-1
Characteristics of Atherosclerotic Plaques

Description	Location	Composition	Consequence
FATTY STREAKS			
Earliest lesion; typically smooth and flat	Within the intima, commonly at the branch points of vessels	Focal accumulations of lipid-filled macrophages and smooth muscle cells	No occlusion
FIBROUS PLAQUE			
Proliferative, intimal plaque; foamlike appearance	Usually in the main stem coronary arteries in the epicardial portion of the vessel	Lipid, macrophages, smooth muscle cells, and connective tissue underlying a fibrous tissue cap	Degeneration, which causes occlusion
COMPLICATED PLAQUE			
Degenerative, complex lesion; gruel-like or pasty consistency	In one, two, or three coronary vessels	Fibrous tissue, fibrin, lipid, calcium, and extravasated blood; often an encapsulated core of necrotic debris	Hemorrhage or degeneration of the core causing possible occlusion or vasospasm as a result of rupture of the intima and aneurysm formation or platelet and fibrin mural thrombus formation

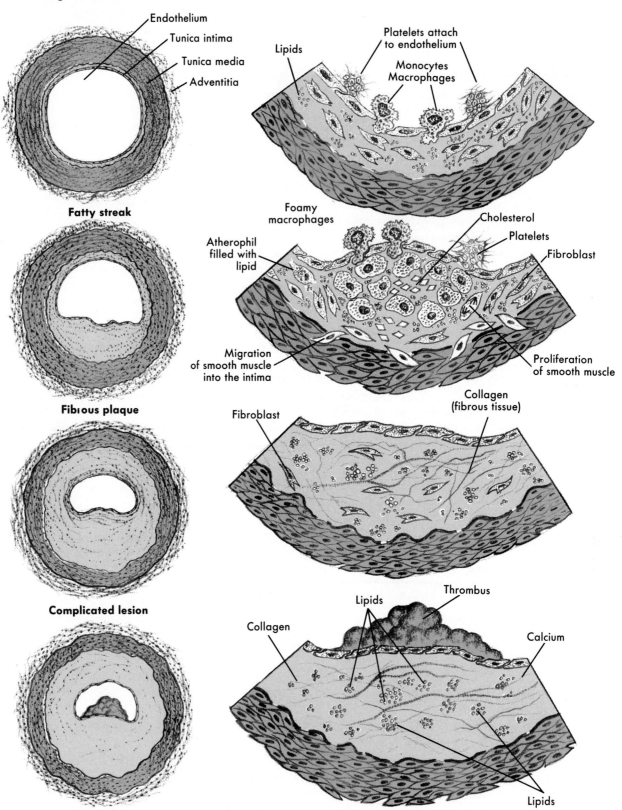

Damaged endothelium

Endothelium
Tunica intima
Tunica media
Adventitia

Lipids
Platelets attach
to endothelium
Monocytes
Macrophages

Fatty streak

Foamy
macrophages
Atherophil
filled with
lipid
Migration
of smooth muscle
into the intima
Cholesterol
Platelets
Fibroblast
Proliferation
of smooth muscle

Fibrous plaque

Fibroblast
Collagen
(fibrous tissue)

Complicated lesion

Collagen
Lipids
Thrombus
Calcium
Lipids

FIG. 9-2 Progression of atherosclerosis.
From McCance LM and Huether SE: Pathophysiology: the biologic basis for disease in adults and children, St Louis, 1990, The CV Mosby Co.

the fatty streak, the fibrous plaque is rich in cholesterol, but the principal ester is linoleic acid.

Complicated plaques are most frequently associated with symptoms of angina. Occlusion and stenosis result from gradual thickening, calcification, necrosis, and ulceration of the plaque with thrombus formation and weakening of the arterial wall. As foam cells continue to accumulate, some near the center of the lesion necrose. The accumulation of disintegrating cells within pools of lipid give the lesion's center a pasty or gruel-like consistency (the term *atheroma* comes from the Greek word *ather* meaning "gruel-like"). The progressive advancement of the atheroma eventually causes destruction of the media and may extend into the adventitia. Although a single epicardial trunk may be affected, frequently two or all three coronary vessels are involved. Depending on the number of vessels involved, coronary atherosclerosis is graded as one, two-, or three-vessel disease. Approximately one third of individuals have single-vessel disease, one third have two-vessel disease, and one third have three-vessel disease.[29]

ATHEROGENESIS AND VESSEL OCCLUSION

Over the years, various theories have been proposed to explain the development and progression of atherosclerotic lesions (Fig. 9-2). There is still controversy about which is correct. The *response-to-injury hypothesis* currently is the most encompassing.[86] Other theories are reviewed in Table 9-2. Ross[109-111] believes that several mechanisms or a combination of theories are responsible for the different lesions. An underlying assumption in all of the theories is that the process is initiated by injury to or change in the structural integrity of vascular endothelium (see Chapter 8).

Endothelial cell injury is the central component of the response-to-injury hypothesis. Endothelial cells forming the intima of coronary vessels (and other arteries) are continually exposed to chemical, mechanical, or immunologic injury. Injury to the endothelium may be subtle (with no morphologic alteration) or gross. Gross injury may stimulate endothelial cell proliferation, migration of monocytes (macrophages) to the subendothelium, and increased platelet attachment. Platelets release *thromboxane A_2*, a potent vasoconstrictor and recruiter of platelets. Platelet adherence and aggregation may produce thrombi large enough to cause occlusion. Fibrous platelet plugs may also disintegrate to enter the circulation as emboli.

The proliferation and accumulation of smooth muscle cells may be triggered or enhanced by toxic substances such as cholesterol or trauma from hypertension. Endothelial cells, macrophages, and platelets may release chemoattractants for smooth muscle cells that move from the media to the intima. They may also release growth factors that contribute to proliferation of smooth muscle cells. Direct stimulation of growth factor production by endothelial

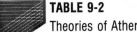

TABLE 9-2
Theories of Atherogenesis

Theory	Mechanism
Lipogenic or insudation theory	Lipids (low-density lipoprotein [LDL] and cholesterol) from the blood accumulate into smooth muscle cells of the intima, which have migrated from the media.
Thrombogenic or encrustation theory	Platelets and fibrin are deposited at the site of fibrous or complicated plaque because of intimal erosion or vasospasm, which contributes to plaque progression when thrombi become part of the plaque.
Monoclonal hypothesis	Atherosclerotic plaque develops from proliferation of a single smooth muscle cell. It is similar to benign tumor cells with cellular accumulation of lipid.
Focal clonal senescence	Intimal smooth muscle cells that proliferate to form an atheroma are controlled by a mitotic inhibitor secreted by smooth muscle cells in the media. With aging, the feedback control system fails as the controlling cells die, and the unsuppressed cells proliferate and accumulate lipid.
Lysosomal theory	Increased deposition of lipid in smooth muscle cells occurs as a consequence of a deficiency of lysosomal cholesterol hydrolase.

cells with migration and proliferation of smooth muscle cells is also proposed. This cause of atherosclerosis may be more important in persons with diabetes or hypertension and persons who smoke cigarettes than in persons with primary hyperlipidemia (see Chapter 8).

The proliferating smooth muscle cells deposit a fibrous connective-tissue matrix and accumulate lipid. As they degenerate, macrophages migrate to the area to engulf and encapsulate them, thus promoting plaque formation. Lipid deposition is enhanced with hyperlipidemia.[127] As the lesion progresses, shearing forces on the endothelial cell increase, further complicating the extent of the lesion.

Spasm of the coronary arteries with significant luminal narrowing has been associated with angina, MI, and sudden death.[68,108,144] The exact mechanism of spasm is unknown, but vasoactive substances, including histamine, catecholamines, prostaglandins, and thromboxane A_2, are thought to be implicated.[50] There may also be spasm of smooth muscle in segments of the coronary vessel wall that are free of atherosclerosis, which leads to dynamic vessel occlusion and ischemia.[64]

TYPES OF ANGINA

Types of angina pectoris include stable, unstable, and Prinzmetal's or variant. Myocardial ischemia also can be present in the absence of clinical symptoms, a state known as *silent myocardial ischemia*. Symptoms such as dyspnea and fatigue that are precipitated by myocardial ischemia but not accompanied by chest pain are described as *anginal equivalents*.[72,73,112]

Stable angina pectoris

Angina pectoris is stable (classic, exertion-induced, fixed-threshold) when the pattern of intensity, frequency, duration, precipitating activity, exertion level, and ease of relief is consistent for at least 2 months.[72,112] Symptoms are absent when the patient is at rest or doing ordinary activity; however, exertion above a certain level predictably precipitates symptoms. The typical symptoms of pressing or constricting substernal chest pain that radiates to the chest and left arm begin during exertion.[72,112] The pain usually does not last more than 5 minutes with cessation of exertion or treatment with vasodilators. More commonly, symptoms are experienced in the morning.[79] The majority of patients with stable angina have normal resting electrocardiograms (ECGs), particularly when there is no pain.[72] ST-segment depression is the usual pattern when there is pain indicating subendocardial ischemia.[118] Although vessel occlusion of less than 70% is not expected to cause symptoms, about 25% of individuals with a history of stable angina have normal or minimally occluded coronary arteries when studied with angiography.[73,112]

Unstable angina pectoris

Angina is unstable when it initially occurs; occurs at rest; increases in intensity, frequency, or duration as compared with a previously stable pattern; or follows a recent acute myocardial infarction (AMI).[119] The imbalance between myocardial oxygen supply and demand that leads to unstable ischemia results from multiple factors, including progressive atherosclerosis with increasing vessel occlusion, erosion or rupture of an atherosclerotic plaque with mural thrombus formation, platelet aggregation and activation with progressive occlusion and release of vasoconstricting agents such as thromboxane A_2, and intermittent or prolonged coronary artery vasospasm.[54]

Symptoms may occur at rest (spontaneously) or with exertion. The pattern of chest pain is characterized by increased ease of provocation, less predictability (variable threshold), and accelerated severity of symptoms (crescendo) when compared to stable angina pectoris.[72,112] The symptoms of unstable angina may mimic AMI. Chest pain is severe and often associated with nausea, vomiting, and diaphoresis. The pain may radiate to adjacent areas, and the discomfort is not easily relieved by sublingual nitro-

glycerin. If left untreated, the symptoms may last from 20 minutes to several hours. In most cases, however, individuals fear that they are having heart attacks and seek medical attention. Sometimes this syndrome is referred to as *preinfarction angina* or *acute coronary insufficiency*, although the ischemia falls short of producing an infarction. Whether the symptoms are new or reflect a change in a stable exertional anginal pattern, they should be regarded as a serious cardiac event because sudden death or MI may occur within a few days, weeks, or months.[73]

Postinfarction angina refers to anginal pain that follows MI. Episodes of anginal pain can occur immediately after a MI, or days or weeks may pass without pain before the episodes begin. In either case the angina represents myocardial ischemia and a serious imbalance of myocardial oxygen supply and demand. The patient is at considerable risk for additional MI.[72,112]

Prinzmetal's or variant angina pectoris

Prinzmetal's or variant angina is the result of vasospasm in partially occluded or normal coronary arteries. It is characterized by recurring attacks of anginal pain at rest and is associated with transient ST-segment elevation (in contrast to the ST-segment depression of stable angina) on the ECG. Pain usually occurs early in the morning and may demonstrate circadian, weekly, and monthly patterns of variation.[5,136,144] Sometimes this type of angina is referred to as *spontaneous* or *variable-threshold*.[72,112] MI can result from prolonged coronary artery spasm and myocardial ischemia.[100,144]

Some individuals experience angina while reclining *(angina decubitus)*, and others are awakened with angina at night *(nocturnal angina)*. The cause of these patterns is probably related to the increase of intrathoracic (circulating) blood volume associated with recumbency and the related increases in ventricular wall tension and myocardial oxygen demand.

Silent myocardial ischemia

Silent (painless, ambulant) myocardial ischemia is a transient imbalance of myocardial oxygen supply or demand unaccompanied by angina or equivalent symptoms. Silent myocardial ischemia is indicated when the patient has no symptoms, although ST-segment depression is recorded on ECG during exercise. Three groups of patients with silent myocardial ischemia have been described.[6,116] Type I patients have no history of angina or MI, but evidence of myocardial ischemia is found during a screening exercise test. Type II patients have a history of MI, and type III patients have a history of symptomatic angina.

The diurnal pattern of ST-segment depression is similar to that described for MI and sudden death, with a higher incidence rate shortly after waking and at noon, a plateau in the afternoon, and low rates at night and in the early morning.[92,140] Studies have shown that patients with silent myocardial ischemia are at risk for further progression of coronary atherosclerosis, development of angina pectoris, and serious cardiac events (sudden death or MI).[6]

Myocardial ischemia, both silent and painful, may be associated with coronary artery stenosis related to a dynamic rather than a fixed obstruction.[99] Changes in smooth muscle tone, platelet aggregability, and stressors such as emotion, mental activity, smoking, exercise, and cold exposure may alter vessel lumen size or increase myocardial oxygen demand above a level that can be met by coronary flow. The dynamic obstruction view modifies the more traditional view that myocardial ischemia is evoked by an increasing myocardial demand that exceeds a fixed myocardial oxygen supply.

Myocardial stunning, previously known as *acute coronary insufficiency* or *threatened MI,* occurs when an acute vessel occlusion subsequently reopens and reperfuses the myocardium. A more chronic reduction in blood flow is described as *hibernating myocardium.* In these instances the myocardium decreases its function to match oxygen supply.[98] Myocardial stunning can result in contraction abnormalities with wall thinning and bulging. The causes are unknown but may be related to decreased adenosine triphosphate levels or oxygen-free radicals.[16,103]

Nursing Process

Case study. Mr. B., a 57-year-old automobile mechanic, came to the emergency department with a chief complaint of chest pain. He described the discomfort as a "heavy sensation." He stated, "It feels like a battery is sitting on the middle of my chest." The discomfort radiated to his neck, left shoulder, and left side of the jaw and was accompanied by nausea, nervousness, and diaphoresis. The episode began 30 minutes before his arrival, while he was working with his arms raised above his head. It decreased but did not stop entirely when he rested in a chair. Sublingual nitroglycerin and morphine sulfate administered in the emergency department gave him complete relief.

Mr. B. explained that he had experienced similar chest pain 1 week before while working underneath an automobile. The episode lasted about 2 minutes and resolved spontaneously. He again experienced substernal chest discomfort 2 days later while carrying an automobile battery. The discomfort lasted longer but stopped when he put the battery down. The pain did not radiate nor was it accompanied by nausea, vomiting, shortness of breath, or diaphoresis. For the past several days, Mr. B. had noticed chest pain once or twice a day that lasted 2 or 3 minutes. He did not seek medical care because the pain lasted such a short time.

Mr. B.'s only prior medical problem was hypertension, detected 5 years before in a screening clinic and treated with hydralazine. He stated that he usually took his medications, although he sometimes forgot. His family did not have a history of heart disease, hypertension, or diabetes. He had smoked 2 packs of cigarettes a day for 35 years.

The physical examination was performed while Mr. B. was having pain. He was a well-developed, well-nourished man in moderate distress. His vital signs were blood pressure, 150/100 mm Hg; pulse,

96 per minute; respirations, 20 per minute; and temperature, 36.4° C (97.6° F). Grade II retinopathy was found during the eye examination. The cardiac examination revealed a point of maximum impulse at the fifth intercostal space, midclavicular line; normal first and second heart sounds; a third heart sound (ventricular gallop); and no audible fourth heart sound, murmurs, or pericardial rub. Pulmonary, neurologic, gastrointestinal, and genitourinary examinations were normal.

The ECG was recorded while pain was present and revealed a normal sinus rhythm; normal QRS, PR, and QT intervals; and an axis of +30 degrees. There were ST and T wave abnormalities in leads II, III, aV_F, V_3, and V_4 that were suggestive but not diagnostic of myocardial ischemia. Cardiac enzymes were within normal limits. The chest x-ray film showed a normal cardiac silhouette and no infiltrates in the lung fields.

Mr. B. was admitted to the coronary care unit (CCU) with a medical diagnosis of unstable angina pectoris and possible MI. For the first 24 hours, bed rest with commode privileges was prescribed. He continued to have frequent episodes of chest pain requiring sublingual nitroglycerin and morphine sulfate for relief. ECGs performed during these episodes revealed significant ST-segment depression and T-wave inversion diagnostic of myocardial ischemia. These changes reverted to a nondiagnostic state after the pain resolved. Nitroglycerin ointment was administered in an effort to prevent the episodes of chest pain. The frequency and intensity of the episodes diminished slightly. Isosorbide dinitrate (Isordil) was also prescribed.

Nifedipine and then propranolol were added to the therapeutic regimen on the second day, when the episodes of pain continued. Because of his unstable chest pain pattern, Mr. B. had a cardiac catheterization with angiography on the third day. The findings included an ejection fraction of 60%, left ventricular end-diastolic pressure of 8 mm Hg, 90% narrowing of the RCA, and 85% narrowing of the LAD branch. Both lesions were in the proximal portions of the vessels, and percutaneous transluminal coronary angioplasty (PTCA) was carried out successfully. Mr. B. was returned to the CCU with the arterial and venous sheaths still in place.

The next several days were uneventful for Mr. B. Bed rest in the CCU was prescribed until the sheaths were removed. He had no episodes of pain or bleeding, and his vital signs were stable. He was transferred to the telemetry unit and began the cardiac rehabilitation program. ECGs and cardiac enzyme evaluations showed no evidence of myocardial ischemia or infarction. A radionuclide scan showed no myocardial necrosis. During a low-level exercise test, he exercised for 3 minutes at 1.7 mph and did not experience fatigue, dyspnea, or chest pain. His vital signs and ECG remained within normal limits. He was discharged with a referral to the outpatient cardiac rehabilitation program.

Nursing assessment

The diagnosis of angina pectoris is suspected initially when an individual (especially a man in his mid-50s) is seen with a complaint of substernal chest discomfort. The discomfort of angina is not uniform,[129] and the taking of a careful history is of prime importance in determining the cause and appropriate management. If angina is suspected, the patient is further evaluated with other diagnostic methods. Physical examinations, ECGs, blood chemistry studies, and diagnostic tests are used to confirm the underlying cause and to determine the extent of myocardial ischemia. The nurse must perform a holistic assessment[62] of the patient's responses to the discomfort of angina pectoris and to the underlying chronic disease and its management.

Feeling and moving patterns

The Feeling and Moving Patterns are closely associated with each other in patients with angina pectoris because these patients usually seek health care for discomfort related to activity. During unstable phases, hospital admission for diagnosis and treatment may be required. Nurses should assess for the patient's state of comfort, usual patterns of discomfort, a recent change in a usual pattern, a comparison of current and past episodes, and level of anxiety associated with the discomfort. It is important to use the patient's words when reporting and recording the information and when asking about relief from subsequent episodes.[70,112,117] The patient's ability to perform activities of daily living should be determined and the angina graded using specific questions (see the box below).

Characteristics of anginal discomfort are summarized in the box on p. 229. Angina may be distinguished from chest pain of other origins[124] by asking specific questions

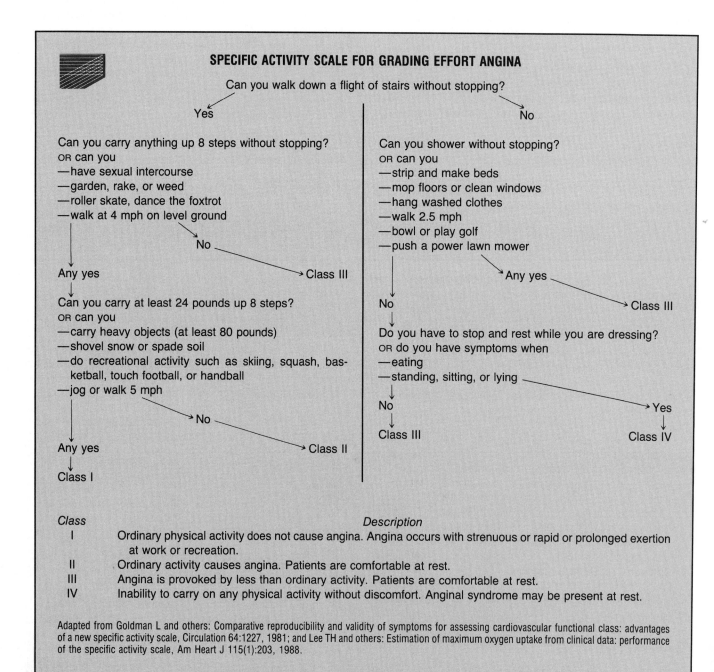

SPECIFIC ACTIVITY SCALE FOR GRADING EFFORT ANGINA

Can you walk down a flight of stairs without stopping?

Yes → / No →

Can you carry anything up 8 steps without stopping?
OR can you
—have sexual intercourse
—garden, rake, or weed
—roller skate, dance the foxtrot
—walk at 4 mph on level ground

Any yes ↓ / No → Class III

Can you carry at least 24 pounds up 8 steps?
OR can you
—carry heavy objects (at least 80 pounds)
—shovel snow or spade soil
—do recreational activity such as skiing, squash, basketball, touch football, or handball
—jog or walk 5 mph

Any yes ↓ / No → Class II

Class I

Can you shower without stopping?
OR can you
—strip and make beds
—mop floors or clean windows
—hang washed clothes
—walk 2.5 mph
—bowl or play golf
—push a power lawn mower

Any yes → Class III
No ↓

Do you have to stop and rest while you are dressing?
OR do you have symptoms when
—eating
—standing, sitting, or lying

No ↓ / Yes →
Class III / Class IV

Class	Description
I	Ordinary physical activity does not cause angina. Angina occurs with strenuous or rapid or prolonged exertion at work or recreation.
II	Ordinary activity causes angina. Patients are comfortable at rest.
III	Angina is provoked by less than ordinary activity. Patients are comfortable at rest.
IV	Inability to carry on any physical activity without discomfort. Anginal syndrome may be present at rest.

Adapted from Goldman L and others: Comparative reproducibility and validity of symptoms for assessing cardiovascular functional class: advantages of a new specific activity scale, Circulation 64:1227, 1981; and Lee TH and others: Estimation of maximum oxygen uptake from clinical data: performance of the specific activity scale, Am Heart J 115(1):203, 1988.

designed to elicit differentiating characteristics shown in Table 9-3. Patients do not always characterize the discomfort of angina pectoris as pain; instead they more often describe it as a crushing, squeezing, pressing, smothering, choking, strangling, tight, or heavy sensation. Chest discomfort that is sharp, tingling, stabbing, or fleeting or that changes with inspiration or position alterations probably does not indicate angina pectoris. The duration of angina is usually 3 to 5 minutes. Symptoms that last less than 2 minutes are rarely due to myocardial ischemia.[14] Symptoms lasting longer than 15 minutes may indicate MI.[14]

The location may be indicated by a clenched fist (Levine's sign) or hand laid across the anterior aspect of the chest; the location said to be under or behind the sternum (substernal or retrosternal). Some patients indicate a circle about the size of the fist. Usually, the area cannot be pinpointed with a finger. Areas of radiation may include the neck, jaw, teeth, back, both shoulders, arms, elbows, and wrists. The majority of radiation is to the left chest and arm rather than the right. Associated symptoms such as nausea, vomiting, dyspnea, and diaphoresis may also occur.

Patients who report symptoms that occur with increased physical exertion (especially at a rapid rate), emotional stress, exposure to cold, and eating large meals (the *four Es* that commonly precipitate angina) are experiencing increases in myocardial work. Usually, patients report that symptoms that begin during activity are relieved by rest. During the stable phase, patients can predict the amount of exertion or circumstances that will precipitate discomfort. Their condition may be *fixed-threshold* or *exertion-induced angina* because a predictable amount of activity precipitates symptoms each time the activity is repeated. Patients may report that they can avoid angina by moderating rate and exertion during activity or by taking antianginal agents before engaging in the activity. In the unstable phases, patients report episodes that begin with less-than-usual amounts of activity or have greater duration or intensity.[70,72,112]

Patients who develop symptoms while resting or sleeping are experiencing temporary obstructions to blood flow caused by *coronary artery vasospasm*. These patients may have spontaneous or variable-threshold angina. When activity is not related to anginal episodes, the angina is *spontaneous*. When the amount of activity that can be performed without precipitating angina is not consistent, the term *variable-threshold* is used. Ischemia is precipitated by intermittent vasospasm that limits coronary blood flow. Because patients are already resting, they are unable to obtain relief by decreasing activity.

Vascular tone varies throughout the day, being highest in the early morning hours and lowest in the afternoon.[112,143] As a result, the majority of resting or *nocturnal anginal episodes* are experienced between midnight and 8 AM.[112,145] Diurnal variations in vascular tone also are thought to account for episodes of pain that recur at about the same time each day and seem unrelated to activity.

Patients may report that sometimes they can perform a lot of activity without difficulty, whereas at other times they cannot. Their symptoms may develop shortly after they arise from sleep and persist intermittently through

---

 CHARACTERISTICS OF ANGINA PECTORIS (MYOCARDIAL ISCHEMIA)

QUALITY

Crushing, squeezing, pressing, smothering, burning, choking, strangling, tight, heavy, or aching sensation; rarely sharp, jabbing, knifelike, or stabbing

ONSET

Gradual or sudden; usually during activity rather than after; sometimes during rest or sleep (spontaneous)

DURATION

Usually 3 to 5 minutes, with a range of 2 to 15 minutes, rarely less than 2 minutes (Continuous discomfort lasting longer than 20 minutes indicates that myocardial infarction may be in progress.)

LOCATION

Usually substernal or retrosternal fist-size area, occasionally in radiation areas only; rarely can be pointed to with one finger

RADIATION

Usually to left chest and arm, possibly including neck, jaw, teeth, back, both shoulders, arms, elbows, and wrists

ASSOCIATED SYMPTOMS

Nausea, vomiting, dyspnea, and diaphoresis

PROVOCATION

Exertion or activity (especially at a rapid rate), emotional stress, exposure to cold or hot environment, eating large meals; predictable or unpredictable regarding amount of exertion, circumstances, or time of day; rarely aggravated by respiration or position

RELIEF

Rest or nitroglycerin; rarely affected by body position

TABLE 9-3
Differentiating Characteristics of Chest Pain

Precipitating factors	Character	Relief
CARDIOVASCULAR		
Effort angina		
Exercise, emotion, extreme temperatures, eating heavy meals	Constricting, squeezing, pressure; usually lasting more than 2 minutes and less than 15 minutes	Rest or nitroglycerin
Rest angina		
Spontaneous; possible daily cycle	Like effort angina	Nitroglycerin
Acute myocardial infarction		
Spontaneous	Like angina but more severe, crushing; usually lasting longer than 20 minutes	Narcotic analgesics, rest or nitroglycerin not effective
Pericarditis		
Deep breath, lying down	Sharp, stabbing; continuous	Antiinflammatories, analgesics, sitting up, leaning forward
Hypertrophic cardiomyopathy		
Exercise, stress	Anginal pain associated with lightheadedness, dizziness, syncope	Rest, β-blockers
Mitral valve prolapse		
Spontaneous	Variable in character, possibly migratory	Time
Acute dissecting aortic aneurysm		
Spontaneous	Sudden, severe, tearing pain in center of chest, radiating to back or abdomen	Large doses of analgesics
PULMONARY		
Pulmonary embolism		
Spontaneous; accentuated by dyspnea and pleuritic respiration	Sharp, stabbing, knifelike; continuous	Time
Pleurisy		
History of recent respiratory illness; worse with respiratory movement	Sharp, burning, ache or "catch" on one side of the chest	Time
MUSCULOSKELETAL		
Coughing, deep breath, movement	Sharp, stabbing, tenderness, localized; fleeting or lasting for days	Antiinflammatories, analgesics, time
GASTROINTESTINAL		
Gastric or duodenal ulcer		
Empty stomach	Burning in epigastrium 60 to 90 minutes after eating	Milk or antacids
Esophageal spasm or irritation		
Spontaneous	Burning deep in throat; accompanying weight loss, dysphagia, regurgitation	Nitroglycerin
OTHER		
Emotional stress		
Stress stimulus	Tightness, aching; if accompanied by hyperventilation, possible ST-segment and T-wave changes	Stimulus removal
Mediastinitis or mediastinal tumors		
Spontaneous	Pleuritic, constriction	Time Removal of mass
Tissue rupture or tear		
Blunt injury	Abrupt, sharp	Time, repair

morning hygiene activities such as shaving or bathing. However, they may exercise vigorously later in the day without incident. Patients also might experience angina during an activity, rest until the discomfort subsides, and resume the activity without further discomfort. When activity tolerance is variable, the ischemia is thought to be caused by atherosclerotic plaque and vasospasm.[73,112]

Angina pectoris also may have *atypical features*. The site of pain or discomfort may be limited to the usual radiation locations, and chest pain or discomfort may be absent. The chief complaint may be breathlessness, dyspnea, faintness, fatigue, or exhaustion that begins abruptly and originates in the substernal area. These are considered *anginal equivalents* if the rest of the history is consistent with myocardial ischemia.[14,73]

Exchanging pattern

Observing and examining patients during anginal episodes is important because impaired physiologic exchange and evidence of left or right ventricular failure may be found.[112,119,139] Patients may appear distressed or frightened and short of breath. Their skin may be pale, moist, and cool. Variations in vital signs depend on the intensity of pain, level of anxiety, and degree of ventricular dysfunction. Hypertension or hypotension and tachycardia may occur.

Usually physical examination of patients with angina pectoris is unremarkable when they are not having pain. Evidence of factors contributing to the development of atherosclerosis (for example, obesity, hypertension, or indicators of hyperlipidemia [xanthomas or xanthelasmas]) might be present (see Chapter 8). Physical findings on inspection and auscultation of the heart are generally normal, unless there are valvular dysfunctions such as aortic or mitral stenosis. On palpation, a dyskinetic apical impulse may be found. Auscultation may reveal signs of ventricular failure such as crackles; a systolic murmur of mitral regurgitation, indicating papillary muscle dysfunction; pulsus alternans; paradoxical splitting of the second sound; or a third or fourth heart sound. Symptoms and manifestations present during anginal episodes usually subside with relief of ischemia, which is usually concurrent with pain relief.[15,112,119,139]

Knowing and choosing patterns

The Knowing and Choosing Patterns are closely associated with each other in angina pectoris because the patient's knowledge and choices regarding risk factors are interconnected. The presence of coronary artery disease (CAD) risk factors strongly influences the diagnosis. Major risk factors include cigarette smoking, hypertension, and hypercholesterolemia, although others may be present. The contributing risks of family history of CAD, left ventricular hypertrophy, obesity, and diabetes mellitus, as well as the patient's age, sex, and race, should be identified. The pa-tient's lifestyle should be assessed regarding habits (eating, sleeping, relaxation, and exercise), stressors (emotional and physical), and coping styles (individual and family).[65,97,123] The patient's knowledge and understanding of risk factors, chest pain, angina, and myocardial infarction should be evaluated. Willingness and ability to manage risk factors and comply with a therapeutic regimen also should be explored.[20,40,107,141]

Relating and perceiving patterns

For some patients, a confirmed medical diagnosis of CAD and angina pectoris interferes with role performance and self-concept. These aspects of patient response can be anticipated by reviewing current social relationships, occupational roles, self-concept, and related concerns. Patients with stressful social and occupational roles should be identified. Persons whose occupations make them responsible for the safety of others (e.g., airline pilots and bus drivers) may be prevented from continuing employment after the diagnosis of angina pectoris is made.[73,112] Patients' estimates of the impact of their illness, self-concept, and self-esteem should be assessed.[20,40,107,141] Denial, adjustment to illness, and coping strategies are also assessed.

Diagnostic tests and procedures
Biochemical tests

Serum levels of cardiac enzymes are measured to distinguish angina pectoris from MI. These levels are normal in persons with angina pectoris and elevated in persons with AMI (see Chapters 6 and 10). Hypercholesterolemia and glucose intolerance indicate the presence of CAD risk factors.[73,112]

ECG

At least one half to three fourths of patients with a history of angina pectoris have a normal ECG during rest.[72] Others may have evidence of an old MI such as Q waves of at least 0.04 second or persistent ST-segment elevation. There also may be evidence of left ventricular hypertrophy with a strain pattern (ST-segment depression) that is generally a result of hypertension. Because angina pectoris is the manifestation of myocardial hypoxia, there may be ECG evidence of myocardial ischemia during an anginal attack.[72,112]

The patient should be instructed to report episodes of angina.[72,112,117] It is valuable to obtain a 12-lead ECG during anginal episodes so that ECG changes can be detected and documented. ECGs obtained during anginal episodes most often reveal ST-segment depression, T-wave inversion, or both, which are common ECG representations of myocardial ischemia. These abnormalities may resolve and return to baseline with the resolution of anginal symptoms, or they may persist. Prinzmetal's angina, which is caused by coronary artery spasm, may manifest itself on the ECG as ST-segment elevation during anginal attacks. Elevated ST segments normally return to baseline after symptoms subside.[72,100,112,145]

Exercise ECG

Exercise ECG (Figure 9-3) has become an important prognostic tool in evaluating the patient with angina pectoris.[72,112,119,139] The procedure was developed to stress the heart and reproduce anginal symptoms under controlled, monitored conditions. Common stress tests include the treadmill, bicycle ergometry, and occasionally the master two-step test (see Chapter 6). The patient exercises until a defined end point is reached. These end points include (1) a predicted maximal heart rate (calculated by the patient's age and sex), (2) development of angina pectoris, (3) hypotension, (4) ventricular dysrhythmias, (5) ECG changes consistent with myocardial ischemia (i.e., at least 2 mm of ST-segment depression or downward sloping persisting at least 0.08 second after the J point), or (6) exhaustion.

Exercise electrocardiography is of limited value in determining the presence or absence of CAD.[112,128] The results of the test are used to determine the severity of ischemic heart disease and the patient's prognosis.[31,33,53,128] Patients who develop chest pain and ST-segment depression

at a light level of activity during an exercise test (less than 4 metabolic equivalents [METs]) are much more likely to have subsequent coronary events (i.e., progression of angina, MI, and sudden death) than patients who exhibit only ST-segment depression or those who have pain and ST-segment depression at a heavier workload (greater than 8 to 9 METs).[28]

Atrial pacing during cardiac catheterization also may be used to stress the heart. In this procedure a pacing wire is inserted into the atrium and stimulates the heart to beat at an accelerated rate (up to 180 beats per minute). The procedure is terminated when the predicted heart rate is achieved, anginal symptoms occur, or ECG changes indicating myocardial ischemia are seen.

Nuclear cardiac imaging

Nuclear cardiac imaging is used to identify areas of myocardial ischemia and infarction. The technique combines intravenous injection of radioisotopes with scintigraphic imaging of the myocardium. Several approaches may be used, including thallium perfusion ("cold spot") myocardial scintigraphy with and without exercise; radionuclide cineventriculography (multiple-gated acquisition [MUGA] or first-pass scanning); and technetium ("hot

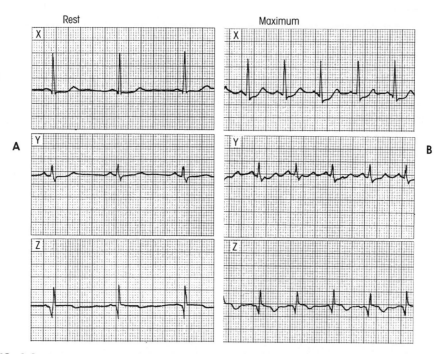

FIG. 9-3 Exercise ECG. **A,** The preexercise tracing shows nonspecific ST-segment depression in leads X and Y. **B,** The postexercise tracing of the same patient shows classic ST-segment depression in leads X and Y and ST-segment elevation in lead Z. These changes are diagnostic of myocardial ischemia.

Courtesy Janet Park and Frankie Kirkwood, Exercise Laboratory, Dallas Veteran's Administration Medical Center, Dallas, Texas.

spot") myocardial infarct scanning (see Chapter 6).[125] In persons with angina pectoris, nuclear cardiac imaging is used to assess myocardial perfusion at rest and during exercise.[133]

Thallium-201, a physiologic analogue of potassium, accumulates in areas of perfused myocardium highlighting normal myocardial tissue. Areas of necrosis or ischemia are represented by a perfusion defect ("cold spot") on the myocardial scintigram. Defects that persist for several hours suggest myocardial necrosis, whereas defects that reperfuse indicate transient myocardial ischemia. Thallium-201 scintigraphy is a useful noninvasive method of evaluating the extent of ischemic heart disease, particularly when used with exercise testing (see Fig. 6-18).

Technetium-99m, a pyrophosphate imaging agent, binds to calcium in acutely and irreversibly damaged myocardial cells to give a visual representation of myocardial necrosis ("hot spot"). Unfortunately the isotope does not redistribute with time in proportion to myocardial mass, so repeated studies must be spaced about a week apart.[128] This isotope is used in radionuclide cineventriculography (MUGA or first-pass scanning) and technetium myocardial infarct scanning.[125] Technetium techniques are especially useful in the diagnosis of recent or acute MI (Fig. 10-7). Other noninvasive radioisotope techniques for evaluating patients with angina pectoris or other ischemic cardiac disease are being developed (see Chapter 6).[128]

Cardiac catheterization and coronary angiography

Cardiac catheterization and coronary angiography are the most invasive diagnostic tests (see Chapter 6). In patients with angina pectoris the purposes of the procedures are to evaluate left ventricular performance, determine the extent of atherosclerotic disease in the coronary arteries, evaluate valvular performance, determine the presence of other cardiac disease, and determine whether the patient is a suitable candidate for percutaneous transluminal coronary angio-plasty (PTCA) or coronary artery bypass graft (CABG) surgery.

Cardiac catheterization is done to assess cardiac chamber pressures, oxygen saturation values, valvular function, and ventricular function and wall motion performance. Coronary angiography is performed to assess the coronary anatomic structures, including the location and degree of coronary artery obstruction (see Figure 6-20). Although they have some risks, these procedures have a low mortality rate[112] (see Chapter 6).

Medical and nursing diagnoses

Patients with the medical diagnosis of angina pectoris are at high risk for developing cardiac dysrhythmias and MI, as well as sudden death. The most common human responses anticipated for a patient with angina pectoris are indicated by the following nursing diagnoses:[21,88]

1. Acute or chronic pain and activity intolerance related to inadequate myocardial tissue perfusion
2. Anxiety related to situational and treatment-related factors
3. High risk for ineffective denial* and high risk for noncompliance† related to knowledge deficit and situational and treatment-related factors

For each diagnosis, the patient outcomes, nursing prescriptions, and evaluation criteria are outlined with a discussion of the factual information that supports the plan and implementation of care.

---

*At the 1990 NANDA Conference the Taxonomic Committee submitted a recommendation that "Ineffective denial" be changed to "Impaired denial." The authors suggest the term *Inappropriate denial.*

†The NANDA Taxonomy uses the term *noncompliance.* Many clinicians object to this label. McFarland and McFarlane[88] indicate that *nonadherence* might be a preferable term. Carey[20] suggests that the attitude and ethical approach of the health professional is most important. Clinicians should use terminology that allows them, patients, and families to set mutual goals.

NURSING DIAGNOSIS 1
Acute or chronic pain and activity intolerance related to inadequate myocardial tissue perfusion (feeling and moving patterns)

PATIENT OUTCOMES	NURSING PRESCRIPTIONS	EVALUATION
Patient will describe pain or discomfort.	Assess for pain or discomfort.	Patient described pain or discomfort.
Patient will not experience prolonged pain or discomfort. Patient will report relief of pain or discomfort.	Administer prescribed antianginal agents and analgesics to provide optimal therapeutic and prophylactic pain relief.	Patient reported that antianginal agents and analgesics reduced, relieved, or prevented pain.
Patient will institute measures to avoid, modify, or control pain or discomfort.	Assess and prevent, reduce, or eliminate factors that decrease pain tolerance or increase pain; including activity, emotional stress, fatigue, eating heavy meals, and cold or hot environment.	Patient identified factors related to the pain experience and instituted measures to avoid, modify, or control their influence; factors include activity, relaxation exercises, rest, diet, and environmental control.
Patient will demonstrate and report improved activity tolerance.	Institute measures to reduce myocardial work and oxygen demand.	Patient reported improved activity tolerance.
Angina will not be precipitated by activity.	Reduce activity below anginal threshold.	Patient reported that angina was not precipitated by activity.
A higher level of activity will be tolerated after patient participates in a therapeutic activity and rest program.	Institute a therapeutic activity and rest program to improve activity tolerance.	Patient tolerated a higher level of activity after participating in the program.
Patient will demonstrate and report fewer episodes of angina after therapy.	Educate about measures to improve myocardial perfusion; including medications, PTCA, CABG surgery.	Patient reported fewer episodes of angina after therapy.

Plan and intervention for acute or chronic pain and activity intolerance

The major symptoms of angina pectoris, pain or discomfort and activity intolerance, are caused by inadequate myocardial tissue perfusion. If symptoms persist, it is assumed that acute coronary insufficiency is continuing, and complications such as cardiac dysrhythmias or MI could ensue. The foremost goals of relief and prevention of pain and activity intolerance are accomplished by restoring adequate myocardial tissue perfusion. Management of the person with angina pectoris* includes measures that increase coronary blood flow (oxygen supply) and measures that decrease myocardial work load (oxygen demand). Medications such as nitroglycerin, morphine, β-adrenergic blockers, and calcium-channel blockers, as well as modification of activity levels, are used to correct the imbalance between myocardial oxygen supply and demand. Reducing CAD risk factors to reverse, halt, or retard the progression of atherosclerosis (see Chapter 8) and treating other underlying disease is important. If drug therapy, activity modification, and risk factor reduction fail to produce an ac-

ceptable angina-free state, PTCA or myocardial revascularization may be indicated.

Angina should be regarded as a chronic illness, and techniques that assist the patient to cope with the symptoms and other stressors should also be instituted.* Relaxation and education are important interventions that assist in pain management.[21,88,105]

Medications

The goals of drug therapy in angina are to decrease the duration and intensity of pain during acute anginal episodes, prevent or decrease the frequency of attacks, and improve work capacity although angina may occur.[35,71,89] Achieving these goals may prevent or delay cardiac dysrhythmias, MI, and sudden death (see Appendix C).

Nitrate therapy. Nitrates or nitrites are a class of drugs that relax most of the smooth muscles in the body, including those of the vascular system. Relaxation of vascular smooth muscle results in vasodilation. The efficacy of the nitrates is thought to result from the hemodynamic effects of vasodilation in the coronary arteries and peripheral ves-

---

*References 8, 18, 19, 89, 125, 133, and 134.

*References 8, 18, 19, 89, 125, 133, and 134.

sels. Dilation of the coronary arteries increases and redistributes coronary blood flow and thus improves myocardial oxygen supply. In the peripheral circulation, dilation of the venous capacitance vessels causes blood to pool in the peripheral veins. This reduces venous blood return to the heart and cardiac preload. Dilation of peripheral arterioles reduces systemic vascular resistance and cardiac afterload, resulting in decreased myocardial work load and oxygen demand. Thus nitrates aid in balancing myocardial tissue perfusion by increasing oxygen supply and decreasing oxygen demand.[35] Multiple-dose forms are available, allowing therapy to be tailored to the individual. The onset and duration of action varies with the form.

Short-acting nitrate preparations, nitroglycerin, are available for administration by the inhalation, intravenous, buccal, and sublingual routes. Sublingual nitroglycerin is most often used for acute episodes. Headache, the result of cerebral vasodilation, is the most common adverse effect. It is usually transient, lasting 5 to 20 minutes. Headaches that last longer usually can be controlled by lowering the nitrate dosage or by prescribing mild analgesics, acetaminophen, or aspirin. The patient should be instructed to sit or lie down when taking the medication because hypotension and syncope may occur because of the reduction in vascular resistance.

Long-acting preparations, nitroglycerin and isosorbide dinitrate, are available for administration by the buccal, oral, topical, and transdermal routes. Long-acting nitrates are of little value in relieving acute attacks of angina pectoris, but they do appear to be beneficial in preventing and reducing the duration of attacks.[42] Long-acting nitrate therapy usually is instituted for the person with angina pectoris, especially if there is an unstable pattern.*

Morphine sulfate. When nitroglycerin fails to relieve anginal pain, morphine sulfate may be administered. The use of morphine raises the pain perception threshold, reduces anxiety and fear, induces sleep, causes venous pooling, and decreases myocardial oxygen requirements.[26,89]

β-adrenergic blockers. β-adrenergic blocking agents act by blocking catecholamine stimulation of the β-adrenergic receptors. β_1-receptors are located in the myocardium and kidney. β_2-receptors are located in the bronchioles and arterial smooth muscles. Blocking β_1 receptors reduces the myocardial response to stimulation by the sympathetic nervous system. This results in decreased heart rate and myocardial contractility (reduced oxygen demand) and alleviates anginal symptoms. Blocking β_2 receptors limits relaxation of arterial and bronchiole smooth muscle. There are numerous β-adrenergic blockers under investigation. In the United States, atenolol (Tenormin), metoprolol (Lopressor), nadolol (Corgard), and propranolol (Inderal) are available and approved for use in angina pectoris.[26,84,89]

There is no clear difference in their antianginal effects. Those that are selective for β_1 sites are less likely to cause pulmonary or peripheral vascular side effects. Those that are less lipid soluble are less likely to cause central nervous system side effects. Of the drugs listed, atenolol is the only one that is less lipid soluble and β_1 selective.

Most of the adverse effects of the β-blockers stem from their blockade of β-receptors. Careful monitoring of the patient is necessary because bradycardia, left ventricular dysfunction, hypotension, and congestive heart failure may result from β-blockade in the heart. β-blockers are contraindicated in patients with asthma and obstructive pulmonary disease because blockade of β_2-receptors in the lungs may compromise pulmonary function. Lethargy, weakness, fatigue, mental depression, psychosis, and sexual dysfunction may result from effects on the central nervous system.[41,112]

Generally, doses of the β-blockers are adjusted to meet the needs of individuals. As the dose increases, β_1 medications lose their selectivity and affect β_1- and β_2-receptors. The dose is considered appropriate if heart rate is 55 to 60 beats per minute at rest and does not exceed 90 to 100 beats per minute with exercise.[41,112] β-blocking agents are usually more successful in relieving activity-induced myocardial ischemia than that induced by vasospasm. Combined nitrate and β-adrenergic blockade therapy may improve myocardial perfusion and reduce ischemia more than either drug used alone.*

Calcium-channel blockers. Calcium-channel blocking agents block the passage of calcium ions across myocardial cell membranes to cause vasodilation of the coronary arteries and collateral vessels, vasodilation of the peripheral arteries, decrease of the contractile force of the myocardium, and decrease of cardiac workload. Coronary blood flow is increased and myocardial oxygen demands are decreased with the institution of these drugs. Calcium-channel blockers are more successful than β-blockers in alleviating vasospasm, so they are often prescribed for patients with unstable and Prinzmetal's angina. Calcium-channel blockade combined with nitrate therapy or β-blockade may produce more beneficial effects at lower doses than either drug used alone. However, the use of several therapeutic agents also increases the likelihood of adverse effects.[84]

Verapamil (Isoptin, Calan), nifedipine (Procardia), and diltiazem (Cardizem) have been approved by the Food and Drug Administration for the treatment of angina pectoris. Although they have similar results, they act in slightly different ways, and one or the other may be preferred for an individual (see Appendix C). Adverse reactions of bradycardia, heart block, and congestive heart failure are less likely to occur when nifedipine is used. Hypotension, flush-

*References 26, 84, 89, 102, 112, 119, 134, and 139.

*References 26, 84, 89, 102, 112, 119, 134, and 139.

ing, and headache are less likely with diltiazem or verapamil.[112]

Activity

Myocardial ischemia is caused by levels of activity that increase the myocardial workload so that myocardial oxygen demand exceeds the available oxygen supply. When anginal symptoms result, patients have exceeded the anginal threshold. Patients will need to tailor or adjust their activity levels to relieve or avoid the myocardial ischemia and pain or discomfort.[12]

During acute episodes of pain, activity should be reduced to bed or chair rest. Most patients are not comfortable lying flat and prefer to have the head of the bed elevated or sit in a chair. Emotional and environmental stress are decreased by a quiet, dimly lit, comfortably warm room and reduced traffic from professionals and overanxious visitors. Relaxation exercises should be used to reduce anxiety initially and on a regular basis. Sleep should be promoted if fatigue was a precipitating factor, and light, low-fat meals should be served.

Patients may find that they can avoid pain by taking nitroglycerin before engaging in activities that usually precipitate angina. During activity, they should avoid hurried paces and extreme cold or hot environmental temperatures. They should also participate in a therapeutic program designed to improve body conditioning and exercise tolerance.

Revascularization

Myocardial revascularization is indicated when drug therapy, activity modification, and risk factor reduction fail to produce an acceptable angina-free state.[112,138] PTCA and CABG surgery are two approaches to myocardial revascularization. Not all patients can benefit from these techniques that increase coronary blood flow by dilating or bypassing obstructions in the coronary arteries. If PTCA or CABG surgery are planned, the nurse must provide support and teaching. The patient should be aware of the nature of the procedure, the risks, and the benefits. In addition, the patient must be aware that neither method is a curative; they are only palliative. The patient must understand that the resolution of symptoms does not indicate that the atherosclerotic process has been stopped. CAD risk factors still must be altered, exercise must be encouraged, stress must be reduced, and dietary habits must be changed to reduce accelerated progression of the disease process. A confident, knowledgeable approach should be used to convey this information to the patient.

Angioplasty

PTCA is a procedure that has been introduced as an alternative to CABG surgery for selected patients. The optimal PTCA candidate has a short history (less than 1 year) of angina that is refractory to medical therapy and has

compressible, noncalcified, concentric, discrete (less than 1 cm in length) atherosclerotic plaques in the proximal portions of the coronary arteries. During the procedure, a balloon-tipped catheter is maneuvered so that the balloon lies within the lumen of the coronary lesion. The balloon is then inflated to compress the lesion against the arterial wall.

It is not clear whether dilation of the vessel results from compression and redistribution of the atherosclerotic plaque or disruption of the intima with stretching of the media and adventitia. Several mechanisms probably come into play. Compression of the atheroma may occur,* but a controlled injury with splitting of the atheromatous plaque, intimal disruption, and endothelial desquamation[10,11,23,96] has also been demonstrated.[83,104,121] The healing process is thought to contribute to successful dilation, with development of local aneurysm and an autoimmune response that produces reabsorption and retraction of damaged material.[83] (Fig. 9-4).

History of the procedure. Transluminal angioplasty began with the work of Dotter and Judkins in 1964.[39] They developed a percutaneous technique that used coaxial catheters of increasing sizes passed over a guide wire to successfully dilate the atherosclerotic segments of peripheral arteries. During the 1970s, Gruntzig, Senning, and Siegenthaler[58] developed a miniaturized balloon-catheter system and performed the first human PTCA in September 1977. By July 1979, they had completed 50 PTCA procedures, reporting a 66% success rate.[58] The National Heart, Lung, and Blood Institute (NHLBI) recognized the impact of this procedure and established a registry to help evaluate its merits. The Early Registry enrolled more than 3000 patients from 1979 to 1981. The data showed a primary reperfusion success rate of 68%, with restenosis occurring in 30%. Failure to cross or dilate the lesions were the major reasons for lack of initial success. Complications included emergency CABG surgery (6.1%), nonfatal MI (4.9%), and death (1.3%).[37,121] Catheters were redesigned, and the NHLBI opened a Late Registry in 1985. Data demonstrated an increase in success to 91%, with restenosis remaining 25% to 30%.[7,34,121]

There have been few long-term studies of the efficacy of PTCA.[47,69] A long-term follow-up study[59] of 133 patients successfully treated in Zurich, showed that at 10 years 90 patients (68%) had no symptoms and that only 5 cardiac deaths (4%) had occurred. Repeat angioplasty was done in 27 patients, and CABG was done in 19 patients. A 5 year follow-up study[130] of 427 patients treated at Emory University Hospital revealed that 79% were free of cardiac events and 97% were still alive. Two randomized trials funded by the National Institutes of Health are underway. The Emory Angioplasty Study Surgery Trial

---

*References 7, 10, 39, 57, 58, 67.

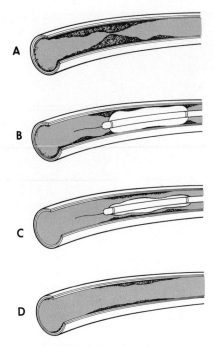

FIG. 9-4   Effect of PTCA on atherosclerotic lesions. **A,** Plaque before PTCA. **B,** Inflation of angioplasty balloon. **C,** Plaque after PTCA. **D,** Six months after PTCA, the plaque has retracted even farther.

From Beare PG and Myers JL: Principles and practice of adult health nursing, St Louis, 1989, The CV Mosby Co.

(EAST) began in 1987. A multicenter trial by the Bypass Angioplasty Revascularization Investigation (BARI) began in 1988. Both studies compare angioplasty and CABG surgery.[77]

Patient evaluation. Candidates for PTCA are carefully selected and screened. All candidates must have disabling angina pectoris that does not respond to maximal medical therapy. Objective evidence of angina is documented to facilitate follow-up evaluation. A complete history and physical examination, ECG, exercise ECG, and coronary angiography are performed. The extent of the disease and exact location of the lesion determine whether PTCA is the treatment of choice. Patients with lesions in the left main stem are usually not offered PTCA. In the past, only patients with single-vessel disease were considered good candidates. With advances in technique, physicians in many centers are successfully performing PTCA on patients with multiple lesions.[83,112]

Procedure. During the procedure a balloon-tipped catheter is guided into the coronary artery lesion so that the balloon lies in the lumen of the lesion. Then the balloon is inflated briefly so that the atheromatous material is compressed against the vessel wall. In this manner, the coronary artery stenosis is reduced and myocardial perfusion is improved directly without the need for CABG surgery.

Patients undergoing PTCA are brought to the cardiac catheterization laboratory, where the femoral or brachial area is prepared and a local anesthetic is administered. A venous catheter with a cardiac pacemaker lead is usually inserted in the vein and advanced to the right side of the heart or the pulmonary artery. This catheter is used as an anatomic marker during the procedure (Fig. 9-5, *A*), for cardiac pacing if necessary and to monitor pressures on the right side of the heart.

Two arterial catheters, a guiding catheter and a dilating catheter, are used during PTCA. The guiding catheter is preshaped to engage the ostium of the coronary artery requiring dilatation. At the tip of the catheter is a short, highly flexible, soft wire that guides the dilating catheter through the artery, preventing injury to the arterial wall. The dilating catheter is a double-lumen, polyvinylchloride, inflatable but nondistensible balloon-tipped catheter. The balloon is 2, 3, or 3.7 mm in diameter and 20 mm in length. This catheter also contains two distal side ports for monitoring pressure or infusing medications or contrast media.

After the venous catheter is in place, the guiding catheter is inserted into the artery. It is advanced retrogradely through the ascending aorta and into the ostium of the right or left coronary artery. Angiography is performed to ensure that the lesion has not changed in a manner that would contraindicate PTCA. The dilating catheter then is inserted through the guiding catheter into the coronary artery and manipulated into the stenotic area of the artery. Angiograms are taken at frequent intervals to identify the exact location of the catheter and lesion. Minute amounts of contrast material are used to make the artery barely visible angiographically. Continuous pressure monitoring reduces the risk of occluding the coronary artery ostium and allows measurement of the pressure gradient across the lesion. As the catheter enters the lesion, the pressure measured at the tip of the catheter falls, yielding the distal coronary perfusion pressure.[7,30,58,83]

The balloon is then inflated with a mixture of 50% contrast medium and 50% saline for 3 to 5 seconds and then deflated (Fig. 9-5, *B* and *C*). Inflation is controlled by a pressure pump, which allows selection of pressures from 3 to 6.5 atmospheres. The pressure across the lesion is again measured to determine the pressure gradient after dilation. The number of dilations can vary, depending on the response of the distal perfusion pressure to successive increases in inflation pressure.

Angiography is repeated at the end of the procedure to evaluate the effect of angioplasty.[7,58,83] Successful PTCA yields a 20% or greater decrease in the degree of coronary stenosis and a decrease in the pressure gradient across the lesion.[75,101] After the procedure, arterial and venous sheaths are left in place for a period of time in case complications occur and emergency vascular access is required.

A

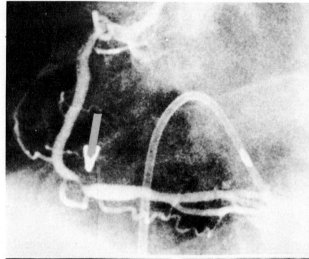

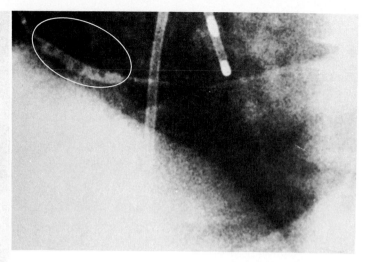

B

C

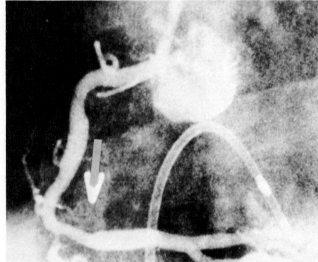

FIG. 9-5 Arteriograms during PTCA. **A,** High-grade lesion of right coronary artery *(arrow)* before balloon inflation; transvenous cardiac pacemaker lead *(left of arrow)* is used as an anatomic marker. **B,** Balloon catheter is inserted through the lesion, and the balloon is inflated. **C,** Same lesion *(arrow)* viewed after balloon inflation and catheter removal.

Nursing care. Nursing care of the PTCA patient must be individualized and goal directed.[74,133] A holistic approach, beginning with a thorough biopsychosocial assessment, is essential. Special attention should be given to the cardiovascular system and any physical or psychologic process that may complicate recovery after PTCA. A complete data base must be gathered and recorded to facilitate the identification of individual problems and needs.

Patient education needs are acute because this procedure is usually carried out as an emergency. Many new concepts must be understood by these patients before they will be able to give their informed consent. About 7% of these patients will require emergency CABG surgery, and appropriate preoperative teaching is required.[37,121]

After the patient's readiness to learn and current knowledge and perceptions related to the procedure are assessed, several areas specific to PTCA should be discussed. The physician should describe PTCA thoroughly with special attention to the procedure, statistics, complications, alter-

natives, and follow-up care. The nurse should reinforce these areas and be prepared to answer questions that the patient might have. Anticipatory guidance is used to ensure a thorough understanding of all aspects of the procedure and care. Because of the necessity to gather long-term statistical information, the patient usually is asked to return for a medical evaluation. The importance of follow-up evaluation must be explained thoroughly to gain the support of the patient. The patient will have many questions, and the nurse needs to anticipate and prepare for them.

Close monitoring and astute observational skills are a necessity after the procedure because major complications can develop suddenly. Nursing care includes monitoring, detecting, and reporting the complications shown in Table 9-4. Chest pain or other anginal symptoms should not occur if PTCA was successful. Therefore if these symptoms appear, they should be evaluated and reported to the physician quickly because they require emergency intervention. Complications of the cannulated limb also require rapid

TABLE 9-4
Complications of PTCA

Complications	Signs and symptoms	Usual management
Abrupt coronary artery reclosure Coronary artery rupture Myocardial ischemia or MI	Chest pain and anginal symptoms ST-segment depression or elevation Cardiac tamponade signs and symptoms Hypotension Tachycardia Dysrhythmias	Depending on cause: medications, intravenous fluids, recatheterization, intraaortic balloon pump, or emergency CABG surgery
Bleeding at the catheter insertion site	Bleeding Swelling Hematoma Pain Hypotension Tachycardia Shock signs and symptoms	Manual pressure held on the site (30 minutes or more) until all evidence of bleeding has subsided Avoidance of flexion of the hip for several hours
Occlusive thrombus at the insertion site Ischemia of cannulated extremity	Diminished or absent pulses Numbness or pain Pallor	Heparin Embolectomy

treatment. Emotional status must be assessed after successful or unsuccessful PTCA, and appropriate psychologic support should be given to the patient.

Discharge planning should include teaching the patient about take-home medications, CAD risk factor intervention, management if symptoms recur, and follow-up assessment. There is usually no activity restriction after discharge.

Follow-up. Results of PTCA are evaluated primarily by monitoring clinical symptoms. If PTCA is successful, the patient will not have anginal symptoms. Return of chest pain or other anginal discomfort indicates abrupt reclosure or restenosis. Exercise testing combined with thallium imaging and radionuclide ventriculography are used to objectively measure myocardial perfusion. Patients are not routinely followed by angiography, although the procedure may be needed in high-risk patients, airline pilots, and bus drivers.[7,101] Successful PTCA avoids the discomfort, lengthy hospital stay, and risk of complications associated with CABG surgery. The cost to the patient is reduced substantially.

Complications. Complications occur during or immediately after the procedure in about 10% of patients.[112] Minor complications include emergency recatheterization, side-branch closure, blood loss requiring transfusion, and femoral artery damage requiring repair. Abrupt reclosure may result in the need for emergency CABG surgery, major complications such as AMI, or death.[112]

Because complications that require emergency CABG surgery may arise, all candidates for PTCA must be acceptable candidates for CABG surgery and accept this as the alternative treatment in case PTCA fails. Patients are asked to sign consent forms for surgery, as well as for PTCA, and the entire open-heart surgical team must be on standby in the hospital during PTCA procedures.[77] The likelihood of complications is increased in patients who are women, have left ventricular damage, have few collateral vessels distal to the stenosis, have long eccentric or irregular lesions, or have calcified plaques.[112,119]

Abrupt reclosure may occur immediately or within 24 hours of dilation due to dissection, vasospasm, or thrombosis and cause prolonged angina leading to MI or sudden death. Efforts to recanalize the vessel begin with emergency recatheterization and intracoronary infusion of calcium-channel blocking or thrombolytic agents. Placement of a *coronary artery shunt catheter* may be done as a temporary measure to protect the myocardium while the patient is transported to the operating room for revascularization. Emergency CABG surgery is required if the coronary artery does not reopen, dissects, or ruptures. Various medications, including nifedipine, heparin, dipyridamole, low-molecular-weight dextran, and nitroglycerin, as well as investigational medications, are used prophylactically in efforts to avoid abrupt reclosure.

Data from the NHLBI registry indicates that, although primary success is achieved in 91% of patients, restenosis occurs within 6 months in 25% to 30% of patients.[7,77,121] Repeat PTCA is recommended as the treatment of choice. Some patients may require three or four dilation procedures before long-term patency is secured.[7] If restenosis does not develop within 6 months of dilation, it is unlikely to do so in future years.[47] However, anginal symptoms may recur resulting from progression of disease at other sites.[7,101]

Techniques that reduce the incidence of restenosis and abrupt closure such as laser angioplasty, coronary atherectomy, and intravascular stents are currently under investigation and may be combined with balloon angioplasty.[7,63,121] A laser may be used to vaporize the contents of the atheromatous lesion or to thermally weld the internal portion of the lesion. In *coronary atherectomy,* the plaque is stripped from the vessel. *Intravascular stents* may be placed to hold the coronary artery lumen open.*

Laser angioplasty

Lasers (light amplification by stimulated emission of radiation) are being used for various cardiovascular applications, including recanalization of occluded vessels before balloon angioplasty, sealing of intimal aberrations after balloon angioplasty, promotion of revascularization of the myocardium, ablation of aberrant conduction pathways, and resection of stenotic valves or hypertrophic myocardium.[113]

Lasers emit monochromatic (single-wavelength) light energy that is selectively absorbed by cardiovascular tissue, thus creating the thermal effects of coagulation or vaporization, depending on the dose of light emitted. The light can be transmitted via a flexible optical fiber, and because they are of small diameter (i.e., 600 microns) and because the monochromatic light can be focused to a very small spot size, the vaporizing effect can be used like a "light knife" to precisely ablate tissue. The bare fiber can be passed percutaneously for a transluminal approach to recanalize obstructed coronary vessels or to remodel structures within the heart chambers using a *direct beam of laser light.* The major complication using a bare fiber is vessel wall perforation. Perforations may occur when the fiber is passed through bends in thin walled vessels, the fiber is not centered coaxially in the arterial lumen, or there are nonuniform thermal effects along the vessel wall.

In addition to the direct-beam technique, laser energy can be used to *heat a metal or sapphire tip* attached to the end of the fiberoptic catheter. The tipped catheter is directed through an arterial catheter and used as a probe to recanalize atherosclerotic plaque in occluded vessels. This technique has resulted in less-frequent vessel perforation. *Laser-assisted balloon angioplasty* also holds promise for alleviating obstructed coronary arteries. Conventional balloon angioplasty is followed by use of a laser to "seal" the vessel lumen, leaving a smoother, less thrombotic surface.

Improving fiberoptic guidance through arterial vessels will assist in improving safety and increasing efficacy. Fluoroscopic guidance is commonly used, but other techniques such as angiographic, ultrasonic, or spectroscopic guidance may offer more precision. Several different wavelengths of lasers are being evaluated for their effects on recanalization and prevention of restenosis; these include argon (Ar, 488 to 514 nanometers [nm]—blue green), carbon dioxide (CO_2, 10600 nm—far infrared), neodimium-yittrium aluminum garnet (Nd-YAG, 1060 nm—near infrared), and excimer (308 nm—ultraviolet). The potential of using percutaneous lasers to open occluded vessels appears promising and less costly, with fewer complications than CABG surgical procedures.

An alternative approach to revascularization of the myocardium is the formation of *transmural left ventricular conduits.* Preliminary results indicate that direct revascularization using a carbon dioxide laser is a viable alternative for individuals with diffuse or small vessel disease and those who have had previous bypass procedures with poor results. The procedure is performed during open heart surgery and may be combined with CABG surgery. Carbon dioxide laser-light energy is used to create channels from the left ventricular cavity into ischemic myocardial tissue. This frequency of laser energy is highly absorbed by water in biologic tissues, and the tissue can be precisely removed without manipulation or damage to surrounding tissue. Bleeding after the procedure is not a problem because there is coagulation of vessels in the zone immediately around the channel. The laser energy does not adversely affect contractility, heart rate, arterial pressure, or electrical activity.[94] Although other techniques for creating myocardial conduits have resulted in premature closure by fibrosis and scarring,[80,85] channels created with the carbon dioxide lasers have endothelialized and remained patent for up to 2 years.[90,91]

CABG surgery

CABG surgery consists of bypassing significant obstructive lesions in the coronary arteries with the internal mammary artery or with saphenous vein bypass grafts. Any number of diseased major vessels or their branches may be bypassed, depending on the surgeon's preference and experience, the caliber of the diseased vessels, and the location of the lesions (see Chapter 17). The principle of myocardial revascularization is to increase coronary blood flow to the myocardium, which increases the myocardial oxygen supply and prevents angina pectoris. Patients whose symptoms are predominantly caused by vasospasm, heart failure, and diffuse poor left ventricular contraction are unlikely to benefit from revascularization.[112,138]

Results of angina pectoris. Most patients experience major relief of angina pectoris symptoms and improved physical and sexual function after CABG. However, improvement in activity tolerance and return to full employment has been disappointing.[3,112] Approximately half of patients return to presurgery levels of household activity. Factors indicating that the patient may not return to full employment are increasing age, postoperative angina, and unem-

---

*References 7, 63, 76, 114, 115, 121.

ployment or disability before surgery.[112] Enthusiasm for CABG surgery is tempered by observations that approximately 50% of saphenous vein grafts are no longer patent 10 years after surgery. In addition, although symptoms and exercise tolerance are improved 5 years after surgery, 10 years after they are similar to patients treated medically.[112]

Substantial attention has been given to medical versus surgical intervention for the treatment of angina pectoris. Investigations have compared immediate and long-term survival, as well as symptom relief and quality of life.[112,138] Three major randomized trials have been conducted. The Veterans Administration Randomized Trial established the superiority of surgery over medical management for left main coronary artery disease, although the study was criticized for some of its conclusions.[93,138] The European Cooperative Trial confirmed the advantage of surgical intervention in patients with left main coronary artery disease and in those with symptomatic three-vessel disease.[44,138] The Coronary Artery Surgery Study (CASS)[22] consisted of a randomized group of patients and a registry of patients. Initially, the study concluded that surgery did not offer advantages over medical management in mild stable angina pectoris.[138] Subsequent criticism of the study's design and conclusions related to the small number of patients who were randomized and the exclusion of severely symptomatic patients.[138] Further follow-up of patients in the registry has indicated that those with compromised left ventricular function and three-vessel disease benefit from CABG surgery in terms of survival and quality of life.[138]

Observational studies comparing medically and surgically treated patients have been conducted by the Seattle Heart Watch Group and Duke University. The Seattle Heart Watch Group has concluded that surgery is beneficial to patients with coronary artery disease of the left main coronary artery and two or three vessels, as well as patients with compromised left ventricular function.[138]

Duke University initiated their study in 1969.[138] In 1984, they concluded that survival after surgery exceeded survival after medical treatment, regardless of left ventricular function. They also noted that changes in medical and surgical treatment over the years had resulted in improved survival rates in surgical patients but little change in survival with medical therapy. When interpreting results of studies comparing therapy, it is important to see that patients with similar disease are included in both groups.

Coronary angiography and myocardial revascularization (PTCA or CABG surgery) are recommended for patients who have unstable angina pectoris despite optimal medical therapy, anatomically bypassable coronary artery lesions in the left main vessel or two or three other vessels, and depressed left ventricular function (ejection fractions of 15% to 35%).[112,138] Because graft patency declines after surgery to 50% at 10 years and reoperation is associated with higher operative risk, patients with normal ventricular function and mild-to-moderate symptoms are encouraged to postpone surgery.[138]

Postoperative patency of bypass grafts is a major concern. Graft occlusion early in the first year after surgery (18% in the first month) is usually due to thrombosis. By the end of the first year, 16% to 47% of grafts are no longer patent as a result of thrombosis, intimal hyperplasia, or fibrosis. Development of atherosclerosis in the grafts and its progression in the distal coronary arteries contributes to late closure of the graft (after the first year).[112,138] Antiplatelet therapy (dipyridamole or aspirin) has been shown by some investigators to be beneficial in maintaining graft patency.[24,51] The internal mammary arteries may be used to bypass atherosclerotic plaque. Their patency rate is more satisfactory when compared with the rate of patency for vein grafts.[56,120,138] For details of the preoperative and postoperative nursing care of the CABG surgical patient, see Chapter 17.

NURSING DIAGNOSIS 2   **Anxiety related to situational and treatment-related factors (feeling pattern)**

PATIENT OUTCOMES	NURSING PRESCRIPTIONS	EVALUATION
Patient will not experience severe anxiety or panic and will report a reduced anxiety level. Patient's pain will not increase as a result of anxiety.	Assess anxiety and institute measures to reduce anxiety; including reassurance, orientation to environment and therapeutic regimen, decreased sensory stimulation, and medications.	Patient did not experience severe anxiety or panic and reported a reduced anxiety level. Pain did not increase as a result of anxiety.
Patient will institute measures to reduce anxiety levels.	Use behavioral and cognitive strategies to guide the patient in relaxation, imagery, and music.	Patient used relaxation, imagery, and music to reduce anxiety.
Patient will cope effectively with anxiety.	Discuss possible concerns with patient, including fear of death, changed self-concept, and feelings of apprehension, anger, or hostility.	Patient discussed fears of death and changed self-concept and negative feelings.

Plan and intervention for anxiety

Anxiety

Anxiety is a normal reaction and subjective feeling of apprehension to unspecified or consciously unknown threats.[46] Anxiety is experienced psychologically, physiologically, and behaviorally according to the individual's perception of danger.[21,52,88] Individual coping mechanisms vary from person to person. Anxiety and coping are adaptive when arousal is appropriate to the situation and problem solving proceeds without difficulty. When inappropriate behavioral patterns, exaggerated responses, and decreased role performance are seen, anxiety and coping are maladaptive.[21,52,88]

Angina and anxiety

Anginal attacks provoke anxiety because they are stressful and threatening to patients. Patients in this situation often perceive the angina and accompanying diagnosis of CAD as a threat to bodily health, self-concept, and role performance. Diagnostic and therapeutic procedures separate patients from significant others and place them among strangers in a scary, unfamiliar environment.[25,27,61] The goals in management of anxiety are to avoid severe or panic levels, to reduce the anxiety to a mild level, and to avoid problems caused by anxiety.[21,88] Chest pain and other anginal symptoms, conversely, may be provoked or made worse by anxiety. In addition, patients with severe or panic levels of anxiety have distorted perceptions and impaired problem-solving abilities. Because anginal symptoms recur, the long-term management of anxiety during and between attacks must be learned by patients. Short- and long-term goals are accomplished by helping patients change their perceptions of the threats associated with angina pectoris and CAD.[21,88,107]

Persons with angina pectoris may feel helpless and fear that life is coming to an end. *Physiologic responses* to stress vary with severity and include increased heart rate and respirations, hypertension, temperature shifts, peripheral vasoconstriction, increased perspiration, dilated pupils, and dry mouth.[27,61] Patients with angina pectoris receive no hemodynamic benefit from anxiety, especially if the anxiety level is high enough to cause panic. Psychologic

---

INTRODUCING RELAXATION TECHNIQUES

Nurse: What do you feel like when you're having an angina attack?

Patient: It's pretty scary. I think sometimes I make it worse because I get so scared.

Nurse: When people get anxious, they forget to breathe in a relaxed way. Do you ever try to relax when you feel an attack coming on?

Patient: No. All I can think about is taking a nitroglycerin tablet and wondering whether I'm having a heart attack. When this last one happened, I think I was so scared I didn't breathe very much.

Nurse: May I share some simple relaxation exercises with you?

Patient: Boy, I could sure use some.

Nurse: I would like to tell you about some simple things you can begin to practice that will help you relax while you're awake.

Patient: Super, I'm ready for that.

Nurse: The places where we carry tension are varied in each of us. For a few minutes, I'll act as a guide and give you some suggestions to help you relax. I'll ask you to breathe in a slow, relaxed manner. As you breathe in, allow your stomach to blow up like a balloon. As you breathe out, pull your stomach back to your spine. This might seem difficult at first, but this is the nice, relaxed breathing that you and I do every night before we fall asleep. The second thing I'll ask you to do is relax the muscles around your mouth, jaws, and shoulders. You might want to be aware of your teeth not touching and letting go of the muscles of your tongue. You can even let your lips be apart a little bit. The third suggestion is to concentrate on a number such as *one* or a word such as *relax* or *calm* as you breathe out.

Patient: I'll think of *calm.*

Nurse: Terrific. Keep in mind, I'm a guide, and you're the one changing your tension to deep relaxation. (The exercise then took place over 10 minutes.)

Patient: Boy, that was something. I've never been aware of how I can relax myself. You know, I go all day long at work and then at home.

Nurse: Something to think about doing is taking time out once or twice a day to relax. By doing this, you practice and increase your relaxation skills. Then when you get tense, anxious, or tired, you can relax instead of increasing that tense state, because you really know how to relax. While you're recuperating in the hospital is a good time to start practicing. I'll check with you tomorrow to see if you have any questions about relaxation. At that time I'll share some more information about relaxation.

manifestations usually are reflected in behavioral patterns such as withdrawal, muteness, hyperactivity, swearing, excessive talking and joking, verbally or physically striking out, and fantasizing, complaining, and crying.[27,61]

Therapeutic environment

The patient requires reassurance, understanding, and support from the nurse. Reassurance is gained by the physical presence of the calm, alert, interested, and empathic nurse (therapeutic use of self).[27] Orienting the patient to the environment, routines of the care unit, and therapeutic regimen reduces fear of the unknown and promotes comfort. Explanations of the cause and meaning of symptoms may reduce anxiety levels associated with an anginal event. Communication should be simple, clear, and direct in a calm, relaxed voice.[132] Decreasing sensory stimulation by providing a warm, comfortable, quiet environment is also beneficial. Administering a prescribed mild sedative or anxiolytic medication may be necessary to reduce the anxiety; however, nonpharmacologic approaches also are required for acceptable long-term management of anxiety levels. Management of anxiety is incomplete without a discussion of the patient's concerns. The nurse should discover the meaning and significance that the patient attaches to symptoms.[20,52,107] Misconceptions or misapprehensions should be corrected. Nursing intervention is considered effective in reducing anxiety when the patient does not experience severe anxiety or panic during episodes of angina, reports a reduced anxiety level, does not experience increased pain resulting from anxiety, discusses concerns, and uses relaxation, imagery, and music to reduce anxiety.

Relaxation, imagery, and music

Relaxation, imagery, and music are used to reduce stress and induce the relaxation response, which in turn helps mitigate anxiety and the pain experience.[1,2,32,38,60] Initially, the nurse should direct patients in relaxation and imagery exercises that are acceptable to them (see Chapter 5). As patients become familiar with the exercises, they can perform them alone. Teaching patients relaxation and imagery techniques will enable them to reduce their anxiety levels during and between attacks. The box, p. 242, demonstrates how the nurse can introduce such techniques.

NURSING DIAGNOSIS 3 **High risk for ineffective denial and noncompliance related to knowledge deficit and situational and treatment-related factors (choosing pattern)**

PATIENT OUTCOMES	NURSING PRESCRIPTIONS	EVALUATION
Patient will avoid inappropriate denial as indicated by correct interpretation of symptoms and verbalization of when to seek health care.	Offer guidance and information about the meaning of symptoms. Instruct patient about when and how to access health care.	Patient interpreted symptoms correctly and verbalized when and how health care should be sought.
Patient will verbalize an understanding of angina (causes, symptoms, and risk factors) and the prescribed therapeutic regimen and its purpose.	Teach patient about angina (causes, symptoms, and risk factors) and the prescribed therapeutic regimen and its purpose.	Patient verbalized an understanding of anginal causes, symptoms, and risk factors and the prescribed therapeutic regimen and its purpose.
Patient will verbalize a willingness to comply with the prescribed therapeutic regimen.	Assess patient's willingness to comply with prescribed therapy, including activity, medications, CAD risk factor modification, and follow-up care.	Patient verbalized willingness to comply with activity, medications, CAD risk factor modification, and follow-up care.

Plan and intervention for ineffective denial and noncompliance

Coronary artery disease and associated angina pectoris are chronic diseases that patients must manage for the rest of their lives. Patients may deny the meaning of their symptoms and delay seeking medical care, which may have detrimental effects on their health.[48,66] They also may not comply with the prescribed therapeutic regimen, although they say that they intend to do so.[107] Many factors play a role in placing patients at high risk for developing these problems. All patients experience changes in bodily health, self-concept, and role performance and treatment-related problems (hospitalization and prolonged therapy) sometime during their extended illness.[107] If these problems are resolved satisfactorily, patients are unlikely to be at high risk for developing these diagnoses. The goals are for patients to maintain or improve their health status by complying with the therapeutic regimen and avoiding denial, which is detrimental to their health. Teaching and counseling assist in increasing compliance when the topics include the meaning of patients' signs and symptoms, times and ways to access health care, methods to reduce anxiety, CAD risk factor reduction, and the purpose and details of the prescribed therapeutic regimen. The therapeutic relationship between health care providers and the patient,[20,40,107,141] as well as family support,[122] are also important in achieving compliance.

Denial is a coping strategy used by patients to manage anxiety.[27] It is adaptive and beneficial as long as it does not interfere with effective problem-solving or required action.[52,82,88,131] When patients' health is impaired as a result of the inability to take appropriate action, the denial becomes maladaptive, inappropriate, or ineffective.[48,66] Knowledge deficit is a factor for patients who do not know the risk factors, signs, or symptoms of CAD and therefore fail to recognize them.[106] Patients who recognize that their signs and symptoms could indicate cardiac disease and impending premature death may not acknowledge these implications in an effort to reduce the anxiety evoked by this situational threat. Taking action requires seeking treatment and choosing among unattractive alternatives related to adoption of the sick role and changing lifestyles (reducing CAD risk factors [e.g., changing dietary habits, stopping smoking, or beginning an exercise program], a change

---

STANDARD INSTRUCTIONS FOR PATIENTS WITH ANGINA PECTORIS

Relieve anginal attacks when they occur.
  Carry nitroglycerin at all times.
    Keep nitroglycerin in a tightly closed, dark glass container.
    Replace with new tablets every 3 months.
    If potent, nitroglycerin should cause slight burning when placed under the tongue.
    Do not mix with other pills in the same container.
  When taking needed medication, use an important ritual.
    As you hold the nitroglycerin tablet under your tongue, feel the power and immediate action as it dissolves in the saliva and is absorbed into the mucous membranes under your tongue.
    Say to yourself, "The medicine is in my body and working."
    Take the time to practice deep breathing exercises and relaxing your jaw.
    If you feel a rush of the medicine in your body or feel a pounding sensation in your head, you know the medicine is in your body and working. If the pounding sensation is not relieved shortly, take slow, relaxed deep breaths. Stroking your temples with a light circular movement also helps relieve the pressure.
  Take nitroglycerin prophylactically to avoid pain.
  If angina occurs, at the first sign of symptoms, stop your activity and take sublingual nitroglycerin.
    Place nitroglycerin under the tongue and rest.
    Allow medication to be absorbed through mucous membrane. Do not swallow saliva until the tablet is completely dissolved.
    If quick action is desired, bite the tablet between the front teeth, and slip it under the tongue to dissolve.
    Repeat the dosage at 5-minute intervals until relief is obtained. Do not use more than three tablets.
  If angina persists, seek medical attention promptly.

Avoid angina-provoking situations.
  Avoid emotional upsets, undue fatigue, and stressful confrontations.
  Avoid overeating.
  Avoid exposure to extreme temperatures.
  Avoid beverages that contain caffeine.
Follow recommended pharmacologic management of angina.
  Take long-acting nitrates.
  Take β-adrenergic blockers.
  Take calcium-channel blocking agents.
Engage in a regular program of physical activity.
  Perform normal daily activities that do not provoke angina.
  Avoid strenuous activity that produces angina, dyspnea, or fatigue.
  Avoid isometric activity such as lifting heavy objects.
  Engage in a regular program of gradual progressive exercise. Do not exercise so hard that pain occurs.
Reduce factors that contribute to the development of atherosclerosis.
  Modify attitude and lifestyle to adapt to stress.
  Avoid foods that are high in saturated fat and cholesterol.
  If you are overweight, reduce body weight.
  If you smoke, stop smoking.
  If you are hypertensive, reduce sodium intake and take prescribed medication.
  If you are diabetic, comply with medical therapy to control your blood glucose.
Integrate stress management strategies each day to increase the quality of your daily living (see Chapter 5).
  Frequently remind yourself that you are doing a very good job in your recovery.
  Set simple and realistic goals.
  Practice and use relaxation skills.
  Practice and use imagery skills to help integrate healthy lifestyle behaviors.

of environment [clinic, emergency department, or hospital], and painful procedures [venipuncture, exercise testing, cardiac catheterization, or myocardial revascularization]).[107]

Compliance or adherence to a therapeutic regimen usually requires the patient to adopt and perform a new role.[40,107] Patients who see themselves as ill or at risk are motivated to behave and act differently. They also must understand the purpose and details of the regimen and believe that it will be safe and effective. Aspects of therapy associated with *noncompliance* include regimens that are complex, expensive, or prolonged; unpleasant or unacceptable side effects; lack of rapport between patient and health care provider; and professional advice that conflicts with the patient's health beliefs and practices.[20,21,40,88,107]

Teaching is important in patient management[106,126] and may be done individually or in a group. A calm, relaxed atmosphere facilitates interaction between patient and nurse and builds a therapeutic relationship.[20] It also allows incorporation of exercises that use the right side of the brain, such as relaxation, imagery, or music therapy. This increases active participation. Cardiac education should teach experiential (right-brain) as well as intellectual (left-brain) information to patients and families. Standard instructions[8,18,19,74,133] are shown in the box, p. 244.

Lifestyle change is an important factor in maintaining an angina-free state. It helps to remember the "four Es" when teaching patients about angina: exertion, emotion, eating, and extreme temperatures. Patients should be instructed to avoid activities that provoke angina, such as climbing stairs or standing for prolonged periods; working in a hot or cold environment; fatigue; sudden bursts of activity after long rest; and people, places, or situations that cause anxiety. Regular rest periods should be included in the daily routine.[41,72,112]

CAD risk factor reduction is a necessary part of patient management and involves changes in patients' health beliefs and practices[55,97,112,135,137] (see Chapter 8). Discussing the detrimental effects of smoking on the cardiovascular system and offering substitutes are useful measures to promote cessation of this habit. Behavior modification programs also may help. Hypertension should be monitored carefully and treated appropriately. Diuretics, β-adrenergic blockers, and vasodilator agents are useful in treating the disorder. Frequent blood pressure determinations are needed to ensure compliance and drug efficacy. Diabetes mellitus also should be controlled and may require dietary restrictions and oral hypoglycemic agents or insulin. Self-monitoring of blood glucose levels allows better control. If this method is not used, regular glucose and acetone determinations should be made from the urine. Obesity and serum lipid concentration should be managed by limiting the intake of saturated fats, carbohydrates, dairy products, and sweets.[123]

Although physical activity is beneficial to cardiac performance, activity prescribed for patients with angina pectoris should be monitored closely. Isometric exercise, which greatly increases myocardial oxygen demand, should be avoided. Patients should maintain and adjust their activity levels to avoid provoking anginal symptoms. Patients must learn to pace themselves throughout their daily routine. Activity should be reduced in the morning and immediately after meals. Situations that provoke angina should be avoided if possible. However, when this is not feasible, nitroglycerin should be used prophylactically to prevent pain. When anginal symptoms occur, patients should cease the activity in which they are engaged, rest, and take sublingual nitroglycerin for relief of symptoms. Patients should seek medical attention if symptoms persist or occur with increasing frequency.

Sexual activity is often a concern of the patient and partner.[87] Both may fear that intercourse will precipitate an anginal attack or even death. However, normal sexual relations usually can be maintained if the patient controls risk factors, takes medication appropriately, and engages in sexual activity when rested and free of emotional stress such as anger or hostility. Nitroglycerin may be taken before intercourse as a prophylactic measure. Counseling may be necessary to facilitate a healthy sexual relationship between the patient and partner. An atmosphere of openness, honesty, and realism will help resolve the conflicts and fears of engaging in sexual activity for these individuals.

KEY CONCEPT REVIEW

1. Angina pectoris may occur during:
   a. Strenuous exercise
   b. Rest or sleep
   c. Emotional stress
   d. All of the above
2. The immediate cause of all types of angina pectoris is:
   a. Decreased oxygen supply
   b. Inadequate myocardial perfusion
   c. Increased oxygen demand
   d. Decreased myocardial contractility
3. Which of these events occurs during the development of atherosclerotic plaques?
   a. Injury to arterial endothelium
   b. Smooth muscle cells migrating from the media to the intima
   c. Lipid deposition in lesions of the artery
   d. All of the above
4. Which of the following symptoms most accurately describes the characteristic discomfort of angina pectoris?
   a. Sharp, stabbing pain in the left side
   b. Pain in the chest that gets worse during deep breathing

c. Heavy substernal sensation that radiates to the left arm
d. A feeling of indigestion and nausea in the stomach

5. The most important data to obtain when assessing the person with angina pectoris is the:
   a. Electrocardiogram
   b. Cardiac enzyme levels
   c. Patient history
   d. Physical examination

6. Which of the following diagnostic tests is *least* valuable in evaluating patients with CAD?
   a. Echocardiography
   b. Exercise electrocardiography
   c. Coronary angiography
   d. Thallium-201 scintigraphy

7. Common medications used to treat the patient with angina pectoris include all of the following *except:*
   a. Nitroglycerin
   b. Calcium-channel blockers
   c. β-adrenergic blockers
   d. Warfarin

8. CAD risk factors that cannot be reduced or modified include:
   a. Family history
   b. Hypertension
   c. Smoking
   d. Glucose intolerance

9. The patient with CAD and angina pectoris should be taught relaxation exercises to reduce:
   a. Atherosclerosis
   b. Anxiety, stress, and pain
   c. Myocardial necrosis
   d. Anxiety

10. The patient outcome of improved activity tolerance can be achieved by:
    a. Participating in a graded exercise program
    b. Using nitroglycerin prophylactically
    c. Reducing stress during activity
    d. All of the above

11. The diagnoses of "noncompliance" and "ineffective denial" are avoided by:
    a. Patient education
    b. Medication
    c. PTCA
    d. CABG surgery

12. During PTCA, a balloon-tipped catheter is used to:
    a. Monitor cardiac pressures
    b. Compress atherosclerotic lesions
    c. Interrupt coronary vasospasm
    d. Pace the atria

13. Patients are considered candidates for PTCA if they:
    a. Are also acceptable candidates for CABG surgery
    b. Have single-vessel disease
    c. Have chronic angina refractory to medical therapy
    d. All of the above

ANSWERS

1. d	4. c	6. a	8. a	10. d	12. b
2. b	5. c	7. d	9. b	11. a	13. d
3. d					

REFERENCES

1. Achterberg J and Lawlis F: Bridges of the bodymind: behavioral approaches to health care, Champaign, Ill, 1980, Institute for Personality and Ability Testing, Inc.
2. Achterberg J and Lawlis F: Imagery and health intervention, Top Clin Nurs 3:55, 1982.
3. Allen JK: Physical and psychosocial outcomes after coronary artery bypass graft surgery: review of the literature, Heart Lung 19:49, 1990.
4. American Heart Association: 1990 heart and stroke facts, Dallas, 1989, The Association.
5. Araki H and others: Diurnal distribution of ST-segment elevation and related arrhythmias in patients with variant angina: a study by ambulatory ECG monitoring, Circulation 67:995, 1983.
6. Assey ME: The recognition and treatment of silent myocardial ischemia. In Hurst JW and Schlant RC, editors: The heart, arteries, and veins, ed 7, New York, 1990, McGraw-Hill, Inc.
7. Baim DS: Interventional catheterization techniques: percutaneous transluminal balloon angioplasty, valvuloplasty, and related procedures. In Braunwald E, editor: Heart disease: a textbook of cardiovascular medicine, ed 3, Philadelphia, 1988, WB Saunders Co.
8. Beare PG and Myers JL: Principles and practice of adult health nursing, St Louis, 1990, Mosby–Year Book, Inc.
9. Berne RM and Levy MN: Physiology, ed 2, St Louis, 1988, The CV Mosby Co.
10. Block PC: Percutaneous transluminal coronary angioplasty, Am J Radiol 135:955, 1980.
11. Block PC, Fallon JT, and Elmer D: Experimental angioplasty: lessons from the laboratory, Am J Radiol 135:907, 1980.
12. Braun LT and Holm K: Preservation of ischemic myocardium through activity management, J Cardiovasc Nurs 3:39, 1989.
13. Braunwald E, editor: Heart disease: a textbook of cardiovascular medicine, ed 3, Philadelphia, 1988, WB Saunders Co.
14. Braunwald E: The history. In Braunwald E, editor: Heart disease: a textbook of cardiovascular medicine, ed 3, Philadelphia, 1988, WB Saunders Co.
15. Braunwald E: The physical examination. In Braunwald E, editor: Heart disease: a textbook of cardiovascular medicine, ed 3, Philadelphia, 1988, WB Saunders Co.
16. Braunwald E and Kloner RA: The stunned myocardium: prolonged, postischemic ventricular dysfunction, Circulation 66:1146, 1982.
17. Braunwald E and others, editors: Harrison's principles of internal medicine, ed 11, New York, 1987, McGraw-Hill, Inc.
18. Brunner LS and Suddarth DS: The Lippincott manual of nursing practice, ed 4, Philadelphia, 1986, JB Lippincott Co.
19. Brunner LS and Suddarth DS: Textbook of medical-surgical nursing, ed 6, Philadelphia, 1988, JB Lippincott Co.
20. Carey RL: Compliance and related nursing actions, Nurs Forum 21:157, 1984.
21. Carpenito LJ: Nursing diagnosis application to clinical practice, ed 3, Philadelphia, 1989, JB Lippincott Co.

22. CASS Principal Investigators and Their Associates: Coronary artery surgery study (CASS): a randomized trial of coronary bypass surgery: survival data, Circulation 68:939, 1983.

23. Castaneda-Zuniga WR and others: The mechanism of balloon angioplasty, Radiology 135:565, 1980.

24. Chesebro JH and others: Effect of dipyridamole and aspirin on late vein-graft patency after coronary artery bypass operations, N Engl J Med 310:209, 1984.

25. Chyun D: Patient's perceptions of stressors in intensive care and coronary care units, Focus Crit Care 16:206, 1989.

26. Clark JB, Queener SF, and Karb VB: Pharmacological basis of nursing practice, ed 3, St Louis, 1990, Mosby–Year Book, Inc.

27. Clark S: Nursing diagnosis: ineffective coping. I. A theoretical framework. II. Planning care, Heart Lung 16:670, 1987.

28. Cole JR and Ellestad MH: Significance of chest pain during treadmill exercise: correlation with coronary events, Am J Cardiol 41:227, 1978.

29. Cotran RS, Kumar V, and Robbins SK: Robbins pathologic basis of disease, ed 4, Philadelphia, 1989, WB Saunders Co.

30. Cowley MJ and Block PC: Percutaneous transluminal coronary angioplasty, Mod Con Cardiovasc Dis 50:25, 1981.

31. Dagenais GR and others: Survival of patients with a strongly positive exercise electrocardiogram, Circulation 65:452, 1982.

32. Davis-Rollans D and Cunningham SG: Physiologic responses of coronary care patients to selected music, Heart Lung 16:370, 1987.

33. Deering TF and Weiner DA: Prognosis of patients with coronary artery disease, J Cardiopulmon Rehabil 5:325, 1985.

34. Detre K and others: Percutaneous transluminal coronary angioplasty in 1985-1986 and 1977-1981: The National Heart, Lung, and Blood Institute PTCA Registry, N Engl J Med 318:265, 1988.

35. Dix-Sheldon DK: Pharmacologic management of myocardial ischemia, J Cardiovasc Nurs 3:17, 1989.

36. Dorland's illustrated medical dictionary, ed 24, Philadelphia, 1965, WB Saunders Co.

37. Dorros G and others: Percutaneous transluminal coronary angioplasty: report of complications from the National Heart, Lung, and Blood Institute PTCA Registry, Circulation 67:723, 1983.

38. Dossey BM and others: Holistic nursing: a handbook for practice, Gaithersburg, Md, 1988, Aspen Publishers, Inc.

39. Dotter CT and Judkins MP: Transluminal treatment of arteriosclerotic obstruction: description of a new technique and a preliminary report of its application, Circulation 30:654, 1964.

40. Dracup KA and Meleis AI: Compliance: an interactionist approach, Nurs Res 31:31, 1982.

41. Dunagan WC and Ridner ML, editors: Manual of medical therapeutics, ed 26, Boston, 1989, Little, Brown and Co.

42. Eberts MA: Advances in the pharmacologic management of angina pectoris, J Cardiovasc Nurs 1:15, 1986.

43. Enger EL and Schwertz DW: Mechanisms of myocardial ischemia, J Cardiovasc Nurs 3:1, 1989.

44. European Coronary Surgery Study Group: Prospective randomized study of coronary artery bypass surgery in stable angina pectoris, Lancet 2:491, 1980.

45. Factor SM: Pathophysiology of myocardial ischemia. In Hurst JW and Schlant RC, editors: The heart, arteries, and veins, ed 7, New York, 1990, McGraw-Hill Inc.

46. Fadden T, Fehring RJ, and Kenkel-Rossi E: Clinical validation of the diagnosis anxiety. In McLane AM, editor: Classification of nursing diagnoses: proceedings of the seventh conference, St Louis, 1987, The CV Mosby Co.

47. Faxon DP, Ruocco N, and Jacobs AK: Long-term outcome of patients after percutaneous transluminal coronary angioplasty, Circulation 81(suppl IV):IV-9, 1990.

48. Fields KB: Myocardial infarction and denial, J Fam Pract 28:157, 1989.

49. Friesinger GC: The natural history of atherosclerotic heart disease. In Hurst JW and Schlant RC, editors: The heart, arteries, and veins, ed 7, New York, 1990, McGraw-Hill Inc.

50. Ginsberg R and others: Studies with isolated human coronary arteries: some general observations, potential mediators of spasm, role of calcium antagonists, Chest 78:180, 1980.

51. Goldman S and others: Effect of anti-platelet therapy on late graft patency after coronary artery bypass grafting: VA Cooperative Study No. 207, Abstract 37, Annual Scientific Session, American College of Cardiology, J Am Coll Cardiol 11(3)(Suppl A):152A, 1988.

52. Gomez EA, Gomez GE, and Otto DA: Anxiety as a human emotion: some basic conceptual models, Nurs Forum 21:38, 1984.

53. Gordon DJ and others: Predictive value of the exercise tolerance test for mortality in North American men: the Lipid Research Clinics Mortality Follow-up Study, Circulation 74:252, 1986.

54. Gottlieb SO and Gerstenblith G: Assessing the total ischemic burden in the management of unstable angina: a review, Am J Med 81(suppl 4A):7, 1986.

55. Gotto AM: AHA conference report on cholesterol, Circulation 80:1, 1989.

56. Grondin CM and others: Comparison of late changes in internal mammary artery and saphenous vein grafts in two series of patients 10 years after operation, Circulation 70(suppl I):208, 1984.

57. Gruntzig A and Kumpe DA: Technique of percutaneous angioplasty with the Gruntzig balloon catheter, AJR Am J Roentgenol 132:547, 1979.

58. Gruntzig AR, Senning A, and Siegenthaler WE: Nonoperative dilatation of coronary artery stenosis: percutaneous transluminal coronary angioplasty, N Engl J Med 301:61, 1979.

59. Gruntzig AR and others: Long-term follow-up after percutaneous transluminal coronary angioplasty: the early Zurich experience, N Engl J Med 316:1127, 1987.

60. Guzzetta CE: Effects of relaxation and music therapy on patients in a coronary care unit with presumptive acute myocardial infarction, Heart Lung 18:609, 1989.

61. Guzzetta CE and Forsyth GL: Nursing diagnostic pilot study: psychophysiologic stress, ANS 1:27, 1979.

62. Guzzetta CE and others: Clinical assessment tools for use with nursing diagnoses, St Louis, 1989, The CV Mosby Co.

63. Halfman-Franey M and Levine G: Intracoronary stents, Crit Care Nurs Clin North Am 1:327, 1989.

64. Hangartner JRW and others: Morphologic characteristics of clinically significant coronary artery stenosis in stable angina, Br Heart J 56:501, 1986.

65. Helgeson VS: The origin, development, and current state of the literature on type A behavior, J Cardiovasc Nurs 3:59, 1989.

66. Herlitz J and others: Delay time in suspected acute myocardial infarction and the importance of its modification, Clin Cardiol 12:370, 1989.

67. Hill JA and others: Coronary arterial aneurysm formation after balloon angioplasty, Am J Cardiol 52:261, 1983.

68. Hillis LD and Braunwald E: Coronary artery spasm, N Engl J Med 299:695, 1978.

69. Holmes DR and Vlietstra RE: Balloon angioplasty in acute and chronic coronary artery disease, JAMA 261:2109, 1989.

70. Hurst JW: Atherosclerotic coronary heart disease: historical benchmarks, methods of study and clinical features, differential diagnosis, and clinical spectrum. In Hurst JW and Schlant RC, editors: The heart, arteries, and veins, ed 7, New York, 1990, McGraw-Hill Inc.

71. Hurst JW: Methods of treating atherosclerotic coronary heart disease. In Hurst JW and Schlant RC, editors: The heart, arteries, and veins, ed 7, New York, 1990, McGraw-Hill Inc.

72. Hurst JW: The recognition and treatment of specific subsets of patients with atherosclerotic coronary heart disease. In Hurst JW and Schlant RC, editors: The heart, arteries, and veins, ed 7, New York, 1990, McGraw-Hill Inc.

73. Hurst JW and Schlant RC, editors: The heart, arteries, and veins, ed 7, New York, 1990, McGraw-Hill Inc.

74. Johanson BC and others: Standards for critical care, ed 3, St Louis, 1988, The CV Mosby Co.

75. Kent K and others: National Heart, Lung, and Blood Institute: percutaneous transluminal coronary angioplasty (PTCA): update from NHLBI registry (abstract), Circulation 62(suppl III):160, 1980.

76. King SB: Vascular stents and atherosclerosis, Circulation 79:460, 1989.

77. King SB and Douglas JS: Percutaneous transluminal coronary angioplasty. In Hurst JW and Schlant RC, editors: The heart, arteries, and veins, ed 7, New York, 1990, McGraw-Hill Inc.

78. Kinney M and others: Comprehensive cardiac care, ed 7, St Louis, 1991, Mosby–Year Book, Inc.

79. Lambert CR and others: Influence of beta-adrenergic blockade defined by time series analysis on circadian variation of heart rate and ambulatory myocardial ischemia, Am J Cardiol 64:835, 1989.

80. Lary BG: Effect of endocardial incisions on myocardial blood flow, Arch Surg 88:82, 1963.

81. Lee KT, editor: Atherosclerosis, Ann NY Acad Sci 454:1, 1985.

82. Levenson JL and others: Denial and medical outcome in unstable angina, Psychosom Med 51:27, 1989.

83. Loan T: Nursing interaction with patients undergoing coronary angioplasty, Heart Lung 15:368, 1986.

84. Malseed RT and Harrigan GS: Textbook of pharmacology and nursing care using the nursing process, Philadelphia, 1989, JB Lippincott Co.

85. Massimo C and Boffi L: Myocardial revascularization by a new method of carrying blood directly from the left ventricular cavity into the coronary circulation, J Thorac Surg 34:257, 1957.

86. McCance KL and Huether SE: Pathophysiology: the biologic basis for disease in adults and children, St Louis, 1990, Mosby–Year Book, Inc.

87. McCann ME: Sexual healing after heart attack, Am J Nurs 89:1133, 1989.

88. McFarland GK and McFarlane EA: Nursing diagnosis and intervention. planning for patient care, St Louis, 1989, The CV Mosby Co.

89. McKenry LM and Salerno E: Mosby's pharmacology in nursing, ed 17, St Louis, 1989, The CV Mosby Co.

90. Mirhoseini M, Fischer JC, and Cayton MM: Myocardial revascularization by laser, Lasers Surgery Med 3:241, 1983.

91. Mirhoseini M, Shelgikar S, and Cayton M: New concepts in revascularization of the myocardium, Ann Thorac Surg 45:415, 1988.

92. Muller JE, Tofler GH, and Stone PH: Circadian variation and triggers of onset of acute cardiovascular disease, Circulation 75:395, 1989.

93. Murphy ML and others: Treatment of chronic stable angina: a preliminary report of survival data of the randomized Veterans Administration Cooperative Study, N Engl J Med 297:621, 1977.

94. Naprstek Z and Rockwell RJ: Some laser application in cardiovascular research, International Congress of Medical Engineering Session 34(6):1, 1969.

95. National Center for Health Statistics: Vital statistics of the United States, 1987, vol II, mortality, part A, Hyattsville, MD, 1990, US Public Health Service.

96. Pasternak RC and others: Scanning electron microscopy after coronary transluminal angioplasty of normal canine coronary arteries, Am J Cardiol 45:591, 1980.

97. Pearson TA: Multiple risk factors for coronary artery disease: behavioral factors in preventive cardiology, Am J Cardiol 60:74, 1987.

98. Pepine CJ: New concepts in the pathophysiology of acute myocardial infarction, Am J Cardiol 64(4):2B, 1989.

99. Pepine CJ: New concepts in the pathophysiology of acute myocardial ischemia and infarction and their relevance to contemporary management, Cardiovasc Clin 20:3, 1989.

100. Perchalski DL and Pepine CJ: Patient with coronary artery spasm and role of the critical care nurse, Heart Lung 16:392, 1987.

101. Popma JJ and Dehmer GJ: Care of the patient after coronary angioplasty, Ann Int Med 110:547, 1989.

102. Pratt CM and Roberts R: Pharmacologic therapy of atherosclerotic coronary heart disease. In Hurst JW and Schlant RC, editors: The heart, arteries, and veins, ed 7, New York, 1990, McGraw-Hill Inc.

103. Przyklenk K and Kloner RA: Superoxide dismutase plus catalase improve contractile function in the canine model of the "stunned" myocardium, Circ Res 58:148, 1986.

104. Przybojewski JZ and Weich HFH: Percutaneous transluminal coronary angioplasty: a review of the literature, S Afr Med J (special issue) January 1984.

105. Radwin LE: Autonomous nursing interventions for treating the patient in acute pain: a standard, Heart Lung 16:258, 1987.

106. Raleigh EH and Odtohan BC: The effect of a cardiac teaching program on patient rehabilitation, Heart Lung 16:311, 1987.

107. Riegel B: Social support and psychological adjustment to chronic coronary heart disease: operationalization of Johnson's behavioral system model, ANS 11:74, 1989.

108. Roberts WC and others: Sudden death in Prinzmetal's angina with coronary spasm documented by angiography: analysis of 3 necropsy patients, Am J Cardiol 50:203, 1982.

109. Ross R: The pathogenesis of atherosclerosis: an update, N Engl J Med 314:488, 1986.

110. Ross R: The pathogenesis of atherosclerosis. In Braunwald E, editor: Heart disease, ed 3, Philadelphia, 1988, WB Saunders Co.

111. Ross R: Factors influencing atherogenesis. In Hurst JW and Schlant RC, editors: The heart, arteries, and veins, ed 7, New York, 1990, McGraw-Hill Inc.

112. Rutherford JD, Braunwald E, and Cohn PF: Chronic ischemic heart disease. In Braunwald E, editor: Heart disease, ed 3, Philadelphia, 1988, WB Saunders Co.

113. Sakallaris BR: Laser therapy for cardiovascular disease, Heart Lung 16:465, 1987.

114. Sanborn TA: Laser angioplasty: what has been learned from experimental studies and clinical trials? Circulation 78:769, 1988.

115. Schatz RA: A view of vascular stents, Circulation 79(2):4, 1989.

116. Schiro AG and Curtis DG: Asymptomatic coronary artery disease, Heart Lung 17:144, 1988.

117. Schneider AC: Unreported chest pain in a coronary care unit, Focus Crit Care 14(5):21, 1987.

118. Scientific American: Ischemic heart disease: angina pectoris. In Scientific American Medicine: Cardiovascular medicine, 1988.

119. Selwyn AP and Braunwald E: Ischemic heart disease. In Braunwald E and others, editors: Harrison's principles of internal medicine, ed 11, New York, 1987, McGraw-Hill, Inc.

120. Singh RN, Sosa JA, and Green GE: Internal mammary artery versus saphenous vein graft: comparative performance in patients with combined revascularization, Br Heart J 50:48, 1983.

121. Sipperly ME: Expanding role of coronary angioplasty: current implications, limitations, and nursing considerations, Heart Lung 18:507, 1989.

122. Sirles AT and Selleck CS: Cardiac disease and the family: impact, assessment, and implications, J Cardiovasc Nurs 3:23, 1989.

123. Smith A: Physiology, diagnosis, and life-style modifications for hyperlipidemia, J Cardiovasc Nurs 1:15, 1987.

124. Smith CE: Assessing chest pain quickly and accurately, Nurs 88 18(5):52, 1988.

125. Solomon J: Introduction to cardiovascular nursing, Baltimore, 1988, Williams & Wilkins.

126. Steele JM and Ruzicki D: An evaluation of the effectiveness of cardiac teaching during hospitalization, Heart Lung 16:306, 1987.

127. Steinberg D and others: Beyond cholesterol: modifications of low-density lipoprotein that increase its atherogenicity, N Engl J Med 320(14):915, 1989.

128. Steingart RM and Scheuer J: Assessment of myocardial ischemia. In Hurst JW and Schlant RC, editors: The heart, arteries, and veins, ed 7, New York, 1990, McGraw-Hill Inc.

129. Sylven C: Angina pectoris: clinical characteristics, neurophysiological and molecular mechanisms, Pain 36:145, 1989.

130. Talley JD and others: Clinical outcome 5 years after attempted percutaneous coronary angioplasty in 427 patients, Circulation 77:820, 1988.

131. Thomas SA, Sappington E, and Gross HS: Denial in coronary care patients: an objective reassessment, Heart Lung, 12:74, 1983.

132. Thompson EA: Anxiety: a mental health vital sign. In Longo DC and Williams RA, editors: Clinical practice in psychosocial nursing, ed 2, Norwalk, Conn, 1986, Appleton and Lange.

133. Thompson JM and others: Mosby's manual of clinical nursing, ed 2, St Louis, 1989, The CV Mosby Co.

134. Underhill SL and others: Cardiac nursing, ed 2, Philadelphia, 1989, JB Lippincott Co.

135. Vitello-Cicciu J, Stewart SL, and Griffin EL: Coronary artery disease. In Kinney MR, Packa DR, and Dunbar SB: AACN's clinical reference for critical-care nursing, ed 2, New York, 1988, McGraw-Hill, Inc.

136. Waters DD and others: Circadian variation in variant angina, Am J Cardiol 54:61, 1984.

137. Wenger NK and Schlant RC: Prevention of coronary atherosclerosis. In Hurst JW and Schlant RC, editors: The heart, arteries, and veins, ed 7, New York, 1990, McGraw-Hill Inc.

138. Whalen RE and Hurst JW: The surgical treatment of atherosclerotic coronary heart disease. In Hurst JW and Schlant RC, editors: The heart, arteries, and veins, ed 7, New York, 1990, McGraw-Hill Inc.

139. Willerson JT: Angina pectoris. In Wyngaarden JB and Smith LH, editors: Cecil textbook of medicine, ed 18, Philadelphia, 1988, WB Saunders Co.

140. Willich SN and others: ISAM Study Group: increased risk of myocardial infarction in the morning (abstract), J Am Coll Card 11:28A, 1988.

141. Woods N: Conceptualizations of self-care: toward health-oriented models, ANS 12:1, 1989.

142. Wyngaarden JB and Smith LH, editors: Cecil textbook of medicine, ed 18, Philadelphia, 1988, WB Saunders Co.

143. Yasue H: Pathophysiology and treatment of coronary arterial spasm, Chest 78:216, 1980.

144. Yasue H, Ogawa H, and Okumura K: Coronary artery spasm in the genesis of myocardial ischemia, Am J Cardiol 63:29E, 1989.

145. Yasue H and others: Cardiac variations of exercise-induced coronary arterial spasm, Circulation 59:938, 1979.

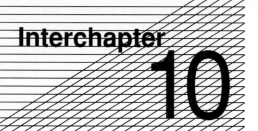

Interchapter 10

The Value of Denial and Illusion

Denial as a helper may sound like a paradox, but it does save lives in some cases.[1] For example, Hackett[2] has shown that the higher a patient's denial within the first 24 hours following an acute myocardial infarction, the lower the mortality. When denial is present, stress is reduced, and thus the level of adrenalin and other stress-induced hormones in the blood are lowered, which decreases the sensitivity of the injured myocardium to the development of potentially fatal dysrhythmias. Those patients who give the appearance of minimal worry, who deny the seriousness of their acute illness, or who deny being frightened survive the coronary care unit experience in larger numbers than those patients who are worried and frightened.

Denial, however, also can cause death in those patients who deny their severe chest pain and delay seeking medical advice. An example of how denial kills is when a person with chest pain says "This can't be chest pain. I'm too young to have a heart attack," or "This awful pain is just bad indigestion." Denial contributes to the 50% percent mortality of patients with acute myocardial infarction who never reach the hospital.[2] As Hacket and Rosenbaum[3] observed "While denial can play the role of the enemy to the myocardial infarction victim in delaying his arrival in the emergency room, it can also serve as his ally in the CCU."

If denial seems to work toward survival in the first hours following AMI, should we encourage patients to use denial? This presents a paradox. One cannot suggest to another person to use denial. Likewise, a person cannot say "I think I am going to deny this situation." When denial is consciously chosen, it is no longer a genuine response.

Taylor[5] studied many forms of illusion, one of which is denial in cardiac and cancer patients, rape victims, and others with catastrophic illness or life-threatening situations. She has shown that when a life situation becomes too difficult, a person will adopt a coping strategy based on illusion. Taylor[6] states, "The effective individual in the face of threat . . . seems to be one who permits the development of illusions, nurtures those illusions, and is ultimately resorted by those illusions. . . ."

Taylor's use of the word *illusion* does not imply that a person believes a lie. Rather the person takes the facts of a situation and views them with a different meaning so that a positive rather than a negative outcome results. For example, many cancer and cardiovascular patients describe their illness as positive because the disease has caused them to reappraise their lives. Taylor[6] suggests that the readjustment process following the crisis focuses around three themes: (1) a search for meaning in the experience; (2) an attempt to regain mastery over the event in particular; and (3) an effort to enhance one's self-esteem in the midst of crisis.

Ornish's[4] research has demonstrated that these three themes also are part of the readjustment process with cardiac patients and are essential components that must be explored for a cardiac patient to reverse coronary artery disease. His work with cardiac patients has shown that a frequent receptive image (see p. 104) is the image of a wall or fortress around the heart. Metaphorically the heart is the organ that is most associated with our feelings. Over the years it is possible to protect ourselves from emotional pain that occurs in our relationships with family, friends, and colleagues, and to create barriers in our communication with others. Ornish suggests that healing frequently manifests as we explore our dialogue and recognize the walls or barriers that have been erected around our heart. This allows for "opening" of feelings and emotions and the reintegration of ourselves leading to greater intimacy between us and others. It also leads to a fundamental kind of intimacy with ourselves that we have walled off or disowned. The following is an adapted version of Ornish's[4] inner heart imagery exercise:

Imagine your heart in any way as it comes to you . . . it may look like an anatomical drawing or quite different. . . . When that image comes . . . introduce yourself as if you were meeting a person for the first time . . . You will find that your heart has its own voice . . . it may be the same as yours or it may be a different voice. . . . You can communicate with your heart with images, sounds, or feelings. . . . You will know the best way. Think about its rhythm, its beating continually since you were born, for keeping you alive . . . listen to the reply. . . .

Once you are able to receive messages from your heart . . . ask your heart what it needs in order to be healed. You may begin by physical healing . . . listen to the answer. It may be specific such as diet or exercise. Next ask for emotional and spiritual healing . . . listen to the inner wisdom. . . .

Allow yourself to feel the love for your heart, and to experience the love that your heart has for you. . . . Finally, ask your heart how you can get in touch with it again. . . .

This imagery exercise evokes varied responses from people. Many find a fortress that has been erected over years, both protecting and isolating it. It is suggested that if the person imagines an obstruction, begin a dialogue with it and listening to the reply. Then ask the wall to let the other side to be seen, allowing that the wall can come back instantly if it is needed.

REFERENCES

1. Dossey L: Meaning and medicine: a doctor's stories of breakthrough and healing, New York, 1991, Bantam.
2. Hackett TP and others: The coronary care unit: an appraisal of its psychogical hazards, N Engl J Med 279: 1365, 1968.
3. Hackett TP and Rosenbaum JF: Emotions, psychiatric disorders, and the heart. In Braunwald E, editor, Heart disease: a textbook of cardiovascular medicine, Philadelphia, 1980, WB Saunders, 1923-1943.
4. Ornish D: Dr. Dean Ornish's program for reversing heart disease, New York, 1990, Random House.
5. Taylor SE: Adjustment to threatening events: a theory of cognitive adaptation, Am Psych 11:1161, 1983.
6. Taylor SE: Positive illusions: creative self-deception and the healthy mind, New York, 1989, Basic Books.

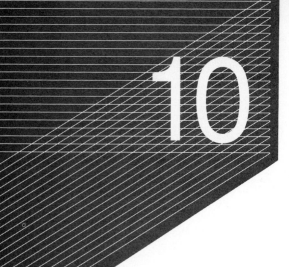

10

The Person with Myocardial Infarction

Sandra W. Haak
Sue E. Huether

LEARNING OBJECTIVES

1. Describe the pathophysiologic changes that accompany acute myocardial infarction.

2. Compare and contrast the four types of acute myocardial infarction.

3. Identify the major signs and symptoms of acute myocardial infarction.

4. Examine the major areas of nursing assessment for patients with acute myocardial infarction.

5. Analyze specific modalities to improve myocardial perfusion in the patient with acute myocardial infarction.

6. Explain specific interventions to reduce the patient's and family's anxiety after acute myocardial infarction.

7. Discuss the major complications of patients with acute myocardial infarction.

8. Describe specific nursing interventions for each complication of acute myocardial infarction.

9. Evaluate components of holistic health that must be considered in cardiac rehabilitation.

Acute myocardial infarction (AMI) results when severe, prolonged myocardial ischemia causes death and necrosis of the heart muscle.[49,52] In the majority of patients, atherosclerosis, vasospasm, and thrombosis reduce blood flow by narrowing and ultimately occluding the coronary arterial lumens.[3,52,137,140] The consequent profound myocardial ischemia results from reduction in myocardial perfusion to critical levels.[49,52] Irreversible cell injury and infarction begin within 20 to 40 minutes of onset[128] and progress if perfusion is not re-established in a timely manner. The typical initial clinical manifestation is pain, which is severe, intolerable, crushing, pressing, or constricting; is located in the substernal area of the chest; begins at rest after exertion or during exertion; lasts more than 20 minutes; radiates to the neck, jaw, or left arm; is associated with nausea, vomiting, and diaphoresis; and is relieved by narcotic analgesics rather than rest or nitroglycerin.[128,136,137,213] The therapeutic focus is on reperfusion and limitation of infarct size; prevention, detection, and treatment of complications; and patient and family education.[10,88,128,137] The major complications, cardiac dysrhyth-

mias and ventricular failure, develop suddenly and are life threatening.[128,137] Therefore nurses must be able to rapidly assess signs, symptoms, and complications of AMI; make accurate decisions; and anticipate or initiate appropriate treatment quickly and accurately.[10,88,206]

INCIDENCE

AMI remains the leading cause of death in the United States despite healthier lifestyles, advances in medical treatment, and declining mortality rates.[6,130,190] More than 5 million people in the United States have a history of MI, angina, or both. Approximately 1.5 million people in the United States have an AMI each year, and 35% (more than 500,000) die.[6,136] Half or more of the deaths attributed to AMI occur during the first 1 to 2 hours,[64,137] and about half of AMI patients delay seeking health care for 2 hours or more, and consequently many die before they are hospitalized.[6,84] The majority of inhospital deaths occur during the first 24 hours.[64] Of patients discharged from the hospital, approximately 10% die within a year.[64,137] Data from the Framingham Heart Study[6] indicates that 45% of all AMIs occur in persons under age 65 and that 5% occur in persons under age 40. In the age range, 45 to 64, 76% of AMIs occur in men and 24% in women. However, in persons 65 and older, the rate drops to 54% for men and rises to 46% for women. Hazzard[79] proposes that these differences in mortality rates can be explained by differences in hormonal influence on lipoprotein metabolism.

MYOCARDIUM

The adult heart is about the size of a fist and weighs less than 1 pound. Three layers of tissue, pericardium, myocardium and endocardium, compose the heart walls. The *pericardium* is a connective tissue sac with two membranes that enclose the myocardium. The *visceral pericardium* (also known as the *epicardium*) is in contact with the myocardium and forms the inner layer. The *parietal pericardium* is the outer layer and is composed of mesothelium over a thin layer of connective tissue. The space between the visceral and parietal layers contains approximately 10 to 30 ml of pericardial fluid, which provides lubrication for movement of the membranes as the heart beats. Pain receptors and mechanoreceptors within the pericardium detect reflex changes in blood pressure and heart rate. The pericardium prevents displacement of the heart and provides a protective barrier against inflammation and infection.[11,118]

The *myocardium* is composed of cardiac muscle and is anchored to the fibrous rings of the heart valves. The myocardium varies in thickness, depending on the amount of resistance that the muscles must overcome to pump blood from the chambers. (Myocardial contraction and relaxation are discussed in Chapters 6 and 7.) The trabeculae carneae are folds and ridges on the inner surface of the myocardium. The cone-shaped papillary muscles project from the myocardium into the ventricular chambers and attach to the cusps of the atrioventricular (AV) valves via strong fibrous bands called *chordae tendineae*. The papillary muscles contract during ventricular systole, holding the valves closed and preventing regurgitation.[11,118]

The myocardium is lined by the *endocardium*, which is composed of connective tissue and an inner layer of squamous cells. Folds of the endocardium form the cardiac valves. The endocardium of the heart is continuous with the endothelial lining of the systemic arteries.[11,118]

ETIOLOGY AND PRECIPITATING FACTORS

The direct cause of AMI is severe myocardial ischemia that persists long enough to cause irreversible cell injury and death.[3,52] Precipitating factors for profound myocardial ischemia are total occlusion of the related coronary artery, a major reduction in blood flow to portions of the myocardium, and insufficient increase in blood flow relative to

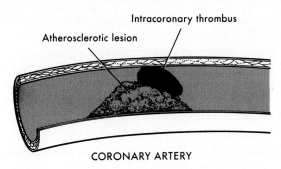

FIG. 10-1   Coronary atherosclerosis complicated by thrombosis. From Beare PG, Myers JL: Principles and practice of adult health nursing, St Louis, 1990, The CV Mosby Co.

myocardial oxygen demand.[52,137,213] In 90% of patients with AMI, coronary atherosclerosis narrows vessel lumens and limits blood flow (see Chapter 9) before total occlusion by thrombosis occurs (Fig. 10-1).*

Over the last decade, much information on risk factors for coronary artery disease (CAD) has been accumulated (see Chapter 8).[74,106,211] The American Heart Association[6] has identified the following factors commonly found in people with AMI:

1. A family history of atherosclerosis
2. Male gender
3. Increasing age
4. Cigarette smoking
5. Hypertension
6. Hypercholesterolemia
7. Diabetes mellitus
8. Obesity
9. Sedentary lifestyle
10. Excessive stress

The three major CAD risk factors that can be changed are cigarette smoking, hypertension, and hypercholesterolemia.† The more risk factors an individual has, the greater the chance of developing atherosclerosis. Modification of established lifestyles can reduce the impact of risk factors.[138,211] Educating parents and children about risk factors may prevent development of unhealthy lifestyles.[211]

The use of *oral contraceptives* containing estrogen, especially if the woman smokes and is older than 35, increases the risk of AMI.[137] Oral contraceptives affect the coagulation process through increased platelet counts, increased platelet adhesiveness, shortened thromboplastin time, elevation of various clotting factors, and decreased clearance of clotting factors. In addition, contraceptives may decrease glucose tolerance and increase high blood pressure, triglyceride, and low-density lipoprotein (LDL) levels.

*References 49, 52, 117, 137, 213, and 214.
†References 6, 73, 74, 177, 184, 187, and 211.

AMI can occur in people without significant atherosclerosis.[89,137] Less common causes of AMI include coronary artery embolism, inflammation, malformation, sclerosis, and trauma; decreased cardiac output resulting from dysrhythmias, cardiomyopathy, valvular disease, hemorrhage or fluid shifts; decreased coronary perfusion resulting from systemic hypotension or hypertension; decreased blood oxygen content or availability resulting from hypoxemia, anemia, or carbon monoxide poisoning; or hypermetabolic states resulting from fever, allergic reactions, or endocrine disorders.[52,137]

CORONARY THROMBOSIS

There has been controversy regarding the role of thrombosis in AMI. It is now recognized as a causative factor in coronary occlusion.* Although atherosclerosis, plaque rupture, vasospasm, intimal injury, and platelet activation interact to cause thrombosis,† the precise pathophysiologic sequence is not well understood. In a normal coronary artery, the endothelium regulates smooth muscle function through the release of endothelium-derived relaxation factors that cause vasodilation and prevent platelet aggregation. In atherosclerosis, thrombi form at sites of severe narrowing (Fig. 10-1) because this protective endothelial function is lost. A cycle of vasospasm, endothelial injury, and platelet aggregation is promoted.[140]

Vasospasm alone and with atherosclerosis (see Chapter 9) has been implicated in decreasing blood flow, leading to ischemia.[137,140,219] Spasm may initiate endothelial injury or make it worse.[137] Platelets gathering at the site of injury may release vasoconstricting substances such as thromboxane A_2 to enhance, maintain, or initiate spasm. Release of platelet-activated growth factor may further compromise lumen diameter.[33,58] Leukocytes appear to play a role in the development of thrombosis through the release of leukotrienes and other factors that enhance blood coagulation and stimulate cell migration.[107] High sheer stress associated with high velocity flow through partially occluded coronary vessels may also further damage the endothelium.[140]

Atherosclerotic plaque rupture and fissures have also been identified with vessel occlusion.[52,56] Plaque rupture may initiate the clotting cascade by releasing tissue thromboplastin, stimulating platelet aggregation, or mechanically occluding the vessel. Vasomotion of smooth muscle cells within the plaque may cause its rupture.[52,53]

COLLATERAL CIRCULATION

Normal hearts do not have microvascular connections at the boundaries between regions perfused by separate large

---

*References 3, 52, 128, 137, 139, and 140.
†References 3, 52, 137, 139, 140 and 158-160.

coronary arteries.[20,34,52,54] However, significant connecting vessels between coronary arteries, called *collaterals,* are located in the epicardial layers. Collateral vessels and circulation increase in patients with long-standing CAD and gradual arterial obstruction. When coronary arteries are almost totally obstructed, collateral vessels enlarge over several weeks and appear to become functional.[20] However, collateral blood flow may be inadequate to fully meet myocardial metabolic needs when sudden total occlusion occurs. Infarction of the entire distribution of the occluded artery ensues unless collateral circulation meets some energy requirements of the jeopardized myocardium and thus limits infarct size.[20,34,52]

EFFECTS OF CORONARY OCCLUSION

Infarction does not occur instantly or simultaneously. Instead, it is a progressive process and occurs with injury and ischemia for at least the first 4 to 6 hours. The final size of the infarct is determined in part by the duration and severity of vessel occlusion, oxygen demand at the time of ischemic occlusion, and the amount of collateral blood supply to ischemic tissue.

Myocardial ischemia begins immediately after total occlusion of a coronary artery.[3] Cell injury follows ischemia and is reversible for a time if perfusion resumes naturally or therapeutically. Irreversible injury and infarction do not usually begin until 20 to 40 minutes after cessation of blood flow.[128] Cells in the subendocardial portion of the artery's distribution are affected first, whereas cells in the epicardial portion are affected last (see Chapter 9).[3] The infarcted zone usually progresses from the subendocardium to the subepicardium and is surrounded by zones of injured and ischemic cells (Fig. 10-2). During the first 4 to 6 hours, clinicians consider the infarct to be evolving because progression and the final size of infarction can be limited by reperfusion of the ischemic and injured areas.[16,90] After 6 hours of total ischemia, the infarct is considered completed.[128]

The extent of necrosis determines whether the infarction includes the endocardial, subendocardial, myocardial, subepicardial, or epicardial layers of the ventricular wall (Fig. 10-3). Infarctions that extend through the myocardium from the subendocardium to the subepicardium are termed *transmural* (Q-wave) *infarctions.*[16,90] Necrosis restricted to the subendocardium produces *subendocardial* (non-Q-wave) *infarctions,* which are smaller and have a better short-term prognosis. The long-term prognosis for both types is similar.[64]

The local and systemic catecholamine release and sympathetic response to coronary occlusion produces metabolic, mechanical, electrical, and psychologic effects.[3,20] These effects are part of the normal adaptive psychophysiologic stress response.[77] However, in an individual with AMI, they can be detrimental to the body (the ischemic myocardium), as well as to the mind and spirit.

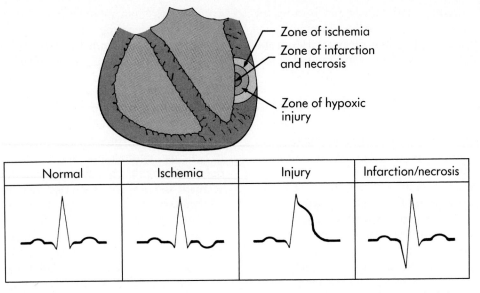

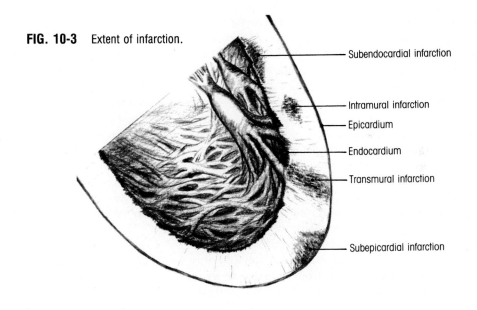

FIG. 10-2 Electrocardiographic alterations associated with the three zones of myocardial infarction.

From McCance KL and Huether SE: Pathophysiology: the biologic basis for disease in adults and children, St Louis, 1990, The CV Mosby Co.

FIG. 10-3 Extent of infarction.

Metabolic effects

The metabolic effects result from inefficient energy production. Under normal aerobic conditions, myocardial cellular energy comes from conversion of free fatty acids (FFA) to high-energy phosphates. Adenosine triphosphate (ATP) provides most of the energy for muscle contraction. Creatine phosphate is another energy source found in small amounts in the cardiac muscle. With the onset of myocardial ischemia, stored ATP is depleted within seconds, and myocardial cells begin to produce it by anaerobic metabolism of glucose. Unfortunately, anaerobic glycolysis only produces 65% to 70% of the energy required to maintain the sodium-potassium pump. Sodium extrusion is decreased, resulting in cellular accumulation of sodium, inhibition of calcium entry, release of potassium, swelling and decreased contractility. Potassium released from ischemic tissues contributes to electrical abnormalities by causing *hypopolarization* of the affected cells. With hypopolarization, calcium shifts occur, and dysrhythmias may be produced. Lactic acid, a product of anaerobic metabolism, accumulates and lowers the intracellular pH because the poorly perfused myocardium has a reduced buffering capacity. Acidosis further compromises the myocardium and increases vulnerability to damage from lysosomal enzymes.[3,20,52,75,137]

Mechanical effects

Normal contraction of ischemic cells declines rapidly with loss of energy-rich phosphates and ceases entirely 15 to 90 seconds after interruption of blood flow.[3] In adjacent cells, contraction is reduced while normal cells attempt to compensate with hyperfunction. The ejection fraction is reduced when 10% of the myocardium contracts abnormally. Elevation of left ventricular end-diastolic pressure (LVEDP) and volume occur with 15% involvement. Stroke volume and resting cardiac output are significantly reduced when 20% to 25% of the myocardium is dysfunctional. Elevated pulmonary pressures and clinical evidence of heart failure develops when 25% or more of the myocardium is lost. Cardiogenic shock, usually fatal, develops in patients with infarction of 40% or more of the myocardium.[3,64] These factors encourage clinicians to attempt to limit the size of the infarcted and ischemic area.[3,20,52,137,140]

Diastolic function is also affected. The myocardium becomes stiffer and less compliant because of interstitial edema and leukocyte infiltration immediately and in the early stage of AMI. During healing, stiffness is a consequence of fibrous tissue formation.[3,20,52,137,140]

Electrical effects

Electrical instability results from disturbed metabolic and mechanical function. It is manifested by changes in the electrocardiogram (ECG) pattern and a wide variety of dysrhythmias.[60,136] Impaired ATP production, dysfunction of the sodium-potassium pump, release of potassium, and calcium shifts cause changes in polarization, conduction, and the refractory period. Released metabolic products such as FFAs, lactic acid, and catecholamines can alter automaticity. Mechanical stretch from dilation can interfere with impulse propagation. Consequently, dysrhythmias are caused by reentry, reexcitation, and increased automaticity[3,20,137,140] (see Appendix B).

Dysrhythmias are estimated to occur in all patients with AMI but are observed in 72% to 96%.[137] Life-threatening dysrhythmias include sustained ventricular tachycardia, ventricular fibrillation, and heart block. Heart block occurs in about 20% of individuals with MI.[103] Ventricular tachycardia and fibrillation occur more often in individuals with larger infarcts.[137] Patients with anterior MI complicated by ventricular fibrillation have a greater risk of sudden death in the first yeart after MI.[170] Premature ventricular contractions (PVCs) have been considered a warning sign and predictor of ventricular tachycardia and fibrillation. How-

ever, studies[137] have shown that ventricular fibrillation occurs without warning in 40% to 83% of patients. Furthermore, patients with frequent and complex PVCs do not always develop ventricular fibrillation. Cardiac arrest is more common in older individuals and in patients with Q-wave and larger infarcts as documented by creatine kinase (CK) values.[70]

The ECG records changing potentials of aggregate cardiac cells (see Chapter 6). Potentials are altered or absent in ischemic, injured, and infarcted cells, which is reflected in leads facing the area. Repolarization, reflected in the ST segment and T wave, is affected first (Fig. 10-4). *Ischemia* is manifested by ST-segment depression and T-wave inversion. *Injury* is manifested by ST-segment elevation. Severely injured and infarcted cells have no potentials and do not depolarize (Fig. 10-2). If a large number of cells have no electrical activity, the QRS complex changes, and significant Q waves develop *(Q-wave infarction)*. If only a small number of cells are affected, Q waves do not develop *(non-Q-wave infarction)*. With healing, ST-segment and T-wave changes usually return to normal, but Q waves persist for a variable period of time. Because each individual is unique, changes related to AMI are best identified by comparing a series of ECGs.[3,20,60,189]

Psychologic effects

There are circular interrelationships among the psychologic and physiologic effects of AMI. A person's psychologic state can precipitate life-threatening dysrhythmias[31,44,45,151] and affect outcome.[135,153] The psychologic effects of AMI include fear of death or dependency, as well as anxiety, denial, and depression.[95,110,135] Fatigue, altered sleep patterns, monotony, change of environment, and previous mental illness may contribute to psychologic responses to AMI. Blue-collar workers experience more anxiety than professionals.[142,217] Depression after AMI is reported to be more severe among individuals with type A personalities.[93]

The process of *adjustment* during recovery consists of four stages.[95] The first stage, *defending oneself,* begins when patients first develop symptoms and continues as long as 7 days; patients try to maintain a sense of control and use the coping strategies of denial and distancing. During the second stage, *coming to terms,* patients struggle with a perceived loss of control by facing their mortality, making sense of the event, facing limitations, and looking to the future. It may begin as early as 3 days or as late as 8 days after an AMI. Patients may return to this stage when faced with setbacks and unmet expectations. The third stage, *learning to live,* involves the struggle to reestablish a sense of control. Patients seek lifestyles that they can maintain and tolerate and begin to trust their own abilities. In the process, they endeavor to preserve a sense of self, minimize uncertainty, and establish guidelines for living. Patients who are unsuccessful in reestablishing control abandon the struggle and become invalids. Those who are successful

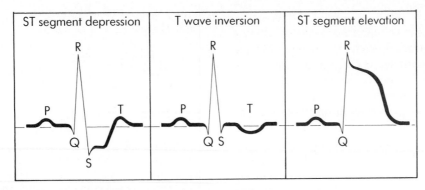

FIG. 10-4   Electrocardiographic alterations associated with ischemia.
From McCance KL and Huether SE: Pathophysiology: the biologic basis for disease in adults and children, St Louis, 1990, The CV Mosby Co.

reach the fourth stage, *living again,* in which they accept limitations, refocus on other aspects of living, and attain mastery.[95]

LOCATION OF INFARCTION

The location and size of infarction are determined by the distribution of the occluded coronary arteries and extent of necrosis. These factors have a direct bearing on complications and the prognosis of AMI.[64,128,137] Depending on the coronary artery occluded, infarcts are described as *right* or *left ventricular* and *anterior, posterior, inferior,* or *lateral.* The left main coronary artery has two branches, the left anterior descending and the left circumflex (Fig. 9-1) (see Chapter 9). *Anterior MI* occurs with occlusion of the left anterior descending branch (40% to 50% of AMIs) and can involve the anterior left ventricle, anterior interventricular septum, bundle of His, right bundle branch, anterior fascicle of the left bundle branch, posterior fascicle of the left bundle branch, and left ventricular apex. Heart failure, AV block, mural thrombosis, and late aneurysms are associated with MI in this location, which has a high mortality rate. *Lateral MI* occurs with occlusion of the left circumflex branch (15% to 20% of AMIs) and can involve the lateral and posterior left ventricle, posterior interventricular septum, posterior division of the left bundle branch, left atrium, AV node (10%), and sinoatrial (SA) node (45%). *Anterolateral MI* occurs with occlusion of the left main stem and can involve tissues supplied by both branches. *Inferior* and *posterior MIs* occur when the right coronary artery is occluded (30% to 40% of AMIs) and can involve the inferior and posterior left ventricle, posterior interventricular septum, bundle of His, right ventricle, right atrium, SA node (55%), and AV node (90%). Complications include atrial dysrhythmias, SA block, and AV block.[34,64,128,137] Studies have shown 14% to 40% of all patients suffering AMI have associated *right ventricular infarction.* The incidence is 37% to 52% when only transmural infarctions of the inferior wall are considered.[156]

PATHOLOGIC CHANGES AFTER AMI

Pathologic changes in the myocardium do not appear immediately after coronary occlusion because it takes time for biochemical reactions to cause morphologic changes.[34]

Nonreperfused myocardium

About 6 hours after cessation of blood flow, a thin, wavy fiber pattern of irreversibly injured cells can be seen under a microscope.[34,80,137] Nonreperfused myocardium examined 18 to 24 hours after AMI shows a gross, pale gray-brown, patchy surface in the region of infarction. Microscopic changes include minimal neutrophilic infiltrates. This pattern is termed *coagulation necrosis,* and the white or pale color results from the complete absence of blood flow. At 48 to 72 hours after infarction, reddish purple focal areas appear around the yellow-brown area of necrosis. Moderate neutrophilic infiltrates are accompanied by necrotic muscle fibers and interfiber hemorrhage. About 4 days after infarction, the infarcted areas consist of a soft region with central fatty changes and regions of hemorrhage, surrounded by a hyperemic border. Microscopic examination shows dense neutrophilic infiltrates and severe muscle necrosis. At 10 days, there are well-developed yellow necrotic changes with a red-brown, soft, vascularized border. Fibrotic scar tissue begins to form, beginning with revascularization.

At 2 weeks, the thickness of the myocardial wall at the infarcted site and tensile strength of the wound has decreased. Microscopic examination reveals predominantly mononuclear cells and obvious granulation tissue with some collagen strands. At 4 weeks the infarcted area has become red-purple from newly formed blood vessels with prominent granulation tissue and collagen. Over the next month, this area becomes pale gray. Microscopic examination reveals disappearance of mononuclear cells, with collagen replacing the granulation tissue. At 3 months, a firm, white scar is apparent in the infarcted area.[34,80,137]

Reperfused myocardium

Infarcted myocardium can be reperfused by blood flow of collateral vessels or in association with reperfusion therapy. With reperfusion, hemorrhage occurs within the subendocardial portion of the infarct because microvascular injury has developed with necrosis. The area of injury may be expanded by reperfusion as a result of myocardial cell swelling and microvascular and cell membrane disruption. Liberation of free-oxygen radicals, accumulation of mitochondrial calcium, and formation of *contraction band necrosis* are characteristic of reperfusion injury.[13,14,208] The necrosis appears red because restored flow causes blood to hemorrhage into the interstitial spaces of infarcted myocardium.[34,80,137]

Nursing process

Case study. Mr. D., a 50-year-old engineer, and his wife came to the emergency department shortly after eating breakfast at home. Mr. D. complained of excruciating, crushing, substernal chest pain that had lasted 1 hour. The pain began suddenly while he was reading the newspaper, radiated down both arms, and was accompanied by nausea, vomiting, and shortness of breath. He appeared anxious and distressed, with gray, diaphoretic skin. His vital signs were blood pressure, 140/90 mm Hg; temperature, 36.4° C (97.6° F); pulse, 140 per minute; and respirations, 20 per minute. Mr. D. explained he had never experienced chest pain or heart problems before, his usual blood pressure was 120/80 mm Hg, and his weight was 165 lbs (75 kg).

Oxygen at 3 L/min by nasal cannula and an infusion of 5% dextrose in water were begun. A total of 10 mg of morphine sulfate given intravenously over 20 minutes was required to relieve his pain. His breath sounds were clear. His heart sounds included soft S_1 and S_2, as well as S_3 and S_4 but no rubs or murmurs. A 12-lead ECG showed sinus tachycardia and ST-T changes consistent with acute anterior myocardial ischemia and injury. Blood was drawn for a serum CK level test. Thrombolytic therapy was begun with tissue plasminogen activator (tPA).

Mr. D. was transferred to the coronary care unit (CCU) immediately after the tPA infusion began. As he was admitted, his pain returned. His vital signs were blood pressure, 135/85 mm Hg; temperature, 36.4° C (97.6° F); pulse 110 per minute; and respirations 15 per minute. The ECG monitor showed sinus tachycardia with 6 to 10 PVCs per minute and ST-segment elevation. Another intravenous line was started, a lidocaine bolus of 75 mg was given, and a lidocaine drip at 2 mg/min was begun. While giving intravenous morphine, nurses used therapeutic touch, relaxation, and imagery to help calm Mr. D. They also explained the CCU routines and equipment. This was effective, and an hour later, Mr. D. fell asleep. The bedside monitor then showed normal sinus rhythm without ectopy at a rate of 90 per minute. The ST elevation had reduced somewhat.

When Mr. D. awakened, the nurse continued a holistic assessment. Mr. D. said he had no pain but was worried about his heart and an important report that was due at work. He felt the future of his career depended on the quality of the report, so he had been working on it 12 hours a day for the past week. His work was a source of stress. The company that employed him had recently

merged with another because of financial difficulties. The new management style was very different and not to Mr. D.'s liking. Mr. D. knew about CAD risk factors, including family history. He hoped to avoid his father's fate, death at age 60 from a heart attack, because he exercised regularly and did not smoke. His mother, age 70, was still living. He and his wife of 25 years lived in an old farm house with their three adolescent children. When asked how he thought this hospitalization might change his life, he replied that he was worried it would cause him to lose his job.

When all the tPA had infused (60 mg the first hour, then 10 mg/hour for 4 hours), Mr. D. was given a heparin bolus of 5000 units, and a heparin drip was begun at 1000 units/hour. The nurse explained he would be receiving the heparin for several days. That evening, several hours after the tPA had infused, Mr. D. had a burst of ventricular tachycardia. This was interpreted as a reperfusion dysrhythmia. A 25-mg bolus of lidocaine was given, and the lidocaine drip rate was increased to 3 mg/min. He had no further dysrhythmias.

The next morning, the nurse noted that his heart sounds included S_1, S_2, S_4, and a pericardial friction rub. His breath sounds were clear. Mr. D. said he felt very tired but had no pain or discomfort in his chest. He asked if he could be discharged later in the day so that he could go home and finish his report. The nurse explained that although he would not be discharged for several days, his activity could increase from bed rest to chair rest. The nurse reviewed the results of the serum CK levels drawn every 8 hours since admission. In the emergency department, 1 hour after his symptoms began, the total CK level was 90 units/L. At 8 hours the total CK level was 800 U/L, and the CK-MB level was 40%. At 16 hours the total CK level was 400 U/L, and the CK-MB level was 20%. At 24 hours the total CK level was 100 U/L. The nurse recognized that this rapid rise and fall was related to the tPA therapy. Serial 12-lead ECGs done at admission, the first evening, and next morning showed elevated ST segments and inverted T waves that resolved. However, deep QS waves developed, indicating that some infarction had occurred despite tPA therapy.

Denial, anxiety, and anger were some of Mr. D.'s feelings during his hospitalization. Denial was overt during the first 36 hours. He told his wife and nurse, "I'm not sick, now that the pain is gone." His sister, who lived in another state, came to visit. Mr. D. said he wished she had waited to visit until he "was out of the hospital and could show her the sights in a few days." Later, while his wife and children were visiting, he stated, "I need to get out of here; nothing is wrong with me." Mr. D.'s anger was revealed in several ways. He did not comply with bed or chair rest much of the time. Periodically he refused to have vital signs taken. He was verbally abusive and made sexual advances to the nurses. The nursing staff held team conferences to develop a plan for consistent care and peer support.

Mr. D. was transferred to a telemetry unit on the third morning, where he began to ambulate. He began the cardiac rehabilitation program and was discharged 7 days after admission. About 2 weeks after discharge, Mr. D. told the phase II cardiac rehabilitation nurse that he felt his progress was extremely slow and he was very discouraged. During the next month, through discussion, caring, empathy, and multidisciplinary rehabilitation, Mr. D. began to accept the events in his life. He had viewed himself as a dying old man who would never return to work. The cardiac rehabilitation team helped him shift to a positive focus by teaching him to relax while visualizing himself as a healthy man fishing at his favorite lake. He returned to work 2 months after discharge in a new position.

Nursing assessment

The diagnosis of evolving AMI is suspected when a person (especially a middle-age man) is seen with a complaint of substernal chest pain that has lasted more than 20 to 30 minutes and less than 4 to 6 hours.[64,137] To be effective, interventions to limit infarct size must be instituted promptly, usually before confirming evidence of AMI from diagnostic tests is available. Therefore diagnosis and decisions to intervene are made primarily on the basis of the history.[46,128,137] Physical examinations, ECGs, blood chemistry studies, and diagnostic tests are used to confirm the diagnosis and to evaluate the effect of interventions.

In this case, nursing assessment is continuous. A patient may be completely stable for several hours and then quickly develop ventricular fibrillation, complete heart block, severe congestive heart failure, or cardiogenic shock. Initial assessment of patients admitted to the CCU with chest pain or AMI should include subjective data (pain, anxiety, and history of present illness) and objective data (general appearance, vital signs, cardiac rhythm, and physical assessment). Ischemic chest pain, ventricular dysrhythmias, and cardiac failure must be identified and relieved quickly because 70% to 80% of deaths from AMI occur in the first 24 hours[64] and are due to ventricular fibrillation or cardiac failure.*

Nurses should begin to alleviate the patient's and family's anxiety by introducing themselves and offering simple explanations about monitoring equipment and routines of patient care. Initial assessment should be followed by a more thorough and holistic evaluation[78] of the patient's and family's response to AMI, CAD, and their management.

Feeling pattern

The majority of patients with AMI have chest pain or discomfort. Chest pain in AMI actually represents myocardial ischemia and indicates that infarction is imminent or progressing.[128,137] Specific characteristics of chest pain can be used to differentiate between causes (Table 9-3).[10,100,128,137,178] In contrast to stable angina pectoris (see Chapter 9), the pain of AMI begins spontaneously, is similar in character but more intense, lasts longer, has more associated symptoms, and is not relieved by rest or sublingual nitroglycerin. Most patients report that the pain begins while they are resting.[46,89,137,216] In some patients, pain begins during or after exertion. It is usually described as *constricting, crushing, squeezing,* or *compressing,* although some say it is *stabbing, boring,* or *burning.* Intensity can vary but is usually rated as severe and the worst pain the patient has ever experienced. The midsternal or retrosternal area is the usual location. Radiation can include both arms,

the fingers, shoulders, neck, jaws, and back. Occasionally, patients experience pain only at referral locations. Associated symptoms include nausea, vomiting, diaphoresis, abdominal distention, shortness of breath, and overwhelming fatigue. Patients may change position, belch, or walk to try to relieve the pain. A feeling of impending doom may be expressed through statements such as, "I think I'm going to die." Narcotic analgesia (morphine) is usually required for pain relief.[10,17,100,128,137]

The term *silent myocardial infarction* refers to the 12% to 30% of AMIs that are not accompanied by chest pain.[89,128,137,166] Atypical symptoms seen in this group include respiratory difficulties, extreme fatigue, nausea, vomiting, abdominal pain, and syncope. Elderly, hypertensive, and diabetic patients are more likely to be in this group.[128,137]

Within the Feeling Pattern, the patient's emotional status should also be assessed.[78] Feelings related to illness and hospitalization such as anxiety, fear, anger, sadness, and depression should be elicited and managed. Patients entering the hospital with chest pain are usually anxious and may fear that they will die.[95] They experience fears of the unknown because of separation from family and admission to a technical and foreign environment. The unfamiliar personnel, noises, equipment, and procedures can make patients feel insecure and out of control, thus increasing anxiety. Patients may be distressed by ambiguity and uncertainty because confirmation of AMI diagnosis is delayed until serial ECGs and enzymes are obtained. They may fear that parts of their body will no longer work properly or that they will lose their jobs. Anxiety and fear will increase pain, heart rate, blood pressure, and dysrhythmias, which can be detrimental.[16,45,90]

Anxiety is an interpersonal event[71] and may be transferred between patients and families.[62] Families should be kept well informed of patients' status and allowed to visit frequently to reduce their anxiety and enable them to support patients.[131,193]

The nurse should ask patients about recent stressful life events because many of them experience AMI after or during a period of stress.[137,149] Patients may initially not recognize significant changes in their lives or understand the relationship of these changes to their current health problem. To elicit such information, the nurse might ask patients to describe their lives during previous years.

Exchanging pattern

The general appearance of patients with AMI can range from gravely ill to healthy with no apparent symptoms. Patients usually have a characteristic ashen-gray pallor, but they may have normal skin color. The skin may be warm or cool and dry or clammy. Most patients prefer to sit in a chair or in the semi-Fowler's position and are uncomfortable lying flat.[18,128,137]

---

*References 64, 94, 128, 137, 180, and 199.

Vital signs. The pulse is frequently rapid (100 to 110 beats per minute) and irregular, although it may be profoundly bradycardic.[137] The rate is affected by sympathetic and parasympathetic stimulation, the systemic metabolic response, and pain and anxiety. The irregularity is often due to PVCs.[137] PVCs occur in 95% to 100% of patients evaluated early after the onset of AMI.[128,137]

Blood pressure is usually not outside the normal range, although there may be a slight decrease in systolic and increase in diastolic pressure.[137] Some patients become hypertensive because of catecholamine release secondary to pain, anxiety, and agitation.[137] Patients with hypertension may become normotensive. Hypotension (systolic pressure less than 90 mm Hg) does not always signify cardiogenic shock. However, the presence of peripheral hypoperfusion with hypotension does indicate cardiogenic shock (see Chapter 11).[137] Early signs of peripheral hypoperfusion include clouded mentation; cold, clammy, mottled skin; and a low urine output.[10,23,88]

The respiratory rate may be elevated as a result of pain and anxiety. If the patient has no heart failure, the respiratory rate will return to normal with relief of pain and psychophysiologic stress.[137] If the patient has left ventricular failure, the respiratory rate usually correlates with the degree of failure.[137]

Most patients develop a fever within 24 to 48 hours after the onset of AMI as a result of tissue necrosis.[137] Oral temperatures may reach 38° C (101° F). Usually, the fever resolves in 1 week. Fever may also be secondary to the inflammation of acute pericarditis.

Jugular venous and carotid pulses. When only the left ventricle is infarcted, the jugular venous pulse and pressure are normal. If the patient has had a right ventricular infarction, there may be marked jugular venous distention because of rises in right atrial and ventricular pressure related to right ventricular dysfunction. If papillary muscle necrosis is present in the right ventricle, there are tall *p* waves of tricuspid regurgitation. If cardiogenic shock develops, the jugular venous pulse is usually elevated. The *carotid pulse* should be examined because it reflects left ventricular stroke volume. A weak, thready pulse indicates a reduced stroke volume. A brief, sharp pulse upstroke may indicate a left-to-right shunt, mitral regurgitation, ruptured ventricular septum, or aortic insufficiency.[137]

Breath sounds. It is essential to do baseline assessments of breath sounds. Early in AMI it is common for symptoms of left-sided heart failure to be absent. Over time, as ventricular dysfunction increases, varying symptoms of decreased cardiac output may develop. An early sign of left ventricular failure is a dry, hacking cough.[137] Patients may request cough syrup and say they are "coming down with a cold." Crackles in the lung bases are heard in patients with left ventricular failure. The size of the area in which crackles are heard is a prognostic indicator.[99,137] Diminished sounds, wheezes, and rhonchi may also be heard in left ventricular failure and pulmonary edema.[137]

Heart sounds. Early in AMI, heart sounds are often soft and muffled. As healing occurs, sounds are more easily heard. A fourth heart sound is almost always present in patients with AMI but has little significance. It is best heard between the left sternal border and the apex. Fourth heart sounds may reflect reduction in left ventricular compliance and are associated with an elevated LVEDP, even when acute heart failure is absent (see Chapter 3).

A third heart sound is significant and demonstrates extensive left ventricular dysfunction, decreased compliance, and ventricular dilation. The mortality rate for patients with a third heart sound during the acute phase of infarction is 40%, compared with 15% in patients without a third heart sound.[137] The third heart sound is best heard at the apex when patients are in the left lateral recumbent position. It is more common in patients with a transmural anterior wall MI than in patients with other types of infarction.

A new systolic murmur is significant and may indicate mitral regurgitation secondary to papillary muscle dysfunction or rupture.[89] A transient pericardial friction rub is audible in at least 20% of patients with AMI and is more common in patients with transmural infarction than in patients with other types of infarction. Friction rubs are most audible on the second or third day after infarction along the left sternal border or just inside the point of maximal impulse.[18,137]

Relating and perceiving patterns

Responses to and effects of AMI are not confined to the patient but also extend to the family.* Patient and family relationships, as well as perceptions of the illness and expectations of therapy, must be assessed. Sudden, unexpected hospitalization and subsequent lengthy recovery from life-threatening illness challenge roles, relationships, and coping skills of the patient and family.[31,95,132,135,153] As the patient adopts the sick-role, family members are suddenly required to assume roles formerly filled by the patient such as decision-maker and wage earner. Family members may also take on new care giver roles. The patient's and family members' self-esteem and self-concept may be threatened by role changes that require redefinition of relationships. The sudden, unexpected nature of the illness causes the entire family to perceive a loss of control. In an effort to maintain equilibrium, they may appear to deny illness or risk by resisting or avoiding role changes.[95,131,132,135] Assessment should include the family as a support system; physical and mental energy requirements related to the patient's usual occupational and family roles; perceptions of patient and family related to the illness' effects on roles, relationships, and self-concepts; and perceptions of loss of control.[78,95]

---

*References 25, 35, 131, 132, 135, and 153.

Knowing and choosing patterns

Significant family members, particularly spouses, should be included when the nurse assesses the Knowing and Choosing Patterns.[132,153] As soon as possible, the nurse should determine patients' and families' methods of coping and problem-solving. This information is helpful if patients' decision-making abilities are impaired and consent for life-support or other therapy must be obtained from families. Inquiry regarding knowledge of current health status, illness, and therapy should include patient and family expectations of therapy. Thus the nurse can correct misconceptions or unrealistic expectations. Patients' stages in the process of adjustment and readiness to learn should be determined. Spouses may be ready to learn earlier than patients because they seek information as a coping strategy during the acute phase,[132] whereas patients attempt to distance themselves from the meaning of the event.[95] Many patients use *denial* as an initial coping mechanism,[95] and some studies show that patients who deny the event for the longest period and with the most fervor have a better outcome.[59,108,153] Patients should be given opportunities to discuss their concerns; however, their need to deny should be respected[192] (see Interchapter 10).

Discussion of CAD risk factors and compliance with past health care regimens may help patients and spouses make sense of the illness, but it also may induce guilt.[95,132] Therefore sensitivity should be used when attempting to discover willingness and ability to comply with future health care regimens.[31]

Diagnostic tests and procedures

Definitive diagnosis of AMI requires at least two of the following criteria:

1. A history of characteristic chest discomfort
2. Evolutionary ECG changes
3. Elevated cardiac enzymes.[46]

In a few patients, radionuclide studies are the most useful diagnostic indicators because ECGs are negative or enzyme levels are normal. If dysrhythmias or conduction disturbances distort the appearance of the ECG, diagnosis is based on the history and cardiac enzyme levels, with support from physical examinations and myocardial scans.[89]

Cardiac enzyme levels. Myocardial infarction is associated with release of intracellular contents into the interstitial spaces. They are drained by the lymphatics into the plasma, where they can be measured by serologic testing.[154] After approximately 20 minutes of sustained ischemia, cell membrane integrity is impaired, and enzymes move from intracellular to interstitial fluid.[20,52] The delay between cellular injury onset and appearance of enzyme elevation in the blood depends on enzyme molecular size, regional myocardial blood flow, lymph flow, and the concentration gradient between blood, lymph, and interstitial fluid. Three enzymes have been used to diagnose myocardial infarction, specifically, aspartate aminotransferase (AST), formerly known as serum glutamic-oxaloacetic transaminase (SGOT); lactate dehydrogenase (LDH); and CK. AST is present in many organs and is least sensitive and nonspecific, so it is no longer used in diagnosis of AMI.[89,137,154]

The enzyme most useful for confirming diagnosis of AMI is CK and its MB isozyme (CK-MB). CK is involved in the production, storage, and transfer of energy. It is found primarily in skeletal and heart muscle, although it is also present in brain and visceral tissues. Elevation of total CK levels occurs during myocardial infarction and other situations, including myopathic conditions, trauma, intramuscular injections, cerebral disease, cardiac catheterization, electrical cardioversion, defibrillation, stroke, surgery, pulmonary embolism, and extensive third-degree burns.[89,154]

CK can be fractionated into its isozymes: CK-MM (muscle), CK-MB (heart tissue), and CK-BB (brain tissue and smooth muscle). In cardiac muscle, the MM isozyme predominates; however, about 15% of CK is MB. Because very little CK-MB is found in other organs, a rise in the CK-MB level is considered specific for myocardial release of the isozyme. In skeletal muscle, CK is almost entirely CK-MM. CK elevation from skeletal muscle is usually associated with elevation in the CK-MM fraction. Thus isozyme analysis of elevated total CK levels can be used to differentiate myocardial and nonmyocardial injury.[89,137,154]

Usually AMI produces elevated total CK and CK-MB levels. The plasma CK-MB is the most sensitive enzyme indicator for myocardial injury. When therapeutic reperfusion is not used, plasma CK-MB activity increases 4 to 6 hours after onset of symptoms, peaks at 12 to 24 hours, and returns to normal in 48 to 72 hours (Fig. 10-5).[89,154] Because peak CK-MB levels correlate with infarct size, they

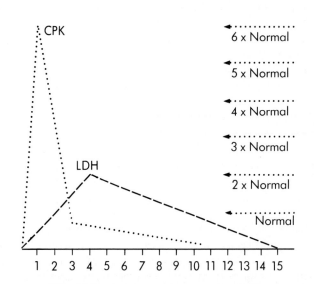

FIG. 10-5 Cardiac enzyme levels after AMI.

are used to predict complications and outcome. Therapeutic or spontaneous reperfusion causes CK-MB levels to peak earlier and renders estimation of infarct size less accurate.[137] The use of time-to-peak and peak level of CK-MB has been suggested as an alternate means to estimate infarct size.[87,137]

Reliance on only CK-MB levels to confirm AMI may be inadequate if more than 24 to 48 hours have passed since the onset and if myocardial damage has been minimal. LDH isozyme analysis and/or myocardial scans may then be used for more specific documentation of AMI because CK levels have already peaked. LDH enzyme catalyzes the reversible reaction of lactate to pyruvate and has five isozymes. The level of isozyme predominant in the heart, LDH_1, elevates 8 to 12 hours after AMI, peaks in 3 to 4 days, and returns to normal in 10 to 14 days. Normally, the level of LDH_1 is less than that for LDH_2. A rise in the level of LDH_1 greater than that of LDH_2 can be used to confirm the diagnosis of AMI.[89,137,154]

There are other markers of myocardial injury. *Myoglobin*, a heme-containing protein, has been investigated as a market for AMI.[89,137] It is abundant in skeletal and cardiac muscles, where it is a reservoir for oxygen. Elevations of serum myoglobin occur as early as 1½ hours after infarct and return to normal within 24 hours. However, this marker is not used clinically because it is not specific for myocardial damage, does not correlate as well with infarct size as CK-MB levels, and requires too much time for immunoassay.[137]

Other biochemical tests

Other biochemical tests may reveal the numerous manifestations of the inflammatory response accompanying AMI. They are not generally used in confirming the diagnosis, but awareness of their appearance is important to avoid misdiagnosis of other problems. Elevated blood glucose levels frequently occur immediately and for several weeks after AMI. Serum lipid levels generally remain at baseline levels for 24 to 48 hours after infarction and then fall. They do not restabilize until 8 weeks have elapsed. The erythrocyte sedimentation rate (ESR) is increased, as is the white blood cell (WBC) count. Leukocytosis develops within 2 hours of symptoms onset, peaks at 2 to 4 days, and declines to normal in 7 days. Peak WBC levels range from 12,000 to 15,000 per cubic millimeter.[137]

ECG evidence of AMI

The occurrence and location of AMI are indicated by characteristic changes in ST segments, T waves, and QRS complexes of leads facing the infarction (Fig. 10-6). More than one surface of the heart may be involved, and a combination of the abnormalities shown may be seen.

Evidence of AMI is seen on the ECG in evolving phases.[20,60,189] The sequence of changes is predictable, although time periods vary from patient to patient and features of one phase may overlap with the next. Changes in the ECG pattern depend on the location and size of the infarction and on therapy. Patients with small infarcts and those who receive thrombolytic therapy may not proceed through all phases.

During the *hyperacute phase*, T waves first become taller and more peaked. This immediate, transient change is rarely recorded because it usually occurs before the patient obtains medical care.[60,189] Next, within minutes to hours, elevated ST segments (greater than 1 mm) and tall, upright T waves are seen in the leads facing the infarction (indicative changes). ST-segment depression and inverted T waves are seen in leads opposite the infarction (reciprocal changes). Subtle widening of the QRS complex may be seen. Recognition of the hyperacute phase is important because serious ventricular dysrhythmias occur most often during this phase.[60,189] The *fully evolved phase* is characterized by ST-segment elevation, deep T-wave inversion, and the appearance of significant Q waves within hours to days. To be significant, Q waves must be 0.04 second in duration or more than 25% of the R wave amplitude.[206,213] During the *resolution phase*, ST segments return to baseline, usually within 2 weeks. T waves return to normal within months to a year. During the *stabilized chronic phase*, diagnostic Q waves will probably remain permanent.[60,189]

Q-wave and non-Q-wave infarction. Two types of MI, Q-wave and non-Q-wave, can be distinguished by comparing serial 12-lead ECGs.[140] In the past, transmural infarction was assumed when Q waves developed, and subendocardial or nontransmural infarction was assumed when ST-segment elevation and T-wave inversion occurred, but Q waves did not appear. However, autopsy findings have not supported these distinctions and assumptions.[60,137] It is still useful to distinguish between them because significant Q waves are quite specific for infarction. ST-segment and T-wave changes, however, may occur in a variety of conditions, such as stable and unstable angina pectoris, acute pericarditis, myocarditis, ventricular hypertrophy, digitalis toxicity, and electrolyte and metabolic disturbances. Probable infarction is identified by observing evolution of ST-T changes in specific leads.[60,137]

Anterior infarction. Q waves are seen in leads V_3 and V_4 (Fig. 10-6, *A*). (Q waves also may appear in leads I and aV_L.) ST-segment elevation and T-wave inversion may be seen in leads V_2 to V_5. Reciprocal changes may occur in leads II, III, and aV_F.

Anteroseptal infarction. Q waves are seen in leads V_1 to V_4. ST-segment elevation and T-wave inversion may be seen in leads V_1 to V_5. Reciprocal changes reflecting anteroseptal injury may *not* be seen in standard leads.

Anterolateral infarction. Q waves are seen in leads I, aV_L, and V_3 to V_6 (Fig. 10-6, *B*). (Q waves also appear in leads V_1 and V_2 if the AMI is extensive.) ST-segment elevation and T-wave inversion are visible in the same leads. Reciprocal changes may occur in leads II, III, and aV_F.

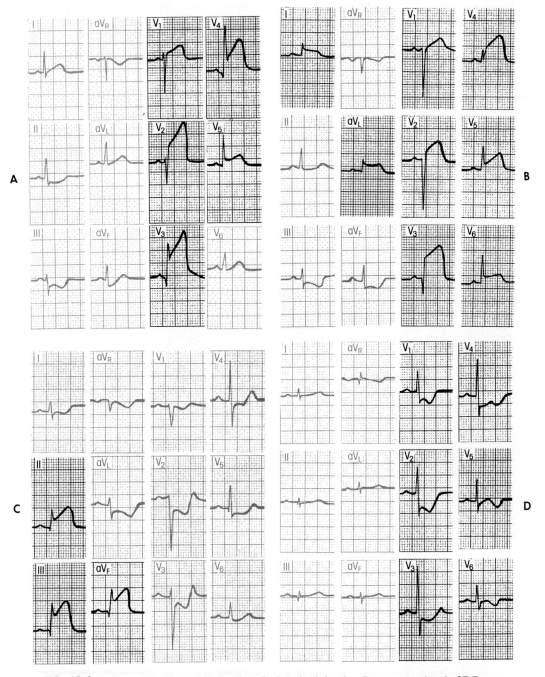

FIG. 10-6   Hyperacute phases of infarction. **A,** Anterior infarction (hyperacute phase). ST-T–wave elevation in V₁ to V₅ with appearance of diagnostic Q waves in V₃ and V₄. Reciprocal changes are seen in leads II, III, and aVF. **B,** Anterolateral infarction (hyperacute phase). Elevated ST segment in I, aVL, V₂ to V₆ with diagnostic Q waves in V₁, V₂, and V₃. Reciprocal changes are seen in leads III and aVF. **C,** Inferior (diaphragmatic) infarction (hyperacute phase). Elevated ST segments in II, III, and aVF with Q waves in II, III, and aVF. Reciprocal changes are seen in I, aVL, and V₁ to V₅. **D,** Posterolateral infarction (hyperacute phase). Depressed ST segments are seen in V₁ to V₅. Increased R waves are seen in V₁ and V₂, with wider T waves in V₁ to V₃.

Inferior (diaphragmatic) infarction. Q waves, ST-segment elevation, and T-wave inversion are visible in leads II, III, and aV_F (Fig. 10-6, *C*). Reciprocal changes may occur in leads V_1 to V_3.

Posterior infarction. None of the conventional leads is oriented to the posterior heart surface. Infarction is inferred from changes (reciprocal) occurring in the anterior leads. Diagnosis of true posterior infarction is made when there is an R-wave:S-wave ratio of greater than 1 and an increase in R-wave height in leads V_1 and V_2 (Fig. 10-6, *D*).[60] In early posterolateral MI, the ECG shows lateral and inferior wall involvement, ST-segment depression in leads V_1 to V_4, and an inverted, widened T wave in lead V_1. ST-segment elevation with widening of the T wave in lead V_6 is evidence of lateral wall involvement. Widening of the T wave with ST-segment elevation in standard leads II, III, and aV_F is evidence of inferior wall involvement. Inferior MI is often associated with true posterior MI. A fully evolved true posterior infarction with inferolateral extension shows increased R-wave amplitude in leads V_1 to V_3 (the inverse change of pathologic Q wave) and upright, widened, symmetrical T waves in leads V_1 to V_3 (the inverse change of the inverted T wave). Posterior infarctions are easily missed when there are lateral inferior changes, as well.

Right ventricular infarction. Right ventricular infarction is difficult to diagnose, presumably because right ventricular mass is small compared with left ventricular mass. ST-segment elevation in V_1 and V_3R to V_6R is a relatively sensitive marker. Development of Q waves and T-wave inversion is inconsistent. Right ventricular infarction occurs almost exclusively as a complication of a transmural inferoseptal left ventricular infarction. Approximately 50% of this group of patients may have associated right ventricular involvement.[57,136,188]

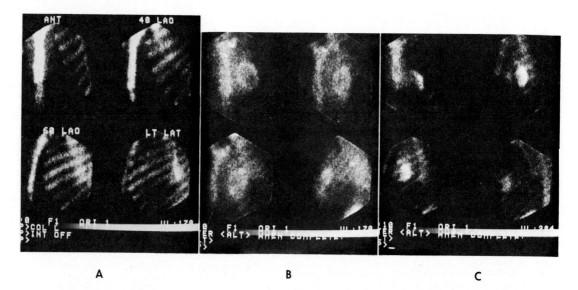

A   B   C

FIG. 10-7 Myocardial isotope scans. **A,** Normal technetium-99m pyrophosphate scan is shown with four standard views after administration of the isotope. The views are anteroposterior projection (ANT), 40 degrees left anterior oblique (40 LAO), 60 degrees left anterior oblique (60 LAO), and left lateral (LT LAT). Normal uptake is seen by the vertebrae in the dorsal spine, the ribs, and the sternum. The intensity of uptake increases over the first 24 to 48 hours and then progressively diminishes over the next several days. No significant cardiac uptake is evident in this normal scan because the isotope is bound only to ionic calcium, which is present in significant quantities in the heart only when AMI occurs. **B,** The four standard views of ANT, 40 LAO, 60 LAO, and LT LAT are shown. Uptake of technetium-99m pyrophosphate is seen near the sternum in each view. In the 60 LAO projection, there is a circular uptake evident, the so-called donut effect. These findings indicate anterolateral MI. The intensity of the uptake is moderate, is considered 3+ on a 4+ scale, and is referred to as a "hot spot." **C,** Again, the standard four views are shown. There uptake is very intense, with a "hot spot" of 4+. The technetium-99m pyrophosphate is located next to the dorsal spine. This is best seen in the 40 LAO projection. The patient has had a transmural posterior and posterolateral MI.

Chest x-ray examination

The incidence of atelectasis and congestive heart failure after AMI is high. Chest x-ray films are obtained at admission to establish a baseline and assess the presence of pulmonary edema. Arterial calcification, underlying pulmonary disease, or other complicating features also may be revealed.[89,137]

Radionuclide studies

All major forms of nuclear cardiac imaging are useful in detecting AMI, in assessing infarct size and jeopardized myocardium, in determining ventricular function, and in establishing prognosis (see Chapter 6).[89,137] *Thallium-201* scanning differentiates ischemic from normal or infarcted muscle (see Chapters 6 and 9).

Technetium-99m pyrophosphate isotope scanning is used to detect AMI (Fig. 10-7, *A* to *C*). The isotope binds to calcium in acutely and irreversibly damaged myocardial cells and appears as a "hot spot" because normal tissue does not take up the isotope. The isotope is injected into a peripheral vein, and scanning is done 1 to 3 hours afterward. The scan is negative for the first 24 hours after AMI, with peak uptake occurring around 48 hours. At 4 days the image begins to fade. By day 7 to 10 after MI, the scan is probably negative. All types of infarcts can be located because views from various positions are taken—anterior, left anterior oblique, and lateral. The scan is most helpful when the ECG does not confirm an MI, when the patient has complete left bundle branch block, when an old MI is present on the ECG, when enzyme levels are unreliable (such as after cardiac surgery), or when pacemaker activity distorts the evolutionary changes of infarction. Computed tomography allows cross-sectional views of the heart from base to apex, including areas that can be hidden by isotope uptake of the ribs, sternum, and spine.[46]

Echocardiography

Two-dimensional echocardiography is a valid method for identifying abnormal ventricular wall movement and mechanical complications in AMI. Because ischemic and infarcted tissue cannot be distinguished, infarct size tends to be overestimated using this technique[137] (see Chapter 6).

Cardiac catheterization and angiography

Cardiac catheterization and angiography are performed in patients with AMI when there is recurrent chest pain or other evidence of ongoing ischemia.[89,186] Patients who develop papillary muscle or septal rupture also are candidates

for the procedure.[89] The purpose is to determine whether revascularization or surgical repair can be done (see Chapters 6 and 9).

Medical and nursing diagnoses

The medical diagnosis is AMI. Complications develop in 80% to 90% of patients[34] and may be anticipated by knowing the specific location and evolutionary stage of the infarction. The major complications are dysrhythmias (75% to 95% of patients), cardiac failure (60%), thromboembolism (15% to 40%), cardiogenic shock (10%), and rupture of free wall, septum, or papillary muscle (1% to 5%).[34]

The most common human responses anticipated for a patient with AMI are indicated by the following nursing diagnoses:[27,120]

1. Acute pain and activity intolerance related to inadequate myocardial tissue perfusion
2. High risk for decreased cardiac output related to
   a. Electrical factors (rate, rhythm, and conduction)
   b. Mechanical factors (preload, afterload, and inotropic state)
   c. Structural factors (papillary muscle dysfunction, interventricular septal rupture, ventricular aneurysm, and ventricular rupture)
3. High risk for altered comfort related to systemic response of AMI (nausea, vomiting, and hiccuping; gastrointestinal tract problems; genitourinary tract problems; thromboembolism; pericarditis; Dressler's syndrome)
4. Anxiety (patient and family), ineffective coping (patient and family), and altered role performance (patient and family) related to pathophysiologic, situational, and treatment-related factors
5. High risk for noncompliance* and altered sexuality related to knowledge deficit and situational and treatment-related factors

For each of these diagnoses, patient outcomes, nursing prescriptions, and evaluation criteria are outlined with a discussion of the factual information that supports the plan and implementation of care.

---

*The NANDA Taxonomy uses the term *Noncompliance*. Many clinicians object to this label. McFarland and McFarlane[120] indicate that *Nonadherence* might be a preferable term. Carey[26] suggests that the attitude and ethical approach of the health professional is most important. Clinicians should use terminology that allows them, patients, and families to set mutual goals.

NURSING
DIAGNOSIS 1

Acute pain and activity intolerance related to inadequate myocardial tissue perfusion (feeling and moving patterns)

PATIENT OUTCOMES	NURSING PRESCRIPTIONS	EVALUATION
Patient will report and describe pain and discomfort.	Assess pain and discomfort.	Patient reported and described pain and discomfort.
Patient will report relief of pain and discomfort and not have any new episodes of pain.	Institute measures to relieve pain, including prescribed analgesic and antianginal agents and holistic measures.	Patient reported that analgesics and antianginal agents relieved pain and that no new episodes of pain occurred.
Patient will not have complications from therapeutic measures.	Institute measures to improve myocardial perfusion and reduce myocardial work and oxygen demand.	Patient demonstrated no complications related to therapeutic measures.
Patient will tolerate light activity at discharge.	Gradually increase patient's activity.	Patient demonstrated tolerance of light activity before discharge.

Plan and intervention for acute pain and activity intolerance

The priorities in managing the patient with AMI are pain relief, improvement of myocardial oxygenation, continuous cardiac monitoring for detection of dysrhythmias and conduction disturbances (see Appendix B), anxiety reduction, detection of complications, and sleep and rest.[10,23,88,199] An infusion of 5% dextrose in water is started as soon as possible for rapid intravenous access if complications occur and medications are required.

The patient with suspected AMI is admitted to the CCU or telemetry unit, depending on the initial presentation, ECG, and CK level.[24,68,137] Vital signs should be checked hourly until the patient is stable and free of pain and then are checked every 4 hours. Oral temperatures should also be taken every 4 hours unless the patient has cardiogenic shock; then rectal temperatures are more accurate. Cardiovascular and pulmonary assessment continues throughout the patient's hospital stay and should always include lung and heart sounds, urinary output, and mental state.[10,23,88] The length of stay in a specialty unit for patients who suffer no complications is 24 to 48 hours.[128,137]

Pain management

Pain accompanying AMI represents ongoing myocardial ischemia and causes increased autonomic nervous system activity that results in negative psychophysiologic responses. Treatment is aimed at reducing pain promptly.[10,22,23,88,199] Before giving pain medication, the nurse should know the patient's baseline vital signs to assess whether the agents give effective pain relief. Other baseline parameters are anxiety level, body gestures showing pain, and statements of pain or discomfort by the patient. For additional comfort, the patient should be placed in a comfortable position with the head of the bed elevated. The patient is instructed to inform the nurse immediately if the pain continues or returns after being relieved. The patient also must be observed for pain behaviors because pain may not be reported.[4,167]

Medications. Morphine sulfate (2 to 8 mg) is administered intravenously at 5- to 15-minute intervals until pain relief occurs. Morphine sulfate also reduces anxiety, dilates vascular beds, reduces the work of breathing, and slows heart rate, which are added benefits during AMI.[30,114,121] Patients may require and usually tolerate large cumulative doses (2 to 3 mg/kg).[137] It is perferable to give small, frequent doses (2 mg at 5-minute intervals) to avoid the side effects of hypotension and respiratory depression. Confining the patient to bed after morphine administration can minimize hypotension. Respiratory depression (respiratory rate of less than 8 breaths per minute) is an unusual complication but may occur. Maximum risk is approximately 7 minutes after injection. Naloxone (0.1 to 0.2 mg), given intravenously at 15-minute intervals, can reverse this complication.[137] For the person who has a hypersensitivity to morphine, meperidine, 50 to 150 mg intravenously over the same period of time, may also be used. Meperidine is less effective and more likely to cause side effects such as tachycardia.[137] These medications are given intravenously instead of intramuscularly to enhance absorption and prevent elevation of CK-MM levels.[128,137]

If a patient is not hypotensive and the pain is not relieved by morphine sulfate and large doses of sublingual nitroglycerin, an intravenous infusion of nitroglycerin may be started. Intravenous administration allows maintenance of a constant, controlled blood level. Nitroglycerin relaxes vascular smooth muscle and dilates the venous and arterial beds. Such vasodilation decreases preload and afterload, reducing myocardial oxygen consumption and demand. The dosage is started at 5 to 10 μg/minute and then titrated to the patient's needs. During titration, doses are usually increased by 5 μg/minute every 3 to 5 minutes. Intravenous nitroglycerin has no maximum or optimum dosage, but doses greater than 100 μg/min are unusual. Nitroglycerin is titrated with an end point of pain relief but is stopped or decreased if severe headache, tachycardia, or symptomatic hypotension occurs. Therefore the patient's blood pressure and heart rate must be monitored carefully when the drug is titrated to achieve the appropriate dosage for the patient's condition and to prevent toxicity.[41,128,137,181]

Studies have shown that early use of intravenous nitroglycerin in AMI may favorably affect early and long-term morbidity and mortality rates.[181] Although nitroglycerin does not possess intrinsic antidysrhythmic properties, the favorable relationship between oxygen supply and demand established by nitrates accounts for the reduction in early and late PVCs, as well as a decreased incidence of ventricular tachycardia and fibrillation. Optimally, the patient should have arterial and pulmonary artery catheters in place for evaluation of response to therapy. Nitroglycerin should be used cautiously in patients with inferior wall and right ventricular infarction because they are very sensitive to its effects.[137] β-blocking agents and calcium blockers may be used in some patients to augment pain control[46,128,137] (see Chapter 9 and Appendix C).

Holistic techniques in pain relief. Patients with chest pain are anxious and sometimes fearful that they will die during the acute event.[95] All persons with pain have a contracted or constricted time sense. A few minutes of chest pain may seem like hours to AMI patients. Nurses need to do more than give pain medication to AMI patients in pain.[4,148] They must also intervene to reduce anxiety and alter patients' perceptions of pain and time.

After receiving morphine or other narcotic analgesics, it is not uncommon for patients to say, "That medicine helped me forget where I was" or "I lost track of time." Such statements suggest that altered time perception is one of the hidden benefits of narcotic analgesic therapy. Mental states can evoke actual changes in brain physiologic states that alter pain perception. The human brain produces *endorphins*, which have potent pain-relieving properties. CCU nurses can and must use bedside techniques to elicit the *placebo effect* and expand patients' time sense during the acute event. Investigative data on biofeedback, imagery, meditation, and self-hypnosis show that patients can achieve physiologic self-control. Through these techniques, nurses can help patients set in motion complex biochemical events in their bodies, which can be subjectively experienced as time expansion and analgesia via natural endorphin release[4] (see Interchapters 3, 4, and 13).

Response to pain is an individual matter that is difficult to measure or compare. Pain is emotionally and physically draining. Nurses can help patients enhance their own pain relief through imagery and relaxation. When chest pain is frequent or lasts a long time, anxiety and fear are increased. Patients should be taught proper breathing techniques and ways to relax their jaws and neck. When this is done, time perception is altered, and they can benefit more from the medication they receive. They also gain a sense of control. If pain relief is not immediate, nurses must give more pain medication, stay with patients, and guide them in relaxation. Soft music can help the process.[4,37,76,148]

Every nursing intervention, whether it involves drug administration, treatment, or teaching of relaxation and imagery exercises, has *placebo* aspects.[43] When helping relieve a patient's chest pain, the nurse should maximize the placebo effect of the drug. The elements that contribute to a positive placebo response are using convincing stimuli, focusing attention on the symptoms, explaining the intent of the pain relief measure, and having the drug administered by a trusted expert. When convincing stimuli are used, the patient understands the pain-relieving treatment. For example, when administering intravenous morphine, the nurse should explain how rapidly the medication will traverse the patient's system and relieve the pain. The patient should watch the administration of the medication. Some patients believe that an intramuscular injection is the best route. The nurse should correct this misconception. If the nurse focuses attention on the symptom, the patient perceives the nurse's concern, which helps elicit the placebo response. Inquiring about the patient's history at this time disrupts the focus of attention on pain relief and interferes with the placebo effect. Some statements that explain the intent of the pain relief measure are: "This medicine is extremely effective in getting rid of chest pain" and "Giving this medicine through your vein is the best way to relieve your chest pain." Trust or faith in the person giving the medicine is important. Reinforcing the patient's faith in the physician also enhances the placebo effect.[4]

Infarct extension. Extension, or progressive infarction, occurs in 7% to 31% of patients, depending on the measures instituted. It is recognized by continued or new ECG changes or elevation of CK levels. Persistent or recurrent pain indicates that infarction is likely to extend and requires prompt, aggressive treatment. Ischemic pain is most likely to return after 24 hours in patients with multiple vessel disease, non-Q-wave infarctions, and previous histories of angina. Left ventricular failure and other complications are more likely to develop in patients with extension. Inhospital death may also occur. Emergency PTCA or myocardial revascularization may be necessary.[8,128,137,169,212]

Oxygen therapy

Hypoxemia is common among patients with AMI. In some centers, oxygen via nasal cannula is routinely given at 3 to 5 L/min for the first 24 to 48 hours. However, increasing inspired oxygen does not benefit and may harm patients who are not hypoxemic. Therefore arterial oxygen tension should be measured at admission, and oxygen is administered only if necessary.[137]

Physical activity

Physical activity is modified to decrease myocardial oxygen consumption and physical stress on the infarcted area. The nurse must consider the most effective measures to modify physical activity to decrease myocardial work.[15] These include positions for activities of daily living such as rest, elimination, eating, and bathing. After admission, bed rest with commode privileges is prescribed for the patient. Studies of toileting[15] have shown that using a bedside commode requires less energy than using a bedpan. Although a bowel movement is not necessary for the first 3 to 5 days, a stool softener is commonly given to prevent constipation. The patient should be told not to strain with bowel movements. Male patients may be allowed to stand at the bedside to void.

Studies have varied in their assessment of the energy cost of bathing.[15] Showering requires more energy than bed or tub baths. The common practice is to give bed baths during the first 3 to 5 days and then allow tub baths or showers if no dysrhythmias, heart failure, or recurring chest pain occur.[15,210] In patients with CAD, the postural difference between standing to shower and sitting for bed or tub baths may cause hemodynamic and metabolic changes after AMI.[96] Usually, male patients may shave themselves on the fourth day.[128]

If the patient has no complications, after 24 to 36 hours, activity may be progressed to chair rest for 30 to 60 minutes twice daily. Chair rest is beneficial because it promotes a feeling of well-being, requires less myocardial work, and avoids the adverse effects of prolonged bed rest.[15,128,137,146] An alternative to chair rest is propping the patient comfortably in a semi-Fowler's position and suggesting some rhythmic lower-extremity exercises.

The AMI patient is allowed limited ambulation in the room on the third or fourth day. Exercise continues in a progressive fashion, with specific instruction on exercise stages by the nurse and physical therapist involved in the cardiac rehabilitation program (see Chapter 19). Activity is usually kept within 1 to 3 metabolic equivalents (METs) during the hospital stay.[10,210] Activity should be stopped or decreased if the patient develops signs or symptoms of intolerance; these include cardiac discomfort or breathlessness; dizziness, confusion, faintness; marked pallor; cold sweat; ataxia; severe fatigue; heart rate greater than 110 beats per minute; a decrease or no change in heart rate with increasing physical activity; a fall in systolic pressure of 10 mm Hg or more; an increase in systolic pressure of 40 mm Hg or more; ST-segment displacement of 1 mm or more; or the appearance of new cardiac rhythm disturbances.[10,15] If the patient has complications, activity is increased more slowly, and discharge from the CCU occurs later.

In the past, traditional *coronary precautions* were taken to prevent vagal or sympathetic stimulation of the heart. Physical activities that were avoided included rectal temperature and backrubs. There is little data indicating that rectal temperature measurements should not be taken. It is anatomically and physiologically impossible to induce vagal stimulation with the normal method of taking rectal temperatures. The best reason not to take rectal temperatures is that it is embarrassing and less aesthetic. Turning the patient in bed produces more physiologic effects than the actual temperature-taking.[101] Also no data support the avoidance of backrubs. A gentle backrub can enhance deep relaxation and is a powerful way to shift a patient's perception of time, as well as convey care and compassion.[4,101]

Sleep and rest

Sleep and rest are extremely important for recovery but are difficult for patients to achieve in the hospital and CCU setting.[162] Sleep is a state of rest that occurs for sustained periods. The reduced consciousness during sleep provides time for repair and recovery of the mind and body. Sleep restores energy and feelings of well-being. People at rest are free from physical and mental exertion. They feel mentally and physically relaxed and calm. Patients on bed rest are actually not at rest if they are anxious and worried. Nurses must create the conditions for proper rest, which include physical comfort, freedom from worry, and sufficient sleep. Factors that affect the quality of sleep and rest include patients' mental states, severity of illness, metabolic function, medications, environment, and interruptions for medical and nursing care.[88,143]

There are five stages of sleep: stages 1, 2, 3, 4 (referred to as *non-rapid eye movement* or NREM) and *rapid eye movement* or REM. During NREM sleep (stages 1 to 4), the body repairs and renews epithelial and specialized cells. Release of growth hormone in stage 4 stimulates protein synthesis, tissue repair, and bone growth. During REM sleep, metabolic activity, hormone release, and autonomic function are increased. REM sleep is important for memory, learning, and behavioral adaptation. The dreams of REM sleep are believed to be functionally important in reviewing the day's events, clarifying emotions, and preparing for the next day. Periods of stress, worry, and intense new learning increase the need for REM sleep.[118,143]

It usually takes 10 to 30 minutes or more for a person to fall asleep and enter stage 1. A person moving through natural sleep progresses from stage 1 through stage 4, then back through stage 3 to stage 2, and then into REM sleep. When the REM stage is over, they have completed the first full sleep cycle and reenter stage 2 to begin the next cycle. It takes 90 to 120 minutes to complete an entire cycle and a typical night's sleep consists of 4 to 6 cycles. The time spent in each stage varies. Stage 4 shortens, and REM lengthens progressively with each cycle. The first REM cycle lasts only a few moments. Most stage-4 sleep occurs early in the night, and most REM sleep occurs early in the morning.[118,120,143] Increased morbidity and mortality rates are associated with unusually short (less than 4 to 6 hours) and long (more than 9 to 10 hours) sleep lengths.[199]

Considering the time involved in falling asleep and completing a sleep cycle, patients need a minimum of 2 to 3 hours of uninterrupted sleep. Nurses should try to identify patients' stages of sleep to let them complete an entire cycle before awakening them.[143] In stages 1 and 2, light sleep, persons are easily aroused by noise and light. In stages 3 and 4, deep sleep, persons are difficult to arouse and rarely move because their muscles are completely relaxed. Vital signs are lower during stage 4 than in waking periods. People usually change body positions at the end of stage 4 and REM sleep. REM sleep is recognized by rapid eye movement, which can be seen through closed eyelids. There is also complete relaxation of the lower jaw, slight muscular twitching, profound muscular relaxation, dreams, and in males, penile erection. Blood pressure and pulse and respiration rates normally become irregular and variable during REM sleep.[118,143]

In the CCU, patients are frequently awakened by noise, lights, pain, anxiety, and procedures.[171] When sleep is interrupted, persons start over at stage 1 after they have fallen asleep again. As a result, patients experience more stage-1 sleep with each sleep interruption. A significantly greater number of PVCs occur in stage 1 than in other sleep stages. Heart rate, a determinant of myocardial oxygen consumption, is highest during waking states and lowest in deep sleep. Thus sleep interruption increases myocardial oxygen consumption and may precipitate myocardial ischemia and increase PVCs.[42] In addition, interruptions often prevent patients from reaching the deeper stages of sleep (NREM stages 3 and 4 and REM). Persons deprived of REM sleep become confused and suspicious. Repeated nights of REM deprivation are implicated as a cause of ICU psychosis.[171] Persons deprived of stage-3 and stage-4 sleep feel withdrawn and physically uncomfortable.[143]

Other adverse effects of sleep deprivation are irritability, anxiety, fatigue, restlessness, increased sensitivity to pain and discomfort, apathy, lack of alertness, exhaustion, hallucinations, and migraine headaches. Disruption of biologic rhythms, metabolic functions, and hormone release can have a detrimental effect on patients' stress responses and healing processes.[88,143] During recovery from sleep deprivation, there is a significant increase (rebound) in the total time spent in the deprived sleep stage. REM rebound periods are frequently accompanied by nightmares and unpleasant dreams that can further interrupt sleep and contribute to cardiac stress.[82]

Sleep is a priority for AMI patients and should receive the same emphasis as other aspects of care. Procedures, tests, vital signs, medications, and other nursing care should be planned to allow uninterrupted 2- to 3-hour periods for sleep. The more consecutive, uninterrupted

sleep cycles patients have, the more they are assured of sleep that promotes recovery.[88,171]

Many hypnotic, tranquilizing, and sedating drugs suppress REM sleep. Common REM-suppressant drugs given in CCU are flurazepam (Dalmane), triazolam (Halcion), glutethimide (Doriden), pentobarbital sodium (Nembutal), and methyprylon (Noludar). Diazepam (Valium), chlordiazepoxide (Librium), and chloral hydrate (Noctec) also have a REM-suppressant effect. One of the more prominent cognitive effects of these drugs is a reduction in the ability to learn new information. Triazolam (Halcion) is particularly implicated in this effect.[46,165]

Diet

Patients may receive liquid diets during the first 24 hours because of the increased risk of nausea and vomiting. There is also an increased incidence of cardiac arrest, during which aspiration of food might occur. The liquid diet is then frequently followed by a 1200- to 1800-calorie soft diet with no added salt and a low-fat content.[46,128,137,199]

Traditional *coronary dietary precautions* include avoidance of beverages with ice or stimulants.[101] A recent report[102] indicates that universal restriction of iced beverages is not needed. Only 6 of 89 patients were found to have clinically detectable ST-segment and T-wave changes within 3 minutes of drinking 200 ml or 400 ml of ice water. The investigators recommend that newly admitted patients be monitored in several leads for 3 minutes while drinking ice water. Baseline tracings should be compared for shifts in ST segments and T waves. Beverages with ice should not be given to patients with significant shifts.

Caffeine is a cardiac stimulant and should generally be restricted; beverages that contain caffeine include coffee, tea, and cola.[101,128,137] However, patients' previous consumption should be considered. Those with large previous intakes should be observed for withdrawal symptoms. Gradual reduction may be preferred.

Measures to improve myocardial perfusion

Infarction does not occur simultaneously or immediately after arterial occlusion.[214] The most effective means of reversing ischemic injury is to increase the myocardial blood supply. Myocardial tissue can be salvaged for at least 2 to 3 hours and possibly 6 to 24 hours after coronary occlusion.[47,109,128,141]

Thrombolytic therapy. Thrombolytic therapy improves coronary blood flow by lysing clots that occlude coronary arteries.[41,48] It is effective in reperfusing reversibly injured myocardium (in 40% to 80% of patients), thereby reducing infarct size, left ventricular dysfunction, and mortality rates.* Nursing responsibilities include assessment before infusion, proper administration of the agent, monitoring of the response to therapy during and after infusion, and

---

*References 19, 21, 91, 98, 113, 168, 169, and 200.

monitoring and detection of complications during and after infusion.*

Patients are selected for thrombolytic therapy on the basis of the presence of indications and the absence of contraindications (see the box). Indications for thrombolytic therapy are persistent anginal chest pain lasting 30 minutes or longer and not relieved by nitroglycerin, onset of pain less than 6 hours before beginning thrombolytic therapy, and ST-segment elevation of 0.2 millivolts (mV) or more in at least two ECG leads overlying adjacent areas of the myocardium. Some centers also require the patient to be less than 70 to 75 years old.[134,157] Contraindications for thrombolytic therapy include active internal bleeding; history of cerebrovascular accident; recent (within 2 months) intracranial or intraspinal surgery or trauma; intracranial neoplasm, arteriovenous malformation, or aneurysm; bleeding diathesis; and severe uncontrollable hypertension.[48] Major surgery within the last 10 days, CPR trauma, infective endocarditis, significant valvular disease, or any risk of hemorrhage are also considered contraindications.[46] Patients with circulating streptococcal antibodies are at risk for allergic reaction to streptokinase and therefore recent streptokinase therapy or streptococcal infection is a relative contraindication.[48] If patients meet the selection criteria, written informed consent for thrombolytic therapy is obtained.*

Nursing responsibilities during the preinfusion period include providing usual care for patients with AMI, explaining procedures to patients and families, performing baseline physical assessments, obtaining baseline laboratory studies and ECGs, ensuring intravenous access at two or three sites, and administering prophylactic medications such as steroids, antihistamines, or lidocaine, if ordered. A coagulation profile and blood type and cross-match and the usual laboratory studies are done. Different vascular access sites are needed to infuse the thrombolytic agent, to administer emergency medications, and to sample blood for laboratory studies.*

During the infusion, nurses are responsible for properly administering the agent, monitoring patient response, and detecting complications. *Urokinase* (Abbokinase), *streptokinase* (Streptase, Kabikinase), *tissue plasminogen activator or tPA (Activase)*, and *anisoylated plasminogen streptokinase activator complex (APSAC) (anistreplase, Eminase)* are approved for coronary thrombolysis.[122] Another agent, single-chain urokinase-type plasminogen activator (scu-PA, prourokinase), is under investigation.[32] Because research on thrombolytic therapy is still being done, protocols vary among institutions. Nurses should check the policy at the institution for which they work.

Only the intracoronary route is used for urokinase. Other agents may be administered by intracoronary or

---

*References 23, 30, 48, 94, 114, 121, 203, and 207.

INDICATIONS AND CONTRAINDICATIONS FOR THROMBOLYTIC THERAPY

INDICATIONS

Chest pain, consistent with myocardial ischemia lasting 30 minutes or longer and not relieved by nitroglycerin

Onset of chest pain less than 6 hours before beginning thrombolytic therapy

ST-segment elevation of 0.2mV or more in at least two adjacent leads of the ECG

CONTRAINDICATIONS

Active or recent internal bleeding

Bleeding disorder or anticoagulant therapy

Evidence of aortic dissection

History of cerebrovascular accident, especially a recent one

Intracranial neoplasm, arteriovenous malformation, or aneurysm

Known or suspected pregnancy

Recent, prolonged cardiopulmonary resuscitation causing obvious chest trauma

Recent surgery or trauma, including invasive procedures

Terminal cancer

---

intravenous infusion. The intracoronary route is used in the cardiac catheterization laboratory or operating room during coronary angiography, percutaneous transluminal angioplasty (PTCA), or surgical intervention. Intravenous administration is advantageous because the delay in assembling personnel, transporting patients to the cardiac catheterization laboratory, and performing angiography can be avoided.[46] The intravenous route may be used in centers without cardiac catheterization facilities, as well as in the field.[40,116,185]

Urokinase is a naturally occurring human protease derived from renal parenchymal cells. It directly converts plasminogen into plasmin and is not clot specific. Urokinase is more expensive than streptokinase and causes fewer allergic reactions. Drug dosages vary but intracoronary administration may consist of a bolus of 10,000 to 30,000 units (U) followed by continuous infusion at 2000 to 24,000 U/min.[48,111,157,161,195]

Streptokinase is an enzyme derived from β-hemolytic streptococci that activates conversion of plasminogen to plasmin. Its action is not confined to the clot because it is not fibrin specific. Systemic consumption of fibrinogen and other clotting factors creates a hypocoagulable state that may persist for 18 to 24 hours.[48,157] Current dose recommendation is 1.5 million U given intravenously over 60 minutes. When the intracoronary route is used, the dose is a 25,000 to 50,000 U bolus followed by infusion of 2000 to 4000 U/min for 60 minutes. Compared with other agents, streptokinase is more likely to cause allergic reactions, including fever, chills, rashes, and anaphylaxis. To prevent these side effects, patients are usually given steroids and antihistamines before infusion.[111,169]

tPA is a naturally occurring human protease secreted by the vascular endothelium. This thrombolytic factor is synthesized artificially using recombinant DNA techniques.[48,124,157] It is thought to be relatively clot specific because it acts on fibrin bound rather than circulating plasminogen. Braunwald,[19] in examining data from the TIMI[28,196] and European Cooperative Study Group[204,205] trials, found tPA to be more effective than streptokinase. Collen[32] also reviewed studies of thrombolytic therapy and came to the same conclusion. Current intravenous dosage recommendation is a total of 100 mg delivered as a 10-mg bolus, then 50 mg over 1 hr, then 10 mg/hr for 4 hrs.[169] In some centers, the medication is given by weight.[48]

APSAC is an inactive derivative of plasminogen.[112,127,169] It is injected as a bolus, 30 units intravenously over 2 to 5 minutes, and thus is more convenient to administer.[122] Theoretically, it is selective for fibrin, concentrates at the site of thrombus, and has a sustained local action. In practice, systemic fibrinolysis has been noted, although significant hemorrhage has been rare.[127] Allergic reactions are possible because the compound contains streptokinase. Therefore some centers administer antihistamines and steroids before APSAC.[48] Reperfusion rates have been similar to other agents. Comparison studies with tPA and streptokinase are planned.[127,169]

Thrombolytic therapy is successful when reperfusion occurs within 30 to 90 minutes of administration. Abrupt cessation of chest discomfort, rapid fall in ST-segment elevation, early peaking of CK levels, and appearance of reperfusion dysrhythmias are clinical indicators of reperfusion. However, reperfusion dysrhythmias are less-reliable indicators than the others. After the thrombolytic infusion is complete, nursing care consists of continuing to monitor for complications and usual care for patients with AMI.*

There are obvious benefits to dissolving a clot in a coronary artery. However, there may be complications such as bleeding (65% incidence), dysrhythmias (38% to 45%), and reocclusion (20% to 45%).[179] Monitoring and management of complications (Table 10-1) is needed during and after infusion.† The usual cause of bleeding is disruption of natural clotting processes and lysis of protective hemostatic clots. The cause of *reperfusion dysrhythmias* is debated and poorly understood. They are usually ventricular (PVCs, ventricular tachycardia, and accelerated idioventri-

cular rhythm), although sinus tachycardia is also seen.[48] *Reocclusion* is a significant problem associated with thrombolytic therapy. Heparin, aspirin, or another anticoagulant is commonly used as an adjunct to prevent new clot formation after thrombolytic therapy.* Reocclusion is indicated by chest pain and elevation of ST segments. The cause may be vasospasm or formation of a new thrombus.[48,203]

PTCA. PTCA can be used to achieve reperfusion in patients with AMI. It is used instead of thrombolytic therapy, when thrombolytic therapy was unsuccessful, or when severe stenosis remains after successful thrombolysis.[8,38,137,175] The procedure improves blood flow to the ischemic myocardium by compressing atherosclerotic plaque and dilating the stenosed segment of the coronary artery (see Chapter 9). The results of the Thrombolysis and Angioplasty in Myocardial Infarction (TAMI) trials[197] indicate that thrombolytic therapy followed by elective angioplasty can be advantageous.

Surgical myocardial revascularization. Surgical revascularization in the AMI patient is controversial. Most authorities agree that an established infarct of 48 hours or more is a relative contraindication for myocardial revascularization.[128,137] Emergency myocardial revascularization has been tried as a means to reduce infarct size.[137,206] Although it seems to be effective, when carried out within 4 hours of onset, it is unlikely to be adopted as a routine approach because of the logistic difficulties involved. In patients who are already in the hospital waiting for surgery, it is the treatment of choice.[128] It also benefits patients with recurrent pain indicating incomplete or stuttering infarction.[137] Rapid coronary revascularization has implications for nursing because patients may go from the acute anxiety of an MI to facing open heart surgery in a matter of minutes or hours. Skillful preoperative teaching is vital because learning is compromised by high anxiety levels. Teaching that incorporates imagery and relaxation may be more effective (see Chapter 5).[115,147]

Intraaortic balloon counterpulsation

Theoretically, counterpulsation with the intraaortic balloon pump (IABP) is useful in decreasing infarct size.[137] At present, little data support its use in place of other therapies with lower complication rates. Consequently, it is reserved for patients who are hemodynamically compromised by mechanical or structural failure. The IABP has been successful in maintaining patients who are in cardiogenic shock or as preparation for emergency surgery (see Chapter 11).

Medications to alter myocardial metabolism

The size of infarction may be reduced by improving or reducing myocardial metabolism.[137]

---

*References 23, 30, 48, 94, 114, 121, and 203.
†References 23, 48, 51, 195, 199, and 203.

*References 9, 19, 46, 48, 67, and 72.

TABLE 10-1
Complications of Thrombolytic Therapy

Monitoring	Prevention or management
BLEEDING	
Perform baseline assessment before infusion: history, vital signs, skin color and integrity (punctures, incisions), and extremities (pulses, color, sensation).	Screen patients for contraindications.
Review coagulation profile and laboratory data.	Maintain infusions at prescribed rate.
Monitor vital signs and neurologic status.	Keep involved extremity straight.
Inspect skin and injection sites for bleeding and hematoma at infusion site.	Draw all blood from arterial catheter.
Monitor for signs of concealed bleeding (test emesis, nasogastric drainage, urine, and stool for occult blood).	Give all medications by previously existing intravenous lines.
Monitor extremity pulses, sensation, and color.	Apply firm pressure to infusion site for 30 to 45 minutes after catheter is removed.
Monitor for signs and symptoms of pericardial tamponade.	Apply firm pressure to bleeding site for at least 30 to 45 minutes.
Continue observation for bleeding after the infusion until laboratory test values return to normal.	If needed, administer prescribed blood products, anticoagulant antidote, and histamine$_2$ antagonists.
DYSRHYTHMIAS	
Record baseline ECG before infusion.	Administer prophylactic lidocaine if ordered.
Monitor cardiac rhythm continuously.	Treat dysrhythmias according to usual protocol.
Observe response to dysrhythmias by monitoring vital signs and neurologic status.	Administer vasopressors as needed to maintain blood pressure.
REOCCLUSION	
Observe for complaints of chest pain, pain behavior, and other signs and symptoms of myocardial ischemia.	If pain occurs, notify physician and document patient status.
Compare character of new chest pain with previous ischemic episodes.	Administer morphine, oxygen, nifedipine, or nitroglycerin, if prescribed.
Record 12-lead ECG and compare ST segments and T waves with baseline tracing.	Prepare patient for coronary angiography, further thrombolysis, PTCA, or intraaortic balloon pumping.
Continue to monitor for several hours after infusion is complete.	

Glucose-insulin-potassium infusion. Glucose-insulin-potassium (GIK) infusion, a metabolic therapy, has been used in the management of AMI.[20,126,137,199] It enhances anaerobic glycolysis and reduces the toxic effects of FFAs. In the ischemic zone, glycogen stores are rapidly depleted. The GIK combination increases the transport of glucose into myocardial cells, which provides a needed, continuous fuel supply in anaerobic glycolysis. The additional glucose may also aid aerobic metabolism. Potassium entry into the cells is enhanced by this infusion, thereby restoring ionic gradients and reducing ventricular dysrhythmias. Insulin is believed to improve myocardial perfusion and contractility. GIK is thought to work best if started within the first 6 hours after onset of AMI and infused for 48 hours. Serum glucose and potassium levels are monitored to detect latent diabetes mellitus or renal insufficiency. Hemodynamic monitoring is not required, and therapy does not interfere with the use of other drugs such as vasodilators, diuretics, analgesics, narcotics, and antidysrhythmic medications. No definitive effect on infarct size or long-term mortality rates has been described in a prospective, controlled, randomized trial.[137]

β-adrenergic blockade. During AMI, increased circulating catecholamines and sympathetic nervous system activity cause increases in heart rate and contractility. β-adrenergic blockade can counteract these effects.[104,137,145] Studies have shown reduced mortality rates with β-blockers.[86] However, reduction in infarct size is not consistent.[128] Indications are that patients with evolving AMI and evidence of increased sympathetic activity (tachycardia or hypertension) should receive β-adrenergic blockade therapy.[128,137,144] Pasternak, Braunwald, and Sobel[137] recommend metoprolol because it is cardioselective and does not have intrinsic sympathomimetic effects. Propranolol also has been used successfully, and other agents are being investigated. Heart rate and arterial pressure should be measured by cuff or indwelling arterial catheter. If there are no side effects, intravenous administration is followed by oral therapy. The heart rate is kept at 50 to 65 beats per minute, and the systolic blood pressure is kept at about 95 mm Hg.

NURSING DIAGNOSIS 2

High risk for decreased cardiac output related to electrical factors (rate, rhythm, conduction), mechanical factors (preload, afterload, inotropic state of the heart) or structural factors (papillary muscle dysfunction, interventricular septal rupture, ventricular aneurysm, and ventricular rupture) (exchanging pattern)

PATIENT OUTCOMES	NURSING PRESCRIPTIONS	EVALUATION
Patient will demonstrate hemodynamic stability and no decrease in cardiac output. Patient will maintain optimal rate and rhythm without conduction abnormalities.	Assess vital signs, cardiac rhythm, peripheral perfusion, and hemodynamic monitoring parameters. Monitor for bradydysrhythmias; tachydysrhythmias; bundle branch blocks; ectopy; aberrancy; first-, second-, or third-degree AV heart block; and atrial, junctional, or intraventricular conduction abnormalities.	Patient demonstrated hemodynamic stability and no decrease in cardiac output. (State specifics.) Patient did not sustain a cardiac rate, rhythm, or conduction disturbance. (State specifics.)
If rate, rhythm, or conduction disturbances occur, the patient will respond appropriately to prescribed therapy.	As needed for dysrhythmias, administer antidysrhythmic medication safely and in a timely manner as needed for dysrhythmias, according to standing or specific physician orders; and evaluate patient response.	If required, patient responded appropriately to the antidysrhythmic medication and did not experience side effects. (State specifics.)
If conduction or rate disturbance or symptomatic bradycardia occurs, the patient will respond appropriately to prescribed therapy. If cardioversion or defibrillation is required, patient will not experience complications.	If required by conduction or rate disturbances or symptomatic bradycardias, assist with temporary artificial cardiac pacing. If indicated for cardiac dysrhythmia, cardiovert or defibrillate the patient safely and in a timely manner.	If required, patient responded appropriately to pacemaker therapy and did not experience complications. (State specifics.) If required, patient responded appropriately to the cardioversion or defibrillation and did not experience complications. (State specifics.)
Patient will maintain normal mechanical function, including normal preload, afterload, and contractility.	Assess patient for evidence of mechanical dysfunction, including hypotension, hypoxemia, pain, shortness of breath, dyspnea, tachypnea, orthopnea, pulmonary crackles, S_3 gallop, a diffuse point of maximal impulse, neck vein distention, hepatic enlargement, and peripheral edema.	Patient demonstrated normal mechanical function, including normal preload, afterload, and contractility. (State specifics.)
Patient will respond to appropriate therapies to maintain mechanical function.	Administer oxygen, diuretics, fluids, analgesics, vasodilators, vasopressors, and IABP therapy safely in a timely manner, according to standing or specific physician orders to maintain mechanical function.	If required, patient responded appropriately to oxygen, diuretics, fluids, analgesics, vasodilators, vasopressors, and IABP therapy and experienced no complications.
Patient will maintain a balanced intake and output without significant weight change. Patient will not demonstrate complications from diagnostic test and procedures.	Monitor intake and output balance and weight changes. Evaluate patient's mechanical function by analyzing the results of diagnostic tests and procedures (electrolytes, BUN, and creatinine levels; specific gravity; chest x-ray films; ECG; echocardiogram; or radionuclide studies).	Patient maintained a balanced intake and output without significant weight change. Patient had no complications from diagnostic tests and procedures.

Continued.

NURSING
DIAGNOSIS 2

High risk for decreased cardiac output related to electrical factors (rate, rhythm, conduction), mechanical factors (preload, afterload, inotropic state of the heart) or structural factors (papillary muscle dysfunction, interventricular septal rupture, ventricular aneurysm, and ventricular rupture) (exchanging pattern)—cont'd

PATIENT OUTCOMES	NURSING PRESCRIPTIONS	EVALUATION
Patient will not demonstrate signs and symptoms of cardiogenic shock.	Assess for signs and symptoms of cardiogenic shock (hypotension, tachycardia, urine output below 30 ml/hour, mental confusion, decreased peripheral perfusion, and abnormal blood oxygen tension).	Patient showed no signs and symptoms of cardiogenic shock. (State specifics.)
Patient will not demonstrate complications from hemodynamic monitoring.	If indicated, monitor mechanical function using invasive hemodynamic techniques (arterial, pulmonary artery, and cardiac output catheters).	Patient had no complications from hemodynamic monitoring.
Patient will not demonstrate cardiac structural failure.	Assess for murmurs, signs of heart failure, pulmonary edema, and cardiogenic shock.	Patient did not demonstrate murmurs, heart failure, pulmonary edema, or cardiogenic shock.
If structural failure occurs, patient will respond appropriately to therapy.	If indicated, support mechanical function of the patient's heart.	If required, patient responded appropriately to mechanical support of the heart.
Patient will verbalize an understanding of diagnostic procedures or surgery.	If diagnostic procedures or surgery are required, explain the indications and preparation involved.	If required, patient demonstrated an understanding of the indications and preparation involved in cardiac catheterization, coronary angiography, or surgery.
Patient will not demonstrate signs and symptoms of papillary muscle rupture or dysfunction.	Assess for systolic murmurs, left-sided heart failure, and pulmonary edema.	Patient demonstrated absence of papillary muscle rupture or dysfunction.
Patient will not demonstrate signs and symptoms of interventricular septal rupture.	Assess for pansystolic murmurs, hypotension, and heart failure.	Patient demonstrated absence of interventricular septal rupture.
Patient will not demonstrate signs and symptoms of ventricular aneurysm.	Assess for persistent S_3 gallops, outward systolic impulses medial or superior to the point of maximal impulse, and activity intolerance.	Patient demonstrated absence of ventricular aneurysm.
Patient will not demonstrate signs and symptoms of ventricular rupture.	Assess for sudden development of electromechanical dissociation, intractable heart failure, and cardiogenic shock.	Patient demonstrated absence of ventricular rupture.

Plan and intervention for decreased cardiac output

Major complications

The major complications of AMI associated with decreased cardiac output[201] include:

1. Dysrhythmias (see Appendix B)
2. Heart failure (see Chapter 11)
3. Cardiogenic shock (see Chapter 11)
4. Cardiac arrest

Factors that contribute to the development of these complications include changes or failure in electrical, mechanical, or structural function of the heart. The nurse's responsibilities include monitoring, detecting, and reporting loss of function and decreased cardiac output; collaborating with physicians in management and support of cardiac output; and explaining procedures and events to patients and families.[88,201]

Electrical factors and cardiac output

Cardiac rate, rhythm, and conduction patterns are frequently altered in AMI, resulting in dysrhythmias that decrease cardiac output. Immediate treatment is necessary for most dysrhythmias, and vigorous treatment is mandatory for impaired hemodynamic states. Precise recognition of dysrhythmias is necessary (see Appendix B). Dysrhythmias are observed in 75% to 95% of patients who have had an AMI.[137,206]

The following factors must be considered in managing dysrhythmias and conduction disturbances:

1. The oxygen transport system, including the heart and circulation
2. The effect of the dysrhythmia on the individual
3. The exact nature of the dysrhythmia
4. Previous episodes of the dysrhythmia and patient response

Nurses should remember that they are observing and treating persons with dysrhythmias and not the dysrhythmias themselves. Patients should be encouraged to discuss their condition. Often they can give valuable information to the physician and nurse.

Nurses should observe patients' ECG patterns for dysrhythmias and ST-segment changes. The life-threatening dysrhythmias—ventricular fibrillation, ventricular tachycardia, asystole, and progressive or complete heart block—should be treated promptly according to the standing protocol or specific physician orders. Dysrhythmias that change or persist should be reported to the physician. Careful assessment of the patient who has a dysrhythmia includes detecting changes in blood pressure, heart rate, apical pulse, respiratory rate, skin temperature, color, mental status, and urine output.[88,206,215]

Ventricular dysrhythmias. Ventricular dysrhythmias are the most common of all the rhythm disturbances after AMI. These appear to come in three phases—early, intermediate, and late.[20] The *early phase* occurs within the first 3 to 30 minutes after coronary occlusion. Dysrhythmias are thought to be due to immediate effects on the ventricular muscle, which are increased automaticity and shortening of the action potential duration and refractory period in ischemic cells. The disparity between conduction in normal and ischemic cells creates the conditions necessary for reentry. PVCs are thought to arise from the increased automaticity, whereas ventricular tachycardia and fibrillation are related to reentry.[20] The *intermediate phase* begins 6 to 9 hours after occlusion and lasts 24 to 72 hours. Most patients are in a monitored setting during this period. Increased automaticity causes spontaneous polymorphic ventricular rhythms, but ventricular fibrillation is uncommon.[20] In the *late phase,* which begins 72 hours after occlusion, disparity between injured and healthy tissue again allows the reentry mechanism to produce ventricular extrasystoles, tachycardia, and fibrillation. Electrophysiologic abnormalities persist for long periods after myocardial infarction and may be responsible for the risk of sudden death during the first year.[20]

In some centers, lidocaine is administered prophylactically to prevent dysrhythmias, although this use remains controversial.[128,137] Studies of ventricular dysrhythmias have indicated that PVCs do not reliably predict development of ventricular tachycardia or fibrillation.[128,137] Fur-

thermore, lidocaine has adverse effects. Some recommend, however, that prophylactic lidocaine be given to selected patients during the first 24 hours after AMI for the prevention of ventricular fibrillation.[46,128,136] Patients who are particularly eligible for lidocaine prophylaxis include those under age 50 who are experiencing their first AMI and who are seen within 6 hours of onset.[128] Patients who are over age 70 and are seen more than 6 hours after onset should be excluded because they have a low incidence of ventricular fibrillation and a high incidence of lidocaine toxicity. AMI patients who have cardiogenic shock, severe right or left ventricular failure, heart block, and sinus bradycardia should also be excluded. These patients already have depressed myocardial automaticity, and further suppression with lidocaine may lead to ventricular standstill and death. If lidocaine must be used in patients who have suffered congestive heart failure or in patients with cardiogenic shock or hepatocellular disease, the loading dose and infusion rate are reduced by 50%. The plasma half-life of lidocaine increases by a factor of about 2 after 24 hours. Thus the infusion rate may have to be decreased.[46,128,136] The treatment algorithm for ventricular ectopy as recommended by the American Heart Association is outlined in the box on p. 276.[5]

Lidocaine is metabolized less effectively by the liver when given with cimetidine because the latter agent can depress liver metabolism. Many patients in the CCU receive *cimetidine* to decrease upper gastrointestinal tract symptoms secondary to the stress of hospitalization. Patients who receive lidocaine and cimetidine simultaneously may develop toxic side effects.[46,128,136] Researchers recommend avoiding administration of cimetidine to patients receiving lidocaine unless serum lidocaine levels are being monitored.[46,128,136] The antidysrhythmic dosage should be adjusted to counterbalance the enhanced or potential toxic effects of the drug combination. If patients require therapy for gastrointestinal tract upsets, antacids should be considered first, along with relaxation techniques.

Accelerated idioventricular rhythm (AIVR) is common in inferior AMI and as a reperfusion dysrhythmia. It occurs as an escape rhythm at a rate of 60 to 120 per minute when the sinus node slows. Because it is an escape rhythm and is protective, it should not be abolished with lidocaine. If the patient's hemodynamic status is compromised, atropine should be used to speed the SA node and overdrive the rhythm. If atropine is not effective, temporary cardiac pacing may be required.[46]

Sinus bradycardia. Sinus bradycardia occurs in 15% to 40% of patients with AMI and is more frequent in patients with inferior or posterior wall infarction. This may result from decreased blood flow to the SA node or enhanced vagal stimulation. It can be a protective mechanism because the decreased rate of SA node discharge reduces the myocardial oxygen needs of the heart after AMI. However, it can also be a detriment, because it is more possible

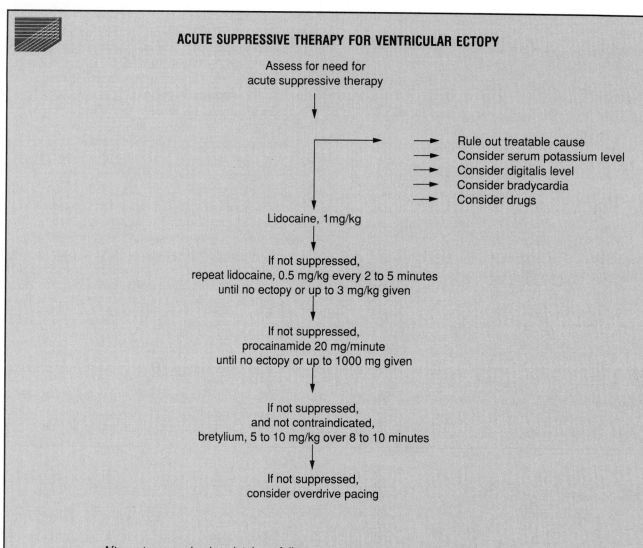

ACUTE SUPPRESSIVE THERAPY FOR VENTRICULAR ECTOPY

Assess for need for
acute suppressive therapy

→ Rule out treatable cause
→ Consider serum potassium level
→ Consider digitalis level
→ Consider bradycardia
→ Consider drugs

Lidocaine, 1mg/kg

If not suppressed,
repeat lidocaine, 0.5 mg/kg every 2 to 5 minutes
until no ectopy or up to 3 mg/kg given

If not suppressed,
procainamide 20 mg/minute
until no ectopy or up to 1000 mg given

If not suppressed,
and not contraindicated,
bretylium, 5 to 10 mg/kg over 8 to 10 minutes

If not suppressed,
consider overdrive pacing

After ectopy resolved, maintain as follows:
    After lidocaine, 1 mg/kg...Lidocaine drip, 2 mg/ minute
    After lidocaine, 1 to 2 mg/kg...Lidocaine drip, 3 mg/minute
    After lidocaine, 2 to 3 mg/kg...Lidocaine drip, 4 mg/minute
    After procainamide...Procainamide drip, 1 to 4 mg/minute (check blood level)
    After bretylium...Bretylium drip, 2 mg/minute

This sequence was developed to assist in teaching how to treat a broad range of patients with ventricular ectopy. Some patients may require therapy not specified herein. This algorithm should not be construed as prohibiting such flexibility.
From McIntyre KM and Lewis AJ: Standards and guidelines for cardiopulmonary resuscitation and emergency cardiac care, JAMA 255:2841, 1986.

for PVCs, ventricular tachycardia, and ventricular fibrillation to develop with a slow rate.[137] The treatment algorithm for symptomatic bradycardia is outlined in the box at right.

Conduction disturbances. Ischemic injury can interfere with normal sinus impulse transmission at any level of the conduction system. Blocks may occur in the SA node, AV node, bundle of His, and bundle branches.[137] Conduction abnormalities can be transient and cause no harm. They also may result in slow ventricular rates, decreased cardiac output, hypotension, complete ventricular standstill, and death if not treated.

First-degree AV heart block (a PR interval greater than 0.20 second) occurs when impulse conduction through

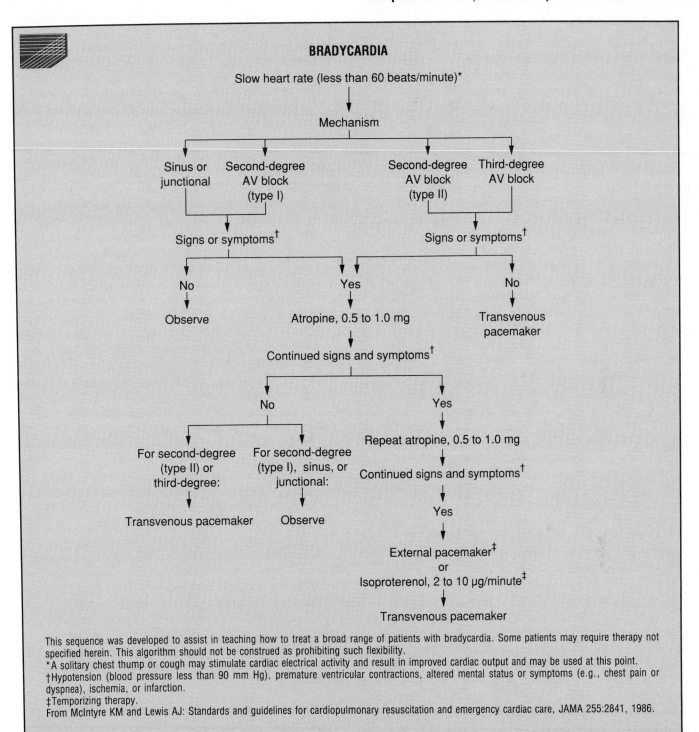

BRADYCARDIA

Slow heart rate (less than 60 beats/minute)*

This sequence was developed to assist in teaching how to treat a broad range of patients with bradycardia. Some patients may require therapy not specified herein. This algorithm should not be construed as prohibiting such flexibility.
*A solitary chest thump or cough may stimulate cardiac electrical activity and result in improved cardiac output and may be used at this point.
†Hypotension (blood pressure less than 90 mm Hg), premature ventricular contractions, altered mental status or symptoms (e.g., chest pain or dyspnea), ischemia, or infarction.
‡Temporizing therapy.
From McIntyre KM and Lewis AJ: Standards and guidelines for cardiopulmonary resuscitation and emergency cardiac care, JAMA 255:2841, 1986.

the AV node is delayed. In patients with AMI, 4% to 14% experience first-degree block, which generally does not require specific treatment. It should be monitored carefully because it may progress to a higher degree of block.[137]

Second-degree AV heart block occurs in two types. *Mobitz type I* (Wenckebach) is the most common form and appears in 4% to 10% of patients with AMI. It is recog-

nized by progressive lengthening of the PR interval between at least two or more consecutive beats followed by a P wave that is not accompanied by a QRS complex. It occurs more commonly in patients with inferior infarction and rarely progresses to complete heart block. It is usually transient and does not last more than 72 hours. These blocks occasionally require temporary cardiac pacing because of a slow ventricular rate.[137] *Mobitz type II* is seen in only 1% of patients with AMI but requires specific therapy with a temporary cardiac pacemaker because it often progresses suddenly to complete heart block and ventricular standstill. It is recognized by constant PR intervals on conducted beats and multiple blocked P waves. The QRS complexes may be widened. It occurs more frequently in patients with anterior rather than inferior AMI.[137]

Third-degree (complete) heart block occurs in approximately 5% of patients with AMI.[137] Because not all blocks are located in the AV node, the term *complete heart block* is more appropriate than *complete AV block*. Its significance depends on the location of the block and size of the infarct. With inferior infarctions, conduction problems are usually limited to the AV node, and the mortality rate is 15%. With anterior infarctions, the block is usually below the bundle of His, and the mortality rate is 70% to 80%. With inferior AMI, complete heart block may resolve in a week, whereas with anterior AMI, it is usually permanent.[137] Some patients may have stable escape rhythms, but the majority require cardiac pacing. These blocks can have a sudden onset, and the nurse must be alert to this possibility.

Intraventricular conduction system disturbances, bundle branch blocks, make up 10% to 20% of conduction problems in AMI patients.[137] Not all can be attributed to infarction because almost half are seen on the first ECG. *Right bundle branch block* is a problem in 2% of AMI patients. This form of heart block is frequently associated with complete heart block and has a high mortality rate (46%). Blocks of the anterior fascicle of the left bundle branch, *left anterior hemiblock,* occur alone in 3% to 5% of AMI patients and in association with right bundle branch block in another 5%. Blocks of the posterior fascicle of the left bundle branch, *left posterior hemiblock,* occur in 1% to 2% of AMI patients, usually with a large infarction.

About 45% of AMI patients who develop blocks in two fascicles will develop complete heart block. The most common bifascicular block is right bundle branch block and left anterior hemiblock. Physicians should always be notified of the development of intraventricular blocks, even when the patient has no symptoms because complete heart block may develop. A temporary cardiac pacemaker may be inserted prophylactically when right bundle branch block and left anterior hemiblock are present, or an external pacemaker may be kept ready at the bedside. In addition to being alert to development of complete heart block, nurses should be aware that patients with intraventricular conduction defects account for the majority of patients who develop ventricular fibrillation late in their hospital stay.[137]

Supraventricular tachydysrhythmias. Almost one third of patients with an AMI develop sinus tachycardia during the first few days.[137] In part, this is compensatory for the reduced stroke volume; however, contributing causes are anxiety, persistent pain, and left ventricular failure. Other supraventricular tachycardias that may develop are premature atrial contractions (PACs), atrial fibrillation, atrial flutter, and paroxysmal supraventricular tachycardia. These supraventricular dysrhythmias are far more common in patients with extensive infarction. They may indicate incipient or persistent heart failure. Atrial flutter and fibrillation have an increased mortality rate in patients with anterior wall infarction. Treatment must be prompt because tachycardias increase myocardial oxygen consumption, which is undesirable in patients with AMI. Verapamil, digitalis, and β-adrenergic blockers may be used in management of tachydysrhythmias.[137] The treatment algorithm for paroxysmal supraventricular tachycardia is outlined in Appendix D.

Cardiac arrest. Cardiac arrest is the gravest complication of AMI and requires prompt cardiopulmonary resuscitation and advanced cardiac life support. Ventricular fibrillation, asystole, and electromechanical dissociation will render the patient unconscious almost instantaneously. Respiratory arrest soon follows. Ventricular tachycardia and complete heart block may be tolerated for a short period before cardiac arrest occurs. CCUs with their careful continuous cardiac monitoring, prompt treatment of dysrhythmias, and rapid resuscitation are credited with reducing the inhospital mortality rate of AMI.[5,137]

All nurses working with cardiac patients must be certified in basic life support (BLS). Nurses also must know the principles, revisions, and performance skills of advanced cardiac life support (ACLS). Because of the high performance skills that must be maintained, the reader is referred to the American Heart Association Subcommittee on Emergency Cardiac Care for standards and guidelines on training, certification, and recertification in BLS and ACLS.[5]

Ventricular fibrillation, sustained ventricular tachycardia, and paroxysmal supraventricular tachycardia are treated with defibrillation or cardioversion (see Appendix D for treatment algorithms and details on defibrillation and cardioversion). Asystole and electromechanical dissociation also require prompt and immediate treatment.[5,137] The treatment algorithms for asystole and electromechanical dissociation are outlined in the boxes on p. 279.

Mechanical factors and cardiac output

Mechanical function in the maintenance of cardiac output is influenced by preload, afterload, and the inotropic state of the heart (see Chapters 7 and 11). The majority of inhospital deaths are attributed to cardiac failure and shock.[137] Left ventricular function is a powerful determinant of postmyocardial infarction outcome.[64] The presence of *cardiac failure* is indicated by hypotension, crackles, jugular venous distention, low urine output, fluid weight gain, and change in mental status.[10] The goals for management are reducing myocardial work, increasing cardiac output and myocardial contractility by manipulating preload and afterload, and decreasing retention of salt and water.[88]

Left ventricular failure. Because of loss of contracting myocardial cells, preload, afterload, and contractility can be altered by AMI. Because AMI usually involves the large muscle mass of the left ventricle, heart failure after AMI usually occurs on the left side. Ineffective cardiac pumping is found in 40% to 50% of AMI patients admitted to the CCU[137] and in 60% of patients within 24 to 48 hours after admission.[61] An abnormally increased LVEDP in the first 5 days after an AMI is common and is a result of decreased compliance in the area of infarction. The injured myocardium loses its ability to stretch and creates increased resistance to filling, which causes the LVEDP to rise. This is associated with an S_3 gallop and pulmonary crackles.[128]

Development of crackles in left ventricular failure complicating an AMI results from the increased LVEDP and subsequent sequential rises in left atrial, pulmonary venous, and capillary pressures.[61,137] Thus an elevated pulmonary artery wedge pressure (PAWP) reflects the increased LVEDP. When the increased pulmonary capillary hydrostatic pressure elevates the interstitial hydrostatic pressure above normal levels, fluid moves into the interstitial lung spaces because the plasma protein oncotic pressure is no longer great enough to reabsorb the interstitial fluid. Treatment of AMI patients with left ventricular failure should begin with rest in a semi-Fowler's position[169] and attention to oxygenation. Hypoxemia must be avoided.[137]

Preload is adjusted with volume, diuretics, and vasodilators. It is common for elderly, vomiting, or diaphoretic patients to become hypovolemic. Crystalloid or colloid

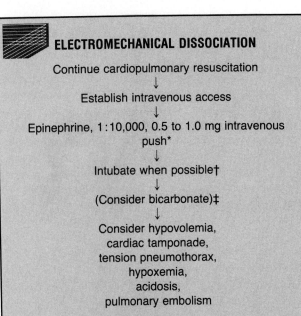

ELECTROMECHANICAL DISSOCIATION

Continue cardiopulmonary resuscitation
↓
Establish intravenous access
↓
Epinephrine, 1:10,000, 0.5 to 1.0 mg intravenous push*
↓
Intubate when possible†
↓
(Consider bicarbonate)‡
↓
Consider hypovolemia,
cardiac tamponade,
tension pneumothorax,
hypoxemia,
acidosis,
pulmonary embolism

This sequence was developed to assist in teaching how to treat a broad range of patients with electromechanical dissociation. Some patients may require care not specified herein. This algorithm should not be construed to prohibit such flexibility. Flow of algorithm presumes that electromechanical dissociation is continuing.
*Epinephrine should be repeated every 5 minutes.
†Intubation is preferable; if it can be accomplished simultaneously with other techniques, then the earlier the better. However, epinephrine is more important initially if the patient can be ventilated without intubation.
‡Value of sodium bicarbonate is questionable during cardiac arrest, and it is not recommended for the routine cardiac arrest sequence. Consideration of its use in a dose of 1 mEq/kg is appropriate at this point. Half of original dose may be repeated every 10 minutes if it is used.
From McIntyre KM and Lewis AJ: Standards and guidelines for cardiopulmonary resuscitation and emergency cardiac care, JAMA 255:2841, 1986.

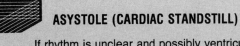

ASYSTOLE (CARDIAC STANDSTILL)

If rhythm is unclear and possibly ventricular fibrillation, defibrillate as for ventricular fibrillation if asystole is present*
↓
Continue cardiopulmonary resuscitation
↓
Establish intravenous access
↓
Epinephrine, 1:10,000, 0.5 to 1.0 mg intravenous push†
↓
Intubate when possible‡
↓
Atropine, 1.0 mg intravenous push (repeated in 5 minutes)
↓
(Consider bicarbonate)§
↓
Consider pacing

This sequence was developed to assist in teaching how to treat a broad range of patients with asystole. Some patients may require care not specified herein. This algorithm should not be construed to prohibit such flexibility. Flow of algorithm presumes asystole is continuing.
*Asystole should be confirmed in two leads.
†Epinephrine should be repeated every 5 minutes.
‡Intubation is preferable; if it can be accomplished simultaneously with other techniques, then the earlier the better. However, cardiopulmonary resuscitation and use of epinephrine are more important initially if patient can be ventilated without intubation. (Endotracheal epinephrine may be used.)
§Value of sodium bicarbonate is questionable during cardiac arrest, and it is not recommended for the routine cardiac arrest sequence. Consideration of its use in a dose of 1 mEq/kg is appropriate at this point. Half of original dose may be repeated every 10 minutes if it is used.
From McIntyre KM and Lewis AJ: Standards and guidelines for cardiopulmonary resuscitation and emergency cardiac care, JAMA 255:2841, 1986.

fluids are used to increase circulating volume.[137] Preload reduction can be accomplished with only diuretics or with diuretics and vasodilators.[137] Intravenous nitroglycerin may be used to reduce preload in AMI patients.[88,114] In patients who exhibit left ventricular failure and elevated PAWP secondary to AMI, nitroglycerin produces a reduction in right and left ventricular filling pressures. There is decreased cardiac work because of a lower preload and afterload. Reduced preload is the result of a decrease in the blood volume returning to the right ventricle and to the pulmonary system and left ventricle.

Vasodilators are also useful in reducing *afterload*. Studies have compared intravenous nitroglycerin with nitroprusside.[137,181] Although these drugs have similar actions, nitroglycerin primarily decreases preload. Nitroprusside has a balanced effect in decreasing preload and afterload. Nitroglycerin is preferred in managing AMI patients.[128,137,181] If intravenous vasodilators are used, hemodynamic monitoring is necessary to accurately assess arterial pressure and PAWP.[46,136] These pressures give accurate guidance to preload levels and allow the levels to be as low as possible while maintaining arterial pressure adequate for good peripheral perfusion.

Myocardial contractility may be augmented with dopamine or dobutamine. When used in low doses, these agents stimulate primarily β_1 receptors. With increasing doses, above 5 µg/kg/min, they stimulate α receptors and cause peripheral vasoconstriction and increased afterload.[46,137] Digitalis is not the primary inotropic agent for treatment of heart failure in the AMI patient.[137] In the first 72 hours, the ischemic, impaired heart is extremely sensitive to digitalis, and the usual therapeutic dosage of digitalis may be toxic. Therapeutic dosages of digitalis are hard to determine after infarction. If heart failure persists longer than 4 days, digitalis may be given with caution; however, it is best reserved for tachydysrhythmias.[137]

Cardiac failure in right ventricular infarction. Distinction between right and left ventricular infarctions is necessary when discussing heart failure because the pathophysiologic mechanisms, the treatment, and perhaps the prognosis are different. Although right ventricular infarction rarely occurs without left ventricular infarction, the clinical presentation reflects right ventricular failure rather than left.[199] Consequently, jugular venous distention rather than pulmonary congestion is present in patients with cardiac failure and right ventricular infarction. Impaired contractility of the right ventricle results in inadequate filling of the left ventricle. Inadequate preload affects left ventricular performance. Hemodynamic monitoring helps accurate assessment of right and left ventricular performance.

The goal of therapy is to improve left ventricular filling to enhance cardiac output and improve peripheral perfusion. With a dysfunctional right ventricle, an increased right ventricular filling pressure will allow passive flow into the left ventricle if the pressure gradient between the two

ventricles is great enough. After the diagnosis of right ventricular infarction is made, attention must be given to hemodynamic measurements of right atrial pressure (RAP) and PAWP so that volume status and left ventricular filling can be determined for proper management. The usual approach is volume expansion with judicious use of vasodilators and inotropic agents.[199] Diuretics are contraindicated because they would further decrease right ventricular filling pressure and lead to further decreases in blood pressure and cardiac output.[199]

Cardiogenic shock. Cardiogenic shock develops in 10% to 20% of AMI patients who are hospitalized.[99,137] Nurses frequently are the first to identify this complication.[155] The early signs are hypotension (systolic pressure below 90 mm Hg), poor peripheral perfusion, oliguria, mental obtundation, sweating, pallor, and tachycardia. Cardiogenic shock is due to depression of ventricular function, which occurs when 40% of the left ventricular muscle is lost.[128,137] If the patient develops cardiogenic shock, special hemodynamic monitoring of intraarterial pressure, PAWP, blood oxygen tension, and urinary output is required. Treatment is aimed at improving myocardial contractility without increasing myocardial work, raising the mean arterial pressure to obtain adequate coronary blood flow, and lowering peripheral vascular resistance without decreasing renal perfusion (see Chapter 11).

Dopamine is commonly used to raise blood pressure and increase renal blood flow because it selectively causes β-adrenergic and dopaminergic stimulation to reduce afterload and dilate renal arteries. Dobutamine may be more useful than dopamine because of its consistent ability to reduce total peripheral resistance. Therapy with only vasodilators is hazardous because they reduce coronary perfusion pressure. Some authors[137] recommend maintaining arterial diastolic pressure above 50 to 60 mm Hg to adequately perfuse the myocardium. Support with the IABP may be required. The prognosis for a patient with cardiogenic shock remains poor (see Chapter 11).[99,128,137]

Structural factors and cardiac output

Structural defects that decrease cardiac output and complicate recovery of the patient with AMI are papillary muscle dysfunction, ventricular aneurysm, and rupture of papillary muscles, interventricular septum, or ventricular wall (Fig. 10-8).

Papillary muscle dysfunction and rupture. Papillary muscle dysfunction (Fig. 10-8, *A*) with AMI is suggested by an apical systolic murmur. It frequently radiates to the axilla and occasionally is associated with a thrill. Papillary muscles receive their blood supply from the terminal portions of the large penetrating branches of the coronary arteries. When this coronary artery flow is impaired, papillary muscles become susceptible to injury.

When AMI involves papillary muscle necrosis, papillary muscle rupture can occur. If a papillary muscle ruptures,

FIG. 10-8   Complications of infarction. **A,** Pericarditis, papillary muscle dysfunction and rupture, and interventricular septum rupture. **B,** Ventricular aneurysm.

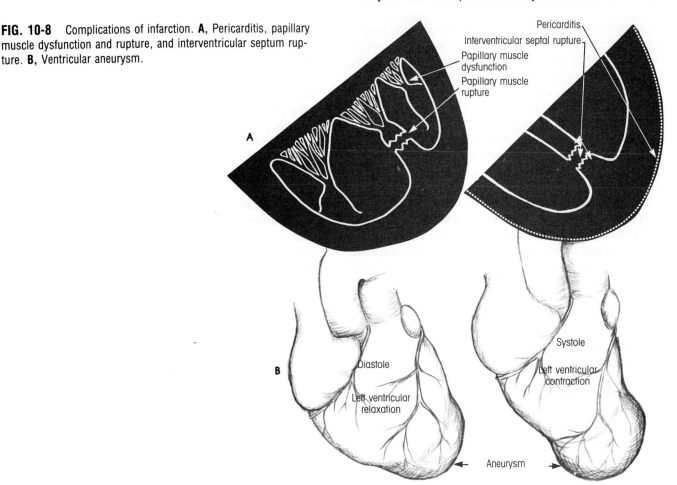

it usually does so within the first week after infarction. A pansystolic murmur is heard, and a thrill is usually present on examination. The patient will most likely have a sudden onset of heart failure associated with dysrhythmias, cyanosis, and fear. Aggressive management involves controlling dysrhythmias and heart failure. The IABP is usually required to enhance forward blood flow. An adequate airway and oxygenation must also be ensured. Without emergency surgical intervention the patient frequently will die within hours or days.[128,137]

Mitral insufficiency secondary to infarction may be due to several anatomic abnormalities, such as papillary dysfunction, ruptured papillary muscle or tip, or annular dilation from left ventricular failure and possible ventricular dilation. This patient may not be as critically ill as the patient with a ruptured ventricular septum. If cardiac catheterization is required for diagnosis, the patient is given digitalis, vasodilators, and diuretics; salt intake is restricted; and the patient also may be placed on the IABP. In cases of mild functional mitral insufficiency, catheterization and IABP would be unlikely. When emergency valve replacement surgery is necessary, complete heart catheterization

and coronary angiography are performed to determine whether the patient is also a candidate for myocardial revascularization.[128,137]

Interventricular septum rupture. Rupture of the interventricular septum (Fig. 10-8, *A*) occurs in 1% to 3% of AMI patients and is most common in the first week after AMI.[128] It can be identified by a loud pansystolic murmur accompanied by a thrill.[137] The murmur is loudest along the left sternal border in the fourth and fifth intercostal spaces. Depending on the size of the defect, the rupture causes congestive heart failure or cardiogenic shock. The diagnosis is confirmed by right heart catheterization. Bedside differentiation by auscultation of a systolic murmur of a ruptured septum and mitral insufficiency is difficult. Catheterization of the right side of the heart can be performed in the CCU by inserting a pulmonary artery catheter via a vein to the right atrium, right ventricle, and pulmonary artery. The catheter can be advanced to obtain a wedge pressure, which can indicate whether mitral insufficiency is present. Oxygen saturation in blood samples from each chamber is determined. The diagnosis of a ruptured ventricular septum is made when there is stepped-

Gastrointestinal tract problems

Abdominal distention, constipation, and fecal impaction can occur during recovery from an AMI. They are usually caused by decreased exercise, decreased roughage in the diet, medications, or potassium depletion after diuresis. A stool softener is commonly prescribed to prevent constipation and straining. The stress reaction of AMI can precipitate gastrointestinal hemorrhage due to stress ulcer formation.[137] It is common for patients to be given cimetidine or another H_2 antagonist to reduce the secretion of hydrochloric acid. If the patient is receiving lidocaine, the physician and nurse must be alert to increased susceptibility to lidocaine toxicity if cimetidine is used (see p. 275).

Genitourinary tract problems

Bladder distention can be a problem in a man with prostatic hypertrophy. Medications, such as atropine, sedatives, and opiates, as well as bed rest, aggravate the distention. Assisting the patient to stand to void may help. If an indwelling urinary catheter is required, urinary tract infection and gram-negative septicemia may develop.[195]

Thromboembolism

Thromboembolic complications of AMI include deep vein thrombosis, pulmonary embolism, mural thrombosis, and systemic embolism. Deep vein thrombosis occurs in about 30% of individuals experiencing AMIs.[128] The risk is greater for individuals with varicose veins, histories of thrombophlebitis, congestive heart failure, obesity, shock, or older age. In most patients, venous thrombi are limited to the calf. Pulmonary emboli originate from these deep vein sites. Early ambulation reduces the incidence of death caused by pulmonary embolus to less than 1%.[128] If pulmonary emboli occur, morbidity rates vary according to the size of the embolus.

Mural thrombus formation is common in large anterior infarctions and ventricular aneurysms. It can be detected with echocardiography only some of the time. Pieces of thrombus can break off and become systemic arterial emboli. They may lodge in peripheral or visceral arteries, causing injury to the extremities, brain, kidneys, spleen, or intestines. Arterial emboli occur in approximately 5% of patients with known infarction, usually within 6 weeks.[169] Cerebral emboli cause changes in the patient's sensorium, whereas sudden pain, pallor, pulselessness, coldness, and numbness of an extremity indicate a peripheral site.[128,137,169]

Treatment depends on the organ or tissue compromised. If the occlusion is significant, surgical removal of the clot may be needed. Anticoagulant therapy with heparin and warfarin (Coumadin) is frequently used if it is not contraindicated.

Precautions such as antiembolic stockings and low-dose heparinization have decreased the incidence of complications. All patients should wear antiembolic stockings and be taught passive rhythmic foot exercises to prevent the complications of bed rest. These stockings should be removed at least once per shift to allow inspection of the lower extremities and pedal pulses. Routine anticoagulation to minimize bed rest complications is recommended by some[137] but not by others.[128] Low-dose heparin schedules, 5000 units subcutaneously every 8 to 12 hours until 2 or 3 days before discharge, decreases leg vein thrombosis by two thirds,[128] but there is no evidence that it reduces AMI mortality rates.[137] All agree that patients at high risk for embolization who have or have had thrombophlebitis, ventricular aneurysm, atrial fibrillation, obesity, or cardiogenic shock should be given anticoagulant therapy. Full-dose heparinization by continuous or intermittent infusion of 10,000 to 20,000 units per day to maintain the clotting time and partial thromboplastin time (PTT) at 1.5 to 2.5 times the normal value may be used for 5 to 7 days. This may be followed by oral anticoagulants, even after hospitalization, depending on the individual.[137]

Pericarditis

Pain during the acute and later stages of MI may be caused by acute pericarditis. Pericarditis is an inflammatory process that accompanies transmural infarction (see Chapter 15). It develops in 10% to 15% of AMI patients 2 to 7 days after infarction. Pericardial effusion is common and may be asymptomatic. Transient pericardial friction rubs are common in the first 48 hours. When they are accompanied by chest pain and ECG changes, pericarditis is suspected. The related chest pain is usually aggravated by deep inspiration and lessened by leaning forward while sitting. Aspirin, indomethacin, or corticosteroids may be prescribed to reduce the inflammation and pain.[169] Relief may not be obtained for as long as 48 hours.[128] Pericarditis is a relative contraindication for anticoagulant or thrombolytic therapy because of the risk of hemorrhage and pericardial tamponade. If therapy must be continued, close attention to clotting parameters and signs of tamponade is warranted.[128,137,169]

Dressler's syndrome

Dressler's syndrome (postmyocardial infarction syndrome) develops 1 to 12 weeks after AMI. This uncommon complication may recur and is characterized by fever, pleuropericardial chest pain, a pericardial friction rub, and left pleural effusion. An autoimmune response is the most widely accepted cause,[169] although a viral etiology has been proposed.[36,85] Aspirin, nonsteroidal inflammatory agents, rest, reassurance, relaxation exercises, and analgesics can help relieve the anxiety and discomfort.

NURSING DIAGNOSIS 4

Anxiety (patient and family), ineffective coping (patient and family), and altered role performance (patient and family) related to pathophysiologic, situational, and treatment-related factors (feeling, choosing, relating patterns)

PATIENT OUTCOMES	NURSING PRESCRIPTIONS	EVALUATION
Patient and family will express anxiety, fears, and concerns. Patient will not experience severe anxiety or panic and will demonstrate reduced anxiety levels.	Assess anxiety, fears, concerns, and coping in the patient and family. Institute measures to reduce anxiety, including reassurance; explanation of illness, CCU environment, and therapeutic regimen; decrease sensory stimulation; medications.	Patient and family expressed their anxiety, fears, and concerns. Patient did not experience severe anxiety or panic, and demonstrated reduced anxiety levels.
Patient will institute effective coping behaviors such as relaxation, imagery, and music. Patient will demonstrate resolution of anxiety, denial, anger, depression, and aggressive sexual behavior.	Guide patient and family in using specific coping strategies (relaxation, imagery, and music). Recognize and accept anxiety, denial, anger, depression, and aggressive sexual behavior as coping behaviors. Provide emotional- and problem-focused support.	Patient used effective coping behaviors such as relaxation, imagery, and music. Patient demonstrated resolution of anxiety, denial, anger, depression, and aggressive sexual behavior.
Patient will not demonstrate increased levels of anxiety on transfer or discharge. Patient and family will express and demonstrate acceptance of changed roles.	Provide structured teaching before transfer and discharge. Assess patient's and family's usual roles. Elicit and discuss changes in role performance and feelings about role changes. Allow patient some control of daily care, including bed bath, hygiene, and visitors. Provide daily private time for patient and family. Facilitate telephone contact with family and friends.	Patient did not demonstrate increased levels of anxiety on transfer or discharge. Patient and family described their usual roles. Patient and family expressed feelings and demonstrated acceptance of changed roles. Patient demonstrated some control of daily care and visitors. Patient and family expressed satisfaction with their level of contact with one another.

Plan and intervention for anxiety, ineffective coping, and altered role performance

An AMI is an unexpected, life-threatening event with an uncertain outcome; it represents a loss to the patient and family members. It is usually disruptive to the patient's and family's relationships because of sudden separation and imposition of changed roles.[131,153,220] The diagnoses presented in this section, as well as Nursing Diagnosis 5, are interrelated. The interventions will aid in meeting more than one goal simultaneously. Rehabilitation success hinges on the family, especially the spouse, but family turmoil is common and lasts long after discharge from the hospital.[176,220] The underlying long-term goal is achievement of psychologic adjustment to chronic coronary heart disease by the patient and family.[153]

Emotional responses

Nurses need to use focused support to help patients and families work through the common emotional *responses to loss* precipitated by the AMI. The same emotions are usually experienced by the patient and family members. However, they may appear separately or simultaneously, in any order, and to different degrees. Family members are likely to experience a different sequence and timing than patients.[88,131,132]

Anxiety. In the critical or early phases of the AMI, anxiety and fear of death are common thoughts.[29,95,131] Anxiety is accompanied by anxious expressions and behaviors, repetitive talking, feelings of powerlessness, restlessness, and sleeplessness.[55,194] Because they are overwhelmed by the event, patients and families have difficulty remembering what they are told. Severe and panic levels of anxiety must be avoided because of their detrimental effects on cardiac performance. Emotion-focused support should include reassurance, the nurse's presence, repeated simple explanations, specific verbal instructions, and written materials at an appropriate reading level.[95,132,135] Although anxiety usually lessens after the first 24 to 48 hours after admission, it may persist a year or longer.[153] Previous experiences with illness, hospitalization, and stress are likely to influence responses to the present situation. Anxiety may be transmitted between family and patient; therefore the health care team must manage anxiety in both the patient and family members.[62] Systematic nursing support can have a significant effect on reducing anxiety and depression in patients and anxiety in their spouses[193] (see also Chapter 9).

Coping behaviors. Coping behaviors may be directed at lessening emotional distress or managing the problem. *Problem-focused behaviors* include strategies such as defining the problem, gathering information, finding alternative solutions, weighing solutions, and deciding on appropriate action. *Emotion-focused behaviors* that are used to defend against anxiety[10,23,88,143] and the threat of AMI include:

1. *Denial.* Symptoms of AMI are ignored, and discussion of AMI is avoided.
2. *Repression.* Persons seem to forget about the illness.
3. *Displacement.* Persons complain about relatively unimportant matters such as noise level, food, or air conditioning.
4. *Projection.* Persons talk about the anxieties of relatives but not about their own.
5. *Rationalization.* Indigestion is blamed for the AMI rather than smoking, obesity, high blood pressure, or known atherosclerotic heart disease to avoid painful lifestyle changes.
6. *Paranoid reaction.* Persons show symptoms of delusions, hallucinations, aggression, and projection (e.g., they may accuse the CCU staff of trying to poison them).

Denial. Denial is a common initial coping response to anxiety and is related to the first stage of adjustment, *defending oneself*.[95,153,192] It may be verbal or acted out and will usually change with time. Unrealistic expectations of the future and cheerfulness are often seen. To assess for denial and the underlying anxiety, the nurse must explore the meaning of the illness to the patient and spouse.[192] The patient's denial usually lasts for 7 days after admission,[95] although it may last longer.[153] The spouse's denial period probably will be much shorter.[131] Studies have shown denial to be protective and associated with a positive outcome,[108,135] whereas clinicians believe it is detrimental.[59,84] During this period, the patient may not report chest pain.[167] Denial may be expressed as outright refusal to comply with the treatment regimen. The patient may get out of bed or exercise to see if pain will occur. The best interventions are directed at reducing anxiety so that the

person does not use destructive forms of denial as a coping mechanism.[88,120]

Anger. Anger appears as the patient and families try to resolve their loss and understand why the patient has had an AMI; they are *coming to terms*.[88] Guilt is closely tied to anger. Anxiety and guilt may be expressed as angry complaints about nursing or medical care. The patient may be hostile to family members.[88,132] Family members may be angry at the patient for disrupting their routine, plans, or role relationships.[143] Some people believe their anger should be controlled, so they do not express it openly and appear depressed. Nurses must facilitate expression so that internalized anger does not hinder recovery. Several steps can be used to help the angry person.[88,173]

First, the nurse should recognize anger by overt and convert signs. Examples are sarcasm, loud voice, insults, angry statements, stiff body posture, throwing of things, depression, fatigue, withdrawal, apathy, angry gestures, overcompliance, noncompliance, and an attitude of being overly agreeable. Second, the nurse should remain in control. A patient who is losing control is frightened. The nurse's posture of being in control is reassuring. Limit setting often provides structure to the patient's experience and lowers the energy that accompanies the anger. It helps to indicate that anger is acceptable but that aggression and loss of control are not.

Third, the nurse should accept, acknowledge, and validate the emotion by remarks such as, "Many people are angry after a heart attack." Some patients and families can be hostile and outright abusive. Openly acknowledging the behavior is better than ignoring it or trying to joke them out of anger.

Fourth, the nurse should listen and help persons *explore* the situation and events that are causing anger. Often angry persons have lost or believe they have lost something of value. The expression of anger gives them a sense of power. When they can identify and express what they are angry about, an effective solution may be self-evident. If they are angry about happenings in the health care setting, a nondefensive posture is best.

Fifth, the nurse and patients should identify and plan constructive outlets for anger and ways for persons to have some control of their situation. Constructively channeling anger is necessary. Relaxation exercises and anxiolytic medication may be required to help them tolerate their changed situation and decreased activity. Reevaluation and modification of the plan will be needed to incorporate changes in mood.[10,173]

Depression. Depression begins 3 to 14 days after admission and may last more than a year.[95,153] It is coupled with the work of coping constructively with loss and *learning to live*. Crying, hopelessness, helplessness, unresponsiveness, and despondency may be seen. The nurse should ask for and listen to the patient's and family's comments about their feelings. Again, the emotions should be accepted, and reassurance that others feel this way should be given. Participation in a support group may prove beneficial.[88]

Depression can have immediate physiologic consequences, such as chest pain, dysrhythmias, and increased blood pressure, as well as, long-term consequences such as cardiac invalidism.[153] Successful adjustment to AMI requires regaining indepenence, self-confidence, and self-worth. Allowing patients to take responsibility for some part of their treatment plan can help reestablish a sense of self.[88] Simply being able to state how they want to organize their daily hygiene and ambulation can be very meaningful.

Aggressive sexual behavior. Occasionally, patients exhibit aggressive sexual behavior in the early days of hospitalization. This is often an expression of anxiety, fear, and anger related to a changed self-concept. The nurse must find out what need or anxiety patients express through this behavior. If patients' lewd or suggestive remarks or gestures make a nurse uncomfortable, patients should be told so simply and directly. When the incidents are dealt with appropriately, a higher level of nurse-patient relationship emerges.

Helping the AMI patient and family cope

Nurses must help the patient and family reduce their anxiety levels and cope with the psychologic aspects of AMI. This is done by reassurance, explanation, a therapeutic environment, and specific interventions such as relaxation exercises, imagery, and music.

Coping patterns. Several coping patterns may be seen in patients and families faced with a crisis. Persons using *unconflicted adherence* choose to continue previous behaviors and coping despite any new information they have received or risk that might be involved. *Unconflicted change* is almost the opposite in that persons indiscriminately follow any new advice or suggestions. *Defensive avoidance* involves the use of defensive behaviors to avoid confronting the stressor directly. *Hypervigilance* may also be viewed as "panic." Persons search for simplistic solutions and make impulsive solutions that are later regretted. *Vigilance* is the most mature and effective pattern. Persons rationally and systematically assess the stressors, consider possible alternatives, decide on appropriate action, and then evaluate the effectiveness of their actions. It is important to recognize that persons may be exercising vigilance and still not follow all medical advice. In other words, persons may be coping effectively and choose not to comply or adhere.[10,92,120,218]

Focused support. The CCU and its personnel are unknown to the patient and family. Helping them to develop trust in the staff is an emotion-focused way of reducing anxiety. The nurse should establish a good rapport with the patient and family. Providing information is a problem-focused way of helping them cope. Anxiety is lessened when CCU routines are explained.[29] Anticipatory guidance for both patients and families[88] should include the following:

1. Explaining bed rest, commode privileges, monitoring, alarm systems, intravenous lines, oxygen, vital signs assessment, diet, and medication
2. Explaining visiting restrictions, their purpose, and the time for visiting hours
3. Instructing patients to report chest pain
4. Instructing patients to avoid sudden physical effort and how to turn from side to side in bed without overexertion
5. Warning patients to avoid straining while defecating
6. Explaining the purpose and steps of the progressive activity program
7. Explaining the specific signs of activity intolerance

The patient's and family's understanding of the information given should be evaluated. Unnecessary information that is not understood may increase anxiety. Nurses should not expect all information to be retained in the first session. More than one repetition will probably be needed. Questions and feedback should be solicited. Everyone's knowledge and prior experience with AMI should be discussed, and misconceptions should be corrected. The nurse must give frequent, specific information and explanations to the patient and family about the patient's progress and present condition. Trite, evasive remarks, such as, "You're okay," should be avoided. "Your blood pressure is 120/80; that's in the normal range," is preferred.[10,88,143]

When a nurse spends time alone with patients during each shift, patients can express their thoughts and feelings. During this time the nurse learns more about patients' concerns, including those expressed without words. Patients' preferences about visitors and daily activities should be determined and accommodated. This can be accomplished by including patients in routine decisions.[29]

Relaxation, imagery, and music for anxiety reduction

After patients have been stabilized, they should be assisted in visualizing themselves in an active role again. They may begin this period with *abreactive responses,* the process of releasing a repressed emotion by reliving in imagination the original experience.[172] *All patients image.*[2] Patients and people who were with them at the time of the AMI review different experiences surrounding the AMI, such as the initial excruciating pain, specific complications, associated anxiety, and the CCU. Many patients and spouses have *negative imagery* during this period, such as seeing the patient's heart as big, overstretched, and ineffective. The more complicated the events surrounding patients' AMI, the greater the degree of negative imagery. This kind of thought keeps patients and spouses anxious and fearful.

Nurses can facilitate the healing process by teaching relaxation skills and assisting with positive imagery. These activities are helpful in shifting patient's and family's focus to active mental and physical participation in the healing process (see Chapter 5).[88] Effective and positive activation of thoughts can cause psychophysiologic change. Relaxa-

GUIDE TO STRUCTURED PRETRANSFER TEACHING

1. Average length of stay in CCU is 2 to 3 days; average length of hospitalization is 5 to 7 days. Patient will convalesce at home and return to part-time work and former activities in 6 weeks.
2. Learning relaxation, imagery, and stress-management techniques and new health behaviors will lead toward a successful recovery (see Chapter 5).
3. Transfer or discharge is a sign of progress. Such a decision usually occurs during morning rounds, and the transfer usually occurs in the early afternoon. (Intravenous infusions are discontinued during the transfer. Patients go by wheelchair and are shown telemetry equipment and the new floor, meeting the new staff and roommate. Patient and family members are told telemetry visiting hours.
4. Medical supervision of care will continue on telemetry.
5. Telemetry nurses have specialized training in care of patients with AMI. CCU nurses are available for consultation; the nurse/patient ratio changes.
6. After the transfer:
   a. Monitoring by telemetry is usually continued for 3 to 5 days.
   b. Rest is still important.
   c. Activity progression will continue (cardiac rehabilitation stages and activity level are explained in writing).
   d. Many patients feel anxious or depressed; these feelings are normal.
7. The patient should report to the telemetry nurse:
   a. Chest pain
   b. Shortness of breath
   c. Questions
   d. Problems with roommate or roommate's visitors
   e. Request for change in number of visitors
   f. Requests to contact physician

Modified from Toth JC: Effect of structured preparation for transfer on patient anxiety on leaving coronary care unit, Nurs Res 29:28, 1980.

---

tion is a prerequisite to working on a patient's imagery.[1,43] An example of how to introduce relaxation and imagery at the bedside is given in Chapter 9.

Biofeedback is any procedure in which an external sensor is used to provide persons with an indication of the state of any bodily process, usually in an attempt to effect a change in the measured quantity.[10] The CCU nurse may not use actual biofeedback equipment but can still use biofeedback principles. The three principles of biofeedback are helping patients to develop awareness about a particular aspect of themselves, shaping a particular response, and transferring the newly shaped response to real situations.

Music can be used alone or with relaxation techniques to reduce stress.[37,76] In fact, patients and families may already have music that they listen to during stressful times. They should be helped in using this coping strategy, and their musical preference should be considered.

Altered family processes

Family dynamics can have a positive or negative effect on the AMI patient. As the prime socialization unit, the family is involved in promoting health, illness, and sick role behaviors of members.[176] The following assumptions can be made about the effect of life-threatening illness on the family:

1. The diagnosis of life-threatening illness is a social contract between the patient, family, and health care system.
2. A diagnosis of a life-threatening condition changes the family's life trajectory.
3. Families need to review a life-threatening event.
4. Family members' reactions influence the course of a life-threatening illness.
5. Family members' beliefs about a life-threatening illness influence how they and the patient cope with the situation.

The ultimate goal for the family faced with a life-threatening cardiac illness is to reorganize and stabilize family structure and function as the affected member progresses through the acute, transitional, and rehabilitation phases of recovery. Meeting this goal requires the integration of the biopsychosocial consequences of the illness into an acceptable lifestyle for the family.[176]

To assist with changes in role performance, the nurse must gather some information and, in the process, help the patient and the family solve problems. First, the nurse determines who is in the family, where they live, and what their roles have been in the past. Specific questions about roles such as, "Who usually mows the lawn?" or "What jobs around the house do you usually do?" will gather more useful information than general questions. Second, the nurse asks about changes the family members believe are needed. For example, the family members might believe that someone else will need to do tasks that have been done by the patient. In addition, the nurse needs to ask whether family members believe they must care for the patient after discharge. Third, the nurse assesses whether family members' beliefs are warranted in view of the patient's condition and likely outcome. Fourth, the nurse asks about past experience the family has had with the same or a similar situation. Fifth, the nurse also determines whether there is agreement within the family and the role the patient is willing for the family to play.[143,153,176,195]

The first priority in facilitating family function is to meet the emotional needs of family members. When anxiety lessens, problem-focused, cognitive supports can be received. The majority of patients and families are distressed by the enforced separation.[88,131,132] Spouses should be allowed to help with daily activities if they and patients wish. Visiting hours should be flexible when possible.[88] Private family time should be planned as a part of every day for relationships to be maintained. The nurse should facilitate contact between patients and families for the patient to avoid feeling socially isolated.[88]

The majority of issues related to altered roles surface after hospitalization as the family learns to live together once more. While still in the hospital, they should be referred to a cardiac rehabilitation program that can assist them with these difficulties.[153,176]

Anxiety associated with transfer and discharge

Transfer from the CCU and discharge from the hospital can be stressful for patients and families. Anxiety is a common response when patients and families are prepared, but it is especially difficult when transfer or discharge is perceived as unplanned. Transfer and discharge anxiety are a special form of separation anxiety.[88,125] Patients and families see the CCU with its constant nursing as secure and familiar. The anxiety level of patients who receive pretransfer or predischarge teaching can be significantly lowered.[150,198,199] Information that should be included is presented in the box at left.

Preparation for transfer and discharge should begin during admission, with emphasis placed on CCU and hospital stays being short followed by convalescence at home. Transfer and discharge should be presented as positive and progressive moves toward recovery. Transfer should always be planned to occur in the daytime and not at shift change. Nighttime transfers do not allow adequate time for patients to become oriented to their new surroundings before sleeping. Shift change transfers do not facilitate development of the new nurse-patient-family relationship.

The patient and family should be informed of a transfer before it occurs. Anxiety can be reduced further if the nurse gradually removes CCU paraphernalia before transfer. If possible, a family member should be with the patient at the time of transfer. The CCU nurse should accompany the patient to the new unit and introduce the patient and family to the new nurse. Patient, family, and CCU nurse should take time to say goodbye to one another.[88,164] Cardiovascular signs and symptoms can become unstable and dysrhythmias are most likely to occur within 2 hours after transfer.[125] Thus nurses on the new unit should give prompt attention to anxiety during this time.

NURSING DIAGNOSIS 5	**High risk for noncompliance and altered sexuality related to knowledge deficit and situational and treatment-related factors (choosing and relating patterns)**

PATIENT OUTCOMES	NURSING PRESCRIPTIONS	EVALUATION
Patient will demonstrate an understanding of self-care.	Teach patient about self-care for AMI and angina signs and symptoms, CAD risk factor modification, medications, progressive activity schedule, and relaxation exercises.	Patient verbalized an understanding of self-care for AMI and angina signs and symptoms, CAD risk factor modification, medications, progressive activity schedule, and relaxation exercises.
Patient will indicate willingness to comply with the prescribed therapeutic regimen.	Assess willingness and ability to comply with prescribed therapy.	Patient showed willingness and ability to comply with CAD risk factor modification, medication therapy, progressive activity schedule, and relaxation exercises.
Family members will demonstrate an understanding of patient's self-care.	Teach family about the patient's self-care regimen.	Family members verbalized an understanding of the patient's self-care regimen.
Family members will indicate a willingness to assist patient in compliance with prescribed therapy.	Assess family's willingness and ability to assist patient with prescribed therapy.	Family members showed willingness and ability to help patient comply with prescribed therapy.
Patient and sexual partner will demonstrate an understanding of recommendations relating to sexual activity.	Include content on sexual relations for patient and sexual partner in patient and family teaching.	Patient and sexual partner verbalized a specific understanding of recommendations relating to sexual activity.

Plan and intervention for noncompliance and altered sexuality

Lack of information and the difficulties involved in adjusting to chronic cardiac disease place patients at high risk for noncompliance (see Chapter 9, Nursing Diagnosis 3) and altered sexuality patterns. Cardiac rehabilitation should begin early after admission to the CCU, with explanation, counseling, and activity progression. As patients stabilize and progress, they and their families should be given specific information orally and in writing. When the patient is stable and responding appropriately to medications, progressive discharge activities are planned. Patients usually transfer from the CCU within 2 or 3 days and are discharged from the hospital 5 to 7 days after an uncomplicated AMI. When there have been complications, discharge may be delayed 2 or 4 weeks. Before discharge, the home and family situation should be assessed to make sure the environment will be conducive to continued physical and emotional rest and progressive activity. The patient should be referred to a cardiac rehabilitation program for continued activity progression. The objectives during the first 2 months after discharge are to allow the heart to heal and form scar tissue, gradually increase activity tolerance to a level required for return to work or previous activities, and continue psychologic adjustment to chronic heart disease.[133,210]

Cardiac rehabilitation

Inpatient and outpatient cardiac rehabilitation programs create a setting in which patients and families can ask questions and relieve their anxieties (see Chapter 19). Outcomes to be expected from cardiac rehabilitation are favorable physiologic adaptations, relief of symptoms, a sense of well-being, and preservation of patients' roles in the family and society. Less certain outcomes are retardation of atherosclerosis, protection against further cardiac complications, and prolonging life.[133] Each patient and family in a cardiac rehabilitation program has different needs, and an individualized approach is needed. The process is a joint venture, with the cardiac rehabilitation team, patient, and family working together.[63]

Retention of information in the acute phase of the illness is variable but can be enhanced with structured content and distribution of written materials at an appropriate reading level.[150,182] Inhospital teaching is more effective for immediate postdischarge experiences than for long-term behavioral change.[182] Continued instruction after discharge is needed on medication, progression of physical activity, resumption of sexual activity, weight reduction, managing chest pain and shortness of breath, and CAD risk factor reduction.[63,210] If booklets and other printed material on these topics are provided during hospitalization, patients and families can refer to them when more information or reinforcement is needed. A group of investigators found that patients and families have the most questions during the first 6 weeks after discharge, and this may be the most receptive instruction period.[163]

Nurses who care for cardiac patients should consider ways to enhance the education process after discharge, especially for those who do not enter formal cardiac rehabilitation programs. Many hospitals have established "sharing and caring" programs in addition to the cardiac rehabilitation program. Special focus is placed on discussion of the emotional aspects of the past and present events surrounding cardiac disease.[176]

The integration of physical exercise training with professionally led psychodynamic group meetings can lower patient anxiety levels and reduce the number of emergency room visits and hospitalizations caused by a suspected recurrence of AMI.[138] Patients who receive *behavioral counseling* with a standard cardiac rehabilitation program have a lower recurrence rate of acute cardiac events and suffer fewer cardiac fatalities than do patients who do not receive behavioral counseling.[81] Cardiac rehabilitation programs are being increasingly recommended to enhance beneficial physiologic, psychologic, and social effects.[133,135,210] Patients report that cardiac rehabilitation programs assist them in making needed lifestyle changes.[63] Spouses are also thought to benefit from cardiac rehabilitation programs.[123,210]

Early in cardiac recovery the major areas that present adjustment difficulties are daily events, lifestyle changes, family dynamics, and readjustment to work. These are predicted areas of difficulty; all require discussion during recovery. Discussion should take place when it is appropriate. Open discussion helps patients and families become aware of normal events and ways to cope effectively.

Discussion of readjustment to work frequently involves self-image, self-confidence, job description, peer groups, superiors, subordinates, and conflictive relationships. Patients are uncertain of their ability for optimal performance on the job again. In many situations, patients realize that something about their work responsibility must shift for a while, and they need support in asking for help from colleagues. The overall rate of return to work ranges from 62% to 90%. Patients less likely to return to work are women working outside the home; blue-collar workers, especially those with physically strenuous jobs; and persons with emotional problems.[174]

Specific teaching about CAD risk factors

Teaching about reduction of specific CAD risk factors can result in retardation, stabilization, or regression of the CAD process (see Chapters 8 and 9). Patient or family education should not be assumed to be successful on the basis of statements of intent to change certain lifestyle behaviors. Family support and assistance are needed to make these difficult changes because the entire family group will be affected. Nurses can influence patients and guide them in pacing the changes.[63]

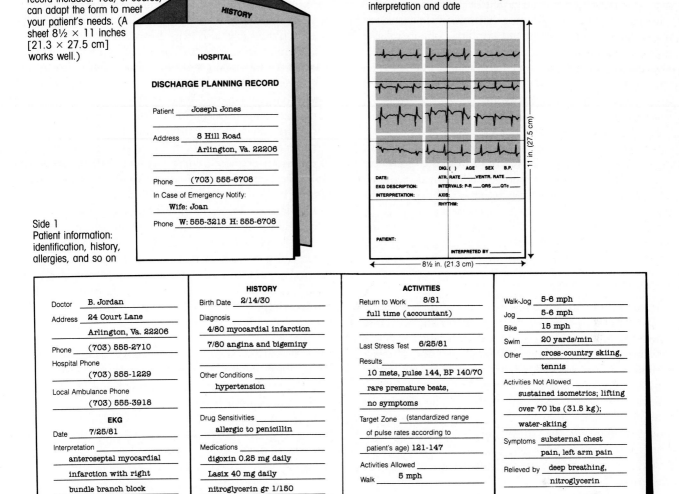

FIG. 10-9   Pocket discharge record.
From Glover JC: Reducing discharge planning with a pocket-size discharge planning record, Nurs 81 11(12):50, 1981.

Family stress

Because the patient is part of a family system, a change in one perpetuates and causes change in another. This can be particularly dramatic when the patient with AMI is the head of the household. Family stress is related to uncertainty about dependence and independence, future of the family unit, role divisions, sexuality, and the possibility of conflict in relationships. The spouse may become overprotective of the patient. The patient struggles with the necessity of periods of dependence and at the same time tries to remain independent. The younger the patient with an AMI, the more concerns he or she may have about family future and job. During the early recovery phase the patient is unable to participate in activities such as sports and brisk family outings. This can cause feelings of conflict, inadequacy, disappointment, and guilt. These feelings can perpetuate destructive effects on family dynamics.[95,135]

A patient who has had one AMI is likely to have another.[64] The stress and anxiety that result from this expectation can be detrimental to adjustment. Receiving instruction in BLS can give family members some feeling of control. Cardiac rehabilitation programs can assist the patient and family in dispelling myths and misconceptions about prospective life expectancy, desirable and undesirable behaviors, and lifestyle changes after the acute event. Regular and informal group meetings with a specific structure and teaching goals can assist in achieving positive adjustments.

Spouses of AMI patients

Spouses of AMI patients can benefit from group discussion sessions during the adjustment period. Their purpose is to help spouses clearly view family dynamics, gain awareness and insight about feelings and conflicts, obtain reliable information and guidance about the disease and rehabilitation process, and express and share feelings, examine their behavior, and receive advice and reinforcement from a professional and other spouses in the same situation.[172] The most frequent topics in these sessions are insecurity and guilt, simple day-to-day habit changes, and the weakness and regression of some patients, which causes parental and overprotective behavior reactions from the spouses.[220]

The patient and spouse should be informed of the results possible from cardiac rehabilitation. When both are involved, a plan of action can be developed and agreed on to modify lifestyle and maximize health care.[133,210] Spouses and significant others play a crucial role in psychosocial adjustment and return to work after AMI.[135,153]

Altered sexual patterns

Resumption of sexual activity may present difficulties for the patient and partner because they do not know what to expect and are afraid intercourse will cause sudden death. Sexual counseling should be an integral part of the cardiac rehabilitation process.[7,137] It requires an understanding of human sexuality and cardiovascular disease.[119] A patient with uncomplicated AMI can usually resume intercourse within 5 to 8 weeks. Nurses involved in sexual counseling should consult with the patient's physician to obtain specifics about the patient resuming sexual activity. The nurse should also know the physician's general advice about sex after AMI.[119]

Some activities that will help couples maintain and resume sexual intimacy are touching, such as during personal care, and taking daily walks together. Reminding them that energy required for sexual activity is similar to other daily activities may also help. Research[105,119,133] has shown that cardiovascular demands of sexual activity in the cardiac patient are of modest severity. Patients and partners can assess readiness for sexual activity by taking a brisk walk or climbing two flights of stairs (20 steps) in 10 seconds.[119] If patients remain symptom free, they are likely to be ready for sexual intercourse. Partners may be more comfortable if patients take responsibility for initiating sexual activity. Positions that conserve energy are lying side-to-side, sitting in a chair, and lying with patients on the bottom. Patients should be instructed to avoid intercourse in a hot or cold environment, after heavy meals, when angry or emotionally upset, when tired, and after drinking alcohol. Patients should be cautioned that more energy may be required in performing sexually with a new partner or in an extramarital relationship. Also, if the patient participates in anal intercourse, stimulation of the vagus nerve may diminish cardiac output and precipitate chest pain.[119]

Discharge record

Patients need a useful discharge record (Fig. 10-9 on p. 291). Original records can be kept at the hospital, and patients can have photocopies of them. The advantages of such records are that they are ready at discharge, contain detailed information, and can be carried in wallets at all times. They free the nurse to spend more time teaching patients at discharge.[69]

KEY CONCEPT REVIEW

1. Local metabolic alterations in the zone of infarction include:
   a. Accumulation of lactic acid
   b. Reduced ATP production
   c. Change to anaerobic glycolysis
   d. All the above
2. Mechanical alterations in AMI include:
   a. Reduced contractility in the ischemic zone
   b. Hyperfunction in the normal zones
   c. Cessation of contractility in the infarcted zone
   d. All of above
3. Which of the following descriptors of location and size may be applied to AMIs?
   a. Anterior, inferior, posterior, or lateral
   b. Q wave or non-Q-wave
   c. Transmural or subendocardial
   d. All of the above
4. Which of the following correctly contrasts AMI pain with angina pectoris pain?
   a. Pain of AMI is relieved by rest.

   b. Pain of AMI is related to exertion and stress, as is angina.
   c. AMI pain lasts longer than that of angina.
   d. AMI pain is relieved by leaning forward.
5. In AMI with documented ST-T changes, pain that continues or returns may indicate:
   (1) Infarction is complete.
   (2) Ischemia is continuing and extension is likely.
   (3) Ulcer disease is a more likely cause.
   (4) Pericarditis may be developing.
   a. 1 and 4
   b. 2 and 4
   c. 3 only
   d. 4 only
6. Initial nursing assessment for patients with AMI should include:
   a. Pain, anxiety, and history of present illness
   b. Vital signs and physical assessment
   c. Evidence of dysrhythmias and heart failure
   d. All of the above

7. Ongoing nursing assessment for patients with AMI should include:
   a. Dysrhythmias
   b. Activity tolerance
   c. Evidence of heart failure
   d. All the above
8. Thrombolytic therapy is effective in improving myocardial perfusion after AMI because it:
   a. Lyses the clot occluding the related artery
   b. Dilates stenosed coronary arteries
   c. Alters myocardial metabolism
   d. All the above
9. PTCA is effective in improving myocardial perfusion after AMI because it:
   a. Lyses the clot occluding the related artery
   b. Dilates stenosed coronary arteries
   c. Alters myocardial metabolism
   d. All the above
10. Which of the following interventions are likely to be effective in reducing the patient's and family's anxiety after AMI?
    a. Relaxation and imagery exercises
    b. Music
    c. Explanation and information
    d. All the above
11. The major complications of AMI patients are:
    (1) Ventricular dysrhythmias
    (2) Cardiac failure
    (3) Dressler's syndrome
    (4) Pericarditis
    a. 1 and 4
    b. 1 and 2
    c. 1, 2, and 3
    d. 1, 2, 3, and 4
12. PVCs are usually suppressed with lidocaine because:
    a. They indicate ventricular irritability.
    b. They often precede supraventricular tachycardia.
    c. They have a profound effect on cardiac output.
    d. They are uncomfortable for the patient.
13. Nitrates are used in the management of heart failure because:
    (1) They dilate the arterial bed, thereby reducing afterload.
    (2) They have a positive inotropic effect.
    (3) They dilate the venous bed, thereby reducing preload.
    (4) They reduce impedance to left ventricular emptying.
    a. 1, 2, and 3
    b. 1, 2, and 4
    c. 1, 3, and 4
    d. 2, 3, and 4
14. Important components of cardiac rehabilitation are:
    a. Inclusion of family, especially the spouse
    b. CAD risk factor reduction
    c. Graded, progressive exercise
    d. All of the above

ANSWERS

1. d	4. c	7. d	9. b	11. b	13. c
2. d	5. b	8. a	10. d	12. a	14. d
3. d	6. d				

REFERENCES

1. Achterberg J and Lawlis F: Bridges of the bodymind: behavioral approaches to health care, Champaign, Ill, 1980, Institute for Personality and Ability Testing, Inc.
2. Achterberg J and Lawlis F: Imagery and health intervention, Top Clin Nurs 3:55, 1982.
3. Alpert JS: The pathophysiology of acute myocardial infarction, Cardiology 76:85, 1989.
4. Altice NF and Jamison GB: Interventions to facilitate pain management in myocardial infarction, J Cardiovasc Nurs 3:49, 1989.
5. American Heart Association: Standards and guidelines for cardiopulmonary resuscitation and emergency cardiac care, JAMA 255:2841, 1986.
6. American Heart Association: 1990 heart and stroke facts, Dallas, 1989, The Association.
7. Baggs JG and Karch AM: Sexual counseling of women with coronary heart disease, Heart Lung 16:154, 1987.
8. Baim DS: Interventional catheterization techniques: Percutaneous transluminal balloon angioplasty, valvuloplasty, and related procedures. In Braunwald E, editor: Heart disease: a textbook of cardiovascular medicine, ed 3, Philadelphia, 1988, WB Saunders Co.
9. Bang NU, Wilhelm OG and Clayman MD: After coronary thrombolysis and reperfusion, what next? J Am Coll Cardiol 14(4):837, 1989.
10. Beare PG and Myers JL: Principles and practice of adult health nursing, St Louis, 1990, The CV Mosby Co.
11. Berne RM and Levy MN: Physiology, ed 2, St Louis, 1988, The CV Mosby Co.
12. β-Blocker Heart Attack Trial Research Group, Bethesda, Md: A randomized trial of propranolol in patients with acute myocardial infarction, JAMA 247:1707, 1982.
13. Black S, Coombs VJ, and Townsend SN: Reperfusion and reperfusion injury in acute myocardial infarction, Heart Lung 19:274, 1990.
14. Bodwell W: Ischemia, reperfusion, and reperfusion injury: role of oxygen-free radicals and oxygen-free radical scavengers, J Cardiovasc Nurs 4:25, 1989.
15. Braun LT and Holm K: Preservation of ischemic myocardium through activity management, J Cardiovasc Nurs 3:39, 1989.
16. Braunwald E, editor: Heart disease: a textbook of cardiovascular medicine, ed 3, Philadelphia, 1988, WB Saunders Co.
17. Braunwald E: The history. In Braunwald E, editor: Heart disease: a textbook of cardiovascular medicine, ed 3, Philadelphia, 1988, WB Saunders Co.
18. Braunwald E: The physical examination. In Braunwald E, editor: Heart disease: a textbook of cardiovascular medicine, ed 3, Philadelphia, 1988, WB Saunders Co.
19. Braunwald E: Thrombolytic reperfusion of acute myocardial infarction: resolved and unresolved issues, J Am Coll Cardiol 12:85A, 1988.
20. Braunwald E and Sobel BE: Coronary blood flow and myocardial ischemia. In Braunwald E, editor: Heart disease: a textbook of cardiovascular medicine, ed 3, Philadelphia, 1988, WB Saunders Co.
21. Brooks-Brunn J: Thrombolytic intervention and its effect on mortality in acute myocardial infarction: review of clinical trials, Heart Lung 17:756, 1988.

22. Brunner LS and Suddarth DS: The Lippincott manual of nursing practice, ed 4, Philadelphia, 1986, JB Lippincott Co.

23. Brunner LS and Suddarth DS: Textbook of medical-surgical nursing, ed 6, Philadelphia, 1988, JB Lippincott Co.

24. Brush JE and others: Use of the initial electrocardiogram to predict in-hospital complications of acute myocardial infarction, N Engl J Med 312:137, 1985.

25. Caine RM: Families in crisis: making the critical difference, Focus Crit Care 16:184, 1989.

26. Carey RL: Compliance and related nursing actions, Nurs Forum 21:157, 1984.

27. Carpenito LJ: Nursing diagnosis application to clinical practice, ed 3, Philadelphia, 1989, JB Lippincott Co.

28. Chesebro JH and others: Thrombolysis in myocardial infarction (TIMI) trial, phase I: a comparison between intravenous tissue plasminogen activator and intravenous streptokinase, Circulation 76:142, 1987.

29. Chyun D: Patient's perceptions of stressors in intensive care and coronary care units, Focus Crit Care 16:206, 1989.

30. Clark JB, Queener SF, and Karb VB: Pharmacological basis of nursing practice, ed 3, St Louis, 1990, The CV Mosby Co.

31. Clark S: Nursing diagnosis: ineffective coping. I. A theoretical framework. II. Planning care, Heart Lung 16:670, 1987.

32. Collen D: Coronary thrombolysis: streptokinase or recombinant tissue-type plasminogen activator? Ann Intern Med 112:529, 1990.

33. Conti CR and Mehta JL: Acute myocardial ischemia: role of atherosclerosis, thrombosis, platelet activation, coronary vasospasm, and altered arachidonic acid metabolism, Circulation 75(suppl V):V-84, 1987.

34. Cotran RS, Kumar V, and Robbins SK: Robbins' pathologic basis of disease, ed 4, Philadelphia, 1989, WB Saunders Co.

35. Cray L: A collaborative project: initiating a family intervention program in a medical intensive care unit. Focus Crit Care 16:213, 1989.

36. Crispell KA, Maran JN, and Warren EC: Postmyocardial infarction syndrome: a case study, Focus Crit Care 14:67, 1987.

37. Davis-Rollans D and Cunningham SG: Physiologic responses of coronary care patients to selected music, Heart Lung 16:370, 1987.

38. de Bono DP: The European Cooperative Study Group trial of intravenous recombinant tissue-type plasminogen activator (rt-PA) and conservative therapy versus rt-PA and immediate coronary angioplasty, J Am Coll Cardiol 12(6):20A, 1988.

39. Dhurandhar RW and others: Bretylium tosylate in the management of recurrent ventricular fibrillation complicating acute myocardial infarction, Heart Lung 9:265, 1980.

40. Dillon J and others: Rapid initiation of thrombolytic therapy for acute MI, Crit Care Nurs 9:55, 1989.

41. Dix-Sheldon DK: Pharmacologic management of myocardial ischemia, J Cardiovasc Nurs 3:17, 1989.

42. Dohno S and others: Sleep-waking changes in cardiac arrhythmias in a coronary care patient, Psychosom Med 39:39, 1977.

43. Dossey BM and others: Holistic nursing: a handbook for practice, Gaitherburg, Md, 1988, Aspen Publishers, Inc.

44. Drew BJ: Cardiac rhythm responses. I. An important phenomenon for nursing practice, science, and research, Heart Lung 18:8, 1989.

45. Drew BJ: Cardiac rhythm responses. II. Review of 22 years of nursing research, Heart Lung 18:184, 1989.

46. Dunagan WC and Ridner ML, editors: Manual of medical therapeutics, ed 26, Boston, 1989, Little, Brown & Co.

47. Ellis SG: Interventions in acute myocardial infarction, Circulation 81(Suppl IV):IV-43, 1990.

48. Emde KL and Searle LD: Current practices with thrombolytic therapy, J Cardiovasc Nurs 4:11, 1989.

49. Enger EL and Schwertz DW: Mechanisms of myocardial ischemia, J Cardiovasc Nurs 3:1, 1989.

50. The E.P.S.I.M. Research Group: A controlled comparison of aspirin and oral anticoagulants in prevention of death after myocardial infarction, N Engl J Med 307:702, 1982.

51. Erickson DE and Kleven M: Addendum: a standardized nursing care plan for the acute myocardial infarction patient receiving tissue-type plasminogen activator, Heart Lung 16:794, 1987.

52. Factor SM: Pathophysiology of myocardial ischemia. In Hurst JW and Schlant RC, editors: The heart, arteries, and veins, ed 7, New York, 1990, McGraw-Hill Inc.

53. Factor SM and Cho S: Smooth muscle contraction bands in the media of coronary arteries: a post-mortem marker of antemortem spasm? J Am Coll Cardiol 6:1329, 1985.

54. Factor SM and others: The microcirculation of the human heart: end-capillary loops with discrete perfusion fields, Circulation 66:526, 1982.

55. Fadden T, Fehring RJ, and Kenkel-Rossi E: Clinical validation of the diagnosis anxiety. In McLane AM, editor: Classification of nursing diagnoses: proceedings of the seventh conference, St Louis, 1987, The CV Mosby Co.

56. Falk E: Plaque rupture with severe pre-existing stenosis precipitating coronary thrombosis: characteristics of coronary atherosclerosis plaques underlying fatal occlusive thrombi, Br Heart J 50:127, 1983.

57. Felblinger D: Right ventricular infarction. In Sommers MS: Difficult diagnoses in critical care nursing, Rockville, Md, 1989, Aspen Publishers, Inc.

58. Feldman RL: Coronary thrombosis, coronary spasm and coronary atherosclerosis and speculation on the link between unstable angina and acute myocardial infarction, Am J Cardiol 59:1187, 1987.

59. Fields KB: Myocardial infarction and denial, J Fam Pract 28:157, 1989.

60. Fisch C: Electrocardiography and vectorcardiography. In Braunwald E, editor: Heart disease: a textbook of cardiovascular medicine, ed 3, Philadelphia, 1988, WB Saunders Co.

61. Foster SB and Canty KA: Pump failure following myocardial infarction: an overview, Heart Lung 9:293, 1980.

62. Frederickson K: Anxiety transmission in the patient with myocardial infarction, Heart Lung 18:617, 1989.

63. Frenn MD and others: Life-style changes in a cardiac rehabilitation program: the client perspective, J Cardiovasc Nurs 3:43, 1989.

64. Friesinger GC: The natural history of atherosclerotic heart disease. In Hurst JW and Schlant RC, editors: The heart, arteries, and veins, ed 7, New York, 1990, McGraw-Hill, Inc.

65. Frishman WH and Miller KP: Platelets and antiplatelet therapy in ischemic heart disease, Curr Prob Cardiol 11(2):73, 1986.

66. Furberg CD: The secondary prevention trials: lessons learned, questions raised, Postgrad Med 83(special report):83, Feb 29 1988.

67. Fuster V and others: Antithrombotic therapy after myocardial reperfusion in acute myocardial infarction, J Am Coll Cardiol 12:78A, 1988.

68. Gheorghiade M and others: Risk identification at the time of admission to coronary care unit in patients with suspected myocardial infarction, Am Heart J 116:1212, 1988.

69. Glover JC: Reducing discharge planning with a pocket-size discharge planning record, Nurs 81 11:50, 1981.

70. Goldberg RJ and others: Outcome after cardiac arrest during acute myocardial infarction, Am J Cardiol, 59:251, 1987.

71. Gomez EA, Gomez GE, and Otto DA: Anxiety as a human emotion: some basic conceptual models, Nurs Forum 21:38, 1984.

72. Gordon DJ and others: Predictive value of the exercise tolerance test for mortality in North American men: the Lipid Research Clinic's Mortality Follow-Up Study, Circulation 74:252, 1986.

73. Gotto AM: AHA conference report on cholesterol, Circulation 80:1, 1989.

74. Gotto AM and Farmer JA: Risk factors for coronary artery disease. In Braunwald E, editor: Heart disease: a textbook of cardiovascular medicine, ed 3, Philadelphia, 1988, WB Saunders Co.

75. Guyton AC: Textbook of medical physiology, ed 7, Philadelphia, 1986, WB Saunders Co.

76. Guzzetta CE: Effects of relaxation and music therapy on patients in a coronary care unit with presumptive acute myocardial infarction, Heart Lung 18:609, 1989.

77. Guzzetta CE and Forsyth GL: Nursing diagnostic pilot study: psychophysiologic stress, ANS 1:27, 1979.

78. Guzzetta CE and others: Clinical assessment tools for use with nursing diagnoses, St Louis, 1989, The CV Mosby Co.

79. Hazzard WR: Why do women live longer than men? biologic differences that influence longevity, Postgrad Med 85:271, 1989.

80. Healy BP: Pathology of coronary atherosclerosis. In Hurst JW and Schlant RC, editors: The heart, arteries, and veins, ed 7, New York, 1990, McGraw-Hill, Inc.

81. Helgeson VS: The origin, development, and current state of the literature on type A behavior, J Cardiovasc Nurs 3:59, 1989.

82. Hemenway JA: Sleep and the cardiac patient, Heart Lung 9:453, 1980.

83. Hennekens CH: Role of aspirin with thrombolytic therapy in acute myocardial infarction, Chest 97(4 Suppl):151S, 1990.

84. Herlitz J and others: Delay time in suspected acute myocardial infarction and the importance of its modification, Clin Cardiol 12:370, 1989.

85. Hirsch AT: Postmyocardial infarction syndrome, Am J Nurs 79:1240, 1979.

86. Hjalmarson A: International beta-blocker review in acute and postmyocardial infarction, Am J Cardiol 61:26B, 1988.

87. Horie M and others: A new approach for the enzymatic estimation of infarct size: serum peak creatine kinase and time to peak creatine kinase activity, Am J Cardiol 57:76, 1986.

88. Hudak CM, Gallo BM, and Benz JJ: Critical care nursing: a holistic approach, Philadelphia, 1990, JB Lippincott Co.

89. Hurst JW: Atherosclerotic coronary heart disease: historical benchmarks, methods of study and clinical features, differential diagnosis, and clinical spectrum. In Hurst JW and Schlant RC, editors: The heart, arteries, and veins, ed 7, New York, 1990, McGraw-Hill, Inc.

90. Hurst JW and Schlant RC, editors: The heart, arteries, and veins, ed 7, New York, 1990, McGraw-Hill, Inc.

91. ISIS-2 (Second International Study of Infarct Survival) Collaborative Group: Randomized trial of intravenous streptokinase, oral aspirin, both, or neither among 17,187 cases of suspected acute myocardial infarction: ISIS-2, J Am Coll Cardiol 12:3A, 1988.

92. Janis I: Stress, attitudes, and decisions: selected papers, New York, 1982, Praeger Publishers.

93. Jefferson RH: Biologic treatment of depression in cardiac patients, Psychosomatics 26(suppl 11):31, 1987.

94. Johanson BC and others: Standards for critical care, ed 3, St Louis, 1988, The CV Mosby Co.

95. Johnson JL and Morse JM: Regaining control: the process of adjustment after myocardial infarction, Heart Lung 19:126, 1990.

96. Johnston BL, Watt EW, and Fletcher GF: Oxygen consumption and hemodynamic and electrocardiographic responses to bathing in recent post-myocardial infarction patients, Heart Lung 10:666, 1981.

97. Kay JH: Emergency operation for complications of myocardial infarction, Heart Lung 11:40, 1982.

98. Kennedy JW: Streptokinase for the treatment of acute myocardial infarction: a brief review of randomized trials, J Am Coll Cardiol 10(5):28B, 1987.

99. Killip T and Kimball JT: Treatment of myocardial infarction in a coronary care unit: a two-year experience with 250 patients, Am J Cardiol 20:457, 1967.

100. Kinney M and others: Comprehensive cardiac care, ed 7, St Louis, 1991, Mosby–Year Book, Inc.

101. Kirchhoff KT: An examination of the physiologic basis for "coronary precautions," Heart Lung 10:874, 1981.

102. Kirchhoff KT and others: Electrocardiographic response to ice water ingestion, Heart Lung 19:41, 1990.

103. Klein RC, Vera Z, and Mason DT: Intraventricular conduction defects in acute myocardial infarction: incidence, prognosis, and therapy, Am Heart J, 108:1007, 1984.

104. Lambert CR and others: Influence of beta-adrenergic blockade defined by time series analysis on circadian variation of heart rate and ambulatory myocardial ischemia, Am J Cardiol 64:835, 1989.

105. Larson JL and others: Heart rate and blood pressure responses to sexual activity and a stair climbing test, Heart Lung 9:1025, 1980.

106. Lee KT editor: Atherosclerosis, Ann NY Acad Sci 454:1, 1985.

107. Lets G: Leukotrienes: role in cardiovascular physiology. In Mehta JL and Conti CR, editors: Cardiovascular clinics, thrombosis and platelets in myocardial ischemia, Philadelphia, 1987, FA Davis Co.

108. Levenson JL and others: Denial and medical outcome in unstable angina, Psychosom Med 51:27, 1989.

109. Leya F: Acute myocardial infarction: options on arrival at the hospital, Postgrad Med 85:131, 1989.

110. Lloyd GG: Myocardial infarction and mental illness: a review, J R Soc Med 80:101, 1987.

111. Loscalzo J: Thrombolysis in the management of acute myocardial infarction and unstable angina pectoris, Drugs 37:191, 1989.

112. Loscalzo J: An overview of thrombolytic agents, Chest 97(4 Suppl):117S, 1990.

113. Maggioni AP and others: GISSI trials in acute myocardial infarction: rationale, design, and results, Chest 97(4 Suppl): 146S, 1990.

114. Malseed RT and Harrigan GS: Textbook of pharmacology and nursing care using the nursing process, Philadelphia, 1989, JB Lippincott Co.

115. Mandle CL and others: Relaxation response in femoral angiography, Radiology 174(3 Pt 1):737, 1990.

116. Mark DB and others: Administration of thrombolytic therapy in the community hospital: Established principles and unresolved issues, J Am Coll Cardiol 12:32A, 1988.

117. Maseri A: Pathogenetic components of acute ischemic syndromes: focus on acute ischemic stimuli, Circulation 81(Suppl I):I-1, 1990.

118. McCance KL and Huether SE: Pathophysiology: the biologic basis for disease in adults and children, St Louis, 1990, The CV Mosby Co.

119. McCann ME: Sexual healing after heart attack, Am J Nurs 89:1133, 1989.

120. McFarland GK and McFarlane EA: Nursing diagnosis and intervention: planning for patient care, St Louis, 1989, The CV Mosby Co.

121. McKenry LM and Salerno E: Mosby's pharmacology in nursing, ed 17, St Louis, 1989, The CV Mosby Co.

122. Anistreplase for acute coronary thrombosis, Med Lett 32:156, 1990.

123. Miller PJ and Wikoff R: Spouses' psychosocial problems, resources, and marital functioning postmyocardial infarction, Prog Cardiovasc Nurs 4:71, 1989.

124. Milligan KS: Tissue-type plasminogen activator: a new fibrinolytic, Heart Lung 16:69, 1987.

125. Minckley BB and others: Myocardial infarct stress-of-transfer inventory: development of a research tool, Nurs Res 28:4, 1979.

126. Misinski M: Role of conventional management and alternative therapies in limiting infarct size in acute myocardial infarction, Heart Lung 16(6 Pt 2):746, 1987.

127. Monk JP and Heel RC: Anisoylated plasminogen streptokinase activator complex (APSAC): a review of its mechanisms of action, clinical pharmacology, and therapeutic use in acute myocardial infarction, Drugs 34:25, 1987.

128. Morris DC, Walter PF, and Hurst JW: The recognition and treatment of myocardial infarction and its complications. In Hurst JW and Schlant RC, editors: The heart, arteries, and veins, ed 7, New York, 1990, McGraw-Hill, Inc.

129. Moss AJ and Benhorin J: Prognosis and management after a first myocardial infarction, N Engl J Med 322:743, 1990.

130. National Center for Health Statistics: Vital statistics of the United States, 1987, II. Mortality. Part A. Hyattsville, Md, 1990, US Public Health Service.

131. Nyamathi AM: The coping responses of female spouses of patients with myocardial infarction, Heart Lung 16:86, 1987.

132. Nyamathi AM: Perceptions of factors influencing the coping of wives of myocardial infarction patients, J Cardiovasc Nurs 2:65, 1988.

133. Oberman A: Rehabilitation of patients with coronary artery disease. In Braunwald E, editor: Heart disease: a textbook of cardiovascular medicine, ed 3, Philadelphia, 1988, WB Saunders Co.

134. Ornato JP and Smith M: Thrombolytic therapy in acute MI, Patient Care 24:76, 1990.

135. Owen PM: Recovery from myocardial infarction: a review of psychosocial determinants, J Cardiovasc Nurs 2:75, 1987.

136. Pasternak RC, Braunwald E, and Alpert JS: Acute myocardial infarction. In Braunwald E and others, editors: Harrison's principles of internal medicine, ed 11, New York, 1987, McGraw-Hill, Inc.

137. Pasternak RC, Braunwald E, and Sobel BE: Acute myocardial infarction. In Braunwald E editor: Heart disease, ed 3, Philadelphia, 1988, WB Saunders Co.

138. Pearson TA: Multiple risk factors for coronary artery disease: behavioral factors in preventive cardiology, Am J Cardiol 60:74J, 1987.

139. Pepine CJ: New concepts in the pathophysiology of acute myocardial ischemia and infarction and their relevance to contemporary management, Cardiovasc Clin 20:3, 1989.

140. Pepine CJ: New concepts in the pathophysiology of acute myocardial infarction, Am J Cardiol 64(4):2B, 1989.

141. Peterson JE and Emmot WW: Therapies to limit infarct size: timing, dosage, and effectiveness, Postgrad Med 86(3):54, 1989.

142. Philip AE and others: Personal traits and the physical, psychiatric and social state of patients one year after a myocardial infarction, Int J Rehabil Res 2:479, 1979.

143. Potter PA and Perry AG: Fundamentals of nursing: concepts, process, and practice, ed 2, St Louis, 1989, The CV Mosby Co.

144. Pratt CM and Roberts R: Pharmacologic therapy of atherosclerotic coronary heart disease. In Hurst JW and Schlant RC, editors: The heart, arteries, and veins, ed 7, New York, 1990, McGraw-Hill, Inc.

145. Prichard BNC: Beta-blockade therapy and cardiovascular disease: past, present, and future, Postgrad Med 83(special report):8, Feb 29, 1988.

146. Quaglietti SF, Stotts NA, and Lovejoy NC: The effect of selected positions on rate pressure product of the postmyocardial infarction patient, J Cardiovasc Nurs 2:77, 1988.

147. Quirk ME and others: Evaluation of three psychologic interventions to reduce anxiety during MR imaging, Radiology 173:759, 1989.

148. Radwin LE: Autonomous nursing interventions for treating the patient in acute pain: a standard, Heart Lung 16:258, 1987.

149. Rahe RH and others: Recent life changes, myocardial infarction, and abrupt coronary death, Arch Intern Med 133:221, 1974.

150. Raleigh EH and Odtohan BC: The effect of a cardiac teaching program on patient rehabilitation, Heart Lung 16:311, 1987.

151. Reich P: Psychological predisposition to life-threatening arrhythmias, Annu Rev Med 36:397, 1985.

152. Relman AS: Aspirin for the primary prevention of myocardial infarction, N Engl J Med 318:245, 1988.

153. Riegel B: Social support and psychological adjustment to chronic coronary heart disease: Operationalization of Johnson's behavioral system model, ANS 11:74, 1989.

154. Roberts R: Diagnostic assessment of myocardial infarction based on lactate dehydrogenase and creatine kinase isoenzymes, Heart Lung 10:486, 1981.

155. Roberts SE: Nursing care study: a patient with myocardial infarction, Nurs Times 78:190, 1982.

156. Robison JS: Acute right ventricular infarction: recognition, evaluation, and treatment, Crit Care Nurs 7:42, 1987.

157. Rodriguez SW and Reed RL: Thrombolytic therapy for MI, Am J Nurs 87:632, 1987.

158. Ross R: The pathogenesis of atherosclerosis: an update, N Engl J Med 314:488, 1986.

159. Ross R: The pathogenesis of atherosclerosis. In Braunwald E, editor: Heart disease, ed 3, Philadelphia, 1988, WB Saunders Co.

160. Ross R: Factors influencing atherogenesis. In Hurst JW and Schlant RC, editors: The heart, arteries, and veins, ed 7, New York, 1990, McGraw-Hill, Inc.

161. Rutherford JD and Braunwald E: Thrombolytic therapy in acute myocardial infarction, Chest 97(4 Suppl):136S, 1990.

162. Sanford S: Sleep and the cardiac patient, Cardiovasc Nurs 19(5):19, 1983.

163. Scalzi C and others: Evaluation of an inpatient educational program for coronary care patients and families, Heart Lung 9:846, 1980.

164. Schactman M: Transfer stress in patients after myocardial infarction, Focus Crit Care 14:34, 1987.

165. Scharf MB, Fletcher K, and Graham JP: Comparative amnestic effects of benzodiazepine hypnotic agents, J Clin Psychiatry 49:134, 1988.

166. Schiro AG and Curtis DG: Asymptomatic coronary artery disease, Heart Lung 17:144, 1988.

167. Schneider AC: Unreported chest pain in a coronary care unit, Focus Crit Care 14(5):21, 1987.

168. Schreiber T: Review of clinical studies of thrombolytic agents in acute myocardial infarction, Am J Med 83(suppl 2A):20, 1987.

169. Schroeder SA and others: Current medical diagnosis & treatment 1990, Norwalk, Conn, 1990, Appleton & Lange.

170. Schwartz PJ and others: Effect of ventricular fibrillation complicating acute myocardial infarction on long-term prognosis: importance of the site to infarction, Am J Cardiol 56:384, 1985.

171. Sebilia AJ: Sleep deprivation of biological rhythms in the critical care unit, Crit Care Nurs 1:19, 1981.

172. Seger H and Schlesinger Z: Rehabilitation of patients after acute myocardial infarction: an interdisciplinary, family-oriented program, Heart Lung 10:841, 1981.

173. Self PR: Four steps for helping a patient alleviate anger, Nurse 80 10:66, 1980.

174. Shanfield SB: Return to work after an acute myocardial infarction: a review, Heart Lung 19:109, 1990.

175. Sipperly ME: Expanding role of coronary angioplasty: current implications, limitations, and nursing considerations, Heart Lung 18:507, 1989.

176. Sirles AT and Selleck CS: Cardiac disease and the family: impact, assessment, and implications, J Cardiovasc Nurs 3:23, 1989.

177. Smith A: Physiology, diagnosis, and life-style modifications for hyperlipidemia, J Cardiovasc Nurs 1:15, 1987.

178. Smith CE: Assessing chest pain quickly and accurately, Nurs 88 18(5):52, 1988.

179. Sobel BE and others, editors: Tissue plasminogen activator in thrombolytic therapy, New York, 1987, Marcel Dekker, Inc.

180. Solomon J: Introduction to cardiovascular nursing, Baltimore, 1988, Williams & Wilkins.

181. Sorkin EM, Brogden RN, and Romankiewicz JA: Intravenous glyceryl trinitrate (nitroglycerin): a review of its pharmacological properties and therapeutic efficacy, Drugs 27:45, 1984.

182. Steele JM and Ruzicki D: An evaluation of the effectiveness of cardiac teaching during hospitalization, Heart Lung 16:306, 1987.

183. Stein B and others: Platelet inhibitor agents in cardiovascular disease: an update, J Am Coll Cardiol 14:813, 1989.

184. Steinberg D and others: Beyond cholesterol: modifications of low-density lipoprotein that increase its atherogenicity, N Engl J Med 320(14):915, 1989.

185. Steinberg EP and others: Cost and procedure implications of thrombolytic therapy for acute myocardial infarction, J Am Coll Cardiol 12:58A, 1988.

186. Steingart RM and Scheuer J: Assessment of myocardial ischemia. In Hurst JW and Schlant RC, editors: The heart, arteries, and veins, ed 7, New York, 1990, McGraw-Hill, Inc.

187. Stone NJ and Van Horn LV: Controlling cholesterol levels through diet, Postgrad Med 83:229, 1988.

188. Sunquist JM and others: Right ventricular infarction: recognition, treatment, and nursing considerations, Heart Lung 9:706, 1980.

189. Sweetwood HM: Clinical electrocardiography for nurses, ed 2, Rockville Md, 1989, Aspen Publishers, Inc.

190. Sytkowski PA, Kannel WB, and D'Agostino RB: Changes in risk factors and the decline in mortality from cardiovascular disease: the Framingham heart study, N Engl J Med 322:1635, 1990.

191. Theroux P and others: Prognostic value of exercise testing soon after myocardial infarction, N Engl J Med 301:341, 1979.

192. Thomas SA and others: Denial in coronary care patients: an objective reassessment, Heart Lung, 12:74, 1983.

193. Thompson DR: A randomized controlled trial of in-hospital nursing support for first-time myocardial infarction patients and their partners: effects on anxiety and depression, J Adv Nurs 14:291, 1989.

194. Thompson EA: Anxiety: a mental health vital sign. In Longo DC and Williams RA, editors: Clinical practice in psychosocial nursing, ed 2, Norwalk, Conn, 1986, Appleton & Lange.

195. Thompson JM and others: Mosby's manual of clinical nursing, ed 2, St Louis, 1989, The CV Mosby Co.

196. TIMI Study Group: The thrombolysis in myocardial infarction (TIMI) trial: phase I findings, N Engl J Med 312:932, 1985.

197. Topol EJ and others: Insights derived from the Thrombolysis and Angioplasty in Myocardial Infarction (TAMI) trials, J Am Coll Cardiol 12:24A, 1988.

198. Toth JC: Effect of structured preparation for transfer on patient anxiety on leaving coronary care unit, Nurs Res 29:28, 1980.

199. Underhill SL and others: Cardiac nursing, ed 2, Philadelphia, 1989, JB Lippincott Co.

200. Van de Werf F: Lessons from the European Cooperative recombinant tissue-type plasminogen activator (rt-PA) versus placebo trial, J Am Coll Cardiol 12:14A, 1988.

201. Vaughn P and Rice V: Complications of myocardial infarction, Crit Care Nurse 2:44, 1982.

202. Vejar M and others: Comparison of low-dose aspirin and coronary vasodilators in acute unstable angina, Circulation 81(suppl I):I-4, 1990.

203. Ventura B: Thrombolytic therapy for MI, Am J Nurs 87:631, 1987.

204. Verstraete M: Thrombolysis after myocardial infarction (letter), Lancet 1:763, 1988.

205. Verstraete M and others: Randomized trial of intravenous recombinant tissue-type plasminogen activator versus intravenous streptokinase in acute myocardial infarction, Lancet 1:842, 1985.

206. Vitello-Cicciu J, Stewart SL, and Griffin EL: Coronary artery disease. In Kinney MR, Packa DR, and Dunbar SB, editors: AACN's clinical reference for critical-care nursing, ed 2, New York, 1988, McGraw-Hill, Inc.

207. Wallace D and Ivey JD: The bifocal clinical nursing model: description and application to the patient receiving thrombolytic or anticoagulant therapy, J Cardiovasc Nurs 4:33, 1989.

208. Weisfeldt ML: Reperfusion and reperfusion injury, Clin Res 35:13, 1987.

209. Wehrmacher WH: Acute myocardial infarction: the race to the hospital, Postgrad Med 85:112, 1989.

210. Wenger NK and Fletcher GF: Rehabilitation of the patient with atherosclerotic coronary heart disease. In Hurst JW and Schlant RC, editors: The heart, arteries, and veins, ed 7, New York, 1990, McGraw-Hill, Inc.

211. Wenger NK and Schlant RC: Prevention of coronary atherosclerosis. In Hurst JW and Schlant RC, editors: The heart, arteries, and veins, ed 7, New York, 1990, McGraw-Hill, Inc.

212. Whalen RE and Hurst JW: The surgical treatment of atherosclerotic coronary heart disease. In Hurst JW and Schlant RC, editors: The heart, arteries, and veins, ed 7, New York, 1990, McGraw-Hill, Inc.

213. Willerson JT: Acute myocardial infarction. In Wyngaarden JB and Smith LH, editors: Cecil textbook of medicine, ed 18, Philadelphia, 1988, WB Saunders Co.

214. Willerson JT and Buja LM: Myocardial cellular alterations during myocardial ischemia and evolving infarction, Postgrad Med 83(special report):69, Feb 29, 1988.

215. Williams SM: Decision making in critical care nursing, Philadelphia, 1990, BC Decker Co.

216. Willich SN and others: ISAM Study Group: increased risk of myocardial infarction in the morning (abstract), J Am Coll Cardiol 11:28A, 1988.

217. Wishnie HA, Hackett TP, and Cassem NH: Psychological hazards of convalescence following myocardial infarction, JAMA 215:1292, 1971.

218. Woods N: Conceptualizations of self-care: toward health-oriented models, ANS 12:1, 1989.

219. Yasue H, Ogawa H, and Okumura K: Coronary artery spasm in the genesis of myocardial ischemia, Am J Cardiol 63:29E, 1989.

220. Young RF and Kahana E: Conceptualizing stress, coping, and illness-management in heart disease caregiving, Hospice J 3:53, 1987.

Interchapter 11

Stressors and Cardiac Illness

It has long been observed anecdotally that stressors are related to an increased incidence of myocardial infarction (MI) and sudden cardiac death. Scientific studies, however, are replacing such personal testimonials. These studies support the notion that a person's psychologic state can actually produce body illness. Since the work of Rahe and Lind,[11] it has been possible to quantify some of the psychologic variables involved. It has been shown, for example, that longevity is affected by events such as recent bereavement and grief, loss in job status, divorce, and financial distress. It is possible to assign such events a value, called a *life-change unit,* and to objectively assess the degree of stress an individual is perceiving.

In one such study, 1279 survivors of MI rated their life changes by assigning such values, as did the spouses of 226 sudden-death victims. The life-change units for these persons were higher during the 6 months preceding MI or sudden death than during the same time interval 1 year earlier. Sudden-death victims had much higher scores than did survivors of MI.[12]

Impressive evidence also exists to document that emotions such as anxiety, fear, and social isolation are associated with coronary artery disease,[2,8,16,20] hypertension,[10,15,21] dysrhythmias,[3,5,9,14] myocardial ischemia,[1,4,6,17] and sudden cardiac death.[13,18] Consider the evidence, for example, supporting the role of mental stress in association with the development of myocardial ischemia. Deanfield and others[4] found that stressful mental activity could trigger episodes of myocardial ischemia in patients as documented by regional abnormalities in myocardial perfusion, ST-segment changes, and anginal events independent of physical exertion. Likewise, Freeman and others[6] reported that a time frame of

high stress was associated with episodes of myocardial ischemia and elevated urinary cortisol and norepinephrine levels in patients with angina pectoris. Rozanski and others[17] reported that different forms of psychologic stress could provoke transient myocardial ischemia in patients with coronary artery disease as evidenced by the development of ventricular wall-motion abnormalities, ST-segment changes, or angina pectoris. Also, Barry and others[1] found that myocardial ischemia could be precipitated by psychophysiologic stress in patients with chronic stable angina. In this study, 22% of ischemic myocardial episodes occurred during intense emotional activities unrelated to physical exertion. Moreover, a direct correlation was discovered between the intensity of the emotional stress experienced and the duration of the myocardial ischemia. The results of these studies provide objective and compelling evidence that mental stress, unrelated to physical exertion, can cause myocardial ischemia in patients with coronary artery disease. The findings also suggest that mental stress may be as critical as physical exertion in triggering the ischemic episodes.[19]

In another study supporting the link between emotions and illness, Ruberman and others[18] reported the findings of a landmark investigation involving 2320 men who were survivors of acute MI. When age, history of acute MI, dysrhythmias, smoking, and treatment were controlled, patients with high stress were found to have 4 times the risk of sudden death than those with low stress. This study points to the causal role of stress in cardiac death independent of other prognostic variables.

These types of studies suggest that the heart is not an isolated organ. It is more than an element of hard wiring, contractile cells, and ions in flux. It is more than a

hydraulic chamber and mechanical pump. It is more like a delicate musical instrument on which persons play the melody of their emotions. These studies also provide conclusive evidence to prove that the body and mind communicate. They provide data to support the conclusions that consciousness can play an important negative and villainous role in matters of illness.

These studies provide many implications for practice. They suggest that we can no longer ignore the effects of the mind on the body and that body illnesses can no longer be treated exclusively with body-oriented therapies. These implications force us to collide with some startling realities.[7] We are struck with the realization that therapies used to reduce emotional stressors may be as important to patient outcomes as the traditional and highly technologic forms of therapies. We are obliged to recognize that mind-oriented therapies must be combined with traditional medical therapies to access and facilitate effective healing in patients.

REFERENCES

1. Barry J and others: Frequency of ST-segment depression produced by mental stress in stable angina pectoris from coronary artery disease, Am J Cardiol 61:989, 1988.
2. Blumenthal J and others: Effects of task incentive on cardiovascular responses in Type A and Type B individuals, Psychophysiology 20:63, 1983.
3. Bove AA: The cardiovascular response to stress, Psychosomatics 18:13, 1977.
4. Deanfield JE and others: Silent myocardial ischaemia due to mental stress, Lancet 1001, Nov 1984.
5. Eliot R and Buell J: Role of emotions and stress in the genesis of sudden death, J Am Coll Cardiol 5:95B, 1985.
6. Freeman LJ and others: Psychological stress and silent myocardial ischemia, Am Heart J 114:477, 1987.

7. Guzzetta CE: The human factor and the ailing heart: folklore or fact? J Inten Care Med 2:3, 1987.

8. Jenkins CD: Behavioral risk factors in coronary artery disease, Annu Rev Med 29:253, 1978.

9. Lown B and others: Basis for recurring ventricular fibrillation in the absence of coronary heart disease and its management, New Engl J Med 294:623, 1976.

10. Pilowski I and others: Hypertension and personality, Psychosom Med 35:15, 1973.

11. Rahe RH and Lind E: Psychosocial factors and sudden cardiac death: a pilot study, J Psychosom Res 15:19, 1971.

12. Rahe RH and others: Recent life changes, myocardial infarction and abrupt coronary death: studies in Helsinki, Arch Intern Med 133:221, 1974.

13. Rahe RH and Romo M: Recent life changes and the onset of myocardial infarction and sudden death in Helsinki. In Gunderson EK and Rahe R, editors: Life stress and illness, Springfield, Ill, 1974, Charles C Thomas.

14. Reich P and others: Acute psychological disturbance preceding life-threatening arrhythmias, JAMA 246:233, 1981.

15. Reiser MF, Burst AA, and Ferris EB: Life situations, emotions, and the course of patients with arterial hypertension, Psychosom Med 13:133, 1951.

16. Rosenman RH and others: Coronary heart disease in the Western Collaborative Group Study: final follow-up experience of 8½ years, JAMA 233:872, 1975.

17. Rozanski A and others: Mental stress and the induction of silent myocardial ischemia in patients with coronary artery disease, N Engl J Med 318:1005, 1988.

18. Ruberman W and others: Psychosocial influences on mortality after myocardial infarction, N Engl J Med 311:552, 1984.

19. Selwyn AP and Ganz P: Myocardial ischemia in coronary disease, N Engl J Med 318:1058, 1988.

20. Williams RB: Type A behavior and elevated physiologic and neuroendocrine responses to cognitive tests, Science 218:483, 1982.

21. Wolff HG: Stress and disease, Springfield, Ill, 1953, Charles C Thomas.

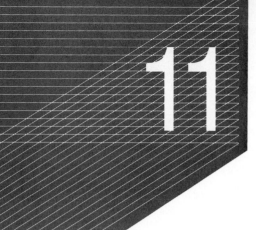

11

The Person with Heart Failure and Cardiogenic Shock

Susan J. Quaal

LEARNING OBJECTIVES

1. Examine the terms *preload, afterload, compliance, contractility, peripheral resistance,* and *impedance.*

2. Examine calcium's role in myocardial contraction.

3. Compare and contrast the major signs and symptoms of left and right ventricular failure and cardiogenic shock.

4. Describe the pathophysiologic changes that occur in heart failure and cardiogenic shock, and relate associated clinical findings specific to the integumentary, respiratory, cardiovascular, gastrointestinal, endocrine, neurologic, and renal systems.

5. Analyze medical treatment for the patient with congestive heart failure and cardiogenic shock.

6. Compare and contrast four methods of mechanical assistance for the patient in cardiogenic shock.

7. Synthesize measures to assist the patient and family in dealing with anxiety and fears related to potential death.

Heart failure

Over the last decade, congestive heart failure (CHF) has rapidly become one of the most important public health problems in cardiovascular medicine. An estimated 3 million people in the United States and 15 million worldwide are afflicted.[156] Whereas most cardiovascular disorders have decreased over the past 10 years, the incidence and prevalence of CHF has increased at a dramatic rate. Nearly 400,000 people in the United States develop CHF each year; this figure will probably increase as greater numbers of patients who might have died of an AMI are surviving but with compromised ventricular function. Consequently, the number of hospitalizations for CHF has increased more than threefold during the past 15 years; this disorder now represents the most common medical discharge diagnosis for patients over the age of 65 years.[115]

Heart failure is not a specific disease but rather the inability of the heart to pump blood commensurate with the metabolic needs of body tissues. Heart failure may be acute or chronic and may be precipitated by unrelated illness or stress. The patient's entire organ system and psychosocial well-being are affected by CHF; therefore a holistic perspective must be used. Interventions must thus extend beyond the physiologic scope (that is, a malfunctioning myocardium). The nurse must also assess for factors that produce fatigue and impaired physical mobility and thus assist the patient with adjusting to a way of life that conserves myocardial work and yet maximizes performance for the best possible quality of life.

SIGNIFICANCE

During the past 15 years, strides have been made in understanding CHF and cardiogenic shock. These advances originated with investigation into myocardial mechanics, which clarified the influence of preload on myocardial fiber shortening.[17] These concepts were then tested in the laboratory, facilitated by invasive monitoring techniques. Further studies suggested that such hemodynamic abnormalities could be partially improved by pharmacologic interventions.[26] Measurement of regional blood flow confirmed the presence of diminished perfusion of vital organs, especially the kidneys.[96] Recent investigations have been directed toward delineating many of the neurohormonal derangements.[90] Through precise measurements of respiratory gas exchange,[48] physiologists also have been able to probe mechanisms underlying exercise intolerance of CHF patients. Based on this impressive research, a variety of pharmacologic approaches that produce short-term and occasionally long-term reversal of specific pathophysiologic events are available to enhance the functional capacity of many CHF patients.[128]

Although many treatments are available, severe myocardial pump failure progressing to cardiogenic shock may not respond to these conventional and experimental pharmacologic therapies. Treatment of cardiogenic shock with pharmacologic agents has a mortality rate of 90% or greater.[142] Mechanical support of the failing heart has therefore evolved into a discipline. The profoundly depressed myocardium is capable of dramatic recuperative powers if temporarily supported by mechanical assistance. Intraaortic balloon pumping (IABP) and ventricular assistance devices (VADs) are therefore a necessary part of cardiogenic shock treatment. The patient awaiting cardiac transplantation may need to use pharmacologic support, temporary mechanical assistance, or a total artificial heart.

MYOCARDIAL MECHANICS

Myocardial ultrastructure, as described by Fawcett and McNutt,[50] is illustrated in Fig. 11-1. The myocardium is composed of a longitudinal series of myocardial cells that interdigitate to form fibers, the *myofibrils,* which lie parallel to one another. Sandwiched between myofibrils are *mitochondria,* the sources of energy for contraction. The myocardial ultrastructure consists of the following organelles within each cell: cell membrane or sarcolemma, intercalated disk, sarcomere, myofibrils, actin, myosin, tropomyosin and troponin protein, and the sacrotubular system.[143]

Sarcolemma (cell membrane)

Intracellular constituents are separated from extracellular fluid by the *sarcolemma* (Fig. 11-1, *A*). Functions ascribed to the sarcolemma are separation of intracellular and extracellular environments, membrane transport activity as necessary for cellular metabolism, active maintenance of the ionic composition of the cells, and transmembrane movement of ions, producing electrical currents that are inscribed on the electrocardiogram (ECG).[49,50]

Intercalated disk

Each cell is separated by an intercalated disk (Fig. 11-1, *B*). Therefore the cells of the working myocardium are not an anatomic *syncytium* (a group of cells in which the pro-

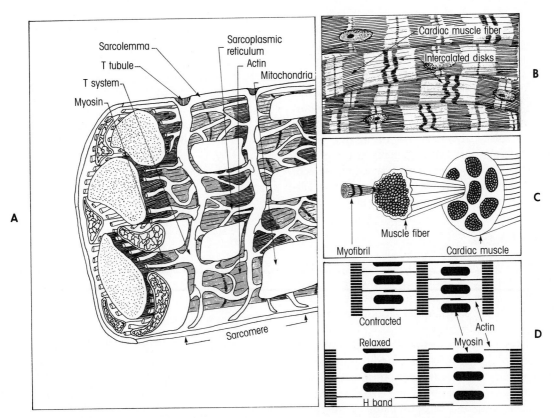

FIG. 11-1   A, The ultrastructure of the heart. **B,** Cardiac muscle fiber and intercalated disk. **C,** Myofibril. **D,** Actin and myosin activity during muscle contraction and relaxation.

toplasm of one cell is continuous with that of adjoining cells). These boundaries, however, offer little electrical resistance, so the myocardium is considered a functional syncytium.[37]

Sarcotubular system

Microtubules, the *sarcoplasmic reticulum* and *T system,* fill interfibrillar spaces. Calcium is thought to be bound within the sarcotubular system (Fig. 11-1, *A*). When an action potential transverses the surface of a cardiac muscle fiber, a wave of depolarization spreads passively along the membranes of the sarcotubular system; this leads to a release of bound calcium.[161]

Myofibrils

Each cardiac muscle fiber contains a group of branching, longitudinal, striated strands approximately 1 mm in diameter; these are termed *myofibrils* (Fig. 11-1, *C*). They exhibit a characteristic pattern of light and dark transverse bands and are subdivided into a series of repeating contractile units, the *sarcomere,* by a dark, transverse line, the *Z band.* Sarcomeres function as the cellular contractile units and are ideally suited to the mechanics of contraction because of their elongated shape. Sarcomeres look like a band because they are composed of two different proteins, *actin* (thin) and *myosin* (thick).[78]

Katz[86] described the properties of myocardial contraction; this theory involves interaction of the myosin heads with the actin to form cross-bridges. Calcium triggers this contractile process. Depolarization causes calcium to be released from its stores into the T tubes and sarcoplasmic reticulum. Calcium then migrates to the thin actin filaments and binds with an actin-protective covering protein called *troponin C.* The physical interaction of myosin cross-bridges, that of sliding onto actin filaments, is the process of contraction. These cross-bridges systematically detach; myosin then returns to its original configuration and reattaches to new, reactive actin filament sites.[79] (Fig. 11-1, *D*).

CARDIAC METABOLISM

The heart functions normally as an aerobic organ, converting metabolic energy to intracardiac pressure that is necessary to produce systolic ejection; the result is perfusion of blood to the myocardium to produce the energy needed during systole.[88]

The high metabolic requirements of the contractile proteins and active processes involved in ion transport require substantial quantities of adenosine triphosphate (ATP). The mechanism by which cells meet these requirements is oxidation of fatty acids and carbohydrates in the mitochondria. Oxidative phosphorylation requires a continual supply of oxygen to the myocardium. Because of this high

aerobic metabolism, *myocardial oxygen consumption* (MVO_2) is believed to reflect the net tissue energy use. Therefore indirect myocardial metabolism studies use changes in MVO_2 as an index of the heart's metabolic state.[161]

MYOCARDIAL DYNAMICS

External and internal work are involved in the myocardial transfer of energy from its metabolic substrate to the pressure developed in contraction. External work is illustrated in Fig. 11-2. During the isovolumic phase of ventricular contraction (*A* to *B*), pressure increases, but volume remains unchanged. Ventricular volume decreases rapidly during ventricular ejection (*B* to *C*), whereas the pressure continues to rise. Ventricular pressure falls rapidly after the aortic valve closes during isovolumic relaxation (*C* to *D*). Finally, ventricular volume rises during ventricular filling, with only a small increase in pressure (*D* to *A*).

The area bounded by loop *ABCDA* represents the heart's pressure-volume *(external work).*[151] *Static external work* refers to the development and maintenance of ventricular pressure before the opening of the aortic valve. *Dynamic work* occurs during ventricular ejection. Little[99] described the static and dynamic components of external work by comparing it to the forces involved in pouring a pail of water over a fence. Static effort is constituted by lifting the pail of water to a height equal to or slightly above the top of the fence. Additional energy (dynamic) must be used to tip the pail so that water pours over the fence.

According to Laplace's formula (P = T/R), pressure *(P)* developed by a particular level of wall tension *(T)* is

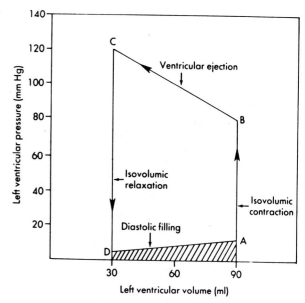

FIG. 11-2 Schematic representation of relationship between left ventricular pressure and volume during the cardiac cycle (see text).

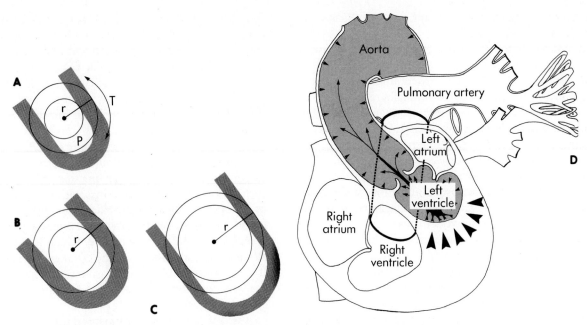

FIG. 11-3   **A,** Laplace's law. Relationship of wall tension to the ventricular systolic pressure. T = P × R: Wall tension = Pressure × Radius. **B,** As wall tension increases, pressure increases, the radius is greater, the wall becomes thinner, and the heart enlarges. T = Pressure × Radius. **C,** Resultant heart failure. **D,** Afterload = Aortic impedance = Peripheral resistance. Impedance is related to the load to eject, or stroke volume, and ejection tension (Laplace's law).

inversely proportional to the radius of the chamber (Fig. 11-3). Applied to the contracting ventricle, Laplace's law indicates that the myocardial tension required to sustain a particular level of intraventricular pressure diminishes as the chamber radius is reduced by ejection. As diastolic volume increases, greater myocardial tension is needed to develop the required level of intraventricular pressure.[1]

EXTRINSIC CIRCULATION CONTROL
Autonomic nervous system

The autonomic nervous system (ANS) comprises the *sympathetic nervous system (SNS)* and *parasympathetic nervous system (PNS)*. Most postganglionic fibers (fibers that innervate a target organ or vessel) of the SNS release *norepinephrine*. These fibers are called *adrenergic fibers,* a term that indicates a relationship to adrenalin. The postganglionic fibers of the PNS release *acetylcholine*. These are called *cholinergic fibers.*

Cardiovascular adrenergic receptor system

Norepinephrine, epinephrine, and sympathomimetic amines stimulate the heart and blood vessels by interacting with macromolecular cell structures called *receptors.*[4] Adrenergic drugs interact with the receptors and elicit a variety of responses as described in the following paragraphs.

α-Adrenergic receptors are most responsive to stimulation by norepinephrine. Most α-adrenergic receptors are located outside of the heart in the peripheral arteries and veins, although some are found in the coronary arteries. Others may exist in the heart. When stimulated, α-receptors produce a vasoconstrictive response.

β-Adrenergic receptors are divided into cardiac β-receptors (β_1) and peripheral β-receptors (β_2). Although β-receptors release norepinephrine at their nerve endings, they are most responsive to stimulation by isoproterenol. Stimulation of β_1-receptors increases heart rate, atrioventricular (AV) node conduction, and myocardial contractility. Stimulation of β_2-receptors produces vasodilation of arterial vessels and bronchodilatation in the lungs, effects that are opposite to those of α-adrenergic receptors.

Dopaminergic receptors are stimulated by low doses of dopamine and have a vasodilating effect in renal, mesenteric, coronary, and intracerebral vessels; this results in increased blood flow.

Neurologic control of peripheral circulation
Vasoconstrictor center

The vasoconstrictor center *(pressor center)* is located in the upper lateral portion of the medulla. It transmits impulses to the heart, arteries, arterioles, precapillary sphincters, and veins through the SNS. These impulses arrive at the terminal nerve endings in the heart and vessels and stimulate release of norepinephrine.[69]

Stimulation of the vasoconstrictor center and release of norepinephrine produces an increase in heart rate and myocardial contractility and vasoconstriction of most vessels. Because the vasomotor center continually releases impulses, resistance vessels (primarily the arterioles composed of vascular smooth muscle) maintain a partial state of contraction (tone) at all times. Maintenance of tone in the arterial system is termed *vasomotor tone,* and maintenance of tone in the venous system is termed *venomotor tone.* Any reflex or hormone that increases stimulation of the vasoconstrictor center increases impulse transmission to the vessels and further increases vessel constriction.

Sympathetic nerve stimulation reduces blood flow by constricting resistance vessels, which reduces capillary hydrostatic pressure and causes tissue fluid to move into the capillaries. Furthermore, it reduces tissue blood volume by constricting capacitance vessels (veins).

During exercise, SNS stimulation causes venous constriction, which mobilizes blood to increase the intravascular fluid volume. This, in turn, increases cardiac filling pressures. During hypotension, SNS stimulation also produces venous constriction, which mobilizes blood and increases the circulating fluid volume. The resistance vessels also constrict to increase arterial blood pressure. However, during arteriolar constriction, the capillary hydrostatic pressure is reduced, thereby reducing tissue volume and further mobilizing extra fluid from tissues.[9]

SNS vasodilatation

Although most peripheral blood vessels have SNS adrenergic vasoconstrictor fibers, resistance vessels of the skeletal muscles also have SNS cholinergic vasodilator fibers. These SNS cholinergic fibers release acetylcholine at their nerve endings and dilate skin and skeletal muscle resistance vessels to increase blood flow to these tissues. Although these fibers are not tonically active normally, they have an important role during exercise, when SNS activity is increased and greater blood flow to the muscles is needed. SNS vasodilatation also can occur during stimulation of β_2-adrenergic receptors in peripheral blood vessels.

Neurologic control of the heart

Cardiac SNS fibers originate in the spinal cord. Norepinephrine released from the SNS postganglionic fibers stimulates β_1-adrenergic receptors in the heart. Effects of SNS stimulation last a long time because the norepinephrine released from nerve endings must be carried away by blood or taken up by the nerve endings before its effects cease.

SNS stimulation increases heart rate and conduction through the AV node. Myocardial performance is also affected by SNS stimulation via increased peak ventricular systolic pressure, augmented rate of isovolumetric con-

traction, and shifting of the Frank-Starling curve to the left. Ventricular filling is enhanced because the strength of atrial contraction is augmented and the rate of rapid ventricular filling during the cardiac cycle is prolonged. Norepinephrine also enhances cell permeability to calcium, thus increasing its availability during the cardiac action potential plateau. Norepinephrine increases the quantity of cyclic AMP.[177]

Cyclic adenosine 5'-monophosphate (AMP) is an intracellular mediator of hormonal and neurotransmitter activity responsible for many cellular functions. When a hormone such as norepinephrine combines with the specific receptor of a target cell, it activates adenylate cyclase, an enzyme found within the cell membrane. *Adenylate cyclase* converts cytoplasmic ATP to cyclic AMP, which is responsible for altering the permeability of the cell membrane to calcium. It also is responsible for increasing the quantity of calcium available for interaction with myofibrils to augment myocardial contractility.[177]

Cardiac PNS fibers originate in the medulla; impulses are mediated through vagi. After acetylcholine is released from the PNS nerve endings, its effects last only a short time because it is quickly destroyed in the tissues by cholinesterase.

PNS stimulation slows the heart rate and conduction through the AV node. It was once generally believed that vagal stimulation did not exert any influence on myocardial performance because parasympathetic fibers were thought not to exist in the ventricles. Currently, however, it is believed that they exist in the ventricles, and vagal stimulation has been found to exert a small depressant effect on myocardial performance.[39] PNS stimulation decreases the peak systolic ventricular pressure and rate of muscle fiber shortening. It shifts the Frank-Starling curve to the right, demonstrating depressed myocardial contractility. Vagal stimulation increases intracellular *guanosine-3',5'-cyclic phosphate (cyclic GMP).*[9] Cyclic GMP in turn hydrolyzes cyclic AMP. (Cyclic AMP, produced during SNS stimulation, may be responsible for enhancing myocardial contractility.) Increasing cyclic GMP reduces the level of cyclic AMP, which may be responsible for depressing myocardial contractility during vagal stimulation.

Because some of the postganglionic parasympathetic nerve endings lie close to the postganglionic sympathetic nerve endings, release of acetylcholine inhibits the release of norepinephrine; this causes further depression of myocardial performance.

Control of heart rate

Heart rate generally is controlled by reciprocal changes in both divisions of the ANS.[9] For example, when heart rate increases, it frequently is the result of a reciprocal increase in SNS stimulation and a decrease in PNS stimulation. Sometimes, however, heart rate is affected selectively by only one division of the ANS.

Under normal conditions, the sinoatrial (SA) node is stimulated at all times by sympathetic and parasympathetic impulses. In normal individuals, parasympathetic tone predominantly influences the SA node. If cardiac sympathetic and parasympathetic fibers are completely blocked so that all autonomic tone ceases, the heart rate tends to be above normal levels, and the *intrinsic heart rate* prevails.

Baroreceptor control

Baroreceptors *(pressor receptors)*[9] are important in the short-term control of blood pressure. Baroreceptors are stretch receptors located in the carotid sinus and aortic arch. Sudden elevation of arterial blood pressure stretches receptors in the carotid sinus and sends impulses up the sinus nerve to the medulla. Stretch receptors in the aortic arch send impulses up through the vagus nerve to the medulla. Stimulation of stretch receptors in the carotid sinus and aortic arch by an acute rise in blood pressure, inhibits the vasoconstrictor center in the medulla and causes peripheral vasodilation. These impulses also stimulate the vagal center, causing bradycardia and reduced myocardial contractility. Stimulation of the carotid sinus and aortic arch causes a rapid reduction in arterial blood pressure. Carotid sinus receptors tend to be more sensitive than aortic arch receptors to rapid changes in blood pressure.

Conversely, if there is a sudden drop in arterial blood pressure, receptors in the carotid sinus and aortic arch are not stimulated (decreased stretch); thereby the number of impulses inhibiting the vasoconstrictor center and stimulating the vagal center are reduced. This increases vasoconstriction and heart rate.

Thus a rise in blood pressure stimulates baroreceptors, and the heart rate reflexively decreases. Conversely, decreased blood pressure inhibits baroreceptor stimulation; thus the heart rate increases. The inverse relationship between arterial blood pressure and heart rate evoked by carotid and aortic baroreceptors is called *Marey's law of the heart.*[1,9]

The response of the baroreceptors is greater with a large pulse pressure than with a low pulse pressure. For example, during hemorrhage, the mean arterial pressure and pulse pressure are low. The lower the pulse pressure, the greater the systemic vascular resistance. Baroreceptor response is minimal in patients experiencing hemorrhage because an increased systemic vascular resistance lowers pulse pressure.

Baroreceptors regulate blood pressure between 50 and 200 mm Hg. These receptors are also useful in reducing moment-to-moment variations in pressure that might be observed during activities of the day, such as going from a laying to a standing position. Baroreceptors also regulate acute blood pressure changes but adapt to chronic elevations in blood pressure; therefore they are not effective for long-term control of blood pressure (as in chronic hypertension).

Manual stimulation of the carotid sinus (carotid massage) produces a fall in blood pressure and lowering of heart rate (via PNS stimulation). In patients who are highly sensitive to carotid sinus pressure, turning the neck or wearing a tight shirt collar can cause severe stimulation of the carotid sinus, producing hypotension, bradycardia, and fainting. This is known as *carotid sinus syncope.* Extreme stimulation of the carotid sinus can cause cardiac arrest. An externally controlled *carotid sinus nerve stimulator,* however, can be effective in lowering the blood pressure and reducing the work of the heart. Reducing the work of the heart decreases myocardial oxygen demand, thereby relieving the pain of angina pectoris.[9]

Baroreceptors located in the lungs, called *cardiopulmonary pressor receptors,* can change peripheral resistance when pulmonary vascular pressures are altered. Other baroreceptors located in the atria and ventricles can inhibit the vasoconstrictor center in the medulla.

Stretching of *atrial receptors* (hypervolemia) causes impulses to inhibit the vasoconstrictor center and stimulate the vagal center to dilate resistance vessels. Dilation of resistance vessels reduces total peripheral resistance, resulting in a drop in blood pressure. It also elevates the capillary hydrostatic pressure, causing fluid to filter out of the capillary and into the tissues to reduce intravascular fluid volume. Dilation of the arteriolar resistance vessels of the kidneys elevates the hydrostatic pressure of the glomerular capillaries. Fluid is filtered into the kidney tubules, thereby increasing urinary output and reducing extracellular fluid volume. Atrial stretch receptors also send impulses to the hypothalamus to reduce the secretion of *antidiuretic hormone (ADH)* by the posterior pituitary to increase urinary output and reduce extracellular fluid volume.

Heart rate is also controlled by atrial stretch receptors. The *Bainbridge reflex* occurs when atrial stretch receptors are stimulated by an increase in atrial pressure. The stretch receptors send impulses to the medulla, which stimulates the SNS to increase the heart rate and the strength of contraction. This reflex helps prevent damming of blood in the atria and pulmonary circulatory system.[9]

Chemoreceptor control

Chemoreceptors are located near the aortic arch and carotid sinus. They primarily are responsible for regulating respiration; they influence the cardiovascular system only during emergencies (such as a decreased arterial oxygen pressure [PaO_2] secondary to a drop in cardiac output). When stimulated by a low PaO_2, a low pH, or a high carbon dioxide pressure ($PaCO_2$), chemoreceptors increase respiratory rate. Chemoreceptor stimulation also results in stimulation of the vasoconstrictor center, producing constriction of resistance vessels. Whether the heart rate is increased or decreased during chemoreceptor stimulation depends on ventilatory status. When ventilation is not controlled, respiratory rate increases during chemoreceptor stimulation; heart rate increases because of excessive ventilatory movements and hypocapnia. If ventilation is controlled, however, and the respiratory rate is not permitted to increase during chemoreceptor stimulation, bradycardia, various degreees of AV heart block, and depression of left ventricular contractility may result from the central nervous system (CNS) ischemic response.

Humoral control

Many humoral substances such as hormones and ions influence the peripheral circulatory system and heart.[14,90,177] Lowering of arterial blood pressure or the serum sodium levels triggers production of angiotensin, which causes arterial and venous vasoconstriction. *Bradykinins,* elevated calcium levels, and vasopressin cause vasoconstriction. Elevated levels of potassium, magnesium, sodium, hydrogen, or carbon dioxide; a lowered pH; increased osmolality; and histamines produce vasodilatation. *Serotonin* and *prostaglandins* may produce vasodilatation or vasoconstriction. The hormones, epinephrine and norepinephrine (released from the adrenal medulla and regulated chiefly by the SNS), constrict resistance vessels and exert a positive inotropic effect on the heart. These actions are identical to the actions produced by the norepinephrine released from the SNS nerve endings.

PATHOPHYSIOLOGIC CAUSES OF HEART FAILURE

Experimental data from studies of isolated cardiac muscle provide a framework for understanding the pathophysiologic cause of heart failure. Shortening of a myocardial muscle fiber depends on the following factors: (1) preload, or the muscle's length at the onset of contraction; (2) afterload, or the tension required during contraction to induce shortening; and (3) contractility, or inotropic state, which depends on intrinsic biochemical parameters.[14,15,69,77]

Preload is proportional to the ventricular volume at end-diastole and is clinically estimated by the left ventricular filling pressure (indirectly reflected by the pulmonary artery wedge pressure [PAWP]). *Contractility* cannot be readily measured in the intact heart because it represents an undefined biochemical state rather than a physical force. A theoretic index of contractility represents the maximum velocity of muscle-fiber shortening with nonafterload and the maximal rate of myosin cross-bridging with actin.

Several hemodynamic parameters, such as the rate of force development or the change in pressure over the change in time (peak dP/dt, and V_{max}) are used to assess inotropic state. Each of these parameters is affected to a variable degree by preload and afterload.[136,145]

As the resting length (preload) of the cardiac muscle is increased, the force that it develops during contraction increases; this fundamental relationship is expressed as the Frank-Starling curve[120] (Fig. 11-4). Depressed contractility, which can occur in myocardial pump failure, shifts the Frank-Starling curve downward and to the right. The administration of an inotropic agent should shift the curve upward and to the left.[31]

Afterload is the amount of resistance to blood flow as the left ventricle ejects into the aorta. This resistance must

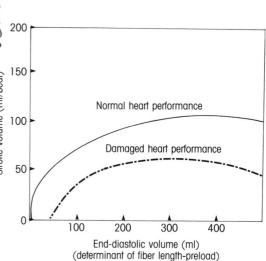

FIG. 11-4   Preload (the volume of blood in the ventricle before ejection) and the Frank-Starling mechanism.

be overcome before ventricular systole can occur. Afterload is primarily a factor of aortic impedance and peripheral vascular resistance. *Impedance* is the amount of mechanical resistance against the stroke volume as it leaves the aortic valve. When blood flows through resistant vessels, the pressure falls. An increase in impedance causes a rise in myocardial oxygen consumption, which increases cardiac work.

Sonnenblick and LeJemtel[164] describe the pathophysiologic cause of heart failure in terms of pump dysfunction and CHF, which results from primary cardiac failure. Cardiac failure is modeled from responses to various forms of work that lead to abnormalities of pump function. When work overload is imposed on the heart, which occurs with high systolic blood pressure or an increased diastolic volume, hypertrophy of myocardial cells occurs to normalize the load. A similarly heavy workload can be created by loss of myocardium, which taxes the remaining myocardium. Such loss of myocardium may be segmental and diffuse, which occurs in the cardiomyopathies.[48,175]

In heart failure, there is also a slowing of the biochemical pumps responsible for calcium sequestration into the myocardial cell. The rate of myocardial contraction is slowed, time-to-peak tension development is prolonged, and a delay in relaxation occurs. Ventricular wall thickening limits ventricular filling, resulting in so-called diastolic dysfunction. Ultimately myocardial contraction force is reduced as excessive hypertrophy progresses and the ejection fraction decreases.[18,146]

Heart failure may be a result of underlying or fundamental causes or precipitating factors. Underlying causes comprise congenital or acquired structural abnormalities of the pericardium, myocardium, cardiac valves, or peripheral and coronary vessels. They lead to myocardial insufficiency or an increased hemodynamic burden that results in heart failure. Fundamental causes include the physiologic or biochemical mechanisms that result in impaired cardiac contraction. Precipitating factors comprise about 50% of heart failure episodes. These include dysrhythmias (i.e., bradydysrhythmias, tachydysrhythmias, and AV dissociation), inappropriate changes in drugs or treatment (e.g., increasing salt intake or gaining weight), systemic infection, pulmonary embolism, stressors (emotional, physical, environmental, or sociocultural), cardiac inflammation and infection, untreated illness (e.g., anemia and hyperthyroidism), or development of a secondary form of heart disease.[35,140]

CAUSE OF HEART FAILURE
Acute syndromes

The most frequent cause of acute CHF is myocardial infarction (MI). Failure of the heart to contract adequately partly is due to intracellular acidosis and partly is due to the accumulation of intracellular phosphates.

Chronic syndromes

Ischemic heart disease and dilated cardiomyopathy are the most frequent causes of chronic CHF. In contrast to acute syndromes, the mechanisms responsible for chronic CHF are unclear. The cause for loss of contractile function in patients with dilated cardiomyopathy is unknown. Abnormal function of the sarcoplasmic reticulum and altered properties of the myofibrils are suggested biochemical causes. Pump failure as a chronic syndrome also may be caused by fibrosis and altered ventricular chamber shape.

Whether the patient develops acute or chronic heart failure depends on how rapidly the syndrome develops after myocardial infarction. A ruptured valve or pulmonary embolus can cause sudden or acute heart failure. Chronic heart failure caused by valvular disease, hypertension, or chronic obstructive pulmonary disease may slowly accelerate over years.[48,51,70,128,164]

FORMS OF HEART FAILURE
Backward versus forward failure

The backward failure hypothesis states that, as the ventricle fails to discharge its contents, blood accumulates and pressure rises in the ventricles and atria and the venous systems that empty into them. This theory has been supported by studies showing that the inability of the cardiac muscle to shorten against a load changes the relationship between ventricular end-systolic pressure and volume so that residual volume rises. The backward theory reflects the Frank-Starling phenomenon in which distention of the ventricle, within limits, helps maintain cardiac output.[48]

The forward heart failure theory suggests that reduced cardiac output diminishes vital organ perfusion. A state of mental confusion results, skeletal muscles become weak, and the kidneys eventually retain sodium and water, thereby augmenting extracellular fluid volume. This, in turn, leads to symptoms that cause congestion of organs.

Both mechanisms occur in the majority of patients with CHF. With an acute condition, both may occur, and rigid distinctions are not necessary. For example, the patient with AMI can have forward failure with a significant reduction of left ventricular output and cardiogenic shock, or the AMI can produce backward failure in which there is a transient inequality of cardiac output between the two ventricles that results in acute pulmonary edema. This is because AMI usually involves the left ventricle.[48,51,70,128,164]

Right versus left ventricular failure

Much emphasis has been placed on the symptom patterns of right versus left ventricular failure. However, after one ventricle has been stressed for a time, the other ventricle also undergoes biochemical changes. Both ventricles share a common wall, the interventricular septum, and their muscle bundles are continuous. Therefore over time an isolated abnormal ventricular load will be responsible for total heart failure if not corrected.[48,51,70,128,164]

Low-output versus high-output failure

The patient with low-output heart failure shows clinical evidence of impaired peripheral circulation and vasoconstriction. Extremities are usually cold, pale, and cyanotic. In later stages, stroke volume decreases, and the pulse pressure narrows. Low-output heart failure occurs in patients with congenital or rheumatic, valvular, coronary, hypertensive, and cardiomyopathic heart disease.

In high-output failure, patients have warm extremities and a widened pulse pressure. High-output states require an increased oxygen supply to the peripheral tissues, which can occur only with an increased cardiac output. In a patient with an already compromised heart, these cardiac demands cannot be met. High-output states that lead to heart failure are thyrotoxicosis, arteriovenous fistula, Paget's disease, anemia, beriberi, or pregnancy.[48,51,70,128,164]

COMPENSATORY MECHANISMS
Frank-Starling regulation

The earliest mechanism that responds to acute left ventricular failure and regulates beat-to-beat variations in venous return is the *Frank-Starling mechanism.* In early heart failure, increased end-diastolic volume maintains an adequate stroke volume on the steep, ascending portion of the Frank-Starling curve (Fig. 11-4). Moreover, small increments in preload (end-diastolic volume) produce substantial increases in stroke volume. As heart failure progresses, thus flattening the curve, larger increases in preload are required to produce smaller increases in stroke volume. Thus the effectiveness of this compensatory mechanism becomes limited.

Two complications result from activation of the Frank-Starling mechanism in heart failure. First, an increase in ventricular diastolic pressure that accompanies ventricular dilation is transmitted retrogradely to the pulmonary vascular system, where it causes pulmonary congestive symptoms. Second, elevations in ventricular preload increase ventricular wall tension, which, in turn, increases myocardial oxygen consumption.[178]

Sympathetic nervous system

Increased SNS activity can respond quickly to depressed cardiac function. Increased levels of circulating catecholamines, such as norepinephrine, have been found in patients with CHF.[28] Elevated norepinephrine levels increase contractility and heart rate to preserve cardiac output, elevate peripheral vascular resistance, increase venous tone, and redistribute cardiac output away from nonessential organs via selective alterations in peripheral arterial tone.

Circulating catecholamine levels are increased in patients with CHF but myocardial norepinephrine levels are depleted.[29,126]

Renal compensations: renin-angiotensin-aldosterone response

Blood flow to the kidneys proportionally diminishes with decline in cardiac function. Consequently, vasoconstriction of the renal arterioles occurs, and the capacity to excrete sodium, chloride, and water is reduced. Homeostatic adaptations occur within the renal system to compensate for reduced arterial blood pressure associated with heart failure (Fig. 11-5). Increased renin secretion occurs from the kidney in response to hypoperfusion and possibly to the increased distention of the atria and large veins.[48,71,179]

Renin acts on a substrate in the blood to release the peptide, *angiotensin I,* which is converted to *angiotensin II* by the action of the converting enzyme that is primarily found in the lungs and to a lesser amount in blood vessels and kidneys. Angiotensin II produces vasoconstriction of arteriolar smooth muscle; it is the most potent pressure substance released by the body (i.e., 10 times more potent than norepinephrine).[48] Angiotensin II is an important stimuli to cause adrenal secretion of *aldosterone,* which acts on the distal tubules and collecting ducts of the kidney to increase tubular reabsorption of sodium, chloride, and water in exchange for potassium and hydrogen ions.[72]

Evidence suggesting that the renin-angiotensin-aldosterone system is overly active in heart failure has been suggested by administering an *angiotensin-converting enzyme inhibitor* such as captopril, which has resulted in an increase in cardiac output and a reduction in PAWP. Controlled studies have shown improved exercise tolerance in such patients, suggesting that counteracting the excessive rise in angiotensin II can benefit patients with chronic CHF.[49]

Myocardial metabolism

There has been considerable argument about whether there is depression of mitochondrial function during heart failure. Some investigators have demonstrated that there is no difference in the mitochondrial activity.[163] Others have shown marked reduction in mitochondrial function.[165] Another study suggests that cardiac mitochondria respond to failure in a biphasic manner. In the early, compensatory, hypertrophic stages of failure, mitochondrial function is normal or even hypernormal, but it decompensates during the later states.[98] Normal cellular concentration of ATP have been recorded from patients with CHF. ATP levels have also returned to normal at the onset of failure but decreased as CHF worsened.[127,167,168]

Although mitochondria are the heart's principle source of ATP production, current theory[80,81,102,105] suggests that

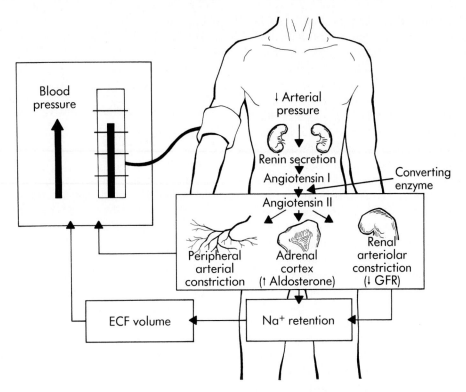

FIG. 11-5   Renin-angiotensin mechanism in heart failure. As systemic pressure drops, blood flow to the kidney decreases proportionately with resultant renal vasoconstriction. Renin is secreted by the kidney in defense of hypotension, which acts to release angiotensin I from the blood; angiotension I is converted to angiotensin II (a potent vasoconstrictor). Angiotensin II prompts release of aldosterone from the adrenal glands. *ECF,* Extracellular fluid; *GFR,* glomerular filtration rate.
From Quaal SJ: Comprehensive intra-aortic balloon pumping, St Louis, 1984, The CV Mosby Co.

ATP produced by mitochondria is probably not the ATP used during contraction. Rather, ATP produced by oxidative phosphorylation is rapidly converted to phosphocreatine by the mitochondria enzyme, creatine kinase. Phosphocreatine then diffuses to the energy-using enzymes and is converted back to ATP by another creatine kinase isoenzyme. The phosphocreatine level is reportedly reduced in the failing heart, which may represent a compensatory effort to maintain normal ATP levels.[87,170] Therefore a failing heart may continue to supply the cell with adequate amounts of ATP, which will not affect the myocardium's inotropic state.

β-Adrenergic receptor down regulation

Subdivision of adrenergic receptors into subtypes of α and β was originally postulated by Ahlquist.[4] Three adrenergic receptors, β_1, β_2 and α_1 are found in the human heart. Nonfailing human ventricular myocardium contains 80% β_1-receptors and 20% β_2-receptors.[22] Stimulation of these β-receptors by an adrenergic compound such as norepinephrine causes increased production of adenylate cyclase and generation of cyclic AMP, which is the carrier compound needed to move calcium from its stores to the site of actin-myosin interaction (see p. 304).[19,92,94] Thus these myocardial receptors have positive inotropic properties because, in health, stimulating them will result in a greater myocardial contraction. Norepinephrine, which is adrenergic or stimulatory to these receptors, has an affinity for β_1-receptors, which is 10 times higher than α_1 norepinephrine affinity and 30 to 40 times greater than the affinity of norepinephrine β_2-receptors.[21,22]

β_1-Receptor density decreases in the failing heart to about 60%, but β_2-receptor density remains about the same. Therefore the ratio changes to approximately 60% β_1 and 40% β_2 compared with β receptor density in the healthy heart. Because of this loss of β_1-receptors, the failing myocardium is markedly subsensitive to β_1 stimulation; adenylate cyclase response is decreased by about 60% to 70%.[97,107] The mechanism that accounts for this β_1-receptor *"down regulation"* is not clear, but it is believed to be related to the receptors' exposure to increased levels of catecholamine, which is produced in excess secondary to sympathetic overstimulation in heart failure.[20]

Despite the fact that β_2-receptor density is maintained in heart failure, the adenylate cyclase response is significantly decreased. This decrease in pharmacologic responsiveness of the β_2-receptor pathway despite unchanged receptor density suggests that β_2-receptors in failing hearts are "uncoupled" from their pharmacologic pathways.[19] The nature of this uncoupling is not fully understood, but it is believed to be correlated with an increase in activity of inhibitory G protein, which interferes with uptake of adenylate cyclase. An increase in G protein activity is quantitatively similar to the decrease in β_2-receptor sensitivity.[109]

The human heart apparently does not contain spare β-adrenergic receptors. If receptors were present in excess of the amount required to produce a maximal response, the loss of these excess receptors would lead to a rightward shift in adenylate cyclase and a decrease, but not a drastic one, in contraction. Research in this area suggests that a 50% reduction in β-receptor density produces a similar degree of reduction in hormone-stimulated adenylate cyclase activity and myocardial muscle contraction.[89]

Alterations in coronary flow

The stimulus for changes in metabolism of the cell may result from a decrease in coronary perfusion that accompanies heart failure.[72] CHF secondary to acute ischemic or myopathic disease is usually associated with a global decrease in mechanical function. In most cases, this results from a decrease in contractility that is reflected in a lowered cardiac output. The response of the systemic circulation is increased vasoconstriction in an attempt to maintain arterial pressure. This vasoconstriction increases left ventricle burden or load. Impedance to ejection results in an increase in wall stress.[73] According to Laplace's law, the stress in the wall will be greater at the endocardial surface than at the epicardial surface. Left ventricular end-diastolic pressure will also be elevated. Ohm's law describes coronary flow as proportional to the difference between the pressure gradient in the walls of the vessel and the coronary perfusion pressure; therefore there will be a decrease in endocardium perfusion.[77]

Release of atrial natriuretic factor

Specific atriopeptide granules, termed *atrial natriuretic factors* (ANFs) have been found in atrial but not in ventricular tissue. This polypeptide has natriuretic (increased excretion of sodium), vasorelaxant, and aldosterone-inhibiting properties.[38] The granules are more abundant in the right as compared with the left atrium.[59,75] Stretching of the atrial wall by increased atrial volume or pressure is a well-documented stimulus for the release of ANF.[63,100] With the development of radioimmunoassay for human ANF, it is possible to study the release of this peptide in humans. In normal persons, the basal plasma levels of ANF range from 10 to 70 mg/ml.[93] Several studies in humans have demonstrated that patients with CHF have elevated circulating plasma concentrations of ANF, which increase during CHF from 5 up to almost 20 times those of control values in healthy subjects.[45] Patients with CHF with demonstrated high levels of ANF also have peripheral vasoconstriction and oliguria, suggesting a lack of physiologic response to the excess production of ANF.[52]

Nursing process

Case study. At 8 AM, Mr. J.L., a 56-year-old business executive, was admitted to the coronary care unit (CCU) after experiencing 2 hours of chest pain and dyspnea at home after arising from a restless night. He felt totally exhausted. At admission his skin was warm and dry. ECG revealed changes consistent with an AMI of the anterior wall with 4 to 6 unifocal premature ventricular complexes per minute. On examination, he had pulmonary crackles bilaterally at both lung bases, an S_3 gallop, and an elevated jugular venous pressure estimated to be 12 cm H_2O.

His initial care consisted of 3 to 5 mg of intravenous morphine every 5 minutes for a maximum of 12 mg, oxygen administered at 4 L/min, ECG monitoring, complete bed rest, frequent cardiac assessment, reduction in anxiety, monitoring of intake and output, and a quiet environment. Other medications ordered were 80 mg of intravenous furosemide and an intravenous bolus of 50 mg of lidocaine, followed by a lidocaine infusion at 2 mg/min.

Nursing assessment
Exchanging pattern

Signs and symptoms. The box, p. 313, lists signs and symptoms of left and right ventricular failure.

Dyspnea. A cardinal manifestation of left ventricular failure is dyspnea. The failing left ventricle causes a rise in pulmonary venous pressure, which results in pulmonary congestion. As the lungs become less compliant, there is also an increase in airway resistance. The increased work of breathing results in symptoms of breathlessness. There are several types of dyspnea, including exertional dyspnea, orthopnea, paroxysmal nocturnal dyspnea, and dyspnea at rest.

In *exertional dyspnea,* patients feel breathless during certain activities, such as climbing stairs. A cough is often overlooked as a symptom of left ventricular failure; it is usually related to dyspnea caused by pulmonary congestion that occurs during exertion or while the patient is recumbent. Patients may complain of a dry, hacking cough and may link it with stress, exercise, or sleep. A cough may severely interfere with sleep, resulting in fatigue and insomnia.

Dyspnea that occurs at rest and in the recumbent position is referred to as *orthopnea*. Patients with orthopnea usually sleep on several pillows at night. It is common for their heads to slip off the pillows during the night and for them to wake up suddenly very short of breath. They may start walking around and open windows or doors for fresh air to reverse the breathlessness. Sitting up with the legs

SIGNS AND SYMPTOMS

LEFT VENTRICULAR FAILURE
Early: dyspnea on exertion or effort

Block dyspnea (after walking 1 block)
Flight dyspnea (after climbing a short flight of stairs)
Shortness of breath 15 minutes after retiring
Dyspnea with usual activity in the house, office, or
    yard

Intermediate

Paroxysmal nocturnal dyspnea 1 to 2 hours after
    sleep
        Sitting on the edge of the bed after awakening
        Sleeping on several pillows
        Nightmares and wild dreams
Nonproductive new cough for 3 weeks or more
Crackles, wheezes, or pleural effusion
Nocturia

Late

Wheezing
Cyanosis
Cheyne-Stokes respirations
Acute pulmonary edema

RIGHT VENTRICULAR FAILURE

Neck vein engorgement
Positive hepatojugular reflux
Hepatomegaly
Splenomegaly
Ascites

dependent relieves the symptoms. Patients may prefer to sleep while sitting. Some patients may have a new nonproductive cough.

Paroxysmal nocturnal dyspnea is a specific symptom of left ventricular failure. It typically occurs after prolonged recumbency. Patients fall asleep, awaken abruptly hours later, sit upright, dangle their feet, and feel as though they will suffocate.

Dyspnea at rest can occur without patients being aware of it. Patients may tell you that they are not short of breath; however, they may interrupt themselves in midsentence to take a breath. With increasing severity of heart failure, patients may become extremely aware of not being able to carry out most activities because of breathlessness.

Pulmonary edema, a physical finding and not a symptom, gives rise to the most severe form of dyspnea. It can develop spontaneously in patients with left ventricular failure; it occurs at rest, after exercise, or during excitement or stress. Observe for complaints of smothering, anxiety, agitation, and tachycardia. Pulmonary edema may also be

manifested by a cough and pink, frothy sputum, which results from an intraalveolar mixture of fluids, red blood cells, and air.[178]

Differentiate cardiac dyspnea from dyspnea caused by anxiety neurosis. Persons with *cardiac dyspnea* have a rapid, shallow breathing pattern. Patients with *anxiety neurosis and dyspnea* exhibit deep, sighing breaths to the point of hyperventilation. These patients feel, no matter how hard or deeply they breathe, that their need for air remains. It is possible for patients to have both types of dyspnea.

Urinary symptoms. Nocturia can be annoying and frequent, interrupting sleep and contributing to fatigue. It can be an early manifestation of heart disease. While the patient is upright and active, urine is suppressed, and there is a redistribution of blood flow away from the kidneys to other organs. At night, when the patient is supine, the deficit in cardiac output in relation to oxygen demand is lowered, renal vasoconstriction diminishes, and urine formation increases.

Cerebral symptoms. Headache, confusion, impairment of memory, bad dreams, and insomnia can occur in patients experiencing severe heart failure. These symptoms are more pronounced in older patients with cerebral atherosclerosis.

Edema and ascites. Systemic edema is a manifestation of right ventricular failure. Have patients at home record their morning nude weights on a bathroom scale before breakfast or liquids. In the normal individual, if daily weighing is done at the same time and in the same manner, there is relatively little real weight-gain errors. Therefore fluid retention is easy to detect if a patient suddenly gains 3 to 5 pounds. Patients also may become aware of dependent edema in ankles, feet, and hands. They may observe impression marks from rings, shoes, socks, or garters. Dependent edema is found over the sacrum rather than in the legs in patients for whom bed rest has been prescribed. It is usually detected during the physical examination by the nurse or physician because patients are unaware of its presence. Diaphoresis, caused by the increased adrenergic activity associated with CHF may be present.

Patients with ascites may feel their clothes tightening around the waist and may feel bloated. If massive, it can affect breathing by forcing the diaphragm upward while the patient is recumbent. The most severe edema is *anasarca,* which involves the whole body.

Abdominal symptoms. Observe for complaints of hepatic pain in the epigastric or right upper quadrant from acute distention of Glisson's capsule (the outer lining of the liver, a pain-sensitive tissue) resulting from hepatomegaly of right ventricular failure. This pain can occur at rest or with activity or when a rise in systemic venous pressure distends the liver further.

Physical findings
Respiratory system. Obtain a baseline for the presence of adventitious sounds. Fine crackles are produced by intraalveolar fluid. Coarse crackles are caused by fluid within

the lumens of bronchioli and bronchi. Dyspnea is caused by pulmonary interstitial edema. Wheezes result from the narrowed lumen of bronchiolus. Crackles can be unilateral but are generally bilateral. Detect pleural effusion during physical examination by palpating the chest; it can also be detected by chest x-ray studies. Pleural effusion can be unilateral or bilateral; however, it is seldom just in the left side of the chest.

Heart. Increased heart size is common in patients with CHF. There is a displacement of the apical impulse to the left, which can be felt by palpation unless pericardial effusion coexists.

Jugular venous pulses are a reliable means of estimating venous pressure. Internal jugular vein–filling height is an index of right atrial pressure. Assess the *hepatojugular reflux* with the jugular venous pulse. Compress the abdomen firmly but gradually to prevent the patient from straining or holding the breath, which also will cause the jugular venous pressure to rise. When the abdomen of a patient experiencing right ventricular failure is compressed, there is an increase in forward flow of blood to the right atrium, and a rise in jugular venous pressure is noted.[24]

Auscultation may disclose an S_3, which is an indication of a pathologic condition in adults over 30. Labeled a *ventricular gallop,* an S_3 usually signifies loss of ventricular compliance. Lack of myocardial distensibility produces the vibration heard during passive filling. An S_3 is accentuated by listening, using the bell of the stethoscope, with the patient in the left lateral position. The S_4 or atrial gallop is not a sign of failure but reflects a decrease in ventricular compliance. It occurs after atrial contraction as blood is ejected into the noncompliant left ventricle. The fourth heart sound is heard immediately before S_1 and is frequently heard in patients with AMI and angina. An S_4 may also appear in patients with coronary artery disease, hypertensive cardiovascular disease, cardiomyopathy, and aortic stenosis.[10]

Abdomen. Assess for hepatomegaly, hepatic pulsations, ascites, and splenomegaly. Carefully perform the examination because the patient may complain of discomfort when touched (see section on *abdominal symptoms*).

Extremities. Check the extremities for edema caused by gravity when the patient is upright during waking hours. Capillary hydrostatic pressure rises, causing fluid to transfer from capillaries to interstitial tissues. Grade peripheral edema on a scale of 1 to 4 (from minimal to severe). Also record the height and extent of edema in the extremity (see Chapter 3).

Diagnostic studies. Before beginning treatment, serum electrolyte levels are usually normal in patients with CHF. Because patients with severe heart failure are treated with diuretic therapy and sodium restriction, shifts in electrolyte levels occur and must be managed; hyponatremia is not uncommon. Although serum potassium levels are usually normal, potassium replacement is necessary to avoid hypokalemia when potent diuretics are administered. Hy-

perkalemia can occur in patients who show a significant reduction in glomerular filtration rate and inadequate sodium delivery to the sodium-potassium exchange sites in the distal tubules. This is more of a problem in patients who are receiving aldosterone antagonists. Many tests may be abnormal because of kidney dysfunction in patients with severe heart failure. Proteinuria, a high specific gravity of urine, and elevated blood urea nitrogen (BUN) and creatinine levels result from end-stage renal dysfunction. Elevated bilirubin, serum glutamic-oxaloacetic transaminase (SGOT), and lactate dehydrogenase (LDH) levels result from hepatic congestion. A complete blood count may show a mildly elevated white blood cell count with an increased hematocrit. Arterial blood gas analyses usually show a low PaO_2, normal or decreased $PaCO_2$, and mild respiratory alkalosis. Pulmonary function tests are nonspecific and usually demonstrate airway disease.

The ECG helps in assessing left atrial and left ventricular hypertrophy and dysrhythmias. A chest x-ray screening test is invaluable. The size and shape of the cardiac silhouette varies according to the underlying heart disease. Cardiothoracic ratio and heart volume seen on x-ray films help in indirectly determining the left ventricular end-diastolic volume and ejection fraction. A lung x-ray film can reveal varying degrees of heart failure. Prominent congested upper lobe pulmonary veins may be manifested.[73,166]

Capillary hydrostatic pressure increases as left atrial pressure rises; interstitial and alveolar edema develops. These changes are most prominent at the lung bases because pulmonary capillary hydrostatic pressure is greater in this area. When it is slightly elevated (approximately 13 to 17 mm Hg), the pulmonary veins of the lower lobe are compressed. There is pulmonary vascular redistribution when pressures reach 18 to 23 mm Hg, leading to further constriction of the vessels of the upper lobe. On x-ray films, interstitial pulmonary edema appears as fluid-filled subsegmental fissures producing *Kerley's B lines.* These appear as sharp, linear densities. As pulmonary capillary hydrostatic pressures reach 20 to 25 mm Hg, interstitial pulmonary edema becomes more severe. These changes are seen on x-ray films as a loss of sharpness of central and peripheral vessels with blurred mediastinal margins. X-ray films of the lungs also may show patchy and spindle-shaped infiltrates. As pulmonary capillary hydrostatic pressure exceeds 25 mm Hg, alveolar edema and large pleural effusions can occur.[178] Effusions are usually right sided or bilateral but rarely are isolated to the left side of the chest. Pleural effusion usually reflects biventricular failure and seldom is observed in pure left ventricular failure.

Echocardiography is used in diagnosing specifics of ventricular hypertrophy, pericardial effusion, or cardiac valvular changes. Findings assist in detecting early chamber enlargement and cardiac dysfunction.

After stabilization of CHF, cardiac catheterization and angiography may be required if there are suspected underlying coronary abnormalities. Ventricular function also is studied in patients requiring cardiac surgery. CHF is always treated medically unless there is rupture of a valve or septum.

Moving pattern

Evaluate the extent to which the patient with CHF can move and perform activities of daily living. Focus on performance of daily activities, exercise capabilities, sleep pattern disturbances, and situations causing boredom and excitement.

Signs and symptoms. Patients may not be aware of dyspnea or activity intolerance; yet both may be observed during assessment. Some patients may report limitations to only very exertional activity, such as shortness of breath when jogging or dancing fast. Other patients may report shortness of breath when walking against a wind or raising their arms up over their heads to shampoo. Certain activities of daily living, such as vacuuming, carrying groceries, or maneuvering a car into a tight parking spot, may initiate fatigue and shortness of breath. Sleep patterns may be interrupted if the patient is awakened with dyspnea. Activities may also be curtailed because the patient is taking diuretics; the patient must therefore stay close to a bathroom during the diuretic period. The patient may complain of dyspnea or activity limitations during hot or muggy weather, when at higher elevations, or with increased air pollution[124] (see Nursing Diagnosis 6).

Weakness and fatigue. Exhaustion in a patient with CHF probably results from a disturbance in sleep and rest patterns, as well as a reduction in cardiac output. Patients may complain of chronic weakness, fatigue, or a heaviness in the arms or legs because the reduction in cardiac output causes poor perfusion of skeletal muscles. Another common cause of these complaints is the use of diuretics, which can result in sodium depletion, decreased potassium levels, and hypovolemia when given in improper dosages. Fatigue can result from the excessive work of breathing that occurs during activity or at rest; this generally worsens as the day progresses.

Symptoms that occur while patients sit in a chair and converse with the nurse are most revealing. If patients are dyspneic while conversing, they obviously have activity limitations. Physical symptoms of limitations to moving are ascertained mostly from patients' histories and descriptions of factors that limit activity.

Activities that induce dyspnea and fatigue (limit moving) can be tested by patients outside the hospital or clinic. A low-level treadmill may help if the patient reports symptoms only with heavy exercise. Quantifying the exact level of METs at which patients become symptomatic can be useful in prescribing activity guidelines (see Chapter 19).

Feeling pattern

Signs and symptoms. The impact of stress and strain on CHF patients needs additional study so that the full effect of heart failure on human function can be better

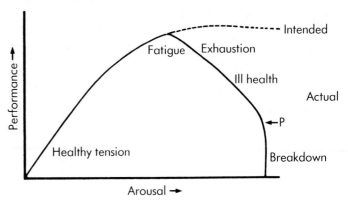

FIG. 11-6   The human function curve. *P*, the point at which even minimal arousal may precipitate a breakdown.
Courtesy Dr. P.G.F. Nixon.

understood. The *human function curve* (HFC) (Fig. 11-6) provides a useful method of assessing the effect of CHF on patients.

The process of arranging aspects of human behavior in the natural order of their passage from health to breakdown originated with Starling's law of the heart. Starling showed that the energy causing contraction of the heart depended on the stretch of muscle fibers.[120] Increasing the stretch increases performance, but if the fibers are overstretched, deterioration in myocardial function occurs. Human function can be described by using a comparable curve wherein human function is plotted against arousal (the ability to be stirred into action). In healthy function, increasing the arousal increases human performance. However, if the person becomes fatigued, deterioration in function occurs. Finally, persistence of arousal leads to exhaustion and can deteriorate into CHF, which is labeled as 'breakdown' in Fig. 11-6.

Synthesis of moving and feeling patterns related to the HFC

In healthy function, individuals feel well. Their manner is relaxed; physical recreation brings pleasure and does not cause guilt. Burdens and pressures that cause loss of happiness and health are rejected. Increasing arousal enhances performance. The originality, vigor, expansion, and capacity for sustained effort are abundant.

"Acceptable" fatigue is felt when an individual acknowledges and shows it, does not deny it, and takes steps to recover as soon as possible. Maladaptive habits that waste time and energy can be modified, and unessential drains on the energy can be stopped or deferred. Performance can increase with arousal, but more effort is required.

In the state of exhaustion, individuals commonly make strong declarations of health and virility that are at odds with behavior observed by the nurse. They may reject the need to maintain a reasonable balance between high endeavor and relaxation and may see no need to modify, balance, and gradually increase exercise tolerance. Excessive burdens and pressures disruptive of health and happiness are accepted as inevitable because exhaustion reduces the ability to distinguish the essential from the nonessential.

Sleep becomes inadequate, increasing exhaustion, promoting high anxiety levels, and producing a cycle of deterioration. Biochemical changes associated with exhaustion and a high level of arousal may be seen, usually manifested as signs of sympathetic overactivity. Catecholamine secretion can reach high levels. Packer and others[115] suggest these high catecholamine levels may exert a deleterious effect on survival of patients with CHF.

After patients are taught the concepts of the HFC, they can assess their own positions on the curve. Patients and significant others can compare days of placing high on the HFC with days when they place themselves at the point of deterioration with worsening signs and symptoms of CHF. Then patients are asked about specific differences between those days. For example, patients might place themselves lower on the HFC and, when asked why, might respond that they drove to the outpatient clinic in a snowstorm. Patients can then be counseled to use good judgment in avoiding situations that cause deterioration in human responses.

Despite the invasive and noninvasive techniques available in a modern cardiovascular laboratory, the most useful tests for impending cardiac dysfunction are patients' own skillfullness in recognizing behavior changes that represent feelings and abilities to detect deepening exhaustion.

Medical and nursing diagnoses

The medical diagnoses are acute or chronic heart failure. The most common human responses anticipated for a patient experiencing CHF are indicated by the following nursing diagnoses:

1. Decreased cardiac output related to mechanical factors (preload, afterload, or inotropic state of heart) and electrical factors (rate, rhythm, and conduction)
2. Impaired gas exchange related to pulmonary congestion
3. Impaired physical mobility related to decreased cardiac output
4. Fatigue related to limited cardiac reserve
5. Anxiety related to acute or chronic illness
6. Knowledge deficit related to complex pathophysiologic illness

For each of these nursing diagnoses, the patient outcomes, nursing prescriptions, and evaluation criteria are outlined with a discussion of the factual information that supports the plan and implementation of care.

Case study, cont'd. About 2 hours after admission, Mr. J.L. did not show clinical improvement. Thus hemodynamic monitoring through a pulmonary artery catheter was begun to assess his status and to monitor his response to therapy. His blood pressure was 100/70 mm Hg, his skin was cool and diaphoretic; PAWP was 30 mm Hg, heart rate was 140 beats per minute, and cardiac index was 1.7 L/min/m².

Despite conventional therapy, there was no improvement, so a nitroprusside infusion was begun. Mr. J.L. showed gradual improvement measured by the disappearance of crackles and jugular venous distention. After 6 hours of nitroprusside treatment, the hemodynamic measurements were blood pressure, 124/80 mm Hg; PAWP, 14 mm Hg; cardiac index, 2.8 L/min/m², and heart rate, 100 beats per minute.

About 36 hours after admission, Mr. J.L. regressed from a normotensive state to one of acute pulmonary edema in a matter of minutes. He awoke and stated that he was short of breath. He was placed in a high-Fowler's position. He appeared in acute distress. His skin was cold and clammy, and his blood pressure was 80/50 mm Hg, with a heart rate of 120 beats per minute and a pattern of sinus tachycardia. He had wheezing respiration and bubbling pink, frothy sputum. Bilateral crackles were auscultated over both lung fields. Oxygen therapy was changed from nasal cannula to a face mask because he was breathing through his mouth. Physician orders included administration of 4 mg of intravenous morphine, 100 mg of intravenous furosemide, 0.25 mg of intravenous digoxin, a sodium nitroprusside infusion of 5 μg/kg/min, and a dopamine infusion at 10 μg/kg/min to keep his systolic blood pressure at 100 mm Hg. Blood gas and electrolyte analyses were done, revealing a pH of 7.1, a Paco₂ of 88 mm Hg, and a Pao₂ of 60 mm Hg. Mr. J.L. was intubated and supported with mechanical ventilation. An indwelling urinary catheter was inserted to measure hourly urine output, with a return of 60 ml. His PAWP was again 30 mm Hg.

Mr. J.L.'s condition responded over the next 4 hours to therapy. He was extubated 8 hours after the initial onset of his pulmonary edema.

NURSING
DIAGNOSIS 1   **Decreased cardiac output related to mechanical factors (preload, afterload, or inotropic state of the heart) and electrical factors (rate, rhythm, and conduction) (exchanging pattern)**

PATIENT OUTCOMES	NURSING PRESCRIPTIONS	EVALUATION
Patient will demonstrate hemodynamic stability and, at discharge, will demonstrate normal blood pressure, pulse, sinus rhythm, and S_1 and S_2; absence of S_3 and S_4; normal apical impulse and breath sounds without crackles and wheezes; warm, dry skin without cyanosis; normal urine output; lack of cough or frothy sputum, dyspnea, orthopnea, paroxysmal nocturnal dyspnea, diaphoresis, jugular venous distention, peripheral or sacral edema, ascites, and hepatic congestion; and normal central venous pressure, PAWP, and cardiac output.	Monitor patient for hemodynamic stability by assessing for normalcy or presence, or absence of blood pressure, pulse, cardiac rhythm, heart sounds, abnormal heart sounds, apical impulse, breath sounds, skin temperature and color, urinary output, cough, dyspnea, orthopnea, paroxysmal noctural dyspnea, diaphoresis, jugular venous distention, edema, ascites, hepatic congestion, and hemodynamic monitoring parameters.	Patient demonstrated normal blood pressure, pulse, sinus rhythm, S_1 and S_2; absence of S_3 and S_4; normal apical pulse; absence of crackles and wheezes; warm, dry skin without cyanosis; normal urine output; lack of cough, dyspnea, orthopnea, paroxysmal noctural dyspnea, diaphoresis, jugular venous distention, peripheral or sacral edema, ascites, and hepatic congestion; normal central venous pressure, PAWP, and cardiac output.
Patient will respond to appropriate therapy and will demonstrate no complications from diuretics, inotropic agents, phosphodiesterase inhibitors, calcium-sensitizing agents, vasodilators, angiotension-converting enzyme (ACE) inhibitors, and β-adrenergic blockade.	Institute appropriate therapy for heart failure; assess response and monitor for complications of diuretics, inotropic agents, phosphodiesterase inhibitors, calcium-sensitizing agents, vasodilators, ACE inhibitors, and β-adrenergic blockade.	Patient responded to and demonstrated no complications from diuretics, inotropic agents, phosphodiesterase inhibitors, calcium-sensitizing agents, vasodilators, ACE inhibitors, and β-adrenergic blockade.
Patient will demonstrate no complications of anxiety from 12-lead ECG, chest x-ray examination, cardiac enzyme assays, electrolyte studies, blood gas analysis, and indwelling urinary catheter.	Explain 12-lead ECG, chest x-ray examination, cardiac enzyme assays, electrolyte studies, blood gas analysis, and indwelling urinary catheter to patient to prevent anxiety.	Patient demonstrated no anxiety from 12-lead ECG, chest x-ray examination, cardiac enzyme assays, electrolyte studies, blood gas analysis, and indwelling urinary catheter.
Patient will demonstrate a reduction in cardiac workload.	Assess patient for a reduction in cardiac workload.	Patient demonstrated a reduction in cardiac workload.
Patient will demonstrate an understanding of measures to reduce cardiac workload, including bed rest with bedside commode, semi- or high-Fowler's position, and rest and relaxation.	Teach the patient about bed rest with bedside commode, semi- or high-Fowler's position, and rest and relaxation.	Patient demonstrated an understanding of measures to reduce cardiac workload, including bed rest with bedside commode, semi- or high-Fowler's position, and rest and relaxation.
Patient will demonstrate no side effects from bed rest.	Assess patient for complications of bed rest.	Patient demonstrated no complications from bed rest.
Patient will experience no daily weight gain.	Weigh patient daily.	Patient showed no daily weight gain.
Patient will demonstrate a positive reaction to vasodilators and no side effects.	Assess response to vasodilators.	Patient demonstrated a positive response to vasodilators.
Patient will demonstrate no side effects from insertion of catheters for measurement of pulmonary artery pressure, PAWP, or cardiac output.	Assess for complications of hemodynamic monitoring.	Patient demonstrated no side effects from insertion of hemodynamic monitoring catheters.

Continued.

NURSING DIAGNOSIS 1   **Decreased cardiac output related to mechanical factors (preload, afterload, or inotropic state of the heart) and electrical factors (rate, rhythm, and conduction) (exchanging pattern)—cont'd**

PATIENT OUTCOMES	NURSING PRESCRIPTIONS	EVALUATION
Patient will maintain normal fluid and electrolyte balance.	Maintain normal fluid and electrolyte balance.	Patient maintained normal fluid and electrolyte balance.
Patient will adhere to a low-sodium diet.	Teach patient about a low-sodium diet.	Patient adhered to a low-sodium diet.
Patient will maintain a normal intake and output.	Maintain accurate intake and output records.	Patient maintained a normal intake and output.
Patient will adhere to fluid restriction if necessary.	Explain the importance of fluid restrictions if ordered.	Patient adhered to restricted fluids.
Patient will respond to diuretics.	Administer diuretics and assess the response.	Patient responded therapeutically to diuretics.
Patient will have no side effects from diuretics such as hypokalemia, hyponatremia, hypovolemia, muscle cramps, lethargy, or postural hypotension.	Monitor for complications of diuretic therapy.	Patient demonstrated no side effects of diuretics. (If they did occur, list specifics, with resolution.)
Patient will respond to mechanical removal of fluid (if required) (e.g., thoracentesis, paracentesis, dialysis, and phlebotomy).	Be prepared to assist with mechanical removal of fluid.	Mechanical removal of fluid was not needed.

Plan and intervention for decreased cardiac output

Diuretics

Retention of sodium and water is an important adverse physiologic response to heart failure. Short-term reversal of fluid retention in heart failure is best accomplished by the use of diuretics. Long-term treatment also incorporates diuretic therapy but usually with vasodilators or inotropic agents. The type of diuretic therapy chosen is often determined by the severity of the CHF. Intravenously administered loop diuretics are preferred for the treatment of pulmonary edema, whereas oral agents are used in more compensated forms of CHF. Two major principles explain the therapeutic action of diuretics: (1) diuretics may retard sodium reabsorption by renal tubular epithelial cells and reciprocally diminish water reabsorption and (2) depending on where the diuretic effects are exerted within the nephron, expected outcomes differ.[57,160]

Weak diuretics. Mannitol, acetazolamide, and potassium-sparing agents are relatively weak natriuretic agents. Osmotic diuretics such as mannitol promote a modest natriuresis, but if not eliminated, they can cause dilutional hyponatremia and extracellular fluid volume expansion.[13]

Spironolactone and triamterene are potassium-sparing and often are used in combination with the more potent loop diuretics. Potassium-sparing diuretics may cause hyperkalemia in patients experiencing CHF.[149,160]

Moderate diuretics. Thiazide-type diuretics are effective at the cortical diluting segment of the loop of Henle and the distal collecting tubule, where they inhibit sodium and chloride reabsorption. Thiazide diuretics are distinguished from one another based on their water solubility. Chlorothiazide and hydrochlorothiazide are moderately water soluble and are primarily distributed in the extracellular fluid space; thus they have a shorter duration of action. Metolazone and chlorthalidone are less water soluble, exhibit a wider tissue distribution, and have a longer duration of action. With the exception of metolazone, thiazide diuretics may become ineffective when the glomerular filtration rate falls below about 30 ml/min.[171]

Potent diuretics. Loop diuretics include furosemide, bumetanide, and ethacrynic acid, which have a rapid onset when given intravenously. These agents may inhibit as much as 25% of the filtered sodium from reabsorption in the ascending limb of the loop of Henle.[40] They cause an increase in systemic resistance resulting from stimulation of the renin-angiotensin-aldosterone mechanism, catecholamines, and ADH. The resulting increase in afterload is transient and is offset by vasodilator prostaglandins, which are then secreted as a result of natriuresis.

Inotropic agents

Digitalis. Reservations have been expressed regarding the potentially harmful effects of inotropic stimulation of the failing heart. Smith[162] summarizes these concerns as follows:

> Generally, the major concern is that an augmentation of contractile state would be anticipated to heighten myocardial oxygen requirements. This could result in a particularly deleterious response in the patient in whom systolic dysfunction is pronounced or exacerbated by ischemic cardiomyopathy. In the normal ventricle, with the initiation of contraction, there is systolic wall thickening, followed by a major reduction in cavity radius during ejection. Wall stress therefore falls during the ejection phase despite the systolic pressure exerted. This normal ejection phase unloading may be deficient in the dilated, poorly contacting ventricle where less prominent systolic thickening and minimal reduction in cavity dimensions are not sufficient to offset the systolic pressure generation. Therefore, although an increase in myocardial oxygen consumption could be anticipated from inotropic stimulation, this direct effect may be balanced by countervailing augmentation of changes in systolic wall thickness and radius reduction. Conceptually, it is quite possible that inotropic stimulation may actually enhance the systolic unloading of the dilated, poorly contracting ventricle and thus may be additive or even synergistic to the actions of peripheral vasodilators.

The mechanism of action of this inotropic action is that of inhibiting the sodium-potassium adenosine triphosphatase mechanism, therefore reducing transport of sodium out of the cell, which results in an increase in intracellular sodium. This creates an environment conducive to a calcium-sodium exchange. More calcium ions are retained in the cell, maximizing the actin-myosin coupling of contraction.[162] The intended result is inotropic, or increased force and velocity of contraction. With therapeutic digitalis levels, parasympathetic effects dominate. Digitalis sensitizes baroreceptors and cardiopulmonary receptors so that afferent input to the central nervous system is enhanced.[108] This results in increased vagal activity (slowing of heart rate) and possibly withdrawal of sympathetic activity. Digitalis exerts a salutary beneficial effect on atrial fibrillation, a dysrhythmia complicating CHF, by decreasing ventricular response mediated by activation of the PNS.[162]

Digitalis in combination with diuretics and vasodilators. Smith[162] suggests that the therapeutic goal of triple therapy with diuretics, digitalis, and vasodilators in patients with chronic CHF is to maintain compensation at an acceptable level of activity with minimum cardiac workload and the greatest possible margin between the dose of each drug administered and the toxicity threshold for each drug. Such combination therapy, however, makes it difficult to distinguish the individual contribution of each form of therapy in the overall clinical response.

In a placebo-controlled comparison of digoxin and captopril therapy in patients with CHF who were also on diuretics, differential responses were observed with respect to alterations in exercise duration and ejection fraction.[162] The ACE inhibitor–treated group exhibited greater prolongation in exercise duration; however, only the digoxin-assigned patients demonstrated an improvement in left ventricular ejection fraction.[54]

Dobutamine. Dobutamine is a synthetic sympathomimetic amine that increases myocardial contracility through stimulation of the β-adrenergic receptors. The isomers of this drug interact with α_1-, β_1-, and β_2-adrenergic receptors. The net effect, however, is that of β_1 selective activity because the vascular effects of the α_1 and β_2 actions counterbalance each other.[41] β-receptor stimulation activates production of adenylate cyclase, a precursor to cyclic AMP that mobilizes calcium from its stores to the site of actin-myosin interaction. As more actin fibers are activated by the binding of calcium with tropomyosin, the peptide preventing actin-myosin interaction, more bridges can be formed through actin-myosin coupling; hence a greater force of contraction exists. Dobutamine also causes vasodilation resulting from β_2-receptor stimulation. The suggested dosage for dobutamine begins at 2 to 5 µg/kg/min, gradually increasing by 5 to 10 µg/kg/min to a maximum dose of 20 to 50 µg/kg/min.[41,174]

Some patients are desensitized to dobutamine after about 72 hours of continuous infusion because of β-receptor "down regulation" (p. 311). Therefore short-term (72-hour) infusions of dobutamine ("dobutamine sprint") have been administered to patients with CHF on a weekly or biweekly basis.[173,174]

This practice led to trials of home infusions of dobutamine.[6,154] Dobutamine depletes plasma potassium levels. In one study, a drop in potassium level persisted for 45 minutes after discontinuing the dobutamine infusion.[64]

Dopamine. Dopamine acts by stimulating α-adrenergic, β-adrenergic and dopaminergic receptors. In low doses of about 4 µg/kg/min, it predominately stimulates the dopamine receptors in renal, splenic, cerebral, and coronary vascular beds, which results in vasodilation and possibly decreased systemic vascular resistance. The clinical benefits of low-dose dopamine are improved renal perfusion, increased glomerular filtration rate, and natriuresis.[64-67]

At intermediate infusion rates of 4 to 8 µg/kg/min, dopamine also stimulates α- and β-adrenergic receptors in the vascular system and myocardium. At high infusion rates, the α-adrenergic effect of dopamine predominates, resulting in increased vasoconstriction.[64,66] Leier and others[95] compared the effects of dopamine and dobutamine in treatment of CHF. Both drugs caused an increase in cardiac index. The increase in heart rate, PAWP, and systemic vascular resistance were greater with dopamine than with dobutamine. These differences primarily reflect the additional stimulation of vascular α-adrenergic receptors by dopamine.

Oral β-agonists. Several oral β-adrenergic agonists have been studied. Some oral agents are relatively selective for the β_1-receptors (prenalterol, butopamine, denopamine, and xamoterol), whereas others are selective for β_2-receptor activity (salbutamol, terbutaline, pirbuterol, and albutamol). Several agents cause improvement in left ventricular hemodynamic performance, but sustained effectiveness has been difficult to demonstrate in patients with CHF. Pharmacologic tolerance may develop during chronic exposure to β-adrenergic stimulation. The effects of pirbuterol and prenalterol disappear after 1 month of therapy. A high incidence of ventricular dysrhythmias has resulted in withdrawal of prenalterol, terbutaline, and pirbuterol from clinical trials. Levodopa and ibopamine are under investigation in clinical trials. Increased diuresis, peripheral vasodilation, and improved contractility have been demonstrated with these agents.[7,58,138]

Phosphodiesterase inhibitors

Phosphodiesterase inhibitors (amrinone, milrinone, enoximone, imazodin, and prioximon) are potent inotropic and vasodilator agents that have undergone extensive recent investigation. These agents increase intracellular calcium availability by increasing cyclic AMP levels. They improve cardiac performance by enhancing contractility, reducing left ventricular afterload, and improving diastolic compliance. Cardiac index is increased by about 50% and is accompanied by marked decreases in PAWP and systemic vascular resistance. Systemic venous pressure and, in some cases, mean arterial pressure also decrease, whereas heart rate increases slightly. Increased cardiac work leads to an increase in myocardial oxygen consumption, but increased coronary flow prevents an imbalance of myocardial oxygen supply and demand. Renal perfusion may increase as a result of the increase in cardiac output.[8,25,31]

Amrinone. Amrinone markedly increases cardiac index and decreases PAWP, pulmonary vascular resistance, and systemic vascular resistance. Heart rate is usually unaffected. It increases myocardial oxygen demand only slightly.[8] Its high incidence of adverse reactions (nausea and vomiting, abdominal pain, anorexia, ventricular dysrhythmias, hepatotoxicity, CNS dysfunctions, and thrombocytopenia), which occurred in 83% of patients in one study, has limited its use to short-term intravenous administration in patients with severe CHF that does not respond to conventional therapy.[33,101]

Milrinone. Positive inotropic effects of milrinone have been well demonstrated.[31,91,106] Hemodynamic improvement is similar to that with amrinone, but the patient tolerates milrinone better. Milrinone can be administered orally and intravenously. Increased fluid retention has been reported. During intravenous administration, there is also a significant increase in forearm venous capacitance, suggesting a venodilator effect.[31] Unlike amrinone, milrinone fails to increase myocardial oxygen consumption.

Enoximone. Enoximone with inotropic and vasodilator effects has been found useful in short-term management of unstable CHF and has demonstrated an additive hemodynamic benefit to dobutamine, dopamine, or both.[84] In one study, 79 patients (18 in class III and 61 in class IV) with CHF were followed for 3 years. The average oral dose of enoximone was 1.7 mg/kg 3 times daily. Improve-

ment of at least one functional class occurred in 55 patients (70%) at 1 month and 27 patients (34%) at 6 months; 19 (24%) maintained their improvement for over 1 year. Investigators concluded that oral doses of enoximone caused an acute and significant improvement in cardiac performance and appeared to provide a sustained clinical benefit to patient with chronic CHF.[84] The European enoximone trial suggested that, if initially tolerated, enoximone appears to be useful in long-term management of patients with chronic CHF.[180] Milrinone and amrinone have FDA approval for treatment of refractory CHF.

Calcium-sensitizing agents

Calcium-sensitizing agents were developed because of known side effects of phosphodiesterase inhibitors, such as dysrhythmias and increased oxygen demand. Calcium-sensitizing agents circumvent these deleterious effects because they do not increase cellular cyclic AMP.[141] Rather, they increase the affinity of troponin C (p. 304) to calcium. Pimobendan and sulmazole are calcium-sensitizing positive inotropic drugs. Both, however, also inhibit phosphodiesterase and therefore increase cyclic AMP levels. Sulmazole was withdrawn from clinical trials because it caused severe gastrointestinal side effects and hepatic neoplasms.[140] Pimobendan has demonstrated favorable effects in trials with patients experiencing CHF.[7,141] It significantly improves myocardial contractility with immediate and prolonged vasodilator effects without producing cardiac dysrhythmias. Its long-term efficacy on exercise tolerance and patient survival has yet to be established.

Vasodilator therapy

Vasodilators have achieved widespread acceptance in the management of heart failure.[32,61,116,117] Vasodilators relax vascular smooth muscle and improve left ventricular function by reducing afterload and preload. Left ventricular diastolic pressures and volumes are reduced as a result of decreased peripheral vascular resistance and increased venous capacitance. As arterioles are dilated, a reduction in afterload occurs. Vasodilators that act equally on the arterial and venous beds are referred to as *balanced vasodilators* (nitroprusside and prazosin). Their actions are intermediate between those of *pure arterial dilators* (hydralazine, minoxidil, and phenoxybenzamine) and *pure venous dilators* (nitroglycerin and isosorbide dinitrate).[53,119,140]

With parenteral vasodilatation, arterial blood pressure may fall unless there is a concomitant increase in cardiac output. For this reason, arterial blood pressure, intracardiac pressures, and cardiac output measurements must be carefully monitored and evaluated. Therefore an arterial line and pulmonary artery catheter should be inserted before beginning intravenous vasodilator therapy.

Sodium nitroprusside. Intravenous sodium nitroprusside produces a balanced and potent vasodilator effect. The intended therapeutic effect is reduction of pulmonary congestion by increasing venous capacitance and reducing the PAWP. Impedance to left ventricular ejection is reduced because of arterial tone relaxation and lowering of systemic vascular resistance. Recommended starting dosage is 3 μg/kg/min for adults and children (range of 0.5 to 10 μg/kg/min). At 3 μg/kg/min blood pressure can be lowered to about 30% to 40% below the pretreatment diastolic levels. To avoid a possible thiocyanate overdose and the possibility of precipitous drops in blood pressure, doses should not exceed 10 μg/kg/min.[111] Symptoms of *cyanide toxicity* include metabolic acidosis and increased tolerance to the drug. These may be associated with dyspnea, headache, vomiting, dizziness, ataxia, and loss of consciousness. Other signs of cyanide toxicity are coma, undectable pulse, absent reflexes, widely dilated pupils, and pink color.[152]

Nitroglycerin. Nitroglycerin may be administered via transdermal patches. An oral form, isosorbide dinitrate, is usually administered in dosages of 20 to 60 mg every 4 hours. Intravenous nitroglycerin has a potent effect on venous tone even at low doses. Arterial dilation occurs at higher doses.[53] It has less of an effect on systemic vascular resistance than sodium nitroprusside. Nitroglycerin also increases flow through collateral coronary beds better than nitroprusside.[112,152]

The initial dose is 5 μg/min, increased by 5 μg/min every 10 min. After a dosage of 20 μg/min is reached, infusion can be increased by increments of 10 μg/min until a hemodynamic response is achieved. Loss of nitroglycerin to polyvinylchloride has been demonstrated. One study[117] reported that the relative absorption of nitroglycerin from polyvinylchloride infusion sets was 41.5%, 62.9%, and 76.0% for the 6, 12, and 24 ml/hr infusion rates. Loss of nitroglycerin was related to the rate of infusion, with slower infusion rates resulting in more nitroglycerin loss. Only minimal loss of nitroglycerin occurred with nonpolyvinyl chloride or polyethylene administration sets, and this loss was not flow related.

Oral vasodilators

Hydralazine. Hydralazine causes vasodilation of the arterial vascular bed, resulting in a lowering of systemic vascular resistance and increased cardiac output. Hydralazine usually has no effect on systemic venous congestion. Oral dosage is 50 to 100 mg every 6 hours. Side effects are usually dose related and include headache, palpitations, and postural hypotension. Long-term therapy is associated with development of a lupuslike syndrome, fluid retention, and a peripheral neuropathic condition.[104]

ACE inhibitors

The role of the renin-angiotensin system in CHF was described on p. 310. During the early compensatory phase of heart failure, this mechanism contributes to sodium and water retention. Expansion of extracellular fluid volume and restoration of blood pressure deactivates the renin-angiotensin system. With profound cardiac failure, such

stabilization may not occur, and the renin-angiotensin system remains activated. The resultant sodium retention and expansion of extracellular fluid volume contribute to increased preload and subsequent edema. Angiotensin is also a powerful renal vasoconstrictor.

The principle action of an ACE inhibitor is to block conversion of angiotensin I to angiotensin II. Angiotensin II is a potent venoconstrictor and aldosterone-releasing agent. It raises blood pressure by increasing venous return, sodium and water retention, and extracellular fluid volume. There is an inverse relationship between plasma renin levels and serum sodium concentrations in patients with CHF. Patients with serum sodium levels less than 130 mg/L are more than 30 times likely to develop symptomatic hypotension during initiation of ACE-inhibiting therapy.[118] As with vasodilators, ACE inhibitors improve the symptoms and hemodynamic measurements of patients with CHF. However, in contrast with vasodilators, ACE inhibitors produce a greater symptomatic improvement during long-term therapy. The recently published Cooperative North Scandinavian Enalapril Survival Study (CONSENSUS)[34] randomly assigned 253 men and women with severe heart failure to treatment with enalapril or a placebo, concomitantly with digitalis, diuretics, and direct-acting vasodilators. Follow-up averaged 188 days. In patients receiving enalapril, the 12-month mortality rate was reduced by 31%. This reduction resulted from the diminished progression to heart failure, whereas no differences were observed in the incidence of sudden cardiac death. This trial suggests that ACE inhibitors prolong the life of patients with chronic CHF who are already being treated with digitalis, diuretics, and conventional vasodilators.[3]

Captopril. Captopril, the first ACE inhibitor to be approved by the Food & Drug Administration (FDA), causes an improvement in pump efficiency by reducing MVO_2. The dosage of captopril for heart failure is 6.25 to 25 mg 3 times a day. It is rapidly absorbed after oral administration. In the fasting state, 60% to 75% of the orally administered dose is bioavailable. With food, only 30%-40% of each dose is absorbed. Serum levels can be detected 15 minutes after ingestion. Peak levels are reached in 30 to 90 minutes. Approximately 25% to 30% of captopril is protein bound. Captopril in the absorbed dose is excreted during the first 4 hours, and 95% of the dose is eliminated over 24 hours.[46]

Enalapril. The second oral ACE inhibitor approved for use in patients with CHF is enalapril. It is relatively weak. The recommended initial dosage is 2.5 to 5 mg. Maintenance doses range from 5 to 40 mg daily. After oral ingestion, approximately 60% to 70% of enalapril is absorbed and bioavailable; absorption is not influenced by food in the gastrointestinal tract. Onset of action is approximately 1 hour after ingestion, and peak ACE inhibition occurs 4 to 6 hours after administration. Over 90% of enalapril is eliminated in the urine; its half-life is approximately 11 hours.[46,157]

β-Adrenergic blockade therapy

Conventionally, β-adrenergic blockers were contraindicated with CHF because it was believed that high-reflex sympathetic tone was necessary to maintain cardiac output.[60] The consequence of catecholamine stimulation is an increase in heart rate and contractility; continued sympathetic stimulation results in β-adrenergic receptor down regulation and possibly a direct toxic effect on the myocardium.[58] Vasoconstriction and release of vasopressin with activation of the renin-angiotensin system with an increase in systemic vascular resistance are untoward side effects of sympathetic overstimulation.[19]

Investigation into the use of β-blockers with CHF began in 1975; later studies showed promising results.[58] The long-term outcome of β-blockers on ventricular function and mortality rates has still not been determined. A large, multicenter, randomized, double-blind investigation organized by the Goteborg, Sweden, group, Metoprolol in Dilated Cardiomyopathy, was initiated in 1986 to address these concerns. Current recommendations are to begin metoprolol at ultra-low doses (5 mg orally twice a day); patient should be observed overnight in an inpatient setting. Dosage titration is performed weekly, increasing up to 50 mg three times a day by day 42. Metoprolol doses are not increased if the heart rate is below 60 beats per minute or systolic pressure is less than 90 mm Hg. Contraindications include a history of asthma, significant AV block, and insulin-dependent diabetes. Fatigue, lightheadedness, and dizziness have been reported, but most patients tolerate the drug well.[36]

NURSING
DIAGNOSIS 2 **Impaired gas exchange related to pulmonary congestion (exchanging pattern)**

PATIENT OUTCOMES	NURSING PRESCRIPTIONS	EVALUATION
Patient will demonstrate absence of dyspnea, orthopnea, cough, paroxysmal noctural dyspnea, sputum (frothy), tachypnea, diaphoresis, tachycardia, apprehension, hypoxemia, and hypercapnia.	Assess patient for signs and symptoms of pulmonary venous congestion, including dyspnea, orthopnea, cough, paroxysmal nocturnal dyspnea, frothy sputum, tachypnea, diaphoresis, tachycardia, apprehension, hypoxemia, and hypercapnia.	Patient demonstrated resolution of pulmonary venous congestion as evidenced by lack of dyspnea, orthopnea, cough, paroxysmal nocturnal dyspnea, frothy sputum, tachypnea, diaphoresis, tachycardia, apprehension, hypoxemia, and hypercapnia.
Patient will respond to oxygen administered by cannula or mask, high-Fowler's position, morphine sulfate, vasodilators, diuretics, and rotating tourniquets.	Initiate therapy for pulmonary venous congestion, including oxygen, high-Fowler's position, morphine sulfate, vasodilators, diuretics, and rotating tourniquets.	Patient responded to oxygen by mask, high-Fowler's position, morphine sulfate, vasodilators, diuretics, and rotating tourniquets.
Patient will demonstrate normal respiratory rate and rhythm and breath sounds without adventitious sounds; lack of jugular venous distention; normal skin color and temperature, good capillary filling, and lack of central or peripheral cyanosis; normal arterial blood gas values, PAWP, and cardiac output; balanced intake and output; and normal sinus rhythm.	Assess patient for normal gas exchange, including respiratory rate and rhythm; breath sounds; jugular venous distention; skin color, temperature, capillary refill, and cyanosis; arterial blood gas values; PAWP; cardiac output; intake and output balance; and cardiac rhythm.	Patient demonstrated normal gas exchange as evidenced by normal parameters, including respiratory rate; breath sounds; lack of jugular venous distention; skin color, temperature, capillary refill, and lack of cyanosis; arterial blood gas values; PAWP; cardiac output; intake and output balance; and normal sinus rhythm.

Plan and intervention for impaired gas exchange

A major complication of heart failure is impaired gas exchange related to pulmonary congestion, which requires quick treatment to reverse severe symptoms. Treatment is usually fairly clear-cut because the usual cause of acute pulmonary edema is acute left ventricular failure. If acute pulmonary edema is superimposed on chronic left ventricular failure, hypervolemia is usually present. With pulmonary edema, patients are anxious and afraid.

General measures

All attempts should be made by nurses and physicians to decrease patients' anxiety. Patients frequently think they may not get another adequate breath or that they may stop breathing. These psychologic feelings are translated to physiologic changes because patients consume more oxygen and produce more carbon dioxide when stressed. Patients with acute pulmonary edema may feel that the medical team is hovering, which also increases anxiety. Procedures should be explained and reinforced in confident, low tones. Intravenous fluids should be given by a microdrip. Hourly output and intake levels should be recorded.

Increasing gas exchange

When there is hypoxemia without hypercapnia, oxygen is given through a face mask at flow rates to raise the oxygen pressure (PO_2) above 60 mm Hg. If arterial oxygen tension cannot be maintained at or near 60 mm Hg with 100% oxygen at 20 L/min or if progressive hypercapnia ensues, intubation and ventilatory management usually are required.[178] A medium concentration mask with a flow rate of 8 to 10 L/min will deliver 40% to 70% fractional inspired oxygen concentration (FiO_2). Higher concentrations can be achieved with a nonrebreathing bag mask. The flow rate is between 6 to 10 L/min. The flow should be adequate to keep the bag inflated. The FiO_2 delivered is from 60% to 95%. Most patients tolerate masks poorly. The patient's face is kept dry under the mask to decrease irritation. With the nonrebreathing bag mask, the bag should never be allowed to collapse completely during inspiration, and a tight seal is maintained between the mask and the patient's face.[181]

The role of mechanical ventilation, when there is progressive hypoxemia without hypercapnia, is to increase mean lung volume during the inspiratory cycle. This opens more alveoli for gas exchange. If hypoxemia is not corrected by ventilatory support or if toxic doses of oxygen are required for extended periods, use of positive end-expiratory pressure may be necessary. Careful management of end-expiratory pressure is necessary to avoid the hazards of high intrathoracic pressures, increasing the lung volume, which can impede venous return and increase right ventricular afterload, thus decreasing cardiac output. Signs of failing cardiac output such as a fall in blood pressure or urine output levels must be recognized. Complications of high pressures can be seen as subcutaneous emphysema, pneumothorax, or pneumomediastinum. If barotrauma results, appropriate decompressive therapy is required. Arterial blood gas levels are measured to monitor treatment and see whether the desired cardiopulmonary effects are being achieved.

Unloading the left ventricle

Unloading the left ventricle involves placing the patient in high-Fowler's position with legs dependent and administering morphine, diuretics, and a vasodilator. The position helps dilate peripheral arteries and veins and causes venous pooling. Dilating peripheral arteries also reduces impedance to left ventricular ejection, and the left ventricular end-diastolic pressure is reduced.

Morphine sulfate

Morphine sulfate can be given safely and is almost always required for patients with pulmonary edema. It is given in small, intravenous, intermittent doses. Morphine helps reduce anxiety, decreases tachypnea, and causes a peripheral pooling of blood, which serves as a pharmacologic phlebotomy.[176] Its circulatory action causes a reduction in preload and afterload. It may cause respiratory depression, so naloxone should be readily available to immediately reverse the situation.

Detrimental effects can occur quickly after morphine infusion. Hypotension occurs within 1 to 2 minutes. This is more common in upright positions and is thought to result from partial inhibition by morphine of baroreceptor vasoconstrictor reflexes. Respiratory depression occurs in approximately 7 minutes.[176] Because of variable absorption rates in the pulmonary edema state, intramuscular morphine is not given because cardiorespiratory depression could be delayed for as long as 1 to 2 hours. Morphine may save lives in patients with acute pulmonary edema, but it can have deleterious effects in patients who have acute respiratory failure or chronic pulmonary disease with carbon dioxide retention. The physician must make the distinction between dyspnea from acute respiratory failure and acute pulmonary edema.

Vasodilators

As previously discussed, vasodilators such as sodium nitroprusside and nitroglycerin are used to unload the left ventricle. Sodium nitroprusside is the preferred vasodilator for treatment of acute pulmonary edema. It reduces pulmonary and ventricular pressures and increases cardiac output, which quickly relieves the symptoms of acute pulmonary edema.

Diuretics

The potent loop diuretics, furosemide and ethacrynic acid, are given to reduce total blood volume and prevent recurrence of pulmonary congestion. These drugs cause a reduction in sodium reabsorption in the loop of Henle and directly affect arterial and venous dilation.

Rotating tourniquets

If the preceding measures do not work, rotating tourniquets may be required. Nursing care for this procedure is very specific. Most authorities suggest using the patient's diastolic presure as a guideline. Inflating the blood pressure cuff to approximately 10 mm Hg below the diastolic pressure will cause fluid loss into the peripheral extravascular spaces. A pressure of 25 to 45 mm Hg usually retards venous return without closing off arterial flow.[56] With an automatic rotating tourniquet machine the tourniquets automatically rotate counterclockwise, filling the deflated cuff as the cuff that has been inflated the longest deflates. Most machines rotate every 15 minutes. The nursing protocol for use with automatic rotating tourniquets is listed in the box. Use of an automatic machine frees the nurse to decrease patient anxiety and deliver emotional support. Because the procedure is done as a last resort, anxiety is usually quite high. Explanations are kept simple, and the patients' comprehension of it is evaluated. Because of their unstable state, patients frequently hear and comprehend only a minimal amount of information, and perceptions of what has been told to them may be wrong.

The most common complications or rotating tourniquets are softening, laceration, or necrosis of tissues and thrombophlebitis caused by the cuff. Patients should not be on the machine longer than 3 to 4 hours at a time. As patients are weaned from the machine, special attention is needed to avoid excessive increases in venous blood volume, which could cause acute pulmonary edema again. As each cuff is removed, it is clamped off; the patient's vital signs, breath sounds, heart sounds, and extremities are evaluated.

NURSING PROTOCOL FOR USE OF AUTOMATIC ROTATING TOURNIQUETS

1. Place the patient in high-Fowler's position and explain the procedure.
2. Record baseline blood pressure, pulses, color of all extremities, and mental status. Mark peripheral pulses with a felt-tip marker.
3. Apply blood pressure cuffs to all extremities in the same position as when taking blood pressure. Make certain that they are snug but that you are able to get two fingers under the cuff. Attach the proper extremity connection (only three of four cuffs will be inflated at any time).
4. Check that the unused cuff is clamped off. Turn on the machine, and let it warm up. Adjust the pressure dial to 10 mm below the level of diastolic pressure.
5. Check all peripheral pulses and the color and temperature of extremities while the machine is operating. Check cuffs for proper inflation and leaks or kinked tubing.
6. Reassure the patient and give emotional support. Include the family, and allow brief visits if possible.
7. When weaning the patient, remove the cuffs one by one in a counterclockwise direction over 45 to 60 minutes. Remove one cuff at a time. Evaluate patient status during weaning.

NURSING
DIAGNOSIS 3 **Impaired physical mobility related to decreased cardiac output (moving pattern)**

PATIENT OUTCOMES	NURSING PRESCRIPTIONS	EVALUATION
Patient will not experience the following complications related to impaired physical mobility:	Reinforce and explain the need for bed rest. Institute the following measures:	Patient did not experience the following:
Skin breakdown	Turn patient every 2 hours.	Skin breakdown
Phlebitis or thromboembolism	Perform range of motion exercises, apply antiembolism stockings, and administer minidose heparin, if ordered.	Phlebitis or thromboembolism
Constipation	Administer laxatives or stool softeners as necessary.	Constipation
Confusion	Orient patient to place, person, time and situation.	Confusion
Discouragement or depression	Point out improvements in the patient's condition, reduce emotional disturbances, guide patient in relaxation techniques, and provide patients with diversional activities.	Discouragement or depression
Pulmonary complications	Assist patient with turning, coughing, and deep breathing.	Secondary pulmonary complications
Patient will participate in supervised cardiac rehabilitation.	Explain inpatient cardiac rehabilitation program and evaluate patient response to progressive activities.	Patient successfully participated in supervised cardiac rehabilitation.

Plan and intervention for impaired physical mobility

The decreased activity associated with bed rest causes many complications. The patient must be encouraged to turn, cough, and breathe deeply to improve muscular tone, aid in venous return to the heart, and prevent skin breakdown, phlebitis, and secondary pulmonary complications. To avoid phlebitis and pulmonary embolism, the patient must understand how to do correct rhythmic extremity exercises and why antiembolism stockings are worn. Patients with severe heart failure or a history of thromboembolic problems may be given minidose heparin to prevent further problems. To avoid straining with a bowel movement, which increases the heart's workload, the patient should be given a stool softener or mild laxative (only if necessary) and should use a bed side commode. The patient must also get psychologic rest. Emotional disturbances can cause increased heart rate, stroke volume, cardiac output, blood pressure, and dysrhythmias at rest; therefore efforts should be made to reduce or eliminate these factors.

The patient with heart failure has limited physical energy and frequently will push beyond the symptom-free threshold. A useful strategy to involve patients in their care within limitation is *contracting*. The nurse and patient have different but equal responsibilities when trying to achieve common goals. The major job of the patient in a contract is adherence to activities. Reinforcements to promote adherence to a contract must be individualized. Contracting helps the patient function as a whole person. It allows the nurse and patient to share all aspects of the recovery process.

All efforts should be made to reduce the patient's depression because of the acute illness by providing some type of appropriate diversional activities. Sitting in a chair instead of lying supine reduces venous return to the heart. At home, patients can be encouraged to sit on a porch or patio and feel the air and see everything around them. However, sitting outside should not be encouraged if the weather is extremely hot, humid, or cold. During recovery, it is important and helpful for the patient to use relaxation and imagery skills, which can result in a positive psychophysiologic response (see Chap. 5). The patient should begin working with a physical therapist as soon as possible in a rehabilitation program. Beginning with very limited activity, such as passive range of motion, provides direction and encouragement. The patient can look forward to a program of gradual improved mobility by mutually setting goals with the therapist.

A physical rehabilitation program that monitors patient progressive physical activity and physiologic responses should be carried out so that activity can be increased according to hemodynamic tolerance. A rehabilitation program can provide encouragement and offer goals of activity thresholds toward which the patient can work. However, the program should set realistic limitations within the cardiac reserve (see Chapter 19).

Case study cont'd. Mr. J.L. steadily improved from his acute episode of congestive heart failure. To achieve and maintain optimal cardiac function, he first had to understand the rationale of and relationship between activity and heart function. Nursing and medical management became a continuous process of setting new goals daily with Mr. J.L. with regard to activity and rehabilitation. Frequently, Mr. J.L. pushed beyond a symptom-free activity level because before activity he exhibited no symptoms. He had to learn how to budget his available energy so that he could participate in his activities of daily living and lead as normal a life as possible. Mr. J.L. began ambulating but complained that each activity from brushing his teeth and eating his meal to slow ambulation left him feeling fatigued.

NURSING
DIAGNOSIS 4   **Fatigue related to limited cardiac reserve (moving pattern)**

PATIENT OUTCOMES	NURSING PRESCRIPTIONS	EVALUATION
Patient will learn to adjust his or her activity level to avoid fatigue.	Place patient in private room when possible.	Patient learned to recognize activities that caused fatigue and ways to adjust activity levels to avoid it.
Patient will learn to take pulse before and after activities.	Record patient's activities to determine which ones elevate heart rate. Teach patient to take pulse before and after activity.	Patient learned to take pulse before and after activities.
Patient will participate in activities known to exacerbate fatigue earlier in the day.	Institute measures known to exacerbate fatigue (such as bathing) earlier in the day.	Patient bathed early in the day to avoid fatigue.

Plan and intervention for fatigue

Placing patients with CHF in private rooms is preferable to placing them in wards because it reduces environmental noise, interference from other patient activities, and nursing interventions administered to other patients. Promoting a restful environment ultimately helps to reduce fatigue. Activities must be evaluated to determine whether any help or hinder cardiac function. Activity is then tailored to minimize fatigue. Data obtained from heart rate response to activities should be used to develop an individualized care plan. If the patient's heart rate increases with bathing, further activities or nursing interventions should be deferred until the heart rate has decreased to preactivity levels. Blood pressure responses to activity should also be evaluated. Raising the arms (isometric exercises) should be avoided to prevent increases in blood pressure and afterload. Fatigue usually increases as the day progresses. Measures that exacerbate fatigue, such as bathing, should therefore be performed early in the day.

NURSING
DIAGNOSIS 5 **Anxiety related to acute or chronic illness (feeling pattern)**

PATIENT OUTCOMES	NURSING PRESCRIPTIONS	EVALUATION
Patient will therapeutically respond to a quiet environment.	Provide quiet, safe environment for patient.	Patient therapeutically responded to a quiet environment.
Patient will verbalize feelings of anxiety or fear.	Assess anxiety and ask patient open-ended questions to elicit worries and fears.	Patient verbalized anxiety and talked about fears.
Patient will not show side effects from medications required to reduce anxiety.	Give antianxiety medication as needed.	Patient did not exhibit side effects from medications.
Patient will use effective coping mechanisms during the course of the illness.	Focus on patient's strengths. Determine ways patient has effectively coped with stress and encourage use of these skills.	Patient used effective coping mechanisms during the illness.
Patient and family or significant others will communicate stressors with each other and the nursing and medical staff.	Continually reassess ways that the patient and family cope with patient's acute illness.	Patient and family communicated stressors to each other and staff.
Patient will demonstrate successful use of relaxation and imagery skills in recovery.	Teach relaxation and imagery skills to decrease anxiety.	Patient successfully demonstrated use of relaxation and imagery skills.

Plan and intervention for anxiety

Nurses must continually reassess the patients' levels of anxiety. The nurse can assist patients in identifying matters that make them anxious and their coping mechanisms. This level of coparticipation is mandatory; the patient and nurse must share perceptions. Open-ended questions with periods of silence can be used to guide patients in verbalizing their stressors. Sitting with the patient and conveying sincerity and interest facilitate patient comfort while talking. Therapeutic touching provides a feeling of security.

When patients are encouraged to interact and take an active role in their daily care, their anxiety also will decrease, and thus a sense of purpose and confidence will be reestablished. Some patients have free-floating anxiety. They may exhibit repetitive behavior for the first time such as shaking a foot nervously, tapping on a table, or pacing. Extremely anxious patients should never be forced to focus on their anxiety. They should be allowed to talk and focus on what they wish. They also should not be left alone. This state may require sedation, as well as the help of the psychiatric clinical nurse specialist, social worker, occupational therapist, or nurse liaison. Nurses also can assist the patient in learning antianxiety techniques such as relaxation, imagery, or music therapy (see Chapter 5).

NURSING
DIAGNOSIS 6   **Knowledge deficit related to complex pathophysiologic illness (knowing pattern)**

PATIENT OUTCOMES	NURSING PRESCRIPTIONS	EVALUATION
Patient will verbalize knowledge about heart failure, signs and symptoms of heart failure, risk factors and ways to modify them, medications (including name, dosage, action, frequency, and side effects), activity level, exercise regimen, diet, and counting of pulse.	Assess patient's readiness and teach appropriate content regarding heart failure, signs and symptoms of heart failure, risk factors and ways to modify them, medications (including name, dosage, action, frequency, and side effects), activity level, exercise regimen, diet, and counting of pulse.	Patient verbalized knowledge about heart failure, signs and symptoms of heart failure, risk factors, medications, activity level, exercise, diet, and counting of pulse.
Patient will describe when to contact the physician for advice.	Teach patient when to contact the physician for advice.	Patient described when to contact the physician.
Patient will state when to return to the outpatient facility for follow-up appointments and advice.	Teach patient when to return for follow-up care.	Patient stated when to return to the outpatient clinic for follow-up care.

Plan and intervention for knowledge deficit

Discharge planning begins at admission. Patients must be taught to listen to their bodies, to minimize fatigue by modifying activity, and to maximize cardiac function. Housework can be a full-time and exhausting job. Questions need to be asked to determine the daily routine of cooking, cleaning, running errands, or caring for children. Patients need assistance regarding ways to get help with tasks that they left unfinished when hospitalized. Nurses should evaluate patients' work-related activities if patients are employed outside the home. Heavy lifting probably will need to be tapered or eliminated. Jobs that require walking up flights of stairs also must be evaluated. If this activity produces dyspnea and fatigue, the approach to it needs to be tailored to patient capabilities. Exhausting sports need to be discontinued, but after patients have stabilized, specific sports can be evaluated. For example, patients might be able to use a golf cart instead of carrying clubs. The New York Heart Association functional classification for heart failure patients is useful in counseling patients about activities after discharge.[110]

Class I	Patients with heart disease who are asymptomatic
Class II	Slight limitation of physical activity; symptoms produced only with more-than-ordinary physical activity
Class III	Significant limitation; symptoms produced with ordinary physical activity
Class IV	Symptoms while patient is resting

Patients in functional classes I and II must learn to avoid tasks that provoke symptoms. As patients approach class III, full-time or even part-time employment in a sedentary job may not be tolerated. Total unemployment is not recommended if at all possible. The patient might be able to work 4 to 5 hours a day or every other day instead of 8 to 10 hours every day.

Specific teaching guidelines for the nursing diagnosis of knowledge deficit are listed below:

1. Environmental factors. Hot weather will make the heart beat faster to pump more blood to the skin for dissipation of heat. Cold weather, especially wind and cold, elevates blood pressure because blood is shunted away from the skin to avoid heat loss, which causes an increase in blood volume and more peripheral resistance for the heart to pump against. The increased water vapor on a humid day restricts evaporation of skin perspiration, which makes heat accumulate in the body. Heart rate will increase. Showering and bathing expose the patient to heat and humidity. The patient should avoid hot showers and baths, as well as a very cold rinse at the end of the shower, which produces a sudden shock to the system. The higher the altitude, the lower the amount of oxygen in the air. The heart therefore has to beat faster to maintain the body's oxygen requirements. Oxygen is also decreased in a polluted environment. Like the situation of increased altitude, the heart must beat faster to maintain body oxygen levels within a polluted environment.

2. Pulse taking. The method of taking a carotid or radial pulse should be taught. If patients are incapable of learning to take their own pulses, significant others should assume this responsibility. Patients need to learn to monitor activities or emotions that increase heart rate. Shortness of breath can be avoided by pacing activities so that the pulse rate stays below the rate at which patients become symptomatic.

GUIDELINE FOR PATIENT EDUCATION

1. Individualize teaching plan for patient, taking into account the patient's and family's readiness to learn, preexisting knowledge, phase of illness, and the patient's major concerns.
2. Develop a scope of content to be discussed. Consider:
   a. Normal anatomic and physiologic condition of the heart and circulatory system
   b. Definition of heart failure
   c. Reasons for signs and symptoms of worsening CHF
   d. Concept of cardiac reserve
   e. Pulse taking
   f. Activity conservation and progression
   g. Times to phone physician
   h. Emergency plans
   i. Dietary restrictions (sodium, fluids, and calories)
   j. Weight management
   k. Rationale for medications
   l. Psychologic aspects of chronic illness
   m. Importance of compliance
   n. Community resources
   o. Follow-up care
   p. Use instructional aids to facilitate learning
   q. Collaboration with other health team members to reinforce teaching content and to ensure consistency of information

Suggested by Doyle B: Nursing challenge: the patient with end-stage heart failure, in Kern L: Cardiac critical care nursing, Gaithersburg, Md, 1988, Aspen Publishers, Inc.

3. Sexual activity. Sexual activity is believed to raise the heart rate to the level that would occur if patients were climbing 60 stairs a minute. This increased rate is usually sustained for 15 to 20 seconds after orgasm. Patients can be taught to minimize the effects of sexual activity on the heart by incorporating several factors. They should avoid extremely warm or cool rooms, which raise the resting heart rate and should wait at least 2 hours after a meal and 1 hour after smoking a cigarette. Sexual activities should be avoided at the end of a long, tiring day; the heart is better able to tolerate the increased heart rate associated with intercourse after a well-rested night. Positions in which patients support themselves on their arms are discouraged. Patients are advised to discuss with their physician the benefit of taking a sublingual nitroglycerin tablet before intercourse. Research has suggested that heart rate may be raised to a higher level when having sex with someone other than the usual partner.[44]

Doyle has nicely summarized items for the nurse to remember, signs and symptoms of heart failure, and guidelines for patient teaching. These recommendations are listed in the box.

Cardiogenic shock

Cardiogenic shock usually presents as a catastrophic complication of AMI, but can result from end-stage cardiac disease of any cause. It may also occur transiently after a cardiopulmonary bypass during cardiac surgery. Despite advances in hemodynamic monitoring and newer pharmacologic agents, the incidence of shock after AMI remains at 10% to 15% and has a mortality rate between 80% and 100%.[168,169] This high mortality rate is chiefly related to a self-perpetuating cycle of progressive ischemic damage culminating in extensive, irreversible myocardial dysfunction. Therefore the success of therapy depends largely on reducing myocardial ischemia and limiting permanent cardiac damage.

SIGNIFICANCE

Cardiogenic shock is a complex clinical syndrome characterized by hypotension, tachycardia, impaired mentation, urinary output level below 20 ml/hour, and peripheral vascular collapse. These symptoms are caused by inadequate delivery of blood to major body organs, particularly the heart, brain, and kidneys. The onset of cardiogenic shock is usually hours to days after the AMI. In patients who develop shock, half do so within the first 24 hours. One sixth develop shock a week or so later. Patients who develop cardiogenic shock usually have sustained damage to at least 40% of the left ventricular muscle mass.[55]

Nurses must be alert for patients at high risk for developing cardiogenic shock because prevention is a key aspect in patient management. If shock occurs, immediate, vigorous correction of cellular and extracellular changes is necessary for patient survival. When a patient has an AMI, prevention of cardiogenic shock involves decreasing the workload of the heart, decreasing oxygen consumption, increasing pump efficiency, and decreasing infarct size. Nurses must understand the cause, compensatory mechanisms, and pathophysiologic states of cardiogenic shock so that they can provide high-level nursing assessment and the best therapeutic plan for the patient. Each patient responds individually to the shock state. Factors that determine the patient's ability to tolerate shock are age, prior health status, presence or absence of other diseases, cause of the shock state, and the duration and severity of shock before therapy.

CAUSE AND PRECIPITATING FACTORS

Cardiogenic shock may be characterized by primary deficiencies or by specific insults. Three causes of cardiogenic shock are myopathic factors, mechanical factors, and dysrhythmias.[169] Myopathic causes are problems of impaired left ventricular contractility, as with AMI, congestive cardiomyopathy, and cardiac amyloidosis. Mechanical factors causing cardiogenic shock are regurgitant lesions, such as acute mitral or aortic regurgitation, ruptured interventricular septum, or massive left ventricular aneurysm, and obstructive lesions of the left ventricular outflow tract such as congenital or acquired valvular aortic stenosis and idiopathic hypertrophic subaortic stenosis. Symptomatic bradydysrhythmias and tachydysrhythmias, as well as conduction disturbances, cause shock over time.

PATHOPHYSIOLOGIC STATES: STAGES OF SHOCK

The physiologic and pathophysiologic changes in response to shock can be divided into four stages. Although the early stages are not easily defined in a clinical setting, they still occur and contribute to a clear picture of the clinical syndrome.[55,169]

Stage I: initial stage

In the initial stage of shock, no signs or symptoms are apparent, but subtle nonspecific changes occur at the cellular level.

Stage II: compensatory stage

In response to declining systemic arterial blood pressure, right ventricular failure, and acidosis, the SNS is stimulated, and the second, or compensatory, stage of shock begins. The compensatory mechanisms brought into action are nervous, endocrine, and chemical homeostatic mechanisms. During this stage cardiac output and blood pressure can be restored and may mask the shock state unless shock is suspected.

Nervous compensatory mechanisms

The nervous compensatory mechanisms are activated as blood pressure and cardiac output fall. Baroreceptors in the carotid arteries and aorta sense hypotension and decrease the impulses sent to the vasomotor center, which thereby remove the inhibition of the vasoconstrictor center in the medulla. This causes SNS stimulation, bringing into play the psychophysiologic stress response to prepare the body for ensuing stress. Heart rate elevates (unless AV block is present) to increase cardiac output and blood pressure. Coronary vessels dilate to increase oxygen supply to the heart. Vasoconstriction occurs to the skin, kidneys, and gastrointestinal tract (shunting blood to heart and brain),

which increases total peripheral resistance. This results in cool, pale skin; decreased urinary output; and decreased peristalsis. The sympathetic cholinergic fibers respond by producing skeletal muscle vasodilation. Other sympathetic responses are an increased rate and depth of respirations to increase alveolar oxygen supply; increased sweat gland activity, causing moist clammy skin; and pupillary dilation in response to stress.

Endocrine compensatory mechanisms

Endocrine compensatory mechanisms also are activated by the SNS. The adrenal medulla releases epinephrine and norepinephrine (Fig. 11-7). Epinephrine stimulates the anterior pituitary gland to release adrenocorticotropic hormone (ACTH). ACTH stimulates the adrenal cortex to release glucocorticoids and mineralocorticoids.

Hydrocortisone (cortisol) is the primary glucocorticoid released. Glucocorticoids increase gluconeogenesis (the conversion of amino acids to glucose) in the liver, elevating the serum glucose level. There is an increase in the transport of amino acids from extracellular fluids to the liver and mobilization of amino acids from extrahepatic tissues, primarily muscle. The uptake of glucose by cells is reduced. Proteins in the cells decrease because there is a depletion of protein stores and a reduction in protein synthesis. Fatty acids are mobilized from adipose tissue, thus increasing their concentration in plasma. Hydrocortisone enhances cellular fatty acid oxidation and shifts the metabolism of cells from glucose to fatty acids for energy. Hydrocortisone also stabilizes lysosomal membranes. Lysosomes contain a hydrolytic enzyme that digests intracellular protein. When lysosomal membranes are stabilized, the destruction of tissues, which usually occurs with inflammation because of the liberation of these enzymes, is prevented.[159]

Aldosterone, the primary mineralocorticoid released, increases reabsorption of sodium at the distal and collecting tubules and loop of Henle; urinary sodium loss is reduced. It also produces an electronegativity in the tubules. Chloride reabsorption is enhanced; hydrogen ions are excreted into the tubules in exchange for sodium. Hydrogen excre-

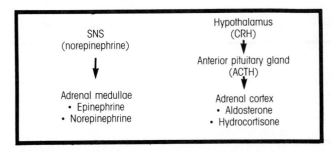

FIG. 11-7   Effects of SNS stimulation. *CRH,* Corticotropin-releasing hormone.

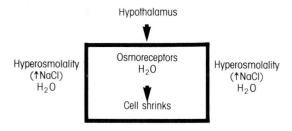

FIG. 11-8 Hyperosmolality and osmoreceptors.

tion may produce a metabolic alkalosis. Likewise, potassium is excreted in the urine, whereas sodium is reabsorbed, which can produce hypokalemia.

Because sodium and chloride are reabsorbed, there is a high plasma sodium chloride concentration, which produces a hyperosmolality that in turn causes the osmoreceptors in the hypothalamus to shrink. This increases impulses transmitted from the osmoreceptors to the posterior pituitary gland, which in turn stimulates the release of ADH (Fig. 11-8). In response to increased ADH, there is an increase in water reabsorption, extracellular fluid volume, cardiac output, and blood pressure and a decrease in serum osmolality to normal.

Adrenal medulla norepinephrine secretion causes renal artery vasoconstriction. The juxtaglomerular apparatus in the kidneys responds by secreting the enzyme, renin. Circulating blood renin reacts with a circulating plasma protein, angiotensinogen, producing angiotensin I. Angiotensin I is changed by angiotensin-converting enzyme in the lungs to angiotensin II, a potent venoconstrictor and aldosterone-releasing agent. Angiotensin II helps raise the blood pressure by increasing venous return, sodium and water reabsorption, extracellular fluid volume, and renal perfusion.[159]

Chemical compensatory mechanisms

The chemical compensatory mechanisms are brought into play as blood flow through the lungs is reduced, resulting in a ventilation-perfusion imbalance. The chemoreceptors in the carotid arteries and aorta sense the low oxygen tension and reflexly increase the rate and depth of respirations. With hyperventilation, carbon dioxide is blown off, and respiratory alkalosis develops. Cerebral vessels sense the fall in carbon dioxide tension and constrict.

Clinical manifestations of compensatory mechanisms

Despite these compensatory changes, abnormal clinical findings become evident. The rate at which they appear depends on the individual response to SNS stimulation and individual factors previously discussed. Blood pressure may be adequate to perfuse vital organs. Heart rate is increased, and the skin is cool, pale, and clammy from peripheral vasoconstriction. Urinary output is decreased by renal vasoconstriction. Level of consciousness is altered

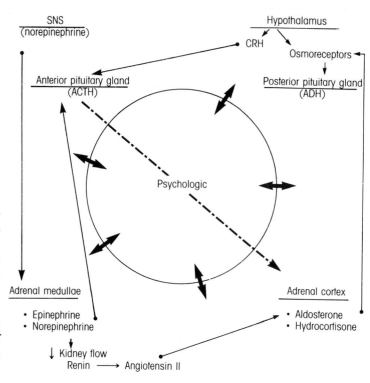

FIG. 11-9 Psychophysiologic stress response. *CRH,* Corticotropin-releasing hormone.

because of sympathetic stimulation, hypoxemia, and hypocapnia. The patient may appear overly anxious, agitated, confused, or restless. Respirations are fast and deep, bowel sounds are decreased, and pupils may be dilated.

As seen in Fig. 11-9, the psychophysiologic stress response is not isolated to physiologic changes. A change in the physiologic mechanism activates psychologic changes. The nurse must know this for critical assessment and proper nursing interventions. Bodymind connections and information flow through the natural systems hierarchy are apparent in this clinical situation. The critically ill patient and the family exhibit differing degrees of anxiety, denial, anger, fear, and increased symptoms from SNS stimulation.

Stage III: progressive stage

If the compensatory mechanisms are not effective in reversing the shock state, they will eventually fail and result in the destructive cellular and systemic changes involved in the progressive stage of shock. Prolonged and severe vasoconstriction causes adverse effects on cellular function, systemic circulation, and specific organ systems. The primary pathophysiologic disturbance in shock is impaired cellular function related to nutritional blood flow.[169] With reduced blood flow, delivery of oxygen and essential nutrients to cells are decreased, causing insufficient ATP production, which is necessary for normal cellular function. Without ATP, anaerobic metabolism occurs, leading to

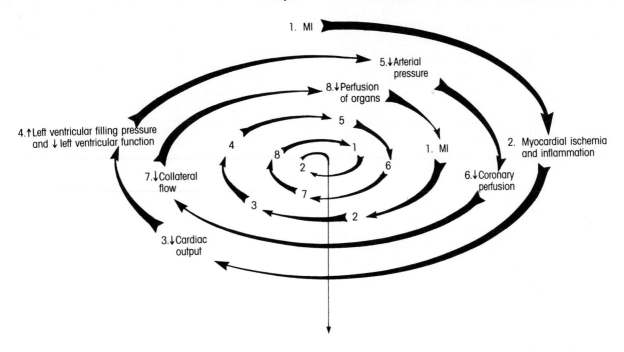

FIG. 11-10   Psychophysiologic events of cardiogenic shock perpetuate a viscious cycle, resulting in progressive and severe circulatory deterioration.

metabolic acidosis. Reduced capillary blood flow also causes a release of toxic substances that localize in tissues, changing their normal state. Precapillary arterioles relax, and the venules constrict secondary to acidosis, trapping blood within the capillaries and increasing capillary hydrostatic pressure. This increased pressure forces fluid from intravascular to extravascular spaces. Local production of histamine can increase capillary permeability, which also facilitates a shift of fluid and protein molecules to the interstitial spaces. A fluid shift produces edema and decreases circulating volume, resulting in increased blood viscosity. Resultant hemoconcentration and capillary slugging may cause diffuse intravascular coagulation.

Specific changes in organ systems occur. The kidneys tolerate prolonged vasoconstriction poorly and lose their ability to filter, excrete, and reabsorb normally. Acute tubular necrosis can occur, resulting in a disproportionate rise in BUN and creatinine levels. Urinary output falls to 20 ml/hour or less. Urinary sodium concentration is high because the kidneys become unable to reabsorb sodium. Urine osmolality drops as the kidneys lose their ability to concentrate urine. Severe vasoconstriction also may cause visceral ischemia, which may lead to ulceration and breakdown of the intestinal mucosa, allowing bacteria and toxins in the gut to enter the circulation. This further aggravates the shock state. The pancreas also suffers detrimental changes from severe vasoconstriction. As pancreatic cells become ischemic and necrotic, they release amylase and lipase into the blood. They also release a proteolytic enzyme that helps in the formation of a polypeptide, *myocardial depressant factor*. This factor further depresses myo-

cardial contractility and increased visceral vasoconstriction. It affects the normal role of calcium in myocardial contractility and electrical excitation.[169]

The heart eventually fails from deprivation of adequate perfusion, which then becomes even more difficult to maintain. Cerebral blood flow is decreased as a result of the reduced cardiac output secondary to the altered capillary dynamics. The nurse sees changes in level of consciousness that range from dulled responses to verbal and painful stimuli to gross personality and behavior changes.

The lungs are severely affected by prolonged vasoconstriction. Decreased pulmonary vascular blood flow causes ischemic and necrotic cellular changes. Damaged cells release toxins such as serotonin and histamine, which increase pulmonary arteriolar vasoconstriction and capillary permeability. Fluid shifts from pulmonary capillaries to pulmonary interstitial spaces, resulting in interstitial edema. The already compromised lungs become wet, stiff, and noncompliant. States of acidosis and hypoxia increase. Perfusion and ventilation are further reduced. The alveoli collapse, and atelectasis worsens because the alveolar cells cannot produce enough surfactant to reduce the alveolar surface tension. The result of these progressive stages is the clincial syndrome of shock.

Stage IV: refractory stage

When death is imminent and the patient in shock no longer responds to any form of therapy, the refractory, or irreversible, stage of shock occurs. As severe vasoconstriction continues, cardiac output falls even further. Buildup of acidosis further impairs respiratory and cerebral function and tissue perfusion. Platelet and red blood cell aggregation occurs because of decreased intravascular blood volume, retarded blood flow, and acidosis. This may lead to disseminated intravascular coagulation. Refractory cardiogenic shock involves all body systems. Vital centers of the brain begin to shut down because of cerebral ischemia. Respiratory arrest and cardiac failure ensue and cause total body system dysfunction and death[159] (Fig. 11-10).

Nursing process

Case study. Mr. J.P., a 62-year-old university physics professor and department chairman, was admitted to the CCU after coming to the emergency room with a history of 20 minutes of excruciating chest pain and dyspnea, unrelieved by three nitroglycerin tablets. On admission to CCU he was awake, alert, and oriented and still experiencing chest pain. His vital signs were stable. All peripheral pulses were bilaterally equal. Mr. J.P.'s heart sounds were normal, and his lung fields were clear on auscultation. His admission ECG revealed elevated ST segments in the precordial leads, suggesting an AMI. Creatine phosphokinase levels at admission were 840 with a 10% MB fraction. Arterial blood gas analyses and chest x-ray studies were unremarkable. An intravenous line of 5% dextrose in water at 30 ml/hour was started in the emergency room. Morphine sulfate was titrated intravenously to control chest pain, and oxygen was administered per nasal cannula at 3 L/minute.

About 10 hours after Mr. J.P.'s admission to the CCU, the nurse noticed some significant changes. He awoke agitated, restless, and confused about where he was. His blood pressure was 70/50 mm Hg, his pulse was 110 beats per minute, his respiratory rate was 28 to 32, and an S_3 was noted. His skin was cool, clammy, and pale.

Mr. J.P. began to have six to eight unifocal premature ventricular contractions each minute. A lidocaine bolus of 100 mg was given intravenously, followed by an infusion of lidocaine at 2 mg/min. Because Mr. J.P.'s blood pressure became inaudible, an ultrasound flowmeter was used and revealed that the pressure was 60 mm Hg. Radial artery and pulmonary artery catheters were inserted. The pulmonary artery pressure was 56/22 mm Hg, and the PAWP was 20 mm Hg. Cardiac index was calculated, at 2 L/min/m², via the thermodilution lumen of the catheter. An indwelling urinary catheter was inserted with only 10 ml of urine measured. He was given a fluid challenge of dextran over the next hour without an increase in blood pressure or urinary output. A dopamine drip was begun at 5 μg/kg/min to maintain a systolic blood pressure of 100 mm Hg. Dobutamine was infused at 8 μg/kg/min for inotropic stimulation. Arterial blood gas analyses revealed hypoxemia and respiratory acidosis. Mr. J.P. showed rapid deterioration and required intubation. He was placed on a volume-cycled ventilator.

Mr. J.P.'s condition deteriorated over the next 2 hours, despite increasing doses of dopamine. The physician then decided to institute intraaortic balloon pump (IABP) therapy, advising the family that the patient would be placed on a left ventricular assistance device (LVAD) if cardiogenic shock did not improve with IABP.

Nursing assessment

In any patient with an AMI, the nurse must be aware of the high risk for developing cardiogenic shock. The longer that a shock state exists unrecognized and untreated, the poorer the patient's prognosis. Perform a complete bio-psycho-social-spiritual assessment on all patients. Organize an assessment that includes the following areas:

1. *Exchanging pattern*
   A. Clinical findings (signs and symptoms)
      (1) Vital signs
      (2) Level of consciousness
      (3) Skin perfusion
      (4) Urinary output levels
      (5) Other signs and symptoms such as fatigue and gastrointestinal problems
      (6) Patient's and family's reaction to the acute situation
   B. Invasive hemodynamic monitoring
      (1) IABP
      (2) Pulmonary artery pressure, PAWP, and right atrial pressure
      (3) Cardiac output
   C. Laboratory tests
      (1) ECG
      (2) Chest x-ray examination
      (3) Blood gas analysis
      (4) Cardiac enzyme and isoenzyme analysis
      (5) Electrolyte tests
      (6) BUN and creatinine clearance level tests
   D. Special studies
      (1) Radionuclide scanning
      (2) Coronary angiography
      (3) Left ventricular cineangiography
      (4) Echocardiography
2. *Perceiving and Feeling Patterns*
   A. Anger
   B. Isolation
   C. Powerlessness
   D. Sensory overload

Exchanging pattern

Vital signs. Decreased blood pressure is a late sign of shock. When taking the blood pressure, get a baseline measurement and evaluate Korotkoff sounds. Clearly hearing all five phases initially with a subsequent decrease of the Korotkoff phases should be a clue to a possible ensuing shock state. Early in shock the blood pressure may be elevated or normal. Systolic pressure may be elevated because of increased stroke volume; diastolic pressure can increase because of arteriolar vasoconstriction. Blood pressure decreases as shock progresses. Pulse pressure decreases related to vasoconstriction and decreased stroke volume. An ultrasound flowmeter may be required to assess an inaudible blood pressure.

Obtain baseline characteristics of arterial and venous pulses for rhythm, rate, amplitude, and duration. Pulsus paradoxus, a sign of poor cardiac output, may be present. In cardiogenic shock, arterial pulses become weak, thready, rapid, and short in duration. Venous pulses may be fuller because of high right-sided heart filling pressures. Early in preshock states, temperature may be elevated related to the inflammation of acute myocardial infarction. Cardiogenic shock may produce a subnormal temperature related to decreased cellular metabolism.

Assess baseline respiratory patterns, and auscultate breath sounds. Cardiogenic shock frequently is complicated by CHF manifested by dyspnea and tachypnea. Auscultation of lung fields reveals varying degrees of adventitious sounds (crackles, rhonchi, and wheezes) as air moves through narrowed air passages, fluid, and mucus. Early in shock, respirations are increased and deep. With the progression of shock, toxic metabolic by-products and inadequate energy production cause generalized muscle weakness and subsequent hypoventilation. The patient begins to show signs of respiratory distress, using accessory muscles in the neck, shoulders, chest, and abdomen with flaring of nostrils, gasping, and fighting for air.

Heart sounds will be abnormal with an S_3, S_4, or both, indicating ventricular noncompliance. A shift of the point of maximum impulse or a strong left ventricular thrust reflects an ineffective cardiac muscle.

Level of consciousness. Recognize subtle changes in the patient's level of consciousness because frequently it is a first sign of impending shock. Early in shock the awake, alert, oriented patient can quickly become confused, agitated, and restless. Other changes may be a sleep pattern disturbance, a personality change, poor judgment, or paranoia, which result from inadequate cerebral blood flow.

As shock progresses, the brain has less oxygen supply, and thus the patient can move through stages of lethargy and drowsiness. Response to verbal stimuli can decrease to states of stupor and coma. In severe shock states the patient usually does not respond to any stimuli.

Skin perfusion. Assess the temperature, color, turgor, texture, and moistness of regions of skin stretched over bones where there is minimal muscle. Palpation of the skin of the arm and thigh can be misleading because of heat from skeletal muscle circulation.

Assess the patient's skin for adequate capillary refill by applying pressure over a nailbed until blanching occurs. The rate at which blanching disappears is an indication of perfusion. In shock states, capillary refill occurs slowly (usually more than 3 seconds) because perfusion is reduced. Assess the skin for edema. As the heart becomes an ineffective pump, interstitial fluid accumulates in dependent areas because of increased venous pressure. Clinical signs of peripheral circulatory collapse are cool, pale, clammy, mottled skin, which indicates collapse of the dorsal veins of the hands and feet. Assess mucous membranes for signs of peripheral or central cyanosis. Peripheral cyanosis is caused by decreased blood flow, which is easily observed in the nailbeds or earlobes. Central cyanosis is related to oxygen deficiency, which

can be noted by a bluish discoloration of the skin around the lips, mouth, nose, and mucous membranes and beneath the tongue. Central cyanosis is present when there is approximately 5 g/dl of unoxygenated hemoglobin in the circulation.[29]

Urinary output. Assess hourly urinary output levels and specific gravity via an indwelling urinary catheter and urinometer readings for accuracy. In shock states, urinary output falls, and the specific gravity rises related to hormonal compensation. Initially the kidneys conserve water by concentrating urine. As shock progresses, renal function drastically deteriorates, with urinary output falling below 20 ml/hour and the specific gravity dropping because the kidneys are unable to concentrate urine and excrete toxic waste products. The decreased hourly output also can indicate decreased visceral blood flow.

Other signs and symptoms. Any type of exertion may require exaggerated effort by patients. They will experience varying degrees of generalized muscle fatigue and weakness secondary to reduced energy production. Ascites increases abdominal girth. Tenderness or pain in the right upper quadrant may appear from liver involvement related to increased venous pressure and right ventricular failure. Bowel sounds may be absent or diminished because of decreased peristalsis and redistribution of sympathetic blood flow. Patients may have nausea, anorexia, constipation, or abdominal distention from gastrointestinal stasis.

Perceiving and feeling patterns

If patients are conscious, they may verbalize feelings of hopelessness, anger, isolation, or powerlessness. Sensory overload also is a common problem, particularly when a lot of technical equipment is being used.

Anxiety and fear levels of patients and families must be assessed in the physiologic, psychologic, sociologic, and environmental domains. Because levels of consciousness vary in shock, patients frequently do not comprehend what they are told.

Medical and nursing diagnoses

The medical diagnosis is cardiogenic shock. The most common human responses anticipated for a patient in cardiogenic shock are indicated by the following nursing diagnoses:

1. Severely decreased cardiac output related to mechanical factors (preload, afterload, and inotropic state of the myocardium) and electrical factors (rate, rhythm, or conduction)
2. Anxiety and fear related to severity of condition, family distress, or threat of death

For each of these diagnoses, the patient outcomes, nursing prescriptions, and evaluation criteria are outlined with a discussion of the factual information that supports the plan and implementation of care.

NURSING
DIAGNOSIS 1

Severely decreased cardiac output related to mechanical factors (preload, afterload, or inotropic state of the myocardium) and electrical factors (rate, rhythm, or conduction) (exchanging pattern)

PATIENT OUTCOMES	NURSING PRESCRIPTIONS	EVALUATION
Patient will demonstrate increased ventricular performance and hemodynamic stability as indicated by systolic blood pressure of 90 to 110 mm Hg; diastolic blood pressure of 60 to 80 mm Hg; pulse pressure within normal limits; palpable pulses; respirations of 10 to 20 breaths per minute; PAWP of 12 to 15 mm Hg; adequate tissue perfusion (skin warm and dry, temperature normal); urinary output of 30 ml/hour or greater; electrolyte and BUN levels, creatinine clearance, and specific gravity within normal limits; normal orientation and lack of restlessness, confusion or psychosis; and normal neurologic status and level of consciousness.	Assess patient's ventricular performance and hemodynamic stability by assessing blood and pulse pressure; peripheral pulses; respirations; PAWP; skin temperature and color; urinary output level; electrolyte and BUN levels, creatinine clearance, and specific gravity; orientation, level of consciousness, and neurologic status.	Patient demonstrated systolic blood pressure of 90 to 110 mm Hg; diastolic blood pressure of 60 to 80 mm Hg; normal pulse pressure and pulses; respirations between 10 to 20/min; PAWP between 12 to 15 mm Hg; normal, warm and dry skin; urinary output of 30 ml/hour or greater; normal electrolyte and BUN levels, creatinine clearance, and specific gravity; normal orientation and ability to communicate; and normal neurologic status.
Patient's circulating blood volume will respond to an intravenous fluid challenge as demonstrated by an increased PAWP and pulmonary artery pressure.	Monitor PAWP and pulmonary artery pressure before, during, and after intravenous fluid challenges.	Patient's PAWP and pulmonary artery pressure returned to normal after a fluid challenge.
Patient will demonstrate no complications from the intraarterial line, including lack of erythema at insertion, intact radial pulse, and pink nail beds without impaired capillary refill.	Monitor arterial line insertion site for signs of erythema and normal radial pulse, nail bed color, and capillary refill.	Patient demonstrated no complications from the intraarterial line.
Patient will demonstrate no complications from hemodynamic monitoring of pulmonary artery and right atrial pressures and PAWP, including lack of dysrhythmias and infection at insertion site.	Observe pulmonary artery catheter insertion site for signs of infection and watch for dysrhythmias that might be caused by pulmonary artery catheter placement.	Patient demonstrated no complications from the pulmonary artery catheter.
Patient will demonstrate increased cardiac output and improved peripheral perfusion in response to sympathomimetic drugs.	Administer sympathomimetic drugs (dopamine, norepinephrine, isoproterenol, neosynephrine, and epinepherine) as ordered and record drug dose, volume infused, and patient response.	Patient demonstrated improved cardiac output and lowered peripheral resistance in response to sympathomimetic drugs.
Patient will be free of pulmonary edema as evidenced by lack of dyspnea and orthopnea and a PAWP between 15 and 20 mm Hg.	Monitor patient for signs of pulmonary edema, including dyspnea, orthopnea, and an elevated PAWP.	Patient did not demonstrate signs of pulmonary edema.
Patient will be free of dysrhythmias.	Monitor patient for dysrhythmias.	Patient demonstrated no dysrhythmias.
Patient will maintain balanced intake and output levels.	Monitor hourly intake and output levels.	Patient maintained balanced intake and output levels.

NURSING
DIAGNOSIS 1 **Severely decreased cardiac output related to mechanical factors (preload, afterload, or inotropic state of the myocardium) and electrical factors (rate, rhythm, or conduction) (exchanging pattern)—cont'd**

PATIENT OUTCOMES	NURSING PRESCRIPTIONS	EVALUATION
Cardiac output will be adequately maintained as evidenced by adequate VAD flow; normal vital signs; adequate urine output; warm, pink and dry skin; lack of dysrhythmias; and normal cerebral function.	Institute the following: Monitor blood pressure, right atrial and pulmonary artery pressure, PAWP hourly. Monitor indicators of perfusion, including urine output; skin color and temperature; cardiac rhythm; and sensorsium. Monitor VAD flow (L/min) and communicate with VAD team regarding any signs and symptoms of VAD dysfunction. Compute thermodilution cardiac output (CO) for left VAD (LVAD) patient and Fick CO for right VAD (RVAD) patient every 4 hours. Observe for volume depletion and replace as ordered with blood, fluid, and colloids. Observe for sign and symptoms of cardiac tamponade. Assess daily patient's intrinsic ventricular function with VAD team. Monitor indicators of perfusion when VAD flow is decreased. Observe arterial pressure waveform for dicrotic notch for LVAD patient and pulmonary artery dicrotic notch for RVAD patient.	Patient maintained adequate cardiac output as evidenced by adequate VAD flow; normal vital signs; warm, pink and dry skin; lack of dysrhythmias; and normal cerebral function.
Patient will maintain satisfactory oxygenation and respiratory status.	Institute the following: While patient is intubated and on ventilator, follow unit procedure for ventilator checks and arterial blood gas and mixed venous oxygen measurements. Verify endotracheal tube placement by chest x-ray film. Suction every 2 hours and as necessary. Auscultate breath sounds every 2 hours.	Patient maintained satisfactory oxygenation and respiratory status.
Patient will maintain hemostasis with normalization of blood clotting factors.	Institute the following: Observe for bleeding from any source (chest tubes, urine, stool, and gastrointestinal tract.) Observe dressing sites for bleeding. Evaluate daily hematologic profile, thromboplastin time, activated clotting time, reticulocyte count, and fibrinogen and fibrin split products. Keep extra set of VAD tubing and clamps at bedside.	Patient maintained hemostasis with normalization of blood clotting factors.

Continued.

NURSING DIAGNOSIS 1   **Severely decreased cardiac output related to mechanical factors (preload, afterload, or inotropic state of the myocardium) and electrical factors (rate, rhythm, or conduction) (exchanging pattern)—cont'd**

PATIENT OUTCOMES	NURSING PRESCRIPTIONS	EVALUATION
Patient will exhibit no evidence of thrombi formation.	Institute the following: If VAD flows are decreased, be aware that patient is susceptible to thrombi formation. Check with physician regarding anticoagulation therapy before decreasing flows. Observe device hourly for thrombus formation. Administer anticoagulation therapy as ordered.	Patient exhibited no evidence of thrombi formation.
Patient will not exhibit evidence of infection related to multiple invasive lines. There will be no sign of redness or drainage from cannula and invasive lines of VAD. Temperature and white blood cell count will be normal.	Institute the following: Observe for redness or drainage from VAD cannula and invasive lines. Monitor temperature. Evaluate the white blood cell count daily. Use strict aseptic technique.	Patient exhibited no evidence of infection.

Plan and intervention for severely decreased cardiac output

Providing care for the patient experiencing cardiogenic shock is one of the most challenging situations in critical care. The psychodynamics of this syndrome and treatment of the whole person must be foremost in the nurse's and physician's minds. The clinical setting and constant monitoring required can be psychologically devastating to patients and families. Patients' conscious thoughts, images, and emotions must be assessed, monitored, and dealt with by the nurse just as carefully as the drugs required in the treatment plan. Because shock can progress to a critical state in a matter of minutes, patients, as well as family members, must receive simple, concise, accurate information; realistic reassurance; and eye contact from the nurse as information is conveyed.

General comfort is vital. Patients should be placed in as comfortable a position as possible. A supine position facilitates venous return. Frequently the patient is more comfortable at a 30-degree angle, especially when dyspnea or pulmonary edema is present.

Nursing assessments and interventions are performed continuously to determine and deal with any change in patient status. Vital signs, skin perfusion, hourly outputs, change in sensorium, absence or stabilization of dysrhythmias, hemodynamic monitoring measurements, anxiety level, absence of signs and symptoms of pulmonary edema,

blood gas and electrolyte levels, and the patient's pain level should be continuously assessed and evaluated.

Invasive hemodynamic monitoring

Because of the rapidly changing physiologic states that occur in shock, invasive hemodynamic monitoring should be done when possible to evaluate the effects of therapy (see Chapter 7). Because arterial blood pressure is difficult to assess in shock states, an indwelling arterial catheter inserted in the radial artery is an accurate method for assessing blood pressure and evaluating the patient's blood gas level and response to pharmacologic agents. PAWPs and cardiac index measurements are critical indicators of the effects of therapy. Fiberoptics have been added to the pulmonary artery catheter to allow a continuous display of mixed venous oxygen saturation (SvO_2). The adequacy of oxygen supply and use by the tissues is assessed by measuring SvO_2. Measures to improve oxygen supply, reduce oxygen demand, or both, may then be matched to the physiologic profile characteristics of the patient's cardiogenic shock syndrome.[182]

Major principles of medical management

In cardiogenic shock the major principles of medical management follow[68]:

   1. Increasing ventricular performance by adjustment of left ventricular filling pressure

2. Pharmacologically increasing myocardial contractility, reducing peripheral vascular resistance, or both
3. Aggressively treating dysrhythmias
4. Reversing hypoxemia and metabolic acidosis
5. Controlling electrolyte disturbances
6. Mechanically increasing myocardial contractility, reducing peripheral vascular resistance, or both

Increasing ventricular performance. The initial priority in treating cardiogenic shock patients is to expand the circulating blood volume with intravenous fluids. Cardiogenic shock from AMI almost always requires intravenous fluids for several reasons. Usually there is a low circulating blood volume, which causes shock with the AMI. Also, a mild volume overload may help the patient because an increased volume return to the infarcted left ventricle may improve myocardial contractility.

The type of fluid used depends on the clinical situation. If the patient's PAWP is not abnormally low, 5% dextrose in water is used. However, if the patient's PAWP or pulmonary artery end-diastolic pressure is abnormally low or clinical signs or laboratory data suggest sodium loss (because of vomiting, diarrhea, diuretic therapy, or prior vasoconstrictor therapy), isotonic saline, half-isotonic saline, low-molecular-weight dextran (dextran 40), or plasma may be used.

Ventricular performance is determined primarily by preload, afterload, and contractility. Therefore in patients with cardiogenic shock a fluid balance needs to be obtained to optimize cardiac output without causing or exacerbating pulmonary edema.

Obtaining serial readings of PAWP or pulmonary artery end-diastolic pressure is the most helpful and reliable way of determining whether a fluid challenge is needed in the cardiogenic shock patient. This approximates the diastolic pressure within the left ventricle and can determine whether the circulating blood volume needs to be expanded. A low or normal PAWP indicates the need for intravenous fluids. A low PAWP or pulmonary artery end-diastolic pressure with signs of pulmonary congestion in the patient still indicate that intravenous fluids are needed, although they should be administered cautiously.

Pharmacologically increasing contractility and reducing peripheral vascular resistance. Sympathomimetic drugs should be used to increase myocardial contractility and reduce peripheral vascular resistance. The goal of drug therapy is to increase cardiac output and raise the systolic blood pressure to 90 to 100 mm Hg. To reach effective doses of these drugs as quickly as possible, institution-approved guidelines for the preparation and titration of the drugs offer a quick, reliable reference for nursing management of the patient in shock. Following such guidelines prevents periods of underaggressive or overaggressive therapy. These guidelines should include generic name, drug action, dosage, preparation, administration, selected side effects, special information, references, and signature of approval from medical and nursing directors for that institution.

Sympathomimetic drugs (see Table 11-1) are frequently used in the medical management of the patient with cardiogenic shock. Adrenergic drugs act in five ways on the cardiovascular system (see p. 305).

Catecholamine drugs most frequently used in cardiogenic shock are dobutamine, dopamine, norepinepherine or levarterenol, epinephrine, metaraminol, and isoproterenol. In patients with cardiogenic shock these drugs may be given in combination because of their different effects. For example, dopamine at very low doses increases renal blood flow but has minimal inotropic effects. It may be given with norepinephrine (levarterenol) to increase cardiac inotropy. These drugs should be given through a central venous line for accurate delivery and to avoid localized sloughing of the tissue should they infiltrate.[137]

Cardiac output is greatly reduced in the patient with cardiogenic shock, and peripheral vascular resistance is elevated. Reducing peripheral vascular resistance can enable the left ventricle to eject blood more easily, thus improving cardiac output. Vasodilator therapy therefore is useful in augmenting cardiac output and in improving tissue perfusion. Because vasodilator therapy can produce hypotension, however, it is not recommended for patients with a systolic blood pressure under 90 mm Hg. The use of combined inotropic agents and vasodilators can be more effective in increasing left ventricular function than either type of drug used alone.[104]

Treating dysrhythmias. Cardiac monitoring should be continuous because dysrhythmias may occur with cardiogenic shock. Bradydysrhythmias may cause hypotension with an AMI. When cardiogenic shock is associated with bradydysrhythmias, cardiac output may be decreased. Intravenous atropine, 0.4 to 0.6 mg, may be given to increase heart rate to maintain cardiac output.

Reversing hypoxemia and metabolic acidosis. The patient should be assessed for an adequate airway. Arterial blood gas analysis is done to ascertain pH and oxygen status. Initially, in the shock state, common complications are metabolic acidosis, hypotension, and tissue ischemia from decreased perfusion. When a patient is in shock, a Venturi mask at low flow rates usually does not raise the PaO_2 to the appropriate level. The PaO_2 should be maintained at 70 to 120 mm Hg (normal is 100 mm Hg). If the PaO_2 is lower than 50 mm Hg, intubation and assisted or controlled respirations with a volume-cycled ventilator is necessary. Metabolic acidosis should be treated with sodium bicarbonate according to the results of blood gas analyses until the pH is corrected. Maximal oxygenation and improved systemic perfusion also help increase aerobic metabolism, thus decreasing lactic acidosis. In rare situations, extracorporeal oxygenation with use of the membrane lung has been used successfully to treat patients with shock lung.[142]

TABLE 11-1

Sympathomimetic Amines Commonly Used in the Treatment of Shock

Drug	Dysrhythmogenic potential	Usual intravenous dosage*	Adrenergic effects			Comments
			Dosage	α	β (cardiac)	
Dopamine (Intropin)	Moderate to marked	2-10 µg/kg/min	Small Large	Minimal Marked	Minimal Moderate	Exhibits a unique "dopaminergic" effect, increasing renal blood flow at dosages of less than 6 µg/kg/min; may cause nausea and vomiting
Dobutamine (Dubutrex)	Minimal	2.5-10.0 µg/kg/min	Predominantly stimulates myocardial β-receptors responsible for inotropy			Has minimal chronotropic and peripheral vasoconstrictor effects; is especially useful in cardiogenic shock
Norepinephrine (levarterenol) (Levophed)	Moderate	2-8 µg/min	Small Large	Moderate Marked	Minimal Moderate	Despite β-adrenergic effects, may cause reflex slowing of heart rate because of increase in blood pressure
Metaraminol (Aramine)	Moderate	8-15 µg/kg/min	Small Large	Minimal Moderate	Minimal Moderate	Appears to act in part by activating release of endogenous catecholamines
Methoxamine (Vasoxyl)	None	8-15 µg/kg/min	Pure α-receptor stimulation			Is of particular value in patients with shock who have a good cardiac function and low peripheral resistance
Phenylephrine (Neo-Synephrine)	None	5-20 µg/min	Predominantly α-receptor stimulation			
Isoproterenol (Isuprel)	Marked	2-20 µg/min	Pure β-receptor stimulation			May cause tremor, anxiety, and lethal dysrhythmias
Epinephrine (Adrenalin)	Marked	1-4 µg/min	Small Large	Minimal Moderate	Moderate Marked	May cause tremor and anxiety

*The usual objective of therapy is to raise the systolic blood pressure to 90 to 100 mm Hg; larger or smaller dosages may be required in any given case.

From De Sanctis RW: Shock. In Rubenstein E and Federman P, editors: Cardiovascular medicine III, 1983, Scientific American Medicine.

Controlling electrolyte disturbances. The most common electrolyte disturbance in patients with AMI and cardiogenic shock is hyponatremia, which is caused in part by low-sodium diets, poor-to-minimal eating, and low-sodium liquids such as water and ginger ale. When crackles are present, patients frequently receive thiazide or loop diuretics, causing sodium ion loss. With AMI, there is also associated stress, causing excess ADH secretion and a retention in body water, thereby diluting the remaining serum sodium. The hyponatremic state can be further aggravated when cardiogenic shock develops. Sympathomimetic drugs produce vasoconstriction, which causes excess transudation of fluid from the vascular system to the interstitial tissues; thus circulating blood volume decreases. Hyponatremia can be corrected by administering dextrose in isotonic saline or dextran 40 instead of 5% dextrose in water.[159]

Mechanically increasing contractility and reducing peripheral vascular resistance. Limitations exist in the capacity of pharmacologic agents to reduce myocardial oxy-

gen demands and improve cardiac output. Mechanical assistance is therefore an essential component of the armamentarium for advanced cardiac therapies. IABP is the first line of cardiac assist devices that may further reduce oxygen demands and enhance circulation. This counterpulsation device is, however, contingent on a left ventricle that is able to contract and sustain the circulation in part. If the left ventricle is severely depressed and needs to be totally but temporarily relieved of the workload associated with left ventricular contraction, an LVAD may be used. Biventricular assistance may be required, which can be provided by some designs of VADs or a total artificial heart.

IABP. The intraaortic balloon (IAB) is a distensible (adult capacity ranges from 20 to 60 cc), nonthrombogenic balloon mounted on a vascular catheter, which is most commonly inserted percutaneously through the femoral artery using Seldinger technique. The balloon is passed retrogradely up the descending thoracic aorta to a position of rest in situ, just below the origin of the left subclavian artery. Inflation of the balloon occurs during diastole with a light, inert gas such as helium; the balloon is deflated during isovolumetric contraction (Fig. 11-11). Despite clinical evidence supporting the beneficial effects of IABP, the underlying mechanisms and basis for hemodynamic improvements are not clearly understood.[27] Balloon inflation during diastole augments intraaortic pressure; blood volume in the aorta is actively displaced proximally and distally. *Volume displacement* is an intended physiologic benefit. Arterial perfusion can be improved by blood volume displacement secondary to balloon inflation. Balloon inflation in diastole also augments the intrinsic *Windkessel effect*, which describes the principle whereby the majority of peripheral run-off or systemic perfusion actually occurs during diastole.[9] Systolic ejection requires a tremendous amount of energy just to move the load of stroke volume out through the aortic valve and into the descending aortic arch. Energy accompanying systole is stored in the elastic aorta as potential energy until diastole, when the elastic aorta releases this energy in the form of kinetic or usable energy; this propels the distal run-off of blood to the periphery (Windkessel effect) (Fig. 11-12).

Coronary perfusion is "potentially" increased with balloon inflation, but it depends on the degree of autoregulatory vasodilatation already in place. Myocardial ischemia is a potent stimulus for increasing blood flow and oxygen delivery to the myocardium through the autoregulated process of vasodilatation. If the coronary arteries are already maximally dilated, little improvement in coronary flow occurs with balloon inflation in diastole.[30]

Autoregulatory vasodilatation of coronary vessels is, however, impaired by atherosclerosis. Augmentation of coronary perfusion pressure by balloon inflation in diastole may therefore cause some improvement in coronary perfusion through atherosclerotic coronary arteries. Balloon inflation also facilitates collateral pathways of perfusion.[131]

Deflation of the IAB during isovolumetric contraction can reduce aortic end-diastolic pressure. Such action lowers the impedance to left ventricular ejection. Thus the afterload of cardiac work is decreased, thereby lowering myo-

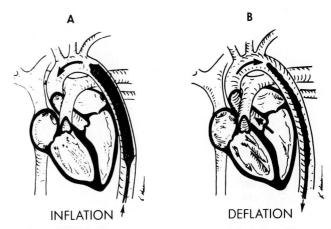

INFLATION ↑   DEFLATION ↓

FIG. 11-11   Counterpulsation effects of IABP. **A,** During diastole, the balloon is inflated with helium. **B,** During isovolumetric contraction, preceding systolic ejection, the balloon is deflated.
From Quaal SJ: Comprehensive intra-aortic balloon pumping, St Louis, 1984, The CV Mosby Co.

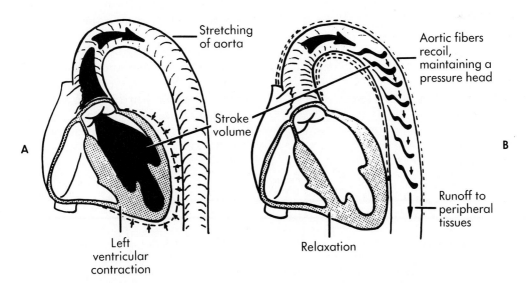

FIG. 11-12   Windkessel effect. **A,** During systole, the elastic proximal aorta and large arteries stretch to accommodate cardiac stroke volume. The force imparted to blood by ventricular contraction is stored as potential energy in the elastic arterial wall. **B,** During ventricular diastole, the fibers in the aorta recoil, maintaining a pressure head. Runoff into peripheral tissues continues in diastole under this pressure head created by stored elastic energy in the aorta.
From Quaal SJ: Comprehensive intra-aortic balloon pumping, St Louis, 1984, The CV Mosby Co.

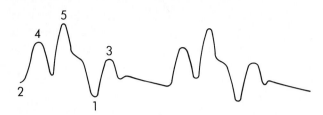

FIG. 11-13 Arterial pressure waveform as impacted by IAB counterpulsation. *5*, Peak diastolic inflated pressure; *3*, assisted systole; *4*, patient systole; *1*, assisted aortic end-diastolic pressure; *2*, patient aortic end-diastolic pressure.

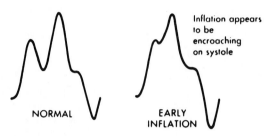

FIG. 11-14 Early balloon inflation. Inflation appears to encroach on the previous systole.

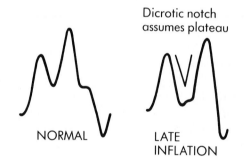

FIG. 11-15 Late balloon inflation. A ledge appears at the dicrotic notch.

cardial oxygen consumption. Akyurekli[5] studied the afterload-lowering effects of balloon deflation during isovolumetric contraction, independent of diastolic augmentation. IAB counterpulsation decreased afterload only in normotensive patients. A plausible explanation for this lack of afterload reduction in hypotensive states is that the aortic wall becomes compliant and loses its tone or supportive structure (secondary to hypotension). During IAB inflation, the aortic wall simply gives way or moves with balloon inflation. This mechanism impairs the expected elevation of aorta pressure during balloon inflation.[23,30] If intraaortic pressure is not elevated with balloon inflation, volume displacement does not occur. Failure to achieve volume displacement with balloon inflation prevents the needed afterload reduction at IAB deflation.

Aries, Division of St. Jude Medical (Chelmsford, Mass), Datascope Corp. (Montvale, NJ), Kontron (Everett, Mass), and Mansfield (Mansfield, Mass) manufacture balloon pump consoles that are user friendly. The nurse can easily learn the skills required to interact with the pump console. It is critical that the nurse understand the correct *"timing"* of inflation-deflation, which is achievable only by assessment of arterial pressure waveforms. Therefore, IAB counterpulsation should *never* begin without a reliable arterial pressure line in place. Percutaneous balloons also include an inner-pressure monitoring line, which allows for immediate recording of invasive blood pressure when the balloon is placed in the descending thoracic aorta.

Balloon counterpulsation has an impact on arterial pressure waveforms. For "timing," the patient should be placed on an assist ratio of 1:2. Diastolic augmented (balloon inflation) pressure is the highest pressure generated in the cardiac cycle, hence the term *peak diastolic augmented pressure.* Balloon inflation displaces blood in the aorta proximally and distally. Pressure in the aorta decreases as blood is displaced. Therefore on deflation, the aortic end-diastolic pressure is lower than the aortic end-diastolic pressure not preceded by balloon inflation. A difference in the arterial pressure waveforms exists when the balloon inflates and deflates with every other heartbeat (Fig. 11-13).

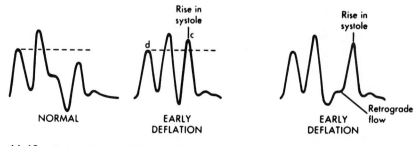

FIG. 11-16 Early balloon deflation. Assisted systole *(c)* appears higher than patient systole *(d)*, and a plateau may appear on the ascending limb of assisted diastole, indicating retrograde perfusion.

Hemodynamically, the aortic valve closes before the appearance of the dicrotic notch on the subclavian, balloon inner-cannula, or radial artery pressure monitoring lines. This delay is approximately 40 milliseconds (msec). To compensate for this delay, inflation needs to occur approximately 40 msec before the midpoint of the dicrotic notch. This earlier, compensated inflation is achieved when the dicrotic notch assumes a U shape as contrasted with its natural V shape. Proper deflation is recognized by two landmarks on the arterial pressure waveforms (Fig. 11-13). Assisted systole must be lower than patient systole, and assisted aortic end-diastolic pressure must be lower than patient aortic-end diastolic pressure.

Early inflation is illustrated in Fig. 11-14. Balloon inflation seems to encroach on the previous systole. The dicrotic notch is no longer visible because of the early rise of augmented pressure as the balloon inflates. Early inflation can raise the pressure of the aorta, thus closing the aortic valve prematurely which impedes complete emptying of the ventricle. Regurgitation of blood may occur into the left ventricle, cardiac output may decrease, and intraventricular volume (preload) and pressure may increase. Fig. 11-15 illustrates late inflation that occurs well after the aortic valve closes. A plateau appears at the location of the dicrotic notch. Diastolic augmented pressure may be lowered because of late inflation.

Early deflation (Fig. 11-16) is marked by an assisted systole that is higher than patient systole. Afterload reduction occurs but it is too soon to benefit the next systole. Thus the premature drop in assisted aortic end-diastolic pressure is nonphysiologic. Because of the time delay before the next systolic ejection, retrograde flow may occur from the coronary, cerebral, or renal arteries in the attempt to restore the aortic end-diastolic pressure to its baseline. Retrograde perfusion may also be identified by a plateau on the upstroke of the next assisted systole.

Late deflation (Fig. 11-17) does not produce a lowering of assisted aortic end-diastolic pressure, which may be higher than patient aortic end-diastolic pressure. The left ventricle must eject against the impedance of a balloon, which is still partially inflated. Myocardial oxygen consumption is increased. The rate of rise of assisted systole (dp/dt) may be prolonged because of the increase in resistance. However, one study suggests that late deflation may be therapeutic in some patients because of an active transfer of energy from the balloon to the ejecting column of blood.[172]

Ventricular assist devices. Hemodynamic criteria for application of VAD therapy apply to patients with cardiogenic shock who have a cardiac index less than 2 L/min/m², systolic blood pressure less than 90 mm Hg, left or right atrial pressure greater than 20 mm Hg, urine output level less than 20 ml/hour, and elevated systemic vascular resistance greater than 2100 dyne-seconds-cm^{-5} despite the use of maximal pharmacologic therapy and IAB support. Patients who meet these criteria should be excluded if they have renal failure (BUN level greater than 100 mg and creatinine clearance greater than 4.0 mg), chronic lung disease, metastatic cancer, chronic liver disease, sepsis, or neurologic deficits.[121]

Roller-pump VADs. The VAD roller pumps are occlusive in design, compressing blood at a manually set point and forcing it forward. The occlusion setting must be high enough to maintain satisfactory blood flow. Blood is evacuated from the left atrium into the roller pump circuit, which intermittently occludes the tubing; this provides the momentum to return flow back through the aortic cannula.

Hemolysis has been a recurrent complication of roller-pump VAD assistance. Factors known or believed to influence hemolysis on a roller pump include occlusions, roller settings, rotary speed (revolutions per minute [rpm]), number of rollers in the pump, tubing material, and tubing diameter.[74] All of these variables have been studied. Results do not suggest any optimum geometric shapes or ratio's of sizes to minimize blood trauma; each variable contributes independently to the presence or absence of hemolysis. At the extreme range of underocclusion, however, hemolysis is minimal regardless of roller or tubing size.[113] If postoperative bleeding is not great, patients receive 250 to 750 units of heparin per hour for 4 to 6 hours after the operation. The activated clotting time is maintained between 150 to 250 seconds.[144]

A 28 to 32 French (Fr) venous cannula is inserted through a purse-string suture into the left atrium through the left atrial appendage or the right superior pulmonary vein. A 5- to 6-mm arterial cannula is inserted through a purse-string suture into the ascending aorta. The tips are advanced beyond the left subclavian artery to decrease the potential for cerebral embolization. Cannulas are brought out through the sternotomy or through a separate parasternal incision.

Centrifugal VADs. Bio-medicus, Inc. (Eden Prairie, Minn) and Sarns, Inc./3m (Ann Arbor, Mich) centrifugal

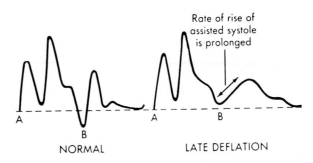

FIG. 11-17   Late balloon deflation. Assisted aortic end-diastolic pressure *(B)* is higher than patient aortic end-diastolic pressure *(A)*.

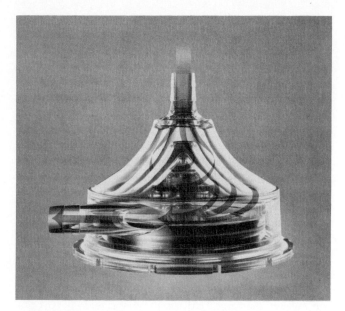

FIG. 11-18 Bio-Medicus vortex certrifugal VAD disposable pump head.

Courtesy Bio-medicus Co, Eden Prairie, Minn.

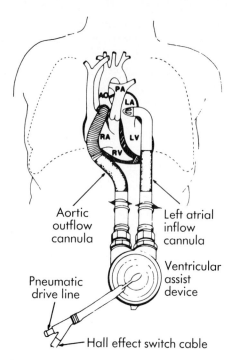

FIG. 11-19 Pierce-Donachy VAD with the inflow cannula receiving blood from the left atrium and the outflow cannula returning blood to the ascending aorta.

From Farrar DJ: Clinical modes of a ventricular assist device, IEEE Engineering in Medicine and Biology Magazine 6:19, 1986.

pumps are FDA approved for use as VADs. These vortex pumps are constructed of nonthrombogenic acrylic magnetic cones, which couple and rotate to propel blood forward in a circular motion, generating centrifugal force, pressure, and flow (Fig. 11-18).[12] Centrifugal pumps are nonocclusive; therefore high negative pressures cannot develop. Flow is controlled by adjusting the rpm of the motor. The flow path of the pump is designed to eliminate turbulence and cavitation, thereby reducing damage to blood elements. Thus the pump is relatively atraumatic to blood. Centrifugal devices can capture the entire left or right atrial blood flow and can pump up to 10 L/min using continuous nonpulsatile flow.[134]

Aortic cannulation is via the right superior pulmonary vein or into the roof of the left atrium at its junction with the right superior pulmonary vein. Aortic cannulation is performed low in the ascending aorta with a standard aortic cannula. The cannulas are held in place with purse-string sutures and tourniquets.

Pneumatic VADs. Pneumatic (air-driven) pumps[97,125] provide pulsatile flow by puffs of air that compress a sac-type device that delivers a set volume of blood to the patient. The Pierce-Donachy (Thoratec Laboratories Corp, Berkeley, Calif) is a paracorporeal pneumatic device constructed of a machined polycarbonate housing containing an inner, flexible, seamfree, segmented polyurethane sac. The VAD uses Bjork-Shiley inlet and outlet valves and has a stroke volume of 65 ml with a dynamic ejection fraction of 0.75. A separate diaphragm is positioned between the side of the housing that receives the air and the blood sac, which thus isolates the blood sac

from the driving air (Fig. 11-19). The atrial cannula is a 51 Fr Sarns venous cannula coated with polyurethane and shaped to a right angle. The aortic cannula is a large-bore, wire-bound, segmented polyurethane tube. A pneumatic power unit provides the compressed air—driving pressure needed to expand the blood-containing sac and to apply vacuum to allow the sac to collapse during filling.

The Pierce-Donachy VAD can be operated under three control modes: (1) fixed rate, asynchronous to the heart rate; (2) full to empty; and (3) synchronous R wave. Fixed-rate asynchronous mode is not synchronized to the ECG. This variable stroke-volume method is the simplest control mode. It is useful for initiating support and for weaning patients from the device when less-than-maximal flow rates are desired. It is also used as a backup mode in case other synchronization signals are lost. The full-to-empty asynchronous method is offered in response to the blood flow needs of the body and, at the same time, provides a consistent washing of all blood-contacting surfaces in the blood pump to minimize the possibility of thrombus formation. A magnet (Hall switch) is used to determine when the blood pump is full; when the pump is full, a driving console initiates the ejection phase. Ejection then proceeds for a preset time. After completing ejection, the drive system switches back to a filling cycle to wait for another signal from the Hall switch, which indicates that the blood pump is again ready for ejection. R-wave synchronous counterpulsation synchronizes VAD to the intrinsic heart rate, resulting in a variable rate and stroke-volume control mode. The R wave of the ECG signals the drive console to end ejection. Pump filling coincides with biologic systole. Ejection then follows the biologic diastole (counterpulsation), which ends with the next R wave. The advantage of this mode is that a greater reduction in left ventricular pressure and volume is achieved and myocardial oxygen consumption is reduced. Disadvantages include difficulty with controlling filling and ejection with irregular heart rhythms. Also, a full VAD stroke volume may not be achieved, which inhibits complete washing of the blood-contacting surfaces of the blood pump. A predilection for thrombus formation therefore exists.[97,123]

Anticoagulation of patients with pneumatic and centrifugal VADs. Methods and degrees of anticoagulation vary for patients with pneumatic and centrifugal VADs.[85,103] Agents include heparin, dipyridamole, aspirin, warfarin, or dextran. High blood flow through the VAD (more than 1.5 to 2.0 L/min) is one of the best strategies to prevent clot formation. Anticoagulants may not need to be used during maximum flow periods. However, during VAD weaning and periods of decreased flow, anticoagulants are needed to decrease the predilection for clot formation.

McGovern, Sang, and Maker[103] demonstrated that the centrifugal vortex VAD could be used for up to 144 hours without anticoagulation. However, a group of panelists representing the Society of Thoracic Surgeons reported that the activated clotting time should be kept at 1.5 to 2 times normal with full heparin started when the chest flow output is less than 100 ml in 3 hours. Devries cautioned that platelets have a significant vasoactive effect, resulting in dilation of the vasculature with extreme reduction of systemic vascular resistance; this may lead to the appearance of hemostasis when in fact it may result from the low perfusion pressure and not true hemostasis.[121]

Bleeding has also been controlled by using fresh frozen plasma, autotransfusion, and platelets. Combined administration of prostacyclin analog and protease inhibitor (nafamstat mesilate) also has been effective in maintaining coagulation, hemolysis, and fibrinolysis at minimal levels.[122]

Biventricular assist devices. Approximately 50% of patients who need VAD support require biventricular support.[122] Ventricular assist can be implemented for the right or left ventricle, but failure can occur in the unassisted ventricle. Failure of the unsupported ventricle can occur immediately after the first ventricle is assisted or days later. Pennington and others[122] have demonstrated that patients with reversible myocardial injury benefit from temporary biventricular assistance because chemical and functional integrity can then return to the injured myocardial cells. Myocardial ischemia can severely deplete ATP levels and

produce myocardial depression. Creatine phosphate stores are exhausted, and metabolites of ATP[83] such as adenosine, hypoxanthine, and inosine, accumulate. Reibel and Rovetto[139] demonstrated that myocardial function remains depressed until the pool of ATP used directly in the contractile process returns to normal. Functional recovery is not instantaneous, and the use of biventricular assist devices is often required from several hours to several days. During this reperfusion period, high-energy phosphate levels increase, but myocardial edema is reduced, thus improving ventricular compliance.

Right ventricular failure can also occur as a consequence of increased pulmonary resistance rather than failure of the right ventricle's ability to contract. Injections of prostaglandin E_2 have been administered directly into the pulmonary artery to reduce pulmonary vascular resistance and the need for biventricular assistance.[121]

Novacor VAD. An implantable LVAD using an electromechanically driven dual pusher-plate blood pump has been employed in a multiinstitutional trial as a bridge to cardiac transplantation.[129,130,158] The device derives power and control from an external console via a percutaneous lead. Implanted in the left upper quadrant within the anterior abdominal wall, the blood pump is connected between the left ventricular apex and ascending aorta (Fig. 11-20). The blood pump consists of a seamless polyurethane

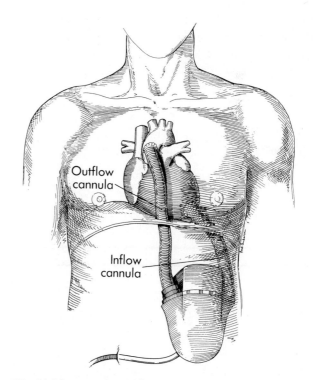

FIG. 11-20   Novacor LVAD.
From Smith SL: Issue and organ transplantation, St Louis, 1990, The CV Mosby Co.

sac bonded to dual, symmetrically opposed pusher plates and to a lightweight housing that incorporates valve fittings.

The pump has a smooth blood-contacting surface and uses pericardial tissue valves with custom silicone flanges (Baxter Healthcare Corp, Edwards Division, Santa Ana, Calif). The pump's geometric configuration was designed for optimal flow patterns without areas of stasis, flow separation, or turbulence. Maximum achievable stroke volume is 70 ml, with a pumping capacity of 10 L/min. It is very responsive, synchronously tracking heart rates as high as 240 beats per minute. The control console provides electrical power and continuously monitors the critical patient and LVAD variables. A physiology monitor incorporated within the console simultaneously displays the patient's ECG, left ventricular and systemic pressure waveforms, and pump volume tracings. A cathode-ray–tube terminal displays beat-by-beat digital information on device performance.

Patients receive minimal amounts of anticoagulants, typically intravenously administered low-dose heparin, platelet-modifying drugs, or both. The Novacor system is intended for left ventricular assistance only. Total support of the systemic circulation and substantial left ventricular unloading has been achieved with synchronous counterpulsation for up to 90 days in 20 patients.[130]

Hemopump. One of the newest VADs, the Johnson and Johnson Hemopump[2,150] is a catheter-mounted device that is the size of a pencil eraser. It consists of a minature turbine mounted inside a catheter. The device can propel 3.5 L/min of blood from the left ventricle into the aorta.

An impeller (rotor blade) rotates at high speeds, drawing blood from the left ventricle into the cannula. The thrust generated by this impeller propels blood into the descending aorta.

The Hemopump consists of the pump assembly, purge assembly, and the control console (Fig. 11-21). The pump assembly is inserted into an arterial femoral cutdown and is advanced retrogradely up the aorta, across the aortic valve into the left ventricle. A rotor acts as a propeller that turns at high speeds within this tightly fitting cylinder (catheter). A lifting action occurs, imparting a velocity to the blood drawn up from the left ventricle through the catheter, escaping through exit ports located more distally in the aortic catheter. An axial flow pump powered by an electromagnetically coupled motor is positioned in the descending aorta. A rotating magnet is connected to a flexible drive cable, which in turn is connected to the pump. The pump can generate 0.5 to 3.0 L/min of nonpulsatile, continuous blood flow up to 25,000 rpm.[148]

Lubrication is delivered to the pump and drive cable by 40% dextrose in water through a multiple lumen sheath, which also houses the drive cable. This dextrose-lubricating fluid infuses through the outer lumen of the multiple lumen sheath and is returned to a collection bag through central lumen. A 25-pound control unit provides power to the motor, which causes the magnet in the pump assembly to spin. The roller pump is responsible for controlling the delivery and collection of the 40% dextrose solution. Several clinical trials are in progress in the United States for patients in cardiogenic shock. Sixty-seven percent of patients in these trials have been weaned from the machine.[148,150]

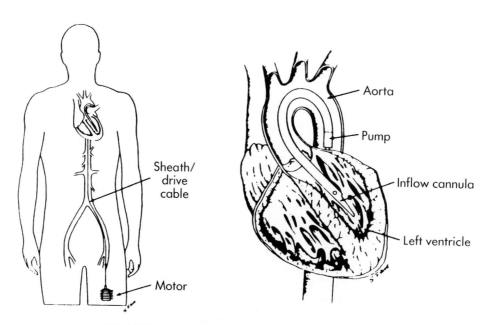

FIG. 11-21 Hemopump placement with femoral introduction.
Courtesy Johnson & Johnson, Rancho Cardova, CA.

Total artificial heart. Pneumatic total artificial hearts have been used successfully as temporary mechanical supports until cardiac transplantation occurs but have not been too successful as permanent cardiac replacements. An ellipsoidal, pneumatically driven diaphragm total artificial heart is now commercially available as a bridge to transplant device (Fig. 11-22). The Jarvik-7 is fashioned from components that consist of right and left hemispheric ventricles; Dacron connections to the remnant atria, pulmonary artery, and aorta (called *quick connects*); and four mechanical tilting-disk prosthetic valves, which ensure laminar flow. Inflow and outflow tracts are angled to provide correct alignment with the native vascular structures and to maintain good laminar flow without turbulence or stagnation.[76,82,132]

All four native heart valves and the ventricles are excised during the surgical procedure. Connection of the prosthetic ventricles to the native atria is then made by the Dacron felt cuffs, or *quick connects*. Attachment components to the great vessels, also called *quick connects,* are made of Dacron vascular prosthetic grafts. Suturing the total artificial heart as a unit directly to the native vascular structure would be impossible because the confines of the adult mediastinum limit anatomic exposure. Careful positioning of the implanted prosthetic ventricles allows their flat bases to be aligned adjacent to one another and to form a nearly spherical configuration. A small, circular patch of Velcro is attached to the housing of each ventricle to hold the two halves in position.[47]

The outer ventricular housing is molded from polyurethane reinforced with Dacron mesh; the base of each ventricle is made from aluminum or plastic. Interior surfaces are formed from segmented polyurethane, which is molded as one piece to eliminate seams and potential thrombus formation. Each ventricle is pneumatically powered by compressed air driven through silicone rubber tubing. An external heart-driver system controls the driveline pressure of compressed air that is pneumatically but intermittently pulsed through the ventricular air chambers at adjustable rates of 40 to 120 beats per minute.[133]

Each ventricle contains a flexible blood chamber—a diaphragm—that separates the air space from the blood-occupying space (Fig. 11-23). As air is intermittently pulsed in and out of the artificial ventricle, the diaphragm synchronously expands and deflates, allowing for filling of blood in diastole and forward ejection during systole. During diastole, the diaphragm collapses in direct proportion to the volume of blood that enters through the inflow port from the atria. As more blood enters the artificial ventricle's diaphragm, the bladder-type sac collapses in increasing amounts until the maximum bladder volume capacity is achieved.[133]

The base of each artificial ventricle is fitted with a tubular connector that attaches to a flexible polyurethane tubing or the driveline (Fig. 11-24). This 8-foot driveline connects at its origin to the outlet of an electropneumatic

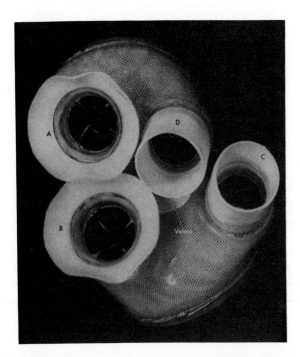

FIG. 11-22 The total artificial heart. Four mechanical tilting disk valves are used in the artificial heart. "Quick connects" for the atria (*A* and *B*) incorporate a cuff of polyurethane-covered felt. Quick connects for pulmonary artery *(C)* and aorta *(D)* consist of short pieces of Dacron-woven graft rather than a cuff.
Courtesy Brad Nelson, Medical Illustrations, The University of Utah, Salt Lake City, Utah.

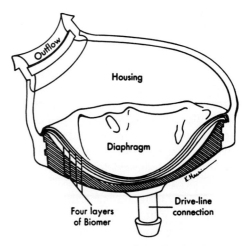

FIG. 11-23 Cross section of Jarvik-7 Symbion pumping diaphragm. Four layers of segmented polyurethane (Biomer) are used to fabricate this component of the artificial ventricle. Each layer is 0.006 inch thick. Dry graphite is placed between layers of Biomer for lubrication.
From Quaal SJ: Comprehensive intra-aortic balloon pumping, St Louis, 1984, The CV Mosby Co.

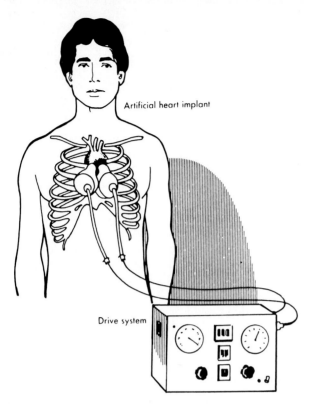

FIG. 11-24   Schematic drawing illustrating the total artificial heart implant with 8-foot drivelines attached to the Utah Heart Driver.

From Quaal SJ: Comprehensive intra-aortic balloon pumping, St Louis, 1984, The CV Mosby Co.

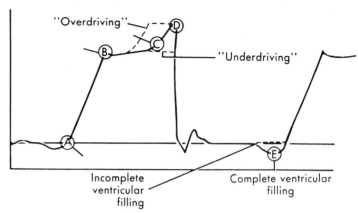

FIG. 11-25   Artificial ventricle driving pressure waveform. Solid line represents ideal pressure waveform. Significant landmarks of pressure waveform are identified. Distortions in pressure waveform that occur with overdriving and underdriving are labeled. *A,* End of diastole, *B,* Beginning of aortic flow, *C,* End of effective ejection, *D,* Peak driving pressure, *E,* Full filling of ventricle.

From Quaal SJ: Comprehensive intra-aortic balloon pumping, St Louis, 1984, The CV Mosby Co.

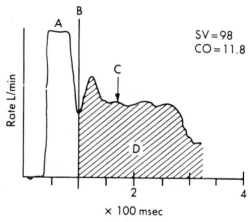

FIG. 11-26   Normal COMDU tracing. *A,* Initial elevation represents earliest portion of diastole, when exhaust valve opens and pressure equilibrates between ventricle and atmosphere. No air has yet left the ventricle. *B,* Vertical line displays where computer begins its calculation of stroke volume by measuring area under the curve. *C,* Line that represents flow of air from ventricle during diastole. *D,* Area beneath this curve, beginning at vertical calibration line, is equal to volume of blood entering ventricle and subsequently ejected (stroke volume).

From Quaal SJ: Comprehensive intra-aortic balloon pumping, St Louis, 1984, The CV Mosby Co.

control unit called the *heart driver.* This unit controls the influx of compressed air through the driveline, thus expanding the artificial ventricle in systole, and controls the exhaust of compressed air via a vacuum in diastole, thus collapsing the diaphragm.[133]

Driving pressures are recorded graphically (Fig. 11-25). Characteristic landmarks that the nurse must learn to recognize are onset of mechanical systole, ventricular ejection and aortic blood flow, end of ventricular ejection, peak driving pressure and end of mechanical systole, full emptying of the ventricle, and complete filling of the ventricle. Driving pressures are adjusted to the lowest value that completely empties the ventricle.[133]

Measurement of cardiac output is most valuable in assessing performance of the total artificial heart. *The cardiac output monitoring and diagnostic unit (COMDU)* provides continuous and reliable calculation of stroke volume and cardiac output. A computer senses the amount and rate of air exiting the right and left ventricles of the total artificial heart during diastole. Air displaced during diastole is equal to the volume of blood filling the diaphragm during the same period. This exhaust airflow signal is displayed on the television screen of the computer (Fig. 11-26). A cal-

ibration constant is used to convert the area under the exhaust air curve to volume in milliliters, or cardiac stroke volume.[183]

Presbyterian-University Hospital of Pittsburgh reported their experience with 16 patients who received total artificial hearts as bridges to transplantation. Postoperative anticoagulation therapy (heparin and dypyridamole) was designed to keep the partial thromboplastin time between 2 and 2.5 times normal. In all cases the function of the total artificial heart was adequate to support the needs of the recipient, and there were no mechanical difficulties with the device or drive system. The average time of implantation was 9 days. The reported limiting factor of the total artificial heart is the strikingly high incidence of mediastinitis.[70]

NURSING
DIAGNOSIS 2   **Anxiety and fear related to severity of condition, family distress, or threat of death (feeling pattern)**

PATIENT OUTCOMES	NURSING PRESCRIPTIONS	EVALUATION
Patient will demonstrate an understanding of reasons for ongoing assessment and management of anxiety, including: Quiet environment Explanations of all personnel, procedures, and equipment Touch and reassurance by nurse Relaxation skills	Continue to reassess states of anxiety and provide ways to decrease anxiety. Provide quiet environment. Explain all interventions. Offer reassurance. Teach relaxation and imagery skills.	Patient demonstrated an understanding of the reasons for assessment and management of anxiety.
Patient will verbalize feelings of anxiety and will talk spontaneously about fears. (If patient is intubated, specific communication codes will be used by nurse and patient.)	Provide quality time for patient to share worries and fears. Use common symbols for communication if patient is intubated.	Patient verbalized anxiety and fears.
Patient will use effective coping mechanisms during course of illness.	Focus on patient's strengths	Patient used effective coping mechanisms during course of illness. (List specific examples.)
Family will communicate stressors associated with patient's illness to staff.	Allow time for family to express worries and fears.	Family communicated stressors to staff.
Patient will verbalize fears of death.	Be present with patient and allow time for patient to talk about fears of dying.	Patient talked of death.
Family will verbalize fears that the patient may die.	If death seems eminent, be with patient and family to assist them through the death.	Patient's family acknowledged the impending death and shared feelings about death.
Family will receive support from nurses and clergy.	Provide spiritual support for patient through presence, life review, prayer, talking, and handholding. Allow family to be with patient. Call clergy for assistance, if requested.	Family received spiritual support and talked to nurses and clergy.

Plan and intervention for anxiety and fear

With the critically ill patient in cardiogenic shock, the situation is life threatening and can be psychologically devastating. Compounding the patient's stress are many types of mechanized equipment producing a variety of noises. Intubation, IABP, and VADs may require patient restraints. Helping the patient cope with this equipment is important to decrease feelings of anxiety, loss of control, and powerlessness.[11]

Increasing communication

Continuous assessment of the patient's anxiety level is essential and also difficult because of an altered level of consciousness from the shock state. In this situation, numerous barriers impede patient communication. Therefore nonverbal communication skills must be used to help decrease anxiety and fear. Touch by the nurse is a powerful form of communication that can convey attitudes and feelings of gentleness, caring, and understanding. Hand holding can be a regular therapeutic intervention to increase non-verbal communication. To enhance the therapeutic results, hand holding must be done with serious intent and at the appropriate time.[155]

A meeting between the physician, nurses, and patient's family should take place as soon as possible after admission to the CCU. This meeting helps enormously in communicating concern for the family, as well as in establishing a cooperative, trusting relationship. The family should be well informed about the patient's status. The staff should listen closely to the family and identify their feelings and coping ability. This enables them to enlist the family as an effective patient support system, as well as giving them guidelines for actively participating in the patient's care when appropriate.

Frequently, relatives need as much or more emotional support than the patient.[114] The nurse observes their behavior patterns to see whether they appear frantic or restless. They may need to be involved in the patient's care. This can reduce their anxiety and help them in dealing with the suffering and grief if the patient dies. They should be allowed help with simple procedures such as bathing, feeding, giving back rubs, caring for the mouth, and turning. If possible, and without compromising safety, the patient and family should have time alone with one another.

The dying patient and family

Many patients in cardiogenic shock do not recover. With the dying patient and family, the nurse moves from a cure-care model to a care model. The nurse has many responsibilities in helping patients achieve a peaceful death. The nurse considers personal beliefs about death, as well as the sociocultural views of the patient and family. Critically ill persons become distraught, depressed, and even terrified when they cannot make their needs known. Such feelings become even more complicated in our culturally integrated society.

The nurse should become aware of the values of patients and family, including their orientation to time, their attitudes toward death ("bad" or part of a natural order), and their concept of family. Cultural differences and priorities should be understood, as should role expectations. Religious beliefs should also be determined. The nurse must assess attitudes toward pain and bereavement, grief, and mourning practices. Nurses encounter many people with contrasting lifestyles and belief systems but must learn to cultivate cultural sensitivity, incorporate patient's beliefs into care plans, and help patients and families realize that life and death experiences are a part of personal and cultural values.

Despite an impressive array of therapeutic modalities, many patients in cardiogenic shock die. Nurses need to elicit from the patient or family coping strategies that have adequately sustained the patient in previous times of crisis. These include aspects of faith that can help in a crisis. The nurse determines whether faith can help the patient find answers.

Of all the health care professionals, the nurse has the highest degree of contact with dying persons and their families. When patients are in the end stages of cardiovascular dysfunction, there are specific therapeutic interventions that can be used. A powerful process is called *life review*.[43] To participate in this process, patients must be conscious and able to communicate. Even for unconscious patients, however, the process can be implemented with the family to assist them in coping with the impending death. Using the life review, the nurse helps patients and families reduce feelings of psychologic isolation, deal with unresolved conflicts, maintain self-esteem, and emphasize positive aspects of their lives. These benefits should be discussed with the patient and family before beginning the life review to enhance the outcomes of the process.

When the nurse has quiet time with the patient and feels that the moment is right for the life review, it can begin. There are no clear-cut steps. Responses are based on a sense of where the process is leading the patient. A question is asked about some significant people in the patient's life, or cues are taken from the patient's conversation or environment, such as pictures or personal objects. The response may be easy for the patient or difficult. If the question elicits memories of stressful events, the nurse helps the patient identify previous coping mechanisms. The patient is encouraged to review special events at different phases in life and to look at decisions such as the kind of treatment or care received, the wish to die at home or in the hospital, or special requests at the time of death. The patient is aided in dealing with unresolved dilemmas such as belief in an afterlife, higher guiding powers, or connections with others. The process might involve one session or many; these sessions vary in length, depending on the amount of exploring that the patient wants to do.

To facilitate the life review process, the nurse (1) encourages self-expression by the patient, (2) involves family members, (3) helps the patient identify satisfaction in life, (4) keeps the information and process confidential, (5) begins when the patient has enough physical strength and is in a mood of openness, (6) listens with focused attention, (7) uses touch when appropriate, and (8) allows the patient periods of silence and time to repeat if needed. This is an active imagery process in which the nurse and patient become inwardly focused.

Meditative techniques also help the patient decrease fear and tension if the patient is conscious and able to participate. The patient can be guided in relaxation imagery scripts involving opening up to death, letting go, finishing business, working with physical and emotional pain, healing and dying, conscious dying, the moment of death, and exploring the afterdeath experience, (see Chapter 5).

When death seems imminent and there is nothing else that can be done, the family is allowed to be at the patient's bedside if it is their desire. The nurse checks to see whether they need anything and stays in the room if they ask; however, the nurse allows privacy and intimacy. The nurse does not need all the answers to talk to the patient or family. The nurse is honest with them and says, "I don't know when death will come." This type of response demonstrates care and concern. In this situation, it is important to have a willingness to listen and a determination to be honest.[153] Patients or families are allowed to talk of death on their own terms (that is, when they are ready). The nurse never denies how sick a patient is but tries to say what seems right at the moment; if the nurse does not know what to say, it is admitted.

Death is painful for the family. When death occurs, the word, *death,* is used. This is not cruel but may help the family begin to face reality. A family member may be present at the time of death and still not be aware of it. A death can leave family members disorganized and unable to collect thoughts. The nurse helps them with basic tasks such as finding money to dial a telephone or finding a quiet conference room in which to stay as long as they need.

The family may want to be isolated from their deceased member, or they may wish to touch, hug, and kiss the patient's body. Death has the potential for evoking tremendous grief in the family, and family members handle their grief about death in many ways. The nurse should not be judgmental when some scream, swear, angrily attack the nursing staff, or show no emotion.

Working through nurses' grieving process

Taking care of the cardiogenic shock patient causes stress for the nurse, too. Nurses must handle their own emotional grief when they realize that death is imminent.

Each death experience is analyzed to find its meaning. This is an essential step in being able to deal with dying patients and their families effectively, honestly, and caringly. Grief is a part of life. Problems arise when nurses refrain from crying or asking for help when they grieve.

Death is not the enemy; suffering is the enemy. Grief can be handled by alleviating the suffering. Nurses should observe colleagues and learn how to recognize hurting. They should allow time to hug, laugh, talk, or cry together.

If the cardiogenic shock patient gets well, the staff members are jubilant. However, when the patient gets worse and dies, the effects on the nursing staff may include frustration, guilt, or anger. If staff nurses base their performance and self-worth on the patient's survival, death is seen as a failure on their part. Stressful work situations such as this must be modified by regularly scheduled meetings for expressing feelings, stressors, and ways to cope more effectively. Group support, relaxation training, stress management education, and counseling services also must be available. Nurses need to identify ways to work most effectively in such high-stress situations. Nursing requires emotional involvement with patients, families, and colleagues. However, nurses also have needs that must be met. They must be assertive and learn how to get those needs met.

Most patients die in hospitals, and the majority of nurses also still work in hospitals. As they care for dying cardiovascular patients, nurses are conditioned by past experiences with dying patients, cultural experiences, and personal experiences. Self-education about death and dying must be a continuing developmental process for all nurses. When patients die, nurses are affected, and conflicts frequently surface. With each experience of birth, wellness, or death, nurses should try to gain a better understanding of the process so that they can interact more humanely and meaningfully with patients, families, colleagues, and selves.

KEY CONCEPT REVIEW

1. Mr. R.C., age 64, developed congestive heart failure with an elevated PAWP. Which factors increase PAWP?
   a. Decreased total blood volume and decreased preload
   b. Increased total blood volume and increased left ventricular afterload
   c. Decreased preload and increased afterload
   d. Decreased total blood volume and increased preload
2. Which of the following factors increase myocardial wall tension?
   a. Decreased afterload, decreased preload, and decreased ventricular radius
   b. Decreased afterload, increased preload, and increased ventricular radius
   c. Increased afterload, increased preload, and increased ventricular radius
   d. Decreased afterload, increased preload, and decreased ventricular radius
3. During the *early stages* of heart failure, the end-diastolic length of each ventricle's fibers:
   a. Increases past the optimal point
   b. Increases to the optimal point
   c. Decreases past the optimal point
   d. Decreases to the optimal point
4. During the *late stages* of heart failure, the end-diastolic length of each ventricle's fibers:
   a. Increases past the optimal point
   b. Decreases past the optimal point
   c. Increases to the optimal point
   d. Decreases to the optimal point
5. The afterload of the left ventricle can be reduced by:
   a. Increasing overall arteriolar resistance

b. Increasing overall PAWP

c. Decreasing PAWP

d. Decreasing overall arterial resistance

6. Sodium nitroprusside is used in heart failure because:
   a. It is a balanced vasodilator.
   b. It increases arterial capacitance.
   c. It decreases arterial capacitance.
   d. It enhances myocardial contractility.

7. Which of the following are prominent signs of left ventricular failure?
   a. Paroxysmal nocturnal dyspnea, ascites, and hepatomegaly
   b. S_3, frequent new cough, and crackles
   c. Pedal edema, ascites, and hepatomegaly
   d. Tachydysrhythmias, chest pain, and frequent cough

8. Which of the following are signs of right ventricular failure?
   a. Jugular venous distention, ascites, and hepatomegaly
   b. Pulmonary edema, S_3, and tachydysrhythmias
   c. Pedal edema, S_3, and crackles
   d. S_4, crackles, and frequent cough

9. Dobutamine may be given in heart failure to:
   a. Increase α-adrenergic response
   b. Block β-adrenergic response
   c. Cause β-adrenergic response
   d. Increase the sensitivity of α_2-receptors

10. The dopaminergic effects of dopamine are most effective at the following dosage:
    a. 1 to 2 μg/kg/min
    b. 4 to 5 μg/kg/min
    c. 10 to 12 μg/kg/min
    d. 18 to 20 μg/kg/min

11. The newer drug given to interfere with the production of angiotensin II in heart failure is:
    a. Isordil
    b. Enoximone
    c. Esmolol
    d. Captopril

12. Enoximone is given in heart failure because it is a:
    a. β-blocker
    b. ACE inhibitor
    c. Phosophodiesterase inhibitor
    d. α-adrenergic drug

13. The primary pathophysiologic mechanism in cardiogenic shock is:
    a. Cardiac failure and respiratory insufficiency
    b. Change in pressoreceptors
    c. Impaired cellular function related to inadequate nutritional blood flow
    d. Increased metabolic acidosis related to anaerobic metabolism

14. The key to success in treatment of cardiogenic shock is:
    a. Early recognition
    b. Pinpointing of the cause
    c. Immediate vigorous treatment
    d. All of the above

15. The primarily intended therapeutic effect of IABP in cardiogenic shock is:
    a. Volume displacement during inflation and enhancement of the intrinsic Windkessel effect
    b. Antagonizing the intrinsic Windkessel effect
    c. Inflation in midsystole
    d. Deflation during diastole to reduce the Windkessel effect

16. A VAD differs from balloon pumping in that it:
    a. Requires removal of the natural heart
    b. Requires placement of two IABs into the aorta
    c. Requires that the heart work harder than in IABP
    d. Totally replaces the work of left ventricular pumping

17. The Novacor Hemopump has been successful for treating cardiogenic shock; its mechanism of action is to:
    a. Divert flow to an external pump that assumes the work of systole
    b. Oxygenate the blood in place of the lungs
    c. Replace right ventricular workload
    d. Withdraw blood from the left ventricle through a catheter and eject it out into the aorta ahead of left ventricular systole

ANSWERS

1. b	4. a	7. b	10. a	13. c	16. d
2. c	5. d	8. a	11. d	14. d	17. d
3. b	6. a	9. c	12. c	15. a	

REFERENCES

1. Abel FL and McCutcheon EP: Cardiovascular function, Boston, 1979, Little, Brown, & Co.
2. Abou-Awdi N and others: New support for the failing heart, Am J Nurs 91: 38-41, 1991.
3. Ader R and others: Immediate and sustained hemodynamic and clinical improvement in chronic heart failure by an oral angiotensin converting enzyme inhibitor, Circulation 61:931, 1980.
4. Ahlquist RP: A study of the adrenotropic receptors, Am J Physiol 53:586, 1948.
5. Akyurekli MD: Effectiveness of intra-aortic balloon counterpulsation on systolic unloading, Can J Surg 23:122, 1980.
6. Appelfeld MM and others: Intermittent continuous outpatient dobutamine infusion in the management of congestive heart failure, Am J Cardiol 51:455, 1983.
7. Baumann G, Ningel K, and Permanetter B: Clinical efficacy of pimobendan (UDCG 115 BS) in patients with chronic congestive heart failure, J Cardiovasc Pharmacol 14:(suppl II):S23, 1989.
8. Benotti J and others: Hemodynamic assessment of amrinone: a new inotropic agent, N Engl J Med 299:1373, 1978.
9. Berne RM and Levy MN: Cardiovascular physiology, ed 5, St Louis, 1986, The CV Mosby Co.
10. Bethell HBN and Nixon PGF: Understanding the atrial sound, Br Heart J 35:229, 1973.
11. Boeing M and Mangera C: Powerlessness in critical care patients, Dimens Crit Care Nurs 8:273, 1989.
12. Boman RM III and others: Circulatory support with a centrifugal pump as a bridge to cardiac transplantation, Ann Thorac Surg 47:108, 1979.
13. Borges HF, Hooks J, Kjellstrand CM: Mannitol intoxication in patients with renal failure, Arch Intern Med 142:63, 1982.
14. Braunwald E: Regulation of the circulation, N Engl J Med 290:1124, 1974.
15. Braunwald E: Determinants and assessment of cardiac function, N Engl J Med 296:86, 1977.

16. Braunwald E: Clinical manifestations of heart failure. In Braunwald E, editor: Heart disease, Philadelphia, 1980, WB Saunders Co.

17. Braunwald E, Ross J, and Sonnenblick EH: Mechanisms of contraction of the normal and failing heart, ed 7, Boston, 1976, Little, Brown & Co.

18. Breish EA and others: Myocardial blood flow and capillary density in chronic pressure overload of the feline left ventricle, Cardiovasc Res 14:469, 1980.

19. Bristow MR, Ginsburg R, and Fowler M: Beta$_1$- and Beta$_2$-adrenergic receptor subpopulations in normal and failing human ventricular myocardium: coupling of both receptor subtypes to muscle contraction and selective Beta$_1$ receptor down-regulation in heart failure, Circ Res 59:297, 1986.

20. Bristow MR and others: Decreased catecholamine sensitivity and beta-adrenergic receptor density in failing human hearts, New Engl J Med 307:205, 1982.

21. Bristow MR and others: Beta-adrenergic receptor pathways in the failing human heart, Heart Failure 5:77, 1989.

22. Brodde OE: Molecular pharmacology of Beta-adenoreceptors, J Cardiovasc Pharm Suppl 4:516, 1986.

23. Brown GB: Diastolic augmentation by intra-aortic balloon: circulatory hemodynamics and treatment of severe, acute left ventricular failure in dogs, J Thorac Cardiovasc Surg 53:798, 1967.

24. Capasso JM and others: Control and peripheral components of cardiac failure, Am J Med 80:2, 1986.

25. Chatterjee K: Newer oral inotropic agents: phosphodiesterase inhibitors, Crit Care Med 18:S34, 1990.

26. Chatterjee L and Parmley WW: The role of vasodilator therapy in heart failure, Cardiovasc Dis 19:301, 1977.

27. Chatterjee S and Rosenzweig J: Evaluation of intra-aortic balloon counterpulsation, J Thorac Cardiovasc Surg 61:405, 1971.

28. Chidsey CA, Braunwald E, and Morrow AG: Catecholamine excretion and cardiac stores of norepinephrine in congestive heart failure, Am J Med 39:442, 1965.

29. Chidsey CA and others: Norephinephrine stores and contractile force of papillary muscle from failing human heart, Circulation 33:43, 1966.

30. Chillian WM and Marcus ML: Phasic coronary blood flow velocity in intramural and epicardial coronary arteries, Circ Res 50:775, 1982.

31. Cody RJ and others: Identification of the direct vasodilator effect of milrinone with an isolated limb preparation in patients with chronic congestive heart failure, Circulation 73:124, 1986.

32. Cohn JN and others: Effect of vasodilator therapy on mortality in chronic congestive heart failure: results of a Veterans Administration Cooperative study, New Engl J Med 314:1547, 1986.

33. Colucci WS, Wright RF, Braunwald E: New positive inotropic agents in the treatment of congestive heart failure: mechanisms of action and recent clinical developments, N Engl J Med 314:290, 1986.

34. CONSENSUS Trial Study Group: Effects of enalapril on mortality in severe congestive heart failure: results of the Cooperative North Scandinavian Enalapril Survival Study (CONSENSUS), N Engl J Med 316:1435, 1987.

35. Covinsky JO and Willett MS: Congestive heart failure. In DiPiro JT and others, editors: Pharmacotherapy: a pathophysiologic approach, New York, 1989, Elsevier Science Publishing Co, Inc.

36. Currie PJ and others: Oral beta-adrenergic blockade with metoprolol in patients with chronic congestive heart failure, N Engl J Med 311:819, 1984.

37. Dawamura K and James TN: Comparative ultrastructure of cellular junctions in working myocardium and the conduction system under normal and pathologic conditions, J Mol Cell Cardiol 3:31, 1971.

38. De Bold AJ and others: A rapid and potent natriuretic response to intravenous injection of atrial myocardial extract in rats, Life Sci 28:89, 1987.

39. DeGeest H and others: Depression of ventricular contractility by stimulation of the vagus nerves, Circ Res 17:222, 1965.

40. Dikshit K and others: Renal and extrarenal hemodynamic effects of furosemide in congestive heart failure after acute myocardial infarction, N Engl J Med 288:1087, 1973.

41. Dobutrex Solution: Dobutamine Hydrochloride injection, Package Insert, Eli Lily & Co., Penn 7363 AMP, 1989.

42. Dole WP: Pathophysiology and management of cardiogenic shock, Clin Cardiol Pract 1:23, 1984.

43. Dossey B: Dying in peace. In Achterberg J, Dossey B, and Kolkmeier L, editors: Rituals of healing, New York, 1992, Bantam Books.

44. Doyle B: Nursing challenge: the patient with end-stage heart failure. In Kern L, editor: Cardiac critical care nursing, Rockville, MD, 1988, Aspen Publishers, Inc.

45. Dramer HJ and Lichardus B: Atrial natriuretic hormones: thirty years after the discovery of atrial volume receptors, Klin Wocheshr 64:719, 1986.

46. Dzau VJ and Creager MA: Progress in angiotensin-converting enzyme inhibition in heart failure: rationale, mechanisms, and clinical responses, Cardiol Clin 7:119, 1989.

47. Elzy PS and Marsh LC: Artificial heart implantation, AORN J 42:171, 1985.

48. Factor SM and Sonnenblick EH: The pathogenesis of clinical and experimental cardiomyopathies: recent concepts, Prog Cardiovasc Dis 27:395, 1985.

49. Fawcett DW: Physiologically significant specializations of the cell surface, Circulation 26:1105, 1962.

50. Fawcett DW and McNutt NS: The ultrastructure of the cat myocardium: capillary muscle, J Cell Biol 43:1, 1969.

51. Feldman MD and others: Deficient production of cycle AMP: pharmacologic evidence of an important cause of contractile dysfunction in patients with end-stage heart failure, Circulation 75:331, 1987.

52. Fife MA and others: Hemodynamic and renal effects of atrial natriuretic peptide in congestive heart failure, Am J Cardiol 65:211, 1990.

53. Flaherty JT: Comparison of intravenous nitroglycerin and sodium nitroprusside on ischemic injury during acute myocardial infarction, Circulation 65:1072, 1982.

54. Folkow B and Neil E: Circulation, New York, 1973, Oxford University Press.

55. Foster S and Canty R: Pump failure following myocardial infarction: an overview, Heart Lung 9:293, 1980.

56. Frantz A and Galdys M: Keeping up with automatic rotating tourniquet, Nurs 78:8:31, 1978.

57. Franuisco LL and Ferris TF: The use and abuse of diuretics, Arch Intern Med 142:23, 1987.

58. Frishman WH and Sonnenblick EH: Beta-adrenergic blocking drugs. In Hurst W: The Heart, ed 6, New York, 1986, McGraw-Hill, Inc.

59. Genest J and Cantin M: Atrial natriuretic factor, Circulation 75:118, 1987.

60. Gerber JG and Niew AS: Beta-adrenergic blocking drugs, Annu Rev Med 36:145, 1985.

61. Ghidsey CA, Braunwald E, and Morrow AG: Catecholamine excretion and cardiac stores of norepinephrine in congestive heart failure, Am J Med 39:442, 1965.

62. Giles D: Principles of vasodilator therapy for left ventricular congestive heart failure, Heart Lung 9:2, 1980.

63. Goetz KL and others: Effects of atriopeptin infusion versus effects of left atrial stretch in awake dogs, Am J Physiol 250:R221, 1986.

64. Goldberg IF and others: Effect of dobutamine on plasma potassium in congestive heart failure secondary to idiopathic or ischemic cardiomyopathy, Am J Cardiol 63:843, 1989.

65. Goldberg LI: Cardiovascular and renal actions of dopamine: potential clinical applications, Pharmacol Rev 24:1, 1972.

66. Goldberg LI: Dopamine: clinical uses of an endogenous catecholamine, N Engl J Med 291:707, 1974.

67. Goldberg LI and Rajfer SI: Dopamine receptors: application in clinical cardiology, Circulation 72:245, 1985.

68. Goldschlager RR: Treating cardiogenic shock during the heart attack, J Resp Dis 5:21, 1984.

69. Green GF: Determinants of systemic blood flow. In Guyton AC and Young DB, editors: International review of physiology: cardiovascular physiology, Baltimore, 1979, University Park Press.

70. Griffith BP: Interim use of the Jarvik-7 artificial heart: lessons learned at Presbyterian-University Hospital of Pittsburgh, Ann Thorac Surg 47:158, 1989.

71. Guyton A: Textbook of medical physiology, ed 8, Philadelphia, 1990, WB Saunders Co.

72. Haber E: The role of renin in normal and pathological cardiovascular homeostasis, Circulation 54:849, 1976.

73. Hammermeister K: Relationships of cardiothoracic ratio and plain film heart volume to late survival, Circulation 59:89, 1979.

74. Heal, LR and others: Operation of roller pump for extracorporeal circulation, J Thorac Cardiovasc Surg 39:210, 1960.

75. Hedner R and others: ANP: a cardiac hormone and a putative central neurotransmitter, Eur Heart J 8:87, 1987.

76. Henker RA and Brown D: Cardiac assist device. In Clochesy JM, editor: Advanced technology in critical care nursing, 1989, Gaithersburg, Md, Aspen Publications, Inc.

77. Honig CR: Modern cardiovascular physiology, Boston, 1981, Little, Brown & Co.

78. Huxley HE: The mechanism of muscular contraction, Science 164:1356, 1969.

79. Huxley HE and Hanson J: Changes in the cross striation of muscle during contraction and stretch and their structural interpretation, Nature 173:973, 1964.

80. Jacobus WE: Respiratory control and the integration of heart high-energy phosphate metabolism by the mitochondrial creatine kinase, Ann Rev Physiol 47:707, 1985.

81. Jacobus WE: Theoretical support for the heart phosphocreatine energy transport shuttle based on the intracellular diffusion limited mobility of ADP, Biocem Biophys Res Comm 133:1035, 1985.

82. Jarvik RK: The total artificial heart, Sci Am 244:74, 1981.

83. Jennings RB and others: Relation between high-energy phosphate and lethal injury in myocardial ischemia in the dog, Am J Pathol 92:187, 1978.

84. Jessup M and others: Effects of low dose enoximone for chronic congestive heart failure, Am J Cardiol 60:80C, 1987.

85. Joist H and others: Bleeding and anticoagulation panel: conference on ventricular assistance devices. Society of Thoracic Surgery, St Louis, Mo, February, 607, 1988.

86. Katz AM: Physiology of the heart, New York, 1977, Raven Press.

87. Keller AM and others: Nuclear magnetic resonance study of high energy phosphate stores in models of adriamycin cardiotoxicity, Magn Reson Med 3:834, 1986.

88. Korner PI: Present concepts about the myocardium, Adv Cardiol 12:1, 1974.

89. Krause SM: Metabolism in the failing heart, Heart Failure 3:267, 1988.

90. Kubo S: Neurohormonal activity in congestive heart failure, Crit Care Med 18:39, 1990.

91. Kubo SH and others: Acute dose range study of milrinone in congestive heart failure, Am J Cardiol 55:726, 1985.

92. Lang RM and others: Role of adrenoceptors and dopamine receptors in modulating left ventricular diastolic function, Circ Res 63:126, 1988.

93. Larose P and others: Radioimmunoassay of atrial natriuretic factor: human plasma levels, Biochem Biophys Res Commun 130:553, 1985.

94. Lee HR: Alpha$_1$ adrenergic receptors in heart failure, Heart Failure 5:91, 1989.

95. Leier CV and others: Comparative systemic and regional hemodynamic effects of dopamine and dobutamine in patients with cardiomyopathic heart failure, Circulation 58:466, 1978.

96. Leithe ME and others: Relationship between central hemodynamics and regional blood flow in normal subjects and in patients with congestive heart failure, Circulation 69:57, 1984.

97. Ley J: The Thoratec ventricular assist device: nursing guidelines. AACN's Clin Issues Crit Care Nurs 2:529, 1991.

98. Lindenmayer GE, Sordahl LA, and Schwartz A: Reevaluation of oxidative phosphorylation in cardiac mitochondria from normal animals and animals in heart failure, Circ Res 23:439, 1968.

99. Little RC: Physiology of the heart and circulation, ed 3, Chicago, 1989, Year Book Medical Publishers, Inc.

100. Luft FC and others: Cardiovascular and renal effects of atrial natriuretic factor, Adv Nephrol 16:37, 1987.

101. Masie B and others: Long-term oral administration of amrinone for congestive heart failure: lack of efficacy in multicenter controlled trial, Circulation 72:963, 1985.

102. McClellan G, Weisberg A, and Winegrad S: Energy transport from the mitrochondria to myofibril by a creatine phosphate shuttle in cardiac cells, Am J Physiol 245:C423, 1983.

103. McGovern GJ, Sang BP, Maker TD: Use of a centrifugal pump without anticoagulants for postoperative left ventricular assist, World J Surg 9:25, 1985.

104. Meinertz T, Drexler H, and Just H: Therapeutic advances in heart failure, CV Drugs Ther 2:413, 1988.

105. Meyer RA, Sweeney HL, and Kushmerick MJ: A simple analysis of the 'phosphocreatine shuttle', Am J Physiol 246:C365, 1984.

106. Monrad ES and others: Effects of milrinone on coronary hemodynamics and myocardial energetics in patients with congestive heart failure, Circulation 71:972, 1985.

107. Motomura S and others: On the physiologic role of beta$_2$ adrenoceptors in the human heart: in vitro and in vivo studies, Am Heart J 119:608, 1990.

108. Nakamura M: Digitalis induced augmentation of cardiopulmonary baroreflex control of forearm vascular resistance, Circulation 71:11, 1985.

109. Neumann J and others: Increase in myocardial G-proteins in heart failure, Lancet 22:936, 1988.

110. New York Heart Association: Functional and therapeutic classification of patients with diseases of the heart: nomenclature and criteria for diagnosis of diseases of the heart and great vessels, Boston, 1973, Little, Brown, & Co.

111. Nitropress: Sodium Nitroprusside, USP package insert, North Chicago, IL 60064, March, 1987, Abbott Laboratories.

112. Nix DE, Tharpe WN, and Francisco GE: Intravenous nitroglycerin delivery: dynamics and cost considerations, Hospital Pharmacy 20:230, 1985.

113. Noon GP and others: Reduction of blood trauma in roller pumps for long-term perfusion, World J Surg 9:65, 1985.

114. O'Keefe B and Gilles CL: Family care in the coronary care unit: an analysis of clinical nurse specialist intervention, Heart Lung 17:191, 1988.

115. Packer M: Prolonging life in patients with congestive heart failure: the next frontier, Circulation 4:75:IV-1, 1987.

116. Packer M: Do vasodilators prolong life in heart failure? New Engl J Med 316:1471, 1987.

117. Packer M: Vasodilator and inotropic drugs for the treatment of chronic heart failure: distinguishing hype from hope, J Am Coll Cardiol 12:1299, 1988.

118. Packer M, Medina N, and Yushak M: Relations between serum sodium concentration and hemodynamic and clinical response to converting enzyme inhibition with captopril in severe heart failure, J Am Coll Cardiol 3:1035, 1984.

119. Parmley W and Rouleu J: Vasodilators in heart failure secondary to coronary artery disease, Am Heart J 103:625, 1982.

120. Patterson SW and Starling EH: On mechanical factors which determine output of ventricles, J Physiol 48:357, 1914.

121. Pennington DG and Swartz MT: Selection of circulatory support devices, Heart Failure 4:5, 1988.

122. Pennington DG and others: Long-term follow up of postcardiotomy patients with profound cardiogenic shock salvaged by ventricular assist devices, Circulation 72(Suppl II): 11, 1985.

123. Pennington DG and others: Use of the Pierce-Donachy ventricular assist device in patients with cardiogenic shock, Ann Thorac Surg 47:130, 1989.

124. Perloff J: The clinical manifestations of cardiac failure in adults. In Braunwald E, editor: The myocardium: failure and infarction, New York, 1974, HP Books.

125. Pierce WS and Myers JL: Frontiers of therapy: left ventricular assist pumps and the artificial heart, J Cardiovasc Med 42:667, 1981.

126. Pierpont GL and others: Heterogeneous myocardial catecholamine concentrations in patients with congestive heart failure, Am J Cardiol 60:316, 1983.

127. Pool PE and others: Myocardial high energy phosphate stores in cardiac hypertrophy and heart failure, Circ Res 21:365, 1967.

128. Poole-Wilson PA: Current therapeutic principles in the acute management of severe heart failure, Am J Cardiol 62:4c, 1988.

129. Portner PM and others: An implantable permanent left ventricular assist system for man, Trans Am Soc Artif Intern Organs 24:98, 1978.

130. Portner PM and others: Implantable electrical left ventricular assist system: bridge to transplantation and the future, Ann Thorac Surg 47:142, 1989.

131. Powell WJ Jr: Effects of intra-aortic balloon counterpulsation on cardiac performance, oxygen consumption and coronary blood flow in dogs, Cir Res 26:753, 1970.

132. Quaal SJ: The artificial heart. In Quaal SJ, editor: Comprehensive intra-aortic balloon pumping, St Louis, 1984, The CV Mosby Co.

133. Quaal SJ: The artificial heart, Heart Lung 14:317, 1985.

134. Quaal SJ: Centrifugal VADs: AACN's Clin Issues Crit Care Nurs 2:515, 1991.

135. Quaal SJ: Pathophysiology of heart failure. In Copstad LE, editor: Pathophysiology, Philadelphia, WB Saunders Co. (In press.)

136. Quinones MA, Gaasch WH, and Alexander JK: Influences of acute changes in preload, afterload, contractile state and heart rate on ejection and isovolumic indices of myocardial contractility in man, Circulation 53:293, 1976.

137. Rabinowitz B: Intravenous isosorbide dinitrate in patients with refractory pump failure and acute myocardial infarction, Circulation 65:771, 1982.

138. Rajfer SI and others: Beneficial hemodynamic effects of oral-levodopa in heart failure: relation to the generation of dopamine, N Engl J Med 310:1357, 1984.

139. Reibel DK and Rovetto JJ: Myocardial ATP synthesis and mechanical function following oxygen deficiency, Am J Physiol 234:620, 1978.

140. Remme WM: Congestive heart failure: pathophysiology and medical treatment, J Cardiovasc Pharmacol suppl I:S36, 1986.

141. Remme WJ and others: Hemodynamic effects of intravenous pimobendan in patients with left ventricular dysfunction, J Cardiovasc Pharmacol 14(suppl II):S41, 1989.

142. Resnehov L: Cardiogenic shock, Chest 6:893, 1983.

143. Robertson JD: The molecular structure and contact relationships of cell membranes, Prog Biophys Mol Biol 10:343, 1960.

144. Rose DM and others: Technique and results with a roller pump left and right heart assist device, Ann Thorac Surg 47:124, 1989.

145. Ross J Jr and Peterson KL: On the assessment of cardiac inotropic state, Circulation 47:435, 1973.

146. Ross J Jr and others: Diastolic geometry and sarcomere lengths in the chronically dilated canine left ventricle, Circ Res 28:49, 1971.

147. Rouleu J: Alteration in left ventricular function and coronary hemodynamics with captopril, hydralazine, and prazosin in chronic ischemic heart failure: a comparative study, Circulation 65:671, 1982.

148. Rountree WD: The Hemopump temporary cardiac assist device, AACN's Clin Issues Crit Care Nurs 2:562, 1991.

149. Rowe G and others: Systemic and coronary hemodynamic effects of triameterene, Proc Soc Exp Biol Med 10:27, 1982.

150. Rutan RM and others: Initial experience with the Hemopump, Crit Care Nurs Clin North Am 1:527, 1989.

151. Sagawa K: The ventricular pressure-volume diagram revisited, Circ Res 43:677, 1978.

152. Saxon SA and Silverman ME: Effects of continuous infusion of intravenous nitroglycerin on methemoglobin levels, Am J Cardiol 56:461,1985.

153. Scanlon C: Creating a vision of hope: the challenge of palliative care, Oncol Nurs Forum 16:491, 1989.

154. Schactman M, Vinsant M, and Crawford M: Dobutamine rescue for intractable CHF, Am J Nurs 88:1642, 1988.

155. Schoenhofer SO: Affectional touch in critical care nursing: a descriptive study, Heart Lung 18:146, 1989.

156. Schwartz DW and Piano MR: New inotropic drugs for treatment of congestive heart failure, Cardiovasc Nurs 26(2):7, 1990.

157. Sharpe DN and others: Enalapril in patients with chronic heart failure: a placebo-controlled, randomized double blind study, Circulation 70:271, 1984.

158. Shinn J: Novacor left ventricular assist system, AACN's Clin Issues Crit Care Nurs 2:575, 1991.

159. Shoemaker WC, Dram HB, and Appel PL: Therapy of shock based on pathophysiology, monitoring and outcome prediction, Crit Care Med 18:S19, 1990.

160. Sica DA and Gehr T: Diuretics in congestive heart failure, Cardiol Clin 7:87, 1989.

161. Simpson FO: The transverse tubular system in mammalian myocardial cells: sarcolemma invaginations and transverse tubular system, J Cell Biol 12:91, 1962.

162. Smith TW: Digitalis: mechanisms of action and clinical use, New Engl J Med 318:358, 1988.

163. Sobel BE and others: Normal oxidative phosphorylation in mitochondria from the failing heart, Circ Res 21:355, 1967.

164. Sonnenblick EH and LeJemtel TH: Pathophysiology of congestive heart failure, Am J Med 87:885, 1989.

165. Sordahl LA and others: Mitochondria and sarcoplasmic reticulum function in cardiac hypertrophy and failure, Am J Physiol 224:497, 1973.

166. Spindola-Franco H: Plain film diagnosis of congestive heart failure, J Med Soc 75:783, 1978.

167. St Cyr J and others: Myocardial high-energy phosphate levels in cardiomyopathic turkeys, J Surg Res 41:256, 1986.

168. Stower CD, Ressalt MM, Sirak HD: Oxidative phosphorylation in mitochonria isolated from chronically stressed dog hearts, Circ Res 23:87, 1968.

169. Strobeck JE: Cardiogenic shock, Heart Failure 1:13, 1985.

170. Swain JL and others: Derangements in myocardial purine and pyrimidine nucleotide metabolism in patients with coronary artery disease and left ventricular hypertrophy, Proc Natl Acad Sci USA 79:655, 1982.

171. Tilstone WJ and others: Pharmacolkinetics of metolazone in normal subjects and in patients with cardiac or renal failure, Clin Pharmacol Ther 16:322, 1974.

172. Tyson GS, Davis JW, Tankin JS: Improved performance of the intra-aortic balloon pump in man, Surg Forum 37:214, 1986.

173. Unverferth DV and others: Improvement of human mitrochondria after dobutamine: a quantitative ultrastructural study, J Pharmacol Exp Ther 215:527, 1980.

174. Unverferth DV and others: Long-term benefit of dobutamine in patients with congestive cardiomyopathy, Am Heart J 100:622, 1980.

175. Unverferth DV and others: The role of subendocardial ischemia in perpetuating myocardial failure in patients with nonischemic congestive cardiomyopathy, Am Heart J 105:176, 1983.

176. Vismara L and others: The effects of morphine on venous tone in patients with acute pulmonary edema, Circulation 54:335, 1976.

177. Wallace AG and Sarnoff SJ: Effects of cardiac sympathetic nerve stimulation on conduction in the heart, Circ Res 14:86, 1964.

178. Waters DD and Forrester JS: Diagnosis and management of congestive heart failure and pulmonary edema. In Elliot RS, Forker AD, and Saenz A: Cardiac emergencies, Mt Kisko, New York, 1983, Futura Publishing Co, Inc.

179. Watkins J Jr: The renin-angiotensin-aldosterone system in congestive failure in conscious dogs, J Clin Invest 57:1606, 1976.

180. Weber KT, Janicki JS, and Jain MC: Enoximone (MDL 17, 043) a phosphodiesterase inhibitor, in the treatment of advanced unstable chronic heart failure, J Heart Transplant 5:105, 1986.

181. Weber KT and others: Oxygen utilization and ventilation during exercise in patients with chronic cardiac failure, Circulation 65:1213, 1982.

182. White KM: Completing the hemodynamic picture: SvO_2, Heart Lung 14:272, 1985.

183. Wilshaw P and others: A cardiac output monitor and diagnostic unit for pneumatically driven artificial hearts, Artif Organs 8:215, 1984.

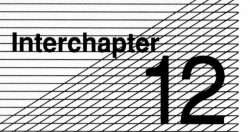

Wellness and Living With Barlow's Syndrome

"Click, click": a young woman, usually tall and thin, has chest pain, a variety of murmurs and clicks, and various neurotic symptoms because of Barlow's syndrome (floppy mitral valve or mitral valve prolapse). Chordae tendineae are longer than usual and mitral leaflets are deformed and cause the clicking sound as they billow like small sails caught in the currents of blood flow.

I'm too young to die—I'm a mother. I have small children. I am a nurse. I've read everything I can find on the situation, and all the references conclude with an estimate of the chances of sudden death. How much of this can I share with my family? I want them to understand why I feel the way I do, but I don't want them to have to come to grips with the possibility of sudden death. One of us working on that is more than enough. How can I ask for sympathy without scaring them? I'm seeing a cardiologist, therefore something is wrong with my heart. He understands; he even lets me cry out my fears in his office. Sometimes he is my best friend.

Some days while working at the hospital, I can go for an hour or more without having my attention pulled back to my heart by crazy dysrhythmias. Is this an R-on-T phenomenon I'm feeling again? How long can I stay in bigeminy and still function? Should I get someone to cover for me while I run over to cardiology and get Pat to run a rhythm strip? Probably not; last time I did that she told the doctors and they doubled my Pronestyl. I'm tired of drugs. I'm tired of being so tired that I have to think about breathing.

Inderal, 10 mg qid—a laughably small dose according to this new cardiologist. "It can't possibly be making you feel that dragged out, silly girl." Why can't they understand I'm an individual, not a diagnosis and application in the *PDR*. Why don't they

believe me when I point out that the joint pain and lupus-like symptoms may be a side effect of the Pronestyl? It says so right there in their own *PDR*. Don't pat me on the head; level with me and help me figure out what we're going to do about it.

Right before Christmas, "Let's try the prednisone and see if the joints go down." Have to buy a bigger purse to carry all this stuff. Forgot to take my third dose today. Things just got too busy. Now I understand "compliance problems" because I have one. One of the kids gets chickenpox and the doctor on call tells me to stop the prednisone cold turkey. I know better than that. You have to wean down on that stuff. I weaned myself down over the weekend until I could talk to my *real* doctor on Monday. . .

That's the first time he's yelled at me. I didn't know that I could have caught the kid's chickenpox and gotten them all over my pericardium, kidneys, and meninges. Now we try Dilantin to calm the dysrhythmias. My medicine cabinet looks like that of an old woman who is falling apart. But I'm young and falling apart. On the Dilantin, I turn bright red and bumpy all over and end up in the hospital on the teaching service for New Year's.

The tenth student, resident, intern, or whatever says I'm a "good historian." Not only am I a good historian but I'm also an "interesting case." They gather around me with their fresh book knowledge and "on call" fatigue. We measure my height and "wing span" against the wall like some rare butterfly.

Slowly I begin to stabilize and feel a bit better. But the ECG and clinical picture suggest pulmonary hypertension. Off to the lab for a cardiac catheterization as I recall the postoperative mitral valve replacement patients I have cared for and wonder if I would trade what I have and know for their un-

knowns. The catheterization shows nothing—no prolapse, no hypertension, and very healthy coronary arteries. Maybe I'm crazy. The cardiologist assures me (he thinks) by telling me there are four ways to diagnose mitral valve prolapse: by auscultation, by echocardiogram, by phonocardiogram, and by cardiac catheterization, and none of them is any good. I take my flip-flopping heart and go home.

Okay guys, you've had 3 years of my life to play with and now it's my turn. I think I know as much about your methods and medicines as you do and I certainly know a lot more about myself than you ever will. If these medicines are supposed to be controlling the dysrhythmias, they're not doing a very good job. If they're supposed to cause side effects, they're doing a superb job. Slowly, but surely, and with tacit approval, I begin to decrease the medication while making some changes in my life. Fatigue heightens my awareness of the dysrhythmias, so I arrange for more rest time in my schedule. I have chest pain when I lie on my left side at night, so I start out sleeping on my right and ease over onto my left sometime in the night. I get a new position at work doing in-service—exciting and challenging but also allowing me some flexibility in my schedule and requiring less time on my feet doing "patient-heavy" work. Aspirin eases the joint pain and may also help decrease clotting, another benefit. I take a community college course in biofeedback and become entranced with the possibilities offered by self-regulation skills.

Slowly over the next several months, I increase my relaxation skills and begin to incorporate them into my day. The rush of adrenaline that used to accompany every run of tachycardia and every PVC is now replaced by an internal voice saying, "The old heart muscle is irritable and kicking up its heels. Maybe I need to get to bed early tonight and let some of the tension out of my shoulders." I have discovered my own internal biofeedback device, and I'm beginning to perfect its use.

I find that exercise obliterates the dysrhythmias for the duration of the exercise time, and, although the dysrhythmias may become more frequent during the cool-down period, I still feel better for having worked hard. Over the next 2 years, I seriously work up an aerobic sweat 2 to 4 times a week and find myself feeling better, stronger, and healthier month by month.

As my relaxation skills improve, I begin teaching them to my patients, letting them in on the little tricks I have learned the hard way—how to deal with a chronic situation and how to decrease the feelings of helplessness and fear. As they learn and begin to use the skills themselves, my confidence and enthusiasm grow. A wonderful cycle has begun.

Finally I go back to the cardiologist for a check-up. It has been 4 years since I decided to take care of myself—4 years of growing confidence and acceptance accompanying a feeling of wellness and a decrease in dys-

rhythmias. Yes, says the cardiologist, you still have the clicks and murmurs of mitral prolapse and mitral regurgitation. Nothing much has changed. Indeed, nothing may have changed from his point of view, but he will never begin to imagine what has changed for me.

LESLIE KOLKMEIER

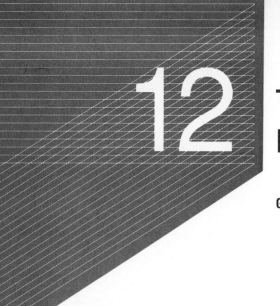

12

The Person with Valvular Heart Disease

Gail A. Oswald Cavallo

LEARNING OBJECTIVES

1. Analyze the physiologic dynamics inherent in each type of valve disease.

2. Describe the physical manifestations possible with each type of valvular involvement.

3. Identify and describe the major aspects of nursing assessment for patients with valvular disease.

4. Synthesize the important areas of teaching to be emphasized with valvular disease patients and their families.

5. Identify the medical and nursing diagnoses for patients with valvular heart disease.

6. Discuss patient outcomes, nursing prescriptions, plan, interventions, and evaluation for each diagnosis listed for patients with valvular heart disease.

The medical community has gained a vast amount of knowledge about the pathophysiologic changes, diagnosis, and therapy of cardiac valvular disease since the advent of cardiac catheterization in the 1960s. Much has been learned since the first cardiology textbooks published 40 to 50 years ago discussed mitral stenosis at length but barely mentioned mitral regurgitation.[17] Since that time the treatment of valvular disease has been altered dramatically by the development of prosthetic and biologic valve replacements, as well as by the use of certain antimicrobials and other pharmaceutical agents.

Abnormal sounds made by the four valves of the heart have puzzled and tantalized physicians since René Laënnec's stethoscope became available in 1817.[47] These sounds are congenital or acquired; acquired lesions often are the result of rheumatic fever. In this instance valvular deformity occurs most frequently in the mitral and aortic valves because of the trauma they receive during valvular action under the higher pressures inherent in the left side of the heart. Valvular deformities of rheumatic origin are seen with less frequency in the tricuspid valve and almost never in the pulmonary valve.[23,46]

Despite the use of improved antimicrobial agents that have decreased the incidence of rheumatic valvular disease, valvular disease of nonrheumatic origin still is a prevalent medical problem. Because people are living longer, senescent and degenerative valve disease has increased and will continue to do so as long as the elderly population gets larger. In addition, valve disease from staphylococcal endocarditis that is caused by intravenous drug addiction leads to valvular dysfunction in younger people. Advances in Doppler echocardiography also have made detection of valvular dysfunction easier, leading to greater numbers of recognized cases, which in turn seems to have led to an apparent increase in the incidence of the disease.[14]

Doppler and transesophageal echocardiography (see Chapter 6) are extremely important advances in the diagnosis of valvular heart disease and enable highly accurate evaluation of these patients. Thus medical practitioners can better plan and prescribe medical and surgical therapy for patients with this condition.[4]

Even though the development of penicillin in the latter part of the 1940s dramatically decreased the occurrence of acute rheumatic fever, several unexplained outbreaks have recently occurred among white people in rural areas. A resurgence of particularly rheumatogenic group A streptococcus strains may be the causative agent.[41,45]

Regardless of their cause, lesions of the cardiac valves can cause the following two different types of stress on the heart; (1) increased afterload (pressure overload), usually the result of valvular stenosis, and (2) increased regurgitation or insufficiency.[20]

Although the coexistence of varying degrees of stenosis and regurgitation is most often seen in the same valve, severe stenosis and severe regurgitation do not coexist. Regardless of the lesion, the cardiac chamber behind the affected valve exhibits some degree of dilatation or hypertrophy.[20,23] As time passes, this situation becomes progressively more hemodynamically unstable until pump failure, disability, and death eventually occur.

LEFT-SIDED VALVULAR SYNDROMES
Mitral valve disease
Mitral stenosis

Etiology. The most prevalent cause of mitral stenosis is rheumatic fever. The valvulitis of rheumatic fever leads to fibrosis, thickening, and adhesion of the valve commissures and chordae tendineae, thus impeding blood flow through the valve. Two thirds of the victims of this condition are women.[11] Mitral stenosis resulting from rheumatic fever results in 25% of all patients having pure mitral stenosis and an additional 40% having mitral stenosis and regurgitation.[36] A nonrheumatic cause of this disorder, although far less frequent in occurrence than rheumatic fever, is congenital malformation of the mitral valve. Unusual causes of mitral stenosis are systemic lupus erythematosus and rheumatoid arthritis. Other causes are thrombus formation, bacterial vegetation, calcium accumulation, and atrial myxoma (a primary cardiac neoplasm arising most commonly in the left atrium and resembling an organized mural thrombus). It is felt, although yet unproved, that several viruses, especially coxsackie could cause chronic valvular disease, including mitral stenosis.[11]

Pathophysiology. The stenosis of the mitral valve resulting from rheumatic fever results from fusion of the commissures, cusps, and chordae tendineae, as well as fusion of one, two, or all of these structures. Most commonly the cusps of the mitral valve fuse along their edges, and the chordae fuse together, shortening and becoming thickened. The resultant stenotic mitral valve has a characteristic funnel shape, and its orifice has a "fish mouth" or buttonhole appearance. Deposits of calcium in the valvular leaflet can become so advanced that the valvular ring is involved. The thickening of the ring and leaflets can be so pronounced that normal opening and shutting is prevented, reducing the intensity of the S_1 and leading to combined mitral stenosis and mitral regurgitation.[48]

Blood flows through the normal mitral valve orifice, which is 4 to 6 cm^2 and through the spaces between the chordae tendineae, which form multiple secondary orifices. When stenosis reduces the valvular orifice to 2 cm^2, mild mitral stenosis exists. Blood flow from the left atrium to left ventricle requires an abnormally high pressure gradient.

When the opening across the valve is reduced to 1 cm^2, critical mitral stenosis exists, and an even higher AV pressure gradient is essential to maintain a normal resting cardiac output.

The rise in left atrial pressure is not without untoward results. The elevated mean left atrial pressure (LAP) and volume cause dilation and hypertrophy of the chamber. The increased pressure is reflected backward like a row of falling dominoes, elevating pulmonary venous and capillary pressures.

As the pressure in the pulmonary capillaries increases and exceeds the oncotic pressure of the plasma proteins in the blood, fluid is forced out of the capillary bed and cannot be reabsorbed. If this rate of transudation exceeds the rate of lymphatic drainage of the lung tissue, exertional dyspnea and pulmonary edema develop (Fig. 12-1).

Hyperplasia and hypertrophy of the pulmonary arterioles develops in response to the backward transmission of the chronically elevated LAP. This leads to pulmonary hypertension and ultimately right ventricular hypertrophy (RVH), dilation, and heart failure. Left ventricular function eventually deteriorates in response to the reduced left ventricular diastolic filling from the left atrium. Reduction of cardiac output varies greatly among patients with mitral stenosis. The variance of hemodynamic response to a given degree of stenosis ranges from a normal cardiac output and high AV pressure gradient to a significantly reduced cardiac output and a low AV pressure gradient.

Even though some patients with mild-to-moderate mitral stenosis are able to maintain a normal cardiac output at rest, exercise can exacerbate hemodynamic abnormalities. The decreased rate of blood flow across the mitral orifice can result in further elevation of the LAP, possibly causing pulmonary congestion and dyspnea. Although the cardiac output of some patients may rise with exercise, in the majority of cases, exercise fails to increase cardiac output or reduces it. Right-sided heart failure and the left ventricular impairment that results from the stenotic mitral orifice can further reduce cardiac output during exercise. Also the tachycardia that accompanies exertion further lowers cardiac output by shortening the period of diastole and left ventricular filling. Tachycardia increases the pressure needed for blood to flow across the valve, further elevating the LAP. The associated rise in the LAP reflected backward can cause so much congestion in the pulmonary capillary bed that pulmonary edema develops rapidly, even in patients who previously had no symptoms. Atrial fibrillation with a rapid ventricular response can have the same result.

Clinical manifestations. Although the symptoms of severe mitral stenosis generally develop during a minimum of 2 years from the first attack of acute rheumatic fever, many patients have no symptoms for some time, especially those living in the temperate climates. Symptoms may not develop in the population for 10 or more

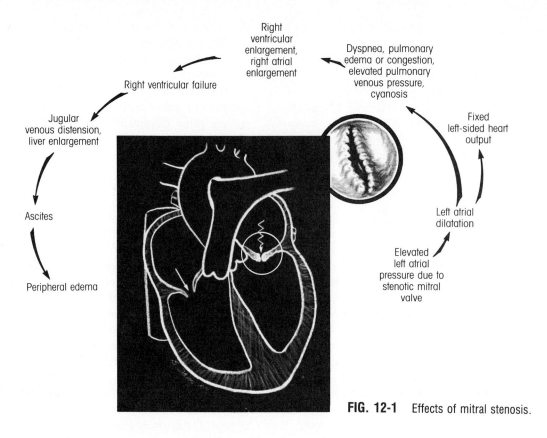

Right ventricular enlargement, right atrial enlargement

Right ventricular failure

Dyspnea, pulmonary edema or congestion, elevated pulmonary venous pressure, cyanosis

Jugular venous distension, liver enlargement

Fixed left-sided heart output

Ascites

Left atrial dilatation

Peripheral edema

Elevated left atrial pressure due to stenotic mitral valve

FIG. 12-1 Effects of mitral stenosis.

years, although mild mitral stenosis in older people is being identified more commonly.[6] However, as the degree of stenosis and valvular dysfunction becomes more pronounced, commonly in the third or fourth decade, complaints of dyspnea, fatigue, palpitations, cough, and hemoptysis are common. In addition, the patient can have dysphagia, hoarseness, chest pain, seizures, or a cerebrovascular accident.[39]

Dyspnea is the most frequent complaint and is attributable to pulmonary venous hypertension resulting from engorged pulmonary vessels and interstitial edema due to an elevated LAP. Precipitating events can include atrial fibrillation with a rapid ventricular response, physical exertion, emotional upsets, fever, severe anemia, paroxysmal tachycardia, sexual intercourse, thyrotoxicosis, and pregnancy.[11,39] Atrial fibrillation is a particularly difficult problem in mitral stenosis. Because atrial contraction adds 30% to the thrust of blood flow across the mitral valve, elimination of the kick that results from atrial fibrillation reduces cardiac output. A rapid ventricular response increases the pressure gradient across the mitral valve, leading to further elevation of the LAP, which augments associated pulmonary problems. As dyspnea worsens, daily activities become progressively limited. Orthopnea and paroxysmal nocturnal dyspnea occur when the patient assumes the recumbent position at night because blood is shifted from the trunk and lower extremities.

Patients experience a cough that can result from bronchial irritation developing when the left main bronchus is lifted by an enlarged left atrium. Dysphagia can result from posterior displacement of the esophagus by the enlarged left atrium. Hoarseness results from pressure exerted by an enlarged pulmonary artery on the left recurrent laryngeal nerve. A very frightening but seldom fatal symptom of mitral stenosis is hemoptysis. It may be related to exertion and is not associated with pulmonary edema. It is usually the result of a thin-walled bronchial vein rupturing because of pulmonary hypertension.

In addition to these pulmonary complications, extensive alveolar wall fibrosis and thickening of the pulmonary capillaries are common in mitral stenosis. This leads to a reduction in oxygen uptake, vital capacity, and total lung capacity. Pulmonary infections are also a problem for many patients. These lung changes are partly the result of the elevated pulmonary capillary pressure increasing the transudation of fluid into alveolar spaces. With such a combination of pulmonary function alterations, especially the decrease in pulmonary compliance, the reason that the patient with mitral stenosis suffers from episodes of dyspnea is evident. In patients with severe mitral stenosis, frank pulmonary edema can be precipitated by situations that increase the flow of blood across the stenotic valve. Such situations include physical exertion, respiratory infection, fever, emotional stress, pregnancy, sexual intercourse, or atrial fibrillation with a rapid ventricular response.[11]

Embolic phenomena are a problem. Arterial thrombi formed in the left atrium because of ineffective atrial contractions often embolize to the brain, liver, spleen, and kidneys. Patients with atrial fibrillation and reduced cardiac output are most at risk for this complication. The presence of atrial fibrillation accounts for 80% of systemic emboli in patients with mitral stenosis.[1] Pulmonary emboli tend to occur late in the course of the disease and generally in patients with right-sided failure and greatly increased pulmonary vascular resistance.

In severe mitral stenosis, systemic changes can be quite uncomfortable. As pressure increases in the left atrium, it is reflected backward into the pulmonary system. The elevated pulmonary vascular resistance is reflected backward to the right side of the heart, leading to increased right ventricular systolic pressures and eventually to right ventricular failure. This in turn is reflected backward into the systemic venous circulation, causing hepatic congestion with resultant abdominal discomfort and distention, fatigue, weakness, and ankle edema. Atrial dysrhythmias, such as premature atrial contractions (PACs), paroxysmal atrial tachycardia (PAT), atrial flutter, and atrial fibrillation also are frequently seen in mitral stenosis.

Physical findings. When performing a physical assessment of a patient with severe mitral stenosis, a nurse is likely to find a resting tachycardia, which is irregular if atrial fibrillation is present; an increased respiratory rate; and a narrow pulse pressure resulting from reduced cardiac output and peripheral vasoconstriction. The patient may exhibit *mitral facies,* with a pinched facial expression, malar flush, and peripheral and sometimes facial cyanosis. The neck veins are distended if right ventricular function is impaired. There is a prominant *a* wave in the jugular venous pulse because of vigorous right atrial systole if the patient has severe pulmonary hypertension and is in sinus rhythm. However, with atrial fibrillation the jugular pulse shows only a single systolic expansion, a *c-v* wave. The systemic arterial pressure is normal or possibly low. The lungs sound clear on auscultation unless pulmonary edema has developed.

On inspection of the precordium, the apical pulse may be absent, but systolic activity may be appreciable along the left sternal border due to RVH. Palpation may reveal a diastolic thrill at the apex, especially if the patient is lying on the left side.[3] Auscultation in mitral stenosis generally reveals an accentuated apical first heart sound (S_1) and an opening snap (OS) followed by a diastolic rumble.[40] The S_1 is accentuated and delayed because the mitral valve cannot close until the left ventricular pressure rises to match the elevated LAP. Then the valve ring is pushed upward rapidly and forcefully.

The OS of mitral stenosis is caused by the forceful opening of the rigid mitral valve because of the elevated LAP or by a sudden tensing of the valve leaflets by the chordae tendineae after the valve cusps have opened.[2,27] It is heard best in early diastole with the diaphragm of the stethoscope at the apex. It is often audible along the left sternal border at the base of the heart. If mitral stenosis is severe with a high LAP, the valve is forced open rapidly, moving it closer to the second heart sound (S_2). This causes the OS to be mistaken on occasion for a ventricular gallop (S_3).

A low-pitched, rumbling diastolic murmur generally follows the OS. It can best be detected with the bell of the stethoscope at the apex when the patient is lying on the left side or has exercised. The rumbling of the murmur is caused by the flow of blood across the narrowed orifice as the valve leaflets begin to close despite continued flow. The rumbling diastolic murmur and the OS are usually reduced during inspiration and accentuated during expiration.

The electrocardiogram (ECG) may exhibit a normal QRS complex, even when stenosis is very severe. The left atrial enlargement found in this disorder produces a broad, notched P wave, predominantly in lead II. A right axis deviation can be observed as pulmonary hypertension becomes severe, and tall R waves can be found in the right precordial leads as RVH worsens. Atrial fibrillation occurs in more than one third of the patients with mitral stenosis.[20]

The changes evident on the chest x-ray film are the effects of left atrial hypertension and include left atrial enlargement, an altered pulmonary venous pattern, prominent pulmonary arteries, and an enlarged right ventricle.[40] An M-mode echocardiogram is usually done because it defines abnormal movement and thickening of the valve leaflets, left atrial enlargement, symmetric motion of anterior and posterior leaflets, and stages of right ventricular enlargement. Two-dimensional echocardiography is valuable because it provides quantification of the mitral valve area; the entire orifice can be imaged in diastole. Exercise testing is sometimes done to evaluate the symptomatic response, enhance auscultatory events, and assess functional capacity. Doppler ultrasound is used to measure the rate of flow across the stenotic orifice. Higher rates of flow indicate more severe degrees of stenosis.

Radionuclide studies can be done during rest or exercise, usually before and after mitral valve surgery to quantitatively document exercise-induced changes in cardiac performance, such as heart rate, ejection fraction, end-diastolic volume, stroke volume, cardiac output, and diastolic filling rate.[34] Cardiac catheterization frequently is done on these patients to assess the severity of the stenosis and its other effects on the heart. Cardiac output, the diastolic pressure gradient between the left atrium and left ventricle, the area of the mitral valve orifice, right ventricular pressure, and pulmonary vascular resistance via mean pulmonary artery pressure are determined with this procedure.[22]

Treatment. The medical treatment of mitral stenosis is actually more prevention than cure oriented because only surgical intervention (see Chapter 17) can alter the obstruction of flow through the stenotic valve. Prophylactic antibiotic treatment is usually given to prevent recurrence of rheumatic fever in a person with no symptoms and to prevent endocarditis. If the patient exhibits symptoms, improvement can be expected with the use of diuretics, restriction of sodium intake, and avoidance of symptom-producing activities.

If disturbances in atrial rhythm occur, digitalis glycosides may control the ventricular response and slow the heart rate. Digitalis is also helpful in advanced mitral stenosis for reducing the manifestations of right-sided heart failure. Antidysrhythmic preparations such as quinidine may prevent recurrent atrial fibrillation but are used after digitalis. If atrial fibrillation is of short duration, electrical cardioversion is sometimes used to restore sinus rhythm, and digitalis and quinidine are used to prevent further fibrillation. Patients with rheumatic heart disease who also have congestive heart failure or atrial fibrillation refractory to cardioversion should be placed on anticoagulant therapy to prevent venous thrombosis and pulmonary embolism. Digitalis does not improve the hemodynamic problems of mitral stenosis, except when atrial fibrillation occurs. β-adrenergic blocking agents may be useful in slowing the ventricular response in atrial fibrillation. These drugs may improve exercise tolerance by reducing heart rate even if the patient is in sinus rhythm.[30]

Symptoms of pulmonary venous congestion are treated with bed rest, salt restriction, diuretics, and use of the sitting position. If systemic or pulmonary emboli occur, anticoagulation is indicated.

Until 5 years ago, *balloon valvuloplasty* of stenosed adult mitral valves, whether from acquired rheumatic or calcific processes, was not accepted as a desirable treatment option. The reasons for this are that such lesions tend to be more rigid in adults, adult stenotic mitral valves tend to be coated with debris that could embolize when the commissures are opened by the balloon, and severe, uncontrollable regurgitation could result after balloon inflation because the procedure is done with the chest closed.

In 1985, however, valvuloplasty was done on young adults with rheumatic mitral stenosis. The results in this population were so promising that it was used on older adults with more rigidly calcified lesions. Use of balloon valvuloplasty in young and older adults with rheumatic or calcific mitral stenosis has produced physiologically and hemodynamically suitable enlargement of the mitral orifice. Despite prior concern to the contrary, increase in the severity of mitral regurgitation or evidence of systemic embolization has not occurred. However, patients must be screened for left atrial thrombi before the procedure.[11]

From a technical standpoint, mitral balloon valvuloplasty is relatively simple and can be performed in the cardiac catheterization laboratory with local anesthesia. The intraatrial septum is punctured and the site enlarged with a small dilation catheter to allow for the passage of the larger valvuloplasty balloon through the system and ultimately across the stenotic mitral valve. When the balloon is inflated, the fused commissures are separated in a manner very similar to open or closed mitral commissurotomy done in the operating room under general anesthesia.

After the procedure, approximately one third of patients have a small left-to-right atrial shunt resulting from puncture of the septum, but it has not generally been a hemodynamically significant problem. Follow-up studies done 6 to 12 months after valvuloplasty have shown preservation of the enlargement of the mitral orifice. Physiologic improvements similar to those seen after surgical treatment of mitral stenosis, such as a fall in filling pressures and pulmonary vascular resistance, remain evident 6 to 12 months after valvuloplasty. Long-term restenosis rates (around 5 to 10 years) are not available yet to compare the success of balloon valvuloplasty with the success of surgical mitral commissurotomy (see Chapter 17).[11]

Mitral regurgitation

Etiology. In the past, rheumatic heart disease was considered the major cause of isolated mitral regurgitation. However, with the decline in the incidence of rheumatic fever, nonrheumatic causes have been reported as leading causative factors. The list of nonrheumatic causes of mitral regurgitation is lengthy and include systemic lupus erythematosus, scleroderma, Marfan's syndrome, myxomatous degeneration of the valvular leaflets, calcification of the mitral valve annulus, infective endocarditis, and hypertrophic cardiomyopathy.[41]

When involvement of the valve leaflets is the cause of mitral regurgitation, it occurs more commonly in men than women. In this situation, incomplete valvular leaflet closure is caused by shortening, rigidity, deformity, and retraction of one or both cusps of the mitral valve with additional shortening and fusion of the chordae tendineae, papillary muscles, and commissures.[18]

Regurgitation of the mitral valve is often seen with mitral stenosis. Through the widespread use of Doppler and two-dimensional echocardiography, mitral leaflet prolapse has been found to be the most common mechanism for mitral regurgitation in adults.[12]

Other causes of mitral regurgitation are coronary artery disease and left ventricular dilation from any condition that causes enlargement of the chamber and displaces the papillary muscles, resulting in distortion of the valve leaflets.

Dysfunction of the papillary muscle is also a cause of mitral regurgitation. Ischemic heart disease can lead to rupture or fibrosis of a papillary muscle. Abnormal anchoring of the papillary muscle also can be caused by myocardial infarction or a ventricular aneurysm at the base of the papillary muscle. This can occur during periods of myocardial and papillary muscle ischemia in connection with angina pectoris. The papillary muscles are significantly affected by myocardial ischemia because the posterior papillary muscle is supplied by the right coronary and the left circumflex arteries.

Chronic mitral regurgitation is often caused by calcification of the mitral annulus in the elderly. Calcific mitral regurgitation is more commonly seen in women than in men. Chronic mitral regurgitation can also result from a connective tissue disease that abnormally elongates the chordae tendineae and leads to prolapse of the cusps into the left atrium during systole. This is often referred to as the *floppy mitral valve syndrome* (see next section). Mitral regurgitation can also be a congenital anomaly.

The mechanisms involved in acute mitral regurgitation include rupture of the chordae and papillary muscle and mitral valve leaflet perforation. Infective endocarditis, mitral leaflet prolapse, spontaneous rupture, and trauma can cause rupture of chordae tendineae. Acute myocardial infarction is the most common cause of papillary muscle rupture, and infective endocarditis can cause perforation of the mitral valve.

Pathophysiology. Mitral regurgitation occurs as a systolic event. When blood is propelled forward into the aorta, it is also ejected backward into the left atrium through an incompetently closed mitral valve. This backward flow of blood causes left atrial and left ventricular hypertrophy. The left atrium dilates and hypertrophies in response to the large volumes of blood it receives during systole, which is propelled back from the left ventricle. The left ventricle, in turn, tries to compensate for the large amount of blood lost to the left atrium during systole with dilation and hypertrophy for more effective systolic emptying and maintenance of cardiac output. The progressive dilation of the left atrium causes the posterior mitral leaflet to be displaced inferiorly and posteriorly, resulting in increased mitral regurgitation. The dilation of the left ventricle is a progressive phenomenon that eventually results in left ventricular failure.

The amount of blood propelled backward into the left atrium depends on the size of the incompetent valvular orifice and the pressure gradient between the left ventricle and atrium. Systolic pressure in the left ventricle and thus the left ventricular–left atrial gradient are labile in that they depend on systemic vascular resistance and forward stroke volume. When the valvular annulus is not calcific, conditions that increase left ventricular size and enlarge the annulus increase regurgitant flow. Increases in preload and afterload and diminished contractility can intensify mitral regurgitation by enlarging left ventricular dimensions.[51]

Although mitral regurgitation ultimately results in negative effects on the left ventricular myocardium, it can be tolerated by the ventricle, allowing it to sustain large regurgitant volumes for many years while normal forward cardiac output levels are maintained. This is because the regurgitation reduces the wall tension developed in the left ventricular myocardium, permitting the velocity of myocardial fiber shortening to increase. Thus the decreased left ventricular load and increased fiber shortening allow the left ventricle to increase its total output. However, as mitral regurgitation persists over time, the function of the left ventricle can no longer compensate, and left ventricular end-diastolic volume increases progressively, enlarging the ventricle and the size of the orifice so that mitral regurgitation becomes more pronounced.[12]

The flow of regurgitant blood into the left atrium also causes a rise in the LAP. This is reflected backward (Fig. 12-2), resulting in increased pulmonary venous and arteriolar pressure, right ventricular hypertrophy, and eventually right-sided heart failure. As the left atrium dilates, atrial tachydysrhythmias, especially atrial fibrillation, tend to develop. Blood tends to stagnate in the dilated left atrium, and systemic embolization can develop.

Clinical manifestations. By itself, mitral regurgitation does not produce symptoms. Patients with mild mitral regurgitation have no symptoms their entire lives.[44] However, when the left ventricle fails and cardiac output falls, fatigue, exertional dyspnea, orthopnea, and paroxysmal nocturnal dyspnea can occur. When the condition is acute, severe dyspnea, signs of pulmonary congestion, and pulmonary edema manifest rapidly. Because the time course of mitral regurgitation tends to be less intense and dramatic than mitral stenosis, irreversible left ventricular dysfunction may be present when symptoms caused by decreased cardiac output and pulmonary congestion appear.

Mitral regurgitation differs from mitral stenosis because changes in the mean pulmonary capillary pressure are less exaggerated, reducing the episodes of symptoms. Pulmonary edema is rare, and systemic emboli and hemoptysis are infrequent in mitral regurgitation as opposed to mitral stenosis.

When cardiac output is greatly reduced, however, fatigue, weakness, exhaustion, weight loss, and cachexia frequently occur. If the patient with mitral regurgitation also has associated pulmonary vascular hypertension, then right-sided heart failure, distended neck veins, ankle edema, painful hepatic congestion, ascites, and tricuspid regurgitation are common (see Fig. 12-2).

Physical findings. The assessment of the patient with mitral regurgitation may reveal normal vital signs, atrial fibrillation, or changes in heart rate and respiration characteristic of left ventricular failure. The apical pulse becomes forceful and displaced to the left and downward as left ventricular hypertrophy becomes evident. As the left

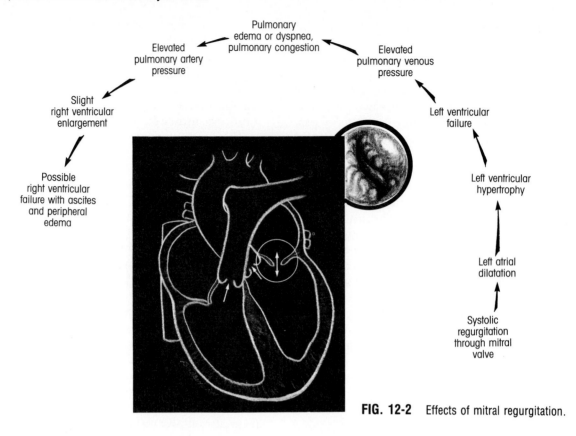

Pulmonary
edema or dyspnea,
pulmonary congestion

Elevated
pulmonary artery
pressure

Elevated
pulmonary venous
pressure

Slight
right ventricular
enlargement

Left ventricular
failure

Possible
right ventricular
failure with ascites
and peripheral
edema

Left ventricular
hypertrophy

Left atrial
dilatation

Systolic
regurgitation
through mitral
valve

FIG. 12-2 Effects of mitral regurgitation.

atrium dilates, atrial fibrillation often occurs. However, because the chronic left atrial volume overload may be tolerated for some time before the symptoms of heart failure develop, heart rate and blood pressure can remain normal in many patients. When right-sided heart failure occurs secondary to left-sided decompensation, neck veins become distended and there are abnormally prominent *a* waves in the jugular venous pulse. There is a characteristic sharp upstroke of the arterial pulse, even though the arterial pressure is usually normal. Inspection of the chest may reveal a rocking motion with each cardiac cycle, which is produced by left ventricular retraction and right atrial expansion during systole.

Auscultation may reveal a diminished or absent first heart sound. Splitting of the second sound is common, with wide splitting occurring in severe mitral regurgitation. Severe regurgitation often exhibits a third heart sound, and acute severe mitral regurgitation characteristically exhibits a fourth heart sound.

The murmur of mitral regurgitation is heard best at the apex with radiation to the left axilla. Because it starts with the isometric phase of ventricular systole (interval between the start of ventricular systole and the opening of the semilunar valves),[4] the murmur is typically pansystolic (throughout systole). The sound of the murmur is produced as blood is regurgitated into the atrium across the incompetent valve during ventricular systole. If the chordae

tendineae rupture, the murmur produces a sound often described as having a cooing or *seagull* quality.

A patient with acute mitral regurgitation exhibits physical findings different from those of a patient with a chronic form of the disease. Acute pulmonary edema, tachycardia, tachypnea, and occassionally lowered blood pressure are seen in this state. If right ventricular function is depressed by pulmonary system overload, the neck veins will be distended, and pulmonary crackles will be diffuse.

In chronic mitral regurgitation the ECG may be normal. As the condition progresses, signs of left ventricular hypertrophy (LVH), as well as left atrial dilation, appear. Left atrial enlargement produced by chronic, severe mitral regurgitation is usually associated with atrial fibrillation.

Although mitral regurgitation does not produce characteristic echocardiographic changes, M-mode and two-dimensional echocardiography can help in determining the cause of mitral regurgitation such as thickening of the valve, valvular prolapse, or calcification of the mitral anulus; it also helps in assessing hemodynamic consequences rather than determining the severity of the regurgitation.[20] Doppler and color-flow Doppler echocardiography can be used to determine the severity of the regurgitant flow.[25,50] The chest x-ray film usually reveals an increased cardiac shadow that indicates left ventricular and atrial enlargement when mitral regurgitation is significant. The left atrium sometimes can enlarge to extend into the right side of the chest, compressing the right bronchus and causing atelectasis.

Radionuclide studies are sometimes performed to measure the ejection fractions in the ventricles. Exercise testing is sometimes used to evaluate the functional reserve and assess symptoms of chronic mitral regurgitation. A decline in exercise tolerance is seen as left ventricular performance deteriorates. Cardiac catheterization usually is performed to determine the degree of mitral regurgitation and to assess left ventricular function.

Treatment. The type of medical treatment depends on the severity of mitral regurgitation. Physical activities that produce extreme fatigue and dyspnea are restricted. A low-sodium diet and appropriate diuretics are used to alleviate congestive failure symptoms. Digitalis is an important part of the therapeutic regimen because it enhances the output of the overburdened left ventricle, thus decreasing ventricular size even if the patient is in sinus rhythm. Because atrial fibrillation tends to be a recurrent problem in mitral valve lesions, these patients are often digitalized to slow the ventricular rate. Quinidine also is used after digitalization to restore sinus rhythm in atrial fibrillation.

Vasodilator therapy often is used for mitral regurgitation. Increased systemic vascular resistance or hypertension increases regurgitation of blood into the left atrium. The regurgitant volume is decreased when blood pressure or peripheral resistance is decreased via vasodilators. These drugs also help in the treatment of left-sided heart failure by reducing afterload. Anticoagulant therapy is needed in the late stages of the disease to decrease the occurrence of emboli. Surgical therapy for the patient with mitral regurgitation may include valve repair such as annuloplasty or mitral valve replacement (see Chapter 17).

Mitral valve prolapse

Etiology. Idiopathic mitral valve prolapse has been called the most common valve disease in adults, probably affecting 5% to 10% of the population. Various terms and names have been proposed for this syndrome: *billowing mitral valve syndrome, systolic click–late systolic murmur syndrome, Barlow syndrome, redundant cusp syndrome,* and *floppy mitral valve syndrome,* with the latter term generally being reserved for advanced forms of the syndrome associated with severe mitral insufficiency. When the pathologic changes in the valve are caused by myxomatous degeneration, the term *Read's syndrome* is often applied.[37]

Sometimes mitral valve prolapse is seen as an isolated abnormality. However, there are a number of other conditions with which it can be associated. Among these are endocarditis, coronary atherosclerosis, myocarditis, trauma, periarteritis nodosa, systemic lupus erythematosus, Wolff-Parkinson-White syndrome, muscular dystrophy, acromegaly, and cardiac sarcoidosis. It has been suggested that mitral valve prolapse may be an inherited disturbance of connective tissue because its association with other abnormalities, such as atrial septal defects, patent ductus arteriosus, ventricular septal defects, and skeletal abnormalities, including pectus excavatum and pectus carinatum.

Mitral valve prolapse also occurs in Marfan's syndrome, an inherited disorder with abnormalities of the connective tissue, and in Ehlers-Danlos syndrome, which is characterized by hyperelastic skin, hyperextensible joints, friable connective tissue, and a bleeding diathesis.[20]

The condition is found in people of all ages and both sexes but most commonly in women between the ages of 20 and 50.[26] The condition tends to be familial and may have an autosomal dominant genetic pattern.[20]

Pathophysiology. In mitral valve prolapse, one or both of the valve leaflets, usually the posterior leaflet, bulge into the left atrium during ventricular systole. There is an actual billowing upward and backward (Fig. 12-3). This billowing is caused by a valvuloventricular disproportion or redundancy of the valve tissues wherein the mitral valve is too large for the ventricle. The posterior leaflet is the most common site of this billowing because it comprises approximately two thirds of the mitral orifice circumference. It normally inflates into a C-shaped gasket during systole, which engulfs the anterior leaflet, thus sealing the valvular opening. This billowing is the result of exaggerated posterior leaflet inflation.[16,29]

If mitral valve prolapse is the result of myxomatous degeneration (degeneration within the mucinous layer of the valve), elongation and thinning of the chordae tendineae may be evident. Thickening of the chordae may develop later. If dilation of the mitral valve anulus is present, premature calcification of the anulus may develop. Asymmetric ventricular contraction often occurs in patients with this defect, but any relationship of this to the clinical findings is unclear.

Mitral valve prolapse is often seen with ischemic heart disease and can occur as a consequence of papillary muscle dysfunction resulting from ischemia or infarction. A number of mitral valve prolapse cases develop for the first time after myocardial infarction. Although mitral valve prolapse may be caused by myocardial ischemia, it may conversely cause ischemia related to increased tension at the base of the involved muscle. It is also possible that spasm of a coronary artery may occur as a response to prolapse of the posterior leaflet of the mitral valve. This reflex spasming of the coronary artery with its accompanying ischemia can lead to angina or angina-like pain, myocardial infarction, dysrhythmias, and possible sudden death.[43]

Clinical manifestations. Although many patients have no symptoms, others exhibit variable symptoms such as chest pain, dizziness, syncope, dyspnea, and palpitations. Symptoms are generally mild, but they can become severe and incapacitating.

Chest pain is the most common and potentially most disabling symptom of this syndrome. It can mimic angina pectoris in that it is felt in the left precordium and some-

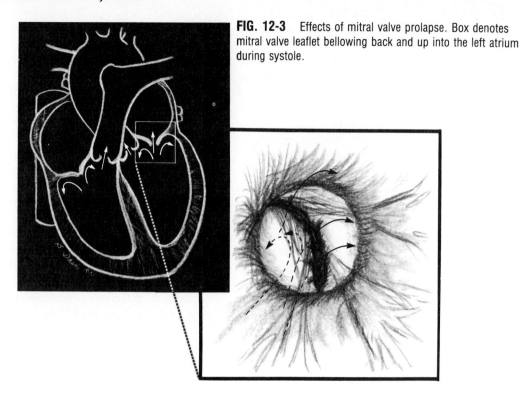

FIG. 12-3   Effects of mitral valve prolapse. Box denotes mitral valve leaflet bellowing back and up into the left atrium during systole.

times radiates to the left arm, back, or jaw. However, unlike angina pectoris, it is unrelated to exertion and is unrelieved by rest or nitroglycerin. The episodes are paroxysmal in nature, and the pain is usually described as *sharp* and *sticking*.

The cause of the chest pain in mitral valve prolapse is not completely understood. It has been attributed to ischemia from the excessive pull of the prolapsed leaflets and their chordae tendineae on the papillary muscles.[43] Under normal conditions the mitral leaflets close tightly together and thus mutually support one another to bear the left ventricular systolic pressure. When the leaflets do not close tightly, the chordae must bear the full thrust of systole, causing excessive pull on the papillary muscles. This excessive pull can adversely affect the blood supply to the papillary muscle. Coronary spasm can result from local trauma caused by stretched papillary muscles.[38,43]

Dyspnea in mitral valve prolapse is not exertional but can have some of the characteristics of the *hyperventilation syndrome* (light-headedness, tingling of the hands, and numbness around the mouth). The pathogenesis of this is uncertain, but it may be psychogenic. Palpitations commonly occur but do not usually correlate with premature beats on the ECG.

It is now felt that the symptoms associated with mitral valve prolapse are due to dysfunction of the sympathetic nervous system, which happens commonly in mitral valve prolapse syndrome. This dysfunction consists of increased excretion and circulating concentrations of epinephrine and norepinephrine that result from accentuated adrenergic tone.[11]

Physical findings. Physically these patients may exhibit pectus excavatum (funnel chest), pectus carinatum (pigeon breast), scoliosis, kyphosis, or the straight back syndrome (spine that lacks the normal curvatures).

On auscultation a nonejection *midsystolic click* or clicks and an apical systolic murmur are common. The click or clicks occur in early midsystole or late systole and are heard best at the apex or along the left sternal border.

The characteristic midsystolic click of mitral valve prolapse is caused by a sudden tensing of the mitral valve leaflet as it reaches its limit while billowing into the left atrium during peak left ventricular systolic pressure. After this a *late* systolic murmur results from regurgitation through the abnormal mitral valve.

The systolic murmur usually is a late systolic phenomenon but also can be pansystolic. The systolic click and murmur can be accentuated or decreased by postural changes. Any change that decreases venous return and left ventricular end-diastolic volume causes the click and the murmur to occur earlier in systole. Sitting, standing, and the Valsalva maneuver are such changes. Maneuvers such as squatting, lying down, elevating the legs, or isometric hand-grip exercises that increase venous return and left ventricular end-diastolic volumes cause the click and the murmur to occur later in systole.

Most commonly, the ECG is normal. However, there can be a number of abnormalities noted on it. Among these are ST-segment depression and inverted T waves, the causes of which are unknown. A slightly prolonged QT interval may be noted, as well. Atrial, supraventricular, and ventricular tachydysrhythmias and PACs and PVCs can occur, but there is no relationship between these and the patient's age, clinical findings, or severity of the condition. Bradydysrhythmias also are noted, including all types of AV blocks and sinus arrest. Continuous ambulatory electrocardiography is usually needed to discover these dysrhythmias.

Echocardiography, especially M-mode echocardiography, is usually used to show the abnormal movement of the posterior mitral valve leaflet. Coronary angiography is usually normal, but blood supply to the papillary muscles is sometimes hampered because of dysfunction of the valve apparatus.

Treatment. The only treatment needed by most of these patients is reassurance that the condition is usually benign, despite the auscultatory, ECG, and echocardiographic findings, as well as its uncomfortable physical effects. Patients with no symptoms and no dysrhythmias and who have normal ECGs and no evidence of serious mitral regurgitation should have follow-up examinations every 2 to 4 years. This examination should include a two-dimensional echocardiogram and a Doppler study for patients who have evidence of mitral regurgitation. Patients with symptoms (i.e., those with palpitations, lightheadedness, dizziness, or syncope) should undergo 24-hour ECG monitoring, treadmill exercise testing, or both. Symptomatic treatment is prescribed for patients with dyspnea, chest pain, and palpitations. Propranolol is used to relieve dyspnea and chest pain and control ventricular dysrhythmias. Antibiotic prophylaxis is used sometimes, although the incidence of infective endocarditis as a complication in mild mitral valve prolapse is low. Prophylactic antibiotics are much more important for patients with more serious mitral valve prolapse and more pronounced regurgitation.[42] Learning relaxation techniques and imagery skills can reduce patient anxiety and relieve symptoms[44] (see Interchapter 12, p. 356).

Aortic valve disease
Aortic stenosis

Etiology. Aortic valve stenosis may be the result of congenital valvular malformation (a unicuspid, bicuspid, tricuspid, or dome-shaped diaphragm valve), rheumatic inflammation of the aortic valve, or idiopathic calcific changes associated with aging. The causes of this valvular abnormality have been influenced by the decline in acute rheumatic fever and an increasing life span among adults. Since the mid-1950s, researchers have suggested that the bicuspid aortic valve is a major cause of aortic stenosis. An aortic valve with a congenital bicuspid formation may not exhibit severe stenosis in childhood, but its abnormal construction tends to make the valve leaflets more susceptible to the normal stresses of cardiac hemodynamics, leading to calcification, rigidity, and narrowing of the orifice.[49]

Aortic stenosis can occur in the supravalvular area, which is rare; the valvular area, which is the most common site; and the subvalvular area, usually termed *subaortic*. It may be caused by hypertrophic obstructive cardiomyopathy (See Chapter 14). Isolated aortic stenosis is the most commonly occurring lesion. When it is found without coincident mitral valve disease, it occurs more commonly in men and is generally congenital or degenerative but not of rheumatic origin.[49] The patient's age when the condition manifests itself usually suggests its cause. When aortic stenosis occurs before the age of 30, it is usually of congenital origin. When it occurs between the ages of 30 and 70, it can usually be attributed equally to a congenital bicuspid valve or rheumatic valvulitis. In patients beyond the age of 70 years, degenerative calcification of a previously normal valve is usually the cause.[4] Although aortic stenosis occurring alone can be rheumatic in origin, rheumatic fever is the usual cause when it occurs with mitral valve disease. Younger men and older women are the two age groups showing the highest incidence of aortic stenosis.[40]

Stenosis develops in the congenitally bicuspid aortic valve, probably because of excessive stress from its abnormal construction. This stimulates the formation of calcium deposits, leading to valvular fibrosis, rigidity, and immobility. Congenitally bicuspid aortic valves remain stenotic unless infective endocarditis develops, which then makes the valve regurgitant. The unicuspid valve is stenotic at birth but is subject to the same stress because of its malformation, leading to the deposition of calcium and further stenosis. Aortic stenosis in the elderly is the result of the stress of wear and tear over many years. The deposition of calcium causes fibrosis and fusion of the valve cusps. The stenosis is caused by calcium deposits that prevent normal systolic valvular excursion. Hypercholesterolemia and diabetes mellitus seem to predispose patients to the development of this form of aortic stenosis.

When aortic stenosis is caused by rheumatic fever, the valvulitis causes adhesions and fusing of the commissures and cusps, which leads to retraction and stiffening of the cuspate borders.[39] Calcific nodules are present on both surfaces, reducing the valvular orifice to a small, round or triangular opening, resulting in regurgitation and stenosis. Patients with severe hypercholesterolemia may have atherosclerotic aortic valvular stenosis, which involves not only the valves but also the aorta and other major arteries.

Pathophysiology. Aortic stenosis is usually not clinically significant until the valvular opening has decreased to one third its normal size.[40] Severe aortic stenosis can exist for many years without causing appreciable disability because the left ventricle can compensate for the stenotic valve. This is in sharp contrast to mitral stenosis, in which

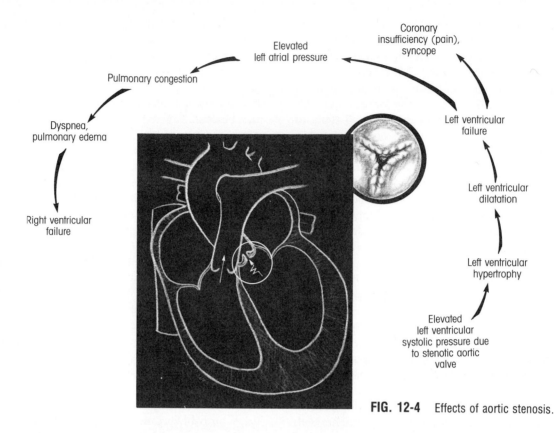

Coronary insufficiency (pain), syncope

Elevated left atrial pressure

Pulmonary congestion

Dyspnea, pulmonary edema

Right ventricular failure

Left ventricular failure

Left ventricular dilatation

Left ventricular hypertrophy

Elevated left ventricular systolic pressure due to stenotic aortic valve

FIG. 12-4 Effects of aortic stenosis.

symptoms are manifested as soon as stenosis becomes severe because the left atrium cannot compensate in the same way.

Aortic stenosis is a systolic event in which obstruction to left ventricular outflow leads to development of a high pressure gradient between the left ventricle and aorta during systolic ejection. Because aortic stenosis develops slowly over several years, the consistently elevated left ventricular pressure causes a pressure overload on the left ventricle, which compensates by a gradual increase in left ventricular wall thickness and left ventricular hypertrophy. This is a concentric hypertrophy of the myocardial muscle fibers without dilation of the chamber, which serves to normalize the systolic force in the ventricular wall for the preservation of the left ventricular ejection fraction and cardiac output at near normal levels.[16]

The left atrium also plays a large part in compensating for the narrowed aortic orifice to maintain normal cardiac output. A strong atrial systole (atrial kick) increases the volume of blood in the left ventricle at the end of diastole, causing an increased left ventricular end-diastolic pressure and increasing left ventricular end-diastolic fiber length. Thus after the Frank-Starling phenomenon, in which increased stretch leads to an increased force of contraction, stroke volume increases. If this regularly timed, vigorous atrial kick is lost, as happens with atrial fibrillation or AV dissociation, it can result in a rapid worsening of symp-

toms. The elevation in left atrial systolic pressure necessary to give the left ventricle an added boost, however, eventually causes enlargement of the left atrium. Through the physiologic mechanisms just described, cardiac output is usually normal at rest in the majority of patients with severe aortic stenosis. However, it does not rise normally in response to physical exertion.

Eventually, severe chronic aortic stenosis leads to depression of the ventricular myocardium as a result of the sustained elevated pressure overload. This leads to dilation of the left ventricle and decreased ejection fraction, cardiac output, and stroke volume. The left ventricular–aortic pressure gradient declines, at which time the mean LAP increases, causing the left atrium to dilate. Again there is a backward reflection of pressure through the cardiopulmonary system. The elevated mean LAP leads to an elevated pulmonary arterial pressure. This pulmonary hypertension is reflected back to the right side of the heart, elevating the right ventricular pressure (Fig. 12-4).

The excessive work of the left ventricle to expel blood against pressure, as well as the hypertrophied left ventricular muscle mass, elevate myocardial oxygen requirements. Because the pressure compressing the coronary arteries exceeds coronary perfusion pressure, there may be interference with coronary blood flow. As a result, symptoms of angina pectoris may develop regardless of whether coronary atherosclerosis is present.

A number of patients with aortic stenosis also have associated mitral valve problems. Aortic stenosis increases mitral regurgitation by intensifying the pressure driving blood from the left ventricle to the left atrium.

Clinical manifestations. If aortic stenosis is the predominant cardiac abnormality, usually patients often do not manifest symptoms until they are between 50 to 60 years of age. During this asymptomatic period, valvular obstruction gradually increases, which in turn increases the myocardial pressure load. The symptoms that develop in response to this pressure are generally angina, syncope, and heart failure. Because cardiac output and stroke volume are usually maintained within normal limits at rest but fail to rise during exercise, exertional dyspnea is common. Valvular obstruction that is not repaired after symptoms begin represents a poor prognosis. For example, the average time interval from the onset of symptoms to the time of death is approximately 2 years in patients with heart failure, 3 years in those with syncope, and 5 years in those with angina. More than half these deaths tend to be sudden.

The angina experienced by patients with critical aortic stenosis is caused by increased oxygen needs by hypertrophied myocardium and reduced oxygen delivery from the coronary vessels caused by excessive compression of the hypertrophied myocardium. Around two-thirds of patients with critical aortic stenosis experience this angina, which is much like the pain seen in patients with coronary artery disease because it starts during exertion and is relieved by rest. About half of all aortic stenosis patients have concomitant significant coronary artery disease.

Aortic stenosis patients commonly experience syncope that is orthostatic and caused by diminished perfusion to the brain during physical exertion when the systemic arterial pressure declines resulting from vasodilation in exercising muscles compounded by a fixed cardiac output. Orthopnea, paroxysmal nocturnal dyspnea, severe exertional dyspnea, and pulmonary edema are symptoms seen in the late stages of the disease as pulmonary venous hypertension worsens.

Because patients with isolated aortic stenosis have no symptoms for many years, symptoms such as marked fatigability, debilitation, and other signs of low cardiac output do not occur until quite late in the course of the syndrome. Severe pulmonary hypertension, atrial fibrillation, and systemic venous hypertension are considered poor prognostic findings.[11]

Physical findings. The patient with aortic stenosis shows hemodynamic alterations in the peripheral pulse and blood pressure. The arterial pulse classically exhibits a slowly rising upstroke that is small and sustained; it is called *pulsus parvus et tardus.* The systemic arterial pressure usually remains normal until the late stages of the illness, when stroke volume declines. At this stage a fall in systolic pressure may occur with a corresponding narrowing of the pulse pressure. Although systemic hypertension is rare in severe aortic stenosis, high systolic pressures can be observed in elderly patients with calcific aortic stenosis and lack of arterial elasticity.

With pure aortic stenosis, the neck veins do not exhibit visible abnormal pulsations. However, the arterial pulse tracing shows a delayed systolic upstroke and an anacrotic notch. *Anacrotic* is an abbreviation for *anadicrotic,* meaning "twice beating on the upstroke." This arterial waveform abnormality is palpable in peripheral arteries (preferably the brachial artery to avoid inadvertent carotid sinus massage) and is attributed to peak turbulence across the aortic valve. In the late stages of the disease, this pulse abnormality is more difficult to appreciate because of narrowing of the pulse pressure.

A systolic thrill generally can be palpated at the base of the heart, in the jugular notch, and along the carotid arteries during expiration with the patient leaning forward. With the patient lying on the left side, a double apical pulse can sometimes be palpated. This reflects the strong atrial kick that is so important to ventricular filling, followed by ventricular systole. A sustained cardiac impulse is seen with left ventricular failure when the ventricle becomes displaced inferiorly and laterally.

The auscultatory findings of aortic stenosis include an aortic ejection sound and the characteristic diamond-shaped, crescendo-decrescendo murmur. This murmur is a systolic phenomenon caused by the flow of blood being forced through a stenotic opening. This characteristically harsh sound is heard best at the base in the second intercostal space to the right of the sternum (the aortic region); it is transmitted upward to the jugular notch and along the carotid arteries. The murmur can be appreciated beginning after the first heart sound with intensity increasing toward the middle of systolic ejection and then decreasing until the aortic valve closure. The aortic ejection sound is heard immediately after S_1 with the diaphragm of the stethoscope and is followed by the murmur.

S_3 can occur when left ventricular dilation and failure develop. The presence of S_4 (atrial gallop) indicates LVH. The lungs are usually clear on auscultation until heart failure and pulmonary venous hypertension develop, at which time characteristics crackles are heard.

The ECG most frequently reveals a regular rhythm with changes produced by LVH. These changes are reflected as large S waves in the right precordial leads and large R waves in the left precordial leads, with depression of the ST segment and inversion of the T waves. Progression of the ST- and T-wave abnormalities is indicative of progressive left ventricular hypertrophy.

First-degree AV heart block and left bundle branch block are sometimes present. In the latter stages of the disease the chest x-ray examination may show left ventricular enlargement and pulmonary congestion. An echocardiogram may reveal thickening, decreased mobility, calcification of the valve cusps, and left ventricular hypertrophy.

Doppler echocardiography can assess noninvasively the severity of valvular obstruction.

Radionuclide studies often are done to assess ventricular function and myocardial perfusion.[10] With this technique the measurement of the left ventricular ejection fraction at rest and during exercise can show left ventricular function deterioration before clinical symptoms have developed. It can also point out impaired perfusion of the myocardium, suggesting underlying coronary artery disease. Cardiac catheterization is done to determine the gradient across the valve and estimate the severity of the stenosis, evaluate left ventricular function, and assess for other valvular lesions; coronary angiography is used to determine the presence of coronary atherosclerosis.

Treatment. Before symptoms develop, the medical treatment of a patient with aortic stenosis involves prophylaxis to prevent infective endocarditis after dental and surgical procedures. Patients who have no symptoms should be reexamined every 6 to 12 months with Doppler echocardiography and ECGs because obstruction tends to progress over time. Patients with critical valvular obstruction are advised to avoid rigorous athletic and physical activities. This does not apply to patients whose valves are only mildly obstructed. These patients have an overall excellent prognosis. When symptoms develop, treatment is aimed at alleviation. However, after symptoms develop, the outlook is poor with only medical management but can improve significantly with surgical replacement of the aortic valve.

When cardiac failure is present, digitalis glycosides, diuretics, a low-sodium diet, and reductions in activity are used to alleviate symptoms. Angina pectoris from coronary artery disease can be alleviated with nitrates, but patients should be cautioned about orthostatic hypotension and syncope. Atrial dysrhythmias can occur in severe aortic stenosis. Loss of atrial kick can cause a fall in cardiac output, serious hypotension, angina, and evidence of myocardial ischemia on the ECG. Prompt treatment with antidysrhythmic medication is essential, and previously undiagnosed mitral value disease should be investigated.[12]

Because of the success of mitral balloon valvuloplasty for acquired mitral stenosis, the treatment is now being used for dilation of calcific aortic stenosis in the adult. Calcific aortic stenosis leads to approximately 20,000 aortic valve replacements yearly in this country. In 1986 alone several hundred patients had benefited from aortic balloon valvuloplasty.[7]

Although the degree of aortic orifice opening is sufficient with aortic balloon valvuloplasty to produce significant improvement in filling pressures, left ventricular function, and overall hemodynamic stability in patients with severe aortic stenosis and pronounced resting symptoms, the results are not as good as with mitral valvuloplasty. However, as with the mitral procedure, significant problems with systemic embolization or worsened aortic regurgitation have not been reported.

Aortic valvuloplasty is usually performed under local anesthesia in the cardiac catheterization laboratory. A balloon catheter is advanced up the aorta until the balloon is within the stenotic aortic valve orifice. A series of catheters of increasing size are used, and each is inflated several times until the desired result is obtained. Although the intraaortic approach is preferred, a few procedures have been performed using the transseptal approach as in mitral valvuloplasty.

Aortic valvuloplasty will probably become the treatment of choice for older patients or those whose physical debility puts them at high risk for surgical valve replacement. However, younger, active patients with severe aortic stenosis will continue to be treated with surgical valve replacement until the valvuloplasty technique is improved so that greater dilation of the aortic valve orifice is achieved[11] (see Chapter 17).

Aortic regurgitation

Etiology. Aortic regurgitation can be caused by the effects of disease on the valvular leaflets or by disease affecting the aortic root. Although improved antimicrobial therapy has decreased the overall incidence of rheumatic fever, it is still a primary cause of aortic regurgitation. Rheumatic fever causes fibrous infiltration of the valve cusps, causing them to retract and preventing cusp closure during diastole, which results in a regurgitant jet into the left ventricle. There can also be fusion of the commissures, resulting in a combination of aortic regurgitation and aortic stenosis. Other causes of aortic regurgitation are infective endocarditis, trauma, and congenital malformations of the valve. Chronic hypertension and arteriosclerosis can cause mild aortic regurgitation.

Diseases that cause dilation of the aortic root can also cause aortic regurgitation. Examples of such diseases are Marfan's syndrome, syphilitic aortitis, ankylosing spondylitis, and rheumatoid arthritis. These conditions cause dilation of the aortic anulus and separation of the leaflets leading to regurgitation. Approximately three fourths of patients with pure aortic regurgitation are men, whereas aortic regurgitation with associated mitral valve problems is more common in women.

Pathophysiology. Aortic regurgitation is a diastolic phenomenon wherein blood is ejected forward into the aorta but also regurgitates backward into the left ventricle through an incompetent aortic valve. This hemodynamic abnormality imposes a volume overload on the left ventricle. In time, dilation and hypertrophy of the left ventricle occur as the work of the left ventricle increases proportionally to the volume of regurgitated blood. Dilation of the mitral valve ring and hypertrophy and dilation of the left atrium can also result over time. As much as 60% of the left ventricular forward stroke volume can be regurgitated.[40] Pockets can form in the endocardium of the left ventricle because of the high pressure impact of the regurgitant jet.

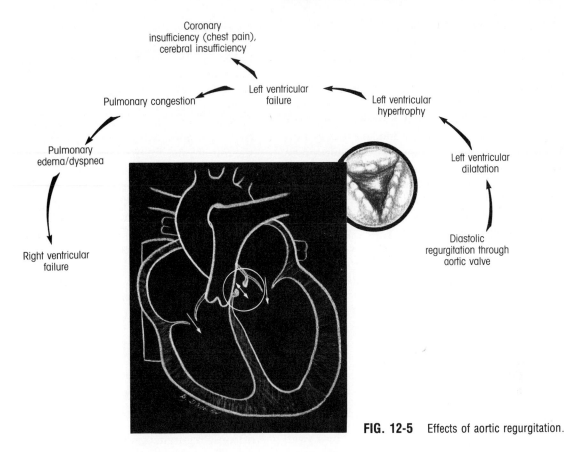

Coronary
insufficiency (chest pain),
cerebral insufficiency

Pulmonary congestion

Left ventricular
failure

Left ventricular
hypertrophy

Pulmonary
edema/dyspnea

Left ventricular
dilatation

Right ventricular
failure

Diastolic
regurgitation through
aortic valve

FIG. 12-5   Effects of aortic regurgitation.

Patients may have severe aortic regurgitation; yet their stroke volume and ejection fraction may be normal, whereas the left ventricular end-diastolic pressure and volume are elevated. The left ventricle dilates, increasing the left ventricular systolic wall tension necessary for the development of systolic pressure needed to maintain normal forward stroke volume and output in accordance with the law of Laplace.[12]

Although chronic aortic regurgitation produces a gradually increased end-diastolic volume as the ventricle receives blood from the left atrium and the aorta, the left ventricular end-diastolic pressure does not increase until heart failure develops. As a compensatory mechanism, total left ventricular stroke volume increases to maintain an effective stroke volume within normal limits. In the early stages of chronic aortic regurgitation, the increased left ventricular stroke volume leads to a normal cardiac output during rest and exercise.[28]

However, as the condition progresses, a gradual decline in the contractile state of the ventricle occurs. In time, the ejection fraction and forward stroke volume decline in the resting state and impaired ventricular emptying occurs. At this point the left ventricular end-diastolic pressure increases, as does the end-diastolic volume. This pressure increase is reflected backward (Fig. 12-5), leading to an elevated LAP and then to pulmonary hypertension and eventually to right-sided heart failure. Peripheral vasodi-

lation often occurs in chronic aortic regurgitation as a compensatory mechanism to decrease afterload, thereby reducing the regurgitant volume. Vasodilation and a warm, flushed appearance are associated with a low diastolic blood pressure.

Myocardial ischemia often occurs in patients with aortic regurgitation because of two main hemodynamic abnormalities. The increased left ventricular dilation elevates myocardial systolic tension, causing increased myocardial oxygen requirements. However, because coronary perfusion may be compromised by low diastolic pressures, the myocardial oxygen supply cannot meet the increased demand, and ischemia develops.

Clinical manifestations. Patients with chronic aortic regurgitation generally have no symptoms for many years because of the compensatory mechanisms of the left ventricle. The first symptoms noticed, usually in the fourth or fifth decade, are the circulatory effects of the increased stroke volume, such as palpitations, prominent neck vein pulsations, and uncomfortable awareness of the heartbeat especially when lying on the left side. Sinus tachycardia or premature ventricular contractions may be notably uncomfortable for these patients because of the greatly increased left ventricular stroke volume causing a great heave of the left ventricle against the chest wall.

As the disease progresses, symptoms of diminished cardiac reserve and left ventricular failure occur, such as increased fatigue, dyspnea, orthopnea, and paroxysmal nocturnal dyspnea. Exertional chest pain occurs as frequently in young as in elderly patients with severe aortic regurgitation. This anginal pain atypically occurs at rest, lasts longer than the ischemia pain of coronary artery disease, and responds unsatisfactorily to sublingual nitroglycerin. Nocturnal chest pain with marked diaphoresis often occurs as well because of a fall in heart rate and an extreme drop in arterial diastolic pressure. Abdominal discomfort may be present with these episodes and is probably caused by ischemia of the splanchnic artery. In the late stages of the disease the symptoms of right-sided heart failure, such as congestive hepatomegaly, ascites, and ankle edema, occur. In general, patients with moderately severe to severe chronic aortic regurgitation have a favorable prognosis, with approximately 75% of patients living for 5 years and 50% for 10 years after diagnosis of the condition. After symptoms occur, the clinical course becomes markedly bleaker. Patients often die within 4 years of developing angina and within 2 years of manifesting symptoms of heart failure. Surgical correction before the irreversibility of these symptoms is very important.[12]

Physical findings. In the early stage of aortic regurgitation, vital signs may remain normal, with the only remarkable finding being the characteristic blowing diastolic murmur. In the later stages of the disease the peripheral pulse exhibits a rapid rise in upstroke followed by a swift collapse of the diastolic pulse (*Corrigan's* or water-hammer *pulse*). The arterial pulse pressure is usually widened, with an elevated systolic pressure and diminished diastolic pressure. Abnormal capillary pulsations, seen as an alternating paling and flushing of the skin at the nailbed root while pressure is applied at the tip (*Quincke's pulse*), are characteristic of aortic regurgitation. The femoral arterial pulse typically exhibits a to-and-fro murmur (Duroziez' sign) and a booming pistol-shot sound when the artery is slightly compressed with the diaphragm of the stethoscope.

Patients with aortic regurgitation may show skin manifestations of the hyperdynamic state with sweating and flushing. An obvious bobbing of the head with each cardiac pulsation can occur (de Musset's sign). The large stroke volume also can be detected in the accentuated pulsatile motion of the carotid arteries. The neck veins are not usually distended unless right ventricular failure has occurred. There often is a diastolic thrill palpable along the left sternal border. The apical beat tends to be displaced laterally and a systolic thrill sometimes can be felt in the jugular notch and along the carotid arteries. S_3 and S_4 commonly are heard.

The classic auscultatory finding of aortic regurgitation is a blowing, high-pitched, decrescendo, diastolic murmur heard best at the second right intercostal space radiating to the left sternal border. It is caused by the backward flow of blood from the aorta to the left ventricle through an incompetent valve. A systolic ejection murmur also can be appreciated as an increased volume of blood crosses the aortic valve. It is heard best at the base of the heart, can radiate to the carotid arteries, is higher pitched than the murmur of aortic stenosis, and does not always mean that aortic stenosis is present. Another auscultatory finding sometimes encountered in aortic regurgitation is the *Austin Flint* murmur. This is a rumbling, diastolic murmur heard best at the apex. It has been attributed to impingement on the mitral valve by the aortic regurgitant flow, creating a functional mitral stenosis.

Chest x-ray examination may reveal cardiac enlargement with left atrial and left ventricular dilation. If heart failure is present, pulmonary venous congestion will be evident. The typical ECG changes of aortic regurgitation are reflections of left ventricular enlargement or hypertrophy. This is manifested by increased QRS amplitude and ST-T—wave depression. Sinus rhythm is usually seen with normal conduction. However, prolonged AV conduction can occur in late stages of the disease. The echocardiogram is useful in detecting ventricular volume overload with increased chamber dimensions. Serial studies with two-dimensional echocardiography can identify early changes in left ventricular function, which can be valuable for determining the most appropriate time for surgical correction. Doppler echocardiography is the most sensitive and accurate technique for detecting even the mildest degree of aortic regurgitation that is not yet evident to auscultation. The amount of regurgitant flow and the size of the regurgitant orifice can be measured using this technique.[33] Radionuclide studies can be used to determine resting and exercise ejection fractions to estimate left ventricular function.

Cardiac catheterization is done in aortic regurgitation to determine the severity of aortic valve incompetence, the degree of left ventricular function, and the presence of other cardiac valve abnormalities; coronary angiography may be used to detect the presence of coronary artery disease.

Treatment. Patients with no symptoms who have only mild or moderate aortic regurgitation and normal or only minimally elevated cardiac dimensions do not require medications but should have yearly echocardiograms. Patients with no symptoms but who have severe chronic aortic regurgitation with normal left ventricular function should be examined every 6 months with echocardiography, ECG, chest x-ray, and radionuclide ventriculography studies. A primary concern with asymptomatic aortic regurgitation is antibiotic prophylaxis against infective endocarditis for all dental procedures and surgery (see Chapter 13). Infections, fevers, and dysrhythmias are poorly tolerated by patients with more severe aortic regurgitation. These patients should avoid heavy exertion and vigorous activities that can result in cardiac decompensation and death.

The use of cardiac glycosides is important for patients with severe aortic regurgitation and left ventricle dilation.

Diastolic hypertension should be controlled because it increases regurgitation. Drugs that decrease left ventricular function (i.e., propranolol) are contraindicated. If left ventricular failure and pulmonary congestion are present, digitalis glycosides, diuretics, vasodilating agents, and sodium restriction are necessary. However, because the defect is mechanical, surgical replacement of the incompetent valve is the only effective long-term corrective measure.

RIGHT-SIDED VALVULAR SYNDROMES
Tricuspid valve disease
Tricuspid stenosis

Etiology. The most common cause of tricuspid stenosis is rheumatic fever. It is an uncommon valvular lesion, not usually occurring alone. It is not often seen with mitral stenosis and sometimes with combined mitral and aortic stenosis. Tricuspid stenosis is sometimes associated with the carcinoid syndrome, endocardial fibroelastosis, endomyocardial fibrosis, and systemic lupus erythematosus. Right atrial myxomas can cause this condition by obstructing the tricuspid orifice. Tricuspid stenosis is often undetected. The typical patient with this abnormality is a woman with mitral stenosis of rheumatic origin between the age of 20 and 60.

Pathophysiology. The typical hemodynamic finding in tricuspid stenosis is a diastolic pressure gradient between the right atrium and right ventricle with an often greatly dilated right atrium. The pressure gradient increases during inspiration as the venous return and transvalvular blood flow rise and decline during expiration when the flow is reduced. Cardiac output is often significantly reduced and does not rise during exertion.

As the mean right atrial pressure (RAP) increases because of the stenotic tricuspid valve, the pressure is reflected backward, resulting in systemic venous congestion, ascites, and edema (Fig. 12-6). The right ventricular output is depressed as a result of elevated RAP and reduced flow across the stenotic valve. Coexisting mitral stenosis influences these hemodynamic abnormalities. Obstruction of the tricuspid valve and reduced right ventricular flow are thought to protect against severe pulmonary hypertension.

Clinical manifestations. The symptoms usually associated with tricuspid stenosis are easy fatigability, effort intolerance from diminished cardiac output, a fluttering sensation in the neck, hepatomegaly, peripheral edema, ascites, and atrial fibrillation in the late stages of the disease. Typically, patients with significant tricuspid stenosis have severe hepatomegaly, ascites, and edema but little dyspnea.

Physical findings. Marked hepatic congestion with resultant cirrhosis, jaundice, malnutrition, severe edema, and ascites are associated with tricuspid stenosis. The jugular veins are distended, and prominent presystolic pulsations in the enlarged liver may be evident in patients with sinus rhythm. The jugular pulse usually exhibits an *a* wave.

Auscultation characteristically reveals a diastolic rumbling murmur heard best at the lower left sternal border. Inspiration markedly accentuates the rumble of tricuspid

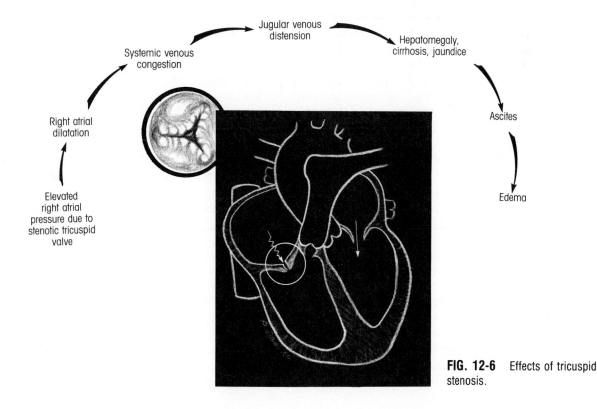

FIG. 12-6   Effects of tricuspid stenosis.

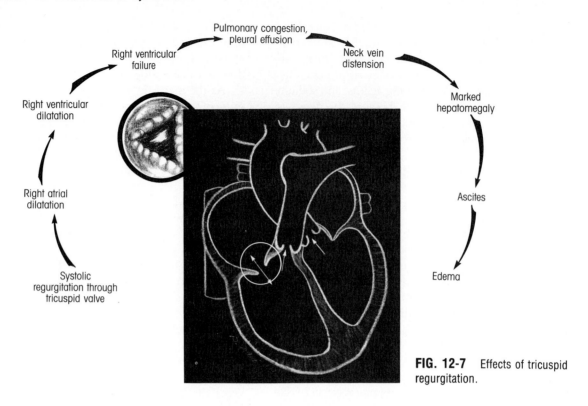

Right ventricular
failure

Pulmonary congestion,
pleural effusion

Neck vein
distension

Right ventricular
dilatation

Marked
hepatomegaly

Right atrial
dilatation

Ascites

Systolic
regurgitation through
tricuspid valve

Edema

FIG. 12-7 Effects of tricuspid regurgitation.

stenosis, differentiating it from the similar murmur of mitral stenosis (Carvallo sign). If tricuspid stenosis is combined with mitral stenosis, the S_1 will probably be split.

The ECG will show tall, peaked P waves (P pulmonale) without signs of RVH if the patient is in sinus rhythm. Also seen commonly is a small RSR' complex in V_1 and V_2 with P waves of larger amplitude than the QRS complex. A prolonged PR interval is also frequently seen. The chest x-ray film usually shows right atrial enlargement when tricuspid stenosis is combined with mitral stenosis. The M-mode echocardiogram usually demonstrates tricuspid valve leaflet thickening. Two-dimensional echocardiography is very helpful in diagnosing tricuspid stenosis by revealing diastolic coning of the leaflets and other restrictive leaflet abnormalities. A cardiac catheterization is necessary to determine the diastolic gradient across the valve.

Treatment. Patients with tricuspid stenosis are usually treated with antibiotic prophylaxis to prevent endocarditis. The marked systemic congestion that accompanies this condition is usually managed with intense sodium restriction, diuretics, and digitalis glycosides.

The treatment of the patient with tricuspid stenosis and other valve lesions usually focuses on the more severe lesion, generally mitral stenosis. Tricuspid commissurotomy is necessary when surgery is performed to correct concurrent aortic or mitral disease if cardiac output is to be improved.[5]

Tricuspid regurgitation

Etiology. Tricuspid regurgitation is generally functional and secondary to right ventricular dilation and failure from any cause. This abnormality can be congenital or caused by rheumatic fever. When rheumatic fever is the cause, it can be associated with tricuspid stenosis or mitral or aortic valve disease. Infective endocarditis, particularly staphlococcal endocarditis as seen in intravenous drug abusers,[4] is the usual cause of isolated tricuspid regurgitation, but this condition is rare. Trauma, prolapsed valve leaflets, congenital abnormalities, and myocardial infarction are less common causes of this condition. However, tricuspid regurgitation can be caused by any condition that produces left ventricular failure or pulmonary hypertension.

Pathophysiology. The RAP is greatly increased in tricuspid regurgitation because of the regurgitant flow of blood from the ventricle into the atrium during systole (Fig. 12-7). The elevated RAP causes increased pressure in the superior and inferior venae cavae and in the hepatic veins. Ascites and peripheral edema develop in response to this. Because only part of the blood is expelled into the pulmonary artery, the workload of the right ventricle increases, and RVH and dilation develop in response to this. Tricuspid regurgitation also causes a decrease in cardiac output.[8]

Clinical manifestations. The symptoms observed in patients with tricuspid regurgitation result from systemic venous congestion and reduced cardiac output. The neck veins are distended and often display a characteristic systolic pulsation as blood regurgitates into the right atrium and superior vena cava. Common symptoms of tricuspid regurgitation include marked hepatomegaly, ascites, pleural effusions, edema, systolic pulsations of the liver, and positive hepatojugular reflux.

Physical findings. Atrial fibrillation is a common finding in tricuspid regurgitation. Right bundle branch block can occur resulting from diastolic overload of the right ventricle. There is often a significant pulsation appreciable at the left parasternal region.

The murmur of tricuspid regurgitation is heard best along the left sternal border in the fourth or fifth intercostal space. It is a blowing pansystolic murmur that characteristically increases during inspiration and decreases during expiration (Carvallo sign) or the Valsalva maneuver. Some patients exhibit a low-pitched early diastolic murmur caused by increased diastolic filling of the right ventricle. The ECG usually shows atrial fibrillation and the chest x-ray examination often reveals right atrial and ventricular dilation.

Two-dimensional color-coded Doppler echocardiography seems to be the most sensitive, accurate, and specific method for the evaluation of tricuspid regurgitation. Cardiac catheterization can identify the severity of regurgitation.

Treatment. Medical management of tricuspid regurgitation usually is aimed at reducing the cause of heart failure. Treatment includes digitalis glycosides, diuretics, and a low-sodium diet. Because functional tricuspid regurgitation is commonly seen in conjunction with mitral stenosis, the condition often improves after mitral valve surgery. Tricuspid valve replacement may be indicated if regurgitation and stenosis are present in the valve.

Pulmonary valve disease

Etiology. Abnormalities of the pulmonary valve are usually congenital; acquired lesions are rare but can be caused by inflammatory lesions of rheumatic fever, carcinoid valvular lesions, tuberculosis, or syphilis. Pulmonary hypertension caused by mitral stenosis, chronic lung disease, or pulmonary emboli can lead to functional pulmonary regurgitation.

Malignant carcinoid tumors can affect the cardiac valves, mostly on the right side of the heart. The valvular lesions associated with the carcinoid syndrome are caused by the effects of serotonin or bradykinins, which are released by the tumor. The pulmonary and tricuspid valves are generally affected and exhibit a pearly white thickening with retraction and fusing of the chordae tendineae.[20]

Pathophysiology. Regurgitation is the most frequent abnormality in pulmonary valvular disease. Pulmonic regurgitation is most commonly caused by dilation of the valvular ring secondary to pulmonary hypertension. The second most common cause is infective endocarditis.[12] Pulmonary regurgitation causes a volume overload in the right ventricle. If pulmonary hypertension is preexistent, this overload is superimposed on the hypertrophied right ventricle, further compounding the problem.

Clinical manifestations. The clinical manifestations of acquired pulmonary valve lesions depend on the severity of valvular impairment and the degree of underlying disease. Patients may not have symptoms for some time with pulmonary regurgitation as an isolated abnormality. Dyspnea, fatigue, and syncope can occur with severe pulmonary hypertension; lesions resulting from inflammatory processes can be associated with fever and lung infections.

If pulmonary valvular problems are associated with the carcinoid syndrome, facial flushing, increased intestinal activity, diarrhea, and bronchial spasms may develop as a result of the effects of serotonin. If the primary lesion is in the abdomen, abdominal pain and weight loss may be a problem.

As right-sided heart failure ensues and the pressure backs up through the systemic circulation, distended neck veins, hepatomegaly, ascites, and peripheral edema may occur (Fig. 12-8).

Physical findings. Because patients with pulmonary valvular disease may have no symptoms for some time, their overall appearance may be normal and healthy. However, if the disease is severe and in its late stages, the symptoms of right-sided and then left-sided heart failure will be evident.

Palpation may reveal a thrusting right ventricular lift extending as far as the apex because of right ventricular enlargement. The classic physical finding in pulmonary stenosis is a systolic thrill heard best in the second intercostal space along the left sternal border. This thrill varies in intensity, depending on the severity of the stenosis. Auscultatory findings in pulmonary stenosis may include a normal S_1 and a split S_2. The sound of pulmonary valve closure may be decreased because of calcification. A systolic ejection click is usually present in the pulmonary area.

The murmur of pulmonary stenosis is characteristically harsh, diamond shaped, and systolic. It radiates along the left sternal border from the pulmonary area and sometimes into the neck. The murmur of pulmonary regurgitation is a moderately pitched, decrescendo, diastolic sound best heard in the fourth or fifth intercostal space at the left sternal border. It can be difficult to distinguish from the murmur of aortic regurgitation (Fig. 12-9).

The ECG may be normal in mild pulmonary stenosis. In severe cases large R waves are evident in V_1, deep S waves will appear in V_6, and T-wave inversion is possible in V_1 through V_4 with right axis deviation. Dysrhythmias are uncommon. Chest x-ray examination frequently shows poststenotic dilation of the main pulmonary arterial trunk and left pulmonary artery, sometimes to aneurysmal proportions. Phonocardiography is another valuable nonin-

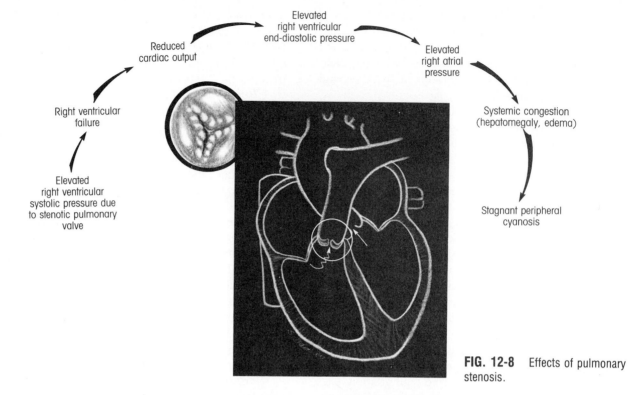

Reduced cardiac output

Elevated right ventricular end-diastolic pressure

Elevated right atrial pressure

Right ventricular failure

Elevated right ventricular systolic pressure due to stenotic pulmonary valve

Systemic congestion (hepatomegaly, edema)

Stagnant peripheral cyanosis

FIG. 12-8 Effects of pulmonary stenosis.

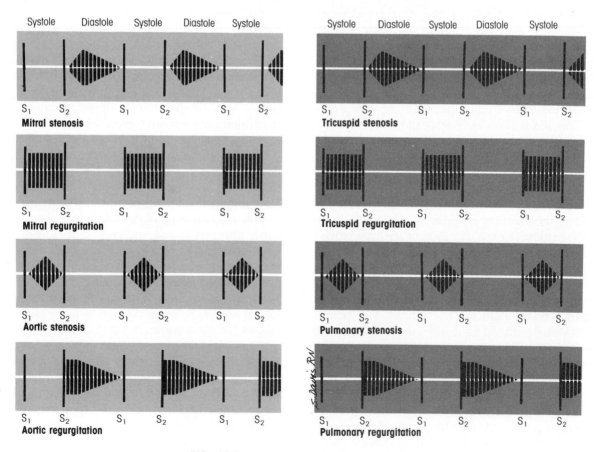

Systole	Diastole	Systole	Diastole	Systole

S_1 S_2 S_1 S_2 S_1 S_2
Mitral stenosis

S_1 S_2 S_1 S_2 S_1 S_2
Mitral regurgitation

S_1 S_2 S_1 S_2 S_1 S_2
Aortic stenosis

S_1 S_2 S_1 S_2 S_1 S_2
Aortic regurgitation

S_1 S_2 S_1 S_2 S_1 S_2
Tricuspid stenosis

S_1 S_2 S_1 S_2 S_1 S_2
Tricuspid regurgitation

S_1 S_2 S_1 S_2 S_1 S_2
Pulmonary stenosis

S_1 S_2 S_1 S_2 S_1 S_2
Pulmonary regurgitation

FIG. 12-9 Valvular heart disease murmurs.

vasive technique for evaluating the severity of pulmonary valve disease. Cardiac catheterization is done to determine the degree of valvular and right ventricular dysfunction.

Treatment. Periodic physical examinations are important for patients with pulmonary valve disease because the appearance of symptoms is an indication for surgical correction. Prophylaxis for infective endocarditis generally is prescribed for these patients. If heart failure is present, it usually is treated with digitalis glycosides, diuretics, and a low-sodium diet. Pulmonary valve commissurotomy may be done to relieve pulmonary stenosis, and valve replacement is rarely necessary.

MULTIVALVULAR DISEASE

Stenosis and regurgitation of significant severity can occur in the same valve. Rheumatic heart disease is the most common cause of these multiple lesions, with concurrent mitral stenosis and aortic regurgitation or aortic stenosis being the most common combinations. Tricuspid stenosis is sometimes seen with mitral or aortic stenosis, but significant problems with all four valves are rare. A functional tricuspid regurgitation is not unusual in the late stages of mitral valve disease.

The clinical manifestations and physical findings of lesions occurring in combination depends on the chronicity and severity of each separate valvular abnormality. However, some concurrent lesions may ease the effects of one another on a chamber. For example, mitral stenosis may prevent the left ventricle from suffering the total effects of aortic valvular disease, and tricuspid stenosis does the same for the right ventricle and pulmonary system when it accompanies mitral stenosis.

The changes on the ECG and chest x-ray film reflect the major hemodynamic stresses of each lesion. The treatment of patients with multivalvular disease depends on the severity of the various lesions and the severity of other myocardial problems.

Nursing process

Case study. Ms. B. C., a 46-year-old housewife, was referred to a cardiologist because of episodes of dyspnea that were becoming increasingly more severe. Ms. B. C. had rheumatic fever at the age of 15 but was not diagnosed as having a heart murmur until the age of 25. Except for mild shortness of breath in the last trimester of her three pregnancies, the patient had no symptoms until the age of 43. At that time, she noticed mild exertional dyspnea, the severity of which remained unchanged until 18 months before seeing the cardiologist. At the time of her referral, she was complaining of shortness of breath on mild exertion to the point where she was unable to perform ordinary household chores. After digitalization, the patient noticed some improvement in exercise tolerance.

During the physical examination, the patient was found to be a well-developed woman who seemed to be anxious but was in no acute distress. The patient's blood pressure was 130/80 mm Hg, the radial pulse was regular at 90 beats per minute, respirations were 24 per minute, and oral temperature was 98.8° F. The neck veins were not distended when the trunk was elevated at 45 degrees, but a prominent jugular *a* wave was noted. The lungs were clear to auscultation and percussion. Palpation revealed a diffuse left parasternal heave, but the apical pulse was discernable. No thrills were noted. There was an accentuation of the S_1 at the mitral area and an OS followed by a low-pitched diastolic rumble at the mitral area. Both components of the S_2 could be heard at the mitral area. The liver edge was palpated 1.0 cm below the right costal margin. The peripheral pulses were present but of low volume, and slight pretibial edema was present.[19]

Nursing assessment

Although the case study and nursing assessment in this section focuses on the patient with mitral stenosis, it is necessary to collect data within the nine human response patterns when assessing a patient suspected of having cardiac valvular disease. The nursing assessment should specifically focus on the Knowing, Moving, Feeling, Exchanging, and Choosing Patterns.

Knowing pattern

When assessing the Knowing Pattern of the patient with mitral stenosis, investigate the history of the present illness to determine the patient's understanding and perceptions of the situation. Investigate when symptoms were noticed by the patient, the way the symptoms have progressed over time, and the reason the patient has sought health care. The patient with valvular heart disease may have become ill at an early age or may have become progressively more disabled over the course of many years. Ask the patient about occurrences of dyspnea on exertion, orthopnea, or paroxysmal nocturnal dyspnea.

Determine any episode of rheumatic fever, when it occurred, and whether the patient has been told of a preexisting heart murmur. Inquire about medical treatment and activity-related restrictions imposed by the illness. Investigate whether a cardiac catheterization has ever been performed, the date it was done, and the results of the procedure. Explore the family's health history, and identify occurrences of valvular or other forms of heart disease or other genetic abnormalities to which the patient may be predisposed.

The patient who has been recently diagnosed with mitral stenosis and the family may need information regarding the cause of the disease, its prognosis, and natural course over time. Their knowledge about the need for prophylaxis against endocarditis should be investigated. Because multiple testing procedures are used to assess, diagnose, treat disease progression, evaluate the patient's and family members' knowledge regarding these procedures (e.g., ECGs, chest x-ray tests, echocardiography, radionuclide testing, and cardiac catheterization), and assess the significance of the information they reveal. Identify signs of readiness to learn (e.g., the patient asking specific questions regarding the illness, testing procedures, and possible outcomes), and determine areas of misconception.

Depending on the severity of the disease process, assess the patient's and family's knowledge regarding medications, dietary restrictions, and activity limitations to reveal areas in which teaching is important. Teach about side effects and proper use of drugs such as digitalis, diuretics, vasodilators, calcium antagonists, antidysrhythmics, and anticoagulants used at various times in the treatment of mitral stenosis. Teach behavior modification regarding activity limitations and dietary restrictions (i.e., sodium).

Moving pattern

Within the Moving Pattern, assess patients' activity tolerance to determine the degree of valvular dysfunction. Patients with mitral stenosis may not have any functional disabilities and may be able to perform all activities of daily living unencumbered by fatigue or dyspnea if the valvular stenosis is not severe. Fatiguability and dyspnea on exertion increase as failure occurs and make activities of daily living difficult to perform. Orthopnea and paroxysmal nocturnal

dyspnea may disturb sleep, accentuate fatigue, and make accomplishment of daily tasks more difficult. Question patients about activities they are able to accomplish and lengths of time before becoming fatigued. Ask about specific activities they are unable to perform and the last time they were able to perform them. Determine patients' sleep patterns and identify whether alterations in normal sleep rest patterns have recently been observed.

Feeling pattern

Depending on the severity of the mitral stenosis, patients may be dyspneic, have uncomfortable palpitations if atrial fibrillation is present, be uncomfortable because of ascites, or be easily fatigued. Patients may have coughs with hemoptysis, which can be frightening to them and families.

However, if patients are in the early stages of the disease and symptoms have not become problematic, they may be anxious about the future. For patients facing cardiac catheterization or valve replacement, fear and anxiety may be significant findings, requiring nursing intervention for teaching and reassurance.[24]

TABLE 12-1
Valvular Heart Disease Symptoms

Mitral stenosis	Mitral regurgitation	Mitral prolapse	Aortic stenosis	Aortic regurgitation	Tricuspid stenosis	Tricuspid regurgitation	Pulmonary valve disease
Dyspnea on exertion	Paroxysmal nocturnal dyspnea	Dyspnea Dizziness; syncope	Exertional dyspnea	Dyspnea Orthopnea	Dyspnea Fatigue	Neck vein distention	Symptoms of right-sided heart failure; then
Orthopnea	Exertional dyspnea	Palpitations	Fatigue	Paroxysmal nocturnal dyspnea	Malnutrition	Pulsating neck veins	Symptoms of left-sided
Paroxysmal nocturnal dyspnea	Weakness and fatigue	Chest pain Atrial tachycardia	Orthopnea Chest pain	Fatigue	Severe hepatomegaly	Pleural effusions	heart failure
Fatigue	Weight loss; cachexia	Ventricular tachycardia	Syncope	Palpitations; awareness of heartbeat	Ascites	Hepatomegaly Ascites	
Palpitations	Atrial fibrillation	Bradydysrhythmias		Exertional chest pain	Edema	Edema	
Cough				Nocturnal chest pain with diaphoresis	Cirrhosis	Hepatic systolic pulsations	
Hemoptysis	Right-sided heart failure			Sinus tachycardia	Jaundice	Positive hepatojugular reflux	
Hoarseness	Ankle edema			Premature ventricular contractions			
Emboli	Ascites			Right-sided heart failure			
Atrial fibrillation	Neck vein distention			Hepatomegaly			
Tachycardia	Tricuspid regurgitation			Ascites			
Narrowed pulse pressure				Ankle edema			
Peripheral cyanosis				Prominent neck vein pulsations			
Neck vein distention							

Exchanging pattern

The symptoms and complications of a patient with valvular heart disease vary (Table 12-1). Identify the specific signs and symptoms to plan and treat the individual effectively at different phases of the illness and during rehabilitation.

Evaluate the degree of altered cardiac output. The presence and severity of the heart murmurs (Table 12-2) and the symptoms exhibited help determine the nursing diagnoses and the interventions for patients with such problems (Table 12-3).

When assessing cardiac output, evaluate patients for resting tachycardia, atrial fibrillation, palpitations, and angina pectoris. Patients' arterial blood pressures may be normal or somewhat low with narrowed pulse pressures. If

TABLE 12-2
Common Murmurs of Valvular Heart Disease

Disease	Timing	Location/radiation	Quality/configuration	Pitch
Mitral stenosis	Diastolic	Apex	Rumbling, crescendo-decrescendo	Low
Mitral regurgitation	Systolic	Apex, radiating to left axillary line	Blowing, pansystolic	High
Aortic stenosis	Systolic	Second right intercostal space to carotid artery	Harsh, crescendo-decrescendo	Low
Aortic regurgitation	Diastolic	Second right intercostal space radiating to left sternal border	Blowing, decrescendo	High
Tricuspid stenosis	Diastolic	Fifth intercostal space, left lower sternal border	Rumbling, crescendo-decrescendo	Low
Tricuspid regurgitation	Systolic	Fifth intercostal space, left lower sternal border	Blowing, pansystolic	High
Pulmonary stenosis	Systolic	Second left intercostal space	Harsh, crescendo-decrescendo	Medium
Pulmonary regurgitation	Diastolic	Third and fourth left intercostal spaces	Blowing, decrescendo	High or low

TABLE 12-3
Medical Treatment of Valvular Heart Disease

Mitral stenosis	Mitral regurgitation	Mitral prolapse	Aortic stenosis	Aortic regurgitation	Tricuspid stenosis	Tricuspid regurgitation	Pulmonary valve disease
Antibiotic prophylaxis	Antibiotic prophylaxis	Reassurance	Antibiotic prophylaxis	Antibiotic prophylaxis	Antibiotic prophylaxis	Digitalis	Antibiotic prophylaxis
Diuretics	Activity limitation	Propranolol	Digitalis	Digitalis	Sodium restriction	Diuretics	Frequent physical examinations
Sodium restriction, sitting position, oxygen	Sodium restriction	Analgesics	Diuretics	Diuretics	Diuretics	Sodium restriction	Digitalis
Avoiding strenuous activity	Diuretics	Antibiotic prophylaxis for more severe prolapse	Sodium restriction	Vasodilators	Digitalis	Oxygen	Diuretics
Digitalis	Digitalis		Activity limitations	Sodium restriction	Oxygen		Sodium restriction
Quinidine	Quinidine		Nitrates	Oxygen			Oxygen
Elective cardioversion	Vasodilators		Oxygen	Activity limitation			
Anticoagulation	Anticoagulation						

severe pulmonary hypertension has developed, there may be prominent *a* waves in the jugular venous pulse. If patients are in atrial fibrillation, the jugular venous pulse may exhibit only a single systolic expansion, called the *c-v* wave.

In mitral stenosis, patients have a rumbling crescendo-decrescendo murmur heard best at the apex after an OS. Palpate the chest to reveal a diastolic thrill at the apex.

Also assess the signs and symptoms of pulmonary venous congestion. Note the degree of dyspnea on exertion and activities with which it is associated. Assess patients' breath sounds; observe for tachypnea, shortness of breath, orthopnea, crackles, and wheezing. Observe patients for "mitral facies," with a pinched, flushed, facial expression, or peripheral or central cyanosis, depending on the severity of the mitral stenosis. In addition, assess patients for dysphagia, hoarseness, seizures, or hemoptysis.

The ECGs of patients with mitral stenosis may have normal QRS complexes with broad, notched P waves. If severe pulmonary hypertension is present, tall R waves in the precordial leads and a right axis deviation may be present.

The chest x-ray films may show an enlarged left atrium and right ventricle with prominent pulmonary arteries if right-sided failure is present. M-mode echocardiography characteristically reveals left atrial enlargement, thickening and limitation of the motion of mitral valve leaflets, delayed diastolic closure of mitral leaflets, and right ventricular enlargement in late stages. Two-dimensional echocardiography can quantify the mitral valve area. Doppler ultrasound can quantify the flow rate across the stenotic orifice. Higher rates of flow signify more-severe degrees of mitral stenosis.

Cardiac catheterization reveals the severity of the mitral stenosis, cardiac output, area of the mitral valve orifice, and condition of the right and left sides of the heart. Radionuclide studies quantitatively reveal changes in cardiac performance produced by exercise. The information from these evaluations can determine if and when valve replacement is necessary.

Communicating pattern

The patient with mitral stenosis might exhibit hoarseness because of pressure on the left recurrent layrngeal nerve by an enlarged left atrium, enlarged tracheobronchial lymph nodes, and a dilated pulmonary artery. The individual may be dyspneic even at rest if pulmonary edema is present. A cough may be present. Thus depending on the severity of the mitral valve disease, the ability to communicate may be impaired.

Valuing pattern

Because mitral valve disease can be present for some time before symptoms appear, these patients may be well motivated to reattain the degree of health they once enjoyed or prevent further deterioration of their condition. How-

ever, if debility has been present for some time, patients may have become resigned to their state of incapacitation or be receiving so much secondary gain from the sick role that there is not much motivation toward wellness-related behavior. Therefore determine whether the patient values a return to a more-healthy state.

Relating pattern

Depending on the degree of mitral stenosis and the severity of symptoms present, these patients may be unable to complete activities of daily living without assistance. Responsibilities around the home and in the family once well within patients' capabilities may now be beyond their physical capacities. Depending on how patients and families or significant others deal with the situation, it may be necessary to use various resources to assist with a healthy adaptation to the situation at present and in the future.

Perceiving pattern

Patients with severe mitral stenosis who are debilitated by heart failure may perceive themselves as burdens on their families or significant others. Self-esteem and self-concept may suffer seriously if patients were the heads of households (i.e., "bread winners") who must now depend on partners or other family members to function in these roles. If fatigue and dyspnea are becoming more pronounced, patients may be feeling a loss of control over their lives because they can no longer function as they once did. Feelings of hopelessness and powerlessness may emerge from the assessment. Self-esteem may be low and cause personal psychologic difficulty for the patient and difficulties within the family unit.

Choosing pattern

For the patient with severe mitral stenosis who has repeated hospitalizations for congestive heart failure, noncompliance with medications and sodium restrictions may be the problem. The patient may not successfully cope with the illness, which is manifested in noncompliance. If the patient is facing surgery, assess the coping mechanisms of all concerned. Expectations regarding the outcome of surgery may give valuable information about how successfully the patient will choose behaviors consistent with postoperative wellness (i.e., compliance with anticoagulant therapy). Assess the patient who has no symptoms for ability and success in choosing to comply with the current medical regimen, the need for regular follow-up care, and endocarditis prophylaxis.

Nursing diagnoses

The medical diagnosis in the case study is mitral stenosis. The most common human responses anticipated for a patient with mitral stenosis are indicated by the following nursing diagnoses:

1. Decreased cardiac output related to (include problem) mitral stenosis
2. Altered protection (emboli and bleeding) related to anticoagulation
3. Impaired physical mobility related to chest pain, dyspnea, and fatigue
4. High risk for valve infection related to hemodynamic valve deformity

5. High risk for noncompliance to the medical regimen related to inadequate health teaching

For each of these diagnoses, the patient outcomes, nursing prescriptions, and evaluation criteria are outlined with a discussion of the factual information that supports the plan and implementation of care.

NURSING DIAGNOSIS 1 **Decreased cardiac output related to (include problem) mitral stenosis (exchanging pattern)**

PATIENT OUTCOMES	NURSING PRESCRIPTIONS	EVALUATION
Patient will appropriately respond to cardioversion or medication to control dysrhythmias and promote adequate cardiac output.	Carefully monitor patient's cardiac rhythm and hemodynamic parameters. Institute therapy such as medications or cardioversion to control dysrhythmias and promote adequate cardiac output.	Patient remained in sinus rhythm without dysrhythmias.
Patient will verbalize the schedule for taking medication and the correct dose, the purpose and importance of medication, and its side effects.	Teach patient medication dose and schedule, purpose and importance of medication, and its side effects.	Patient was able to verbalize appropriate medication dose and schedule, the purpose and importance of the medication, and its side effects.

Plan and intervention for decreased cardiac output

Two major concerns in valvular heart disease are the maintenance of normal cardiac output and sinus rhythm. Atrial fibrillation is common in patients with rheumatic heart disease, especially mitral stenosis and mitral regurgitation.[17] The clinical manifestations of atrial fibrillation depend on the ventricular rate. If the rate is above 150 beats per minute, congestive heart failure or angina pectoris may develop. Congestive heart failure ensues because of the loss of the atrial systolic "booster kick."

Stasis of blood caused by ineffective atrial contractions in mitral stenosis often leads to thrombosis in the left atrium. Serious or lethal embolization can occur when small fragments of these thrombi break off and travel from the left atrium to the systemic circulation or from the right atrium to the pulmonary vasculature in the lungs.

For these reasons it is necessary to attempt to restore sinus rhythm or, if this is unsuccessful, to at least slow the ventricular rate. If the situation is an emergency, digitalis is the drug of choice. The basis for use of this drug in supraventricular tachydysrhythmias such as atrial fibrillation is reflex vagal stimulation, depression of impulse formation at the SA node, and a negative dromotropic effect or impulse conduction through the AV node and bundle branches (negative chronotropic effect). Digitalis also in-

creases the force of contraction by direct effect on the myocardium (promotes passages of calcium, sodium, and potassium ions across the sarcolemma by affecting adenosine triphosphatase). This positive inotropic effect also indirectly slows the ventricular rate.[20,21] The goal of digitalis therapy is to slow the ventricular rate to between 60 and 80 beats per minute. Cardiac output may fall if the ventricular rate falls below 60.

Emergency digitalization is usually accomplished intravenously. It can be done orally if the patient's condition permits. This can be achieved over several days if signs of acute congestive heart failure are absent or if the ventricular rate is approximately 100 beats per minute.

If digitalization slows the ventricular rate but atrial fibrillation does not resolve, quinidine or procainamide may be added to the regimen. These agents are quite similar in their electrophysiologic actions. They decrease myocardial excitability by shifting the threshold potential to less-negative levels and thus increasing the voltage difference between the resting and threshold potentials. Because of this, more current is required to bring the resting membrane potential to threshold potential. Quinidine and procainamide increase the effective refractory period in the muscle fibers of the atria and ventricles and in the Purkinje fibers. The *effective refractory period* refers to the time that must transpire after excitation before another propagated impulse can be initiated.

These drugs slow heart rate by decreasing the conduction velocity in the atrial and ventricular fibers and in the His-Purkinje fiber system. The lowered conduction velocity is the result of quinidine and procainamide acting on the fast sodium channels, ultimately causing the action potential to conduct more slowly or block. Quinidine and procainamide also exert an antiautomatic effect by decreasing the slope of phase 4 diastolic depolarization in Purkinje fibers and in the SA node.

Propranolol or other β-adrenergic blocking drugs can be used with digitalis to increase AV block and slow the ventricular rate. The effect of propranolol on dysrhythmias is the result of β-adrenergic receptor blockade. Restoration of sinus rhythm can be accomplished with a combination of propranolol and quinidine. This is attempted after digitalis has been used to decrease ventricular rate. A maintenance dose of digitalis is administered with the quinidine and propranolol.

Verapamil, a calcium channel–blocking agent, can be given intravenously in an attempt to slow the ventricular rate or restore sinus rhythm. Verapamil prevents rapid and forceful ventricular contractions by preventing the extracellular influx of calcium during the fast-response action potential. The overall effect of this is to reduce electrical excitability and mechanical contractility. Atrial dysrhythmias in particular can be relieved and sometimes prevented in this way. Verapamil also relieves anginal pain caused by coronary artery spasms and reduces peripheral vascular resistance and myocardial oxygen consumption.

When atrial fibrillation is accompanied by a ventricular rate of between 60 and 80 beats per minute and it does not increase above 90 beats per minute with exercise, it is not always necessary to treat the condition. However, when treatment is necessary, the nurse must give the patient and family a thorough explanation of the rationale for and the effects of treatment. The patient and family must be encouraged to ask questions and discuss their feelings. Before patients are discharged, they must be thoroughly instructed in their medication regimen and potential side effects. They should be able to discuss the signs of toxicity of the drugs, as well as what should be done about them. Written instructions should be provided whenever possible (Tables 12-3 and 12-4).

For patients taking digitalis a comprehensive teaching plan should cover the following points:
1. The valvular problem
2. The drug action and dosage schedule
3. Ways to maintain a record of drug administration by checking off the days on a calendar
4. Ways and times when to take a radial pulse reading
5. Daily weight measurement and reporting of a weight gain of more than 3 to 5 pounds per week
6. Diet or fluid restrictions
7. Plans for follow-up care

Signs and symptoms indicative of digitalis toxicity should also be reported; they include nausea, vomiting, anorexia, diarrhea, salivation, fatigue, weakness, visual disturbances, headache, facial neuralgia, confusion, anxiety, apathy, depression, hallucinations, and premature ventricular contractions. Premature ventricular contractures may be described as palpitations, dizziness, faintness, precordial pain, a choking feeling, or a sinking feeling in the stomach.[21]

When quinidine is prescribed, the following points should be included in the teaching plan:
1. The purpose of the drug and its actions
2. The dosage schedule
3. Ways to use a calendar or some other form of recording when the medication is taken
4. Appropriate physical activities with spaced rest periods
5. Appropriate diet and control of weight
6. Factors to avoid, such as excessive fatigue, smoking, alcohol, excessive caffeine, undue stress, heavy meals, and the use of over-the-counter medications without physician approval.

Also include a discussion of the signs of quinidine toxicity that should be reported to the physician. These include visual disturbances, tinnitus, palpitations, breathlessness, and uncomfortable sensations in the chest. Noting the time of occurrence, frequence of occurrence, and duration of these chest sensations must be stressed. The patient must also be taught to report feelings of faintness. This symptom is referred to as *quinidine syncope* and is caused by changes in the ventricular rhythm (tachycardia or fibrillation), which results in a decrease in cardiac output and loss of consciousness.[21]

If procainamide is prescribed, the topics covered in the teaching program for quinidine should be covered because the two drugs are similar in action. The patient is also instructed to report pleuritic pain, arthralgias, fever, skin rashes, or myalgias because procainamide can cause a systemic lupus erythematosus–like reaction. The patient must be taught to be mindful of light-headedness, giddiness, weakness, and syncope because these symptoms may indicate a change in ventricular rhythm. The patient is taught to report and record the date, time, and length of these episodes and is cautioned to avoid driving a car or operating hazardous equipment until all symptoms have resolved. The patient must also be taught to be aware of and report unexplained bleeding or bruising, as well as sore throat, mouth, or gums, fever, or symptoms of a respiratory tract infection, because these are adverse effects that may necessitate discontinuation of the drug. Also discuss the use of over-the-counter medications and instruct the patient to speak with the physician about the continued use of these drugs.

When patients take propranolol (Inderal) and also have diabetes, they must report any and all symptoms of hypoglycemia regardless of how insignificant they may seem. Propranolol can mask the symptoms of insulin overdosage

TABLE 12-4
Drugs Frequently Used in Valvular Heart Disease

Drug	Effects	Side effects
Digitalis	Increases cardiac output by strengthening force of contraction Slows heart rate by decreasing conduction velocity at AV node Prolongs refractory period at AV node directly and through effect on SA node	Anorexia, nausea, vomiting, diarrhea, conduction disturbances. Premature ventricular contractions, supraventricular dysrhythmias, hypotension, fatigue, muscle weakness, hallucinations, agitation, dizziness, paresthesias, stupor, and visual disturbances
Propranolol	Decreases conduction through AV node Increases effective refractory period Has a reentry-blocking effect Reduces heart rate, myocardial irritability, and force of contraction Reduces myocardial oxygen requirements	Nausea, vomiting, diarrhea, abdominal cramps, palpitations, bradycardia, AV heart block, hypotension, acute congestive heart failure, dyspnea, confusion, agitation, hearing loss, visual disturbances, fever, fatigue, and syncope
Diuretics (thiazide and loop)	Enhance excretion of electrolytes and water Decrease plasma volume Lower blood pressure	Hypovolemia, dehydration, hyponatremia, hypokalemia, hypochloremia, metabolic alkalosis, hyperuricemia, postural hypotension, nausea, vomiting, diarrhea, pruritus, urticaria, tinnitus, hearing loss, and hyperglycemia
Quinidine	Depresses myocardial excitability, contractility, automaticity, and conduction velocity Prolongs effective refractory period Blocks vagal stimulation of AV node Causes peripheral vasodilation, resulting in lowering of blood pressure	Diarrhea, abdominal cramps, nausea, vomiting, sweating, palpitations, restlessness, hypotension, congestive heart failure, heart block, fever, and urticaria
Vasodilators (peripheral and coronary)	Relax smooth muscles, especially of blood vessels, resulting in vasodilation Cause pooling of blood in peripheral circulation by venodilation and thus decrease preload and oxygen consumption Cause arterial dilation, thus decreasing peripheral arterial resistance and afterload and oxygen consumption	Headache, dizziness, weakness, orthostatic hypotension, tachycardia, flushing, palpitations, fainting, nausea, vomiting, and rash
Anticoagulants (heparin and warfarin)	Depress synthesis in liver of several factors in the coagulation mechanism Prevent further extension of thrombus but do not directly affect existing thrombus	Anorexia; nausea; vomiting; abdominal cramps; diarrhea; dermatitis; urticaria; alopecia; fever; hematuria; bleeding from skin, mucous membranes, wounds, gastrointestinal tract; and excessive menstrual flow

and prolong hypoglycemic episodes. Patients should not fast longer than 12 hours because it may induce the hypoglycemic effects caused by propranolol. Patients might experience dyspnea, fatigue, weakness, and light-headedness with physical exertion or psychologic stress because propranolol diminishes the adaptive response to exercise and stress. Because of this side effect, it may be necessary to develop individualized activity programs for patients and to caution them against engaging in potentially dangerous activities such as driving cars. Also advise patients

to avoid overindulgence in alcohol, food, and coffee. Caution against smoking because it may induce blood pressure elevation.[20]

When calcium-blocking agents are prescribed, patients are instructed to report symptoms such as dizziness, weakness, fatigue, dyspnea, and light-headedness and are cautioned against driving cars or operating hazardous equipment until their reaction to the drug is known or until symptoms have passed. Patients are taught to report palpitations or uncomfortable sensations in the chest and to weigh themselves daily and report weight gains in excess of 3 to 5 pounds in a week.[35] Sodium restriction should be taught after the physician has been consulted.[20]

If elective cardioversion must be performed to reestablish sinus rhythm, special care must be taken to prepare the patient for the procedure because it can produce anxiety. Patients are told that they will have nothing by mouth after midnight the night before the procedure, unless the situation is urgent. In this case the previous meal will be withheld. Blood work will be done the day before to determine serum levels of digoxin and electrolytes. (Digitalis will not be withheld unless toxicity is suspected.)

Patients should know that cardioversion is usually carried out early in the day. They are assured that the room will be equipped with everything needed and are told that an intravenous infusion will be started for the administration of any necessary drugs, unless a line is already in place. They also should be aware that their blood pressures and ECGs will be monitored during the procedure and afterward.

Patients' most ardent concerns may center on the pain accompanying cardioversion. In some institutions a short-acting anesthetic or sedation and amnesic are given. Patients may also be concerned that they will be burned by the electrical current. Assure patients that the electrodes will be covered with a conductive gel or paste to prevent skin irritation. Patients may be concerned about the possibility of a fatal or serious dysrhythmia being caused by cardioversion; as a result, assure them that the likelihood of ventricular fibrillation being caused by synchronized countershock is rare (less than 5%).[11]

If atrial fibrillation is acute, if the rapid ventricular rate is unresponsive to medical treatment, or if severe congestive heart failure continues despite digitalization, synchronized countershock is the method of choice for cardioversion (see Appendix D). However, if atrial fibrillation is chronic, countershock is contraindicated because of the possibility of embolization from the atria. If the atria are enlarged, sinus rhythm is unlikely to persist after cardioversion because of the conduction disturbances caused by chronic atrial enlargement. Quinidine is administered every 6 hours, beginning 1 or 2 days before cardioversion, in oral doses of 0.3 to 0.4 g. The quinidine is intended to prevent the atrial fibrillation from recurring.

NURSING
DIAGNOSIS 2 **Altered protection (emboli and bleeding) related to anticoagulation (exchanging pattern)**

PATIENT OUTCOMES	NURSING PRESCRIPTIONS	EVALUATION
Patient will respond appropriately to anticoagulants to prevent emboli.	Administer anticoagulants as ordered and evaluate patient for signs and symptoms of emboli.	Patient did not develop emboli.
Patient will verbalize the rationale for the anticoagulant treatment, schedule for taking the drug and the amount to take, complications of the drug therapy (bleeding gums, prolonged bleeding from cuts, rectal bleeding, nosebleeds, and bruising), importance of having frequent coagulation studies, importance of notifying the physician if these complications occur, and precautions to be taken to prevent complications (use of electric razor, careful use of sharp objects, use of soft-bristled toothbrush, filing of nails rather than cutting of them).	Teach patient the rationale for use of anticoagulants, the amount of drug to take and schedule for taking it, complications of anticoagulants, importance of frequent coagulation studies, importance of notifying the physician if bleeding occurs, precautions to prevent complications (use of electric razor and soft toothbrush and care to avoid being cut), and avoiding foods high in vitamin K (green leafy vegetables).	Patient verbalized the rationale for taking anticoagulants, schedule for taking them and the amount to take, complications of therapy, importance of having frequent coagulation studies, importance of notifying the physician about complications, and precautions to be taken to prevent complications.
Patient will not experience complications from anticoagulation (bleeding gums, rectal bleeding, nosebleeds, bruising, and prolonged bleeding from cuts).	Monitor patient for complications of anticoagulant therapy (bleeding gums, rectal bleeding, nosebleeds, and bruising).	Patient did not experience complications from anticoagulant therapy.

Plan and intervention for altered protection related to anticoagulation

Embolic episodes occur in approximately 20% of patients suffering from mitral valve disease. Patients who are at the highest risk for emboli are over 40 years of age and have moderate-to-severe valve disease, enlargement of the left atrial appendage, and atrial fibrillation.[32]

The major source of the embolism in mitral valve disease is atrial thrombosis caused by stasis of left atrial blood. Atrial thrombosis and embolism are most common in rheumatic heart disease when atrial fibrillation is present. The incidence of embolism also increases when the heart rhythm goes back and forth from atrial fibrillation to sinus rhythm.[2]

Research has shown that chronic atrial fibrillation, regardless of whether rheumatic heart disease is present, greatly increases the risk of stroke from emboli. Studies of patients with mitral valve disease have found atrial fibrillation with clot formation in the atrium to be the predisposing factor to embolism.[31,32]

When a patient has valvular disease and chronic atrial fibrillation, anticoagulation is usually part of treatment. The three main groups of drugs used for anticoagulation are classified according to the mechanism by which they prevent clot formation:

1. Coumarin, indanedione derivatives, and heparin prevent the formation of sufficient thrombin to start or propagate a thrombus and thus inhibit the coagulation process.
2. Platelet antiaggregants (aspirin, sulfinpyrazone, dextran) prevent thrombus formation by removing or inhibiting substances necessary for coagulation.
3. Streptokinase, urokinase, and tissue plasminogen activator break down thrombi that have already formed.[16]

The nurse's responsibility to patients taking anticoagulants is to teach them to successfully manage drug therapy and prevent unnecessary complications from medication. If patients are taking coumarin, the prothrombin time must be evaluated at regular intervals. Patients must understand that it is their responsibility to have the test done at the appointed time.

Because vitamin K promotes the clotting of blood, eating many foods with a high vitamin K content can reduce the effectiveness of coumarin. The patient should be instructed to avoid eating large amounts of yellow and dark green vegetables, as well as too many fatty foods, which increase the absorption of vitamin K. Certain nonprescription drugs can increase or decrease the effect of anticoagulants, and all medications containing aspirin should be avoided because they enhance the effect of the anticoagulants. Laxatives with mineral oil should not be used because they facilitate the absorption of vitamin K and decrease the efficacy of the anticoagulant.

Illness accompanied by vomiting and diarrhea can decrease the absorption of the medication and must be immediately reported to a physician. Patients taking anticoagulants should be encouraged to wear gloves when gardening, use an electric razor, and avoid going barefoot. They should also use soft-bristled toothbrushes to prevent bleeding gums and use emery boards rather than scissors or clippers to trim nails.

Participation in any sport in which it is possible to suffer internal injuries or broken skin is discouraged. Because intrauterine devices can cause bleeding and oral contraceptives have been linked to thrombosis formation in some women, women taking anticoagulants should be encouraged to use other methods of birth control.

Any of the following symptoms should be referred to the physician immediately, or the patient should seek emergency attention:

1. Bleeding gums
2. Bleeding from lacerations that will not stop
3. Tarry stools or bright red blood in stools
4. Blood in urine
5. Abdominal pain
6. Headaches that are severe and persistent
7. Unusually heavy menstrual flow
8. Dizziness, faintness, and unusual weakness
9. Nosebleeds
10. Bruises that enlarge

Patients must inform dentists and other health professionals that they are taking anticoagulants. It is also prudent for these patients to wear identification bracelets and carry identification cards stating the name of the drug they are taking.[20,35]

NURSING
DIAGNOSIS 3 **Impaired physical mobility related to chest pain, dyspnea, and fatigue (moving pattern)**

PATIENT OUTCOMES	NURSING PRESCRIPTIONS	EVALUATION
Patient will demonstrate upper and lower extremity range of motion exercises within the limits of cardiac reserve to prevent emboli and stasis ulcers.	Teach and assist patient with upper and lower extremity range of motion exercises.	Patient correctly demonstrated upper and lower extremity range of motion exercises.
Patient will demonstrate coughing, deep breathing, and frequent position change to promote good pulmonary function and proper gas exchange.	Assist patient with turning, coughing, and deep breathing as necessary.	Patient correctly demonstrated turning, coughing, and deep breathing techniques.
Patient will verbalize principles of energy conservation techniques to prevent chest pain, dyspnea, and fatigue. These include spacing household tasks over the entire day and week rather than attempting to do everything at once, allowing for periods of rest between activities, not attempting strenuous activities without assistance, and resting when fatigue or dyspnea is experienced.	Teach patient principles of energy conservation techniques to prevent chest pain, dyspnea, and fatigue.	Patient verbalized principles of energy conservation techniques. (State specifics.)

Plan and intervention for impaired physical mobility

Patients with mitral stenosis may experience altered levels of physical mobility because of related pain, dyspnea, and fatigue. β-Blockers such as propranolol are often used to control chest pain associated with valvular heart disease. Sometimes stronger analgesics such as meperidine (Demerol) or oxycodone (Percodan) are required to alleviate acute pain. Painkillers prevent the uptake of catecholamines at nerve endings, thus interfering with the transmission of nerve impulses at the synapse and blocking pain. However, patients may feel too drugged to function normally while taking these medications. It is essential for the nurse to give reassurance and encourage patients to verbalize fears and frustrations.

Dyspnea, fatigue, and syncope are distressing symptoms experienced by these patients. Syncope can be related to dysrhythmias, but the cause of dyspnea and fatigue is more obscure. They sometimes may be related to pulmonary congestion and decreased cardiac output.

If the patient has a significant decrease in cardiac output and is bedbound or chairbound, range of motion exercises can help prevent emboli formation and stasis ulcers and maintain muscle strength and tone. Making the patient responsible for these exercises promotes feelings of independence and autonomy, which become essential to a person who may be dependent in many other ways. The res-

piratory rate, heart rate, and level of fatigue must be assessed in response to these exercises to ascertain whether they are too strenuous for the patient. Passive range of motion exercises are substituted if the patient cannot tolerate active exercises. Coughing, deep breathing, and frequent turning are also important.

If patients will be bedbound or chairbound for extended periods the nurse helps them find suitable recreational activities. The nurse also encourages family and friends to be supportive in this endeavor. The nurse must help patients cope with their disabilities and make life as rewarding as possible.

Limitations on physical activities may depress and frustrate the patient. Talking to a member of the clergy or spending time with family and friends can help. Reassurance from the nurse is an essential part of the treatment of these symptoms. Again, the opportunity to discuss fears and frustrations is an essential part of care.

Overexertion is dangerous for these patients. The inability of the heart to respond to exercise with an increased cardiac output can result in congestive heart failure or angina pectoris. Therefore thorough education about the disease process and the limitations it places on activities is a priority. However, there may be a serious discrepancy between what patients *want* to do and what their failing hearts *allow* them to do. Careful assessment and reinforcement of the principles of energy conservation are needed.

The nurse should assess how much help the patient will require and can expect at home. Household activities and energy conservation techniques must be reviewed with the patient and family. It may revitalize the person's self-esteem to perform some tasks around the house. The nurse should instruct the patient to intersperse necessary activities with periods of rest to diminish fatigue and shortness of breath. The patient should climb stairs slowly, resting as necessary to avoid dyspnea. Energy conservation techniques, such as completing all tasks on one floor before going to another,

spreading activities over the course of the day or week, and stopping to rest when feeling fatigued, can control dyspnea. Whatever the situation, the patient must change positions slowly to prevent dizziness and refrain from exertion when fatigued or dyspneic.

Relaxation techniques and meditation help to alleviate pain and shortness of breath. Assuming a comfortable position in a relaxed environment; practicing slow, controlled breathing; and deliberately relaxing each area of the body from head to toe can be taught to and practiced by the patient when uncomfortable symptoms are experienced.

NURSING DIAGNOSIS 4   **High risk for valve infection related to hemodynamic valve deformity (exchanging pattern)**

PATIENT OUTCOMES	NURSING PRESCRIPTIONS	EVALUATION
Patient will verbalize the need to take long-term antibiotics to prevent recurrences of rheumatic fever.	Teach patient about the need to take long-term antibiotics to prevent recurrences of rheumatic fever.	Patient verbalized the need to take long-term antibiotics to prevent recurrences of rheumatic fever.
Patient will verbalize and understand the need to take additional prophylactic antibiotic therapy before and after invasive surgical and dental procedures to prevent infective endocarditis.	Teach patient about the need to take additional prophylactic antibiotic therapy before and after invasive surgical and dental procedures to prevent infective endocarditis. Teach the rationale for therapy, schedule for taking the antibiotic, duration of and occasion necessitating antibiotic therapy, and adverse reactions of it.	Patient verbalized an understanding of the need to take additional prophylactic antibiotic therapy before and after invasive surgical and dental procedures to prevent infective endocarditis, and patient was able to verbalize the reasons for therapy, administration schedule, duration of and occasions necessitating antibiotic therapy, and adverse reactions to it.

Plan and intervention for valve infection

If rheumatic fever was the cause of the valvular disease, patients should receive prophylactic antibiotic therapy to protect against a recurrence of rheumatic fever. Long-term continuous antimicrobial prophylaxis, sometimes for life, produces the most effective protection against recurrence of rheumatic fever by preventing recurrent streptococcal sore throat.[35] However, because the risk of exacerbation decreases with the length of time since the last attack, some physicians do not prescribe life-long antibiotic therapy for an older patient. Considering the difficulties with compliance, many factors still must be carefully weighed when deciding whether to prescribe life-long antibiotics. Among these are patients' chances of acquiring streptococcal infections and the possibility and consequences of recurrent infections. Patients most likely to be exposed to strepto-

coccal infections are nurses, physicians, teachers, allied medical personnel, people in military service, parents of young children, and people from lower socioeconomic backgrounds. Patients who are most likely to have a high rate of recurrence are those with rheumatic valvular lesions, those who have recently suffered an attack of rheumatic fever, and those who have suffered several attacks of rheumatic fever.

Monthly injections of 1.2 million units of penicillin G benzathine are most efficient and effective in preventing streptococcal infections.[35] An oral regimen of 1 g of sulfadiazine daily given in one dose or 200,000 units of penicillin G taken twice a day on an empty stomach to ensure optimal absorption are two other options.[35]

Prophylaxis is also appropriate for these patients to protect against infective endocarditis. Preexisting valvular damage can promote localization of circulating organisms because of the hemodynamic abnormalities caused by the deformity. The irregularities of the diseased valve tend to foster precipitation of bacteria from the bloodstream around the valvular base.

For this reason, anything known to facilitate the entry of bacteria into the bloodstream is occasion for antibiotic prophylaxis in these patients, including all dental and sur-gical procedures or instrumentation of the upper respiratory and genitourinary tracts.

The prophylactic regimen for preventing rheumatic fever is different from and inadequate in preventing endo-carditis. Thus for patients on antibiotics to prevent recurrence of acute rheumatic fever, additional antibiotics are necessary when undergoing surgery or other high-risk invasive procedures (see Chapter 13).

NURSING
DIAGNOSIS 5   **High risk for noncompliance to the medical regimen related to inadequate health teaching (choosing pattern)**

PATIENT OUTCOMES	NURSING PRESCRIPTIONS	EVALUATION
Patient will be able to describe the functioning of the heart; function of heart valves; particular valvular abnormality involved; signs and symptoms of the abnormality; pathophysiologic changes that occur with the particular valvular abnormality; and action, dosage, time, and side effects of the med-ications.	Teach the patient and family about the valvular illness. The information should include normal functioning of the heart, functioning of the cardiac valves, particular valvular abnormal-ity involved, pathophysiologic changes that occur, and information about medications (see Nursing Di-agnoses 1 and 2).	Patient was able to describe cardiac function; the abnormality and its signs, symptoms, and pathophysio-logic changes; and the action, dos-age, time, and side effects of the medication.
Patient will verbalize the activities that are or are not allowed before and after discharge.	Discuss restrictions in activities before and after discharge (see Nursing Diagnosis 3).	Patient described permissible activities and limitations.
Patient will describe symptoms that should be reported to the physi-cian for follow-up care.	Discuss symptoms that should be re-ported to the physician.	Patient described symptoms that would require follow-up care.
Patient will state when to see the physician for follow-up care.	Explain when and where to return for follow-up care.	Patient stated when to see the physi-cian for follow-up care.
Patient will obtain a Medic-Alert bracelet.	Refer patient to place where a Medic-Alert bracelet can be obtained.	Patient obtained a Medic-Alert brace-let.

Plan and intervention for noncompliance

Patient teaching can be an important factor in ensuring compliance with the medical regimen and in alleviating the anxiety that usually accompanies valvular abnormalities. Many patients have no symptoms but become very anxious and apprehensive when told they have a heart valve prob-lem. Their concern is understandable, but undue anxiety is inappropriate. Although there are some potentially se-vere complications associated with the disease, the infre-quent occurrence of these symptoms should be stressed.

In patients with symptoms, the perception of pain and its intensity are amplified by anxiety. Patients need to know that the pain and shortness of breath are not life threat-ening. Any fears must be discussed. If patients do not volunteer the information, the nurse must draw them into conversation until they can begin to communicate their fears.

The nurse must give the patient the necessary tools to ensure active participation. These tools are knowledge and understanding. To accomplish this, the nurse must evaluate the patient's level of understanding and ability to compre-hend so that all information can be as easy as possible to assimilate. Instructions should be clearly written whenever appropriate, and family members should be included in teaching sessions. The patient and family should be en-couraged to verbalize concerns and to ask questions. A nonjudgmental attitude is essential to foster open com-munication.

Printed handouts, diagrams, pictures, and other audio-visual aids can be used in the teaching process. After dis-charge, these help as ready sources of information for the patient and family. Patients should be taught about the normal functioning of the heart and heart valves and about the particular valve involved in their illness. They should have an understanding of the pathophysiologic changes that occur with their illness, as well as the signs and symptoms that commonly occur with their particular valve problem. Patients are also taught about their medications (see Nursing Diagnoses 1 and 2) and any restrictions in activities (see Nursing Diagnosis 3).

The patient should be able to state symptoms to report to the physician and should be able to identify when and where to return for follow-up care. If patients are taking anticoagulants, the nurse assists in obtaining a Medic-Alert bracelet and explains the importance of its use.

Patients with valvular heart disease may be on complicated medication schedules and have a very limited level of activity. Such circumstances place patients at high risk for noncompliance. Nurses provide the patient with the necessary knowledge of all aspects of care. Using the approach that the patient is the most vital member of the health care team, nurses teach patients that they are active participants in, rather than passive recipients of, health care.

KEY CONCEPT REVIEW

1. The backward transmission of chronically elevated left atrial pressure due to mitral stenosis results in:
   a. Normal exercise cardiac output
   b. Pulmonary hypertension
   c. Elevated left ventricular pressure
   d. A widened pulse pressure
2. Nonrheumatic causes of mitral regurgitation are:
   a. Myocardial infarction
   b. Calcification of the mitral anulus
   c. Congenital anomaly
   d. All the above
3. The chest pain of mitral valve prolapse is:
   a. Like anginal pain
   b. Triggered by exertion
   c. Relieved by rest
   d. Paroxysmal, sharp, and sticking
4. Aortic stenosis represents:
   a. An obstruction to the left ventricular outflow tract
   b. A valvular disease syndrome that is usually insignificant
   c. A diastolic phenomenon
   d. An association with physical findings such as pectus excavatum and pectus carinatum
5. All of the following are true about aortic regurgitation except:
   a. It can be caused by connective tissues diseases.
   b. It is a systolic phenomenon.
   c. It is often accompanied by myocardial ischemia.
   d. It is accompanied by an elevated left ventricular end-diastolic volume.
6. All of the following are true about tricuspid stenosis except:
   a. Cardiac output is decreased.
   b. When the condition is severe, it can be associated with systemic venous congestion, ascites, and edema.
   c. The most frequently seen symptoms are fatigue and effort intolerance.
   d. It is a commonly found lesion, usually occurring alone.
7. Which of the following is true about tricuspid regurgitation?
   a. It is usually functional and secondary to right ventricular dilatation and failure.
   b. Cardiac output is decreased.
   c. Atrial fibrillation and right bundle branch block often occur.
   d. All of the above are true.
8. A common complication of pulmonary valve disease is:
   a. Clubbing of the fingers
   b. Right-sided heart failure
   c. Anemia
   d. Left ventricular enlargement
9. Antibiotic prophylaxis is used in patients with valve deformities:
   a. To prevent gum infections
   b. To prevent recurrence of rheumatic fever
   c. To prevent bladder infections
   d. None of the above
10. Embolic episodes associated with mitral valve disease:
    a. Occur in approximately 20% of all patients
    b. Necessitate the use of anticoagulant therapy
    c. Occur as the result of clot formation in the atrium secondary to atrial fibrillation
    d. All the above
11. The cause of the pain accompanying mitral valve prolapse is:
    a. Due to coronary artery disease
    b. Imaginary
    c. Thought to be the result of excessive pull on the papillary muscles by the prolapsed valve
    d. Impossible to control
12. The nursing assessment of the Knowing Pattern for the patient with mitral stenosis should include:
    a. When the symptoms were first noticed by the patient
    b. How the symptoms have progressed over time
    c. Whether the patient has experienced dyspnea on exertion, orthopnea, or paroxysmal nocturnal dyspnea
    d. All of the above
13. An important area of teaching for valvular disease patients is:
    a. The appropriate cholesterol level for an adult
    b. Ways to look up medication side effects
    c. The importance of invasive hemodynamic monitoring
    d. The importance of each medication, side effects, and times to take them
14. An appropriate nursing diagnosis for the patient with valvular heart disease is:
    a. Altered mental status related to dyspnea
    b. Altered nutritional status related to nausea
    c. Altered skin integrity related to right-sided heart failure
    d. Impaired physical mobility related to chest pain, dyspnea, and fatigue

ANSWERS

1. b	4. a	7. d	9. b	11. c	13. d
2. d	5. b	8. b	10. d	12. d	14. d
3. d	6. d			

REFERENCES

1. Abernathy WS and Willis PW III: Thromboembolic complications of rheumatic heart disease, Cardiovasc Clin 5:132, 1972.
2. Abrams J: Mitral stenosis. In Essentials of cardiac physical diagnosis, Philadelphia, 1987, Lea & Febiger.
3. Abrams J: Mitral valve prolapse. In Essentials of cardiac physical diagnosis, Philadelphia, 1987, Lea & Febiger.
4. Alpert JS: Clinical evaluation of valvular heart disease, Curr Opin Cardiol 4:206, 1989.
5. Arbulu A and Asfaw I: Tricuspid valvulectomy without prosthetic replacement: ten years of clinical experience, J Thorac Cardiovasc Surg 82:684, 1981.
6. Barnet AL and others: Acute rheumatic fever in adults, JAMA 232:925, 1975.
7. Bell MH and Mintz GS: Mitral valve disease in the elderly. In Frankl WS and Brest AN, editors: Cardiovascular clinics: valvular heart disease: comprehensive evaluation and management, Philadelphia, 1986, FA Davis Co.
8. Berne RM and Levy MN: Cardiovascular physiology, ed 6, St Louis, 1992, The CV Mosby Co.
9. Bisno AL: The concept of rheumatogenic and nonrheumatogenic group A streptococci. In Read SE and Fabriskie JB, editors: Streptococcal diseases and the immune response, New York, 1980, Academic Press, Inc.
10. Borer JS and others: Left ventricular function in aortic stenosis: response to exercise and effects of operation, Am J Cardiol 41:382, 1978.
11. Braunwald E: Valvular heart disease. In Harrison TR, editor: Principles of internal medicine, New York, 1988, McGraw-Hill, Inc.
12. Braunwald E: Heart disease: a textbook of cardiovascular medicine, ed 3, Philadelphia, 1988, WB Saunders Co.
13. Cassling RS, Rogler WC, McManus BM: Isolated pulmonic valve infective endocarditis: a diagnostically elusive entity, Am Heart J 109:558, 1985.
14. Crawford MH: Valvular heart disease: overview, Curr Opin Cardiol 4:189, 1989.
15. Cohn KE and Hultgren HN: The Graham Steel murmur re-evaluated, N Engl J Med 274:486, 1966.
16. Constant J: Bedside cardiology, Boston, 1987, Little, Brown, & Co.
17. Dalen JE and Alpert JS: Valvular heart disease, Boston, 1989, Little, Brown, & Co.
18. Davies MJ: Etiology and pathology of the diseased mitral valve. In Ionescu MI and Cohn LH, editors: Mitral valve disease: diagnosis and treatment, London, 1985, Butterworth Publishers.
19. DePasquale N and Bruno MS: Cardiology case studies, Flushing, NY, 1986, Medical Examination Publishing Co, Inc.
20. Goldberger E: Textbook of clinical cardiology, St Louis, 1989, The CV Mosby Co.
21. Govoni LE and Hayes JE: Drugs and nursing implications, New York, 1988, Appleton-Century-Crofts.
22. Grossman W: Profiles in valvular heart disease. In Grossman W: Cardiac catheterization and angiography, Philadelphia, 1986, Lea & Febiger.
23. Guyton AC: Textbook of medical physical, ed 6, Philadelphia, 1986, WB Saunders Co.
24. Guzzetta CE, and Whitman G: Cardiac surgery. In Dossey BM, Guzzetta CE, and Kenner CV, editors: Critical care nursing: body-mind-spirit, ed 3, Philadelphia, 1992, JB Lippincott Co.
25. Helmcke F and others: Color doppler assessment of mitral regurgitation with orthogonal planes, Circulation 75:175, 1987.
26. Hickey AJ and Wilcken DEL: Age and the clinical profile of idiopathic mitral valve prolapse, Br Heart J 55:582, 1986.
27. Horwitz LD and Groves BM, editors: Signs and symptoms in cardiology, Philadelphia, 1985, JB Lippincott Co.
28. Iskandrian AS, Hakki A-H, Kane-Marsch S: Left ventricular pressure/volume relationship in aortic regurgitation, Am Heart J 110:1026, 1985.
29. Jersaty RM: Mitral valve prolapse, New York, 1986, Raven Press.
30. Klein HO and others: Effects of atenolol on exercise capacity in patients with mitral stenosis with sinus rhythm, Am J Cardiol 56:598, 1985.
31. Kumar A, Sinha M, and Sinha DNP: Chronic rheumatic heart diseases in Ranchi, Angiology 33:141, 1982.
32. Levine HJ: Which atrial fibrillation patients should be on chronic anticoagulation? J Cardiovasc Med 6:483, 1981.
33. Masuyama T and others: Noninvasive evaluation of aortic regurgitation by continuous-wave Doppler echocardiography, Circulation 73:460, 1986.
34. Newman GE and others: Noninvasive assessment of hemodynamic effects of mitral valve commissurotomy during rest and exercise in patients with mitral stenosis, J Thorac Cardiovasc Surg 78:750, 1979.
35. Nurse's reference library: Drugs, Springhouse Publications, 1988, Intermed Communications, Inc.
36. Paraskos JA: Combined valvular disease. In Dlaen JE and Alpert JS, editors: Valvular heart disease, Boston, 1989, Little, Brown, & Co.
37. Perloff JK, Child JS, and Edwards JE: New guidelines for the clinical diagnosis of mitral valve prolapse, Am J Cardiol 57:1124, 1986.
38. Pocock WA: Mitral leaflet billowing and prolapse. In Barlow JB, editor: Perspectives on the mitral valve, Philadelphia, 1987, FA Davis Co.
39. Ptacin M, Sebastian J, and Bamrah VS: Onchronotic cardiovascular disease, Clin Cardiol 8:441, 1985.
40. Rackley CE: Aortic valve disease. In Hurst J, editor: The heart, New York, 1990, McGraw Hill, Inc.
41. Reid CL: Rheumatic fever, endocarditis and thromboembolism, Curr Opin Cardiol 4:191, 1989.
42. Rodbard S: Blood velocity and endocarditis, Circulation 27:18, 1953.

43. Sakuma T and others: Mitral valve prolapse syndrome with coronary artery spasm: a possible cause of recurrent ventricular tachyarrhythmia, Clin Cardiol 8:306, 1985.

44. Stapleton JF: Natural history of chronic valvular disease. In Frankl WS and Brest AN, editors: Cardiovascular Clinics: valvular heart disease: comprehensive evaluation and management, Philadelphia, 1986, FA Davis Co.

45. Stollerman GH: Nephritogenic and rheumatogenic group A streptococci, J Infect Dis 120:25, 1989.

46. Stollerman GH: Acute rheumatic fever and its management. In Hurst J, editor: The heart, New York, 1990, McGraw-Hill, Inc.

47. Vander Cerr JB: Mitral insufficiency: historical and clinical aspects, Am J Cardiol 2:5, 1958.

48. Wald ER and others: Acute rheumatic fever in Western Pennsylvania and the tristate area, Pediatrics 80:371, 1987.

49. Walker BF: Rheumatic and non-rheumatic conditions producing valvular heart disease. In Frankl WS and Brest AN, editors: Cardiovascular Clinics: valvular heart disease: comprehensive evaluation and management, Philadelphia 1986, FA Davis Co.

50. Wautrecht JC, Vandenbiossche JL, and Englert M: Sensitivity and specificity of pulsed Doppler echocardiography in detection of aortic and mitral regurgitation, Eur Heart J 5:404, 1984.

51. Yellin EL and others: In Ionescu MI and Cohn LH, editors: Mitral valve disease: diagnosis and treatment, London, 1985, Butterworth Publishers.

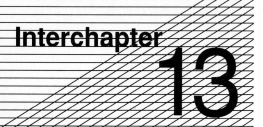

Placebo Response

Placebo means "I will please." The term refers to a medically inert preparation or treatment that has no specific effects on the body and yet can evoke pain relief or dramatically affect symptoms or disease. The placebo effect always has been considered a nuisance and an unreliable factor in medicine. It has been assumed to work only in illnesses that somehow were not real. Those who really understand the placebo effect know that this is not so. For example, the worse the pain or the more stressful the situation, the more effective the placebo pill.[4]

We are beginning to understand the mechanism involved. Recent evidence has shown that the placebo effect can activate the production of endorphins, which are peptide hormones produced and secreted by the brain with opiate properties that are astonishingly powerful and exponentially more potent than morphine (see p. 78). It is thought that endorphins can modify or inhibit pain stimuli transmission throughout the central nervous system.[10]

In an analysis of 15 double-blind studies, for example, placebo medications were found to be effective in pain relief for 35% of patients with postoperative pain.[1] (The placebo effect, however, can be as high as 70% to 100% in some series). These findings were confirmed by an analysis of 11 more recent double-blind studies in which 36% of patients received at least 50% pain relief from placebos.[5] Thus it appears that for over one third of patients, the pharmacologically inert placebo can access and activate body-mind healing mechanisms; this is termed the *placebo response*.[6,8]

The placebo response is not restricted to pain medications. Benson and McCallie,[2] for example, studied angina pectoris and the placebo effect and found success rates up to 90% for operations and drugs that are now shown to have no physiologic effectiveness. They concluded that these results could have come from a placebo response. In addition, the placebo response is present in all the following illnesses and therapeutic procedures, thus implicating that the mind has the ability to produce neurohormonal messenger molecules that alter the autonomic, endocrine, and immune systems:[8]

1. Hypertension, stress, cardiac pain, blood cell counts, headaches, and pupillary dilation (suggesting the mind's ability to alter the autonomic nervous system)
2. Adrenal gland secretion, diabetes, ulcers, gastric secretion and motility, colitis, effects of oral contraceptives, menstrual pain, and thyrotoxicosis (suggesting the mind's ability to alter the endocrine system)
3. The common cold, fever, vaccines, asthma, multiple sclerosis, rheumatoid arthritis, warts, and cancer (suggesting the mind's ability to alter the immune system)
4. Surgical treatments (e.g, for angina pectoris)
5. Readings from biofeedback instrumentation and various medical devices
6. Psychologic treatments such as conditioning (systematic desensitization) and perhaps all forms of psychotherapy

Isolating the effects of the placebo from the effects of an active drug has been the basis of many double-blind research studies investigating the efficacy of new drugs.[9] Thus a new drug is tested against a placebo to determine its effectiveness. Because 35% of patients respond positively to placebos alone, this baseline efficacy must be subtracted from the effectiveness of the active investigational drug.[1]

A person might be able to deduce that some patients respond not only to active drugs but also to the placebo effect, thereby making the active drug even more effective (e.g., the power of morphine is due to its drug effect *plus* its placebo effect). This in fact happens. The degree by which the placebo response augments therapeutic effectiveness for pain medication is uncommonly consistent, averaging about 56%.[5] For example, although morphine is a far more potent analgesic than aspirin, about 56% of the effectiveness of both aspirin and morphine is due to the placebo response.[8]

This 56% effectiveness ratio also is relatively constant for the treatment of other problems.[5] Regardless of the problem or symptom, a 56% effectiveness ratio may be added to many if not all drugs and therapeutic procedures. Thus the placebo response is believed to be a common general mechanism that may occur in all clinical situations.[8] This common general mechanism, called the *general healing response,* is thought to occur because of a communication link between the body and the mind that is mediated by the right cerebral hemisphere[8] (see p. 38).

The placebo response probably is present, more or less, in each person.[7] If it is true that a placebo healing response can occur naturally in all clinical situations,[9] nurses might discover amazing results if they *tried* consciously to enhance its effects. The way that a drug is given or the way a procedure is performed and the person who gives or performs it can influence the outcomes of the placebo response. The placebo response, therefore, is greatly influenced by the faith that the patient has in the caregiver and in the patient's expectation that the drug or therapy will work.[9] Likewise, it is influenced by the faith that the caregiver conveys to the patient regarding the drug or therapy, as well as the trust and rapport established between the two.[6,7]

To enhance the placebo response when administering medications, for example, nurses should make every attempt to discuss with patients facts about the medication's potency and effectiveness. When patients receive intravenous morphine for chest pain, nurses can ask them to visualize the powerful painkilling medicine being injected into their veins and to see the molecules traveling to the source of the chest pain to relieve it. They can suggest that patients work with the medication to enhance its effectiveness by allowing the relaxed, warm, and comfortable feeling associated with the morphine to flow throughout the body. Even mild side effects of drugs or therapy can be used as an opportunity to enhance the placebo response when nurses say, "We know that your nasal congestion and that metallic taste in your mouth are positive signs that the medicine is in your body and working properly."[7,9]

The essence of the placebo response is associated with positive attitudes and emotions.[8] Many of the self-regulation modalities such as imagery, music therapy, relaxation, and biofeedback increase endorphin production. When patients believe they are receiving pain-relief medication and when they believe that they are doing something to enhance healing, endorphin levels rise.[11] Patients therefore can actually influence the course of their own illness and their response to therapy through the impact of their own consciousness.[4] Because basic nursing interventions such as touch, back rubs, preoperative teaching, positioning, and distraction can increase endorphin levels, it is critical that nurses discuss with patients the possible therapeutic benefits of each therapy. When nurses realize that what they say to patients can actually influence the placebo response, then they will develop new communication skills to enhance the healing response in patients and maximize the benefits of all the nursing care given.

REFERENCES

1. Beecher H: The powerful placebo, JAMA 159:1602, 1955.
2. Benson H and McCallie D: Angina pectoris and the placebo effect, N Engl J Med 300:1424, 1979.
3. Cousins N: Anatomy of an illness as perceived by the patient, New York, 1979, WW Norton & Co, Inc.
4. Dossey L: Space, time, and medicine, Boston, 1982, Shambhala Publications.
5. Evans F: Expectancy, therapeutic instructions, and the placebo response. In White L, Tursky B, and Schwartz G, editors: Placebo: theory, research, and mechanism, New York, 1985, The Guilford Press.
6. Frank J: Mind-body relationships in illness and healing, J Intern Acad Prevent Med 2:46, 1975.
7. Perry S and Heidrich G: Placebo response: Myth and matter, Am J Nurs 81:720, 1981.
8. Rossi EL: The psychobiology of mind-body healing: new concepts of therapeutic hypnosis, New York, 1986, WW Norton & Co, Inc.
9. Sandroff R: The potent placebo, RN April, 1980, p 35.
10. West A: Understanding endorphins: our natural pain relief system, Nurs 81 2:50, 1981.
11. Wilson R and Elmassion B: Endorphins, Am J Nurs 81:722, 1981.

13 The Person with Infective Endocarditis

Cathie E. Guzzetta

LEARNING OBJECTIVES

1. Discuss the major microorganisms causing acute and subacute endocarditis.

2. Compare and contrast the pathogenesis of acute endocarditis and subacute endocarditis.

3. Determine patients that are at high risk for developing infective endocarditis.

4. Analyze the major areas of nursing assessment for patients with infective endocarditis.

5. Outline the common nursing diagnoses anticipated for patients with infective endocarditis.

6. Explore patient outcomes, plan, intervention, and evaluation for each diagnosis listed for patients with infective endocarditis.

Infective endocarditis is a microbial infection of the endocardial tissue, which frequently involves the heart valves. Patients admitted to the hospital with infective endocarditis may have subtle influenza-like symptoms or may be in acute distress. As early as 1885, Osler[75] noted that infective endocarditis was a difficult disease to diagnose and treat, and modern medicine has not altered this situation.

Until recently, infective endocarditis was called *bacterial endocarditis. Infective endocarditis* is now preferred because other organisms, in addition to bacteria, have been identified as causative agents. Before the days of antimicrobial medications, infective endocarditis also was categorized according to the length of the patient's survival. Patients with the acute illness were severely ill and usually died within the first 6 weeks, whereas patients with the subacute illness experienced a more chronic course and usually died in 6 to 8 months.

Currently endocarditis is categorized according to the virulence of the infecting organism. In acute endocarditis, the infecting organism is highly virulent, usually affecting normal heart valves and causing rapid and severe hemodynamic and toxic complications. Subacute endocarditis, on the other hand, is caused by an organism of low virulence, generally in patients with preexisting valvular defects. Toxic and hemodynamic complications usually are seen late in the illness.

Patients suffering from infective endocarditis present many medical and nursing challenges. Patients are affected not only by the microorganism but also by the length of treatment, feelings of boredom, knowledge of complications, fear of recurring infection, and the imposed responsibility involved with prophylaxis and prevention of the disease. Thus nurses caring for the person with infective endocarditis are involved not only with the antimicrobial treatment of the infected heart valve but also with the treatment of the psychologic and behavioral responses to the illness.

ETIOLOGY

Infective endocarditis is caused by a variety of organisms. *Staphylococcus aureus* causes most cases of acute endocarditis.[67] It is a highly virulent organism that generally infects normal heart valves, causing rapid and debilitating valvular damage. The enterococcus, such as *Streptococcus faecalis,* is a more virulent strain found in the gastrointestinal and genitourinary tracts.

Gram-negative bacilli and fungi also are known to cause endocarditis. Gram-negative organisms include *Escherichia coli and Klebsiella, Pseudomonas, Salmonella, Bacteroides, and Proteus* organisms.[23] Fungi include *Candida, Histoplasma,* and *Aspergillus* organisms.[15,42] Mixed infections occasionally have been reported.

Streptococcus viridans is the organism responsible for most cases of subacute endocarditis. It is a group of α-hemolytic bacteria commonly found in the oral cavity. *S.*

viridans, an organism of low virulence, classically becomes engrafted on deformed or damaged heart valves to cause endocarditis. Other organisms causing subacute endocarditis include nonhemolytic and microaerophilic streptococci, commonly found in the oral cavity and gastrointestinal, female genitourinary, and respiratory tracts.

PATHOGENESIS

The pathogenesis of acute endocarditis is related to the presence of bacteremia caused by a highly virulent organism. Because 50% to 60% of acute infections occur in patients without previous cardiac valvular deformities,[5,102] several theories have been formulated to explain why some types of bacteria affect normal heart valves. One explanation is that *S. aureus* and other gram-positive bacterium exhibit a unique property that permits them to adhere to the endothelial surface of the heart valve.[32,77] Although the reason for the localization of infection on normal heart valves is not clearly understood, it appears that only a few highly virulent organisms are necessary to establish the infection.

The pathogenesis of subacute endocarditis, in contrast, is more complex. *S. viridans* appears to be a selective organism, affecting only heart valves, apparently because of the following mechanisms involved with the selectivity and localization of the subacute infection[32,102,103]:

1. The presence of preexisting valvular damage or cardiac defects
2. The formation of sterile platelet-fibrin thrombi
3. The presence of bacteremia
4. The development of a high titer of agglutinating antibodies specific for the infecting organism

Preexisting valvular damage or cardiac defects

The first mechanism responsible for the selectivity and localization of subacute infection is the presence of preexisting valvular abnormalities. Valvular damage or cardiac defects commonly are caused by rheumatic, congenital, or degenerative heart disease. The most common problems associated with rheumatic heart disease are mitral and aortic valve deformities, including mitral valve prolapse and mitral stenosis. The congenital defects associated with endocarditis include bicuspid aortic valve, coarctation of the aorta, ventricular septal defect (VSD), tetralogy of Fallot, patent ductus arteriosus, pulmonary stenosis, and hypertrophic cardiomyopathies[15] (see Chapters 12 and 14). Patients with prosthetic heart valves also are highly susceptible to valvular infection.

Because of the abnormal hemodynamics created by valvular abnormalities, organisms can settle out of the circulation and localize around the irregularities of the heart valve.[15] Although the reason for this localization is not clearly understood, Rodbard[87] has developed a hydrodynamic theory to explain the process. This theory is based on three factors: (1) a narrowed valvular orifice, (2) a high pressure gradient between two cardiac chambers, and (3) a rapid blood flow (Fig. 13-1).

Blood flowing through a narrowed cross-sectional area produces an accelerated forward velocity of flow, with a reduced lateral pressure. This situation is illustrated in mitral insufficiency, in which blood is regurgitated back from the left ventricle to the left atrium through an incompetent and narrowed (i.e., not fully and normally opened) valvular orifice. This situation produces an increased forward velocity of blood flow (actually seen as an increased backward velocity) and decreased lateral pressure. Because mitral re-

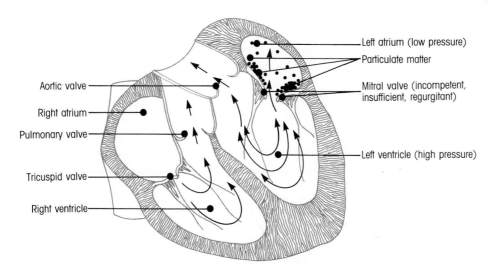

FIG. 13-1   Hydrodynamic theory explaining why lesions localize in subacute endocarditis. In mitral regurgitation, a regurgitant jet occurs during systole from the left ventricle to the left atrium. The jet reduces lateral pressure on the atrial side of the valve, causing the shedding of particulate material and bacteria.

gurgitation occurs during systole (with a high left ventricular pressure and a corresponding low left atrial pressure), a high pressure gradient is established between the two chambers. During systole therefore there is a high velocity regurgitant jet and a reduction in lateral pressure on the atrial side of the valve (Fig. 13-1). If an appropriate bacterium is introduced into the circulation (see later section), organisms are shed from the regurgitant jet and deposited on the atrial side of the valve. The reduced lateral pressure on the atrial side of the valve, in turn, causes the organisms to accumulate locally. Thus the atrium becomes highly susceptible to endocardial lesions. Rodbard's theory[87] may be applied to other valvular deformities, as well (e.g., VSD).[102]

Although infections producing acute endocarditis can develop on abnormal valves, most cases involve normal valves. Thus the abnormal hydrodynamic situation created by valvular deformities, usually seen in subacute endocarditis, is not a necessary mechanism in the development of acute endocarditis.

Sterile platelet-fibrin thrombi

The second mechanism responsible for the selectivity and localization of the subacute infection is the development of sterile platelet-fibrin thrombi.[102] Trauma to the endothelial valvular surface is caused by the inherent valvular disease and turbulent blood flow created by valvular abnormalities. Because the endothelial valvular surface is traumatized, the exposed subendothelial collagen causes local activation of clotting mechanisms, and sterile platelet-fibrin thrombi form on the injured valve leaflets. When an organism is introduced into the circulation, the sterile thrombotic lesions act as foci for infection.

Bacteremia

The third mechanism contributing to the selectivity and localization of the subacute infection involves the development of a bacteremia (fungemia or rickettsemia). Although transient bacteremias occur in individuals with normal heart valves, subacute endocarditis usually does not develop because the endothelial valvular surface of normal heart valves are not traumatized and the organisms causing the subacute infection are of low virulence. When appropriate organisms of low virulence enter the circulation of individuals with preexisting valvular abnormalities, however, the abnormal valve can become infected because of sterile platelet-fibrin thrombi. Because the thrombi are avascular, they are highly susceptible to contamination and permit seeding and proliferation of the microorganism.[4] Some organisms produce a polysaccharide coat that allows them to adhere to the traumatized valvular surface. In addition, fibronectin, a glycoprotein in the plasma that is found on traumatized valvular tissue, also promotes adherence and localization of organisms.[64,93]

Agglutinating antibodies

The fourth major mechanism contributing to the selectivity and localization of the subacute infection is a high titer of agglutinating antibodies. Circulating antibodies, specific for the infecting organism, cause the infection to localize and spread by clumping the organisms. Because the platelet-fibrin thrombi provide a favorable surface for the organisms, agglutinating antibodies further enhance the valvular infection by causing a large number of bacteria to adhere to the thrombotic lesions.[102,105]

PATHOLOGY

Infections forming on heart valves produce endothelial lesions called *vegetations* (Fig. 13-2). Microscopically, the vegetations contain three layers: (1) an inner layer of collagen and elastin, fibrin, neutrophils, lymphocytes, platelets, and red blood cells; (2) a middle layer composed of microorganisms; and (3) an outer layer composed of fibrin and microorganisms.

The vegetations have irregular edges and are easily torn away. Microorganisms lie deep within the platelet-fibrin thrombi and are protected from the individual's normal immune defense mechanisms.[19] Even patients who receive adequate antimicrobial therapy may experience progressive valvular infection because the metabolic activity of the deeply embedded microorganism is reduced, thereby decreasing the effectiveness of most antimicrobial drugs.[77]

In acute endocarditis, especially when caused by fungi, the vegetations develop more rapidly than in the subacute illness. They also tend to be softer, larger, and more easily torn away, causing major embolic complications and leaving ulcerated lesions on the valve surface.

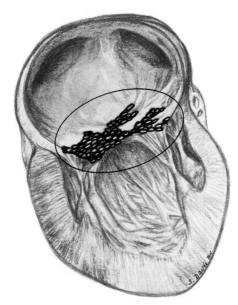

FIG. 13-2 Infective endocarditis vegetations *(circle)* of the mitral valve.

The mitral valve is the site most commonly infected, followed by the aortic valve. Infections of both valves are also common. Infections of the tricuspid valve, and especially the pulmonary valve, are less common. Right-sided valve infections, particularly tricuspid endocarditis, occur more frequently in abusers of parenteral drugs.[20,43]

Aortic valve vegetations generally occur on the ventricular side of the valve, whereas mitral valve vegetations usually occur on the atrial side. With progressive spread of the infection, thinning and destruction of the valve occurs, producing valvular incompetence (regurgitation). Valvular aneurysms may develop, causing the valve to rupture. The infection can erode into the atrial or ventricular myocardium. Erosive and inflammatory complications involving the chordae tendineae, papillary muscles, or conduction system can cause additional hemodynamic abnormalities or dysrhythmias.[102] Without treatment, patients eventually die of heart failure.

When patients are treated with antimicrobial medications, the valvular healing process may take as long as 2 to 3 months.[15] Fibrin is deposited over the vegetations, and granulation tissue grows into the lesions; scarring, calcification, and permanent deformities are common during healing.

NONBACTERIAL THROMBOTIC ENDOCARDITIS

Nonbacterial thrombotic endocarditis—known also as *marantic endocarditis, degenerative verrucous endocarditis, terminal endocarditis,* and *endocarditis simplex*—is a nonbacterial form of endocarditis characterized by sterile platelet-fibrin thrombi on cardiac valves. Patients with preexisting valvular disease are more susceptible to nonbacterial thrombotic endocarditis than patients with normal valves. The mitral and aortic valves are most commonly involved. This type of endocarditis is seen in patients who have a chronic debilitating disease such as cancer.[82] It also occurs in patients with acute disorders such as pneumonia, pulmonary embolism, peritonitis, and glomerulonephritis.[103]

The pathogenesis of nonbacterial thrombotic endocarditis is related to a blood-clotting derangement, a chronic form of disseminated intravascular coagulation that occurs in association with certain underlying disease processes. Chronic disseminated intravascular coagulation is characterized by thrombotic and embolic manifestations, as opposed to acute disseminated intravascular coagulation, which has hemorrhagic manifestations.[82] Chronic disseminated intravascular coagulation, in combination with the valvular trauma and turbulent blood flow found in patients with preexisting valvular disease, provides the setting for sterile platelet-fibrin thrombi to deposit on heart valves and for nonbacterial thrombotic endocarditis to develop. Patients with nonbacterial thrombotic endocarditis also are at high risk for developing infective endocarditis if the patient develops bacteremia. The sterile platelet-fibrin thrombi then become the focus for infection.

Burn patients with an indwelling pulmonary artery or central venous catheter, for example, are at high risk for developing right-sided nonbacterial thrombotic and infective endocarditis.[5,31,40,76,91] Pulmonary artery and central venous catheters can traumatize heart surfaces.[76] Soon after burn injuries, patients have hyperdynamic cardiac function and are in a hypercoagulable state. Because the heart continuously pumps against an indwelling catheter, endocardial and endothelial vessel injury can occur.[31] The endocardial injury and hypercoagulability favor the development of nonbacterial thrombotic vegetations. If the patient develops an intermittent bacteremia, which is common in burn patients, the bacteria can seed these vegetations, and infective endocarditis can result. *S. aureus* is the microorganism frequently involved in tricuspid and pulmonary valve infections.[91]

The benefits versus the risks of using these catheters in burn patients and other critically ill patients should be carefully considered to prevent iatrogenic endocarditis.[31] Shorter central venous catheters positioned outside the heart with the placement verified by chest x-ray films are suggested.[91] Blood cultures should be obtained and catheters changed at least every 72 hours for this group of patients.[91]

The most serious complication of nonbacterial thrombotic endocarditis is caused by the friable cardiac vegetations, which break away easily and produce occlusions and infarctions of various organs. Cerebral emboli are the most common and serious; renal, hepatic, coronary, or splenic emboli also can occur.[82] Currently there is no definitive therapy for this disease, although anticoagulation is useful in preventing recurrent arterial emboli.

LIBMAN-SACKS ENDOCARDITIS

Libman-Sacks endocarditis is a common complication of systemic lupus erythematosus, the most common collagen disease, which produces injury to the vascular system. Libman-Sacks endocarditis is a nonbacterial form that occurs as a late complication in up to 50% of all patients with systemic lupus erythematosus. Patients with Libman-Sacks endocarditis also may have myocardial and pericardial involvement, resulting in conduction disturbances, pericarditis, and pericardial effusion and tamponade.[15]

Nursing Process

Case study. Mr. J.R., a 46-year-old newspaper reporter, was admitted to the coronary care unit (CCU) with chills, an elevated temperature, fatigue, conjunctival petechiae, and hematuria. He remembered that, as a child, he had been told by his family physician that he had a heart murmur. He had no symptoms throughout his life and no restriction in activity. About 2½ weeks before admission he had visited the dentist for a gingivectomy.

On physical examination the patient was found to have a sinus tachycardia of 116 beats per minute and a blood pressure of 106/70 mm Hg. He had normal first and second heart sounds and a grade

3/6 diastolic murmur at the left sternal border. Echocardiography later confirmed the diagnosis of acute aortic regurgitation. All his blood cultures revealed a heavy growth of *S. viridans*. Bed rest, penicillin, and streptomycin were prescribed.

Nursing assessment

The patient's nine human response patterns are thoroughly assessed. The Knowing, Exchanging, Feeling, and Choosing Patterns are particularly important to evaluate in this group of patients with data collection focused on the following areas:

1. Knowing Pattern
   a. Elicit information to determine whether the patient is at high risk for developing infective endocarditis; identify possible portals of entry for the infecting microorganism.
2. Exchanging Pattern
   a. Assess the patient's response to the infection.
   b. Assess cardiac manifestations.
   c. Assess for embolic manifestations.
   d. Assess for immunologic derangements.
   e. Assess laboratory and diagnostic tests.
3. Feeling and Choosing Patterns
   a. Assess the patient's and family's response to the acute illness and coping behaviors.

Knowing pattern

High-risk patients and portals of entry for infection. The boxes, p. 398-399, summarize patients who are at risk for infective endocarditis and the possible portals of entry for the infecting organism. When assessing the patient suspected of having infective endocarditis, focus on this information and include the patient's perception and understanding of risk factors. Thus elicit information to determine whether the patient has a history of endocarditis. Patients who have had endocarditis in the past are at high risk for developing it again. Identify a patient history of congenital or rheumatic heart disease. Query the patient about a history of mitral valve prolapse or a floppy mitral valve, which is a condition that also places the patient at high risk for endocarditis.[22,41,66,77] With mitral valve prolapse, the mitral valve bulges back into the atrium during ventricular systole; it is associated with a midsystolic or late systolic click and a late systolic murmur of mitral regurgitation.[22,28,41,66,77] Patients with hypertrophic cardiomyopathy[77] and nonbacterial thrombotic endocarditis[77,82] also are susceptible to endocarditis (p. 397). All such patients are particularly at high risk when they develop infections remote from the heart or when they are exposed to procedures that traumatize tissues and introduce microorganisms into the circulation.

A common event related to subacute endocarditis among patients with preexisting cardiac abnormalities is a

CONDITIONS THAT PLACE PATIENTS AT HIGH RISK FOR DEVELOPING INFECTIVE ENDOCARDITIS

Infective endocarditis
Prosthetic heart valves
Surgically constructed systemic pulmonary shunts
Congenital heart disease
Rheumatic heart disease
Degenerative heart disease
Mitral valve prolapse
Valvular lesions, cardiac defects
Heart murmurs
Cardiac surgery
Chronic debilitating disease
Nonbacterial thrombotic endocarditis
Intravenous drug abuse
Immunosuppression related to cancer, collagen vascular disease, hepatitis, a burn injury, diabetes mellitus, radiation therapy, prolonged drug therapy (antibiotic, cytotoxic, or steroid medications)

recent history of dental procedures.[39] Because *S. viridans* is found in the mouth, dental disease or dental procedures can cause a transient bacteremia that can result in the development of subacute endocarditis.[53] Therefore query patients about a recent history of dental work. Also determine whether the patient is aware of recent skin lesions, lacerations, or trauma or any recent respiratory, gastrointestinal, or genitourinary tract infections, especially if the patient has a preexisting cardiac abnormality. Also determine whether they have recently undergone surgery or invasive tests involving the ears, nose, or throat or the respiratory, gastrointestinal, or genitourinary tract.

Patients who are immunologically suppressed are a unique subgroup at high risk for developing endocarditis. Immunosuppression can be produced when physiologic resistance is lowered by many types of diseases and therapies. Therefore elicit information from the patient to determine a history of immunosuppression associated with illnesses such as cancer, collagen vascular diseases such as systemic lupus erythematosus or rheumatoid arthritis, hepatitis, diabetes mellitus, and severe burns. Likewise, determine whether patients are receiving prolonged antibiotics, cytotoxic medications, steroids, or radiation therapy that may also place them at risk.[23,39,41] Immunologically suppressed patients who develop endocarditis usually are elderly and more likely to have gram-negative and fungal infections. Right-sided valvular infections are common.

POSSIBLE PORTALS OF ENTRY FOR THE INFECTING ORGANISM

ORAL CAVITY
Recent dental procedures (within 3 to 6 months)

Extractions
Teeth cleaning
Root canal procedures
Bridge work, inlays
Denture procedures
Gingivectomy

Recent dental disease or trauma (within 3 to 6 months)

Gingivitis
Caries
Periodontal disease
Periapical abscess
Recent oral trauma

SKIN

Rashes
Lesions
Lacerations
Trauma
Puncture site from intravenous injections
Abscesses

INFECTIONS

Skin
Respiratory tract (pneumonia)
Gastrointestinal tract
Genitourinary tract (endometritis, septic abortion, use of intrauterine devices)
Central nervous system (meningitis)

SURGERY OR INVASIVE PROCEDURES OR THERAPIES

Ears, nose, and throat (tonsils and adenoids)
Respiratory tract (bronchoscopy)
Gastrointestinal tract (colon, rectal, or hemorrhoidal surgery, endoscopy, and sigmoidoscopy)
Genitourinary or obstetric procedures (uterine dilation and curettage, caesarean section, therapeutic abortion, sterilization procedures, cystoscopy, and indwelling urinary catheterization)
Cardiovascular procedures (arteriovenous shunt or fistulae for hemodialysis, cardiac pacemaker electrodes, arterial catheters, or intravenous catheterization [peripheral, central venous, or pulmonary artery catheters])
Prosthetic valve replacement

The mortality rate associated with this subgroup of patients is high.

Identify a history of parenteral drug abuse. Parenteral drug abusers are highly susceptible to endocarditis[23,32,39,41] because of the use of unsterile equipment and repeated injections of pathogenic microorganisms into the venous circulation. Endocarditis in drug abusers also may be caused by the intravenous injection of their own native microbial skin flora.[43] The microorganisms involved in the infection are frequently *S. aureus,* gram-negative bacilli, or fungi.[32,39,41,67] These patients generally have no known history of valvular disease. There is a high incidence of tricuspid infection, although the aortic or pulmonary valve may be involved. Patients with right-sided endocarditis may exhibit atypical endocarditis symptoms such as a productive cough, hemoptysis, dyspnea, or pleuritic chest pain because bacteria are seeded in the lungs.[24] Embolic complications occur frequently, particularly pulmonary emboli with right-sided heart infection. Congestive heart failure is rare with tricuspid or pulmonary valve endocarditis, and the mortality rate is low.[41] Severe heart failure occurs frequently in patients with left-sided valvular infections and has a high mortality rate.[39,41]

Identify whether the patient is at high risk because of an arteriovenous shunt or fistula used for hemodialysis.[5,41,101] Patients on hemodialysis have high cardiac output states, which results in cardiovascular stress on heart valves. The combination of cardiovascular stress and infected arteriovenous shunts or fistulae producing bacteremia places such patients at high risk for endocardial infection.[5,26,41,101]

Hospital-acquired acute endocarditis caused by *S. aureus,* gram-negative organisms, and fungi is becoming a common problem. Unfortunately with advances in medical science and technology, new medical and nursing problems have been created. Thus elicit information to determine whether the patient recently has had a peripheral intravenous catheter or total parenteral nutrition line, central venous or pulmonary artery catheter, transvenous or epicardial pacemaker electrode, or an intrauterine device that may have been the source of infection.* Patients undergoing myocardial revascularization or cardiac catheterization are not at risk for developing endocarditis unless other cardiac abnormalities also are present.[1]

Identify whether the patient has a prosthetic heart valve. Many patients with rheumatic, congenital, or degenerative valvular disease have been helped to live longer

---

*References 17, 41, 52, 59, 77, 99, 100.

and healthier lives through prosthetic valve replacement. Early prosthetic valve replacement is recommended for many types of patients with valvular disease before significant hemodynamic complications occur. As a result, a large subgroup of patients has one or more prosthetic valves. Although prosthetic valves have enhanced the long-term survival of most of these patients, they also have become the source of various morbid complications, one of which is endocardial infection. It now is known that a disturbingly high percentage of patients with prosthetic valves develop endocarditis.[15,81,101] Prosthetic valve infection can occur during cardiac surgery, during postoperative hospitalization, or any time after discharge. Throughout their lives, prosthetic valve patients who develop bacteremia are predisposed to prosthetic valve endocarditis.

Patients with prosthetic valves or those with surgically constructed systemic-pulmonary shunts are highly susceptible to infective endocarditis if they do not receive prophylactic antibiotics for low risk-procedures (i.e., uncomplicated vaginal deliveries, caesarean section, uterine dilation and curettage, therapeutic abortion, sterilization procedures, barium enemas, and "in-and-out" bladder catheterizations).[1]

The major complication of prosthetic valve endocarditis is detachment of the prosthetic valve, causing severe paravalvular regurgitation and cardiac failure.[41] Occasionally the valve may become obstructed by a large vegetation. The mortality rate associated with prosthetic valve endocarditis is over 50%.[52]

Prosthetic valve endocarditis has been divided into two categories: (1) early prosthetic valve endocarditis, which occurs 2 months or less after surgery, and (2) late prosthetic valve endocarditis, which occurs later than 2 months after surgery.*

Early prosthetic valve endocarditis is a serious problem. During surgery the patient is exposed to many factors that can contaminate. These factors include the cardiopulmonary bypass equipment, sutures, operating room equipment, intravenous solutions and blood products, and the prosthetic valve (porcine or mechanical). During the postoperative period the patient also is exposed to many potential sources of infection, such as intravenous, central venous, arterial, and indwelling urinary catheters, pacemaker wires, endotracheal tubes, ventilatory equipment, and wounds.†

Early prosthetic valve endocarditis is hard to diagnose, is difficult to treat, and has a high mortality rate.[41] Patients have problems with persistent prosthetic valve infection if the microorganisms are seeded before the prosthetic valve has completely endothelialized. In such a case, the microorganisms become deeply embedded in the tissues and supporting structures, thereby making treatment with antimicrobial medications extremely difficult.[39]

When it develops in the early postoperative period, prosthetic valve endocarditis is difficult to diagnose because of the prolonged antibiotics that are given prophylactically for the prosthetic valve surgery and because blood cultures are usually negative due to the antibiotics. Thus the infecting microorganism causing the endocarditis is likely to be resistant to the antimicrobial drugs used for prophylaxis.[41,77] As a result, many cases of early prosthetic valve endocarditis are caused by microorganisms that are highly virulent (e.g., *S. aureus, Staphylococcus epidermidis,* gram-negative bacilli, and fungi), are difficult to eradicate, and cause rapid and severe complications. To avoid this problem, antibiotic therapy should be directed toward staphylococci, and the medication should be started just before the prosthetic valve surgery and continued not longer than 2 days after surgery.[1] It also is recommended that patients with early prosthetic valve endocarditis undergo early reoperation (i.e., prosthetic valve replacement).[23,39,41]

Early prosthetic valve endocarditis should be suspected in a patient who develops chills, fever, and toxemia several days after an operation. Severe congestive heart failure is the most common complication, occurring in 50% of all patients.[39] Cerebral and cardiac emboli frequently occur.[23,39,41]

Late prosthetic valve endocarditis, on the other hand, is caused primarily by a less-virulent organism, the most common of which is *S. viridans.* If the patient develops chills, fever, leukocytosis, or a new murmur later than 2 months after the operation, late prosthetic valve endocarditis should be considered. Although the mortality rate of this disease is lower than that for early prosthetic valve endocarditis, the majority of patients are at risk for developing heart failure or major embolic complications. Early reoperation to eradicate prosthetic valve infection in this group of patients is controversial,[39,41] although it is recommended when associated with heart failure.[57,84]

Exchanging pattern

Patient's response to the infection. The diagnosis of infective endocarditis is suspected in any patient who has a fever of unknown origin and a heart murmur. Patients with subacute endocarditis usually run a low-grade fever ranging from 37.2° to 38.8° C (99° to 102° F).[5,32,39] Patients with acute endocarditis, on the other hand, react more intensely to the infection, with recurrent chills, diaphoresis, and a high-grade temperature ranging from 39.4° to 40° C (103° to 104° F). Evaluate the patient's temperature every 1 to 2 hours, and correlate it with the results of the blood cultures and other laboratory tests.

Frequently patients with infective endocarditis respond to the infection with vague and nonspecific signs and symptoms (see the box). Assess patients for malaise, fa-

---

*References 23, 39, 41, 57, 62, 84.
†References 15, 62, 65, 90, 96, 101.

CLINICAL MANIFESTATIONS OF INFECTIVE ENDOCARDITIS

RESPONSE TO INFECTION

Fever
Anorexia
Chills and diaphoresis
Weight loss
Cough
Headache and backache
Malaise and fatigue

CARDIAC MANIFESTATIONS

New murmur
Change in quality or intensity of old murmur
Congestive heart failure
Pericarditis, pericardial friction rub, or cardiac tamponade
Myocardial infarction
Clubbing

HYPERSENSITIVITY MANIFESTATIONS

Periphery

Petechiae
Splinter hemorrhages
Osler's nodes
Janeway lesions
Roth's spots

Renal system

Focal glomerulitis
Acute or chronic glomerulonephritis

Musculoskeletal system

Arthralgia
Arthritis
Myalgias
Back pain

LABORATORY AND DIAGNOSTIC TESTS

Positive blood cultures
Anemia
Elevated erythrocyte sedimentation rate
Slightly elevated white blood cell count
Thrombocytopenia
Positive rheumatoid factor
Elevated immunoglobulin M and antiimmunoglobulin G
  antibody levels
Low serum complement levels
Albuminuria, pyuria, and hematuria
ECG
  Conduction or rhythm disturbances
  Myocardial ischemic changes

EMBOLIC MANIFESTATIONS

Central nervous system

Transient ischemic attacks
Cerebrovascular accidents
Cerebral mycotic aneurysm and rupture

Signs and symptoms

Confusion and weakness
Reduced concentration
Hallucinations
Sensory impairment
Insomnia
Psychotic behavior
Tremor
Visual field impairment
Pupillary inequality
Hemiplegia, hemiparesis
Paraplegia
Aphasia and dysphagia
Convulsions and coma

Cardiovascular system

Myocardial ischemia or infarction

Signs and symptoms

Chest pain with acute ECG changes

Gastrointestinal system

Splenic or mesenteric infarction

Signs and symptoms

Sudden abdominal pain with radiation to left axilla,
  shoulder, or precordium associated with local rebound tenderness, elevated temperature, chills, vomiting, splenomegaly, leukocytosis, and toxemia

Renal system

Renal infarction

Signs and symptoms

Flank pain with radiation to groin associated with hematuria, pyuria, azotemia, and changes in the results
  of renal function tests

Respiratory system

Pulmonary infarction

Signs and symptoms

Pleuritic chest pain associated with cough and shortness of breath

tigue, headache, back pain, cough, anorexia, and weight loss.[32,39,41]

Cardiac manifestations. Evaluate the patient's cardiovascular status for the rate, regularity, and rhythm of cardiac activity. Some type of cardiac involvement is demonstrated in most patients with subacute endocarditis, with 85% to 95% of patients having heart murmurs.[15,39,41] In contrast, patients with acute endocarditis frequently do not have murmurs in the early stages of the disease. New murmurs may develop during the first few weeks of therapy, or striking changes in the intensity or quality of an old murmur may occur because of destructive valvular complications (i.e., perforation of the valve or torn chordae tendineae). Murmurs usually are absent in patients with right-sided endocarditis, particularly when it involves the tricuspid valve.

The murmurs that develop in endocarditis are usually regurgitant. Assess murmurs for their timing in the cardiac cycle (e.g., systolic or diastolic), pitch, intensity, duration, and radiation (see Chapter 3). Carefully assess the patient throughout hospitalization for a new or changing murmur, which indicates erosive complications of the valve.

Endocardial vegetations can cause perforation, erosion, or rupture of the valve and surrounding tissue to produce congestive heart failure.[39] *Congestive heart failure* is the most common complication of acute and subacute endocarditis. When heart failure occurs, particularly when it is caused by the aortic valve, it has a grave prognosis despite effective antimicrobial therapy. Because heart failure is the most common cause of death in patients with endocarditis, aggressive surgical intervention is advocated[39,41] (see Nursing Diagnosis 1).

Other destructive hemodynamic complications can occur as a result of the erosive and friable vegetations. When the infection extends through the myocardial wall, VSDs, fistulae, abscesses, pericarditis (and pericardial friction rubs), and cardiac tamponade may develop.[27] Myocardial ischemia or infarction, complicated by ventricular dysrhythmias, can occur as a result of obstructive lesions of the coronary ostia or emboli[15,39,41] (see section on diagnostic tests).

Assess the patient for clubbed fingers (Fig. 13-3). Clubbing usually develops late in the disease.[39,51] In clubbing the skin proximal to the nailbed feels spongy, and in some cases the fingertips pulsate and flush. The proximal nailbeds are convex and rise above the flat plane of the finger.[11] The shape of the nailbed frequently returns to normal after the infective endocarditis has been successfully treated.

Embolic manifestations. Arterial embolization is a major complication in up to 50% of all patients with acute and subacute endocarditis.[41,82] Embolic fragments released from the friable endocardial vegetations can produce occlusion in the brain, coronary arteries, kidneys, spleen, lungs, and mesenteric arteries.[53]

Cerebral emboli occur most frequently, causing stroke, delirium, coma, and a variety of neuropsychiatric syn-

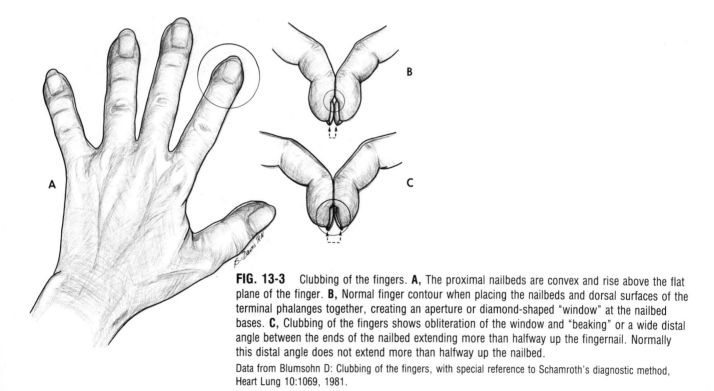

FIG. 13-3 Clubbing of the fingers. **A,** The proximal nailbeds are convex and rise above the flat plane of the finger. **B,** Normal finger contour when placing the nailbeds and dorsal surfaces of the terminal phalanges together, creating an aperture or diamond-shaped "window" at the nailbed bases. **C,** Clubbing of the fingers shows obliteration of the window and "beaking" or a wide distal angle between the ends of the nailbed extending more than halfway up the fingernail. Normally this distal angle does not extend more than halfway up the nailbed.

Data from Blumsohn D: Clubbing of the fingers, with special reference to Schamroth's diagnostic method, Heart Lung 10:1069, 1981.

dromes.[51] Pulmonary emboli are common among drug abusers and immunologically suppressed patients with right-sided endocarditis.[5,51] Emboli that block major arteries, an uncommon event in most bacterial forms of endocarditis, are characteristic of fungal infections.[4] Major embolic complications can occur early in the disease or for weeks to months after effective antimicrobial therapy has been completed.[41,51]

Immunologic derangements. A number of immunologic derangements are associated with infective endocarditis,[94] including rheumatoid factor, hypergammaglobulinemia, reduced complement levels, and cryoglobulinemia.[7] The *rheumatoid factor* (immunoglobulin M and anti-immunoglobulin G antibodies) inhibits the phagocytic action of the polymorphonuclear leukocytes and is found in up to 50% of all patients with infective endocarditis.[18,70,77,103] *Hypergammaglobulinemia* represents stimulation of the humoral immune system by the infection, depression of cellular immune activity, or both.[18,80]

Circulating immune complexes (i.e., cryoglobulins) often are found in patients with infective endocarditis. They produce a *hypersensitivity reaction* that is clinically manifested by an allergic vasculitis in various parts of the body. It was once believed that the peripheral manifestations seen in endocarditis were caused by microemboli. Although the issue is still controversial, it is now believed that the classic peripheral manifestations of endocarditis (e.g., petechiae, splinter hemorrhages, Osler's nodes, Janeway lesions, and Roth's spots) are caused by an allergic vasculitis of the arterioles.[8,18,80,103] With effective antimicrobial therapy, the circulating immune complex titers decline to normal.[18,70,77]

Petechiae (Fig. 13-4, *A*) are one of the most common signs of infective endocarditis and occur in up to 50% of all patients.[51] They occur around the conjunctivae, neck, clavicles, wrists, ankles, and mucous membranes. Petechiae are 1 to 2 mm in diameter, flat, red, and nontender lesions with a white or gray center. They appear in crops and then fade away to brown spots within a few days. However, they are not specifically diagnostic of infective endocarditis. Patients undergoing cardiopulmonary bypass for cardiac surgery, for example, can develop conjunctival petechiae from lipid microembolization.[41]

Splinter hemorrhages (linear subungual hemorrhages) (Fig. 13-4, *B*) may occur in patients with infective endocarditis on the distal third of the nailbed as black longitudinal streaks. They are not a specific sign of endocarditis and also may occur with age, occupational trauma (such as from typing), or mitral stenosis without endocarditis, hemodialysis, or peritoneal dialysis.[41,51]

Osler's nodes (Fig. 13-4, *C*) occur in 10% to 20% of patients with infective endocarditis. They are erythematous, painful lesions with a white center that vary in size from 1 to 10 mm. They are located typically on the pads of the fingers or toes, palms, soles, or thighs. Osler's nodes

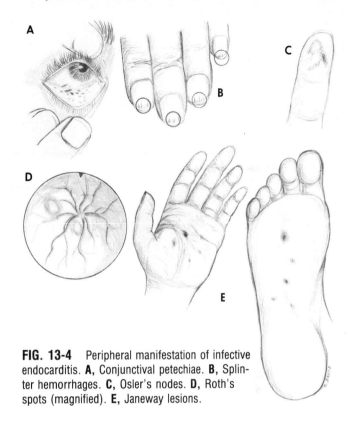

FIG. 13-4   Peripheral manifestation of infective endocarditis. **A,** Conjunctival petechiae. **B,** Splinter hemorrhages. **C,** Osler's nodes. **D,** Roth's spots (magnified). **E,** Janeway lesions.

are not a specific indicator of endocarditis and may occur with a variety of other illnesses.[51]

Janeway lesions (Fig. 13-4, *E*) occasionally are found in patients with infective endocarditis. In contrast to Osler's nodes, Janeway lesions are *nontender* and hemorrhagic lesions 1 to 5 mm in diameter. They occur on the arms, legs, palms, and soles and are accentuated when the extremity is elevated.

Roth's spots (Fig. 13-4, *D*) occasionally occur in patients with infective endocarditis. Funduscopically, Roth's spots are boat-shaped retinal hemorrhages with a pale or white center. They are located near the optic nerve disk and are 3 to 10 mm in diameter. They are also found in patients with a variety of other illnesses, such as anemia, leukemia, septicemia, and thrombotic thrombocytopenia purpura.[41]

Renal disease commonly is associated with infective endocarditis.[5] Renal emboli and infarction were discussed previously. Although focal "embolic" glomerulitis and acute and chronic glomerulonephritis once were believed to be the result of embolic complications, it is now reported that they are secondary to an allergic vasculitis.[41,51,80,94,103] Hematuria, renal failure, uremia, and death can result. Renal disease, associated with immunologic derangements, can be arrested and reversed with early and effective antimicrobial therapy.[8,80] Splenomegaly, probably secondary to continuous antigenic stimulation, also may be observed.

A variety of musculoskeletal manifestations occur in the majority of patients with infective endocarditis. They

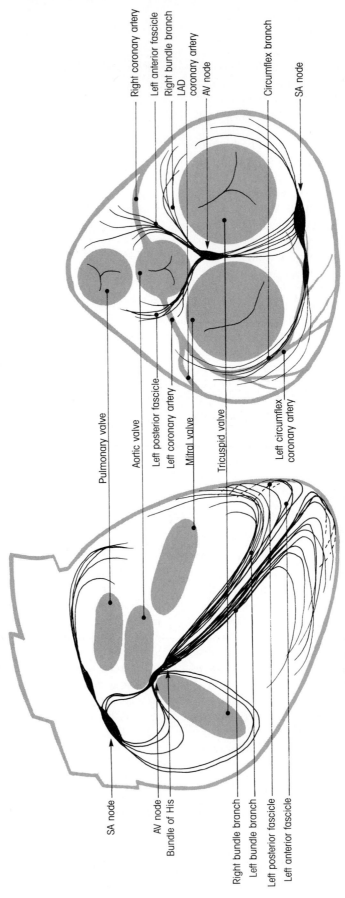

Right coronary artery
Left anterior fascicle
Right bundle branch
LAD
coronary artery
AV node
Circumflex branch
SA node

Pulmonary valve
Aortic valve
Left posterior fascicle
Left coronary artery
Mitral valve
Tricuspid valve
Left circumflex coronary artery

SA node
AV node
Bundle of His
Right bundle branch
Left bundle branch
Left posterior fascicle
Left anterior fascicle

FIG. 13-5 Anatomic relationship among heart valves, conduction system, and coronary arteries.

are probably the result of microemboli that cause a localized immune response. Arthralgias, arthritis, myalgias, and severe lower back pain are common complaints.[41,51,55]

Mycotic aneurysm is a rare but major complication occurring more frequently in subacute than in acute endocarditis. Mycotic aneurysms are associated with immunologic derangements (i.e., immune complexes deposited in the arterial wall) and microembolization, producing inflammation, thinning, dilation, and necrosis of the artery. This process may lead to rupture of the aneurysm months to years after the illness. Rupture of a mycotic aneurysm, particularly in a cerebral artery, can cause intracranial hemorrhage and has a high mortality rate.

Laboratory and diagnostic tests. Assess the patient's laboratory and diagnostic tests. A positive blood culture for the infecting organism is the most important laboratory test in the diagnosis of infective endocarditis. A normochromic, normocytic anemia is found in 60% to 70% of such patients. Leukocyte counts are elevated in acute endocarditis. Erythrocyte sedimentation rates commonly are elevated. A thrombotic thrombocytopenia purpura–like syndrome, associated with a low platelet count, a high titer of circulating immune complexes, and low levels of serum complement, have been reported.[41,51]

Because the right cusp and the noncoronary cusp of the aortic valve lie near the atrioventricular (AV) node and the right and left bundle branches, the endocardial infection can spread from the aortic valve into the myocardium and cause conduction abnormalities[86,103] (Fig. 13-5). As a result, assess the patient's ECG for first-degree AV heart block and left or right bundle branch block or hemiblocks. In contrast, the mitral anulus lies in close proximity to the AV node and bundle of His. Infection spreading from the mitral valve can cause junctional dysrhythmias or first-degree, second-degree, or third-degree AV heart block. Ventricular dysrhythmias occasionally are observed. Also assess the ECG for signs of myocardial ischemic changes caused by emboli.

Transthoracic or transesophageal two-dimensional echocardiography can be helpful in visualizing large valvular vegetations, which characteristically are produced by *S. aureus* or fungi.[5,70,72] Doppler echocardiography can be used to quantitate and confirm valvular lesions. Cardiac catheterization occasionally is done to determine the extent of the infection and identify patients who may require surgical intervention.

Feeling and choosing patterns

Patient's and family's responses to the acute illness. Thoroughly assess the Feeling and Choosing Patterns to determine the patient's and family's responses to the acute illness. The unexpected admission to a CCU and the initial uncertainty of the patient's diagnosis can produce high levels of anxiety for the patient and family.[49] The Cardiovascular Assessment Tool described in Chapter 3 can help in assessing these responses. Synthesize the data from the Exchanging and the Feeling Patterns to identify the patient's psychophysiologic manifestations of anxiety. Also assess the way the patient views the physiologic impact of the illness on the emotional response. Explore the patient's reactions to and perceptions of former illnesses or hospitalizations. Determine whether the patient is accepting or denying the current illness. Investigate coping behaviors that the patient has used during previous crises, and compare this information to the coping behaviors currently manifested. When formulating the plan of care, identify adaptive and maladaptive behaviors so that strengths can be maximized and weakness can be substituted with adaptive behaviors.[30]

Nursing diagnoses

The most common human responses anticipated for a patient with infective endocarditis are indicated by the following nursing diagnoses:
1. Cardiac valve infection related to (include name of infecting organism)
2. Anxiety related to acute illness, diagnostic tests, lengthy hospitalization and treatment, or fear of impending surgery (if indicated)
3. High risk for infective or phlebotic vascular complications related to prolonged intravenous therapy
4. High risk for complications of impaired physical mobility related to prolonged intravenous therapy and restricted activities
5. High risk for valvular reinfection related to insufficient knowledge about illness and future prophylactic care

For each of these diagnoses, the patient outcomes, nursing prescriptions, and evaluation criteria are outlined with a discussion of the factual information that support the plan and implementation of care.

NURSING
DIAGNOSIS 1 **Cardiac valve infection related to (include name of organism when identified) (exchanging pattern)**

PATIENT OUTCOMES	NURSING PRESCRIPTIONS	EVALUATION
Infecting organism will be identified from blood culture studies:	Supervise the drawing of blood cultures:	Patient's infecting organism was identified:
Patient will verbalize the need or rationale for blood culture studies, the frequency of the studies, and a general description of the procedure and amount of blood drawn.	Teach patient the rationale for blood culture studies, the frequency with which they are drawn, the procedure, and the amount of blood drawn.	Patient verbalized the need, frequency, and a general description of the procedure.
Patient will not exhibit a high level of anxiety related to the drawing of blood samples.	Assess patient's level of anxiety as blood samples are drawn.	Patient did not exhibit a high level of anxiety.
Patient will practice relaxation and imagery during the procedure.	Guide patient in relaxation and imagery during the procedure.	Patient practiced relaxation and imagery.
Patient will not experience complications such as redness, swelling, bleeding, or discomfort at the venipuncture site.	Assess venipuncture site for complications and instruct patient to report symptoms.	Patient did not experience complications.
Patient will demonstrate symptomatic improvement as a result of effective antimicrobial therapy:	Administer antimicrobial therapy and evaluate response:	Patient demonstrated symptomatic improvement as a result of effective antimicrobial therapy:
Patient will verbalize the rationale for, the frequency and duration of, and a general description of therapy.	Teach patient the rationale for, the frequency and duration of, and a general description of the therapy.	Patient verbalized the rationale, frequency, duration, and description of therapy.
Temperature will return to normal in 4 or 5 days.	Evaluate temperature daily.	Temperature returned to normal in 4 days.
Appetite will improve.	Assess appetite and provide supplemental feedings and nutritious snacks.	Appetite improved.
Complaints of malaise, fatigue, back pain, and headache will decrease.	Evaluate complaints of malaise, fatigue, back pain, and headache daily.	General complaints related to the infection decreased.
Renal disease will be reversed.	Evaluate results of renal function tests.	Renal disease was reversed.
Clubbing will disappear.	Evaluate degree of clubbing.	Clubbing disappeared.
Blood culture studies will become negative within 1 week.	Evaluate results of blood culture studies after 1 week of antimicrobial therapy.	Blood culture studies were negative in 1 week.
Circulating immune complex titers and erythrocyte sedimentation rate will decline.	Evaluate level of circulating immune complexes and the erythrocyte sedimentation rate.	Circulating immune complexes and erythrocyte sedimentation rate declined.
Rheumatoid factor will disappear.	Evaluate rheumatoid factor laboratory test.	Rheumatoid factor disappeared.
Patient will not experience complications from the antimicrobial therapy such as rash, urticaria, diarrhea, anaphylactic reactions, or other adverse reactions.	Assess for adverse reactions to antimicrobial therapy and instruct patient to report symptoms.	Patient did not experience adverse reactions to antimicrobial therapy.

NURSING
DIAGNOSIS 1 **Cardiac valve infection related to (include name or organism when identified) (exchanging pattern)—cont'd**

PATIENT OUTCOMES	NURSING PRESCRIPTIONS	EVALUATION
Patient will report leakage, pain, or discomfort at the venipuncutre site.	Assess venipuncture site for complications and instruct patient to report symptoms.	Patient had no leakage, pain, or discomfort at venipuncture site.
Patient will not experience major complications associated with infective endocarditis:	Observe for major complications associated with infective endocarditis:	Patient did not experience major complications associated with infective endocarditis:
Patient will not experience hemodynamic deterioration as evidenced by anxiety, restlessness, loss of feeling of well-being, and signs of reduced blood pressure, tachycardia, reduced urinary output, elevated blood urea nitrogen (BUN) levels, or a change in the quality and intensity of the heart murmur.	Assess for hemodynamic deterioration.	Patient did not experience hemodynamic deterioration.
Patient will not experience major recurrent arterial emboli (see p. 401).	Assess for major recurrent emboli.	Patient did not experience major recurrent arterial emboli.
Patient will not experience persistent infection or infection refractory to antimicrobial therapy (see p. 409).	Assess for persistent infection.	Patient did not experience persistent infection.
If patient experiences major complications or if the patient has prosthetic valve endocarditis or left-sided valve endocarditis caused by *S. aureus,* gram-negative bacilli, or fungi, patient will be evaluated as a candidate for prosthetic valve replacement (see Chapter 17).	If patient experiences major complications, help prepare patient for prosthetic valve replacement surgery (see Chapter 17).	Patient was not a candidate for surgery.
If intravenous therapy will be done in the home, patient will prepare for and be able to perform all phases of it.	Assess whether patient is a candidate for home intravenous therapy. Teach necessary techniques for the procedure and evaluate patient's knowledge and skills.	Patient demonstrated the knowledge, readiness, and ability to perform all phases of home intravenous therapy. Home follow-up visits have been scheduled.

Plan and intervention for cardiac valve infection
Identification of the infecting organism

The most important finding in the diagnosis of infective endocarditis is isolation of the causative organism by means of blood cultures.[32,70] The role of the nurse at this stage is primarily to supervise and coordinate the drawing of blood cultures before antimicrobial therapy is initiated and to

help the patient to decrease anxiety. All therapeutic measures should be used to increase patient comfort.

The patient is taught the reasons that blood cultures are done. Serial blood cultures are drawn to demonstrate a sustained or continuous bacteremia. In patients with infective endocarditis, blood cultures remain positive during serial drawings because bacteria are released continuously from the endocardial vegetations into the circulation. In contrast, most bacteria entering the blood from dental procedures or toothbrushing generally cause a transient bacteremia. The bacteria are quickly cleared from the circulation by the reticuloendothelial system, and positive blood cultures will persist for less than 30 minutes.[70] Another important reason for serial blood cultures is to prevent false-negative or false-positive interpretations. Microorganisms commonly causing infective endocarditis also are the ones that frequently contaminate blood cultures.[26] When serial cultures are drawn, the infecting microorganisms usually appear in all cultures, whereas the contaminant appears only in one.[77]

Patients have varied reactions to the blood culture venipuncture sticks. Many patients cannot understand the need for repeated sticks. Others believe that such tests cause a significant reduction in blood volume. Thus the need for serial blood cultures is explained slowly and perhaps repeatedly with each venipuncture stick. The patient should understand that effective antimicrobial therapy depends on identifying the microorganism causing the infection. The nurse emphasizes that blood cultures are drawn serially to demonstrate a continuous bacteremia and rule out a transient infection. The patient should understand the procedure and know that the amount of blood drawn during each venipuncture is generally not more than 1 tablespoon. The patient's reaction to the explanation and procedure are assessed, and the patient is encouraged to verbalize questions or anxieties. The venipuncture sites are checked for signs of complications, and the nurse instructs the patient to report bleeding, pain, or discomfort.

Patients also may become anxious and tense while blood cultures are being drawn. The anticipation of the venipuncture and the expected and perceived discomfort can transiently induce the psychophysiologic stress response manifested by tachycardia and peripheral constriction. Dilated veins are easier to stick than constricted ones. Nurses often use hot packs to peripherally dilate veins before venipuncture. The same results, however, can be elicited by teaching the patient to use relaxation techniques during the procedure to reverse the stress response, lower the heart rate, dilate peripheral vessels, and warm the extremities.[30] The nurse also can guide the patient with imagery during relaxation, suggesting that the patient visualize relaxed, wide open tubes (vessels) in the periphery. Relaxation techniques not only reverse the detrimental physiologic effects of stress but also can induce profound psychologic changes to reduce anxiety, fear, and a feeling of loss of control (see pp. 118-119).

Proper technique must be used when drawing blood cultures. Strict asepsis is needed during the venipuncture and transfer of the blood to the culture tubes to prevent contamination of the cultures. The nurse scrubs the top of the culture tubes and the patient's skin with a 2% solution of iodine in 70% alcohol and removes the iodine after at least a 30-second drying time with 70% isopropyl alcohol.[70]

Because serial blood cultures are needed, the length of time that antimicrobial therapy is delayed while blood culture studies are being drawn depends on the severity of the patient's illness. For the acutely ill patient with rigor, a spiking temperature, and heart failure, three to five blood cultures are drawn at 5- to 10-minute intervals. For the less acutely ill patient, five to six cultures are drawn, usually within 24 to 48 hours.[41] Each tube should be properly labeled and incubated under aerobic and anaerobic conditions. When unusual organisms are suspected or when blood culture studies are negative, the microorganisms should be cultured and incubated for 2 to 3 weeks.[70,77]

Despite proper technique when drawing blood cultures and clinical evidence suggesting that the patient has endocarditis, 15% to 20% of all patients with endocarditis have negative blood cultures.[15,39,79,85] Causes of negative blood cultures include right-sided endocarditis, poor bacteriologic techniques, the presence of unusual organisms, or organisms with special growth requirements (e.g., viruses and fungi or satellite streptococci, which are nutritionally deficient and grow on blood agar only around other bacteria).[41,79,85] The most common cause of negative blood cultures, however, is the prior administration of antibiotics that suppress bacteremia when blood culture samples are drawn.[79] Thus antimicrobial therapy should not be administered until an adequate number of blood cultures have been drawn.

Antimicrobial therapy

After the infecting organism has been identified by blood culture studies, its name should be written on the patient's problem list and care plan (e.g., "cardiac valve infection related to *S. aureus*"). The antimicrobial therapy chosen for the patient with infective endocarditis depends on the microorganism causing the infection. Antimicrobial therapy is administered to kill the microorganism, sterilize the vegetations, reduce symptoms and complications, and prevent a relapse. Frequently antimicrobial medications are administered before the results of the blood culture studies are returned. In such cases, the medication is directed against the microorganism suspected of causing the infection. The antimicrobial agent chosen should have bactericidal action and a narrow spectrum with the fewest possible side effects.[19,77]

After blood culture studies are completed, there should be no delay in administering antimicrobial therapy. Medications should be given intravenously rather than orally to reduce individual variation in absorption and to ensure compliance.[32] Because the vegetations are avascular lesions that contain millions of organisms entrapped within the platelet-fibrin meshwork, high serum concentrations of the medication are needed.[19] Antimicrobial therapy is administered long enough to prevent a relapse and ensure a cure.

A history of allergies to medications must be obtained from the patient. Patients who allege to have penicillin allergies, for example, must be carefully questioned. It is important to establish whether they think they are allergic to penicillin, have a history of rash after penicillin therapy, or have experienced a more severe and immediate reaction, such as hypotension or bronchospasm. It is suggested that patients undergo a skin test before a history of penicillin allergy is accepted.

Most streptococcal infections, with the exception of enterococci, are sensitive to penicillin. Penicillin does not enter the bacterial cell wall, but rather it inhibits the synthesis of the cell wall, thereby making it more susceptible to lysis. Patients with *S. viridans* endocarditis are treated with 10 to 20 million units of parenteral penicillin daily; it is administered as a continuous intravenous infusion or in six equally divided doses.[10,19,77] Penicillin is continued for 4 to 6 weeks.[19,77,83] Such prolonged intravenous therapy can be devastating to many patients. It is important to assist the patient in coping with the length of hospitalization and treatment (see Nursing Diagnosis 2).

Aminoglycosides also are recommended during the first 2 weeks of therapy.[17,83] Streptomycin, 7.5 mg/kg (not to exceed 500 mg), is given intramuscularly every 12 hours, or gentamicin, 1 mg/kg (not to exceed 80 mg), may be given intramuscularly or intravenously every 8 hours. Streptomycin enters the bacterial cell wall and produces changes within the bacteria that impair their survival. Penicillin, when combined with streptomycin, exerts a synergistic bactericidal action that is more effective than penicillin or streptomycin used alone.[83] Six weeks of combination therapy with penicillin and an aminoglycoside is recommended for patients with prosthetic valve endocarditis. For patients with uncomplicated *S. viridans* endocarditis, however, a 2-week course of therapy with penicillin and an aminoglycoside has been successful recently in producing high bacteriologic cure rates.[10]

If an organism is susceptible, penicillin is the drug of choice. However, most strains of *S. aureus*, which cause acute endocarditis, are not sensitive to penicillin. Such bacteria produce penicillinase, an enzyme that inactivates penicillin. Penicillinase-resistant penicillins (i.e., penicillins that are resistant to penicillinase), however, are effective against staphylococcal infections. *S. aureus* is treated with this type of semisynthetic penicillin such as nafcillin or oxacillin generally for 4 to 8 weeks.[19,32,41,77] Gentamicin may be added to the therapy for 3 to 5 days.[19]

The treatment of other microorganisms depends on the culture-proven sensitivity of the infecting organism to the antibiotic. Amphotericin B is used for fungal infections. Vancomycin is given to patients who are allergic to penicillin.[19,32,77]

The nurse explains the reasons for antimicrobial therapy to the patient, including the intravenous procedure, the frequency of administration, the need for tests to monitor serum drug levels, and the duration of therapy. The patient is instructed to report signs of fluid leakage, pain, or discomfort around the venipuncture site (see Nursing Diagnosis 3) and to report any possible allergic reactions to the antimicrobial drugs.

Response to therapy

After antimicrobial therapy is begun, the patient's response to therapy is assessed in terms of clinical improvement, worsening of symptoms, and allergic manifestations. The patient's temperature should drop within a few days of therapy and return to normal within 4 or 5 days. Persistent fever, observed several days after treatment, indicates that the drug selected is inadequate, the dose is too low, or another infection has been superimposed on the original infection. The patient's appetite should improve. Complaints of malaise, fatigue, backache, and headache should decrease. If clubbing is present, the shape of the nailbeds should return to normal. Circulating immune complex titers should decline. Renal disease associated with immunologic derangements should be reversed. Blood culture studies should revert from positive to negative within 1 week. The erythrocyte sedimentation rate should decline, and the rheumatoid factor should disappear.

Several types of clinical manifestations may develop or persist despite effective antimicrobial therapy. These include cardiac manifestations related to destructive and hemodynamic complications (e.g., murmurs, heart failure, and conduction and rhythm disturbances), embolic manifestations, and hypersensitivity manifestations such as petechiae. The nurse assesses the patient for these complications even when antimicrobial therapy is successful.

Allergic reactions to penicillin include mild skin rashes, urticaria, diarrhea, and anaphylactic shock manifested as profound circulatory collapse. If an allergic reaction is noted, the type of allergy and the patient's condition are assessed, and the physician is consulted. If the patient experiences an anaphylactic reaction, the penicillin should be stopped, and intravenous epinephrine, 0.5 mg of a 1:10,000 solution, should be given. The dose is repeated every 5 to 15 minutes until the patient responds. Additionally, cardiopulmonary resuscitation (CPR), intravenous fluids, aminophylline, or hydrocortisone may be needed. Toxic effects of streptomycin may include damage of the eighth cranial nerve, causing dizziness and loss of balance and hearing. Adverse effects of gentamicin include nephrotoxic complications manifested by an elevation of the BUN or creatinine levels or oliguria.[10]

Complications of infective endocarditis

Because of the destructive and erosive complications leading to intractable congestive heart failure, prosthetic valve replacement now is recommended for a select group of endocarditis patients. The patient's hemodynamic status is the most important determining factor in selecting candidates for surgery.[23,105-107] Congestive heart failure, causing severe reduction in cardiac output, is the most common cause of death in these patients. Aortic valve involvement is more likely to lead to severe heart failure and death than mitral valve involvement.[41,67,68] The mortality rate of endocarditis patients with severe heart failure who are treated medically ranges from 50% to 90%.[41,68,77,78,81] As a result, prosthetic valve replacement is recommended for patients with a deteriorating hemodynamic status.[9,37]

Valve replacement dramatically improves the survival in this group of patients.[41,68,77,81] The most important factor in the survival of patients undergoing surgery is their hemodynamic status at the time of operation. Survival is improved if surgery is performed at the first signs of cardiac decompensation rather than after medical therapy has failed and the patient's hemodynamic status is severely impaired.[2,68,77,98] Prosthetic valve replacement is even being done during the active stage of infection. If the patient is acutely ill, valve replacement may be undertaken after only one preoperative dose of antimicrobial medication.[61] Antimicrobial therapy then is continued after surgery.

The aim of surgery for patients with active infective endocarditis is to treat the congestive heart failure that has failed to respond to medical therapy and to eradicate the infection and thus eliminate the source of systemic emboli. During surgery the infected tissue is excised, any abscesses are unroofed, and the valvular lesion is corrected by prosthetic valve replacement.[61,71]

Early prosthetic valve replacement also has been recommended for other subgroups of patients with endocarditis. Because of the toxic fulminant course and the high mortality rate associated with left-sided *S. aureus* endocarditis, surgery has been recommended by some groups[67,68,84] within 2 to 7 days after the diagnosis has been made. Infective endocarditis caused by gram-negative organisms and fungi frequently are resistant to antimicrobial therapy, and patients infected with these organisms often are considered as candidates for surgery. Other indications for prosthetic valve replacement include prosthetic valve endocarditis, large recurrent systemic emboli, the onset of conduction disturbances, and persistent infections or infections refractory to antimicrobial medications.[9,61,68,78]

Other surgical approaches have been recommended for patients who are less severely ill. Tricuspid valve endocarditis, most commonly seen with abusers of parenteral drugs, frequently responds well to antimicrobial therapy and has a good prognosis.[20] Surgical intervention is required, however, in about one quarter of the cases. Patients with right-sided endocarditis who have not responded to antimicrobial therapy can undergo valve reconstruction or reparative approaches, such as valvuloplasty. For patients with well-circumscribed vegetations with little or no valve damage, the local excision of the vegetation, (i.e., vegetectomy) with leaflet repair also has been reported.[33,54]

These procedures are possible because of the low, right-sided intracardiac pressures and the three-leaflet configuration of right-sided heart valves.[109,110]

The nurse should be aware of the indications for surgery in patients with infective endocarditis and should anticipate the immediate objectives of care. The nurse also should be aware of the subgroups of patients who are particularly predisposed to developing acute and severe hemodynamic impairment. These patients must be evaluated frequently. Signs of cardiac decompensation must be reported to the physician immediately.

Signs of cardiac decompensation that result from valve perforation or rupture can occur within hours in the patient with acute endocarditis; they include anxiety, restlessness, loss of feeling of well-being, and signs of reduced cardiac output, such as tachypnea, a changing mental status, decreased blood pressure, tachycardia, decreased urinary output, elevated BUN level, a change in the quality and intensity of the heart murmur, and uncontrolled cardiac decompensation.[67] The nurse plays an important role in helping to evaluate whether the patient is a candidate for surgery before irreversible valve damage occurs.

These patients are confronted not only with the stress of a severe and life-threatening illness but also with the stress of impending and unexpected surgery. The nurse reinforces and clarifies the physician's explanation of the need and rationale for the operation. Patients and families should be encouraged to ventilate their fears and disbeliefs. Relaxation and imagery exercises should be continued and reinforced before and after surgery. The psychophysiologic preparation of patients undergoing cardiac surgery is discussed in Chapter 17.

Home intravenous therapy

A patient with infective endocarditis is allowed an inpatient stay of 18.4 days according to Diagnostic Related Groups (DRGs).[93] As a result, many patients require intravenous antibiotics at home to complete the required 4- to 6-week course of therapy. Some recent reports[21,25,60,97] regarding home intravenous therapy have been published. In developing such programs, it is recommended that a multidisciplinary team, consisting of a nurse, physician, and pharmacist design, implement, and coordinate the home intravenous therapy program. The team should be responsible for assessing each potential candidate after the patient's infection has begun to resolve and the condition has stabilized. Appropriate candidates should have at least 7 days of intravenous therapy remaining (for the program to be cost effective). They should be responding appropriately to therapy without complications and have no need for additional hospitalization except for antimicrobial therapy. The assessment also includes an evaluation of the patient's alertness, emotional stability, cooperation and willingness to comply, history of substance abuse, and the adequacy of manual dexterity necessary to manipulate the equipment and perform the procedures. The home environment also is assessed and a responsible support person should be identified.[25]

The patient should be given a choice to accept or reject the program. If the patient is interested, a nurse and pharmacist should instruct the patient about techniques of self-administered intravenous antibiotics. Before discharge, patients should be assessed regarding their knowledge, readiness, and ability to perform all phases of the procedure. They should be able to discuss potential complications, emergency measures, laboratory testing procedures, physician follow-up appointments, and persons to contact regarding questions or problems.

Patients are sent home with a heparin lock or a Hickman catheter, medications, fluids, and related equipment. A nurse should visit the patient in the home for the first antibiotic administration to provide reinforcement and emotional support and to answer questions. Additional visits should be scheduled on an individual basis. Heparin locks should be changed every 48 to 72 hours by home care nurses[97] or by an intravenous nurse team when patients return to the hospital.[60] Insurance coverage is available for home treatment from most insurance companies.[25]

The conclusions drawn from home intravenous studies[60,97] are dramatic. The savings to patients were reported to be substantial. Hospital beds became available for other patients. In one study of 12 patients receiving home intravenous therapy, hospital stays were reduced by a total of 260 days with a total savings of $109,767 (an average savings of $9,114 per patient). Home intravenous therapy has been shown to be an effective method of administering prolonged intravenous antibiotics with no more untoward effects than in-hospital therapy. Patients were motivated to assume the responsibility of self-care and to learn the necessary techniques. Perhaps most important, home therapy allowed these patients to become active participants and gain tangible control of their therapy. By accepting responsibility for their own care, they were able to return home to a more normal lifestyle. The psychologic impact of this involvement and control undoubtedly is correlated to the patient's physiologic recovery.

Reports of home therapy also point out the essence of communication and cooperation among the health team members. A creative team, sharing ideas, expertise, and knowledge, can achieve dramatic outcomes. Home therapy should be encouraged within hospitals.

NURSING DIAGNOSIS 2   **Anxiety related to acute illness, diagnostic tests, lengthy hospitalization and treatment, or fear of impending surgery (if indicated) (feeling pattern)**

PATIENT OUTCOMES	NURSING PRESCRIPTIONS	EVALUATION
Patient and family will verbalize questions and concerns.	Encourage patient and family to verbalize questions and concerns.	Patient and family verbalized concerns regarding the patient's illness, length of hospitalization, and treatment.
Patient will verbalize an understanding of the illness, diagnostic tests ordered, and need for surgery (if indicated).	During initial admission period, implement teaching regarding the illness, tests, and surgery (if indicated) to reduce anxiety. Keep all explanations brief and concise. Repeat explanations as often as necessary.	Patient verbalized an understanding of the illness and diagnostic test. (Surgery was not indicated.)
Patient (and family) will participate in and practice relaxation exercises.	During initial admission period, teach patient and family relaxation techniques.	Patient and family participated in and practiced relaxation with music twice a day throughout the hospitalization.
Patient (and family) will demonstrate reductions in psychophysiologic stress from baseline observations after relaxation sessions.	Evaluate patient's response to relaxation sessions. Compare heart rates, blood pressures, finger temperatures, and psychologic perceptions before and after the sessions.	Patient successfully lowered the heart rate on an average of 10 beats per minute, raised finger temperatures 5° to 10° F, and reported a relaxed and calm feeling after relaxation sessions.

Plan and intervention for anxiety
Teaching patients who are critically ill or in crises

Most patients admitted to the hospital for an unexpected illness respond to the situation with varying levels of anxiety.[45] Teaching patients during this initial stressful period can have an important psychophysiologic impact. In recent years, however, research has shown that critically ill patients or those in crisis cannot be taught. These research studies have evaluated patient teaching by determining how much patients understand, what they remember, and how well they incorporate this information by changing their behavior or complying with what has been taught. When critically ill patients are evaluated using such criteria, the results have been discouraging. As a result, those in medicine and nursing have come to believe that these patients are too sick or anxious to learn and that learning is not possible during this stressful time.[46]

The author believes, however, that premature conclusions have been drawn about teaching critically ill patients. Most studies investigating patient teaching are based on principles of teaching-learning theories. As a result, the criteria used to evaluate teaching have focused on what the patient should have learned. However, when nurses teach critically ill patients, the use of traditional criteria to measure learning may not be appropriate.[46] Thus researchers may have been evaluating the wrong criteria. The real benefit of teaching these patients probably is not measured adequately by how much they have learned or remember.

Traditional ideas about teaching have permeated the framework of care, which is based on the Cartesian view of the human being as divisible into two parts, body and mind. Nursing and medicine have gradually adopted the primary assumption that essentially it is the body that becomes sick or specifically the heart valve in a patient with infective endocarditis; the mind may be secondarily involved but is seen as a causative factor only in rare circumstances.[30] Thus therapies, procedures, drugs, surgery, and most research are body oriented. Treatment for patients with infective endocarditis, for example, includes antimicrobial agents and intravenous fluids for infected heart valves, antipyretic drugs for fever, and valve replacement surgery for valvular complications. However, holistic nurses clearly understand that although body ailments may be eradicated with body-oriented therapies, the patient's psychologic response to disease may impair the ability to return to full function and may actually interfere with healing.[38]

In a holistic approach to patient care, however, the mind and body are seen as operating on a continuum. Disease is much more than a body process; it involves the whole person. The interconnections of the mind and body, moreover, are reflected in changes of emotion and physiology.[38] Such interconnections may operate at the conscious or unconscious level.

From a holistic framework, it can be deduced that *if the mind is educable, so too must be the body*. This concept is not only startling but also fruitful because it enlarges the nurse's options for effective therapy to include much more than medications, treatments, and surgical procedures. When the nurse teaches the patient, the results can cause body effects as real as those produced by traditional forms of therapy.[46] From this viewpoint, the impact of the teaching process then takes on primary importance and relevance.

The *process* of teaching therefore has value because of its impact on the learner,[46] which is different from measuring the value of teaching from its outcomes, its *products*. Each nurse-patient encounter has therapeutic value and worth. Each time the patient and nurse interact, it can be viewed as a teaching experience; the nurse meaningfully affects the patient's emotions and physiologic status. Each time a nurse answers a patient's questions regarding the illness or procedures or identifies and meets a patient's need, the interaction produces a body-mind response. The nurse who responds to the physical needs of the patient also realizes that such intervention affects much more than the patient's physical function. Each encounter with the patient is a teaching-learning experience affecting the whole patient. This exchange may or may not be remembered by the patient weeks or even minutes later; however, it meets the need at the time and has psychophysiologic effects.

Case study. Mr. J.R. had many concerns and questions about why he had to stay in bed during the early course of his hospitalization. The nurse sat with the patient, explaining briefly and simply that the order for bed rest was important for healing and energy conservation. About 20 minutes later, when the nurse returned to the room, Mr. J.R. was out of bed, with his intravenous lines, looking out the window.

The nurse can evaluate this case study in many ways. If evaluation is based on the *product* of this teaching, one might conclude that the nurse had "failed" in the teaching attempt and that the patient did not remember or understand what he had been told, was denying his illness, or perhaps was an uncooperative or "bad" patient. Such conclusions can produce feelings of frustration and failure and can lead to misunderstandings and power struggles between the patient and nurse.

However, evaluating the situation based on the *process* of teaching reveals that earlier the patient had questions and concerns about the reasons for bed rest. In discussing these concerns with the patient, the nurse met the patient's momentary need, and the experience affected the whole patient. Thus this teaching encounter is successful. When, 20 minutes later, the patient was found out of bed, the situation is viewed as a new teaching experience, a new teaching need that also will have a psychophysiologic impact. The explanations probably will need to be repeated and then repeated again to meet the momentary needs of the patient.

No patient teaching encounter is ever a neutral event. It is a phenomenon that affects the patient and nurse.[46] The effects may be dramatic and measurable or subtle and not quantifiable, but something always happens.

Relaxation and music therapy

The high level of anxiety commonly observed in patients admitted to a critical care unit can negatively alter the patient's psychophysiologic state. The physiologic event (produced by an infection of the heart valve) can produce corresponding psychologic alterations (anxiety), and conversely, the psychologic event associated with illness (the anxiety associated with endocarditis) can produce physiologic alterations (elevations in myocardial oxygen consumption, blood pressure, and heart rate). This example illustrates the negative role that consciousness can play in matters of health and illness. It demonstrates the devastating effects of the mind. The time has come, however, for nurses to intervene in assisting patients to use their consciousness in positively changing their psychophysiologic state to unleash the enormous healing capacity that lies within them.[30]

When nurses incorporate relaxation and music therapy into practice, they provide patients with the techniques to positively change their psychophysiologic state and reduce the stress inherent to most body illnesses.[14] Music therapy is a behavioral science concerned with the use of specific kinds of music and their ability to effect changes in behavior, emotions, and physiologic state.[92] It is used to focus attention, ignore distracting thoughts, and alter perception of time.[13] A major goal is to produce relaxation and a meditative, calm, and hypometabolic state. The immediate impact of such therapy is to influence the mind, which in turn influences the body and leads to positive psychophysiologic outcomes.

Chapter 5 provides the knowledge base for understanding the principles and impact of music therapy. Music therapy can be used for all types of patients. For Mr. J.R., the use of music and relaxation was extremely successful in helping him cope with his lengthy hospitalization and the prolonged intravenous therapy necessary for treating his endocarditis.

There is probably no other more stressful period in a cardiac patient's hospitalization than the first few days in a CCU. Self-regulation therapies are uniquely effective for these patients because of the initial crisis being experienced. This notion is supported by Fenwick, Donaldson, and Gills,[34] who reported that subjects who were highly tense before meditating or listening to music demonstrated greater relaxation responses than did those subjects who were not tense. Thus these techniques may be particularly useful for patients experiencing high levels of psychophysiologic stress.

When practiced twice a day for 15 to 20 minutes, music therapy provides some level of control over the situation and empowers patients to enhance their own recovery. Most patients are receptive to learning such techniques. It gives them a sense of self-responsibility and involvement in their care. The nurse helps patients to realize that they possess a powerful healing potential within themselves.

The kind of music that relaxes one patient may not relax another. Thus the patient's musical preference is an important variable contributing to maximal therapeutic outcomes. Because different types of music create a variety of responses among individuals, musical selections that are calming and meditative to **some** may be disruptive and irritating to others. In addition, music that some individuals identify as relaxing, in fact, may not be psychophysiologically relaxing at all.[49] Although music experts tend to agree that rock music does not evoke relaxation (even if the patient thinks it does), they also agree that soothing classical, spiritual, or popular music also may not be relaxing for some individuals.[49,50] A variety of musical selections should be judged for acceptability and relaxing qualities and made available in a music therapy library for patient use.[47] The Resource List in Chapter 5 provides the names and addresses of companies from whom various types of relaxing and therapeutic tapes can be purchased. Chapter 5 also discusses how to set up a hospital audiocassette library.

Tape recorders and headsets should be available on all hospital units. Headsets, as opposed to earphones, are probably more comfortable for the patient. If the patient's room is quiet, these may be unnecessary. A quiet environment, however, is one element necessary in achieving the relaxation response. In a busy hospital unit where a quiet environment is not possible, headsets have the additional benefit of blocking out distracting and annoying noise.

Several studies have investigated the effects of music therapy on critically ill patients. Intensive care and surgical patients who participated in music therapy had better relief from pain, lower heart rates, and enhanced emotional stability during hospitalization.[12] Another study reported that relaxation and music therapy had an effective cumulative response in lowering apical heart rates, raising peripheral temperatures, reducing cardiovascular complications, and producing positive subjective evaluations of the therapy in CCU patients.[48] Two other studies, however, reported no significant physiologic changes in CCU patients who listened to music,[29,111] although significant psychologic benefits were reported in one.[29]

The effects of various relaxation techniques are frequently measured in research studies using biofeedback equipment. Many CCUs already have such equipment, which could be used for much more than patient monitoring. Cardiac monitors, for example, could be used to measure changes in heart rate and rhythm during relaxation sessions. Likewise, arterial systolic, mean, and diastolic pressures; cardiac output; pulmonary artery pressures; and respirations could be used to measure the effects of such techniques. Inexpensive finger thermistors, used to measure a rise in peripheral temperatures that occurs during relaxation because of vasodilation, can provide the nurse and patient with concrete evidence of the dramatic effects of relaxation (see the Resource List on p. 114).

The box contains a suggested script that can be used (or modified) when guiding patients in music therapy. (Also see Chapter 5 for more details).

SCRIPT FOR MUSIC THERAPY

INTRODUCTION

Discuss the concept of relaxation and music therapy with the patient. If the patient agrees, proceed with the following:
1. Ask patient to select a music tape.
2. Ask patient to urinate, if necessary.
3. Dim lights. Close drapes.
4. Ask patient to remove eyeglasses or contact lenses.
5. Ask patient to lie in supine or semi-Fowler's position. Tell the patient that it sometimes helps to place a small pillow under the knees to relieve lower back strain.

INDUCTION

Give the patient the following instructions:
1. The purpose of the session is to relax in a wakeful state and to have a quiet experience listening to music.
2. First I will guide you in a few exercises to relax.
3. Then I will guide you in how to listen to music (of your choice).
4. Then try to relax for 20 minutes as you listen to the music.
5. Now close your eyes (if you wish).
6. Find a comfortable position:
   a. Hands at side of chest or on body or whatever is most comfortable
   b. Legs uncrossed
7. At any time you may change positions, scratch, or swallow.
8. There may be noises around, but these will not be important if you concentrate on my voice.
9. Now think of relaxation:
   a. Relax the body.
   b. Relax the mind.
   c. Allow yourself to let go of tension.
   d. Allow relaxation to happen.
   e. Do not strain, force it, or resist it.
10. I am going to guide you in relaxing.
11. To begin relaxing, take in three long, deep breaths. Breathe gently with your abdomen. This is the kind of relaxed breathing we do every night as we fall asleep. As you breathe in, let your stomach blow up like a balloon. As you exhale, let your stomach gently fall back to your spine.
12. Feel the relaxation coming over your body.
13. As you begin to relax, focus your attention on the top of your head. Let the muscles go, relax them, feel the relaxation moving in.
14. Let the relaxation flow to your forehead, temples, eyebrows, eyelids, eyes. Let go of the muscles; feel the relaxation and warmth.
15. Let the relaxation flow to your cheeks, lips, chin, and jaw:
   a. Let your jaw drop down a little.
   b. Let your lips part a little.
   c. Let your tongue relax; just let it puddle in your mouth.
16. Relax these muscles; your whole face feels heavy, warm, and relaxed.
17. Let the relaxation flow down your throat, neck, shoulders, upper arms, elbows, lower arms, fingers, and fingertips.
   a. Let these muscles hang heavy, loose, limp, and relaxed.
   b. Notice how heavy and warm both arms feel; these are signs of relaxation. You might even experience a slight tingling, which is also a sign of relaxation.

INDUCTION—cont'd

18. Focus your attention on your back, spine, waist, and buttocks.
    a. Smooth out these muscles, and let go of any tension.
    b. Feel the relaxation and heaviness and warmth. Allow yourself to feel the bed supporting you. Just let go.
19. Let the relaxation flow around to the sides of your chest, abdomen and waist; relax the muscles, and feel the relaxation, warmth, and heaviness.
20. Concentrate on your thighs, knees, calves, ankles, feet, and toes; feel how heavy your legs are, how comfortably heavy, warm, and relaxed.
21. Feel the relaxation from the top of your head to your toes.
    a. Be relaxed, peacefully calm.
    b. Be very quiet, silent, and relaxed.
22. Feel this relaxation flowing through your body. If there are any places in your body that are still tense, move them a little bit, and relax them.

MUSIC TAPES

1. Now, as you continue to relax, I will turn on the music that you have chosen.
2. Listen to the music.
    a. If distracting thoughts occur, let them go and come back to concentrating on the music.
    b. Tell yourself that you would like to go wherever the music takes you.
    c. Allow yourself to follow the music. Let the music suggest to you what to think and what to feel.
    d. Don't try to analyze the music.
    e. Allow the music to relax you even more than you are now.
3. The music will play for 20 minutes, and I will leave the room.
4. I will quietly come back into the room before the music is over.
5. When the music is over, I will guide you in counting from 5 to 1. You will come back into the room easily and quietly. You will feel very relaxed, calm, and peaceful.
6. Now continue to relax your body and your mind; let the music help you.

NURSING DIAGNOSIS 3   **High risk for infective or phlebotic vascular complications related to prolonged intravenous therapy (exchanging pattern)**

PATIENT OUTCOMES	NURSING PRESCRIPTIONS	EVALUATION
Patient will not experience complications from prolonged intravenous therapy as evidenced by thrombophlebitis, cellulitis, and occult intravenous site infection.	Follow standards of practice regarding insertion and care of intravenous lines and prevention of complications. Assess patient for thrombophlebitis, cellulitis, and occult intravenous site infection (erythematous skin over an indurated or tender vein, as well as pus, inflammation, swelling, heat, or bleeding near the insertion site or over the vein).	Patient did not experience complications related to intravenous therapy.
If complications occur, patient will respond to appropriate therapy.	If complications occur, administer appropriate therapy as necessary (removal of the intravenous catheter, blood culture, range of motion (ROM) exercises, warm soaks or heating pad, antipyretics, analgesics, or antimicrobial agents).	

Plan and intervention for preventing infective or phlebotic vascular complications

When administering prolonged intravenous therapy to a patient with an active infection, extreme caution and vigilance are necessary.[58,63,74,95] Intravenous catheters and solutions may cause additional infection and septicemia. Specially trained intravenous teams are recommended to insert, maintain, and replace intravenous needles or cannulas to reduce the complications associated with intravenous therapy.[95] Aseptic technique must be carefully followed. When preparing for the venipuncture or administering intravenous solutions or medications, nurses must thoroughly wash their hands. The patient's skin should be shaved and prepared for the venipuncture by liberally applying tincture of iodine (i.e., 2% iodine in a 70% alcohol solution). After at least 30 seconds of drying, the iodine solution is washed off with 70% isopropyl alcohol. The solutions are applied to the skin with friction, scrubbing from the center of the venipuncture site to the periphery.

When possible, steel (scalp vein) needles should be inserted to help reduce the chance of catheter-related phlebitis and infection. Leg veins should not be used because of the high incidence of catheter-related complications. Traumatic catheter insertions can contribute to the incidence of phlebitis, so they should be charted and the patient observed carefully. Because a needle or catheter that is mobile and allowed to move to-and-fro in the vein can introduce bacteria into the circulation, it must be taped securely to the skin. A topical polyantibiotic ointment and sterile dressing should be applied. The dressing and not the tape should cover the venipuncture site. The use of transparent dressings may be useful so that the site can be inspected without removing the dressing.[63] The needle size, time, date, and the venipuncture site is recorded on the patient's chart or care plan.

Before administering intravenous fluids, all bags or bottles are examined for turbidity or precipitates. Plastic intravenous bags are gently squeezed to check for leaks, and intravenous bottles are examined for cracks. An intravenous bottle that does not have a vacuum when opened should not be used. Infusion pumps should be used when administering a continuous 24-hour antimicrobial solution. Although a terminal membrane filter does not reduce intravenous related infection, one should be used when administering intravenous fluids to block particulate matter.[95]

Single-use or single-dose vials admixtures are used when possible.[95] Before medications are added, the injection port is disinfected. All intravenous solutions should be used as soon as possible after opening. Admixed intravenous fluids that are not used immediately should be refrigerated. Each new intravenous solution is labeled with the patient's name, date of opening, and the name, date, and dosage of additives, the expiration date, and the name of the person mixing the solution.

An accurate intravenous fluid therapy record should be maintained on the patient's chart, and the time and date that each bag or bottle of fluid was started and discontinued, the type of fluid and the dosage of additives, the rate of administration, and the amount of medication and fluid received also is included.

All intravenous solutions are replaced every 24 hours, and the intravenous tubing, extension sets, and administration sets are replaced every 24 hours and when the intravenous solution is changed. All tubing must be changed when the catheter is replaced. All tubings should be changed after the administration of blood, blood products, or lipid emulsions.[95] The new tubing is labeled with the date and time.

The insertion site should be palpated through the intact dressing every 24 hours. If the patient has unexplained fever, pain, or tenderness, the dressing should be removed to inspect for complications such as phlebitis or infection.

Needles or catheters are replaced every 48 to 72 hours; sites should be alternated. If peripheral needles or cannulas remain in place for a longer period of time, the wound is inspected and cleansed with iodine and alcohol, and the sterile dressing is changed after the first 48 to 72 hours. The site should be inspected, antibiotic ointment reapplied, and a new sterile dressing applied every 24 hours thereafter.

To avoid intravenous complications, the intravenous line should not be flushed or irrigated. Blood samples should be withdrawn from the tubing only when it is known that the tubing will be discontinued immediately or in cases of emergencies. At the first sign of infection or phlebitis, a new needle or catheter is inserted, and the old one is removed. This information is charted, and the patient is assessed carefully for additional potential catheter-related complications (e.g., fever, systemic infection, or septicemia).

If an infection related to a plastic catheter is suspected, the tip of the catheter is cultured by thoroughly cleansing the venipuncture site with alcohol and allowing the alcohol to dry. Then the catheter is removed aseptically without touching the skin, the tip of the catheter is clipped off with sterile scissors, and it is placed in a blood culture tube for analysis. If pus or suspicious drainage is observed around the venipuncture site, it is reported to the physician, and it is gram stained and cultured.

If contamination of the intravenous solution is suspected, the solution is discontinued immediately. The bottle should be saved, the solution cultured, and the local health officials, the Center for Disease Control, and the Food and Drug Administration notified.

Increasing patient comfort during intravenous therapy

The patient is instructed about the intravenous routine, the schedule for changing the venipuncture site, and signs and symptoms to report including leakage, heat, pain, or discomfort around the venipuncture site.

When possible, the nurse explores with the physician the feasibility of using a heparin lock to provide periods of activity and rest that are free from intravenous equipment. Active and passive ROM-exercises of the involved extremity should be done on a regular basis. If possible, arms are alternated when changing venipuncture sites. Occasionally the patient may complain of pain with the infusion, which can be corrected by further diluting the medication or administering the infusion more slowly.

If intravenous-related complications occur, appropriate therapy is instituted, depending on the nature and severity of the problem. Warm soaks or a heating pad are applied to the extremity when phlebitis is suspected (after removal of the intravenous line). Elevating the extremity and administering antipyretics, analgesics, or other appropriate antimicrobial medications may be necessary.

NURSING DIAGNOSIS 4   **High risk for complications of impaired physical mobility related to prolonged intravenous therapy and restricted activities (moving pattern)**

PATIENT OUTCOMES	NURSING PRESCRIPTIONS	EVALUATION
Patient will verbalize an understanding of reasons for reduction in activities and bed rest, components of a prolonged progressive activity program, and parameters used to evaluate the response to activity.	Teach patient about the reasons for reduction in activities and bed rest, components of a prolonged progressive activity program, and parameters used to evaluate the response to activity.	Patient verbalized an understanding of reasons for reduction in activities and bed rest, components of a prolonged progressive activity program, and parameters used to evaluate the response to activity.
Patient will participate in activities, keeping in mind the limitations imposed by prolonged intravenous therapy and restricted activities.	Assist the patient to participate in activities of daily living.	Patient participated in activities, keeping in mind the limitations imposed by prolonged intravenous therapy and restricted activities.
Patient will not experience the following complications related to immobility:	Prevent the complications related to immobility:	Patient did not experience complications related to immobility.
Patient will not exhibit respiratory complications.	Prevent respiratory complications by having the patient cough and breathe deeply.	
Patient will not exhibit phlebitis, joint immobility, or loss of muscle tone.	Prevent phlebitis, joint immobility, and loss of muscle tone by using antiembolic stocking and assisting patient to turn independently in bed, perform range of motion exercises, and progress to sitting in a chair, walking in hall, and performing activities with intravenous equipment.	
Patient will not exhibit urinary retention or constipation.	Prevent urinary retention or constipation by encouraging high intake of fluids and increased dietary fiber and roughage.	
Patient will not exhibit nutritional problems.	Prevent nutritional problems by assisting patient to choose a diet high in nutritional value with preferred foods and monitoring actual calorie and food intake.	

Continued.

NURSING DIAGNOSIS 4   **High risk for complications of impaired physical mobility related to prolonged intravenous therapy and restricted activities (moving pattern)—cont'd**

PATIENT OUTCOMES	NURSING PRESCRIPTIONS	EVALUATION
Patient will not verbalize feelings of boredom, role dependency, anxiety, or depression.	Prevent verbalized feelings of boredom, role dependency, anxiety, or depression by guiding the patient in relaxation exercises and providing diversional activities.	
Patient will experience no complications related to progressive activity such as a significant rise or fall in blood pressure, significant rise in pulse or respiratory rate, dysrhythmias, or complaints of weakness, fatigue, dizziness, or angina pectoris.	Assess response to progressive activities in terms of rise or fall in blood pressure, rise in pulse or respiratory rate, dysrhythmias, and complaints of weakness, fatigue, dizziness, or angina pectoris.	Patient did not experience complications related to progressive activity.

Plan and intervention for preventing complications of impaired physical mobility

The nurse must be aware of the potential physiologic hazards of prolonged bed rest, such as decreased stimulus for deep breathing, stasis of respiratory secretions, phlebitis, joint immobility, loss of muscle tone, urinary retention, constipation, and anorexia.[69] Immobility also can produce psychologic hazards, such as feelings of boredom, role dependency, anxiety, depression.

To promote endocardial healing, patients should rest in bed and be taught the reasons for bed rest and principles of energy conservation. The nurse demonstrates and assists the patient in moving and turning in bed with the restrictions imposed by the intravenous equipment. Clear instructions are given about the proper use, movement, and restrictions of the extremity receiving the intravenous solution. If the patient is receiving intermittent antimicrobial therapy, a heparin lock should be used if possible. Initially, the nurse performs passive ROM exercises for the patient. When appropriate, the nurse consults the physical therapist to begin active ROM exercises with the patient. The nurse assists the patient to dangle the feet at the bedside, use the bedside commode, sit in a chair, and walk in the halls. Based on the condition and progress, the nurse encourages independence by teaching patients to transfer the intravenous bottle to a portable stand and to walk without assistance.

Patients must thoroughly understand the many components of a progressive activity program and the ways to evaluate their own response to activity. Patients are taught that activities must be reduced or stopped when the signs of weakness, fatigue, increased respiratory or pulse rates, dyspnea, palpitations, dizziness, or chest pain occur. The nurse should evaluate the patient's response to activity (e.g., blood pressure, ECG changes, ectopy, heart and respiratory rates, shortness of breath, diaphoresis, cyanosis, complaints of weakness, fatigue, angina pectoris, or dizziness).

Patients should be given a restrictive yet progressive activity schedule as their condition improves. A conservative or modified in-hospital acute myocardial infarction activity program can be used as a guideline for the staff. Also patients are given a copy of this program to provide concrete evidence of their progress.

To prevent complications of impaired physical mobility, patients are taught to cough and breathe deeply, drink plenty of fluids (if not contraindicated by heart failure), and eat foods high in fiber and roughage. Patients should understand the importance of nutrition in the healing process. Good skin care, body repositioning, and stool softeners are indicated.

To prevent the psychologic complications associated with immobility and prolonged hospitalization, the nurse explores relaxation techniques with patients. Music therapy, meditation, imagery, and other relaxation techniques can be particularly beneficial for patients undergoing prolonged bed rest (see Nursing Diagnosis 2). An occupational therapist should be consulted to explore various types of diversional activities that may be of interest to patients.

NURSING
DIAGNOSIS 5   **High risk for valvular reinfection related to insufficient knowledge about illness and future prophylactic care (exchanging pattern)**

PATIENT OUTCOMES	NURSING PRESCRIPTIONS	EVALUATION
Patient will verbalize, discuss, or demonstrate:	Teach patient about:	Patient verbalized, discussed, or demonstrated:
Normal function of the heart, valves, and circulation	Normal function of the heart, valves, and circulation	Normal function of the heart, valves, and circulation
Definition of endocarditis	Definition of endocarditis	Definition of endocarditis
Name and location of the valve infected	Name and location of the valve infected	Name and location of the valve infected
Valvular changes that occur with endocarditis	Valvular changes that occur with endocarditis	Valvular changes that occur with endocarditis
Reasons for antimicrobial medications	Reasons for antimicrobial medications	Reasons for antimicrobial medications
Signs and symptoms of endocarditis	Signs and symptoms of endocarditis	Signs and symptoms of endocarditis
Ways to take temperature and the need for daily temperature taking and recording for 1 month after discharge	Ways to take the temperature and how to record daily temperatures for 1 month after discharge	Ways to take temperature and the need for daily temperature taking and recording for 1 month after discharge
Inpatient and outpatient progressive activity schedule (see Nursing Diagnosis 4)	Progressive activity schedule that should be followed in the hospital and after discharge (see Nursing Diagnosis 4)	Inpatient and outpatient progressive activity schedule
Reasons for no strenuous work, sports, or activities for 1 month after discharge	Reasons for no strenuous work, sports, or activities for 1 month after discharge to promote endocardial healing	Reasons for no strenuous work, sports, or activities for 1 month after discharge
Possible portals of entry for the infecting organism	Possible portals of entry for the infecting organism	Possible portals of entry for the infecting organism
Techniques of good oral hygiene and the need for regular dental checkups	Techniques of good oral hygiene, devices that cause gum trauma, and the importance of regular dental checkups	Techniques of good oral hygiene and the need for regular dental checkups
Need for prophylactic antibiotics before and after dental or surgical procedures and manipulations	Importance of prophylactic antibiotics before and after dental or surgical procedures and manipulations and the necessity of informing the dentist or physician about the history of endocarditis	Need for prophylactic antibiotics before and after dental or surgical procedures and manipulations
For women of childbearing age who are at high risk, methods of birth control and antibiotic prophylaxis during labor and delivery	For women of childbearing age, hazards of birth control pills and intrauterine devices and the importance of antibiotic prophylaxis during labor and delivery	For women of childbearing age who are at high risk, methods of birth control and antibiotic prophylaxis during pregnancy
For patients who are abusers of intravenous drugs, high incidence of endocarditis and the need to enroll in a drug treatment program	For patients who are abusers of intravenous drugs, high incidence of endocarditis and the need to enroll in a drug treatment program	For patients who are abusers of intravenous drugs, high incidence of endocarditis and the need to enroll in a drug treatment program

Continued.

NURSING DIAGNOSIS 5 — **High risk for valvular reinfection related to insufficient knowledge about illness and future prophylactic care (exchanging pattern)—cont'd**

PATIENT OUTCOMES	NURSING PRESCRIPTIONS	EVALUATION
Reasons that stress reduction and relaxation techniques should be practiced at home after discharge	Reasons that stress reduction and relaxation techniques should be practiced at home after discharge	Reasons that stress reduction and relaxation techniques should be practiced at home after discharge
Appropriate knowledge and techniques of home intravenous therapy (see p. 410)	Appropriate information and techniques of home intravenous therapy (see p. 410)	Appropriate knowledge and techniques of home intravenous therapy (see p. 410)
Places where and times when to return for medical follow-up and blood testing appointments and the names and telephone numbers of the nurse and physician	Places where and times when to return for medical follow-up and blood testing appointments and the names and telephone numbers of the nurse and physician	Places where and times when to return for medical follow-up and blood testing appointments and the names and telephone numbers of the nurse and physician

Plan and intervention for preventing valvular reinfection

When the patient's condition permits and readiness to learn is demonstrated, a comprehensive teaching program should be started with patients and families. Because all patients with a history of endocarditis are at high risk for valvular reinfection, patients must understand the illness and future prophylactic care.[44,108] Other patients who should be taught about endocarditis and prophylaxis include those with prosthetic heart valves or rheumatic, degenerative, or congenital heart disease that has created valvular deformities or other cardiac defects.

The functions of the heart, heart valves, circulation, and a definition of endocarditis are discussed first using terminology that patients can understand easily. The nurse describes the valve affected by using a heart model and drawings.

Patients should understand the pathophysiologic changes that occur with endocarditis and the rationale and need for a prolonged course of intravenous antimicrobial therapy. The signs and symptoms of endocarditis, such as chills, fever, fatigue, anorexia, weight loss, and diaphoresis, are explained. Patients should understand and demonstrate how to take their temperatures. They are instructed to take it at the same time each day for a month, record it on a calendar, and report elevations to the physician. If a fever is suspected any time after the first month of discharge, the patient should immediately take the temperature and report abnormalities, signs, or symptoms of reinfection to the physician.[104]

Before discharge, the nurse provides patients with a progressive activity program that can be followed at home (see Nursing Diagnosis 4). To promote healing of the endocardium, 1 month of convalescence at home with restriction of strenuous activities, work, and competitive sports is recommended. The nurse explains the possible portals of entry for a future infecting organism. These include sites of dental problems, skin lesions, sites of surgical procedures, sites of invasive tests or manipulation, and infections.

The nurse also discusses good oral hygiene with patients. They should be taught to brush their teeth twice a day with a soft-bristled toothbrush. Trauma to the gums should be avoided by gentle but firm brushing. Any device that causes gum trauma or bleeding, such as dental floss, toothpicks, or a Water Pik, should be avoided. Flossing the teeth, however, promotes good oral hygiene and prevents gum disease, making the recommendation for this precaution somewhat controversial.[56] Instruct patients to visit the dentist routinely for checkups every 6 months to a year. Patients with dentures also require regular dental examinations.

Patients must be aware that antimicrobial medications must be taken prophylactically when undergoing invasive dental manipulations and other procedures listed on p. 399.[1,36,56] Antibiotics usually are given just before the procedure and are usually given after many procedures. Although dentists and physicians should be aware that patients who are susceptible to endocarditis require antimicrobial medications when invasive tests or manipulations are performed, patients should understand that it is their responsibility to inform the dentist and physician about their history of endocarditis or valvular heart disease.

Patients are encouraged to be assertive with physicians and dentists when inquiring about their plan for prophylactic antibiotics for invasive procedures and about whether the antibiotic prophylaxis regimen is in compliance with the American Heart Association's (AHA) guidelines. The AHA publication, *Prevention of Bacterial Endocarditis,*[1] should be given to patients before discharge. This publication describes types of patients that are susceptible to endocarditis, the dental and medical procedures and manipulations that could cause bacteremia, and the recommended dosage for prophylactic antibiotic medications. Patients should understand and be able to discuss this information.

Unfortunately, physician and dentist compliance to the AHA guidelines for prophylaxis against endocarditis has been found to be low.[16,35,73,88,89] Recent studies have documented that dentists, for example, have been inconsistent in following the selection, dosage, and timing of antibiotic prophylaxis as recommended by the AHA.[73,88,89] In another study, only 30% of physicians complied with AHA's antibiotic prophylaxis for prosthetic valve patients undergoing diagnostic or operative procedures.[16] The findings from these studies indicate that many physicians and dentists may not understand the dangers of bacteremia associated with invasive procedures in high-risk patients and the need for appropriate antibiotic prophylaxis. Another factor influencing compliance may be the impracticality of administering prophylactic antibiotics intravenously in the physician's or dentist's office.[6,35] The AHA is currently formulating new guidelines to address this problem, which will probably recommend the use of oral prophylactic antibiotics in the future.

Patients who are currently taking prophylactic antibiotics to prevent recurrences of acute rheumatic fever must understand that the prophylactic regimen for rheumatic fever is different from and inadequate to prevent endocarditis.[1] Thus additional antibiotics are necessary for such patients when they undergo surgery or other invasive procedures (see Chapter 12).

The female endocarditis patient should be told that birth control pills may increase embolic phenomena and are not recommended, particularly if high-dose estrogens are used. Moreover, intrauterine devices may provide a possible portal of entry for the infecting organism. Other forms of birth control should be explored with the patient. The pregnant patient who is at high risk should know that antimicrobial prophylaxis is needed during labor, caesarean delivery, therapeutic abortions, or sterilization procedures.

The incidence of recurrent endocarditis is high in abusers of intravenous drugs.[3] For such patients, the many dangers of drug addiction and their susceptibility of recurrent endocarditis must be completely explained. Every attempt must be made to have the patient enroll in a drug rehabilitation program.

To ensure sterile blood cultures, patients generally have blood cultures drawn every 2 weeks for 6 weeks after antimicrobial medications have been discontinued. Patients should know the importance of this type of follow-up activity and where and when to report for blood tests. Patients are instructed that stress reduction and relaxation also may enhance the healing process and are encouraged to continue practicing relaxation techniques at home.

If patients will continue intravenous therapy at home, they should be able to demonstrate the knowledge and appropriate techniques of home intravenous therapy before discharge (see p. 410). They also should receive the names and telephone numbers of the physician, nurse, and clinic and be instructed to call if they have questions or problems after returning home.

KEY CONCEPT REVIEW

1. Which of the following microorganisms is responsible for most cases of acute endocarditis?
   a. *Streptococcus viridans*
   b. *Staphylococcus aureus*
   c. *Escherichia coli*
   d. *Candida* organisms
2. The pathogenesis of acute endocarditis is primarily related to the presence of:
   a. Preexisting cardiac defects
   b. A microorganism of low virulence in the circulation
   c. A microorganism of high virulence in the circulation
   d. An abnormal hydrodynamic situation between cardiac chambers
3. All the following patients are at high risk for developing infective endocarditis except:

   a. Patients with prosthetic heart valves
   b. Patients with angina pectoris
   c. Patients who are abusers of parenteral drugs
   d. Patients who are immunosuppressed
4. Infective endocarditis can produce which of the following cardiovascular manifestations?
   a. New heart murmurs
   b. Bundle branch blocks
   c. Clubbing of nailbeds
   d. All the above
5. The most common complication of infective endocarditis is:
   a. Congestive heart failure
   b. Pericarditis
   c. Embolic phenomena
   d. Neuropsychiatric manifestations
6. The most common embolic complications occur in the:

a. Spleen
b. Lungs
c. Coronary arteries
d. Brain

7. All the following are related to immunologic derangements *except*:
   a. Petechiae
   b. Splinter hemorrhages
   c. Albuminuria
   d. Arthralgias

8. The most common cause of negative blood cultures in a patient with infective endocarditis is:
   a. Right-sided endocarditis
   b. Poor bacteriologic technique
   c. Presence of satellite streptococci in the blood
   d. The prior administration of antimicrobial medications

9. The treatment of a patient with *Streptococcus viridans* endocarditis includes all the following except:
   a. Restricted activities
   b. Penicillin
   c. Steroids
   d. Streptomycin

10. The most important determinant in recommending surgery for the infective endocarditis patient is:
    a. Deterioration of hemodynamic status
    b. Whether the patient still has an active infection
    c. The administration of antibiotics for at least 72 hours before surgery
    d. The severity of the embolic phenomena

11. Which of the following is true regarding teaching the acutely ill endocarditis patient?
    a. These patients generally cannot be taught because they are too ill.
    b. The process rather than the product of teaching should be evaluated with such patients.
    c. The success of teaching should be based on the outcomes of the teaching-learning experience with such patients.
    d. Both *a* and *c* are correct.

12. Before infective endocarditis patients are sent home, they must be instructed about all the following *except*:
    a. The signs and symptoms of endocarditis
    b. The need for bed rest at home
    c. Ways to take their temperature
    d. The need for prophylactic antimicrobial agents before any invasive test or procedure

ANSWERS

1. b	3. b	5. a	7. c	9. c	11. b
2. c	4. d	6. d	8. d	10. a	12. b

REFERENCES

1. American Heart Association: Prevention of bacterial endocarditis (pamphlet), Dallas, 1985, American Heart Association.
2. Aslamaci S, Dimitri WR, and Williams BT: Operative considerations in active native valve infective endocarditis, J Cardiovasc Surg 30:328, 1989.
3. Baddour LM: Twelve-year review of recurrent native-valve infective endocarditis: a disease of the modern antibiotic era, Rev Infect Dis 10:1163, 1988.
4. Barry J and Gump DW: Endocarditis: an overview, Heart Lung 11:138, 1982.
5. Bayer AS: Staphylococcal bacteremia: distinguishing endocarditis, Am Fam Physician 19:147, 1979.
6. Bayer AS: New concepts in the pathogenesis and modalities of the chemoprophylaxis of native valve endocarditis, Chest 96:893, 1989.
7. Bayer AS and Theofilopoulos AN: Immunopathogenetic aspects of infective endocarditis, Chest 97:204, 1990.
8. Bayer AS and others: Circulating immune complexes in infective endocarditis, N Engl J Med 295:1500, 1976.
9. Becker RM, Frishman W, and Frater RWM: Surgery for mitral valve endocarditis, Chest 75:314, 1979.
10. Bisno AL and others: Antimicrobial treatment of infective endocarditis due to viridans streptococci, enterococci, and staphylococci, JAMA 261:1471, 1989.
11. Blumsohn D: Clubbing of the fingers, with special reference to Schamroth's diagnostic method, Heart Lung 10:1069, 1981.
12. Bonny H: Sound spaces: music rx is proven in the ICU, ICM West Newsletter, 2:2, 1982.
13. Bonny H and Pahnke WN: The use of music in psychedelic psychotherapy, J Music Ther 9:64, 1972.
14. Bonny H and Savary L: Music and your mind, New York, 1978, Harper & Row, Publishers, Inc.
15. Bornstein DL: Bacterial endocarditis. In Conn HL and Horwitz O, editors: Cardiac and vascular diseases, Philadelphia, 1971, Lea & Febiger.
16. Brooks RG, Notariom F, and McCabe RE: Hospital survey of antimicrobial prophylaxis to prevent endocarditis in patients with prosthetic heart valves, Am J Med 84:617, 1988.
17. Bryan CS and others: Endocarditis related to transvenous pacemakers: syndromes and surgical implications, J Thorac Cardiovasc Surg 75:758, 1978.
18. Cabane J and others: Fate of circulating immune complexes in infective endocarditis, Am J Med 66:277, 1979.
19. Cassey JI and Miller MH: Infective endocarditis. II. Current therapy, Am Heart J 96:263, 1978.
20. Chan Pl, Ogilby JD, and Segal B: Tricuspid valve endocarditis, Am Heart J 117:1140, 1989.
21. Christopherson DJ and Sivarajan Froelicher ES: Infective endocarditis. In Underhill SL and others, editors: Cardiac nursing, ed 2, Philadelphia, 1989, JB Lippincott Co.
22. Clemens JD and others: A controlled evaluation of the risk of bacterial endocarditis in persons with mitral valve prolapse, N Engl J Med 307:776, 1982.
23. Cohen PS, Maguire JH, and Weinstein L: Infective endocarditis caused by gram-negative bacteria: a review of the literature, 1945-1977, Prog Cardiovasc Dis 22:205, 1980.
24. Cohle SD and others: Unexpected death as a result of infective endocarditis, J Forensic Sci 34:1374, 1989.
25. Corby D, Schad RF, and Fudge JP: Intravenous antibiotic therapy: hospital to home, Nurs Manage 17:52, 1986.
26. Crespo J: Dialysis-related infections, Heart Lung 11:111, 1982.
27. DaLuz PL: Acute infection of the heart, Heart Lung 2:422, 1973.

28. Danchin N and others: Mitral valve prolapse as a risk factor for infective endocarditis, Lancet 1:743, 1989.

29. Davis C and Cunningham SG: The physiologic responses of patients in the coronary care unit to selected music, Heart Lung 14:291, 1985.

30. Dossey BM, Guzzetta CE, and Kenner CV: Critical care nursing: body-mind-spirit, ed 3, Philadelphia, 1992, JB Lippincott Co.

31. Ehrie M and others: Endocarditis with the indwelling balloon-tipped pulmonary artery catheter in burn patients, J Trauma 18:664, 1978.

32. Everett ED: Infective endocarditis, Mo Med 75:167, 1978.

33. Evora PR and others: Surgical excision of the vegetation as treatment of tricuspid valve endocarditis, Cardiology 75:287, 1988.

34. Fenwick PB, Donaldson S, and Gillis L: Metabolic and EEG changes during transcendental meditation: an explanation, Biol Psychol 5:101, 1977.

35. Finkelmeier BA and others: Implications of prosthetic valve implantation: an 8-year follow-up of patients with porcine bioprostheses, Heart Lung 18:565, 1989.

36. Fleming HA: Preventing infective endocarditis, Br Med J 1:303, 1978.

37. Fowler NO and Van Der Bel-Kahn JM: Indication for surgical replacement of the mitral valve, Am J Cardiol 44:148, 1979.

38. Frank JD: Mind-body relationships in illness and healing, J Intern Acad Prevent Med 2:50, 1975.

39. Garvey GJ and Neu HC: Infective endocarditis: an evolving disease, Medicine 57:105, 1978.

40. Greene JF, Fitzwater JE, and Clemmer TP: Septic endocarditis and indwelling pulmonary artery catheters, JAMA 233:891, 1975.

41. Gregoratos G and Karliner JS: Infective endocarditis: diagnosis and management, Med Clin North Am 63:173, 1979.

42. Grehl TM, Cohn LH, and Angell WW: Management of *Candida* endocarditis, J Thorac Cardiovasc Surg 63:118, 1972.

43. Guzman L: Nursing management of the parenteral drug abuser with infective endocarditis, Heart Lung 10:289, 1981.

44. Guzzetta CE: Infective endocarditis. In Dossey BM, Guzzetta CE, and Kenner CV: Critical care nursing: body-mind-spirit, ed 3, Philadelphia, 1992, JB Lippincott Co.

45. Guzzetta CE: Relationship between stress and learning. ANS 1:35, 1979.

46. Guzzetta CE: Can critically ill patients be taught. In Billie D, editor: Practical approaches to patient teaching, Boston, 1981, Little, Brown, & Co.

47. Guzzetta CE: Music therapy: hearing the melody of the soul. In Dossey BM and others: Holistic nursing: a handbook for practice, Gaithersburg, MD, 1988, Aspen Publishers, Inc.

48. Guzzetta CE: Effects of relaxation and music therapy on patients in a coronary care unit with presumptive acute myocardial infarction, Heart Lung 18:609, 1989.

49. Halpern S and Savary L: Sound health: the music and sounds that make us whole, San Francisco, 1985, Harper & Row, Publishers, Inc.

50. Hamel PM: Through music to the self, Boston, 1979, Shambhala Publishers, Inc.

51. Heffner JE: Extracardiac manifestations of bacterial endocarditis, West J Med 131:85, 1979.

52. Heimberger TS and Duma RJ: Infections of prosthetic heart valves and cardiac pacemakers, Infect Dis Clin North Am 3:221, 1989.

53. Hollanders G and others: A six-year review of 53 cases of infective endocarditis: clinical, microbiological, and therapeutical features, Acta Cardiol 43:121, 1988.

54. Hughes CF and Noble N: Vegetectomy: an alternative surgical treatment for infective endocarditis of the atrioventricular valves in drug addicts, J Thor Cardiovasc Surg 95:857, 1988.

55. Irvin RG and Sade RM: Endocarditis and musculoskeletal manifestations, Ann Intern Med 88:578, 1978.

56. Kaplan EL and others: Prevention of bacterial endocarditis, American Heart Association Committee Report, Circulation 56:139A, 1977.

57. Karchmer AW and others: Late prosthetic valve endocarditis: clinical features influencing therapy, Am J Med 64:200, 1978.

58. Kaye W: Catheter- and infusion-related sepsis: the nature of the problem and its prevention, Heart Lung 11:221, 1982.

59. Khoo DE, Zebro TJ, and English TA: Bacterial endocarditis in a transplanted heart, Pathol Res Pract 185:445, 1989.

60. Kind AC and others: Intravenous antibiotic therapy at home, Arch Intern Med 139:413, 1979.

61. Kinsley RH, Colsen PR, and Bakst A: Emergency valve replacement for primary, infective endocarditis, S Afr Med J 53:86, 1978.

62. Kluge RM: Infections of prosthetic cardiac valves and arterial grafts, Heart Lung 11:146, 1982.

63. Lenox AC: IV therapy: reducing the risk of infection, Nurs 90 March 1990, p 60.

64. Marrie TJ: Infective endocarditis: a serious and changing disease, Crit Care Nurs 7:31, 1987.

65. Maschak BJ: Patient education and prevention of endocarditis, Nurs Clin North Am 11:319, 1976.

66. Mathewson MA: Prolapsed mitral valve syndrome, Am J Nurs 80:1431, 1980.

67. May JM and others: *S. aureus* endocarditis: a review and plea for early surgery, Virol Med 106:829, 1979.

68. McAnulty JH and Rahimtoola SH: Surgery for infective endocarditis, JAMA 242:77, 1979.

69. McFarland GK and McFarlane EA: Nursing diagnosis and intervention, St Louis, 1989, The CV Mosby Co.

70. Miller MH and Cassey JI: Infective endocarditis: new diagnostic techniques, Am Heart J 96:123, 1978.

71. Mills SA: Surgical management of infective endocarditis, Ann Surg 195:367, 1982.

72. Mintz GS and others: Survival of patients with aortic valve endocarditis: the prognostic implications of the echocardiogram, Arch Intern Med 139:862, 1979.

73. Nelson CL and Van Blaricum CS: Physician and dentist compliance with American Heart Association guidelines for prevention of bacterial endocarditis, J Am Dent Assoc 118:169, 1989.

74. Oakley C: Use of antibiotics, Br Med J 2:489, 1978.

75. Osler W: Malignant endocarditis, Lancet 1:415, 1885.

76. Pace NL and Horton WL: Indwelling pulmonary, catheters: the relationship to aseptic thrombotic endocardial vegetations, JAMA 233:893, 1975.

77. Pankey GA: The prevention and treatment of bacterial endocarditis, Am Heart J 98:102, 1979.

78. Parrott JC and others: The surgical management of bacterial endocarditis: a review, Ann Surg 183:289, 1976.

79. Pesanti EL and Smith JM: Infective endocarditis with negative blood cultures, Am J Med 66:43, 1979.

80. Phair JP and Clarke J: Immunology of infective endocarditis, Prog Cardiovasc Dis 22:137, 1979.

81. Rapaport E: Editorial: the changing roles of surgery in the management of infective endocarditis, Circulation 58:598, 1978.

82. Reagan TJ: Cerebral ischemia in nonbacterial thrombotic endocarditis, Curr Con Cerebrovasc Dis 10:13, 1975.

83. Resnick L and Cohen L: Antibiotic treatment of penicillin-sensitive streptococcal endocarditis, JAMA 241:1826, 1979.

84. Richardson JV and others: Treatment of infective endocarditis: a 10-year comparative analysis, Circulation 58:589, 1978.

85. Roberts KB and Sidlak MJ: Satellite streptococci: a major cause of "negative" blood cultures in bacterial endocarditis, JAMA 241:2293, 1979.

86. Roberts NK, Child JS, and Cabeen WR: Infective endocarditis and the cardiac conducting system, West J Med 129:254, 1978.

87. Rodbard S: Blood velocity and endocarditis, Circulation 27:18, 1963.

88. Sadowsky D and Kunzel C: Recommendations for prevention of bacterial endocarditis: compliance by dental general practitioners, Circulation 77:1316, 1988.

89. Sadowsky D and Kunzel C: Usual and customary practice versus the recommendations of experts: clinician noncompliance in the prevention of bacterial endocarditis, J Am Dent Assoc 118:175, 1989.

90. Sande MA and others: Sustained bacteremia in patients with prosthetic cardiac valves, N Engl J Med 286:1067, 1972.

91. Sasaki TM and others: The relationship of central venous and pulmonary artery catheter position to acute right-sided endocarditis in severe thermal injury, J Trauma 19:740, 1979.

92. Schulberg C: The music therapy sourcebook, New York, 1981, Human Sciences Press, Inc.

93. Scrima DA: Infective endocarditis: nursing considerations, Crit Care Nurs 7:47, 1987.

94. Scully R, Galdabini JJ, and McNeely BU: Weekly clinicopathological exercises, N Engl J Med 293:247, 1975.

95. Simmons BP: CDC guidelines for the prevention and control of nosocomial infections: guideline for prevention of intravascular infections, Am J Infect Con 11:183, 1983.

96. Spaccavento LJ and Hawley HB: Infections associated with intra-arterial lines, Heart Lung 11:118, 1982.

97. Stiver HG and others: Intravenous antibiotic therapy at home, Ann Intern Med 89:690, 1978.

98. Stulz P and others: Emergency valve replacement for active infective endocarditis, J Cardiovasc Surg 30:20, 1989.

99. Terpenning MS, Buggy BP, and Kauffman CA: Hospital acquired infective endocarditis, Arch Intern Med 148:1601, 1988.

100. Ward C, Naik DR, and Johnstone MC: Tricuspid endocarditis complicating pacemaker implantation demonstrated by echocardiography, Br J Radiol 52:501, 1979.

101. Watanakunakorn D: Infective endocarditis as a result of medical progress, Am J Med 64:917, 1978.

102. Weinstein L and Schlesinger JJ: Pathoanatomic, pathophysiologic and clinical correlations in endocarditis. I. N Engl J Med 291:832, 1974.

103. Weinstein L and Schlesinger JJ: Pathoanatomic, pathophysiologic and clinical correlations in endocarditis. II. N Engl Med 291:1122, 1974.

104. Welton DE and others: Recurrent infective endocarditis: analysis of predisposing factors and clinical features, Am J Med 66:932, 1979.

105. Williams RC: Subacute bacterial endocarditis as an immune disease, Hosp Pract 6:111, 1971.

106. Wilson WR and others: Valve replacement in patients with active infective endocarditis, Circulation 58:585, 1978.

107. Wilson WR and others: Cardiac valve replacement in congestive heart failure due to infective endocarditis, Mayo Clin Proc 54:223, 1979.

108. Wingate S: Rehabilitation of the patient with valvular heart disease, J Cardiovasc Nurs 1:52, 1987.

109. Yee ES and Khonsari S: Right-sided infective endocarditis: valvuloplasty, valvectomy or replacment, J Cardiovasc Surg 30:744, 1989.

110. Yee ES and Ullyot DJ: Reparative approach for right-sided endocarditis: operative consideration and results of valvuloplasty, J Thorac Cardiovasc Surg 96:133, 1988.

111. Zimmerman LM, Pierson MA and Marker J: Effects of music on patient anxiety on coronary care units, Heart Lung 17:560, 1988.

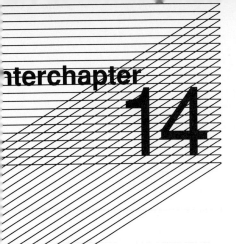

The Meaning of Life and Death

Nothing prepares us completely for our own death or the death of a loved one. In spite of the fact that we will all die, most people have become so accustomed to their bodies that death is often feared or viewed as a tragedy.

If we can learn to accept the reality of our dying, then dying in peace is possible. Our life experiences have no meaning without the complementary role of death. When we stop trying to deny death and admit that the physical body will die, we then are free to recognize that the human spirit is immortal and never dies.[1]

Much emphasis in modern culture is placed on extending life. Medicine's highest duty has become to preserve life at all costs, often despite pain and suffering. Modern medical science can relieve much pain and suffering, but it is limited because there is a part of living where it has no effect. Medicine keeps changing how it treats certain diseases and when it does this it also effects the pattern of dying. When we choose to prolong life we deny death. One's soul may literally die in agony before the physical body dies.

The most common sense of time is that it is the same for everybody—that real time flows and is divisible into past, present, and future. Many hold the notion that life is lived in a linear sequence as a series of episodic events from birth to death, but it has been proven that time is very different from the classical Newtonian model.

When we think of these events as occurring in a linear fashion, we are dependent on an external reality. But the only way we can experience birth, health, illness, and death is by our senses, by our own internal experience. It is our meaning in life that determines our sense of time.[2]

When reflecting on death, what words come to your mind? For most the words are desperate, panic, final, always, ending, or forever. These words create a constricted sense of time, and fear and urgency are inflicted on our experiences. Our experience of time is bound to our senses; it is part of us, not "out there."

An outmoded sense of time is what creates the fears surrounding death. Modern physics can help us to reshape our view of time by proving that time does not flow, that time is now. The healing interventions and rituals discussed in Chapter 5 are a therapeutic reservoir of ways to become familiar with states of awareness in the moment. We can learn to expand time, not constrict it with fear and worries. We can also gain insight from the Eastern world view that approaches life and death as complementary dimensions of the same unified experience. Death is always present and everywhere with life. To experience one is to simultaneously experience the other.

True healing and dying in peace come from releasing one's attachment to the physical body. Learning to let our body-mind-spirit be open to healing comes from within. Although this healing awareness may appear at first to be rare, it is an ordinary and natural event. As we practice living in peace, we enter a healing state where answers to our questions about the complementary nature of living and dying are revealed to us.[3] The insight comes from our own inner wisdom and strength.

REFERENCES

1. Dossey L: Recovering the soul, New York, 1989, Bantam.
2. Dossey L: Meaning and medicine: a doctor's tales of breakthrough and healing, New York, 1991, Bantam.
3. Osborne A: Ramana Maharshi and the path of self-knowledge, New York, 1973, Samuel Weiser Publishers.

14 The Person with Cardiomyopathy or Myocarditis

Sue Wingate

LEARNING OBJECTIVES

1. Define *cardiomyopathy* and *myocarditis*.

2. Describe three types of cardiomyopathies.

3. Compare and contrast three pathophysiologic mechanisms associated with each cardiomyopathy and myocarditis.

4. Analyze the treatment of the three types of cardiomyopathy and myocarditis.

5. Analyze the significance of outflow obstruction in hypertrophic cardiomyopathy and the way it relates to the treatment plan.

6. Outline the steps in establishing an activity plan for the patient with cardiomyopathy or myocarditis.

7. Discuss two specific nursing interventions to help patients overcome hopelessness and powerlessness.

The body of knowledge about heart muscle diseases has greatly expanded over the past several decades. Definitions, etiologies, and functional classifications have changed and evolved with the development of more sophisticated clinical and laboratory techniques.

DEFINITIONS AND CLASSIFICATIONS

Diseases of the heart muscle generally can be divided into two types: those with a specific cause and those with an unknown cause[38] (see the box on p. 428). *Myocarditis,* an inflammation of the myocardium, is a specific heart muscle disease because its cause can be identified. In contrast, *cardiomyopathies* are heart muscle diseases of unknown cause because they are characterized by structural and functional abnormalities of the myocardium not associated with identified heart muscle disease, general system disease, coronary artery disease, systemic hypertension, valvular disease, congenital malformations, or intrinsic pulmonary or vascular disease.[89] The cardiomyopathies can further be divided into three major groups based on their pathophysiologic abnormalities (Fig. 14-1): dilated (formerly congestive), hypertrophic, and restrictive.

The category of *chronic ischemic heart failure* is also included in the box on p. 428. This category includes myocardial diseases caused by chronic ischemia, and thus they are a separate entity from cardiomyopathy. This designation replaces the previous term of *ischemic cardiomyopathy*.[76,89]

The classification in the box, p. 428, is based on the cause of the disease and provides only one type of working framework for understanding the complexities of heart muscle diseases.[76,90,91] Other frameworks may classify heart muscle diseases according to their functional or structural abnormalities (Table 14-1). Regardless of the framework used, it is important to be aware that overlap frequently exists. For example, the specific heart muscle diseases in the box may also be classified into the functional types of cardiomyopathies. Hence amyloidosis may take a restrictive form, and some genetic disorders may take a hypertrophic form. However, most specific heart muscle diseases simulate dilated cardiomyopathy. In the future, with the development of more sophisticated diagnostic techniques, more specific heart muscle diseases will be recognized, and fewer cases of cardiomyopathy will be diagnosed.[76]

426

TABLE 14-1

Functional Classification of Cardiomyopathies

Dilated	Restrictive	Hypertrophic
SYMPTOMS		
Congestive heart failure, particularly left-sided Fatigue and weakness Systemic or pulmonary emboli	Dyspnea, fatigue Right-sided congestive failure Signs and symptoms of systemic disease; amyloidosis, and iron storage disease, etc.	Dyspnea and angina pectoris Fatigue, syncope, and palpitations
PHYSICAL EXAMINATION		
Moderate to severe cardiomegaly, and S_3 and S_4 Atrioventricular (AV) valve regurgitation, especially mitral	Mild-to-moderate cardiomegaly, S_3 and S_4 AV valve regurgitation; inspiratory increase in venous pressure (Kussmaul's sign)	Mild cardiomegaly Apical systolic thrill and heave; brisk carotid upstroke S_4 common Systolic murmur that increases with Valsalva maneuver
CHEST ROENTGENOGRAM		
Moderate-to-marked cardiac enlargement, especially left ventricular Pulmonary venous hypertension	Mild cardiac enlargement Pulmonary venous hypertension	Mild-to-moderate cardiac enlargement
ELECTROCARDIOGRAM (ECG)		
Sinus tachycardia Atrial and ventricular dysrhythmias ST-segment and T-wave abnormalities Intraventricular conduction defects	Low voltage Intraventricular conduction defects AV conduction defects	Left atrial enlargement Left ventricular hypertrophy ST-segment and T-wave abnormalities Abnormal Q waves Atrial and ventricular dysrhythmias
ECHOCARDIOGRAM		
Left ventricular dilation and dysfunction Abnormal systolic mitral valve motion secondary to abnormal compliance with filling pressures	Increased left ventricular wall thickness and mass Small or normal-sized left ventricular cavity Normal systolic function Pericardial effusion	Asymmetric septal hypertrophy Narrow left ventricular outflow tract Systolic anterior motion of the mitral valve Small or normal-sized left ventricle
RADIONUCLIDE STUDIES		
Left ventricular dilatation and dysfunction (RVG*)	Infiltration of myocardium (^{201}TL*) Small or normal-sized left ventricle (RVG) Normal systolic function (RVG)	Small or normal-sized left ventricle (RVG) Vigorous systolic function (RVG) Asymmetrical septal hypertrophy (RVG or ^{201}TL)
CARDIAC CATHETERIZATION		
Left ventricular enlargement and dysfunction Mitral and/or tricuspid regurgitation Elevated left- and often right-sided filling pressures Diminished cardiac output	Diminished left ventricular compliance "Square-root sign" in ventricular pressure recordings Preserved systolic function Elevated left- and right-sided filling pressures	Diminished left ventricular compliance Mitral regurgitation Vigorous systolic function Dynamic left ventricular outflow obstruction

From Wynne J and Braunwald E: The cardiomyopathies and myocarditides. In Braunwald E, editor: Heart disease, ed 3, Philadelphia, 1988, WB Saunders Co.

*RVG, Radionuclide ventriculogram; ^{201}TL, thallium 201.

CLASSIFICATION OF HEART MUSCLE DISEASES

CARDIOMYOPATHY
Heart muscle disease of unknown cause

Acute
Chronic

SPECIFIC HEART MUSCLE DISEASE
Heart muscle disease of known cause or associated with disorders of other systems

Infective myocarditis: bacterial, viral, fungal, and rickettsial conditions
Metabolic: endocrine disorders, nutritional deficiencies, and amyloidosis
General system diseases: connective tissue disorders, infiltrations, and granulomas
Genetic disorders: muscular dystrophy and neuromuscular disorders
Toxins and sensitivity reactions: drugs (especially doxorubicin hydrochloride [Adriamycin]), alcohol, chemicals
Peripartum heart disease

CHRONIC ISCHEMIC HEART FAILURE
Myocardial disease resulting from chronic myocardial ischemia

Myocardial infarction
Hypertension

Data from Shebetai R: J Am Coll Cardiol 1:252, 1983; WHO/15FC Task Force: Br Heart J 44:672, 1980; and Wingate S: Focus Crit Care 11(4):49, 1984.

DILATED CARDIOMYOPATHY
Incidence and precipitating factors

The exact incidence of dilated cardiomyopathy (DC) is difficult to determine because of differing classification systems that may lead to variable disease reporting, especially on death certificates. In 1982, it was estimated that cardiomyopathies were responsible for 46,000 hospitalizations and 10,345 deaths in the United States. Dilated cardiomyopathy comprised the majority of these cases.[36]

By definition, a true idiopathic cardiomyopathy has no known cause; however, several factors have been shown to precipitate or aggravate the development of DC. Three factors commonly associated with the development of DC are alcohol use, pregnancy, and infections. When the contributing factor is definitively diagnosed as the cause of the disease, the classification changes. For example, DC associated with alcohol use will change to "alcoholic heart muscle disease."

Alcohol consumption can lead to cardiac dysfunction and in its severest form may manifest itself as a heart muscle disease with congestive heart failure. Prolonged alcohol consumption causes myocardial damage by direct toxic effects and by nutritional effects associated with thiamin deficiency.[58] Direct toxic effects include changes in mitochondrial activity, alterations in calcium binding and uptake, and disturbances in lipid metabolism, as well as toxic effects related to additives in alcoholic beverages.[79] However, less than 3% of alcohol abusers develop cardiac muscle disease, and those who do develop heart muscle disease usually do not develop alcoholic liver disease.[53] In addition, abstinence from alcohol in the early stages of the disease can increase the ejection fraction and limit or reverse disease progression.[45]

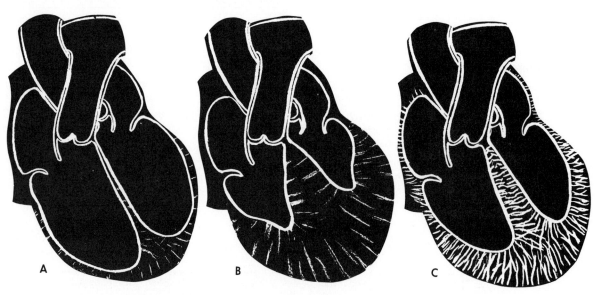

FIG. 14-1 Types of cardiomyopathies. **A,** Dilated (impaired systolic function and cardiac dilation). **B,** Hypertrophic (disproportionate increase in ventricular muscle mass). **C,** Restrictive (marked reduction in diastolic ventricular compliance).

The incidence of cardiomyopathy associated with the *puerperium* varies from one in 3000 to one in 15,000 pregnancies.[78] This cardiomyopathy occurs more commonly in women who are black, over 30 years of age, multiparous, or pregnant with twins or who develop toxemia. For a diagnosis of peripartum heart disease to be made, the following criteria are required:[24]

1. Heart failure must occur between the last month of pregnancy and the fifth postpartum month.
2. Heart failure must be of an undetermined cause.
3. There must be no prior evidence of heart disease.

Prognosis is related to the length of time it takes the heart to return to a normal size. The prognosis is poor if heart size does not return to normal within 6 months after pregnancy. Although a previous history of peripartum cardiomyopathy is not an absolute contraindication to future pregnancies, it may be a relative contraindication, especially for patients whose heart size has not returned to normal.

When an *infectious agent* invades the myocardium and causes an inflammatory process, myocarditis exists. It can be a common precipitating factor of acute or chronic DC. Indeed, the boundary separating myocarditis and DC is unclear, and some investigators purport that myocarditis and DC are stages of the same disease[32] (see later section).

Pathology

The major gross pathologic feature of DC is dilation of both ventricular chambers, although on occasion one ventricle may be more dilated than the other. The atria are usually enlarged also. Intracavity thrombi are common and occur most frequently in the left ventricle. Tricuspid and mitral valve regurgitation occur because of valve dysfunction from chamber enlargement. At autopsy, the heart is increased in weight; however, despite the increased weight, the maximal thickness of the left ventricular free wall and septum is decreased.[89] Coronary arteries are classically normal.

Focal histopathologic results in DC are determined by the course of the disease. Findings may include myocyte hypertrophy, lymphocytes, interstitial fibrosis, endocardial thickening, and myocardial necrosis. The use of endomyocardial biopsy to diagnose DC is controversial because microscopic findings lack specificity. Biopsies are indicated in cases of acute heart failure in an attempt to rule out myocarditis.[7,63]

The exact cause of this pathologic condition is unknown, but research is still being done to determine whether focal rather than diffuse abnormalities are the cause. One group of theorists is exploring the possibility that spasm in the myocardial microcirculation causes focal cellular necrosis that may lead to decreased contractility.[31] Other theorists believe that a decrease in the activity of the sodium-potassium pump may cause intracellular calcium accumulation, mitochondrial calcification, and cell necrosis.[61]

Pathophysiology

Regardless of the cause of DC, the underlying pathologic mechanism interferes with calcium uptake in the mitochondria and impairs myocardial contractility. This inefficient contractile function results in the hemodynamic changes seen in DC patients. With the functional failure of the myocardium, there is a reduction in the rate and degree of muscle fiber shortening. Stroke volume subsequently falls. Initially cardiac output may be maintained as a result of increased heart rate and the Frank-Starling phenomenon (an increase in preload causing an increase in sarcomere length, which increases stroke volume). However, there is minimal reserve during exercise and psychophysiologic stress. In addition, the decreased stroke volume stimulates the sympathetic nervous system and the renin-angiotensin system, which leads to an increased systemic vascular resistance (SVR). This elevated SVR, or afterload, increases the resistance to left ventricular ejection and further depresses cardiac output.

Because of the impaired systolic pump function, there is an increase in ventricular end-diastolic and end-systolic volumes and pressures. Subsequent enlargement and dilation of all four heart chambers occurs, but the ventricles are more dilated than the atria.[92] In addition, the increased end-systolic volume results in stasis of blood and predisposes the patient to mural thrombi.

Left ventricular dilation and a greatly reduced left ventricular ejection fraction are the prominent features of DC. Cardiac output can be normal but usually declines in late stages of illness. The patient's dyspnea and orthopnea are a result of elevated left ventricular diastolic pressure, as well as the increased pressures in the left atrium and pulmonary veins and capillaries. Right ventricular failure usually occurs as a result of chronic elevated pulmonary vascular pressures.

The dilation of the failing ventricle is a compensatory mechanism to increase end-diastolic fiber length and thus increase the velocity of ventricular contraction. Over time, however, this is an inefficient mechanism, as explained by *Laplace's law*:

$$\text{Wall tension (T)} = \frac{\text{Pressure (P)} \times \text{Radius (R)}}{2 \times \text{Hypertrophy (H)}}$$

Thus as dilation increases, the ventricular radius increases, leading to an increase in wall tension, which in turn results in an increased workload and greater myocardial oxygen consumption. As shown in the formula, increased hypertrophy decreases ventricular chamber size and thereby wall tension. The extent of ventricular hypertrophy is a critical factor in DC; patients with more hypertrophy survive longer than those with less hypertrophy, but both groups have the same ejection fraction.

FEATURES OF POOR PROGNOSES IN PATIENTS WITH DILATED CARDIOMYOPATHY

Severity of left ventricular dysfunction
   Increased right atrial pressure
   Increased pulmonary artery wedge pressure
   Increased left ventricular end-diastolic pressure
   Increased left ventricular end-diastolic volume
   Increased left ventricular end-systolic volume
   Decreased left ventricular ejection fraction
Presence of left ventricular conduction delay
Presence of biventricular failure
Decreased amount of ventricular hypertrophy
Older adulthood

Data from Diaz F, Obasohan A, and Oakley CM: Br Heart J 58:393, 1987; Franciosa JA and others: Am J Cardiol 51:831, 1983; Fuster V and others: Am J Cardiol 47:525, 1981; Olshausen KV and others: Am J Cardiol 61:146, 1988; Schwarz FS and others: Circulation 70:923, 1984; Unverferth DV: J Lab Clin Med 106:349, 1985; and Unverferth DV and others: Am J Cardiol 54:147, 1984.

DC typically follows a progressively downhill course characterized by deteriorating myocardial function and repeated episodes of congestive heart failure. Data about the prognosis of patients with DC are influenced by patient selection, diagnostic methods, and the stage of disease.[1] The box lists factors associated with poor survival rates in DC.* Overall the 1-year mortality rate varies from 31% to 35%, and the 5-year rate has been estimated at 50%.[25]

HYPERTROPHIC CARDIOMYOPATHY
Incidence and precipitating factors

Since it was first described in 1907, hypertrophic cardiomyopathy (HC) has been described by various names, the two most frequent being *idiopathic hypertrophic subaortic stenosis* and *hypertrophic obstructive cardiomyopathy*. However, these terms overstate the obstructive element of the disease; thus the current term of choice is *HC* because it emphasizes the predominant increase in ventricular muscle mass. HC affects men and women and occurs commonly in young adulthood, although it has been described in infancy and older adulthood.[23,30]

Early studies noted that most HC patients had a genetic defect transmitted as an autosomal dominant trait. With the advent of echocardiography, however, it was suggested that nongenetic causes may also play a role in precipitating HC.[22] Recent research suggests that the occurrence of HC

may "skip" generations; thus some instances of HC previously judged to be sporadic may indeed be familial.[30a] In addition, work is underway to map the gene for HC with molecular markers.[44a]

Another cause, related to genetics, is an abnormality of myocardial development that occurs in utero. The disorganized myofibril arrangement in HC suggests that the cell type is less well differentiated than that of a fully developed myocardium and resembles that of a primitive or embryonic heart. This abnormal orientation of myofibrils may be caused by an aberration of catecholamine function that occurs in the developing heart.[38,89]

Pathology

The major morphologic alteration in 95% of patients with HC is asymmetric septal hypertrophy, a greater thickening of the ventricular septum than of the left ventricular free wall. Other pathologic changes may include dilated atria, small or normal-sized ventricular cavities, disorganization of myocardial fibers and fibrosis in the ventricular septum, mural endocardial plaque in the left ventricular outflow tract, thickened mitral valve, and abnormal intramural coronary arteries. Histopathologic examination of affected myocardium reveals hypertrophic cells with hyperchromatic and bizarre nuclei and increased amounts of Z-band material.[7,89] Endomyocardial biopsy is not routinely performed in the diagnosis of HC.

Pathophysiology

The predominant impairment in HC is decreased ventricular compliance, which impedes diastolic filling. The left ventricle is too stiff during diastole, partly because of the increased muscle mass, and does not relax adequately to allow for the free inflow of blood. Because of this reduced compliance, there is a marked increased in left ventricular end-diastolic pressure when diastolic filling occurs. In addition, the ventricular filling pattern is disturbed with most patients exhibiting a prolonged isovolumic relaxation period. A forceful atrial contraction in late diastole attempts to compensate for the increased resistance to filling.[22,89]

Systolic function is also disturbed. Left ventricular hypertrophy leads to a hypercontractile ventricle and an exaggerated systole. Ejection fraction is supernormal (approximately 90%) and the majority of the stroke volume is ejected in the first third of the ejection phase.[76] This hyperdynamic state may lead to obliteration of the ventricular cavity during systole.[48] In addition, during systole the anterior leaflet of the mitral valve is pulled toward the hypertrophied septum and thus may narrow the outflow tract of the left ventricle. This abnormality can be increased by mechanisms that increase myocardial contractility or decrease left ventricular volume.

The existence or nonexistence of a narrowed left ventricular outflow tract has led to the classification of HC as

---

*References 34, 35, 64, 72, 84, and 85.

obstructive or *nonobstructive*. Patients with demonstrable pressure gradients across the left ventricular outflow tract (immediately below the aortic valve), either at rest or with provocation, are classified as having *obstructive HC*. Approximately 60% to 80% of patients with HC may exhibit the obstructive type.[22,83] However, it has been questioned whether a true obstruction occurs or whether elimination of the ventricular cavity during systole is the cause of systolic pressure gradients and reduced cardiac output.[76,89]

Although some patients have mild disease and live for many years without symptoms, the natural history of HC is characterized by a slow progression of symptoms. Half of patients die suddenly after no or only very mild symptoms, and approximately 5% die annually. On average, the patient dies at age 40, 5 to 10 years after a period of worsening symptoms.[22] Patients at high risk of *sudden death* are young when diagnosed with HC, have syncope, and have a family history of HC and sudden death.[52]

RESTRICTIVE CARDIOMYOPATHY
Incidence and precipitating factors

Restrictive cardiomyopathy (RC) is the least common type of cardiomyopathy in the Western world; the incidence is unknown. It is characterized by proliferation of the endocardium and reduction in diastolic ventricular compliance. When proliferation becomes quite extensive, an "obliterative" phase, in which the size of the ventricular cavity is reduced and almost entirely obliterated, may occur.

RC may be precipitated by a variety of pathologic processes that affect the myocardium, endocardium, and subendocardium. The most frequent worldwide cause of RC is *endomyocardial fibrosis*. This disorder is manifested in tropical endomyocardial fibrosis and *Löffler's disease,* entities that are now considered to be different stages of the same disease.[89] Amyloidosis, the deposition of an abnormal eosinophilic fibrous protein, is a common cause of RC; however, it does not produce identical hemodynamic effects, and it is usually classified as a specific heart muscle disease. Other causes may be hemochromatosis (a disorder characterized by excessive iron deposition), glycogen deposition, or neoplasm.

Pathology

Gross pathologic examination in end-stage RC reveals a normal heart size overall but a reduced size of the ventricular cavity and extensive thickening of the endocardium. This thickening also involves the papillary muscles and associated valves.[7] The histopathologic structure depends on the course of the disease, and three stages have been identified:[42]

1. The acute necrotic stage characterized by marked eosinophilic inflammatory infiltration
2. The thrombotic stage characterized by extensive thrombi on a thickened endocardium
3. The late fibrotic stage characterized by disappearance of eosinophils and appearance of fibrosis in the endocardium, myocardium, papillary muscle, and chordae tendineae

Pathophysiology

The endomyocardial fibrosis and progressive obliteration of the ventricular cavity produce a noncompliant ventricle that restricts ventricular filling, most markedly in late diastole. Endocardial thickening of the AV valve causes considerable mitral and tricuspid regurgitation. Because diastolic relaxation is impaired, a greater diastolic pressure is required to achieve a given chamber volume. Systolic function usually is preserved, but the altered diastolic function causes higher filling pressures and subsequent pulmonary and/or systemic congestion.[1] These features of RC, as well as its clinical presentation, resemble features of constrictive pericarditis (see p. 433). Although some RCs are benign, the prognosis is generally poor, especially when RC is associated with other specific heart muscle diseases.[1]

MYOCARDITIS
Incidence and etiology

Myocarditis is the process of inflammatory infiltration of the myocardium with degeneration or necrosis of adjacent myocytes not typical of the ischemic damage associated with coronary artery disease.[6] It may be an acute or chronic process. The incidence of myocarditis is not precisely known and may vary with age, sex, season of the year, geographic location, and the availability of public health measures such as immunization and sanitation. The immunodeficient patient is at a high risk.[39,89]

Pathology

Histologic findings depend on the mechanism of myocardial damage, the specific etiologic agent, and the stage of disease when the biopsy is performed. Myocarditis is difficult to study in humans because it frequently remains undiagnosed until cardiac dysfunction is clinically apparent.[39] There is inflammation, primarily of the interstitial tissues. Infiltration of lymphocytes, histiocytes, and polymorphonuclear leukocytes is found between the muscle fibers and perivascular connective tissue. In some types of myocarditis, muscle fiber necrosis may predominate. The key findings that must be present to diagnose myocarditis are lymphocyte infiltration and myocyte necrosis.[6]

Pathophysiology

Most studies of myocarditis in humans and animals have investigated the development of myocardial damage after infection with a virus. Mechanisms for this damage may include viral replication, direct cellular destruction, alteration of cellular energy systems, or activation of an autoimmune response.[88] A viral infection may cause an acute phase of illness from which the majority of people recover without permanent myocardial damage; this is followed by a latent period and the development, in some, of a chronic illness resembling DC.[32,38,39,89] This identification of distinct phases has led researchers to hypothesize that the chronic phase is mediated by an autoimmune response. As a result of the acute viral infection, a new antigen may appear on the myocardium; subsequently, immune cells may activate and attack the antigen and damage the myocardium. This results in cardiac dilation and failure as seen in DC.[32,39] It remains to be proven whether myocarditis and DC are stages of the same disease; however, much evidence is accumulating to support this belief.

Other forms of myocarditis may have variable effects, depending on the causative agent. Myocardial involvement may be focal or diffuse. For example, diphtheria myocarditis is characterized by conduction system abnormalities, whereas Chagas' disease is characterized by generalized cardiomegaly and severe right-sided dilation.[88]

Most patients with myocarditis recover fully. A significant number, however, develop recurrent or chronic myocarditis, and some die from a severe acute illness. Acute myocarditis is not an unusual cause of sudden death in young adults.[88]

Nursing process

Because DC and HC are the two more common types of heart muscle diseases, a case study is presented for each.

Case study 1 (DC). Ms. B.R., a single 20-year-old black woman, was admitted to the coronary care unit (CCU) with the diagnosis of congestive heart failure. She reported a recent onset of severe dyspnea, orthopnea, fatigue, weight gain, and palpitations. The only significant aspects of her medical history were the presence of a "flu-like syndrome" approximately 2 months before admission and the existence of an uncle with chronic heart failure of unknown cause.

While in the CCU, Ms. B.R. underwent invasive hemodynamic monitoring and was treated with oxygen, dobutamine, nitroprusside, and furosemide. Her hemodynamic parameters stabilized, and her initial congestive symptoms subsided. Various tests resulted in the diagnosis of DC. Echocardiography revealed four-chamber dilation and a poorly contracting left ventricle. Cardiac catheterization and angiography showed normal coronary arteries and an ejection fraction of 25%. The ECG revealed sinus tachycardia with frequent premature ventricular contractions (PVCs). Endomyocardial biopsy results were nonspecific but could not definitely rule out myocarditis.

When transferred to the telemetry unit, oral digoxin, captopril, furosemide, potassium, and a low-sodium diet were prescribed for Ms. B.R. She tolerated only minimal activity and thus remained in bed or in a chair most of the time and had to rely on the staff or family members for assistance with daily activities. She frequently verbalized feelings of hopelessness and powerlessness about the insidious, progressive nature of her disease. The staff worked with her and her family to develop mutual daily activity plans and stressed

the importance of her role in following the planned medical regimen. She underwent evaluation for cardiac transplantation (see Chapter 18) and was accepted and placed on a waiting list.

After 3 weeks of evaluation, medication adjustment, and gradual increase in activity levels, Ms. B.R. was discharged. Although she was able to tolerate a short daily walk, she remained despondent over the loss of her prior active lifestyle. She missed the social stimulation of school and work and felt isolated from her friends. Home health care nurses recognized this concern and alerted her family to explain DC to Ms. B.R.'s friends and to encourage them to visit and update her on current events. A tutor was also arranged.

Over the next 6 months, Ms. B.R. was hospitalized twice for exacerbations of congestive heart failure. She was placed on anti-coagulant therapy for mural thrombi and on antidysrhythmic treatment for episodes of symptomatic ventricular tachycardia. About 10 months after the diagnosis of DC, she underwent cardiac transplantation.

Case study 2 (HC). While Mr. J.C., a 28-year-old dentist, and his wife were jogging, he abruptly fell to the ground. His wife began cardiopulmonary resuscitation, and other joggers summoned an ambulance. Mr. J.C. required defibrillation twice before reaching the hospital. He was successfully resuscitated and underwent diagnostic tests to evaluate heart disease.

Mr. J.C. reported no history of heart disease in his family or himself, except for occasional palpitations he attributed to smoking, excessive coffee drinking, and the stress of his dental practice. Mr. J.C.'s stay in the CCU was brief and uneventful. Chest x-ray films, ECG changes, and echocardiographic findings were diagnostic of HC. Mr. J.C. was given propranolol, 40 mg, four times daily.

Early in his recovery, after being confronted with the possibility of death, Mr. J.C. expressed despair about the outcome of having a chronic disease with no real possibility of curative treatment. He was assisted to recognize the cause of his despair and to focus on his strengths rather than the disease's limitations. Future goals regarding family and work were established as a motivational tool for him.

During later recovery, Mr. J.C. was anxious about resuming progressive activity. He became quite concerned about any activity, including sexual activity, that might cause another cardiac arrest. Because of early awareness, Mr. J.C. and his wife received counseling, new information, and insight into how he could again lead a normal life.

About a year after the diagnosis of HC, Mr. J.C. had no more symptoms. He learned to listen to bodily cues of anxiety and used biofeedback as a relaxation technique. He returned to leading an active, healthy life and approached his life with HC as one of prevention rather than of limitation.

Nursing assessment
Knowing pattern

This pattern includes information about the patient's current and past health status and knowledge and perceptions about the illness, symptoms, testing procedures, and treatment.[40] For patients with cardiomyopathy or myocarditis, obtain a detailed patient history to identify possible causes of heart muscle disease. Elicit information about recent illnesses, systemic symptoms, and discomforts. Take a thorough history to identify predisposing factors (such as alcohol, chemotherapeutic agents, viral infection, and a family history) that may be linked with the development of cardiomyopathy or myocarditis.

In patients with DC, symptoms develop gradually. Patients may have no symptoms for months to years because of compensatory mechanisms and still have left ventricular dilation that is discovered only by routine x-ray examination. When symptoms do occur, they usually are left ventricular failure, dyspnea on exertion, fatigue, and weakness. In severe cases, symptoms also may include orthopnea, paroxysmal noctural dyspnea, dyspnea at rest, peripheral edema, and abdominal swelling. Complaints of angina pectoris are unusual but may occur with exertion.[89]

When alcoholic cardiomyopathy is suspected, a history of heavy drinking over many years is often present. In early stages, there may be no symptoms or very mild findings such as decreased exercise tolerance or palpitations. Indeed, the occurrence of paroxysmal dysrhythmias during binge drinking—the "holiday heart" syndrome—may be the first evidence of cardiomyopathy.[51] Some alcoholic patients have no symptoms of heart disease and normal ECG findings and yet have evidence of heart muscle damage when examined by special diagnostic procedures.[80] As the condition progresses, patients may be aware of shortness of breath, fatigue, pedal edema, and palpitations.

The clinical presentation of HC depends on the extent and severity of the disease, the presence of a systolic pressure gradient, and the age of the patient. Exertional dyspnea is the most common symptom of HC. It is caused by elevated pulmonary venous pressure resulting from increased left ventricular diastolic pressure. Syncope may be present as a result of dysrhythmias, sudden reduction in left ventricular filling, or abrupt elimination of the left ventricular cavity during systole.[89] The patient may complain of *graying out*, a term that refers to visual disturbances caused by poor cerebral perfusion. The patient describes a transient darkening of vision or the sensation of a shade being pulled down over the eyes. These presyncopal or near-syncopal spells occur when the patient is erect and are usually relieved by immediately lying down. Fatigue, palpitations, orthopnea, paroxysmal nocturnal dyspnea, ankle edema, and angina pectoris are common signs and symptoms. Angina is caused by an imbalance between the oxygen supply and demand resulting from difficulty in perfusing the increased myocardial muscle mass.[82] Because of this, transmural myocardial infarction (MI) also may occur in the absence of narrowed coronary arteries.[55] Sudden death occurs frequently in this condition and may be the only manifestation of the disease.

The clinical presentation of RC is similar to constrictive pericarditis. Fatigue and exertional dyspnea are the most frequent complaints. These occur as a result of the body's inability to increase cardiac output. Stroke volume is limited by the restriction of venous return to the heart and by the development of a compensatory tachycardia, which further compromises ventricular filling.[92] Peripheral edema, ascites, and hepatic dysfunction usually cause the patient to seek medical attention.[77]

In patients suspected of having myocarditis, there may be no symptoms, or symptoms can range from local inflammation to fatal congestive heart failure caused by diffuse myocarditis. The disease frequently remains undetected until heart failure occurs. Investigate a history of viral or bacterial illness. Frequently an illness may be unrecognized or forgotten because it was of short duration. Patients commonly complain of nonspecific symptoms such as fever, dyspnea, fatigue, and palpitations. Patients may also manifest generalized signs of an infection, as well as symptoms of cardiac disease.

Moving pattern

This pattern is an important component of the initial history, and it involves the assessment of activity, rest, sleep, recreation, environmental and health maintenance, and self-care.[40] For the patient with cardiomyopathy or myocarditis, assessment of activity level is the most important component because dyspnea or exercise intolerance is usually the presenting symptom. Assessment includes the patient's exercise responses, changes in exercise tolerance, and reports of fatigue and inability to perform normal activities.

Because of impaired systolic or diastolic cardiac function, patients may have inadequate energy to perform even activities of daily living. Conversely, patients may have developed compensatory mechanisms that enable them to tolerate daily functions, but because they lack any cardiac reserve, they experience fatigue or dyspnea when extra demands such as exercise or emotional stress are placed on their system. Assessment of activity is critical for these patients because activity prescription is an important part of their treatment plan.

The patient with DC typically experiences a progressive chronic illness with acute bouts of heart failure. Assess the initial activity intolerance that caused the patient to seek health care assistance, and assess the patient's ongoing response to treatment and the therapy's effects on activity status. Frequently, a new onset of activity intolerance signals an exacerbation of DC or inadequate response to therapy. Tools such as the New York Heart Association's functional classification[59] (see p. 327) help to quantify patient responses and determine whether the patient is stable or will deteriorate over time. For the patient in a clinical compensatory state, response to treadmill testing, especially oxygen consumption, also helps in assessing activity levels.[76]

The patient with HC is often a physically active individual who has dyspnea on exertion. In fact, HC is a frequent cause of sudden death occurring in athletes.[75] Exercise, especially strenuous exercise, causes potential problems for the patient with HC. Angina may occur after exercise because of a sudden decrease in blood pressure and venous return that decreases stroke volume.[22] The increased contractility and tachycardia that occur with exercise may also increase the pressure gradient and eliminate the left ventricular cavity. Decreased cardiac output may cause a decrease in cerebral perfusion, resulting in dizziness and syncope.

If patients with RC experience heart failure, their activity assessment is similar to that of patients with DC. Because myocarditis may only be an acute problem with full recovery, assessment of activity levels helps to determine the patient's recovery status. The baseline status is first established, and then determinations are made regarding deterioration, stabilization, or improvement.[39]

Exchanging pattern

The Exchanging Pattern includes physical examination findings and laboratory and diagnostic test results.[40] These components are discussed for each of the cardiomyopathies and for myocarditis (see also Table 14-1).

Patients suspected of having or who have cardiomyopathy exhibit varying degrees of heart failure and cardiac enlargement (Chapter 11). Patients with DC usually have forceful left and occasionally right ventricular impulses. The apical impulse is displaced laterally as a result of left ventricular dilation. S_3 and S_4 may be heard. The pulse is usually rapid and may be irregular because of atrial fibrillation or PVCs. The blood pressure may be elevated, normal, or decreased, depending on the cardiac output and extent of vasoconstriction. Crackles, pulsus alternans, jugular venous distension, hepatomegaly, and peripheral edema often are present in more severe cases. As heart failure increases, tricuspid or mitral regurgitation may appear. Late complications are signs and symptoms of systemic and pulmonary emboli.

Patients with HC usually do not have congestive heart failure in the early stages. However, it may occur if atrial fibrillation develops; this occurs in 5% to 10% of patients. With atrial fibrillation the atrial kick is lost, and ventricular filling and stroke volume are decreased. If the ventricular response is rapid with atrial fibrillation, this further decreases cardiac output. Closely inspect the patient's carotid pulse to identify a brisk and split upstroke, which is opposite of the slow upstroke in valvular aortic stenosis. A double apical impulse, pulsus biferiens, is also present in HC. Jugular pulse inspection usually reveals a large presystolic *a* wave resulting from forceful atrial systole. The heart is enlarged with a firm apical systolic lift caused by ventricular hypertrophy.

An important finding is a systolic ejection murmur heard best at the cardiac apex or left sternal border (grade 3 or louder). The murmur is caused by turbulence as the blood passes through the narrowed left ventricular outflow tract, as well as by the mitral regurgitation that occurs when obstruction is present. A variety of maneuvers can be used to augment or suppress the murmur during the exami-

nation because the murmur is variable in intensity and duration. Ways to increase the murmur include the Valsalva maneuver, suddenly standing upright, or exercise. Ways to decrease the murmur are squatting and handgripping.

In the patient with RC the physical examination most often reveals congestive heart failure, usually right-sided, and systolic murmurs caused by mitral or tricuspid regurgitation. Jugular venous distention, an S_3 gallop, Kussmaul's sign, crackles, an irregular pulse, hepatomegaly, peripheral edema, and a narrow pulse pressure may be present.

Manifestations of myocarditis are variable and depend on the extent and location of the inflammatory process. In fact, the key diagnostic features of myocarditis rarely occur at the height of the illness but rather during convalescence as the systemic infection is subsiding.[88] Physical examination usually reveals mild-to-moderate jugular venous distention, tachycardia (in disproportion to the fever), gallop rhythm, and cardiomegaly. If the case is advanced, findings then may include peripheral edema, hepatomegaly, pulsus alternans, and tricuspid and mitral regurgitation murmurs. If pericarditis is present with myocarditis, the patient may complain of pleural chest pain and have a pericardial friction rub (see Chapter 15). In extreme cases of myocarditis, severe congestive heart failure should be considered to be a result of pericardial effusion with tamponade until proved otherwise.[92]

Laboratory and diagnostic tests. There are no specific tests for diagnosing cardiomyopathies; thus the diagnosis is often made by excluding other disorders that may simulate it, such as coronary artery disease, valvular disorders, hypertension, and pericardial disease.

In DC, the chest x-ray film shows left ventricular enlargement and generalized cardiomegaly. Congestive heart failure may be accompanied by interstitial or alveolar pulmonary edema, pulmonary venous congestion, or pleural effusion. If a pulmonary infarction occurs, atelectasis, scars, or pulmonary infiltrates may be present. In the patient with heart failure, the ECG usually shows sinus tachycardia. ST segments and T waves are frequently abnormal. Intraventricular conduction disturbances, left axis deviation, PVCs, and atrial fibrillation are common.

An echocardiogram is a most useful test in DC and is obtained to assess left ventricular impairment and to rule out concomitant valvular or pericardial disease. With DC, an increased internal dimension of the left ventricular cavity is seen with decreased movement of the left ventricular walls.[3,9] In addition, the other cardiac chambers are dilated, and mural thrombi are sometimes present. Radionuclide ventriculography may be performed to assess ventricular function and to evaluate response to therapy.[20] Elevated end-diastolic and end-systolic left ventricular volumes and a markedly reduced ejection fraction are seen.[92]

Cardiac catheterization and angiography may be performed to assess cardiac filling pressures and the presence and extent of coronary artery disease. Endomyocardial biopsy is not recommended as a routine procedure in DC because findings are usually nonspecific. However, it may be performed to exclude myocarditis and other heart muscle disorders.

With HC, the chest x-ray film is often normal, but it may show an enlarged cardiac silhouette with a prominent left ventricle. The left atrium may also be enlarged. The ECG is usually abnormal. Secondary ST-segment and T-wave changes, pronounced septal Q waves, and ventricular hypertrophy are usually present.[16] Q waves are usually caused by marked septal hypertrophy but occasionally may be the result of transmural infarction.[89] Atrial fibrillation, PVCs, and, less commonly, Wolff-Parkinson-White syndrome may also occur. Over 20% of patients show ventricular tachycardia when ambulatory monitoring is done.[53]

The echocardiogram is the best test for confirming HC. It also is used to follow the patient's progress and course of disease, as well as to screen family members for the disease to identify a genetic cause. Echocardiography shows asymmetrical septal hypertrophy, a small or normal-sized hyperdynamic left ventricle, and the systolic anterior motion (SAM) of the mitral valve anterior leaflet. Doppler studies performed with echocardiography are used to assess subvalvular left ventricular outflow obstruction, mitral regurgitation, and diastolic left ventricular dysfunction. Cardiac catheterization and ventriculography may be performed to determine the exact size of the ventricular chamber and the degree of outflow obstruction and mitral regurgitation. In older patients, it may be important to know whether concomitant coronary artery disease is present.

The diagnosis of RC is made after the exclusion of constrictive pericarditis. Several findings are helpful. Pericardial calcium deposits seen during fluoroscopy usually indicate constrictive pericarditis rather than RC. However, this finding is present in only about one fourth of patients. Abnormalities of depolarization and of AV conduction are more common in RC. Echocardiography or catheterization may demonstrate abnormal pericardial thickness, abnormal right atrial border straightening, and diminished contraction suggesting constriction. Computerized axial tomography may also demonstrate an abnormally thickened pericardium, suggesting the diagnosis of pericardial constriction rather than RC. A left ventriculogram is helpful. Left ventricular end-diastolic pressure is usually higher than right in cardiomyopathy patients. Endomyocardial biopsy also assists in differentiation and may show fibrosis or infiltrative lesions in RC.[77]

The specific diagnosis of myocarditis often is made in association with the symptoms of systemic illness. The cause of myocarditis is determined by identifying a specific virus, bacterium, or fungus found in feces, throat washings, blood, pericardial fluid, and myocardium, as well as by a distinct increase in complement-fixation, virus-neutralizing antibodies or by hemagglutination inhibition titers.[92] The ECG typically shows diffuse ST-segment and T-wave abnormalities, conduction defects, and supraventricular dysrhythmias. Gallium scanning may detect "hot spots" and thereby indicate an inflammatory process.[86] Enomyocardial biopsy provides histopathologic evidence of the diagnosis; however, because of the frequency of sampling errors, a negative biopsy does not rule out myocarditis. Multiple biopsies increase the diagnostic power of this technique.[88]

Perceiving pattern

This pattern involves the reception of information and the way this information is translated meaningfully by patients.[40] It may include self-esteem, meaning of the illness to the patient, and sensory or perceptual deficits. For patients with cardiomyopathy or myocarditis, the most important aspect is assessing the meaning of the illness to patients and their families.

With the exceptions of acute, fully recoverable myocarditis and some HCs, most patients progressively debilitate, have only palliative therapy to control symptoms, and have an uncertain prognosis. Because of this, nurses must assess how patients perceive their situation and whether they remain hopeful about their illness and quality of life. Patients may indeed be confronted for the first time with the possibility of death, and this often affects how they perceive and translate information. Hopeless patients may perceive that there are no alternatives available to them and feel that there is no chance of a favorable outcome. In contrast, hopeful patients may perceive even minor changes in medications as a sign that worsening symptoms may improve.[13] Assess the degree to which patients have hope, as well as mechanisms or strategies (such as spirituality or support systems) that they use to maintain hope.

Patients also may experience powerlessness or a perceived loss of control. Because of the insidious nature of their disease, their frequent lack of decision making in the medical regimen, and their decreased physical activity level, patients often perceive that they have no control or influence over their illness. It is often viewed as a threat to them. Emotional states triggered by hospitalization, medications, or acute illness may influence the ability of the patient to appraise the situation and verbalize their perceptions.

Relating pattern

This pattern involves the establishment of bonds and includes role performance and sexual and social relationships.[40] Assess these areas in the patient with cardiomyopathy or myocarditis. The patient's deteriorating or unstable physical condition frequently disrupts role performance, whether it is as a spouse, parent, employee, or community member.

Elicit the patient's roles before the illness and assess ways they may be affected by the illness and treatment plan. Occupational and leisure roles (such as construction worker or athlete) are important to include because they may depend on physical exertion and thus affect the treatment strategy. The patient's sexuality patterns should also be assessed by determining whether there are any physical difficulties with sex, anxieties about performing sexual activity, and untoward effects of medications on their sexual response. The partner should be included if possible because they frequently express concern about sexual activity and the physical effect it will have on the patient.

Patients' social relationships are assessed by determining their support system and ways this system is used in coping with illness. It is important to include also the quality of their relationships with others. This can be obtained from patients' verbal reports and from observation of the type and amount of contact patients have with members of their support system.

Choosing pattern

The Choosing Pattern involves the selection of alternatives and includes coping style, judgment ability, and level of participation in care.[40] All of these are important in the assessment of the patient with cardiomyopathy or myocarditis. These diseases are characterized by progressive physical deterioration and a poor prognosis. The effort to manage this stressful situation involves the process of coping. Assess the patient's and family's coping response to illness. Include the patient's and family's usual problem-solving methods, strategies for dealing with stress, and existence of support systems. Assess judgment by evaluating the patient's and others' perceptions of their ability to make sound decisions, especially regarding treatment.[40]

Assessment of patients' participation in their care is the most important part of the Choosing Pattern. Treatment of these diseases requires a chronic regimen of complex medical therapies that may exhaust patients' finances and coping abilities. Assess patients' past compliance with health treatment to help determine their commitment to participate in their care. Elicit the reasons (e.g., financial, perceptions, or knowledge deficit) for their past noncompliant behaviors because these greatly affect the treatment plan. Also attempt to determine patients' willingness to comply with the current plan of care.

Nursing Diagnoses

The most common human responses anticipated for patients with cardiomyopathy or myocarditis are indicated by the following nursing diagnoses:

1. Decreased cardiac output related to mechanical (preload, afterload, and inotropic), electrical, and structural factors
2. Activity intolerance related to acute or chronic illness
3. Hopelessness related to unpredictable outcome of acute or chronic illness
4. Powerlessness related to perceived inability to control outcome of disease process
5. Altered sexuality patterns related to physical condition and effects of treatment regimen
6. Impaired social interaction related to physical limitations, anxiety, or hopelessness[14]
7. High risk for noncompliance related to inadequate knowledge about illness and complexity of medical regimen

For each of these diagnoses, the patient outcomes, nursing prescriptions, and evaluation criteria are outlined with a discussion of the factual information that supports the plan and implementation of care.

Decreased cardiac output related to mechanical (preload, afterload, and inotropic), electrical, and structural factors (exchanging pattern)

PATIENT OUTCOMES	NURSING PRESCRIPTIONS	EVALUATION
Patient with DC or RC will demonstrate no signs of ventricular failure, including blood pressure and pulse within normal limits; normal sinus rhythm and S₁ and S₂; absence of S₃ and S₄; normal apical impulse; breath sounds without crackles and wheezes; warm, dry skin; normal urinary output (increased with response to diuretics); absence of cough, neck vein distention, peripheral and sacral edema, ascites, and hepatic congestion; and invasive hemodynamic parameters within normal limits (if performed) (blood pressure greater than 90 mm Hg, pulmonary artery wedge pressure (PAWP) of 12 to 18 mm Hg, and cardiac output greater than 2.2 L/min/m².	Assess parameters to evaluate ventricular function, including blood pressure, pulse, cardiac rhythm, normal and abnormal heart sounds, apical impulse, breath sounds, skin temperature and moisture, urinary output, presence of cough, neck vein distention, peripheral and sacral edema, ascites, hepatic congestion, and hemodynamic monitoring parameters such as blood pressure, PAWP, and cardiac output.	At discharge, patient demonstrated blood pressure and pulse within normal limits; normal sinus rhythm and S₁ and S₂; absence of S₃ and S₄; point of maximum impulse in fifth intercostal space, midclavicular line; absence of crackles or wheezes; warm and dry skin; urinary output within normal limts; absence of cough, neck vein distention, peripheral and sacral edema, ascites, and enlarged liver; and invasive hemodynamic parameters within normal limits (blood pressure greater than 90 mm Hg, PAWP of 12 to 18 mm Hg, and cardiac output greater than 2.2 L/min/m².
Patient with DC or RC will demonstrate a reduction in ventricular failure by responding to inotropic agents, diuretics, and vasodilators.	Institute inotropic, diuretic, and vasodilator therapy to reduce ventricular failure; assess patient response (see Patient Outcome 1).	Patient responded to medications by demonstrating a reduction in ventricular failure (see Patient Outcome 1).
Patient with DC or RC will experience no symptomatic dysrhythmias; if they occur, patient will respond to antidysrhythmic medications, cardioversion, or pacemaker, if needed.	Assess patient for symptomatic dysrhythmias; if they occur, be prepared to institute antidysrhythmic medications or assist with cardioversion or pacemaker insertion.	Patient experienced no dysrhythmias.
Patient with DC or RC will adhere to a low-sodium diet.	Order and explain low-sodium diet. Initiate dietitian referral if needed.	Patient adhered to a low-sodium diet.
Patient with DC or RC will have a balanced intake and output and no weight gain.	Evaluate intake, output, and daily weight measurements.	Patient had balanced intake and output and no weight gain.
Patient with DC or RC will demonstrate successful use of relaxation and imagery exercises.	Guide patient in relaxation and imagery exercises.	Patient successfully used relaxation and imagery skills.
Patient with DC will demonstrate abstinence from alcohol.	Teach patient about importance of alcohol abstinence.	Patient demonstrated abstinence from alcohol.
Patient with DC and family will participate in alcoholic counseling.	Assist patient and family to find alcoholic counseling.	Patient or family participated in alcoholic counseling.
Patient with HC will be free of symptoms of a hypertrophied and noncompliant left ventricle, including dyspnea and angina.	Observe the patient for dyspnea or angina.	Patient did not experience dyspnea or angina.
Patient will demonstrate improved ventricular filling by responding to β-adrenergic and calcium channel blockers.	Institute β-adrenergic and calcium channel blocker therapy to improve left ventricular filling; assess patient response.	Patient demonstrated improved ventricular filling.
Patient will avoid conditions that aggravate outflow obstruction (see the box on p. 440 and text).	Teach patient to avoid conditions that aggravate outflow obstruction.	Patient avoided conditions that aggravate outflow obstruction.

Continued.

NURSING DIAGNOSIS 1   **Decreased cardiac output related to mechanical (preload, afterload, and inotropic), electrical, and structural factors (exchanging pattern)—cont'd**

PATIENT OUTCOMES	NURSING PRESCRIPTIONS	EVALUATION
Patient with HC will demonstrate knowledge of a need for long-term medication therapy. Patient with HC will maintain an optimal cardiac rate and rhythm and not demonstrate atrial fibrillation; if it occurs, patient will demonstrate resolution of atrial fibrillation by responding to aggressive medication therapy or cardioversion.	Teach patient about the need for long-term medication therapy. Evaluate patient for optimal cardiac rate and rhythm, especially assessing for atrial fibrillation; if it occurs, administer the appropriate medication therapy or assist with cardioversion.	Patient or family demonstrated understanding of long-term medication therapy. Patient did not experience atrial fibrillation. (If it did occur, state specific dysrhythmias and treatment.)
Patient with myocarditis will demonstrate resolution of myocarditis by responding to specific antibiotics (depends on causative factors), corticosteroids, and immunosuppressive and antiviral agents. If severely compromised, patient with myocarditis will tolerate hemodynamic monitoring and ventilatory support. Patient with myocarditis will demonstrate no heart failure (see Patient Outcome 1 for patient with DC). Patient with myocarditis will not demonstrate dysrhythmias; if they occur, patient will respond to aggressive medication therapy and temporary pacemaker if needed.	Administer specific antibiotics, corticosteroids, and immunosuppressive and antiviral agents to resolve myocarditis; observe patient response. Assess patient response to hemodynamic monitoring and ventilatory support (if needed). Assess patient for signs of ventricular failure (see Nursing Prescriptions 1 for patient with DC). Assess patient for symptomatic dysrhythmias; if they occur, be prepared to institute antidysrhythmic medications and assist with pacemaker insertion.	Patient responded to antibiotics, corticosteroids, and immunosuppressive, and antiviral agents. If needed, patient tolerated hemodynamic monitoring and ventilatory support. (State specifics.) See Evaluation 1 for patient with DC. Patient demonstrated no dysrhythmias; if they occurred, patient received aggressive medication therapy and transvenous pacemaker if needed. (List specifics).

Plan and intervention for decreased cardiac output
Dilated cardiomyopathy

The major goal of treatment for patients with DC is to improve cardiac output by altering preload, afterload, and contractility.[12,66] The extent and aggressiveness of treatment depend on the degree of heart failure and patients' functional status. If patients are stable or have mild-to-moderate heart failure, they may be treated on an outpatient basis. When patients have severe heart failure, they are admitted to the hospital for therapy. If hemodynamic monitoring and close observation are required, they will be admitted to a CCU. Cardiac parameters and pulmonary artery measurements will be evaluated frequently to guide the appropriate medication and regimen.

Preload. Therapy to reduce preload in the patient with DC includes the use of diuretic agents with a sodium-restricted diet.[45] Furosemide is the diuretic most often used to inhibit the reabsorption of sodium and thereby reduce

vascular congestion. A restricted sodium intake decreases extracellular fluid volume, resulting in a decreased venous return. Medications that cause venodilation also are used to decrease venous return and lower ventricular filling volume. The dilated venous bed causes an increase in venous capacitance, producing a decreased venous return and lowered ventricular filling. With a decreased ventricular end-diastolic volume, there is decreased workload and decreased wall tension with a possible increase in subendocardial perfusion, which causes more efficient myocardial contractions. Nitroprusside (see next section) and prazosin dilate arteriolar and venous beds. Nitrates are primarily venodilators. Long-acting forms, such as nitroglycerin ointment and isosorbide, may be used on a long-term basis.

Afterload. Afterload is reduced by the use of arterial vasodilators and during critical decompensation by the use of the intraaortic balloon pump (see Chapter 11). In the acute setting, nitroprusside is the drug of choice for unloading therapy. This parenteral agent acts rapidly and can be easily titrated to variable patient responses. Nitroprusside dilates arteriolar and venous beds. The arteriolar dilation causes a lowering of SVR and a reduction in the impedance to left ventricular ejection. The ventricles can empty more completely, thereby increasing cardiac output. For the patient with severe heart failure, nitroprusside primarily reduces afterload.[12] The nurse sees this reflected in a decreased PAWP and increased cardiac output. Frequent hemodynamic monitoring and assessment are necessary to achieve the appropriate responses to unloading therapy.[68]

Other agents used to dilate the arterial bed are phentolamine, hydralazine, and minoxidil (arterial dilators); prazosin (venous and arterial dilator); and the angiotensin-converting enzyme (ACE) inhibitors such as captopril, enalapril, and lisinopril (venous and arterial dilators) (see Chapter 11). The *ACE inhibitors* have shown promise as treatment for advanced congestive heart failure because, in addition to decreasing preload and afterload, they exert beneficial effects on coronary and renal hemodynamics and reduce circulating levels of norepinephrine and aldosterone.[15] Vasodilators also may be combined to produce enhanced synergistic effects. For example, hydralazine and isosorbide, in addition to digoxin and diuretics, favorably affect left ventricular function and mortality rates.[19]

Contractility. Positive inotropic drugs are used to enhance myocardial contractility and improve cardiac output. Types of agents used include digitalis glycosides, catecholamines, and phosphodiesterase inhibitors. Digitalis preparations enhance contractility by increasing the amount of calcium available during excitation-contraction coupling. They can be administered parenterally and orally; thus they have been an important part of therapy because of a lack of alternative oral agents for chronic use. There is question, however, regarding the benefits of long-term digoxin therapy in DC. Spodick[81] stated that the global myocardial injury of DC is associated with an early refractoriness to digoxin and that the small, nontoxic doses that are needed will fail to support ventricular function.

Catecholamine agents include epinephrine, norepinephrine, dopamine, and dobutamine. These agents produce a positive inotropic effect by activating β-receptors, which eventually result in elevated intracellular levels of cyclic adenosine monophosphate (AMP).[73] Dobutamine has β$_1$-, β$_2$-, and some α-receptor activity and is the most frequently used catecholamine agent with the DC patient. In addition to increasing contractility, dobutamine also decreases preload and afterload. Hemodynamic responses to dobutamine may vary, however, with the extent of hypertrophy present.[11] Major limitations to the use of dobutamine have been that it requires intravenous administration and thus has not been used on a chronic basis and that tolerance to it develops because of down-regulation of β-receptors (see Chapter 11).[73] To avoid the tolerance problem, *intermittent dobutamine infusions* have been used

to improve the clinical status and exercise capacity of patients with severe heart failure.[49] Infusions are given for 48 to 72 hours every several months, as warranted by the patient's condition. Most often, they are performed in a hospital facility with ECG monitoring. However, the availability of machinery in the outpatient and home setting has prompted investigators to study the possibility of intravenous dobutamine infusions in the *ambulatory setting*. These studies have produced mixed results.[5,26] Proper patient selection is critical, and patients with end-stage heart failure or malignant dysrhythmias may not be candidates for nonmonitored outpatient infusions.

Amrinone and milrinone are examples of *phosphodiesterase inhibitors*. These agents inhibit cyclic-AMP degradation. The resulting cyclic-AMP accumulation elicits a positive inotropic effect and a potent vasodilatory effect. These effects improve hemodynamic parameters and increase myocardial oxygen demand to a lesser degree than dobutamine. Amrinone is approved for short-term intravenous use in patients with severe heart failure that is unresponsive to conventional therapy. Milrinone can be administered orally and intravenously and thus provides an alternative to digoxin for long-term use. However, it is only approved for severe refractory heart failure. Agents that may be available in the future are enoximone, imazodin, and prioximone (see Chapter 11).[73]

Other. Nursing care for patients with acute DC is aimed at continuous hemodynamic assessment, proper administration of medications, maintenance of indwelling catheters, prevention of complications of decreased activity, and psychologic support of the patient and family. Because of decreased activity levels and the potential for venous stasis, the nurse must assist the patient in changing positions at least every 2 hours, guide the patient in passive range of motion exercises, and provide antiembolic stockings. As the hemodynamic status improves, the patient will be weaned from intravenous inotropes and vasodilators, given oral medications for chronic use, and begun on a gradually increased activity regimen.

If the patient has atrial fibrillation, digoxin will usually be prescribed for rate control. Treatment of ventricular dysrhythmias is more complex. Patients with symptoms should receive antidysrhythmics; however, it is controversial whether patients without symptoms should receive antidysrhythmics because of their unproven benefit and potential prodysrhythmic effect in this setting.[87] In addition, in patients with advanced disease, clinicians are reluctant to prescribe conventional antidysrhythmics because of their negative inotropic effects. Amiodarone may offer the best results in this setting.[76]

The use of β-adrenergic blockade in selected patients with DC is under investigation. Studies of β-receptors in the myocardium provide rationale for this therapy. Catecholamine and sympathetic overstimulation causing *down-regulation* of β-receptors have been described as features of DC. If this is true, *up-regulation* of β-receptors by β-blockade could decrease myocardial energy requirements and protect the myocardium. Preliminary studies have shown promising results, but further evidence from prospective trials is needed.[38,76]

The use of corticosteroids in DC is controversial. Prednisone has been used on the basis that DC may be the end-result of an autoimmune response after a viral myocarditis. Results have been mixed, depending on the extent of the heart failure and the biopsy evidence of inflammation.[37] Investigators at the National Institutes of Health conducted a prospective, randomized trial of prednisone for patients with DC.[65] They reported small increases in ejection fraction with administration of 60 mg of prednisone daily; however, this effect was not sustained, and the drug's side effects were problematic. They concluded that this therapy should not be used routinely in clinical practice.

The alcoholic patient must avoid all forms of alcohol.[4,41,70] If the patient discontinues drinking and has not reached an irreversible stage of heart failure, complete recovery is possible. Bed rest may be necessary to allow time for the damaged heart muscle to heal. The period of time is individualized. It may take up to 6 months, depending on the degree of symptoms. Digitalis is used with caution because these patients are more sensitive to it and therefore are more prone to toxicity.

When counseling the alcoholic patient, it is not enough for the nurse or physician to suggest complete abstinence from alcohol. Health care providers must pay particular attention to stressors and identify problematic situations that patients are experiencing. Alcholism is not a simple problem but involves multiple behaviors. Treatment aimed at only the drinking behavior is unlikely to influence the other behaviors. Broad-spectrum cognitive behavioral treatments that involve consciousness and cognition should be used as treatment protocols.[67] Alcoholic patients cannot successfully change drinking behaviors without the support of family and significant others. Alcoholics Anonymous is a very effective support group. Dietary consultation also may help.

Hypertrophic cardiomyopathy

Although there is no known method of preventing HC, certain precautions may aid in averting complications. First, antibiotic prophylaxis to prevent bacterial endocarditis is recommended, especially for patients with obstruction. Second, patients with no symptoms who have mild disease but a normal ECG, no marked septal thickening, no ventricular dysrhythmias, and no family history usually are not treated but are observed closely. Patients who have the same characteristics except who have a definite family history receive propranolol or verapamil in hopes of retarding disease progression.[89] Third, although a woman with HC can bear children without problems, she is observed closely by a cardiologist for worsening symptoms and the need for propranolol therapy, especially in the latter part of the pregnancy. Fourth, factors that increase

FACTORS THAT AFFECT VENTRICULAR OUTFLOW OBSTRUCTION IN HC

INCREASED OBSTRUCTION

Catecholamines
Positive inotropic agents
Vasodilators
Diuretics
Blood loss
Tachycardia
Nonsinus rhythms
Exercise
Valsalva maneuver
Sudden upright position
Dehydration
Stress
Pain

DECREASED OBSTRUCTION

Propranolol
Verapamil
Expansion of blood volume
Squatting or supine position

ventricular outflow obstruction should be avoided (see the box). Thus vasodilators are not indicated, and nitrates are not generally used to treat angina in this population.

The aims of medical therapy in HC are to relieve symptoms, improve ventricular function by enhancing diastolic performance and relieving obstruction, and prevent dysrhythmias and sudden death.[38] Because of the pathophysiologic mechanisms of HC, no single form of treatment is successful in all patients, and several avenues of therapy may be needed before symptom relief is obtained.[10]

β-Adrenergic blocking agents are effective in alleviating symptoms such as dyspnea and angina in about 70% of patients. Nonselective agents such as propranolol are preferred to those with a cardioselective action.[89] Propranolol decreases the outflow gradient, decreases myocardial oxygen consumption, suppresses some atrial and ventricular dysrhythmias, and may enhance left ventricular relaxation. Because it inhibits tachycardia, it allows more time for diastolic filling, thus improving the ventricular volume needed by patients with HC. This is especially important during exercise.

The use of calcium channel blocking agents in HC is increasing; in fact, some investigators now favor verapamil rather than propranolol.[10] Although other calcium-blocking agents have been studied, data are much less extensive than that for verapamil. Verapamil reduces symptoms and improves exercise tolerance in most patients during short-term therapy and causes sustained clinical improvement in 50% of patients during long-term therapy.[10] These beneficial results probably result from verapamil's negative chronotropy, negative inotropy, increased ventricular relaxation, and improved diastolic filling.

Patients with end-stage HC may develop atrial fibrillation. If this occurs, it is treated as a medical emergency because atrial fibrillation with a rapid rate may degenerate into ventricular tachycardia or fibrillation.[22] Cardioversion is indicated for hemodynamically compromised patients. For chronic therapy, patients may require type I antidysrhythmics (see Appendix C), propranolol, or verapamil. Some patients require the judicious use of digitalis to control the ventricular rate adequately. There is also an increased risk of systemic embolization with atrial fibrillation; thus anticoagulants are used as long as the patient has atrial fibrillation.

Ventricular tachycardia is the most common factor associated with sudden death in HC. Patients with sustained or symptomatic ventricular dysrhythmias or those resuscitated from sudden death are usually managed with electrophysiologically guided antidysrhythmic therapy or with amiodarone.[10,76,89] *Amiodarone* decreases heart rate, produces negative inotropy, and enhances left ventricular diastolic performance. Disopyramide also is an effective drug because of its negative inotropic and antidysrhythmic effects. There are uncertainties regarding the management of patients with nonsustained asymptomatic ventricular tachycardia. These patients should be treated with standard antidysrhythmic agents until controlled trials have evaluated the efficacy of amiodarone in preventing sudden death in this population.[10]

Pacemakers have had a limited role in the treatment of HC. They have been used for complete heart block and bradycardia resulting from propranolol therapy. The use of DDD pacing is being explored as a method to improve left ventricular filling and ejection by synchronization of atrial and ventricular activity (see Chapter 16).[38]

Patients who continue to have severe symptoms and demonstrate an outflow gradient of greater than 50 mm Hg while receiving adequate medication are considered surgical candidates. Before surgery, these patients are at high risk for sudden death; thus the nurse must be alert to proceed with emergency care if needed.

Surgical treatment may involve a *myotomy* (incision into the septum) or a *myectomy* (resecting part of the hypertrophied septum). In some cases the mitral valve is replaced to alleviate severe mitral regurgitation or because it may be a significant contributor to the outflow obstruction. Surgery should not be considered a curative procedure because it does not alter the underlying morphologic and pathophysiologic features of HC. However, surgery is often successful in decreasing the systolic pressure gradient and reducing symptoms.

Nursing care after surgery is similar to care of any adult after cardiac surgery (see Chapter 17). The nurse should be alert for postoperative dysrhythmias that may require aggressive drug therapy and cardioversion. Varying de-

grees of heart block also may occur. The hospital mortality rate from the surgical procedure is 8%, with most deaths caused by fatal dysrhythmias.[60] After surgery, some patients may show less-than-optimal cardiac function with signs of continued heart failure. Vasopressors such as dopamine and phenylephrine may be required to maintain adequate cardiac output. Long-term (5 years) postoperative follow-up studies indicate that 70% of patients are alive with substantial improvement in symptoms.[54]

When congestive heart failure develops in the medically or surgically treated patient, treatment becomes difficult. Traditional therapies such as inotropic agents, diuretics, and vasodilators are thought to aggravate the outflow obstruction in HC. Although most patients who develop heart failure lose the outflow tract gradient, this is not consistently so, and these patients present unique problems. Although diuretics theoretically increase the obstruction to outflow, the combination of diuretics and β-blockers is effective in decreasing pulmonary venous pressures and dyspnea in these patients.[10] Cautious use of digitalis is not contraindicated, but its benefits are uncertain.[89]

Restrictive cardiomyopathy

Patients who have RC are treated with positive inotropic agents, diuretics, a low-sodium diet, fluid restriction, and vasodilators to reverse or decrease congestive heart failure. When severely ill, these patients may require hemodynamic monitoring. Patients may receive anticoagulation therapy to prevent mural thrombi.

If endomyocardial fibrosis is extensive, resection of the thickened endomyocardial tissue (*endomyocardiectomy*) may be performed with repair or replacement of the regurgitant AV valves. This procedure may alleviate symptoms for a short period but is unlikely to have long-term success because it does not correct the underlying disease process.[89]

Myocarditis

The treatment of patients with myocarditis is supportive and is aimed at the prominent systemic manifestations of the disease. When an etiologic diagnosis can be made, specific treatment is given with general supportive care. The use of corticosteroids remains controversial. They are not used with early infectious viral myocarditis because they are thought to enhance myocardial damage by increasing tissue necrosis and viral replication. Although corticosteroid use is controversial, it decreases the severity and incidence of subsequent valvular disease. The results of the ongoing Myocarditis Treatment Trial should provide answers to this controversy. The purpose of this clinical trial is to assess the efficacy of immunosuppressive therapy (prednisone and cyclosporine) in active myocarditis.[65]

Patients who develop fungal myocarditis are usually receiving immunosuppressive therapy, chemotherapy, steroids, or radiation therapy. Specific agents such as amphotericin B are used for treatment. For patients who develop bacterial myocarditis, specific antibiotic therapy or, in some cases, antitoxins are given. Symptoms of congestive heart failure are managed as with cardiomyopathy. Some patients may become so severely ill that they require ventilatory support, as well as general supportive measures. A regimen of modified bed rest is important. Myocarditis patients appear to be more sensitive to diuretics and digitalis, and the nurse should be alert for digitalis toxicity. Propranolol is usually avoided because of its negative inotropic action. Dysrhythmias and conduction disturbances are frequent. They can be life threatening and require aggressive drug treatment, temporary or permanent pacing, and cardioversion or defibrillation. Patients with myocarditis are at risk for pulmonary and systemic emboli, particularly when they develop atrial fibrillation and congestive heart failure. Anticoagulant therapy may be administered, but this should be used with extreme caution and observation because of the potential for hemopericardium if pericarditis is present.

General

Cardiac transplantation is the only definitive treatment for cardiomyopathy. Other treatment measures are palliative and do not address the underlying causes of the disease. Research to discover ways to prevent and detect cardiac myocyte dysfunction before decompensation continues.[1,33] Primary prevention efforts include the provision of appropriate genetic counseling and early recognition of cardiotoxins. Secondary prevention to control risk factors for structural damage includes dietary management, vigorous treatment of systemic diseases such as hypertension and diabetes, and avoidance of toxins such as alcohol, cigarettes, cardiotoxic drugs, and radiation.[1]

NURSING
DIAGNOSIS 2   **Activity intolerance related to acute or chronic illness (moving pattern)**

PATIENT OUTCOMES	NURSING PRESCRIPTIONS	EVALUATION
Patient will demonstrate activity below heart-failure threshold and will tolerate an individualized activity schedule.	Assess patient's tolerance to prescribed activity schedule and evaluate whether activity schedule is below heart-failure threshold.	Patient tolerated prescribed activity schedule. (List specific type or level of activity below failure threshold.)
Patient will not experience complications related to decreased activity:	Prevent complications related to decreased activity:	Patient did not experience complications related to decreased activity:
Patient will not demonstrate skin breakdown.	Assess skin (especially pressure points) and assist patient in turning frequently.	Patient did not demonstrate skin breakdown.
Patient will not demonstrate phlebitis or thromboembolism.	Assist patient with passive or active range of motion exercises and antiembolic stockings.	Patient did not demonstrate phlebitis or thromboembolism.
Patient will not demonstrate confusion.	Orient patient to time, place, person, and situation.	Patient did not demonstrate confusion.
Patient will not demonstrate discouragement or depression.	Initiate therapies to prevent or reduce depression, including encouraging family to visit and update patient on family, social, and community news; facilitating involvement in diversional activities; and guiding patient in relaxation and imagery exercises.	Patient did not demonstrate discouragement or depression.
Patient will not demonstrate pulmonary complications.	Assist patient with coughing and deep breathing.	Patient did not demonstrate secondary pulmonary complications. (If any did occur, list specific nursing intervention that corrected the problem.)
Patient with HC will maintain adequate cardiac output during activity. The patient or family will verbalize the physiologic effects of exercise in HC.	Teach patient the physiologic effects of exercise.	Patient or family verbalized the physiologic effects of exercise in HC.
Patient with HC will demonstrate knowledge of schedule, type, and frequency of exercise modification program.	Teach patient the schedule, type, and frequency of an individualized exercise-modification program.	Patient or family verbalized correct steps of exercise-modification program.

Plan and intervention for activity intolerance

Patients with any type of cardiomyopathy or myocarditis require individual activity programs. *Compliance* with an activity schedule is new for patients; therefore adherence may take some time. Frequent explanations regarding the importance of the activity schedule are necessary.

In deciding on the activity schedule, patients must participate in the planning stage. For the best results, the nurse should sit down with patients and write out the activity schedule with them and their families. If patients perceive the importance of the activity schedule and believe they have some input, they are more likely to adhere to the schedule. In doing this, the nurse must keep in mind that the patients' medical diagnosis is the foundation of the nursing care plan. The type of cardiomyopathy or myocarditis dictates the subject matter of teaching and items to include in the activity plan.[57] Goal setting is also necessary. When writing the objective or goal of activity with patients, the nurse should make sure it is specific, measurable, and dated.[50] When patients see it in writing, know what is expected, and know that it is important, adherence is increased. These care plans should be updated frequently as the patient's condition changes.

The degree of left ventricular failure determines the activity schedule for patients with DC, RC, or myocarditis. Patients with moderate-to-severe left ventricular failure may be comfortable with rest or light activity; however, severe symptoms may appear with exercise because patients have no cardiac reserve and are unable to increase cardiac output commensurate with the demands of exercise. The nurse and patient must decide on an activity schedule to avoid unwanted or poorly tolerated symptoms. Bed rest is often prescribed in the acute phase of illness to decrease the workload of the heart, decrease myocardial damage, and promote healing. The efficacy of prolonged bed rest, except in certain cases of alcoholic cardiomyopathy, has yet to be proved by research.[81] As ventricular failure patients approach discharge, a program of bed rest or a modified activity schedule is frequently necessary. The nurse must enlist the help of patients and families in designing the most effective bed rest or activity schedule for home. Information about the home environment is important. Patients may need hospital beds, wheelchairs, bedside commodes, or reclining chairs. If patients need to have their blood pressures checked with activity, then instruction on this procedure and information on ways to obtain blood pressure kits must be given. The temperature in the room must be controlled. Hot or humid environments can adversely affect the heart. Diversional activities involving television, telephone, radio, reading materials, or easy crafts should be discussed. As patients progress back to work and a busier day, the activity schedule again must be reevaluated. A day's schedule should be designed that focuses on activities of daily living—meals, bathing, toileting, rest periods, and interaction with family and friends. The help of a clinic, office, or home health care nurse may be necessary to tailor a bed rest program. Aggressive nursing interventions can facilitate adherence to an activity schedule, thus decreasing the need for readmission and providing a better quality of life for patients and families.

Patients with HC are assessed for level of activity. Some can play tennis, jog, swim, or ski, whereas others, because of severe obstruction, have increased risk of sudden death during or shortly after strenuous activity.

Because HC is an unpredictable disease, it causes different degrees of strain on the patient and family. Nurses should focus on the activity schedule to prevent problems and promote healthy lifestyles rather than as a treatment.[62] Teaching in a positive manner allows patients to accept the disease as something to which they can adjust with a healthy level of acceptance. Explaining the physiologic mechanisms of symptoms related to exercise gives the patient an understanding of any medical restrictions and a basis for planning activities.[22] In some patients, sedentary activities such as reading and listening to music and hobbies such as stamp collecting should be encouraged.

NURSING
DIAGNOSIS 3   **Hopelessness related to the unpredictable outcome of acute or chronic illness (perceiving pattern)**

PATIENT OUTCOMES	NURSING PRESCRIPTIONS	EVALUATION
Patient will talk about fears, stressors, and feelings of hopelessness.	Provide opportunities for patient to express fears, stressors, and feelings of hopelessness.	Patient verbalized fears, stressors, or feelings of hopelessness.
Patient will identify the roots of hopelessness.	Assist patients in identifying the roots of hopelessness.	Patient identified the roots of hopelessness.
Patient will verbalize hope and motivation by identifying strengths and positive coping behaviors, identifying simple daily goals, and demonstrating interest and curiosity in care.	Provide opportunities for hope and motivation, including giving patient feedback on strengths and positive coping behaviors, assisting patients with identifying simple achievable goals, and encouraging patient's interest and curiosity in care and the treatment regimen.	Patient verbalized hope and motivation by identifying strengths and positive coping behaviors, identifying simple daily goals, and demonstrating interest and curiosity in care.

Plan and intervention for hopelessness

Patients with cardiomyopathy or myocarditis with mild to severe heart failure often feel hopelessness. When these behaviors are not recognized, they become internalized, and patients become harder to reach. A simple turn in bed or brushing the teeth brings on acute awareness of the failing heart; patients become short of breath and exhausted. Nurses must try to *reverse states of hopelessness* to states of *hope*. Nurses are not separate entities from patients. Nurses are part of patients' hope and connection with life. As nurses become consciously and actively involved in patients' human struggles, they can exert influence over the course of an illness.

Patients with acute or chronic cardiomyopathy can feel stripped of motivation and hope while in crisis. The nurse should ask simple open-ended questions such as "What do you feel like doing?" or "What do you want to do different from yesterday?" Stated in a slow, easy, sincere manner such questions can often get patients to express some feelings of hope. Hope is increased when daily activities have structure that patients can control and personally affect.[29] Hope grows because patients act, see more options, and can identify goals. Simple decisions about self-care, self-feeding, or sitting in chairs, can be major steps in recovery.

Three major behavioral responses to loss of hope have been identified.[29] First, persons can have average optimism and hope but may lose the capacity to fantasize and resign themselves to fate. Second, with loss of hope persons may withdraw and become isolated to avoid being hurt by more unfulfilled hopes. Third, frustration resulting from lack of ability to meet goals results in destructive behavior.

Nurses must recognize the behavioral responses that patients with cardiomyopathy can exhibit, such as loss of satisfaction with progress, feeling totally out of control, loneliness, powerlessness, withdrawal, silence, and inward anger. Nurses can become aware of these feelings. Nurses are part of patients' lives, and there is information flow whether they realize it or not. If nurses do not recognize hopeless behaviors, they convey a hopeless attitude to patients. Nurses do this by viewing patients as they see themselves. When patients do not effectively interact, the nurse might mutually withdraw. Nurse withdrawal only reinforces patient hopelessness. Dubree and Vogelpohl[29] suggest the following assessment guidelines for dealing with hopeless patients:

1. Try to identify the roots of hopelessness.
2. Focus on the origin or root of hopelessness.
3. Assess family structure, interpersonal relationships, job, and income.
4. Assess the effects of treatments and medications.
5. Assess patients' current situation.

Dubree and Vogelpohl[29] state that the major intervention for hopelessness is attempting to motivate patients. After focusing on the assessment guidelines, the nurse can make appropriate action decisions that should involve the multidisciplinary team, patients, and families. Patients with acute or chronic cardiomyopathy or myocarditis must be provided with strength, hope, and optimism so that some positive alternatives can be identified to move forward. Strengths rather than weaknesses must be identified. Nurses must help patients establish simple and complex goals and identify progress in attaining goals. When a goal cannot be reached, a new one must be made. Hope is a powerful tool that nurses must recognize. It enlarges the nurse-patient relationship.

NURSING
DIAGNOSIS 4   **Powerlessness related to perceived inability to control outcome of disease process (perceiving pattern)**

PATIENT OUTCOMES	NURSING PRESCRIPTIONS	EVALUATION
Patient will verbalize feelings of loss of control and will identify situations in which powerlessness is felt.	Provide opportunities for patient to express feelings about self and illness.	Patient verbalized feelings of loss of control and identified situations in which powerlessness was felt.
Patient will focus on process-oriented events.	Assist patient to become process oriented and focus on situations that can be controlled.	Patient focused on process-oriented events such as diet and daily activities.
Patient will participate in decision making and identify alternatives to the daily schedule.	Facilitate patient decision making in daily activities and in identifying positive alternatives to the daily schedule, activities, diet, rest, relaxation, and sleep.	Patient participated in decision making and identified alternatives to the daily schedule.
	Create an environment to facilitate patient's active participation in self-care and assist patient in meeting self-care needs.	Patient actively participated in meeting self-care needs.
Patient will demonstrate an understanding of the treatment regimen and will have a sense of control over such situations.	Teach patient about the illness and treatment regimen and limit incidents that induce powerlessness.	Patient demonstrated an understanding of the treatment regimen and had a sense of control over such situations.
	Provide information and sensory preparation so that patient is prepared for procedures.	
	Eliminate unpredictable events by informing patient of scheduled tests and procedures.	

Plan and intervention for powerlessness

When persons have a critical illness, they often believe that they have lost control over their bodies, their routines of daily living, and their destinies.[17] Loss of control may increase subjective suffering and impede physical recovery.[44] Patients with cardiomyopathy and myocarditis often struggle to regain a sense of control in their lives.

The concept of control has evolved from research on the sense of mastery. Seligman's learned helplessness model,[74] Langer's perceived control model,[47] and Krantz' control and predictability model[46] are three related frameworks that provide insight into the concept of control and thereby offer guidelines for nursing interventions regarding powerlessness.

Seligman[74] states that *helplessness* is the psychologic state that results when events are uncontrollable; that is, they occur independently of all voluntary responses. Learned helplessness is the phenomenon whereby individuals, faced with an uncontrollable situation, lose their motivation to respond in the future to such situations. They perceive that actions and outcomes are unrelated. An important part of the development of this phenomenon is the attribution individuals make about the first situation. This attribution sets expectations for future situations. Expectations then determine helplessness behaviors.

Three types of attributions may occur in a noncontingent situation:

1. Internal (individual cannot control situation) versus external (individual and relevant others cannot control situation)
2. Global (occur in a broad variety of situations) versus specific (occur in a narrow range of situations)
3. Stable (chronic and long term) versus unstable (transient and short lived)

Based on research with these attributions, Seligman found that depressive or helplessness symptoms were associated with a style of explaining uncontrollable events to internal, global, and stable factors. A treatment strategy was then formulated for individuals to change attributions to more external, specific, and unstable factors.[2] This translates into assisting the individual to evaluate the situation in the following ways: (1) others like oneself could not control the situation, (2) it only occurred in this specific situation, and (3) it is transient and not a chronically recurring situation.

Langer[47] views the illusion of *control* as being the inverse of learned helplessness; that is, there is a perception that actions and outcomes are related. She further states that merely the belief that one has control may be more important than the actual exercise of control and that this perception of control is crucial to psychologic and physical well-being. Langer reports that the process of action, not its outcome, may be the critical factor in providing control. An outcome-oriented individual is goal-directed and may be mindless in performing tasks to reach the goal. A process-oriented individual focuses attention on task performance and feasible solutions rather than only on the goal itself. An individual with a process orientation is significantly more successful at problem-solving than an individual with an outcome orientation.

Krantz[46] contends that adverse reactions to an illness are mediated by feelings of helplessness induced by the illness, as well as by potentially threatening medical procedures. He hypothesizes there are two expectations in his control and predictability model:

1. Cognitive appraisal will be predictably linked to behavioral and physiologic responses.
2. Procedures that enhance the patient's behavioral or cognitive control should facilitate recovery.

These procedures include providing choices, encouraging participation, providing information, and increasing environmental predictability.

The information from these models assists in the development of nursing interventions for patients with cardiomyopathy or myocarditis who perceive loss of control. First, to interrupt the cycle of learned helplessness, nurses can assist patients to make more external-specific-unstable attributions for situations that they perceive to be uncontrollable. For example, if a patient is readmitted to the hospital with congestive heart failure despite following a low-sodium diet, the nurse helps them to realize that this happens to others, it relates only to this admission, and it is a transient event.

Second, to extend the perception of control, nurses can assist patients to become process-oriented rather than outcome-oriented. This entails focusing more on lifestyle changes (diet, activity, and taking medications), which are process events, than on the progression of their disease, which is an outcome event over which they have little control.

Third, nurses should use procedures that enhance patient control. Patients and families should be allowed to participate in their daily care as much as is realistically possible. The nurse focuses on what the patient can do, rather than on restrictions or limitations. Several alternatives are offered for the day's schedule, and patients are allowed to make some decisions about timing of rest and activity periods or personal hygiene requirements. The nurse assists patients to actively solve problems (e.g., ways to follow the sodium-restricted diet when eating out). By shared problem solving, patients are ensured greater control.[69] The nurse provides information about the disease process and treatment regimen so that patients understand the rationale for therapy and realize how essential their participation is to recovery (see Nursing Diagnosis 7). All procedures and equipment are explained, and the nurse introduces all personnel so that patients' environment becomes more predictable and less of a threat.

NURSING DIAGNOSIS 5 **Altered sexuality patterns related to physical condition and effects of treatment regimen (relating pattern)**

PATIENT OUTCOMES	NURSING PRESCRIPTIONS	EVALUATION
Patient and partner will discuss alterations in sexual pattern.	Facilitate discussions with patient and partner to identify alterations in sexual pattern.	Patient and partner discussed changes in sexual pattern.
Patient and partner will state one method for improving their sexual relationship.	Discuss with patient and partner ways for improving their sexual relationship.	Patient and partner stated a method for improving their sexual relationship.
Patient and partner will identify practices that conserve energy during sexual activity.	Teach patient and partner practices that conserve energy during sexual activity.	Patient and partner identified practices that conserve energy during sexual activity.

Plan and intervention for altered sexuality patterns

An altered sexuality pattern is the state in which an individual experiences or is at risk of experiencing a change in sexual health.[14] The expressions of human sexuality, such as fantasy, touching, holding, and intercourse, protect men and women against feelings of isolation.[71] For patients with cardiomyopathy or myocarditis, as with many other patients with heart disease, sexual encounters may be stressful and life threatening. The nurse allays fears by assessing the physical and psychologic status of patients, counseling patients and partners about sexual activities, and referring patients to appropriate sources if more follow-up is needed.

The physical status of the patient and the stability of the disease process are important indicators of the ability to tolerate the energy requirements of sexual activity. Orgasm itself requires approximately five metabolic equivalents (METs), which is roughly equivalent to climbing two flights of steps in 10 seconds. Therefore the decompensated patient with congestive heart failure has a vastly different tolerance limit than the patient with stable HC. The patient's physical status can be assessed by observing the ability to perform daily activities and exercise and by the results of graded exercise testing and ambulatory monitoring. It is important also to assess current medications to determine whether they may affect sexual response. Propranolol and captopril depress the sympathetic nervous system and may cause impotence in men and decreased vaginal lubrication in women. Chronic use of furosemide may also cause impotence.[14]

It is critical to evaluate the psychologic status of the patient and partner because the interrelationship between physiologic and emotional responses is what makes sexual activity so difficult to evaluate in terms of physical impact. Anxiety and depression are common psychologic responses manifested by patients with cardiomyopathy or myocarditis. Anxiety is due to fear of cardiac symptoms or cardiac death occurring during sex. Anxiety may also be caused by a body image disturbance resulting from decreased functional capacity. Depression or a grief response may occur and may cause a decreased libido and impotence. The partner's sexuality is also greatly affected; the partner may be torn between wanting to show love and affection and being afraid of the physical outcome of sexual activity.[71]

Counseling the patient includes: (1) explaining factors that may reduce oxygen consumption and conserve energy during sexual activity,[14,27,69,71] (2) discussing methods to eliminate discomfort during sexual activity, and (3) identifying untoward physical symptoms with sexual activity. The box lists factors that may conserve energy during sexual activity; this list should be individualized. Suggestions to eliminate discomfort during sexual activity include using water-soluble lubricants if vaginal lubrication is decreased,

properly taking prescribed medications before sexual activity to decrease the workload on the heart (vasodilators for heart failure and propranolol for HC), and using relaxation techniques (warm baths, deep breathing, and muscle relaxation exercises) to decrease tension.[14] Patients with severe cardiac impairment may not be able to tolerate the physical requirements of sexual intercourse. For them, alternate means of demonstrating affection such as touching, caressing, and massaging, may be needed.[69] Untoward responses during sexual activity that should be reported include rapid heart rate or breathing that persists 5 minutes after orgasm, feelings of extreme fatigue the day after intercourse, and anginal symptoms during or immediately after sex.[69,71]

Some patients also may need referrals to other health care providers. Sources may include psychiatrists and psychologists for psychologic concerns, marriage counselors for more intense relationship counseling, social workers for financial and occupational concerns that cause tension, and physicians for review and possible modification of medications affecting sexual response.

 ENERGY CONSERVATION MEASURES DURING SEXUAL ACTIVITY

ENVIRONMENTAL

Moderate room temperature
Familiar environment
Supplemental oxygen
Relaxed atmosphere: no time pressure, feelings of relaxation

PERSONAL

Familiar partner
Comfortable position (more decompensated patients may require positions with unrestricted breathing such as side-to-side)
Proper medications: as appropriate, prophylactic nitroglycerin, prescribed vasodilators, or propranolol
Stimulant avoidance: wait 2 to 3 hours after a heavy meal or alcohol and 1 hour after smoking a cigarette

Data from Carpenito LJ: Nursing diagnosis: application to clinical practice, ed 3, Philadelphia, 1989, JB Lippincott Co; Doyle B. In Kern LS, editor: Cardiac critical care nursing, Rockville, Md, 1988, Aspen Publishers, Inc; Rizzuto C. In Michaelson CR, editor: Congestive heart failure, St Louis, 1983, The CV Mosby Co; Scalzi CC and Burke LE. In Underhill SL and others, editors: Cardiac nursing, ed 2, 1989, JB Lippincott Co.

NURSING
DIAGNOSIS 6 **Impaired social interaction related to physical limitations, anxiety, or hopelessness (relating pattern)**

PATIENT OUTCOMES	NURSING PRESCRIPTIONS	EVALUATION
Patient will identify behaviors that disrupt socialization.	Facilitate discussion and provide feedback to patient regarding behaviors that disrupt socialization.	Patient identified behaviors that disrupt socialization.
Patient or family will describe strategies to promote effective socialization.	Assist patient and family to identify strategies to promote effective socialization related to family, occupational, and community roles.	Patient and family described strategies to promote effective socialization.

Plan and intervention for impaired social interaction

Impaired social interaction is the state in which the individual experiences or is at risk of experiencing unsatisfactory, insufficient, or negative responses from interactions.[14] In patients with cardiomyopathy or myocarditis, this impairment may occur because poor cardiac function limits the energy needed to perform social activities or because feelings of anxiety or hopelessness about the illness disrupt the usual role performance. The nurse must recognize aspects of the patient's behavior that are counterproductive to stable, supportive social relationships. This challenge is intensified when the patient is acutely or chronically ill because such a patient often is unable to express emotional needs; thus nurses must be able to assess the patient's behaviors accurately before determining appropriate nursing interventions. Billings[8] offers a model for helping nurses to identify emotional needs. This model is based on Horney's categorizations of "moving toward," "moving away from," and "moving against."[43] It is also based on the theory that a human being has needs that function as energizers through tension states.[56] When needs are met, a patient has more comfortable emotional responses and acceptable constructive behaviors.

Moving-toward behavior occurs when one person reaches out to another to achieve closeness. The effort of satisfying dependency needs is the central theme of this behavior. Typical behaviors include showing friendliness, attracting attention, and seeking interchange and companionship, as well as using demanding actions or seductive overtones, crying, or clinging. When moving-toward behavior is recognized, appropriate nursing intervention specific to dependency needs can begin. Some nursing interventions include increased numbers of nurses having contact with the patient, physical contact by touch or a squeeze of the hand, nurturing, parenting, anticipating requests, and giving praise and encouragement to increase self-confidence and independence.

Moving-away-from behavior occurs when one human withdraws from others. Frequently a patient is reluctant to share feelings until trust is established. Typical behaviors include continual lack of eye contact, denial of feelings, silence, superficial conversations, or avoidance of touch. These behaviors indicate that the patient has safety and security needs. The nurse must recognize these behaviors to intervene and help in the healing and recovery phase. Some specific nursing interventions include decreasing excessive nursing care, spending time with the patient to increase the trusting relationship, and recognizing dehumanizing nursing actions and changing them.

Moving-against behavior occurs when a person needs to remain in control and demonstrate power. Behaviors in this category include desperation, annoyance, anger, frustration, hostility, criticism, sarcastic humor, and frequent competitiveness. Appropriate interventions must be established. If not, the nurse is the one who receives negative behaviors. The nurse may interpret these behaviors as a personal insult, which leads to high levels of stress and a lack of humanistic care. An appropriate intervention might be for the nurse to be a facilitator in getting the patient to verbalize anger and then giving feedback about such feelings. The nurse can offer choices that decrease unnecessary power struggles. The family also must be included in the nursing intervention for all of these behaviors.

For the patient with cardiomyopathy or myocarditis, social impairment can occur in their family, occupational, or community roles. Family roles may include those of child, sibling, spouse, parent, or sexual partner. Difficulties may arise when families try to manage the illness and other aspects of life unrelated to the illness because there may be differences in perceptions of the illness among family members and ways that life goals should be achieved.[18] Corbin and Strauss[21] state that the most important feature of effectively managing the work of chronic illness is the ability to talk about it until an acceptable arrangement is reached. Nurses can promote this sort of collaborative relationship by helping families identify the source of the conflict and by reinforcing the importance of ongoing communication.

The disruption of occupational roles may be temporary or permanent, depending on the acuity and severity of the disease and the patient's physical ability to perform the occupational role. This disruption influences economic status and social relationships. The workplace is a major source of social interactions, which often fade when employment is relinquished.[18] Nurses need to assess the financial and social importance of work to the patient. Referrals can be made to occupational therapists or vocational rehabilitation counselors for job counseling and possible retraining and to social workers for assistance with financial needs.

Community roles may also be disrupted by the patient's lack of energy. The nurse must assess the importance that the patient places on community involvement and plan appropriate interventions. Patients may be encouraged to perform less physically demanding tasks, such as desk work or phone work, or may be referred to occupational or recreational therapists for alternate suggestions for leisure activities.

NURSING DIAGNOSIS 7   **High risk for noncompliance related to inadequate knowledge about illness and complexity of medical regimen (choosing pattern)**

PATIENT OUTCOMES	NURSING PRESCRIPTIONS	EVALUATION
Patient will demonstrate a knowledge base (testing and questioning): including heart function; type of cardiomyopathy and cause if known; causes, signs, and symptoms of heart failure; disease limitations; life style adjustments and ways to modify or eliminate symptoms; diet, weight control, and medications (including name, dosage, action, frequency, and side effects); counting pulse; activity level; exercise regimen, and sleep and rest patterns.	Teach information about the illness and medical regimen to patient and family and evaluate the patient's understanding; information includes heart function; type of illness and cause; causes, signs, and symptoms of heart failure; disease limitations; life-style adjustments and ways to modify or eliminate symptoms; diet; weight control; medications; ways to count pulse; activity level (see Nursing Diagnosis 2); exercise regimen; and sleep and rest patterns.	Patient was able to verbalize, describe, explain, and demonstrate the information in the patient outcome. (Write specific dates and additional comments.)
Patient will demonstrate an understanding of when to report symptoms to physician and when to return for follow-up care and later tests.	Explain to patient symptoms to report to the physician and times to return for follow-up care.	Patient verbalized symptoms to report to the physician and times to return for regular checkup and laboratory tests.

Plan and intervention for noncompliance

As soon as the patient demonstrates a readiness to learn, the nurse should assess the patient's knowledge base. The teaching plan must be individualized. For example, the teaching plan for the patient who has end-stage cardiomyopathy will be different from that of the patient who has HC or minimal symptoms of heart failure. The specific areas to be taught are normal heart function, type of cardiomyopathy and cause if known, heart failure and symptoms, disease limitations, lifestyle adjustments (work, family, and recreation) and alternative choices, diet (salt and perhaps calorie restricted), daily weights (reporting more than a 3- to 5-pound weight gain), medications, counting pulse, exercise and activity schedule (emphasis on oxygen supply and demand during exercise), normal sleep and rest patterns, symptoms to report to the physician or clinic, follow-up care, and hope and motivation for a healthier state (see Nursing Diagnosis 3).

Helping patients with cardiomyopathy adjust to lifestyle changes is a big challenge for the nurse. When such patients are discharged, they are responsible for maintaining as symptom-free a state as possible. All information should be taught from a holistic approach, focusing on the patient's belief system and lifestyle.

For the cardiomyopathy patient to achieve as symptom-free a state as possible, nurses must expand their knowledge and approach to teaching self-care. *Self-care* can be defined as activities concerning health decisions and actions necessary for the patient to maintain a health level supportive of life goals or meaningful activities.[62] It is helpful for the nurse to assess whether the patient possesses the characteristics necessary to actively participate in self-care. These characteristics follow:

1. A health concept that focuses on the importance of self-care and self-responsibility
2. Desire and need to develop a health state that supports life goals and personal philosophy
3. Self-responsibility for the assessment of goals, strengths, and weaknesses that are realistic to attain
4. Establishing priorities, quality health goals, care criteria, and alternatives that are guides in health care
5. Self-responsibility to obtain quality health care

If assessment reveals a patient who cannot maintain a healthy state, the nurse must help the patient search for alternatives. At all times the family and significant others are included in the health teaching. Any change in the patient will also affect the family. Nurses must learn new skills to help challenge the patient in changing perceptions of how to maintain health.

Nurses must see themselves as *facilitators* and *counselors* and not just as educators. Many approaches to patient teaching put patients in passive, recipient positions, which never help them learn self-care. To motivate patients to avoid further devastating bouts of cardiomyopathy or myocarditis, nurses should individualize each teaching session. Adult learners accept only what is relevant to them. Teaching patients specific skills and knowledge helps them comply because the mystery associated with certain drugs, tests, and exercise programs is removed.

The nurse must assess the number of health care providers with whom the patient has had contact during the course of the illness. A patient may receive information from dietitians, physicians, physical therapists, many staff nurses, and clinical specialists. The patient is exposed to different explanations and teaching styles, many of which are contradictory, inconsistent, and sometimes wrong. Many problems of *noncompliance* are directly related to the increased complexity of tests and treatments and the lack of a single, trusted, compatible source for explanations, psychologic support, and counseling.

Having an acute or chronic health problem such as cardiomyopathy or myocarditis can be intellectually and emotionally overwhelming. As they teach patients about lifestyle changes such as diet, exercise, reduction in use of alcohol, weight reduction, and relaxation specific to the illness, nurses must seek information related to "barriers" that keep the patient from making lifestyle changes. When specific barriers are identified, the patient can be helped to find ways and techniques of establishing goals to overcome or decrease these barriers.

Learning specific idiosyncrasies and communication patterns of patients and the patient-family system is helpful when teaching and can be used to help the patient and family cope with change. During patient-family interactions, nurses must recognize that they are not the only educators. The patient and the family members often have a great deal of insight into how to institute a specific health change. Part of the holistic approach to teaching is learning how to be an effective listener (i.e., learning the skills of how to enter into the patient's world). Nurses who listen and question as they teach are most effective because they can integrate more information and perceptions about the patient's bodymind connections.

Four factors have been suggested for consideration in relation to compliance and noncompliance[28]:

1. Patient behavior necessary for performance of a new role
2. Patient's self-concept of moving from sick role or at-risk role
3. Roles played by families, significant others, and health professionals
4. Evaluation of the above roles

After an acute bout of cardiomyopathy or myocarditis, patients have new roles that must be accepted to decrease the risk of recurrence of complications. If patients have chronic cardiomyopathy, compliance behaviors are those of the *at-risk role*. If the patient demonstrates knowledge and competency in the sick or at-risk role, a higher level of health regimen compliance is expected. As nurses counsel and educate patients, they must assess the degree with which patients meet the outcome criteria.

The second important factor for the nurse to recognize is the patient's self-concept. *Self-concept* reflects the patient's life priorities, social and family roles, and sociocultural responses to different degrees of wellness and illness. The patient's compliance is maximized when there is evidence that the sick or at-risk role has been incorporated into self-concept.

The third factor influencing compliance and non-compliance is the *relationship* and behaviors of the patient's family and significant others in complementary roles. Compliance is enhanced when the roles of family and significant others are congruent or complementary with the patient's roles. When significant others reinforce compliant behaviors, compliance increases.

The fourth factor influencing compliance and noncompliance is that *patients have to evaluate their behaviors*. Patients have to view compliant behaviors as having relevance and self-value. For compliance to occur, all four of these factors must be present.[28]

KEY CONCEPT REVIEW

1. Which of the following statements are true about cardiomyopathy?
   1. The cause of the disease is usually known.
   2. It involves a disorder of the heart muscle that may be associated with endocardial or pericardial involvement.
   3. Cardiomegaly and heart failure predominate.
   4. The cause of the disease is unknown or unusual.
      a. 1, 2, and 3
      b. 2 and 3
      c. 2 and 4
      d. 2, 3, and 4

2. In the United States, the most common cause of myocarditis is:
   a. A virus
   b. A bacterium
   c. A fungus
   d. A parasite

3. Cardiomyopathies can be classified into which categories?
   1. Dilated
   2. Hypertrophic
   3. Restrictive
   4. Pericardial
      a. 1 and 2
      b. 1, 2, and 3
      c. 2 and 3
      d. 2, 3, and 4

4. The most common form of cardiomyopathy is:
   a. Dilated
   b. Hypertrophic
   c. Restrictive
   d. Pericardial

5. Which of these statements are true of dilated cardiomyopathy?
   1. It involves impaired contractility.
   2. It interferes with systolic ejection function.
   3. It can cause gross dilation of the heart.
   4. It causes an infiltration of the myocardium.
      a. 1 and 4
      b. 1, 2, and 4
      c. 2, 3, and 4
      d. 1 and 3

6. Which of these statements are true of hypertrophic cardiomyopathy?
   1. There is an enlarged ventricular septum.
   2. The ventricular wall becomes rigid.
   3. There frequently is an obstruction in the left ventricular outflow tract.
   4. The heart becomes enlarged.
      a. 1, 2, and 3
      b. 2, 3, and 4
      c. 1 and 2
      d. 1 and 3

7. Which of the following treatments are used for dilated cardiomyopathy?
   1. Positive inotropic agents
   2. Vasodilator agents
   3. Diuretic agents
   4. Antidysrhythmic agents

   a. 1 and 2
   b. 1, 2, and 3
   c. 2, 3, and 4
   d. 1, 2, 3, and 4

8. Inotropic agents are generally avoided in hypertrophic cardiomyopathy patients because:
   1. They may worsen the patient's obstruction.
   2. They may cause syncope.
   3. They increase the force of myocardial contractility.
   4. They increase end-systolic volume and size.
      a. 1 and 2
      b. 2, 3, and 4
      c. 3 and 4
      d. 1, 2, and 3

9. Patient teaching for a hypertrophic cardiomyopathy patient should include:
   1. Avoiding straining with bowel movements.
   2. Avoiding undue emotional and physical stress.
   3. Allowing rest periods.
   4. Exercising as much as desired.
      a. 1 and 2
      b. 2 and 4
      c. 1, 2, and 3
      d. 2, 3, and 4

10. Interventions to enhance cardiomyopathy patients' sense of control include:
    1. Developing process-oriented strategies
    2. Developing outcome-oriented strategies
    3. Providing information about the disease process
    4. Encouraging decisions about self-care
       a. 1, 2, and 3
       b. 1, 3, and 4
       c. 2, 3, and 4
       d. 1, 2, 3, and 4

ANSWERS

1. d	3. b	5. d	7. d	9. c
2. a	4. a	6. a	8. d	10. b

REFERENCES

1. Abelmann WH: Classification and natural history of primary myocardial disease, Prog Cardiovas Dis 27:73, 1984.
2. Abramson LY, Seligman MEP, and Teasdale JD: Learned helplessness in humans: critique and reformulation, J Abnorm Psychol 87:49, 1978.
3. Agatston A and others: Comparative study of the echocardiographic findings in hypertensive and nonhypertensive cardiomyopathy, Angiology 33:17, 1982.
4. Altman GB: Alcoholic cardiomyopathy, Cardiovasc Nurs 17:25, 1981.
5. Applefeld MM and others: Intermittent continuous outpatient dobutamine infusion in the management of congestive heart failure, Am J Cardiol 51:455, 1983.
6. Aretz HT and others: Myocarditis: a histopathologic definition and classification, Am J Cardiovas Pathol 1:3, 1986.

7. Becker AE: Pathology of cardiomyopathy. In Shaver JA, editor: Cardiomyopathies: clinical presentation, differential diagnosis, and management, Philadelphia, 1988, FA Davis Co.

8. Billings CV: Emotional first aid, Am J Nurs 80:2006, 1980.

9. Bjarnason I and others: Mode of inheritance of hypertrophic cardiomyopathy in Iceland, Br Heart J 47:122, 1982.

10. Bonow RO and others: Medical and surgical therapy of hypertrophic cardiomyopathy. In Shaver JA, editor: Cardiomyopathies: clinical presentation, differential diagnosis, and management, Philadelphia, 1988, FA Davis Co.

11. Borow KM and others: Physiologic mechanisms governing hemodynamic responses to positive inotropic therapy in patients with dilated cardiomyopathy, Circulation 77:625, 1988.

12. Breu C and others: Treatment of patients with congestive cardiomyopathy during hospitalization: a case study, Heart Lung 11:229, 1982.

13. Cardin S and Clark S: A nursing diagnosis approach to the patient awaiting cardiac transplantation, Heart Lung 14:499, 1985.

14. Carpenito LJ: Nursing diagnosis: application to clinical practice, ed 3, Philadelphia, 1989, JB Lippincott Co.

15. Chatterjee K, DeMarco T, and Rouleau JL: Vasodilator therapy in chronic congestive heart failure, Am J Cardiol 62:46A, 1988.

16. Chen C and others: ECG pattern of left ventricular hypertrophy in nonobstructive hypertrophic cardiomyopathy: the significance of the mid-precordial changes, Am Heart J 97:687, 1979.

17. Clark S: Ineffective coping: patient and family. In Kern LS, editor: Cardiac critical care nursing, Rockville, Md, 1988, Aspen Publishers, Inc.

18. Clark S: Quality of life for patients with progressive cardiac disability. In Jillings CR, editor: Cardiac rehabilitation nursing, Rockville, Md, 1988, Aspen Publishers, Inc.

19. Cohn JN and others: Effects of vasodilator therapy on mortality in chronic congestive heart failure, N Engl J Med 314:1547, 1986.

20. Colucci W and others: Chronic therapy of heart failure with prazosin: a randomized double-blind trial, Am J Cardiol 45:337, 1980.

21. Corbin J and Strauss A: Collaboration: couples working together to manage chronic illness, Image 16:109, 1984.

22. Courtney-Jenkins A: The patient with hypertrophic cardiomyopathy, J Cardiovasc Nurs 2(1):33, 1987.

23. Darsee JR and others: Hypertrophic cardiomyopathy and human leukocyte antigen linkage, N Engl J Med 300:877, 1979.

24. Demakis JG and others: Natural course of peripartum cardiomyopathy, Circulation 44:1053, 1971.

25. Diaz RA, Obasohan A, and Oakley CM: Prediction of outcome in dilated cardiomyopathy, Br Heart J 58:393, 1987.

26. Dies F and others: Intermittent dobutamine in ambulatory outpatients with chronic cardiac failure, Circulation 74:II-38, 1986.

27. Doyle B: Nursing challenge: the patient with end-stage heart failure. In Kern LS, editor: Cardiac critical care nursing, Rockville, Md, 1988, Aspen Publishers, Inc.

28. Dracup KA and Meleis AI: Compliance: an interactionist approach, Nurs Res 31:31, 1982.

29. Dubree M and Vogelpohl R: When hope dies—so might the patient, Am J Nurs 80:2046, 1980.

30. Egoville BB: IHSS, Nurs 80 10:51, 1980.

30a. Epstein ND, Lin HJ, and Fananapazir L: Genetic evidence of dissociation (generational skips) of electrical to morphologic forms of hypertrophic cardiomyopathy, Am J Cardiol 66:627, 1990.

31. Factor SM and Sonnenblick EH: Hypothesis: is congestive cardiomyopathy caused by a hyperreactive myocardial microcirculation (Microvascular spasm)? Am J Cardiol 50:1149, 1982.

32. Fallon JT: Myocarditis and dilated cardiomyopathy: different stages of the same disease? In Waller BF, editor: Contemporary issues in cardiovascular pathology, Philadelphia, 1988, FA Davis Co.

33. Firth BG: Southwestern Internal Medicine Conference: Chronic congestive heart failure—the nature of the problem and its management in 1984, Am J Med Sci 288:178, 1984.

34. Franciosa JA and others: Survival in men with severe chronic left ventricular failure due to either coronary heart disease or dilated cardiomyopathy, Am J Cardiol 51:831, 1983.

35. Fuster V and others: The natural history of dilated cardiomyopathy, Am J Cardiol 47:525, 1981.

36. Gillum RF: Idiopathic cardiomyopathy in the United States, 1970-1982, Am Heart J 111:752, 1986.

37. Goodwin JF: The frontiers of cardiomyopathy, Br Heart J 48:1, 1982.

38. Goodwin JF: Overview and classification of the cardiomyopathies. In Shaver JA, editor: Cardiomyopathies: clinical presentation, differential diagnosis, and management, Philadelphia, 1988, FA Davis Co.

39. Grady KL: Myocarditis: review of a clinical enigma, Heart Lung 18:347, 1989.

40. Guzzetta CE and others: Clinical assessment tools for use with nursing diagnoses, St Louis, 1989, The CV Mosby Co.

41. Haughey CW: Alcoholic cardiomyopathy, Nurs 80 10:54, 1980.

42. Herzog CA, Snover DC, and Staley NA: Acute necrotising eosinophilic myocarditis, Br Heart J 52:343, 1984.

43. Horney K: Our inner conflicts, New York, 1945, WW Norton & Co, Inc.

44. Janis IL: Foreword. In Langer EJ: The psychology of control, Beverly Hills, Calif, 1983, Sage Publications, Inc.

44a. Jarcho JA and others: Mapping a gene for familial hypertrophic cardiomyopathy to chromosome 14ql, N Engl J Med 20:1372, 1989.

45. Johnson A and Palacios I: Dilated cardiomyopathies of the adult I. N Engl J Med 307:1051, 1982.

46. Krantz DS: Cognitive processes and recovery from heart attack: a review and theoretical analysis, J Human Stress 5:27, 1980.

47. Langer EJ: The psychology of control, Beverly Hills, Calif, 1983, Sage Publications, Inc.

48. Laurent-Bopp D: Cardiomyopathies and myocarditis. In Underhill SL and others, editors: Cardiac nursing, ed 2, Philadelphia, 1989, JB Lippincott Co.

49. Leier CV and Unverferth DV: Medical therapy of end-stage congestive and ischemic cardiomyopathy. In Shaver JA, editor: Cardiomyopathies: clinical presentation, differential diagnosis, and management, Philadelphia, 1988, FA Davis Co.

50. McConnell E: How nursing care plans help you, Nursing Life 2:55, 1982.

51. McHugh MJ: The patient with alcoholic cardiomyopathy, J Cardiovasc Nurs 2(1):13, 1987.

52. McKenna WJ: The natural history of hypertrophic cardiomyopathy. In Shaver JA, editor: Cardiomyopathies: clinical presentation, differential diagnosis, and management, Philadelphia, 1988, FA Davis Co.

53. McKenna WJ and others: Arrhythmia in hypertrophic cardiomyopathy: exercise electrocardiographic and 48 hour ambulatory electrocardiographic assessment with and without beta adrenergic blocking therapy, Am J Cardiol 45:1, 1980.

54. Maron BJ, Epstein SE, and Morrow AG: Symptomatic status and prognosis of patients after operation for hypertrophic and obstructive cardiomyopathy: efficacy of ventricular septal myotomy and myectomy, Eur Heart J 4(suppl F):175, 1983.

55. Maron, BJ and others: Results of surgery for idiopathic subaortic stenosis, J Cardiovasc Med 5:145, 1980.

56. Maslow AH: Motivation and personality, ed 2, New York, 1970, Harper & Row, Publishers, Inc.

57. Meyer RM and Morris DT: Alcoholic cardiomyopathy: a nursing approach, Nurs Res 26:422, 1977.

58. Mullin CS: The medical consequence of chronic alcohol abuse, Boston, 1980, Division of Alcoholism, Department of Public Health.

59. New York Heart Association: Nomenclature and criteria for diagnosing diseases of the heart and great vessels, ed 6, Boston, 1979, Little, Brown, & Company.

60. Ng L: Nursing aspects of the surgical treatment of idiopathic hypertrophic subaortic stenosis, Heart Lung 11:364, 1982.

61. Norgaard A and others: Relation of left ventricular function and Na$^+$/K$^+$-pump concentration in suspected idiopathic dilated cardiomyopathy, Am J Cardiol 61:1312, 1988.

62. Nowakowski L: Health promotion/self care programs for the community, Top Clin Nurs 2:21, 1980.

63. Olsen EG: Endomyocardial biopsy, Br Heart J 40:95, 1978.

64. Olshausen KV and others: Long-term prognostic significance of ventricular arrhythmias in idiopathic dilated cardiomyopathy, Am J Cardiol 61:146, 1988.

65. Parrillo JE and others: A prospective, randomized, controlled trial of prednisone for dilated cardiomyopathy, N Engl J Med 321:1061, 1989.

66. Pasternac A and others: Pathophysiology of chest pain in patients with cardiomyopathies and normal coronary arteries, Circulation 65:778, 1982.

67. Pattison EM: Behavior modification in alcohol abuse, Behav Med 8:13, 1981.

68. Pierpont GL and others: Congestive cardiomyopathy: pathophysiology and response to therapy, Arch Int Med 138:1847, 1978.

69. Rizzuto C: Psychosocial problems in congestive heart failure: health care implications. In Michaelson CR, editor: Congestive heart failure, St Louis, 1983, The CV Mosby Co.

70. Rubin E: Alcoholic myopathy in heart and skeletal muscle, N Engl J Med 301:28, 1979.

71. Scalzi CC and Burke LE: Sexual counseling. In Underhill SL and others, editors, Cardiac nursing, ed 2, Philadelphia, 1989, JB Lippincott Co.

72. Schwarz FS and others: Determinants of survival in patients with congestive cardiomyopathy: quantitative morphologic findings and left ventricular hemodynamics, Circulation 70:923, 1984.

73. Schwertz DW and Piano MR: New inotropic drugs for treatment of congestive heart failure, Cardiovasc Nurs 26:7, 1990.

74. Seligman MEP: Helplessness: on depression, development, and death, San Francisco, 1975, WH Freeman & Co, Publishers.

75. Shaver JA and others: Clinical presentation and noninvasive evaluation of the patient with hypertrophic cardiomyopathy. In Shaver JA, editor: Cardiomyopathies: clinical presentation, differential diagnosis, and management, Philadelphia, 1988, FA Davis Co.

76. Shebetai R: Cardiomyopathy: how far have we come in 25 years, how far yet to go? J Am Coll Cardiol 1:252, 1983.

77. Shebetai R: Pathophysiology and differential diagnosis of restrictive cardiomyopathy. In Shaver JA, editor: Cardiomyopathies: clinical presentation, differential diagnosis, and management, Philadelphia, 1988, FA Davis Co.

78. Sirignano RG: Peripartum cardiomyopathy: an application of the Roy adaptation model, J Cardiovasc Nurs 2(1):24, 1987.

79. Slutsky R, Berger F, and Garver P: The effect of abstinence on left ventricular performance in asymptomatic chronic alcoholics, Cardiovasc Intervent Radiol 6:153, 1983.

80. Spodick DH and others: Preclinical cardiac malfunction in chronic alcoholism, N Engl J Med 187:267, 1972.

81. Spodick DH: Effective management of congestive cardiomyopathy: relation of ventricular structure and function, Arch Intern Med 142:689, 1982.

82. Sutton MG and others: Angina in idiopathic hypertrophic subaortic stenosis: a clinical correlation of regional left ventricular dysfunction—a videometric and echocardiographic study, Circulation 61:561, 1980.

83. ten Cate FJ and Roelandt J: Progression to left ventricular dilation in patients with hypertrophic obstructive cardiomyopathy, Am Heart J 97:762, 1979.

84. Unverferth DV: Etiologic factors, pathogenesis, and prognosis of dilated cardiomyopathy, J Lab Clin Med 106:349, 1985.

85. Unverferth DV and others: Factors influencing the one-year mortality of dilated cardiomyopathy, Am J Cardiol 54:147, 1984.

86. Uretsky BF: Diagnostic considerations in the adult patient with cardiomyopathy or congestive heart failure. In Shaver JA, editor: Cardiomyopathies: clinical presentation, differential diagnosis, and management, Philadelphia, 1988, FA Davis Co.

87. Vlay SC: How the university cardiologist treats ventricular premature beats: a nationwide survey of 65 university medical centers, Am Heart J 110:904, 1985.

88. Wenger NK, Abelmann WH, and Roberts WC: Myocarditis. In Hurst JW and others, editors: The heart, ed 7, New York, 1990, McGraw Hill, Inc.

89. Wenger NK, Abelmann WH, and Roberts WC: Cardiomyopathy and specific heart muscle disease. In Hurst JW and others, editors: The heart, ed 7, New York, 1990, McGraw-Hill, Inc.

90. WHO/ISFC Task Force: Report on the definition and classification of cardiomyopathies, Br Heart J 44:672, 1980.

91. Wingate S: Dilated cardiomyopathy I. Focus Crit Care 11(4):49, 1984.

92. Wynne J and Braunwald E: The cardiomyopathies and myocarditides. In Braunwald E, editor: Heart disease, ed 3, Philadelphia, 1988, WB Saunders Co.

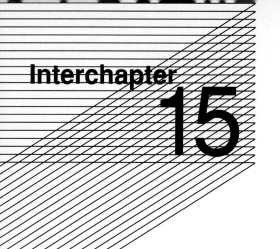

Interchapter 15

Have You Ever Had a Gut Feeling?

Have you ever had a "gut feeling" that your patient was about to have a cardiac arrest? Or develop pulmonary edema? Or cardiac tamponade? Did you listen to that gut feeling? Did it cause you to do anything different for that patient? For example, did you reassess the patient? Recheck the hemodynamic monitoring parameters? Recheck the intravenous drip? Call the physician? Place the crash cart outside the patient's door? These gut feelings are called *intuition*. Intuitive thinking occurs for each one of us. Some of us, however, ignore it. Others try to hide it. Still others value it and try to cultivate the process each day.

Most nurses recognize the importance of the rational, analytical, and verbal (or left brain) way of thinking that surrounds our practice. Many are not aware, however, of the importance of a nonverbal and intuitive (right brain) way of thinking (see The Right and Left Brain, p. 38). Unfortunately, in nursing, we have not placed much value on this intuitive "soft data." Intuitive perceptions have been viewed as opposing the empirical, factual knowledge base of practice.[6] We admit that we are among the many that have shared such a view. In our earlier critical care courses, we stated "We can no longer allow intuition to guide our practice. We need to develop the technical expertise to care for our patients and we must be able to justify our conclusions based on quantifiable data."

Adapted from Dossey BM, Keegan L, Guzzetta CE, and Kolkmeier L: Holistic nursing: A handbook for practice, Gaithersburg, Md, 1988, Aspen Publishing Co. and Guzzetta CE: Research in critical care nursing. In Dossey BM, Guzzetta CE, and Kenner CV: Critical care nursing: body-mind-spirit, ed 3, Philadelphia, 1992, JB Lippincott.

Not only quantifiable data are important in science. Scientific exploration involves analytical thinking, as well as a qualitative yet undefinable process that scientists use to organize fragmented findings into meaningful wholes.[3] This undefinable process is called intuition, or the tacit dimension, which is fundamental to all knowing.[4] It is a process whereby we know more than we can explain.

Clinical intuition has been described as a "process by which the nurse knows something about the patient which cannot be verbalized, or for which the source of the knowledge cannot be determined."[6] It is knowing about something even when there are no "hard data" to support that feeling. It is knowing without consciously using reason.[5] Intuitive perceptions, however, do not conflict with analytical reasoning.[2] Rather, intuition is simply another dimension of knowing. When analytic (left brain) and intuitive (right brain) thinking are used together, whole-brain thinking emerges.

Some exciting "hard data" have been published in the nursing literature to support the notion that intuitive processes are a valid means of conscious knowing and are necessary and desirable perceptions in nursing practice.[5,6] The intuitive experiences of 15 neonatal intensive care nurses, for example, were recently reported.[5] Taped interviews and field notes from the researcher were analyzed to discover factors that impact on intuitive thinking. The first factor identified related to nursing expertise; intuitive thinking occurred more commonly in experienced and technically adept nurses. The second factor involved nurse-patient relationships; intuitive thinking was more likely to occur when a loving, caring, and on-going relationship was established between the nurse

and infant. The third factor identified was the nurse's ability to discern subtle infant cues such as tone, posture, activity, and movement. The fourth factor was associated with the nurse's ability to correlate present perceptions to past experience. This factor is described as a kind of "deja vu" experience wherein nurses are able to link previous experiences to the present situation.

In another study, 75 intuitive events experienced by 41 nurses were analyzed.[6] One of the important outcomes of this study was to define the concept of the *intuitive product,* which is a conclusion or a judgment made because of what is intuitively known or a conclusion that is used to direct the nurse to do something. From this study, it was found that most of the judgments made by nurses from intuitive knowledge were correct. Thus the intuitive cues perceived by nurses culminated in clinical judgments that were useful in deciding on a particular course of action.

From the literature, other factors that facilitate intuitive processes have been identified.[6] Even if an experienced nurse provides ongoing direct patient care, the importance of intuitive perceptions must be recognized for the nurse to be open to intuitive information. Thus intuitive thinking demands that the process be valued. Likewise, nurses need to be receptive and have a desire to "tune in" to subtle cues and feelings that occur between two human beings. Emotionally and physically, they must be able to receive intuitive information. Physical and emotional problems experienced by the nurse reduce this receptivity because energy levels are low during times of stress and illness. In addition, nurses need to develop a sufficient level of self-confidence so that they are able to trust and believe in their intuitive perceptions. With self-confidence, the nurse is able to acknowledge and act on new levels (intuitive) of knowledge without feeling any discomfort about a lack of objective data.[6]

What then can be done to cultivate intuitive thinking in nursing? Although it cannot be taught directly, we can emphasize the value of intuitive thinking in our hospitals, continuing education courses, and nursing curricula.[1,6] We can teach the skills necessary to recognize subjective data and to verbalize feelings, cues, and decisions.[6] Intuitive experiences need to be shared with colleagues and students. Moreover, we must support nurses who have experienced intuitive events and encourage them to review and analyze the process. The usefulness of the cues in identifying problems and in making correct decisions should be evaluated. Finally, inexperienced nurses can be provided with subtle and repeated cue patterns that will assist them in recognizing intuitive information to increase their confidence about interpreting the cues and acting upon their decisions.[6]

Next time you have a "gut feeling," pay attention to your response.

REFERENCES

1. Garrity PL: Perception in nursing: the value of intuition, Holistic Nurs Prac 1:63, 1987.
2. Jung C: Psychological types, New York, Harcourt, Brace, 1959.
3. Polanyi M: Personal knowledge, New York, Harper & Row, 1958.
4. Polanyi M: The tacit dimension, New York, Anchor Press, 1966.
5. Schraeder BD and Fisher DK: Using intuitive knowledge in the neonatal intensive care nursery, Holistic Nurs Prac 1:47, 1987.
6. Young CE: Intuition and nursing process, Holistic Nurs Prac 1:52, 1987.

The Person with Pericarditis, Pericardial Effusion, and Cardiac Tamponade

Suzette Cardin

LEARNING OBJECTIVES

1. Analyze the dynamics of the pericardium.
2. Explain the major symptoms of pericarditis and constrictive pericarditis.
3. Compare and contrast acute pericarditis and constrictive pericarditis.
4. Identify and describe the major areas of nursing assessment for patients with pericarditis by incorporating the human response patterns.

5. Discuss the essential steps in preparing a patient for pericardiocentesis.
6. Formulate the medical and nursing diagnoses for the patient with pericarditis.
7. Evaluate the teaching plan for patients with acute or chronic pericarditis who are discharged while receiving corticosteroids. Make recommendations for nurses and staff for more comprehensive teaching and include families.

8. Evaluate for corticosteroid side effects in patients in a hospital setting. Have patients describe their feelings.
9. Explore patient outcomes, plan, intervention, and evaluation for each diagnosis listed for the patient with pericarditis.

This chapter includes the case of Ms. A.E. and her personal strengths, acute illness, goals, and recovery. Ms. A.E.'s case study reveals a powerful nurse-patient interaction based on consideration of the whole person. As described in Chapter 1 in regard to the bio-psycho-social-spiritual model, nursing care must extend beyond "a woman with an inflamed pericardium from unknown cause," as presented by the traditional medical model. It is easy to focus on the complex pathophysiologic condition and the myriad of laboratory tests and data. These are easily observed. However, when nurses recognize that their own consciousness interacts with the patient's consciousness, a whole new equation in illness and healing evolves.

SIGNIFICANCE

The recognition of pericardial disease dates back to Galen (131 to 200 AD)[1,27,31] who named the pericardium and noted the effects of pericardial effusion on heart motion. Pericarditis is an inflammation of the pericardium, which

may have a variety of causes and clinical circumstances. The pericardium can be primarily or secondarily affected by disorders in many different organ systems. The clinical picture can vary in onset from insidious to abrupt. It can be a benign and self-limited disorder that can be managed without hospitalization or a hemodynamically unstable disorder that can rapidly lead to death. Pericarditis is not just a body process; it is a process that also has an impact on the patient's consciousness.

ANATOMY AND PHYSIOLOGY

The *pericardium* consists of a double-walled sac. The inner serous membrane, the *visceral pericardium,* surrounds the heart and is in contact with the cardiac muscle, forming the external heart surface, or epicardium (Fig. 15-1). The outer fibrous sac, the *parietal pericardium,* is translucent and smooth. This layer is adjacent to the parietal pleura of both lungs. The parietal pericardium also separates the contents of the pericardial sac from other mediastinal structures. Within the pericardium are the heart and central

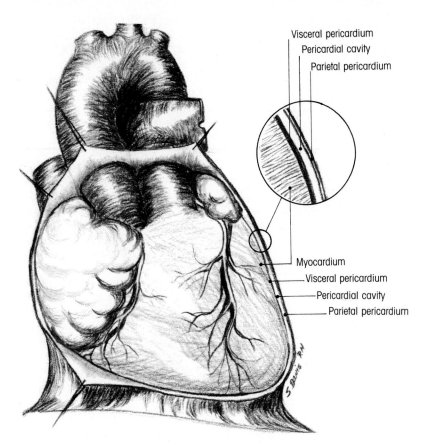

Visceral pericardium
Pericardial cavity
Parietal pericardium

Myocardium
Visceral pericardium
Pericardial cavity
Parietal pericardium

FIG. 15-1 The pericardium is a double-walled sac composed of visceral and parietal layers that create the pericardial cavity.

portions of the great vessels. The sac created by the parietal and visceral pericardium is called the *pericardial cavity* and contains pericardial fluid.

Pericardial fluid is similar in composition to lymph, and there is approximately 15 to 30 ml.[18] This fluid acts as a lubricant and decreases friction that occurs with continuous cardiac movement against the adjacent structures. The dynamics in the pericardial cavity are essentially the same as in the pleural cavity. The pressure within the pericardial cavity is negative. During ventricular filling the pericardial pressure often rises intermittently to a positive value. This process forces excess fluid into lymphatic channels of the mediastinum.

The pericardium limits the degree of outer dilation of the ventricles during exercise and hypervolemia, thus preventing excessive stretching of the myocardial fibers. It holds the heart in a fixed anatomic position and prevents the great vessels from kinking. It also helps decrease the spread of infectious processes from adjoining structures. The pericardium is not essential to life; a person can have congenital or surgical absence of the pericardium without any disturbances of cardiac function or clinical disease.[2,20]

ETIOLOGY AND PRECIPITATING FACTORS

The recognized causes of pericarditis can be classified according to etiology. The most common causes include an idiopathic or viral condition, uremia, bacterial infection, acute myocardial infarction, tuberculosis, neoplasm, and trauma.[18] Etiology is important because a specific therapy often can be designed, such as in malignancies, purulent infections, and parasitoses. Certain etiologic forms of pericardial disease also tend to induce tamponade, pericardial constriction, and effusive-constrictive pericarditis. It is important to obtain a history of previous illness and current or recent ingestion of medications that may include agents that cause or aggravate pericarditis, such as lupus-inducing drugs and anticlotting agents.

CLASSIFICATION OF PERICARDITIS

Pericarditis is the most clinically significant disease process of the pericardium.[18] The clinical spectrum of pericarditis may be considered on a continuum with four major presentations: (1) acute inflammatory; (2) effusive, characterized by an abnormal accumulation of pericardial fluid; (3) effusive-constrictive, a combination of compressive pericardial fluid and fibrinous-constrictive pericardial adhesions; and (4) constrictive with chronic pericardial scarring that surrounds the heart. A sequential evolution from acute inflammatory pericarditis to constrictive pericarditis is not always the norm because of the fact that pericarditis may present at different phases on the continuum, depending on the etiology.

PATHOLOGY

Pericarditis is an inflammation or alteration of the pericardium, regardless of cause. Because few diseases affect the pericardium alone, the cause of associated diseases must be investigated. Many inflammatory processes may involve the pericardium as a secondary complication.

In pericarditis the specific changes and alterations of the pericardium depend on the specific form. For example, viral pericarditis may cause degrees of serous fibrin deposition, dense adhesions, hemorrhage, or calcification. Bacterial pericarditis involves purulent and suppurative fluid and a loss of the transparent smooth surface of the normal pericardium. Tuberculous pericarditis has four stages and results in granulation and fibrinous and calcific changes in the pericardium.

Nursing process

Case study. At 2 PM Ms. A.E., 42-year-old wife, mother, and bank vice-president, arrived on the medical floor. She was anxious, afraid, and trying to remain in control. On that day she had delivered an important speech at a state bank meeting. She had tried to go back to her office to do some work but had started having chest pain and shortness of breath. When she arrived at the hospital, she received meperidine (Demerol), 75 mg intravenously, and oxygen at 3 L/min via nasal cannula. She had never been in the hospital before and was scared that her chest pain meant she was having a heart attack. Her brother was in another hospital's coronary care unit (CCU) with his first heart attack.

She had had a viral respiratory illness 3 weeks before admission that required no medical attention. She said she had not really felt well since that illness. She tired easily and over the past week had noticed exertional dyspnea and orthopnea. She thought these symptoms were related to stress and had planned to rest the following week.

On physical examination Ms. A.E. was found to have a temperature of 38.4°C (101°F), pulse of 136 beats per minute, respirations of 24 breaths per minute, and blood pressure of 124/90 mm Hg. During quiet respiration, she had pulsus paradoxus of 10 mm Hg. The systolic sound diminished as the cuff pressure was lowered to the diastolic level. She had no palpable lymph nodes in her cervical and axillary regions. There were diminished breath sounds and dullness to percussion over the lower third of the left lung posteriorly. Her point of maximum impulse was in the fifth intercostal space at the midclavicular line. She had a loud to-and-fro pericardial friction rub heard best at the lower left sternal border.

Ms. A.E's initial electrocardiogram (ECG) showed sinus tachycardia, low QRS voltage, and inverted T waves in leads II, III, and V_1 to V_6. The chest x-ray examination revealed a large cardiopericardial

silhouette with diminished pulsations on fluoroscopic examination.

Several hours later, her pain had lessened, but with deep breaths and movement, she grimaced, and her anxiety returned. An assessment of Ms. A.E. at this time showed that her personal strengths were intelligence, sensitivity, and ability to verbalize significant insight. She thought that she had probably caused this acute illness at some level because she had been pushing herself without stopping for the last year. The nurse and Ms. A.E. continued to talk with her husband and two teenage daughters who were present. The physical warmth and emotional support from her family was genuine.

During the evening shift of admission day, Ms. A.E. was having more difficulty breathing. She was moved to the CCU for close observation because she was believed to be at high risk for developing cardiac tamponade. After an hour in the CCU, she yelled for help. She was found in acute distress. Assessment revealed a blood pressure of 80/60 mm Hg, a pulsus paradoxus of 20 mm Hg, apical pulse rate of 160 beats per minute, respiratory rate of 36 breaths per minute, and faint heart sounds. Ms A.E.'s neck veins were fully distended on inspiration but collapsed on expiration. She was prepared for a pericardiocentesis and placed in a semi-Fowler's position; an intravenous normal saline infusion was begun to help raise her venous pressure higher than her pericardial pressure. The physician performed a pericardiocentesis, yielding 200 ml of serous fluid. Ms. A.E.'s condition improved immediately. Her cardiac tamponade was due to a rapid accumulation of fluid in the pericardial sac.

Nursing assessment

The nursing assessment of patients suspected of having acute pericarditis should focus on the following areas:

1. Knowing Pattern
2. Feeling Pattern
3. Exchanging Pattern
4. Complications
5. Findings from the diagnostic tests

Knowing pattern

When assessing the Knowing Pattern of the patient suspected of having pericarditis, investigate the history of the present illness not only to identify the causes of pericarditis but also to determine the patient's understanding and perceptions of the current situation. Investigate when symptoms were noticed by the patient, ways the symptoms have progressed over time, and the reasons the patient sought help from health care professionals. Investigate recent upper respiratory tract infections. For example, Ms. A.E. was found to have had a viral illness 3 weeks before admission.

Also assess patient and family knowledge about the illness and determine their understanding about how it is diagnosed and treated. Also identify signs of readiness to learn (e.g., the patient asking specific questions regarding the illness, testing procedures, and possible outcomes) and determine areas of misconception.

Feeling pattern

Patients suspected of having acute pericarditis are assessed for the classic triad of clinical signs and symptoms,[18,29] including precordial pain (assessed under this pattern), pericardial friction rub (assessed under the Exchanging Pattern), and dyspnea (assessed under the Exchanging Pattern). Within the Feeling Pattern, also assess anxiety.

Precordial pain. Precordial pain and pain tolerance vary with pericarditis. Some patients grimace and do not complain, whereas others panic. Patients in pain experience physiologic and psychologic changes. It is a complex example of body-mind-spirit connections.

> **Case study, cont'd.** Ms. A.E.'s pain was stabbing and was most severe with inspiration and when rotating her trunk. On occasion her pain was relieved by leaning forward. With pain medication and corticosteroid therapy, the nurses gave instructions on relaxation and the use of positive imagery (see Nursing Diagnosis 5). After the fourth day in the CCU, Ms. A.E. said that "thinking a peaceful thought" helped her relax and tolerate her pain, which was resolving.

Elicit information about the pain such as location, radiation, quality, quantity, timing, setting, and aggravating and alleviating factors. Precordial pain can be burning, sharp, stabbing, dull, deep, or just a constant ache. It may vary in intensity. Frequently, sharp pain sensations may be caused by pleuritic involvement and be hard to differentiate from precordial pain. As the lower parietal pericardial sac stretches, it may cause deep, dull precordial pain.[3,24,29] Although there are variations in pain, it is characteristically sharp and stabbing. Differentiation must be made between the pain of pericarditis and that of acute myocardial infarction (AMI), which can radiate into the neck and jaws and down both arms. The precordial pain of pericarditis often is aggravated by inspiration, coughing, swallowing, and rotation of the trunk. Sitting up or leaning forward may relieve or eliminate the pain. Typical precordial pain is located in the anterior aspect of the precordium and can radiate to the left shoulder, although the location and referred pain can vary (Fig. 15-2). The pain can be felt in the precordial area, right side of the chest, left shoulder, neck, trapezius muscles, and epigastrium.

The pericardium is innervated by the left phrenic nerve below the fifth or sixth intercostal space. The phrenic nerve is thought to have pain pathways in the left stellate ganglion because left stellate ganglion blockade may relieve severe pericardial pain. The pericardium also is innervated by nerve fibers from the vagus nerve, larynx, and esophageal plexus.[18] Most pericardial pain is caused by inflammation of the adjoining diaphragmatic pleura and structures.[24,25] Only the lower portion of the external parietal pericardium is pain sensitive[29] (Fig. 15-3).

Anxiety and fear. During the initial assessment of the Knowing Pattern, also focus on the patient's perceptions of the illness, as well as the symptoms. Nearly all patients have some degree of anxiety and fear. The degree of anxiety depends on the severity of the illness, patients' perceptions of how ill they are, and patients' past experiences with illness. Patients with pericarditis and pain can be mildly anxious, fearful, or panicked.

> **Case study, cont'd.** Ms. A.E.'s greatest fear on admission was that she was having a heart attack. Listening carefully, assessing her perceptions, and then giving simple explanations of her acute problem and pain medication and corticosteroids helped relieve her fear and anxiety. The nurse did not see her only as a patient with a dysfunctioning body process—an inflamed pericardium—but as an interacting whole.

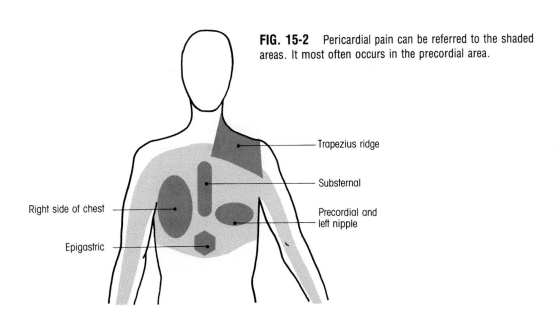

FIG. 15-2 Pericardial pain can be referred to the shaded areas. It most often occurs in the precordial area.

Trapezius ridge

Substernal

Right side of chest

Precordial and left nipple

Epigastric

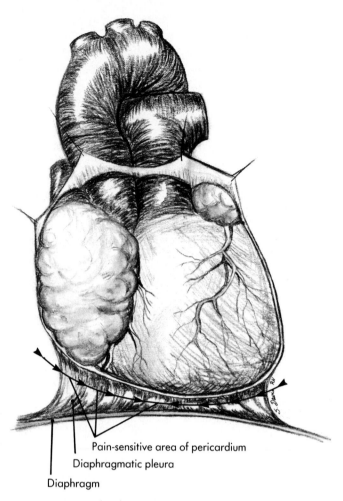

Pain-sensitive area of pericardium
Diaphragmatic pleura
Diaphragm

FIG. 15-3   Only the lower portion of the external parietal area is pain sensitive *(arrows)*, with pain resulting from the inflammation of the adjoining diaphragmatic pleura and structures.

If dyspnea is present, it can exacerbate fear and anxiety. The patient's family or significant others also must be included in explanations regarding pericarditis and its course. Family perceptions of the patient's illness are important assessment parameters. An anxious family can only compound an already stressful situation. Assessment of fear and anxiety should be an ongoing process. Common manifestations of anxiety such as sweaty palms or cold fingers, should be observed. A patient with pericarditis frequently breathes fast. Autogenic suggestions focusing on other parts of the body frequently help the patient (see Chapter 5).

The nurse must be alert to specific behaviors that can occur with different degrees of fear and anxiety, as well as with administration of corticosteroids (see Nursing Diagnosis 6). These activities include frequently turning on the call light, inability to remember or understand simple instructions or information, rapid speech, repetitious questioning, or wringing of the hands. The cause of anxiety may be more than the acute illness. If patients have a eu-

phoric response to corticosteroids, they frequently comprehend little of what is taught and underestimate the seriousness of their illness. Teaching always should involve families of patients receiving corticosteroids.

Exchanging pattern

The symptoms and complications of a patient with pericarditis vary. The nurse must identify the specific signs and symptoms to plan and treat the individual effectively at different phases of the illness and during recovery.

Evaluate the patient for the second and third classical triad of clinical sign and symptoms of pericarditis, which are a pericardial friction rub and dyspnea; also evaluate for systemic symptoms and complications related to pericarditis.

Pericardial friction rub. The most frequent diagnostic sign of pericarditis is a pericardial friction rub, which may or may not be accompanied by pericardial pain. In some cases, pericardial pain related to pericarditis appears before an audible friction rub, or pain may persist and a friction rub may never be heard.[12,30] Some patients may deny having pain even when friction rubs can be heard.[19]

Pericardial friction rubs are best heard during inspiration with the diaphragm of the stethoscope (Fig. 15-4, A). Friction rubs can be described as grating, scraping, squeaking, superficial, leathery, crunching, or scratchy. Because the heart is near the chest wall at the left middle sternal border and there is no pleural tissue to obstruct the sound, friction rubs are loudest and best heard to the left of the sternum in the second, third, or fourth intercostal space or in the mid-clavicular line. Friction rubs frequently change from one examination to the next. They rarely radiate. The sound of the pericardial friction rub results from the release of fibrinous exudate from irritated pericardial cells. This roughens the two pericardial layers, causing increased friction between them as the heart moves in the pericardial sac.[24] It is heard best when there is only a small accumulation of pericardial fluid. When there is extensive inflammation of surrounding structures, friction of the external parietal pericardium also may cause the rub.[18] In some cases it can only be heard if the patient rests on the hands and knees *(Mohammed's sign)*.[15,30] In some patients, respirations make no difference in the audibility of the friction rub.

As the heart moves with systole and diastole, the nurse may hear a *monophasic, diphasic,* or *triphasic* friction rub (Fig. 15-4, B). The triphasic rub is heard most frequently with each heartbeat,[33] producing friction sounds during atrial systole (presystolic), ventricular systole, and early ventricular diastole. The ventricular systole component is the loudest because heart movement is greatest at that time. In some situations rubs and murmurs may be confused. Murmurs radiate in a characteristic fashion, whereas rubs do not. Murmurs of multivalvular disease may be confused with gallop rhythms or friction rubs. Simple maneuvers

FIG. 15-4   A, Pericardial friction rubs are best heard in the second, third, or fourth intercostal space at the left sternal border. **B,** Pericardial friction rubs have presystolic (atrial systole), systolic (ventricular systole), and early diastolic (ventricular diastole) sounds. If all three sounds are heard, it is referred to as a *triphasic pericardial friction rub.*

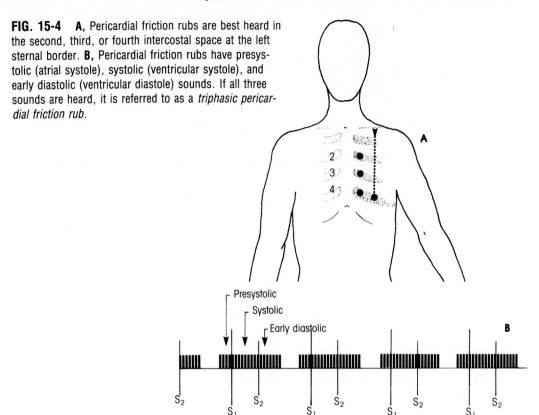

such as having the patient change position or do mild exercise and then auscultating the heart with a stethoscope may help differentiate the sounds.

Dyspnea. It is frightening to patients if they cannot catch their breath. Most patients are acutely aware of their breathing with pericarditis. Dyspnea changes breathing rhythm, and the pericardial pain prevents them from taking adequate relaxed breaths. This creates fear and anxiety, which affects breathing—an example of bodymind connections. The nurse must teach the patient techniques for relaxed breathing during assessment and recovery.

Patients frequently experience dyspnea with acute pericarditis or a moderate-to-large pericardial effusion. This results from compression of the bronchi or the lung parenchyma by the distended pericardium. Dyspnea with chest pain is also a frequent complaint, and patients may start breathing rapidly and shallowly or splinting their chest while breathing or moving. Patients with pericardial effusion frequently find some relief from dyspnea by sitting up and leaning forward. This causes the effusion to move downward from the base of the heart to the inferior heart surface and to the chest wall anteriorly.[18]

Systemic symptoms. It is common for patients to seek medical attention for complaints other than chest pain. They may report fever, chills, fatigue, malaise, nausea and vomiting, skin disease, joint pain, weight loss, and cough with hemoptysis, which may be related to the underlying pathologic cause of the pericardial inflammation. The most common systemic symptoms with pericarditis are chills, fever, and diaphoresis.

Complications of pericarditis. The three major complications of pericarditis are pericardial effusion, cardiac tamponade, and chronic pericarditis.

Pericardial effusion. Pericardial effusion occurs in the course of pericarditis from an accumulation of excess pericardial fluid. The rate of fluid accumulation varies. If it is slow, there may be no hemodynamic changes.[26,32] The rate and not the volume of fluid accumulation determines whether cardiac tamponade ensues. In chronic states in which the pericardium has stretched and adapted to the effusion state, the accumulated fluid can reach 1000 ml before hemodynamic changes occur.[6,13,32]

Cardiac tamponade. Cardiac tamponade exists when accumulated fluid in the pericardial cavity restricts diastolic ventricular filling (Fig. 15-5). This is a cardiac emergency requiring prompt and live-saving procedures (see Nursing Diagnosis 3). This critical state may occur with as little as 100 to 250 ml if the fluid accumulation is rapid. The most common causes of cardiac tamponade are bleeding into the pericardial sac after trauma (i.e., gunshot and stab wounds or iatrogenic trauma such as cardiac perforation during diagnostic procedures) and malignancy, pyrogenic infection, uremia, idiopathic pericarditis, or hemopericardium associated with anticoagulants.[6,9,18,32]

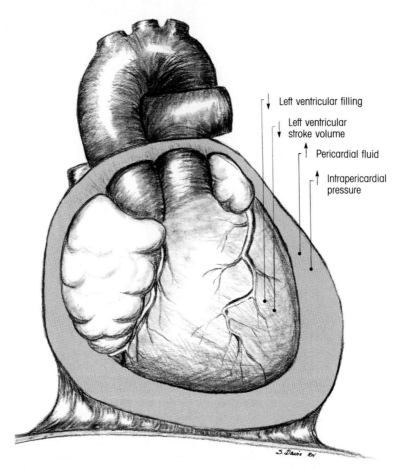

FIG. 15-5 The following hemodynamic effects may occur after pericardial effusion and cardiac tamponade: (1) accumulation of pericardial fluid, resulting in increased pericardial pressure, (2) elevated right atrial pressure, (3) elevated left ventricular end-diastolic pressure, (4) reduced left ventricular end-diastolic volume and cardiac output, and (5) elevated central venous pressure.

Chronic pericarditis. Chronic pericarditis takes the following forms: (1) chronic pericardial effusion, (2) effusive-constrictive pericarditis, (3) constrictive pericarditis, and (4) adhesive pericarditis. *Chronic effusion* may occur after pericardial inflammation. If it is untreated, it may result in constrictive pericarditis. *Effusive-constrictive pericarditis* is caused by a thickened visceral pericardium, resulting in cardiac constriction and effusion between the visceral and parietal layers.[25] When the pericardium becomes scarred, rigid, and unable to stretch, *constrictive pericarditis* exists. The severity of cardiac filling involvement depends on the rate at which the pericardial scarring occurs. In most cases of *adhesive pericarditis,* the entire pericardium and the adjoining mediastinal structures are involved. With adhesive pericarditis, cardiac filling usually is not affected.[14]

The cardiovascular system must compensate when cardiac compression states exist, such as with constrictive pericarditis, to maintain adequate diastolic filling. Systemic and pulmonary venous pressure increases, and an elevated central venous pressure (CVP) is sustained.

Clinical manifestations of complications. Assess the following parameters to evaluate possible ensuing complications of pericardial effusion and tamponade: diminished heart sounds, breath sounds, pericardial friction rubs, quality of the blood pressure, narrowing of the pulse pressure, presence of tachycardia or pulsus paradoxus, presence of Ewart's sign (determined by auscultating for tubular breath sounds and dullness over the left scapula) or Kussmaul's sign (increased neck vein distention on inspiration), or elevated CVP. These assessment parameters, with the physiologic changes, are listed in Table 15-1. More significant changes in these parameters occur with increasingly large pericardial effusion and cardiac tamponade.

Pulsus paradoxus is an exaggerated normal respiratory variation in arterial pressure. In patients without pericardial disease, increased inspiratory venous return to the right ventricle is offset by the huge volume pooled in the pulmonary vasculature. Thus left ventricular stroke volume transiently falls during inspiration. With pericardial effusion the inspiratory increase in blood to the right side of

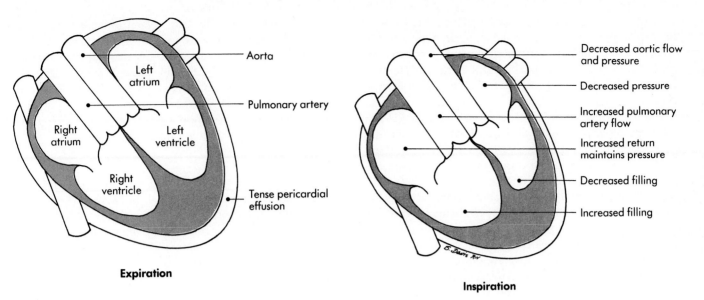

FIG. 15-6 Postulated changes in the ventricular size and hemodynamic changes that result from competitive filling of the ventricles, producing pulsus paradoxus.

the heart is more pronounced, which further restricts ventricular filling. During inspiration the increased capacity in the pulmonary vascular bed reduces pulmonary venous return to the left side of the heart, causing a significant reduction in left ventricular filling, stroke volume, and systolic blood pressure. In cardiac tamponade there is a sharp fall in the mean arterial and pulse pressures during inspiration.

Pulsus paradoxus is a decline of more than 10 mm Hg in systolic blood pressure with normal inspirations[9] (Fig. 15-6). To detect this condition, place a sphygmomanometer on the patient's arm and a stethoscope over the brachial artery. Instruct the patient to breathe normally. Inflate the cuff 20 mm Hg above the systolic pressure. Then listen, slowly deflating the cuff (1 to 2 mm Hg/sec) until the Korotkoff sounds appear only during *expiration*. (Sounds are first heard during expiration and then during inspiration.) Deflate the cuff until the Korotkoff sounds are heard equally well during inspiration and expiration. The *difference* between the level of blood pressure when sounds are first heard during expiration and when sounds are heard on inspiration and expiration determines the degree of pulsus paradoxus. This difference is normally less than 10 mm Hg. In patients whose breathing is normal and not obstructed, a systolic difference greater than 10 mm Hg indicates cardiac compression and possibly tamponade.

Pulsus paradoxus can be found in patients without pericardial disease such as those with congestive heart failure caused by chronic myocardial disease, obstructive lung disease, constrictive pericarditis, restrictive cardiomyopathy, and hypovolemic shock.[5,21] Pulsus paradoxus, an extension of the normal variation of blood pressure that accompanies respiration, may result in pooling of blood in the pulmonary vasculature during inspiration related to lung expansion and increased negative intrathoracic pressure.[18,21]

TABLE 15-1
Physiologic Changes Associated with Pericardial Effusion and Tamponade

Assessment parameter	Physiologic change
Dyspnea Diminished heart sounds Decreased friction rub (may not disappear) Increased anxiety or restlessness	Distention of pericardial sac
Hypotension and decreased pulse pressure Tachycardia	Reduced cardiac output
Pulsus paradoxus Increased CVP ECG changes (dysrhythmias, decreased QRS voltage, or electrical alternans)	Rapid accumulation of pericardial fluid and decreased circulating volume
Kussmaul's sign (increased neck vein distention on inspiration; neck veins normally disappear during inspiration)	Impaired right-sided cardiac filling
Ewart's sign (tubular breath sounds and an area of dullness heard over the left scapular angle)	Compression of the lung

In the left figure (Expiration):
- Aorta
- Left atrium
- Pulmonary artery
- Right atrium
- Left ventricle
- Right ventricle
- Tense pericardial effusion

In the right figure (Inspiration):
- Decreased aortic flow and pressure
- Decreased pressure
- Increased pulmonary artery flow
- Increased return maintains pressure
- Decreased filling
- Increased filling

Assessing for *cardiac tamponade* is a challenge. Be alert for it. The patient may be awake and alert with normal vital signs and then suddenly feel impending doom and panic. When fluid accumulates rapidly, a critical state may be produced with as little as 100 to 250 ml of pericardial fluid.[9,26,32] Physical signs accompanying cardiac tamponade include tachypnea (80% of patients), tachycardia (77%), pulsus paradoxus (77%), pulsus paradoxus with total inspiratory disappearance of the brachial pulse and Korotkoff sounds (23%), pericardial friction rub (29%), hepatomegaly (55%), and diminished heart sounds (34%).[18]

After cardiac injury from a knife wound, the development of a cardiac tamponade may momentarily save the patient from massive blood loss and death. In this situation the pericardial sac traps blood from the wound. This can be only temporary because of the rigidity of the pericardial sac, which results in excessive intrapericardial pressure. This impedes venous return to the heart and lowers stroke volume and cardiac output, and the patient will develop profound cardiogenic shock.

In patients with *constrictive pericarditis*, look for signs of chronic right-sided congestive heart failure. These patients have varying degrees of dyspnea, exertional fatigue, lassitude without paroxysmal nocturnal dyspnea, and orthopnea. Abdominal swelling, hepatomegaly, and peripheral edema also may be present. Over time, pulmonary and systemic venous pressures become equal because the pul-

monary venous system can tolerate these high pressures.[16,32] This is what causes right ventricular failure. Pulsus paradoxus and Kussmaul's signs are not as common as in cardiac tamponade.[9,18] In some patients with constrictive pericarditis a *pericardial knock* (loud and sharp third heart sound) may be heard. Sinus dysrhythmias, specifically atrial dysrhythmias, are common because the sinoatrial (SA) node lies just below the epicardium.

Diagnostic studies

Chest x-ray examination. In limited acute pericarditis the chest x-ray examination is normal. However, when a significant pericardial effusion is present, radiographically the cardiac silhouette is enlarged and may have a globular shape. The chest x-ray examination may help establish the specific cause of the pericarditis. When patients have tuberculosis or idiopathic pericarditis, pulmonary parenchymal changes, transient pulmonary infiltrates, or pleural effusions may help with the etiologic diagnosis.[18] Chest x-ray examination helps support the diagnosis of pericardial effusion when there is a rapid increase in the cardiac silhouette size and clear lung fields (Fig. 15-7).

Specific ECG changes. With acute pericarditis, distinct ECG changes of the ST-T−wave configuration, a decrease in QRS voltage, and the appearance of dysrhythmias occur in up to 80% of patients.[18] The changes in acute pericarditis

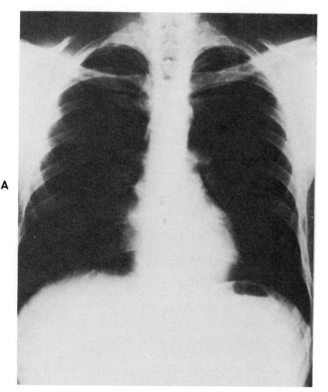
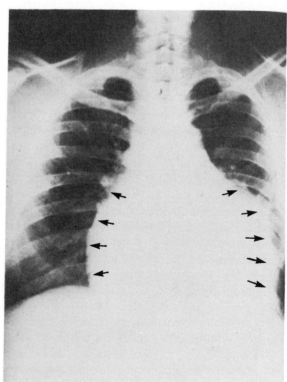

FIG. 15-7 **A,** A normal chest x-ray film. **B,** With pericardial effusion, the cardiac silhouette is enlarged with a globular shape *(arrows).*

are due to inflammation of the myocardium causing ST-T–wave changes and the presence of pericardial fluid or thickened pericardium, which short-circuits impulses and lowers the voltage. These changes must be differentiated from those associated with AMI. In acute pericarditis the ST segment initially is elevated and usually is concave upward (Fig. 15-8, *A*). The T-wave inversion occurs in precordial leads and is usually characteristic. After the acute phase of pericarditis the ST-segment changes return to baseline before T-wave inversion occurs (Fig. 15-9, *A*). There are no Q waves in acute pericarditis.

In contrast, in the early stages of AMI the ST segment is usually convex upward (Fig. 15-8, *B*). Q waves appear after 72 hours and are most always present,[28] Fig. 15-9, *B*, shows an inferior AMI at 4 days with Q waves in leads II, III, and aV$_F$. Although the ST-segment elevation is not as acute as with pericarditis, it does occur simultaneously with T-wave inversion. These are typical evolutionary changes of an inferior AMI.

If low-voltage QRS complexes occur with decreased voltage of every other beat, *electrical alternans* is present.

However, it may be caused by pleural effusion without pericardial effusion. If low voltage remains after aspiration of pericardial fluid, it probably is due to the insulating effect of fibrin in the pericardial sac[18,22] (Fig. 15-10). Two mechanisms of QRS alternans have been proposed: positional oscillation and aberrancy of intraventricular conduction. The mechanism of detection has improved with echocardiography. The concept of oscillation explains the fact that the P-wave alternans is seen predominantly with massive pericardial effusion.[11]

Dysrhythmias may occur with acute pericarditis. Atrial dysrhythmias and atrioventricular (AV) conduction disturbances are caused by SA node irritation because the SA node is near the overlying pericardium and becomes inflamed with the perinodal tissue and the pericardium.[17,23] Sinus bradycardia is the result of vagal stimulation caused by pericardial inflammation.[4] Sinus tachycardia is a common finding and is not directly related to congestive heart failure, fever, or inflammation.[7,8,23]

Laboratory studies. The differential diagnosis of certain causes of pericarditis is determined by specific cultures and

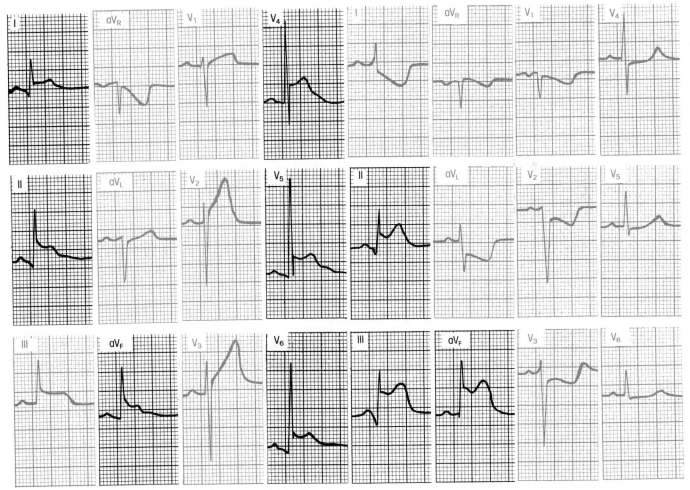

A

FIG. 15-8   **A,** In acute pericarditis, ST-segment elevation is typically upward and concave in leads I, II, aV$_F$, and V$_4$ to V$_6$. **B,** In inferior AMI, Q waves are present after 72 hours in leads II, III, and aV$_F$. ST segments are elevated upward and convex in leads II, III, and aV$_F$.

B

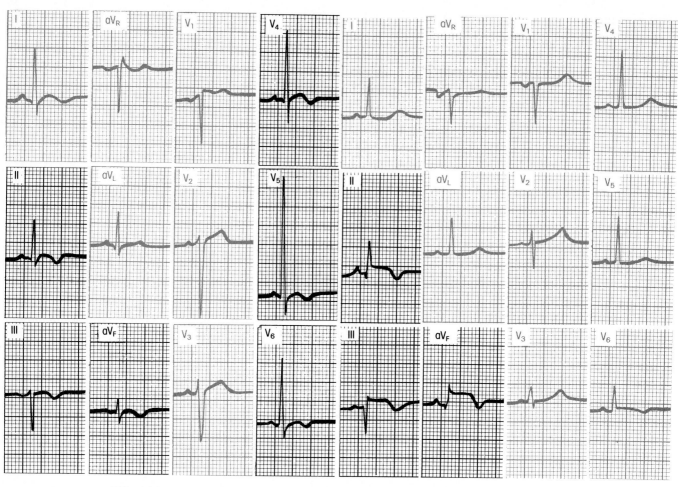

A

B

FIG. 15-9 **A,** The ST-segment elevation in acute pericarditis usually resolves before T-wave inversion (leads I to III and V₄ to V₆). **B,** In a patient with an inferior MI 4 days after admission, there are Q waves in leads II, III, and aV_F and T-wave inversion occurring, whereas ST segments remain somewhat elevated.

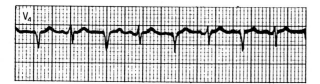

FIG. 15-10 In acute pericarditis and pericardial effusion, low voltage and electrical alternans of the QRS complexes may occur.

stains of different body fluids (Table 15-2). Because there is no specific test for idiopathic pericarditis, the differential diagnosis is made by exclusion of other causes. Some patients may require more extensive diagnostic tests to clarify the possibility of an underlying systemic disease.[18] In certain patients with acute pericarditis, further laboratory studies need to be done (Table 15-3).

Echocardiogram. Echocardiography is used to obtain a more definitive picture of pericardial effusion.[10,18] It is the most sensitive and accurate tool in detecting and quantifying pericardial fluid. The detection of effusion is one of the most useful applications of echocardiography. It helps in establishing specific types of pericardial disease. The echocardiogram outlines the cardiac chamber borders (Fig. 15-11). With a transducer, sound waves across the heart are picked up and recorded as reflections of the waves (echoes) off solid structures in their path.[10,17] A minimum of 20 ml of excess pericardial fluid can be detected by the echocardiogram.[10] Excess accumulation of free fluid in the pericardial sac creates an echo-free space between the ventricular wall and parietal pericardium.

Blood pool scanning. Blood pool scanning is a moderately sensitive test that requires an intravenous injection of albumin-labeled technetium or thallium to show the intracardiac blood pool, perfused myocardium, liver, and lungs simultaneously. If a patient has a pericardial effusion, the blood pool scan reveals an abnormal space between the heart and liver or between the heart and lungs.

TABLE 15-2

Diagnostic Tests for Patients with Acute Pericarditis

Test	Time and frequency	Reason for test
Tuberculin skin test	On admission	To assess previous tuberculosis exposure
Blood cultures	Three separate cultures within first 12 hours	To determine bacterial pathogens
Blood urea nitrogen (BUN) and creatinine levels	On admission and as necessary during clinical course	To investigate uremic cause
Cultures of throat, urine, and blood	On admission and during convalescent period (after 2 weeks)	To determine viral cause
Heterophil test	On admission	To detect infectious mononucleosis
Antinuclear antibody titer	On admission	To assess for systemic lupus erythematosus
Leukocyte and differential blood cell count	On admission and as indicated	To determine leukemic or infectious causes
Cold agglutinin test	On admission	To assess for mycoplasma

Modified from Braunwald E: Heart disease: a textbook of cardiovascular medicine, Philadelphia, 1988, WB Saunders Co.

TABLE 15-3

Additional Diagnostic Tests for Selected Patients with Acute Pericarditis

Tests or procedures	Reason for test	Specific test
Thyroid tests	To determine hypothyroidism if patient's clinical features suggest it	T_3 resin index, T_4 test, and thyroid-stimulating hormone test
Assessment of connective tissue disorders	To determine connective tissue disorders if suggested by patient's clinical features	Lupus erythematosus cell test, complement levels, extractable nuclear antigen test, rheumatoid factor, and skin or muscle biopsy
Pericardiocentesis	To determine bacterial pericarditis	Aerobic and anaerobic cultures, tuberculosis cultures, fungal cultures, cryptococcal antigen test, protein and glucose levels, and blood cell count (fluid saved for further testing)
	To determine therapy with neoplastic pericarditis	All the above, plus cytologic examination
	To determine cardiac tamponade	All the above
Fungal serology tests	To determine type of infection if patient is from endemic region	Coccidioidomycosis tests in Southwest and histoplasmosis tests in Midwest
	To determine type of infection in immunosuppressed patients	Histoplasmosis tests, coccidioidomycosis tests, and *Candida, Cryptococcus,* and *Aspergillus* organism tests

Modified from Braunwald E: Heart disease: a textbook of cardiovascular medicine, Philadelphia, 1988, WB Saunders Co.

Cardiac catheterization. In most patients, pericardial effusion is identified by echocardiographic studies. In cases in which a satisfactory echocardiogram is not obtainable, cardiac catheterization may be necessary. Cardiac catheterization is invaluable in establishing the hemodynamic importance of pericardial effusion. It confirms the diagnosis of cardiac tamponade or pleural effusion, quantitates the magnitude of hemodynamic compromise, and guides pericardiocentesis by documenting that pericar-

dial aspiration is associated with hemodynamic improvement.

Right-sided cardiac catheterization helps identify pericardial effusion by showing degrees of thickness of the pericardial shadow. The catheter tip is pushed along the inner wall of the right atrium. When pericardial effusion or thickening is present, the catheter tip is seen to be separated from the lungs by an opaque band.[2] The atrial wall is normally thin when seen radiographically. Pressure

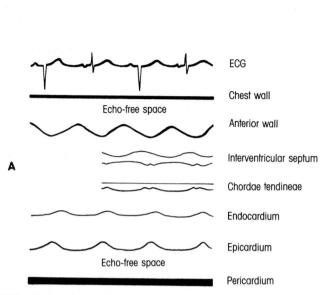

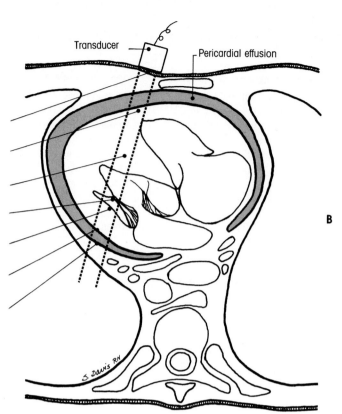

FIG. 15-11   A, Echocardiogram showing pericardial effusion. **B,** Echocardiographic technique for detecting the presence of excess pericardial fluid. After the proper position for the echo beam is established, the weaker echoes can be damped out manually, which allows visualization of a distinct echo-free space between the epicardium and the pericardium.

recordings are taken during the procedure to provide more detail in regard to pericardial effusion.

Medical and nursing diagnoses

The medical and nursing diagnoses associated with acute or chronic pericarditis and the presence of complications are derived from the specific areas of patient assessment previously discussed and the findings from the diagnostic tests.

The medical diagnosis is acute pericarditis and, if present, pericardial effusion or cardiac tamponade. The most common human responses anticipated for a patient with pericarditis are indicated by the following nursing diagnoses:

1. Pain related to pericardial inflammation
2. Decreased cardiac output related to structural factors (changes in the pericardium)
3. High risk for cardiac tamponade related to pericardial effusion
4. Decreased cardiac output related to chronic pericardial disease (Include this nursing diagnosis only if constrictive pericarditis present.)
5. Fear (mild, moderate, or severe) related to inadequate knowledge of disease process or to chest wall pain

6. High risk for noncompliance related to inadequate knowledge about illness and future care

For each of these diagnoses, the patient outcomes, nursing prescriptions, and evaluation criteria are outlined with a discussion of the factual information that supports the plan and implementation of care.

Case study, cont'd. Ms. A.E. started receiving 80 mg of prednisone in the CCU for rapid pain relief. About 5 days after her pericardiocentesis the prednisone was tapered 10 mg/day. (Teaching about corticosteroids was deferred at this time because of her continued acute anxiety; see Nursing Diagnosis 6 for corticosteroid teaching.) She also was taking indomethacin, 50 mg as necessary, for pain relief.

She again complained of pain and was fearful that she might be having another episode like the one before her pericardiocentesis. Assessment at this time revealed no increase in neck vein distention, stable vital signs without pulsus paradoxus, no dysrhythmias, and no change in QRS voltage. She continued to have distant heart sounds and diminished breath sounds. As she described her pain, it occurred again with trunk rotation and was sharp with each inspiration. On further investigation her new pain was not like her pericardial pain but had seemed like it because of fear. It became apparent that, as she had gotten out of bed on her own, she had pulled a back muscle. When she got back in bed, she was given a back rub, which allowed her to relax, slowing her respirations from 24 to 16 breaths per minute. She fell asleep for 3 hours without more medication.

NURSING
DIAGNOSIS 1   **Pain related to pericardial inflammation (feeling pattern)**

PATIENT OUTCOMES	NURSING PRESCRIPTIONS	EVALUATION

Patient will be pain free:
  Patient will verbalize that there is no pain.
  Patient will demonstrate no non-verbal cues of pain.
	Implement techniques for pain relief:
	  Instruct the patient to inform nurse of pain relief.
	  Assess for nonverbal cues of pain.
		Patient experienced no pain:
		  Patient verbalized that there was no pain.
		  Patient demonstrated nonverbal cues demonstrating relaxation and comfort.

Patient will achieve pain relief from pain medication and leaning forward on a bedside table as necessary.	Medicate for pain and provide a bedside table for patient support.	Patient achieved pain relief.
Patient will practice relaxation.	Guide patient in relaxation exercises.	Patient practiced relaxation.
Patient will remain in bed (except for going to the bathroom) until pain and fever are resolved.	Discuss with patient the need for remaining in bed (except for going to bathroom) until pain and fever are resolved.	Patient remained in bed.
Patient will ask nurse for assistance when needed in activities of daily living.	Assist patient in activities of daily living as needed.	Patient asked for assistance with activities of daily living.
Patient will achieve normal sleep and rest patterns.	Teach patient the need for normal sleep and rest patterns and encourage patient to take sleep medication as needed.	Patient slept comfortably 6 to 8 hours each night.
Patient will move in a normal manner during activities of daily living without splinting when breathing or turning.	Teach and assist patient to move in a normal manner during activities of daily living without splinting when breathing or turning.	Patient was able to move and breathe without pain.
Patient will tolerate passive range of motion (ROM) exercises.	Assess patient's tolerance for passive ROM exercises.	Patient tolerated passive ROM exercises.
Patient will be free of fever, chills, and signs of infection before discharge.	Assess for signs and symptoms of infection before discharge.	Patient was free of fever, chills, and signs of infection.
Patient will have decreased complaints of malaise or fatigue within 72 hours.	Assess for decreased complaints of malaise and fatigue within 72 hours.	General complaints related to pericardial inflammation were not elicited after 72 hours.
Patient will demonstrate an understanding of corticosteroid therapy, including action, dosage, schedule, and side effects.	Instruct patient on how to take corticosteroids, including action, dosage, schedule, and side effects (see Nursing Diagnosis 6).	The patient demonstrated an understanding of corticosteroid therapy. (Record specific dosages given and side effects.) (see Nursing Diagnosis 6.)
Patient will demonstrate no pericardial friction rub.	Assess patient for pericardial friction rub.	Patient was free from pericardial friction rub.
Patient's ECG will show normal ST segments and sinus rhythm before discharge. The characteristic ECG changes with pericarditis will resolve before discharge. (T-wave changes may not resolve for weeks to months.)	Assess and document patient's ECG.	Patient had a normal ECG.
Patient will tolerate laboratory studies necessary to rule out different causes (Tables 15-2 and 15-3).	Instruct patient on the necessity of the laboratory studies that need to be done to rule out different causes of pericarditis.	Patient tolerated laboratory studies. (State specific tests patient received and response to them.)

Plan and intervention for pericardial pain

Nurse-patient interactions are powerful events. They can set in motion a host of measurable psychophysiologic responses. In this case listening, touching, and assessing Ms. A.E.'s situation enabled the nurse to identify her fear, which resulted from a pulled muscle instead of more pericardial pain. The nurse's presence, touch, or words have an impact on the patient's consciousness and thus the patient's physiologic condition.

The usual clinical course of acute pericarditis is self-limiting and short term, from 2 to 6 weeks, when it is related to AMI, Dressler's syndrome, postpericardiotomy syndrome, and idiopathic, viral, traumatic, or drug-induced pericarditis. Patients with pericarditis related to idiopathic, viral, and connective tissue disorders may have one or more recurrent episodes of pericarditis over a 6- to 12-month period. If left untreated, there are higher morbidity and mortality rates in patients who have pericarditis related to tuberculosis, fungal or bacterial infections, neoplasms, uremia, or chest wall trauma. Neoplastic and bacterial pericarditis have the poorest prognosis even with appropriate treatment.[18]

Treatment of pericarditis is aimed at the major triad of signs and symptoms: chest pain, pericardial friction rub, and dyspnea.

Pain

Pain is a complex phenomenon perceived physiologically, as well as emotionally. Nurses must use many techniques, including medication, relaxation, distraction, imagery, listening, and touch, to relieve the patient's pain (see Chapter 5).

Pain management is an early focus in the course of the illness. The patient's pain is continually assessed, and clear descriptions from the patient are obtained to help differentiate pericardial pain from other types of chest pain. The nurse asks questions about the onset, quality, quantity, site, radiation, alleviating factors, and precipitating factors (that is, turning the trunk, deep inspiration, or movement). The severity of pain and type of pericarditis determine the type and strength of analgesics given. After pain medication is administered, the frequency of occurrence, description of the pain, and responses to the intervention should be charted and evaluated. Some patients require meperidine or morphine during the acute phase, whereas others may require only salicylates. Most patients receive relief from chest pain with indomethacin, salicylates, or other nonsteroidal antiinflammatory medications. For rapid pain relief, corticosteroids are effective. Patients should be monitored closely if they receive corticosteroids because of a possible relapse when the drugs are discontinued.[18]

During the acute phase, patients frequently develop sleep and rest irregularities from pain, corticosteroids, and many tests. Manipulation of environmental stimuli to provide a calm, soothing atmosphere should be done to increase patients' comfort and normal sleep patterns. It may be necessary to have limited visiting hours and to place a sign on the door stating "Patient sleeping—please do not disturb." During the acute phase, patients frequently get discouraged when they need assistance in activities of daily living. Much reassurance and many explanations about the course of the illness may be necessary to relieve their frustrations.

Pericardial friction rub

Close cardiovascular assessment, specifically of pericardial friction rub, is essential at least every 2 hours or more often if indicated. With the diaphragm of the stethoscope pressed firmly on the patient's chest, the nurse assesses the pericardial friction rub for location, quality, timing (continuous or intermittent), and number of cardiac components (see Figure 15-4).

ECG changes

The patient's ECG is monitored closely to distinguish changes of acute pericarditis from those of AMI (see Figs. 15-8 and 15-9). Specific attention also is given to occurrence of dysrhythmias, change in QRS voltage, or appearance of electrical alternans. These rhythm strips should be placed on the patient's chart and the physician notified of changes because they may warn of impending complications.

General considerations

The nurse monitors all tests and treatment of the underlying disease so that specific management can be undertaken and so that information patients will need to understand can be identified (see Nursing Diagnosis 6). For example, if patients have tuberculous pericarditis, they will need initial tuberculosis therapy and instructions for long-term therapy. These patients are treated with antituberculous drugs (isoniazid, rifampin, pyrazinamide, and streptomycin) and perhaps with corticosteroids if there is persistent cardiac compression.[18] Patients with rheumatic pericarditis receive aspirin and indomethacin and require long-term follow-up care. Corticosteroids may be used with these patients in the acute phase. When long-term steroid administration is needed to control pain and other evidence of inflammation, alternate day therapy should be attempted. Patients in whom steroids cannot be discontinued may tolerate tapering of steroids and weaning to nonsteroidal antiinflammatory agents.[18]

Nursing care is directed toward management of the pain and inflammation and observation of changes that suggest a fall in cardiac output and systemic venous congestion. Vital signs are checked every 4 hours or more often if indicated. A close watch should be kept on chills and diaphoretic patterns. Documentation should reflect whether these occur before or after salicylates are given to help determine the cause of the pericarditis. Some patients may need a warm blanket during a chill, and others may have a fever and require a cooling blanket. To decrease fatigue, malaise, and tachycardia, the patient should be encouraged to gradually increase activity.

Until fever and chest pain have subsided, the patient should remain in bed except to go to the bathroom. Increased activity too early may exacerbate symptoms. Proper positioning of the patient in the acute phase helps. Leaning forward on a bedside table frequently increases comfort.

Patients with acute pericarditis are almost always hospitalized at least for a few days to distinguish it from other problems that can cause acute chest pain. These conditions are AMI, acute pulmonary embolism, pleurisy without associated pericarditis, dissecting aortic aneurysm, mediastinal emphysema, spontaneous pneumothorax, or mediastinitis from esophageal rupture.[18]

NURSING DIAGNOSIS 2 **Decreased cardiac output related to structural factors (changes in the pericardium) (exchanging pattern)**

PATIENT OUTCOMES	NURSING PRESCRIPTIONS	EVALUATION
Patient will show resolution or absence of cardiac effusion or tamponade. As a result, patient will demonstrate hemodynamic stability and will have no dyspnea, diminished heart sounds and friction rub, hypotension (less than 100 mm Hg) and decreased pulse pressure (less than 20 mm Hg), tachycardia, distended neck veins, pulsus paradoxus (greater than 10 mm Hg), increased CVP, Kussmaul's sign, and ECG changes.	Assess patient for signs and symptoms of hemodynamic instability, including dyspnea, diminished heart sounds and friction rub, hypotension (less than 100 mm Hg) and decreased pulse pressure (less than 20 mm Hg), tachycardia, distended neck veins, pulsus paradoxus (greater than 10 mm Hg), increased CVP, Kussmal's sign, and ECG changes.	Patient demonstrated no dyspnea, diminished heart sounds or rub, hypotension or decreased pulse pressure, tachycardia, distended neck veins, pulsus paradoxus, increased CVP, Kussmaul's sign, or ECG changes.

NURSING DIAGNOSIS 3 **High risk for cardiac tamponade related to pericardial effusion (exchanging pattern)**

PATIENT OUTCOMES	NURSING PRESCRIPTIONS	EVALUATION
If pericardial effusion is present, patient will be prepared for special tests to determine the presence and amount of pericardial fluid (ECG, blood pool scan, echocardiography, chest x-ray study to determine heart size, cardiac catheterization, and radioisotope angiography).	Teach patient about the special tests that will be performed (ECG, blood pool scan, echocardiography, chest x-ray study, cardiac catheterization, and radioisotope angiography).	Patient verbalized proper instruction and information regarding specific tests. (Specify tests.)
If cardiac tamponade is present, patient will respond to emergency treatment. Specifically, the patient will demonstrate resolution of cardiac tamponade by responding to rapidly infused saline to increase venous pressure above pericardial pressure and to pericardiocentesis in presence of cardiac tamponade.	Assess for resolution of cardiac tamponade according to patient's response to rapidly infused saline to increase venous pressure above pericardial pressure and to pericardiocentesis in presence of cardiac tamponade.	Patient demonstrated resolution of cardiac tamponade by responding to normal saline infused rapidly, which increased venous pressure, and by tolerating pericardiocentesis without side effects.

Continued.

NURSING
DIAGNOSIS 3 **High risk for cardiac tamponade related to pericardial effusion (exchanging pattern)—cont'd**

PATIENT OUTCOMES	NURSING PRESCRIPTIONS	EVALUATION
If pericardial effusion is present, patient will demonstrate resolution of pericardial effusion by responding to corticosteroids to treat recurrent effusion, as well as antipyretics for fever and pain and specific medication for specific causes of pericarditis.	Teach patient about medications specific for pericardial effusion (corticosteroids) and for pericarditis (antipyretics for fever and pain).	Patient responded to corticosteroids, antipyretics, pain medication, and specific medications for specific causes of pericarditis.
If surgery is indicated, patient will demonstrate adequate understanding of presurgical and postsurgical information.	Assess patient understanding of presurgical and postsurgical information; teach specifics to patient as indicated.	Patient verbalized an understanding of presurgical and postsurgical procedures. (List specifics.)

Plan and intervention for decreased cardiac output and cardiac tamponade

Ms. A.E. was not treated as an object with a sick heart. Caring, touching, and explanations were given to help her clarify her feelings. Nurse-patient bonds are real; the flow of information between the two is omnidirectional and integral.

Medical and nursing management of pericardial effusion and cardiac tamponade is aimed at identification of the cause of the underlying disease process and aspiration or surgical drainage of pericardial fluid as needed. The various causes of pericardial effusions are identified and treated according to standard protocols (Table 15-4). Pericardial effusion with most forms of pericarditis usually resolves spontaneously over time. Oral corticosteroids typically cause a rapid resolution of the effusion. Some patients with effusion who have discomfort but no cardiac filling compromise may not respond to 2 or 3 weeks of oral corticosteroids, so pericardiocentesis may be needed. Instillation of nonabsorbable corticosteroids, as well as insertion of a plastic catheter into the pericardial cavity for further drainage, may be done. If a patient has neoplastic pericarditis, chemotherapy may be used. If there is a continual accumulation of fluid despite these measures, the surgical procedure of a *pericardial window* may be necessary. This is the surgical removal of a segment of the pericardium to establish continuous decompression and drainage.[18] It is rarely necessary in acute pericarditis.

The nursing plan and intervention are aimed at close observation and quick recognition of *subtle* or *drastic* changes in hemodynamic status, as well as managing increasing fear and anxiety (see Nursing Diagnosis 5). When there is a rapid accumulation of pericardial fluid in a short time, it can be an ominous sign and may be a warning of impending cardiac tamponade. The nurse should be alert for the signs of pericardial effusion or cardiac tamponade, recognize them, and know the physiologic changes involved (Table 15-1) and specific nursing actions to alleviate the symptoms. These findings are reported to the physician immediately, and the nurse should be ready to assist the physician in preparing the patient for specific tests and lifesaving procedures.

Rapid accumulation of pericardial fluid causes the intrapericardial pressure to increase from subatmospheric to positive values. The pericardial sac distends and assumes a globular shape. Because increased intrapericardial pressure impairs diastolic filling, venous pressure and right atrial pressure must increase to maintain cardiac filling. Thus distended neck veins and hepatic engorgement are seen. When the heart is surrounded by positive pressure, left ventricular filling is reduced, causing the stroke volume and arterial pressure to decline and the pulse pressure to narrow. Cardiac tamponade, producing hypotension and shock, occurs when the intrapericardial pressure equals the right atrial pressure.

Special tests to determine the presence and amount of pericardial fluid are echocardiography, blood pool scan, cardiac catheterization and angiocardiography, and contrast studies. The patient and family should receive adequate, clear, and simple explanations of all tests and procedures. Specific procedure permits must be signed by the patient or family.

Because of the risk for cardiac tamponade with a large pericardial effusion, equipment for pericardiocentesis must be readily available at all times.[33] Pericardiocentesis may be used for determining the cause or instilling medication

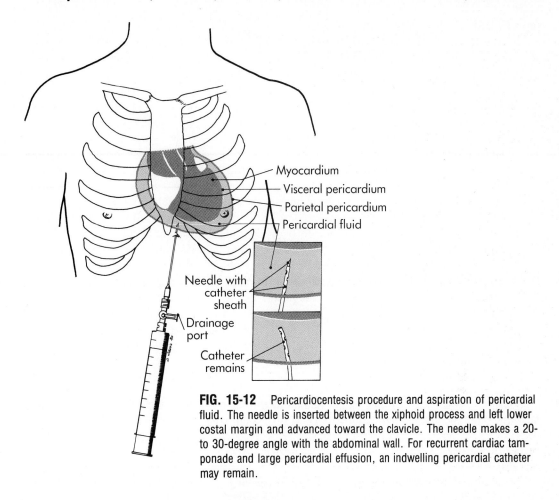

Myocardium
Visceral pericardium
Parietal pericardium
Pericardial fluid

Needle with catheter sheath
Drainage port
Catheter remains

FIG. 15-12   Pericardiocentesis procedure and aspiration of pericardial fluid. The needle is inserted between the xiphoid process and left lower costal margin and advanced toward the clavicle. The needle makes a 20- to 30-degree angle with the abdominal wall. For recurrent cardiac tamponade and large pericardial effusion, an indwelling pericardial catheter may remain.

in the treatment phase, as well as for a life-saving procedure. Regardless of the rationale, it must be done carefully and with constant monitoring because the risk of complications is high.[18]

Patients who are initially seen with cardiac injuries must be monitored closely because of the potentially lethal nature of such injuries. Early detection of cardiac tamponade may be necessary to save the patient's life. The clinical manifestations of cardiac tamponade are a drastic fall in cardiac output and systemic venous congestion. The increased intrapericardial pressure interferes with adequate cardiac filling, which results in a compromised state that is inadequate to support life.

Until the physician is ready to perform pericardiocentesis, the nurse should be ready to rapidly infuse saline or blood (as ordered) to raise the venous pressure above the pericardial pressure. Frequently the physician uses the *rule of 20* as a criterion for pericardiocentesis: pulses paradoxus greater than 20 mm Hg, venous pressure greater than 20 cm H_2O, and pulse pressure less than 20 mm Hg.

Pericardiocentesis procedure

As soon as respiratory distress is recognized or any other signs of cardiac tamponade develop, the patient should be

TABLE 15-4

Additional Management of Certain Types of Pericardial Effusion

Type of pericardial effusion	Specific therapeutic approach
Neoplastic pericarditis	Chemotherapy; injection of
Pericardial metastases	alkylating agents
Bacterial, tuberculous, or fungal pericarditis	Antimicrobial agents
Rheumatic fever, systemic lupus erythematosus, postcardiotomy syndrome, Dressler's syndrome, and benign idiopathic pericarditis	Corticosteroids
Uremic pericarditis	Dialysis

placed in high-Fowler's position (unless the condition requires a supine position); oxygen is administered, and a crash cart is kept ready with emergency drugs. The removal of 25 to 100 ml of fluid may have dramatic results. The patient should receive a tremendous amount of emotional support and simple explanations because this is a frightening experience. While one nurse is assisting the physician with the pericardiocentesis, another nurse should administer medications and intravenous solutions as ordered for pain and dysrhythmias. The pericardiocentesis procedure is as follows (Fig. 15-12 on p. 473).

1. With antiseptic solution, an area to the left of the fifth or sixth intercostal space is prepared at the left sternal margin.
2. A large-bore, short-beveled spinal needle attached to a 50-ml syringe and a lidocaine syringe (if the patient is not allergic to it) for local anesthesia are made available for the physician.
3. The physician will insert the needle between the xiphoid process and left lower costal margin and advance it toward the left clavicle. The needle will make a 20- to 30-degree angle with the abdominal wall. The chest lead is attached to the needle by an alligator clamp.

4. The ECG is watched for changes in ST segment. If the needle touches the epicardium, ST-segment elevation occurs, producing a pattern of injury. The ST segment is normal when the needle is in the pericardial space.
5. The pericardial fluid is checked for color, turbidity, and blood. Specific tests that also may be done are total and differential white blood cell count, bacterial and fungal cultures, cytologic studies, and glucose, cholesterol, hemoglobin, and protein concentration measurements.

Complications of this procedure are laceration of the myocardium or coronary arteries, vasovagal arrest, or ventricular fibrillation.[35] As the procedure is being performed, the patient's blood pressure, ECG, and anxiety level are closely monitored and appropriate intervention given.

For some patients who have recurrent cardiac tamponade and large pericardial effusions, successful medical management may require an indwelling pericardial catheter.[34,35] Corticosteroids, antibiotics, or antineoplastic agents may be instilled with specific types of pericarditis.

NURSING DIAGNOSIS 4	Decreased cardiac output related to chronic pericardial disease (include this nursing diagnosis only if constrictive pericarditis present) (exchanging pattern)	

PATIENT OUTCOMES	NURSING PRESCRIPTIONS	EVALUATION
Patient will demonstrate an absence or resolution of constriction and will not demonstrate evidence of peripheral edema; elevated CVP; fluid retention, abdominal swelling, exertional dyspnea, or lassitude; decreased pulse pressure; pulsus paradoxus; Kussmaul's sign; and ECG changes (low QRS, flattened or inverted T waves, conduction disturbances, or atrial fibrillation).	Assess patient for signs and symptoms of constriction, including peripheral edema; elevated CVP; fluid retention, abdominal swelling, exertional dyspnea, or lassitude; decreased pulse pressure; pulsus paradoxus; Kussmaul's sign, and ECG changes (low QRS, flattened or inverted T waves, conduction disturbances, or atrial fibrillation).	Patient demonstrated absence of constriction.
If there is constrictive pericarditis, patient will tolerate specific tests, including chest x-ray examination, liver function studies, or cardiac catheterization.	Teach patient about specific tests for constrictive pericarditis: chest x-ray examination, liver function studies, or cardiac catheterization.	Patient tolerated special procedures without complications.
Patient will demonstrate an adequate understanding of presurgical and postsurgical information (if surgery is required).	Assess patient's understanding of presurgical and postsurgical information (if surgery is necessary). Teach specifics to patient as indicated.	Patient demonstrated an adequate understanding of presurgical and postsurgical information and instructions.

Plan and intervention for decreased cardiac output with chronic pericardial disease

After the diagnosis of constrictive pericarditis is made with echocardiography, with or without radionuclide scanning, the treatment is aimed at the basic problem, which is mechanical. In some cases the only satisfactory treatment may be pericardiectomy.[18] The severity of symptoms, associated diseases, and the patient's age have to be considered.

In the management of constrictive pericarditis, chest x-ray examinations are used to identify specific calcium deposits, liver function studies are done to evaluate hepatic insufficiency, or cardiac catheterization is done to rule out myocardial and valvular disease. These patients also receive treatment of pain, anxiety, and complications and education (see Nursing Diagnoses 1, 2, 5, and 6).

Preoperative management of candidates for surgery usually includes several weeks of bed rest. Attempts are made to remove large pericardial, pleural, or abdominal effusions by aspiration. This is usually replaced by a similar quantity of intravenous salt-poor albumin or plasma. Complications from these procedures, such as hypotension, bleeding, or pneumothorax, occur. The procedures should be performed by experienced physicians, and the patients are monitored in a critical care setting. Patients with tuberculous pericarditis should receive antituberculous medications for 2 weeks before and then after surgery.

A *complete pericardiectomy* involving removal of the parietal and visceral layers of the pericardium, is indicated for patients with constrictive pericarditis.[18,36] The procedure is performed through a median sternotomy or left thoracotomy, with the cardiopulmonary bypass team "on standby" because of the high risk of blood loss and myo-cardial tear. Complete removal of the pericardium from phrenic nerve to phrenic nerve with a freeing of the venae cavae from fibrous tissue is the most common procedure for constrictive pericarditis. The left ventricle is freed first to avoid acute pulmonary edema; then the right ventricular constrictions are released, which results in increasing pulmonary blood flow. The adhesive process may involve the coronary arteries and veins, and extreme caution is needed to avoid these structures. Care also is taken to avoid the phrenic nerve where it leaves the pericardium and enters the diaphragm. Sometimes calcium may infiltrate the myocardium, and the surgeon may be unable to completely remove the pericardium. Drainage tubes are inserted before closing the incision. Long-term results are best when a total or near-total pericardiectomy is performed.[18]

Case study, cont'd. Ms. A.E. described her hospital recovery as frustrating rather than anxiety producing. She was frustrated because she had work in her hospital room pertaining to her job but she didn't feel like doing it. Also, she had viral pericarditis, which had no specific cure. A question she frequently asked was, "Why couldn't it be bacterial so I could have antibiotics and it would be gone?" She was aware of denying that she really had pericarditis. Although she had a great deal of energy, as a side effect of the corticosteroids, she found that the simple activity of getting out of bed and going across the hall to the nurses' station sent her pulse to 110 beats per minute. She was alarmed at her voracious appetite and feared weight gain.

The nursing care emphasis at this time for Ms. A.E. was periods of rest, gradual activity increases, explanations about medications, and twice during each shift, talks about her anxieties and work on specific goals for her recovery. This was extremely important. She was an intelligent, responsible woman, and the prednisone made her unrealistic about what she was physiologically capable of doing.

NURSING DIAGNOSIS 5	**Fear (mild, moderate, or severe) related to inadequate knowledge of disease process or to chest wall pain (feeling pattern)**	
PATIENT OUTCOMES	NURSING PRESCRIPTIONS	EVALUATION
Patient will demonstrate knowledge about the course of pericarditis and have decreased anxiety.	Teach patient about the course of pericarditis.	Patient demonstrated an understanding of adequate information about the course of pericarditis.
Patient will verbalize fear and talk spontaneously about it.	Assess fear and anxiety; encourage discussion regarding fears and anxiety.	Patient verbalized and talked about fears.
Patient will tell the nurse when pain is occurring.	Teach patient to report any occurrence of pain.	Patient reported chest wall pain.
Patient and family or significant others will communicate stressors of illness with each other and the nursing and medical staff.	Discuss stressors of the illness with patient and family or significant others and have them communicate stressors of illness with each other and the nursing and medical staff.	Patient and family communicated stressors to the nursing and medical staff.
Patient will use coping mechanisms during course of pericarditis.	Assess and encourage coping behaviors during the course of pericarditis.	Patient used effective coping mechanisms.
Patient will practice relaxation and imagery exercises during recovery.	Guide patient in relaxation and imagery exercises during recovery.	Patient used relaxation and imagery exercises during recovery.

Plan and intervention for fear

Nursing is not a neutral event. Taking special time with Ms. A.E., a basic nursing act, became a powerful tool. Although she was receiving corticosteroids, goal setting allowed her to make realistic bodymind connections, which decreased her frustration. As explained in Chapter 1, consciousness affects health and can be a help to nurses. The nurses enlisted the patient's psychologic forces to aid her own healing, even though these forces were altered by medication. Information flow from the psyche is pervasive throughout the body. The bio-psycho-social-spiritual model warns us against the fragmentation of our patients.

During acute episodes of anxiety, nurses must *actively listen* to patients and give clear, concise explanations about what is going on. If possible, nurses should spend at least 10 minutes or longer two or three times a shift to obtain clear perceptions about how patients understand their states. During periods of fear no demands should be made on patients.

Ask questions to facilitate identification of *specific sources* of fear. Family members and significant others should be included whenever possible because they are a part of the information flow for the patient. A worried family member certainly can convey this to the patient, thus increasing the patient's fear. Reinforcing explanations already given is extremely helpful and necessary.

The nurse should be aware of the cause and course of the pericarditis and convey this to the patients to reduce fear. For example, specific information is necessary for patients 3 days after an MI when chest pain and a pericardial friction rub may begin. Otherwise fear may be increased because patients may think they are having another heart attack. Caringly and confidently tell patients that pericarditis after a heart attack usually only lasts several days and is self-limiting, short term, and not a serious problem.[24] The patient is reassured that the pain can be controlled. The nurse guides the patient in relaxation and imagery exercises as discussed in Chapter 5.

Case study, cont'd. Before discharge Ms. A.E. received specific instructions regarding corticosteroids and activity. About 3 months after discharge, she described herself as being in limbo. The corticosteroids were discontinued on two occasions with recurrence of shortness of breath and chest pain. She was still frustrated with her pericarditis and corticosteroids. She had gained 7 kg, her appetite was voracious, she had acne and facial hair growth, and she slept 4 to 5 hours a night. She found herself starting many different projects and completing very few. At times, she felt like an old lady because she could not remember whether she had taken her daily prednisone. She finally poured each dose in individual bottles for a week at a time and labeled them. She had mood swings from euphoria to depression and crying. After 4 months she was given permission from her physician to go to her office for a few hours a day. At first it was frustrating because she did not know what her emotional state would be. Some nights she had bad dreams and did not allow herself to go back to sleep.

Each time the corticosteroids were tapered, she related specific symptoms such as tightness of her heart area, tingling around the mouth, shakiness, depression and crying, and frustration. This would last for 2 or 3 days.

About 6 months after discharge, after not receiving corticosteroids for 2 months, Ms. A.E.'s acne was fading, she had lost 2.5 kg, and she was able to work a normal day. She had made a deal with herself to listen to her body and not push herself so hard. She had the encouragement and support of her family and friends. She attended two relaxation sessions in the cardiac rehabilitation progam and wanted to learn more about her bodymind connection. She is in a high-stress job that she loves. However, she wants to learn how to cope better and is now learning biofeedback skills to increase and use relaxation skills daily.

NURSING
DIAGNOSIS 6

High risk for noncompliance related to inadequate knowledge about illness and future care (choosing pattern)

PATIENT OUTCOMES	NURSING PRESCRIPTIONS	EVALUATION
Patient will verbalize or demonstrate knowledge about pericarditis and prophylactic care, including heart function; definition of pericarditis; signs and symptoms of pericarditis; pathophysiologic changes; medications (action, dosage, frequency, and side effects); reason to avoid exposure to upper respiratory tract infections and report signs and symptoms of cold, cough, or sore throat; activity patterns during recovery and after discharge; times to contact the physician for help; hope and motivation for a healthier state; times to return for follow-up appointments and laboratory tests; and places to obtain Medic-Alert bracelet if discharged while receiving corticosteroids and reasons it is important to wear it.	Teach patient about pericarditis and the methods of prophylactic care, including heart function; definition of pericarditis, signs and symptoms of pericarditis, and pathophysiologic changes; medications (action, dosage, frequency, and side effects); reason to avoid exposure to upper respiratory tract infections and report signs and symptoms of cold, cough, or sore throat; activity patterns during recovery and after discharge; times to contact the physician for help; hope and motivation for a healthier state; times to return for follow-up appointments and laboratory tests; and places to obtain Medic-Alert bracelet if discharged while receiving corticosteroids and reasons it is important to wear it.	Patient verbalized or demonstrated knowledge about pericarditis and prophylactic care, including heart function, definition of pericarditis, signs and symptoms of pericarditis, pathophysiologic changes; medications (action, dosage, frequency, and side effects); reason to avoid exposure to upper respiratory tract infections and report signs and symptoms of cold, cough, or sore throat; activity patterns during recovery and after discharge; times to contact the physician for help; hope and motivation for a healthier state; times to return for follow-up appointments and laboratory tests; and places to obtain Medic-Alert bracelet if discharged while receiving corticosteroids and reasons it is important to wear it.

Plan and intervention for noncompliance

Teaching and evaluating learning are essential for the recovery of patients with pericarditis. *Readiness to learn* always should be evaluated before teaching. Basic concepts of heart function and the definition of pericarditis are the best place to start. When possible, family members should be included in teaching sessions so that they also can understand the illness and help patients adhere to medications, treatments, and a gradual return to activity during recovery. Detailed information should be given to families when patients are discharged while receiving corticosteroids because the medication may cause dramatic side effects (Table 15-5).

The patient must be knowledgeable enough about the symptoms to recognize recurrence of the problem. Evaluating patients' understanding of dyspnea, chest pain, fever, and increased fatigue is essential. Patients should receive additional information about the specific cause of the pericarditis, because this determines the medications and treatments. For example, tuberculous pericarditis would involve antituberculous medications, diet, and evaluation of the family for tuberculosis. If pericarditis patients do not have a private physician, at the time of discharge, the nurse should talk with them about when to return to the clinic or health department for follow-up care, which includes further chest x-ray examinations and specific laboratory studies, depending on the cause of the pericarditis. Some patients may need to be referred to the public health nurse.

Hope and motivation for a healthier state are two important factors in health maintenance. When patients hope for an improvement in health status, the nures is in a better position to help them set realistic goals in altering lifestyles for high-level wellness. Recovering from an illness such as pericarditis may mean changing some daily routines, especially when patients are taking steroids. The side effects are not predictable, and patients need to know when to contact the physician. The nurse should recognize patients' strengths for making change, their emotional state, and ways the stress of the recent illness has been handled. Knowing the interaction of the patients' support systems and including them in the teaching enhances healthy changes during recovery.

TABLE 15-5

Side Effects and Nursing Implications for Patients Receiving Corticosteroids

Side effects	Monitor	Prevention of complications	Patient education
FLUID AND ELECTROLYTE BALANCES			
Sodium retention Fluid retention Congestive heart failure in susceptible patients Potassium loss Hypokalemic alkalosis Hypertension Hypotension or shocklike reaction Calcium and phosphorus loss	Check results of serum sodium. Weigh patient daily. Record intake and output each shift. Observe for edema of feet and sacral area. Check results of serum potassium. Check results of arterial blood gases. Check vital signs each shift. Check results of serum calcium.	Collaborate with physician and dietitian concerning a low-sodium, high-potassium diet. Avoid the use of saline solutions to prepare injectable medications. Collaborate with physician to restrict activity in patients susceptible to congestive heart failure. Collaborate with physician for calcium replacement when indicated.	Explain the need for a low-sodium, high-potassium diet. Explain foods that are acceptable on the diet. Explain the need for restricted activity if ordered. Explain the need for calcium replacement if ordered.
MUSCULOSKELETAL SYSTEM			
Muscle weakness Steroid myopathy Loss of muscle mass Osteoporosis Vertebral compression fractures Aseptic necrosis of femoral and humeral heads	Observe for muscle weakness.	Report complaints of back, hip, or shoulder pain to physician. Encourage patient to follow a routine of ROM exercises. Stress the importance of preventing accidents. Collaborate with physician and dietitian concerning a high-protein diet. Collaborate with physician in obtaining an order for a bed board.	Explain the importance of following an exercise regimen. Teach patient some of the more common accident hazards and ways to avoid them. Explain the need for a high-protein diet. Teach about foods high in protein.
GASTROINTESTINAL SYSTEM			
Peptic ulcer with possible perforation and hemorrhage Pancreatitis Abdominal distention Ulcerative esophagitis	Check all stools and vomitus for blood.	Give all oral steroid preparations after a meal or with milk. Report dyspepsia to the physician. Collaborate with physician for prophylactic antacid. Report complaints of abdominal discomfort to physician.	Teach patient to take oral medications with meals or milk only. Explain the importance of taking antacid therapy if ordered. Teach patient the importance of reporting dyspepsia and tarry stools.
DERMATOLOGIC CONDITIONS			
Impaired wound healing Thin, fragile skin Petechiae and ecchymoses Erythema Increased sweating Burning or tingling, especially in parenteral area after intravenous injection Acne	Check progress of wound healing daily, especially surgical incisions. Inspect skin condition daily.	Advise patient to avoid injury. Collaborate with physician for a topical cream to treat acne. Give meticulous skin care using a desired skin lotion. Provide emotional support especially for women experiencing hirsutism and acne. Use a minimal amount of adhesive tape and always remove it with gentleness.	Explain importance of avoiding injury. If patient experiences parenteral burning after intravenous injection of steroid, explain that this is an expected occurrence. Explain that acne and hirsutism are side effects of the steroid and will disappear when the drug is discontinued.

From Garza CS: Adrenocorticosteroid therapy and documented nursing assessment: a comparison, thesis. Texas Woman's University, Denton, Texas, May 1977.

TABLE 15-5

Side Effects and Nursing Implications for Patients Receiving Corticosteroids—cont'd

Side effects	Monitor	Prevention of complications	Patient education
NEUROLOGIC SYSTEM			
Convulsions Increased intracranial pressure with papilledema Veritgo Headache Insomnia Psychoses	Observe patient for impending psychotic episodes, manic or depressive states, paranoia, a change in sleep patterns, nervousness, and excessive motor acitivity.	Provide environment as indicated by patient's mood.	Teach family that changes in mood are a result of the steroid therapy. Teach family how to deal with patient in the altered mental state.
ENDOCRINE SYSTEM			
Menstrual irregularity Cushing's syndrome Decreased growth (in children) Adrenopituitary suppression Decreased carbohydrate tolerance Latent diabetes Increased requirements for insulin Hypothyroidism	Check blood sugar reports. Do urine sugar and acetone tests each shift. Observe patient for polydypsia and polyuria. During period of decreasing steroid dose, observe patient for signs of adrenal insufficiency, headache, lethargy, weakness, hypotension, and diarrhea.	Collaborate with physician and dietitian concerning a diet low in saturated fats and carbohydrates. Help patient identify stressors, especially during time of steroid withdrawal. Help patient find ways of coping with stressors. Reassure patient that menstrual irregularities may be caused by these drugs.	Teach patient why it is necessary to be on a low–saturated fat, low-carbohydrate diet. Teach patient foods acceptable on the diet. If patient is to go home on a steroid drug, teach: 1. Taking medicine *as ordered* is vital 2. Not to give medication to anyone else 3. To avoid stressful situations 4. To notify the physician at once to have dose regulated if a cold is caught, elevated temperature occurs, or psychologic stress occurs. 5. To wear a Medic-Alert bracelet with the name of the physician, drug taken, the dose, and instructions for emergency situations
OPHTHALMIC			
Posterior subcapsular cataracts Increased intraocular pressure Glaucoma Exophthalmos	Collaborate with physician to order regular tonometry readings.	Check to see if patient has a history of glaucoma and is currently being treated. Collaborate with physician to order glaucoma therapy. Report visual disturbances or eye pain to physician.	If patient has glaucoma, reinforce the need to take eyedrops and to have regular tonometry tests. Teach patient to avoid increasing ocular pressure by avoiding tight collars, straining, lifting, emotional upsets, and excessive fluid intake.

Continued

TABLE 15-5

Side Effects and Nursing Implications for Patients Receiving Corticosteroids—cont'd

Side effects	Monitor	Prevention of complications	Patient education
OTHER			
Hypersensitivity	Observe patient for signs of anaphylactic reaction.	Report complaints of a sore throat or a sick feeling to physician.	Teach patient to report sick feelings.
Thromboembolism			
Mask signs of infection	Check complete blood count for elevated white blood cell count.	Obtain a history of allergies, clotting disorders, and medications that were taken routinely.	Teach patient good hand-washing technique.
Suppression of immune response			Instruct patient to avoid crowds and people with known infections.
Increased appetite due to parenteral therapy	Check urinalysis reports for bacteria.	Encourage patient to exercise legs to prevent blood stasis.	Teach reasons it is necessary to increase vitamin C intake and foods high in vitamin C content.
Hypopigmentation or hyperpigmentation	Check for elevated temperature.	Collaborate with physician and dietitian to increase vitamin C intake.	
Subcutaneous atrophy		Use good hand-washing technique.	
Sterile abscess		Give intramuscular medicines deep in gluteal muscle, not in the deltoid muscle.	
		Discard unused steroid preparations 48 hours after opening.	
		Check compatibility if intravenous medication is to be mixed with other drugs in a solution.	
		Report calf pain or tenderness to physician.	

KEY CONCEPT REVIEW

1. The pericardium is a double-walled sac composed of:
   a. Endocardial and epicardial layers
   b. Visceral and parietal layers
   c. Constrictive and visceral layers
   d. Epicardial and visceral layers
2. The most classic signs of acute pericarditis are:
   a. Orthopnea, electrical alternans, and pericardial effusion
   b. Pain, friction rub, and dyspnea
   c. Dysrhythmias, hypoxia, and shock
   d. Fear, mental confusion, and bradycardia
3. On x-ray film, pericardial effusion is usually associated with:
   a. A decreased cardiac silhouette
   b. Kurley's B lines
   c. An enlarge cardiac silhouette
   d. Normal heart size
4. Clinical manifestations of cardiac tamponade are caused by:
   a. Incompetent cardiac valves and normal heart size
   b. Fall in cardiac output and systemic venous congestion
   c. Coronary artery spasm and tachydysrhythmias
   d. Accumulation of thrombi in intimal chambers

5. The most important complications for the nurse to be aware of while caring for a patient with acute pericarditis are:
   a. Tachycardia, dyspnea, and pulsus paradoxus
   b. Pericardial friction rub, mental confusion, and restlessness
   c. Pericardial effusion, cardiac tamponade, and cardiac dysrhythmias
   d. Congestive heart failure, embolic phenomenon, and neuropsychiatric manifestations
6. The major diagnostic procedures used in diagnosing complications of pericarditis are:
   a. ECG, coronary arteriography, and thallium scanning
   b. Echocardiography, exercise testing, and thallium scanning
   c. Echocardiography, cardiac catheterization, and blood pool scanning
   d. Pyrophosphate scintigraphy, echocardiography, and exercise testing
7. Assessment of anxiety and fear during stages of pericarditis should:
   a. Be ongoing and include psychophysiologic responses to stress
   b. Be done every 2 days and include documenting behaviors
   c. Not include patient's perceptions of illness
   d. Not include family members' responses

ANSWERS

1. b   4. b   6. c
2. b   5. c   7. a
3. c

REFERENCES

1. Alexander J and others: Sensibility of exposed human heart and pericardium, Arch Surg 19:140, 1929.
2. Braunwald E: Pericardial disease. In Petersdorf RG and others: Harrison's principles of internal medicine, New York, 1983, McGraw-Hill, Inc.
3. Capps J and Coleman G: An experimental and clinical study of pain in the pleura, pericardium and peritoneum, New York, 1932, Macmillan Publishing Co.
4. Coffin C and Scarf M: Acute pericarditis simulating coronary artery occlusion, Am Heart J 32:515, 1946.
5. Cohn J and others: Mechanism of pulsus paradoxus in clinical shock, J Clin Invest 46:1744, 1967.
6. Concilus E and Bohachick P: Cancer: pericardial effusion and tamponade, Cancer Nurs 7:392, 1984.
7. Dossey B: Acute pericarditis. In Kenner CV, Guzzetta CE, and Dossey BM: Critical care nursing: body-mind-spirit, Philadelphia, 1985, JB Lippincott Co.
8. Dressler N: Sinus tachycardia complicating and outlasting pericarditis, Am Heart J 72:422, 1966.
9. Estes ME: Management of the cardiac tamponade patient: a nursing framework, Crit Care Nurse 5:17, 1985.
10. Feighenbaum H: Echocardiography. In Braunwald E, editor: Heart disease, Philadelphia, 1988, WB Saunders Co.
11. Fisch C: Electrocardiography and vectorcardiography. In Braunwald E, editor: Heart disease, Philadelphia, 1988, WB Saunders Co.
12. Goldberger E: Acute pericarditis. In Goldberger E, editor: Textbook of clinical cardiology, St. Louis, 1982, The CV Mosby Co.
13. Guberman BA and others: Cardiac tamponade in medical patients, Circulation 64:633, 1981.
14. Hancock E: On the elastic and rigid forms of constrictive pericarditis, Am Heart J 100:917, 1980.
15. Harvey WP: Auscultatory findings of diseases of the pericardium, Am J Cardiol 7:15, 1961.
16. Hiller G: Cardiac tamponade in the oncology patient, Focus Crit Care 14:22, 1987.
17. James TN: Pericarditis and the sinus node, Arch Intern Med 110:305, 1962.
18. Lorell BH and Braunwald E: Pericardial disease. In Braunwald E, editor: Heart disease, Philadelphia, 1988, WB Saunders Co.
19. Lovelys BJ: Complications of acute myocardial infarction. In Underhill E and others, editors: Cardiac nursing, Philadelphia, 1989, JB Lippincott Co.
20. Mangano DT: The effect of the pericardium on ventricular systolic function in man, Circulation 61:352, 1980.
21. McGregor M: Pulsus paradoxus, N Engl J Med 301:480, 1979.
22. McGregor M and Baskind E: Electric alternans in pericardial effusion, Circulation 11:837, 1955.
23. Miles W and Zipes D: Myocardial and pericardial disease. In Andreoli T and others, editors: Cecil essentials of medicine, Philadelphia, 1990, WB Saunders Co.
24. Moore SJ: Pericarditis after acute myocardial infarction, Heart Lung 8:551, 1979.
25. Muirhead J: Pericardial disease. In Underhill and others, editors: Cardiac nursing, Philadelphia, 1989, JB Lippincott Co.
26. Roberts S: Physiologic concepts and the critically ill patient, Englewood Cliffs, NJ, 1985, Prentice-Hall Press.
27. Rogers FB: Historical review of pericardial disease. In Cortes' FM, editor: The pericardium and its disorders, Springfield, Ill, 1971, Charles C Thomas, Publisher.
28. Sawaya J, Muyais S, and Armenian H: Early diagnosis of pericarditis in acute myocardial infarction, Am Heart J 100:144, 1978.
29. Shabetai R: Function of the pericardium. In Fowler NO, editor: The pericardium in health and disease, Mount Kisco, NY, 1985, Futura Publishing Co, Inc.
30. Spodick D: Pericardial rub: prospective, multiple observer investigation of pericardial friction rub in 100 patients, Am J Cardiol 35:357, 1975.
31. Spodick D: The hairy hearts of hoary heroes and other tales: medical history of the pericardium from antiquity through the twentieth century. In Fowler NO, editor: The pericardium in health and disease, Mount Kisco, NY, 1985, Futura Publishing Co, Inc.
32. Spodick D: Pericarditis, pericardial effusion, cardiac tamponade and constriction, Crit Care Clin 5:455, 1989.
33. Stein L and others: Recognition and management of pericardial tamponade, JAMA 225:503, 1973.
34. Wei J and others: Recurrent cardiac tamponade and large pericardial effusions: management with indwelling catheter, Am J Cardiol 42:281, 1978.
35. Wong B and others: The risk of pericardiocentesis, Am J Cardiol 44:1110, 1979.
36. Zucherman J and others: Rational use of operation in pericardial constriction, Int Surg 62:204, 1977.

UNIT IV

THE PERSON UNDERGOING SELECTED CARDIOVASCULAR THERAPIES

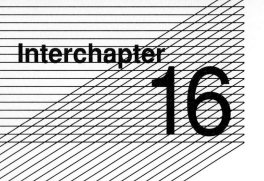

Interchapter 16

Awakening the Inner Healer

As a nurse you have had the privilege of working with many people before, during, and after medical tests and surgical procedures. No doubt you also have noticed when you were most successful in helping patients access their own inner healing resources. Your presence and the skills you teach patients can make the difference of whether patients go to tests and procedures feeling fearful and anxious or confident and relaxed.

What happens when you tell a patient the specifics about medical tests or surgery? Frequently, most patients start thinking about the tests or surgery and create unnecessary anxiety and fear about anesthesia, surgical complications, and maybe even death. Unfortunately, most patients don't share these feelings with anyone, especially nurses or physicians. Their fears create harmful images that are transmitted by the brain's limbic hypothalamic system to the neurotransmitters, the chemical messengers, which then send the message of anxiety and fear to all major body systems. This generates negative physiologic effects on their body (see the critical link between mind and body, p. 78). Any concerns that patients convey must be viewed as real. Most fears can be significantly reduced or completely eliminated when patients are taught to access their own inner healing resources.

People who go into medical tests, procedures, and surgery with high levels of stress experience more depression, have increased complications, require more medication and anesthesia, have suppressed immune function, and take longer to heal.[1,2] Research consistently has shown that people who know how to connect body, mind and spirit before, during and after these situations reduce their stress and complications.[3,4,5] The following contrasting case studies illustrates these facts:

CASE 1

"I worry about my Barlow's syndrome (prolapse of the mitral heart valve)," said Lynn, age 39, to her friend who was a nurse. "I'm excited about my cosmetic surgery and have been looking forward to it for some time. But being excited has an opposite side—questions, fears, and tension. My crazy heartbeats have been acting up, and I know it's related to being anxious about wild heartbeats that might get me into trouble during surgery. My cardiologist said that I shouldn't have problems, which is reassuring. However, I've got to create some ways to calm myself for a successful procedure."

Lynn asked her friend to make her a relaxation and imagery tape. Although Lynn had bought a packaged standard tape on preparing for surgery, she decided that she also wanted to listen to a presurgery–postsurgery tape of her own images and healing suggestions. She gave her friend specific instructions of healing and phrases that she wanted to receive while listening to the tape (e.g., the surgery is going fine, my heart beat is regular and at a normal rate). Lynn listened to the tape twice a day for a week before her surgery and listened to it while in the operating room. Her surgical procedure went flawlessly. She was relaxed and cooperative. Her wound healed quickly without complications.

CASE 2

With a belly laugh, Jack, a robust, athletic, 42-year-old man with cardiac symptoms, says "Doc, I'm afraid of needles." Jack had sweaty palms and was shivering prior to venipuncture before a cardiac catheterization. The cardiologist looked at Jack's normal sinus rhythm, which was marching across the cardiac monitor at about 90 beats per minute. He said, "Are you having chest pain now?" Jack said laughingly "No, I'm just scared. Scared of needles and just scared." The cardiologist said "Relax. You'll do just fine," and began the venipuncture for intravenous fluids and medications. Within seconds there was a significant change in Jack's cardiac rhythm. His heart rate dramatically increased to 200 to 250 beats per minute with frequent PVCs. As cardiac medications were being given, Jack had a cardiac arrest requiring defibrillation. He was resuscitated and the cardiac catheterization was cancelled.

That evening in the coronary care unit when Jack was stable, the cardiologist and nurse who had done the resuscitation procedure spent time exploring the meaning of Jack's fear of needles. Jack once again said, "Doc, I don't know why, but I'm just scared to death of needles." Since the cardiac catheterization was not an emergency, the cardiologist recommended that Jack learn some relaxation, imagery, and biofeedback skills and then return for the procedure. Jack was open to the idea. Over the next 2 weeks, he had six biofeedback sessions with the biofeedback nurse therapist. At the first visit, the nurse explored the origin of Jack's fears. She gave him a piece of paper and crayons and asked him to draw his images, which revealed vicious, gigantic jagged painful needles. Further discussion allowed Jack to remember many painful times 9 years previously. Due to infective endocarditis he had required frequent venipunctures for blood cultures and intravenous antibiotic therapy over a 6 week period. They were often traumatic, since his vessels collapsed as the needle touched the vein.

Jack was eager to learn relaxation and imagery skills. He practiced several times a day during the 2 weeks before his rescheduled cardiac cathetherization. He was able to change his negative imagery of needles to a positive one. His new image was of the "needle being the touch of a tiny light beam against his vein going in easily without trauma or pain." He also had the most success with moving into relaxed states quickly when listening to a music tape that also included ocean sounds.

Jack decided on his healing ritual before the repeat procedure and discussed it with the cardiologist. He would arrive at the hospital and get all the paperwork done and information needed by the cardiologist before the procedure. He would then put on a hospital gown and listen to his music tape for 20 minutes in a small private office near the procedure room. During the procedure he would continue listening to this tape. Jack also asked that the cardiologist and nurse remind him during the procedure to focus on rhythmic breathing and frequently to tell him that he was doing fine. The cardiologist and nurse agreed that it was an excellent plan. The procedure went smoothly with no complications.

One of the great gifts nurses can give patients is to help them access their inner healing resources. The process requires the nurse's presence, authenticity, and active listening skills. Teach patients ways to release their anxiety with relaxation and imagery interventions before, during and after procedures (see Chapter 5). An overview of these interventions follows:

Cue-controlled relaxation: use cue words such as "calm" and "relax" during the procedure.

Affirmations: use positive self-statements, such as "I'm doing fine; I can handle this." Instead of viewing high-tech equipment as frightening, reframe thoughts and perceptions to "state-of-the-art technology that will carefully monitor my condition."

Distraction: distract yourself during the procedure by creating general healing imagery such a pleasant scene, imagining being involved in another activity, or counting your breaths from 1 to 5 or 10 and then starting over.

Relaxation and imagery: Increase your trust in the upcoming events by setting aside time to rehearse the following: overcoming fear, being relaxed to ease necessary procedures (anesthesia, intravenous lines, etc.), minimizing pre-operative and post-operative medications, decreasing blood flow in the operative area or increasing blood flow to extremities to increase relaxation, minimizing infections, wound healing, pain management, aiding in prompt and regular elimination, alleviating nausea and vomiting, early ambulation, and inducing naps and sleep.

REFERENCES
1. Dossey B: The psychophysiology of bodymind healing. In Dossey B and others: Critical care nursing: body-mind-spirit, Philadelphia, 1992, JB Lippincott.
2. Linn BS, Linn WM, and Klimas NG: Effects of stress on surgical outcome, Advances 6(2):21-23, 1989.
3. Munford E, Schlesinger HJ, and Glass GV: The effects of psychological interventions on recovery from surgery and heart attacks: an analysis of the literature, Am J Pub Health 72 (2):141-151, 1982.
4. Achterberg J, Dossey B, and Kolkmeier L: Rituals of healing, New York, 1992, Bantam.
5. Dossey B: Imagery: awakening the inner healer. In Dossey B and others: Holistic nursing: a handbook for practice, Gaithersburg, 1988, Aspen Publishers.

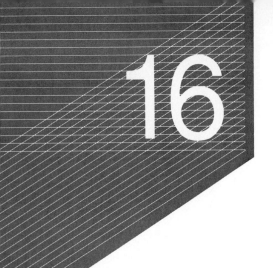

16 The Person with an Artificial Cardiac Pacemaker

Diane Proctor Sager

LEARNING OBJECTIVES

Temporary Pacing

1. Describe the normal process of sinoatrial node function, conduction of its impulse through the heart, and myocardial cell depolarization.

2. Identify the elements that alter this process and the results of such alteration.

3. Discuss the symptoms of conduction disorders and their natural history.

4. Identify the currently accepted indications for temporary cardiac pacing.

5. Describe the basic components and function of the temporary pacing system.

6. Describe the nursing diagnoses, patient outcomes, and nursing prescriptions in the care of the patient requiring temporary pacing.

7. Discuss the possible complications associated with the insertion of the temporary cardiac pacing system.

8. Analyze the forms of temporary pacemaker malfunction and their prevention and management.

Permanent Pacing

1. Discuss the currently used modes of permanent pacing and their indications.

2. Evaluate the uses and hazards of pacemaker programmability.

3. Describe the nursing diagnoses, patient outcomes, and nursing prescriptions in the care of the patient requiring permanent pacing.

4. Describe the types of power sources used for permanent pacing and their implications for patients.

5. Analyze the forms of permanent pacemaker malfunction and complications and their cause, prevention, and management.

6. Evaluate a comprehensive, long-term teaching plan for the person receiving a permanent pacemaker.

SECTION I

 Knowledge base

SIGNIFICANCE AND INCIDENCE

Since the late 1950s the technology of cardiac pacing has expanded rapidly. Before the advent of artificial pacing, persons with severe bradydysrhythmias lived as invalids, and their life spans were drastically shortened. In 1952, Zoll demonstrated the ability to artificially pace the heart by applying electrical current externally to the chest wall. This therapy was painful and impractical for prolonged periods of time. Then in 1957 the technique of applying small amounts of current directly into the right ventricle via a transvenous electrode was shown to be effective and practical. The first permanent, surgically implanted pacemaker was made available in 1960. Since that time, nearly 1 million pacemakers have been implanted world wide for the treatment of not only bradydysrhythmias but also certain tachydysrhythmias.

PATHOGENESIS AND PATHOLOGY
Causes of dysfunction in the conduction system

The tissues of the sinoatrial (SA) node, the conduction system, and the electrically active myocardium are vulnerable to damage in several ways. They depend on oxygen for the production of adenosine triphosphate (ATP) and on the presence of particular levels of electrolytes and substrates, which are provided by an adequate flow of arterial

TABLE 16-1
The NASPE/BPEG Generic Pacemaker Code*

Position	I	II	III	IV	V
Category	Chambers paced	Chambers sensed	Response to sensing	Programmability, rate modulation	Antitachydysrhythmia functions
	0 = None	0 = None	0 = None	0 = None	0 = None
	A = Atrium	A = Atrium	T = Triggered	P = Simple programmable	P = Pacing (antitachydysrhythmia)
	V = Ventricle	V = Ventricle	I = Inhibited	M = Multi-programmable	S = Shock
	D = Dual (A + V)	D = Dual (A + V)	D = Dual (T + I)	C = Communicating	D = Dual (P + S)
				R = Rate modulation	

*Positions I through III are used to describe antibradycardia functions. Positions IV and V are for special functions.
From Bernstein AD and others: Pace 10:794, 1987.
BPEG, British Pacing and Electrophysiology Group.

blood. Therefore any acute or chronic interruption in blood supply to any part of the heart can precipitate dysrhythmias. Additionally, the structures of the conduction system lie close to the cardiac skeleton and the atrioventricular (AV) valves. This anatomic arrangement, coupled with the delicate structure of the conductive tissue, means that conditions that effect changes in valve tissue can disrupt generation and transmission of an impulse, producing bradydysrhythmias and tachydysrhythmias. Other factors that can cause dysrhythmias include infection (viral, bacterial, or fungal), trauma (surgical or accidental), chemical toxicity, collagen diseases, radiation therapy to the chest, and congenital malformations.

ARTIFICIAL PACEMAKER THERAPY

A pacing system, whether temporary or permanent, is simply an electrical circuit composed of an object to receive electrical current, in this case the myocardial cell, connected to a power source by an electrically conductive, insulated wire, or in pacing terms, a lead. In pacing, the power source is a pulse generator, or pacemaker, that is capable of producing timed and measured impulses of electrical current and sensing the presence of natural electrical impulses within the heart. Impulses from the pacemaker are conducted through the lead to and from the heart to the pacemaker to complete the electrical circuit. The basic objectives of pacing are to elicit myocardial cell depolarization and subsequent contraction, to sense intrinsic cardiac rhythm, and to pace the heart only in the absence of sensed intrinsic activity.

Pacemaker nomenclature

To avoid confusion and to define the specific mode of operation of all units, Smyth[72] created an easy but comprehensive nomenclature for pacing called the three-letter

identification pacemaker code. This system, modified by Parsonnet, Furman and Smyth,[59] describes the various modes of temporary and permanent pacing. Revisions have been made in this original code in response to the advent of new modes of pacing.[60,61] The newest version of the code was developed and adapted by the North American Society of Pacing and Electrophysiology (NASPE) (Table 16-1).

Looking at the table, *VVIPO* describes a simple pacing system that paces in the ventricles, senses in the ventricles, responds to a sensed beat by inhibiting output, is programmable (in two functions or less), but has no antitachydysrhythmia function. A VVIR is a rate-modulated VVI pacemaker. The code for an implantable cardioverter-defibrillator would be OOOPS; it does not perform antibradydysrhythmic function but is programmable, and when it senses the presence of ventricular tachycardia or ventricular fibrillation, it releases an impulse of current or shock. Table 16-2 lists other examples.

Pacemaker function

A simple demand pacing system (AAI or VVI) behaves in the following manner (Fig. 16-1). The cycle begins with a pacemaker impulse. An *impulse* is a measured release of current that has a predetermined magnitude and duration. The pulse generator emits the impulse (e.g., 10 milliampere [mA] of current delivered over 1 millisecond [msec] of time) that then produces depolarization of the ventricular or atrial myocardium, or in pacing terms, *capture*.

For a predetermined amount of time after the pacemaker impulse, the pacemaker is in a refractory period and is incapable of sensing incoming signals from the myocardium. This mechanism prevents the pacemaker from sensing its own *afterpotential*, which is the dissipation of the delivered electrical current from the pacemaker through the myocardial tissue,[43] and can be of enough magnitude

TABLE 16-2

Examples of the NASPE/BPEG Generic Pacemaker

Code	Meaning
VOOO or VOOOO	Asynchronous ventricular pacing, no adaptive rate control or antitachydysrhythmia functions (also VOO in clinical use but not in device labeling)
DDDM or DDDMO	Multiprogrammable "physiologic" dual-chamber pacing, no adaptive rate control or antitachydysrhythmia functions
VVIPP	Simple-programmable VVI pacemaker with antitachydysrhythmia-pacing capability
DDDCP	DDD pacemaker with telemetry and anti-tachydysrhythmia-pacing capability
OOOPS	Simple-programmable cardioverter, defibrillator, or cardioverter-defibrillator
OOOPD	Simple-programmable cardioverter, defibrillator, or cardioverter-defibrillator with antitachydysrhythmia-pacing capability
VVIMD	Multiprogrammable VVI pacemaker with defibrillation (or cardioversion, or cardioversion and defibrillation) and antitachydysrhythmia-pacing capabilities
VVIR or VVIRO	VVI pacemaker with escape interval controlled adaptively by one or more unspecified variables
VVIRP	Programmable VVI pacemaker with escape interval controlled adaptively by one or more unspecified variables, also incorporating antitachydysrhythmia-pacing capability
DDDRD	Programmable DDD pacemaker with escape interval controlled adaptively by one or more unspecified variables, also incorporating antitachydysrhythmia-pacing capability and cardioversion (or defibrillation, or cardioversion and defibrillation) functions

From: Bernstein AD and others: Pace 10:794, 1987.

to be sensed by the pacemaker. The QRS complex or T wave theoretically also could be sensed. The refractory period usually lasts for 250 to 350 msec. After the refractory period is the *noise-sampling* phase. If any electromagnetic interference is sensed during this phase, the pacemaker goes into a fixed rate mode of operation and remains in this mode until the source of interference is removed. At the end of the noise-sampling period, the alert period begins, and the cycle starts over. The time in milliseconds between two pacemaker impulses during continuous pacing is called the *automatic interval*. If the pacemaker is set for a rate of 72 pulses per minute (ppm), the automatic interval is 830 msec.

If a premature ventricular contraction (PVC), premature atrial contraction (PAC), or other intrinsic beat occurs during the alert period, the pacemaker will sense it (depending on which chamber the lead is in) and start its cycle over again without emitting an impulse. The *sensitivity* of a pulse generator refers to its ability to see an impulse generated by the heart and is expressed in millivolts (mV). An intrinsic impulse from the heart travels up the pacing lead into the pulse generator. At this point the pacemaker evaluates the incoming signals and permits only those with certain predetermined qualities to enter the sensing circuit for processing; it ignores most extraneous electical signals. The *sensing circuit* uses two dimensions of the intrinsic impulse for deciding whether the incoming signal is a legitimate cardiac impulse: (1) slew rate, or the change in the signal's voltage over time (volts/second), a way of defining the shape of the impulse,[17] and (2) its amplitude in millivolts.

Sensing is illustrated in Fig. 16-2. *Complexes 1* and *2* are paced beats, that is, a pulse generator impulse is followed by a QRS complex (myocardial capture). The distance (time) between *1* and *2* is determined by the programmed rate of the pacemaker. After *complex 2*, an intrinsic beat (*complex 3*) occurs at the same time as the pacemaker impulse. *Complex 3* can be called a *fusion beat*.

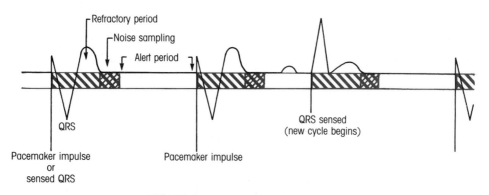

FIG. 16-1 Phases of normal VVI pacing.

Complex 4 is an intrinsic beat (ventricular) that falls within the pacemaker alert period. The electrical impulse generated by this intrinsic beat is sensed. In response to the sensed beat, the pacemaker does not emit a pacing impulse and recycles. This new cycle contains a refractory period and an alert period, followed by *complex 5*, a normal paced beat. The *escape interval* is the time in milliseconds from a sensed beat to the next pacemaker impulse. In some pacemakers the automatic interval and the escape interval are equal; in others the escape interval is longer. The prolongation of the time after an intrinsic beat before the next paced beat is called *hysteresis*. In units with hysteresis, the alert period after a sensed beat is longer than that after a paced beat because the escape interval is longer. If intrinsic beats occur one after another at a rate greater that the set rate of the pacemaker, the sensing circuit will continue to inhibit output.

Complex systems pacing the atria and ventricles, such as DVI or DDD, behave basically the same as the simple VVI. They emit measured and timed impulses, and there are refractory periods, alert periods, sensing, and coordination between the atrium and ventricle. The AV cycle begins with ventricular output, producing a QRS complex followed by the ventricular refractory period and then an atrial alert period. Then if during the alert period there are no sensed intrinsic beats, atrial output occurs, and atrial depolarization is initiated. Next there is a built-in interval called the *A-V delay* to allow a measured pause between the atrial and the ventricular impulses. This delay allows for ventricular filling and can be programmed to meet the patient's needs. After the delay, if there is no intrinsic ventricular beat, the pacemaker fires an impulse into the ventricle, and the cycle begins again. These systems are described in detail in Section III.

Myocardial threshold

A measured amount of current is needed to elicit myocardial depolarization. Inherent in the ability of the pacemaker system to depolarize the myocardium (i.e., to elicit capture) is the myocardial cell's ability to respond to the electrical stimulus. This ability is called *threshold* to pacing and is measured in voltage (mV) or current (mA) of electricity. Thus threshold is the amount of current or voltage required to elicit cell depolarization to produce contraction.

Threshold can vary with the resistance within the pacing equipment to the flow of current in the following locations:

1. Within the leads
2. At the connections between the pulse generator and the leads
3. At the lead electrode-myocardial interface
4. Within the body tissues composing the return circuit of the pacing system

This resistance is usually 500 ohms (range: 300 to 800 ohms). Resistance is also referred to as *impedance* when describing pacing systems, although the terms are not synonymous. Impedance represents the degree of nonconductivity within the system. For simplicity the term *resistance* is used here.

Threshold may vary with the characteristics of the final current to touch the cells, and this depends on voltage and resistance. These characteristics include the current density and the current duration. The current density, which depends on the surface of the electrode touching the cells, is measured in square millimeters; the smaller the surface area, the greater the current density, and thus the less current (or voltage) required to produce depolarization.[17] The duration of the current, measured in milliseconds is also called the *pulse width*; usually the longer the duration, the less current needed to produce depolarization.

The location of the electrode also affects threshold. The threshold is inversely proportional to the square of the distance of the electrode tip to the closest excitable tissue.[81] Capture can take place if the lead tip is slightly displaced off the endocardial surface, but thresholds rise directly with the distance away from the endocardial surface and eventually exceed the output capabilities of the pulse generator if the distance becomes too great. The chamber being paced also affects thresholds. Generally, atrial thresholds are higher than ventricular, and epicardial are higher than endocardial thresholds.

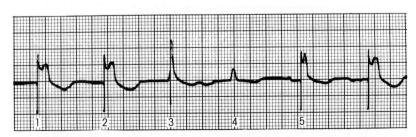

FIG. 16-2   Normal sensing in VVI pacing. *Complexes 1* and *2* are normal, paced beats; *complex 3* is a fusion beat; *complex 4* is an intrinsic QRS that has been sensed and is followed by recycling of the pacemaker and a normal paced beat, *complex 5.*

Finally, the status of the cells in contact with the electrode affects threshold. The ability to depolarize depends on cell oxygenation, acid-base balance, electrolyte balance, and the availability of substrates. If the lead is placed with the electrode tip touching an area of fibrosis or ischemia, the threshold to pacing will be higher than normal. If the threshold is higher than a pacemaker's output the situation is called *exit block*. In cases of endocardial fibroelastosis, endocardial pacing may be impossible because of the abnormal cells in contact with the lead tip. In these cases, epicardial thresholds can be normal. In temporary epicardial pacing, the cells around the pacing wire (electrode) are injured during insertion. Later fibrosis forms around the lead within the myocardium, and the threshold begins to rise within 24 hours of insertion. This change in threshold can interfere with pacemaker function within a week of implant.[72] Also, after cardiac surgery, myocardial excitability may be depressed, resulting in higher thresholds.

Electrocardiogram of pacing

The surface electrocardiogram (ECG) of cardiac pacing appears different from that of normal sinus rhythm in several respects. To begin with, a *pacing artifact* is seen. With atrial pacing a P wave follows the artifact (Fig. 16-3), but

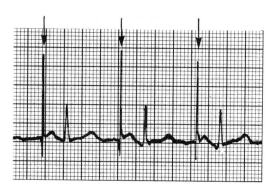

FIG. 16-3 ECG of atrial pacing: AAI, showing the pacemaker impulse followed by a P wave and QRS complex.

in some leads, it may be hidden in the pacing spike afterpotential. Leads II and V_1 are usually the best for deciding whether a P wave has been produced. The QRS complex after an atrial-paced P wave usually appears the same as a nonpaced complex. If bundle branch conduction is normal, the QRS will be narrow.

The QRS complex produced by ventricular pacing appears abnormal (Fig. 16-4). In normal conduction the SA node impulse travels through the AV node and into the ventricular conduction network, with the right and left ventricles receiving this signal almost simultaneously because of the Purkinje system; this produces a consistent, narrow complex. However, in ventricular pacing the stimulating impulse originates in the ventricle itself, in the tip of the right ventricle in endocardial pacing or somewhere on the exterior of the right or left ventricle in epicardial pacing. With right ventricular endocardial stimulation, a pseudo–left bundle branch block (LBBB) with left axis deviation (−30 to −90 degrees) is created.

The impulse travels through the right ventricle and septum to the left ventricle. The paced beat has a deep S wave in leads II, III, V_1, and V_3. If the left ventricle is the site of the electrode, as with epicardial pacing, the QRS complex may look like a right bundle branch block (RBBB) with right axis deviation, depending on the position of the electrode. The QRS complex may be very small or slightly positive in leads II, III, and V_1 because the main vector is posterior. Occasionally a RBBB pattern can be seen with apical right ventricular endocardial pacing.

The ECG is one way that ventricular capture is verified. Usually a QRS complex is seen; however, in some leads only the pacing spike and afterpotential are seen. A large pacing spike and afterpotential are the hallmarks of unipolar pacing and distort the P or QRS complex in some leads. If capture has actually occurred, a T wave always can be identified. Two other ways that capture can be verified are by a palpable pulse and heart sounds. Knowing how a paced complex (pacing artifact with resulting P or QRST) should appear, based on the knowledge of where the impulse is originating, is important in the understanding of malfunctions and monitoring.

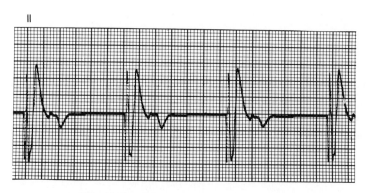

FIG. 16-4 ECG of ventricular pacing: VVI.

Temporary pacing

LEADS

To deliver current to the myocardial cells and collect electrical signals from intrinsic cardiac activity, temporary and permanent pacing leads are placed endocardially within the right atrium or ventricle or epicardially on the atrium or ventricle. These leads are unipolar or bipolar. *Temporary endocardial leads* are usually bipolar and consist of two insulated wires connected to two exposed metal electrodes (the portion of the wire where current is released or picked up) at one end and two terminal pins at the other (Fig. 16-5).

The electrode at the extreme end is called the *distal electrode.* The electrode just above it that is a ring around the lead is called the *proximal* or *ring* (or *indifferent*) *electrode.* The distal electrode is in direct contact with the endocardium, and the proximal electrode is approximately 1 cm above it. When this lead is connected to an external pulse generator with the distal electrode on the negative terminal and the proximal electrode attached to the positive terminal, current flows from the negative (cathodal) pacemaker terminal down the wire to the distal or tip electrode and into the myocardium. The current then seeks the positive (anodal) proximal electrode, reenters the lead, and flows up to the positive terminal of the pulse generator to complete the circuit. Electrical signals from the myocardium can travel from the electrode up the lead and into the pacemaker for sensing. These intrinsic signals are gathered over the same pathway that the pacing current takes.

Temporary bipolar endocardial leads are available for atrial, ventricular, and AV sequential pacing. The temporary atrial lead is J shaped to allow it to be placed in the atrial appendage, where it is less likely to be displaced. Ventricular leads are smooth tipped and straight for placement in the right ventricular apex. They are flexible enough to go around curves in the venous system but rigid enough at body temperature to be wedged and held in the right ventricle. This type of semifloating lead is 3 or 4 French (Fr) in size and can be passed into the heart without fluoroscopy. A similar lead that can be placed without fluoroscopy, in patients who have sufficient blood flow, has a small, latex balloon between the proximal and distal electrodes. This lead is inserted through a percutaneous introducer that has been placed into a large vein, preferably the femoral for ease of insertion and lead stability. The jugular, subclavian, and brachial veins should be avoided if permanent pacing is anticipated. After it is in the vein, the balloon is inflated with sterile saline. Blood flow pushing against the balloon quickly propels the lead into the right ventricle. The balloon then is deflated, and the lead is wedged through the trabeculae and into pacing position in the apex. More rigid 6 or 7 Fr leads are placed with the aid of the fluoroscope. Another type of temporary lead contains both a J-shaped atrial wire and a straight ventricular wire for AV sequential pacing. All these leads are inserted transvenously.

For rapid insertion of a pacing lead during cardiopulmonary resuscitation, when there is no blood flow to carry a lead into place transvenously, a *transthoracic endocardial lead* can be used.[54] This temporary bipolar lead is J shaped to hold it within the ventricular chamber after it has been inserted through the ventricular wall. It is flexible enough, however, to be inserted and removed by gentle pushing or traction. Transvenously placed leads are considered more reliable than the transthoracic lead but are nearly impossible to position during resuscitative measures.

Temporary epicardial leads are used for pacing during the first few days after cardiac surgery when dysrhythmias are common. These leads are simply insulated wires with an uninsulated area at one end that is looped but not tied into the myocardium and acts as a stimulating electrode; a Keith or straight suture needle at the opposite end is connected to the pacemaker terminal. Two wires are used for each chamber to be paced. A bipolar system is created

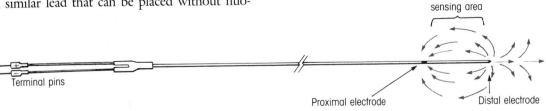

FIG. 16-5 Components of a temporary bipolar transvenous pacing lead.

when one wire is connected to the positive terminal of the pacemaker and the other to the negative. Frequently one wire is connected to the heart and the other to subcutaneous tissue. The wire on the myocardium is connected to the negative terminal of the pacemaker and the other to the positive.

TEMPORARY EXTERNAL PACING

Based on the original device introduced by Zoll in the 1950s, a temporary external pacemaker now is being used to support patients with bradycardia until a pacing lead can be inserted. Enough current to induce myocardial contraction is applied though the chest wall by two flat, round electrodes. Discomfort has been reduced through electrode design. These leads must be carefully placed and maintained to prevent movement or loss of contact with the skin.

TEMPORARY PULSE GENERATOR

The pulse generator may have dial or touch controls with a digital display (Fig. 16-6). In most pulse generators the *rate control* allows the rate of impulses delivered to the myocardium to be varied from 30 to 180 ppm. Pulse generators used for overdrive therapy, in which rapidly delivered pacemaker impulses can be used to control certain tachydysrhythmias, can be set as high as 800 ppm. *Current output*, measured in milliamperes, can be adjusted according to the amount of current needed to elicit myocardial depolarization from as low as 0.1 mA to as high as 20 mA. The current required to produce myocardial depolarization then can define threshold numerically. The voltage generated is internally and automatically regulated by the pacemaker to deliver the set current. The *sensitivity control* on the pacemaker usually goes from 0.5 or 1.0 mV to 20 mV. These numbers represent the millivolt size or amplitude of an R or P wave that the pacemaker is capable of sensing. Thus at a setting of 0.5 mV, the pacemaker is at its most sensitive; at a setting of 20 mV, it may read *asynchronous*, which means the unit is incapable of sensing any intrinsic beat and will function as fixed-rate. The sensitivity control not ony allows the user to adjust for sensing but also gives a numeric definition in millivolts of the size of the R or P wave being seen by the lead. The technique for measuring intrinsic beats is described later. Sensitivity is important so that the pacemaker can avoid competition with the patient's own rhythm, whether that rhythm be normal or ectopic.

In addition to these controls, some external pacemakers also have a *pulse-duration control* that can assist in managing a rising myocardial threshold. When the myocardium will not depolarize at an output of 10 mA and a pulse duration of 0.5 msec, it may depolarize if the pulse duration is increased to 1 msec. Pacemakers without this control are set at a fixed pulse duration of less than 2 msec.

It is important to be familiar with the operation of the on-and-off switch. Some manufacturers have designed this control to be easy to turn on but difficult to turn off to prevent inadvertent loss of pacing. Most temporary units also have a battery test indicator to show whether the batteries are producing an adequate output and may have an indicator to show the percentage of battery life remaining. The pace-sense indicator tells whether the pacemaker has emitted an impulse to pace or has been inhibited by a sensed beat.

Some external pulse generators can pace the atria and ventricles sequentially when used with atrial and ventricular epicardial or endocardial leads. These units have separate controls for atrial and ventricular output. Rate and sensitivity are controllable only in the ventricle. An additional control is the *AV interval*, or time between atrial and ventricular output (measured in milliseconds). The AV interval has an influence on cardiac output; that is, longer AV intervals (250 msec) can promote better ventricular filling from the atria and thus increase cardiac output. Adjustment of this setting is based on cardiac output or arterial blood pressure studies; it is set normally between 150 and 250 msec.

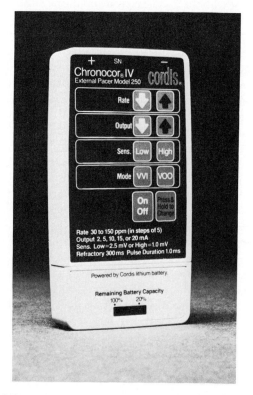

FIG. 16-6 External pulse generator for temporary AAI or VVI pacing. The area to the left of the control buttons gives a visual display of the pacemaker settings. The pacing lead terminals are inserted at the top.

Courtesy Cordis Corp, Miami.

INDICATIONS FOR TEMPORARY PACING

Patients with bradydysrhythmias should be stabilized with temporary cardiac pacing if a slow heart rate is producing symptoms, fostering ventricular irritability, occurring in a clinical situation where it can be potentially lethal, or associated with severe bradycardia or ventricular standstill, such as with complete heart block. This is especially true

---

TEMPORARY PACING INDICATIONS

Sinus dysrhythmias (sick sinus syndrome) when the patient has no symptoms:
   Sinus pauses longer than 2 seconds
   Sinus bradycardia with rates less than 40 beats per minute (bpm)
Slow junctional rhythm with symptoms
Second-degree heart block with symptoms
Complete heart block, congenital and acquired, with symptoms
Atrial flutter or fibrillation with a symptomatic slow ventricular rate (less than 40 bpm)
Recurrent ventricular standstill
Acute myocardial infarction (AMI)
   Inferior or posterolateral AMI with sinus bradycardia, sinus pauses or arrest, high-degree second-degree AV block (usually appearing several days after the onset of the AMI), or complete AV block*
   Anterolateral or anteroseptal AMI with transient or persistent Mobitz I or II second-degree AV block, complete AV block, or new RBBB (a qR pattern in V$_1$) and left anterior and posterior hemiblock, especially if first-degree AV block is also present (complete AV block can ensue suddenly, and asystole is not uncommon)*
   Any AMI with second- or third-degree AV block, increasing PR interval, shifting axis, or widening QRS complex
Tachydysrhythmias that are unresponsive to drugs or are secondary to an element that cannot be removed (pacing will be for overdrive)
High-risk situations such as coronary angiography, major surgery, cardiac surgery, or permanent pacemaker or implantable defibrillator insertion
Syncope without proven cause†
When drugs such as digitalis and propranolol cause symptomatic slowing of heart rate but cannot be discontinued
During permanent pacemaker replacement when the patient has a slow or nonexistent intrinsic rhythm

*Data from Gann D, El-Sherif N, and Samet P: In Samet P and El-Sherif N, editors: Cardiac pacing, ed 2, New York, 1980, Grune & Stratton, Inc, and McIntire K and Lewis J: Textbook of advanced cardiac life support, Dallas, 1981, American Heart Association.
†Mond H: PACE 4:432, 1981.

---

when pharmacologic agents are ineffective, produce undesirable side effects, or are contraindicated. Opinions vary as to when to pace, especially when the patient has no symptoms. The decision must be based on the assessment of the resting ECG, symptoms, predicted prognosis, and general myocardial status (presence or absence of congestive heart failure, ischemia, or hypotension). Age usually is not a factor, but the presence of a terminal disease may be. The situations listed in the box generally are accepted as indications for initial temporary pacing.

Nursing process

Case study. Mr. R. is a 42-year-old accountant with a history of isolated, congenital complete heart block. Until recently, Mr. R. considered himself without symptoms despite the presence of heart block; although he was not athletically active, he did belong to a hiking club and enjoyed dancing. About 1 month before admission, he began experiencing shortness of breath, mild chest discomfort, and fatigue when climbing stairs. At the insistence of his wife, he saw his cardiologist. His ECG showed complete heart block with a ventricular rate of 25 bpm; his usual intrinsic rate had been 50 to 60 bpm before this time. The physician recommended admission to the coronary care unit (CCU) immediately and the insertion of a temporary pacing system. Mr. R. was informed that he would probably need a permanent pacemaker.

On admission, Mr. R. was placed on bed rest. His heart rate was still at 25 bpm, and the patient was complaining of fatigue. He also stated that he was very concerned about the temporary pacemaker insertion procedure and the possibility of needing a permanent device. About 2 hours after admission a temporary transvenous ventricular pacing system was installed via the right femoral vein. At the time of insertion, the patient's intrinsic R wave was measured at 11 mV, and the pacing threshold was low at 0.9 mA at the fixed pacemaker output of 5 mV and a pulse duration of 1 msec. The temporary pacemaker was set at a rate of 60 ppm, an output of 2 mA, and a pulse width of 0.5 msec.

Nursing assessment
Exchanging pattern

Electrocardiographic monitoring must be initiated as soon as possible for patients who exhibit symptoms of slow or rapid heart rates or who are at high risk for developing these dysrhythmias. Monitor continuously, paying attention to heart rate, the status of any existing dysrhythmia, the presence or absence of ventricular irritability, blood pressure and cardiac output when indicated, and the effect of pharmacologic support.

The clinical manifestations of a bradydysrhythmia or tachydysrhythmia vary with the degree of reduction in cardiac output. All body systems should be evaluated for dysfunction related to reduced cardiac output. If the person's heart rate slows, the stroke volume must increase to maintain an adequate output. If stroke volume cannot increase and output decreases, peripheral vascular resistance can increase to maintain arterial pressure and tissue perfusion. Gradual development of a bradycardia may give the body time to compensate, and the patient may have no symptoms. On the other hand, a sudden onset of a slow rate or the presence of myocardial disease may not permit the adaptation just described, and the patient may have symptoms secondary to inadequate perfusion of the brain, heart, lungs, and kidneys. Within the Exchanging Pattern, assess for the following:

1. Central nervous system
   a. Neurologic signs: weakness, fatigue, dizziness, and syncope
   b. Level of consciousness: confusion, stupor, and unresponsiveness
2. Heart
   a. Presence of angina
   b. Arterial pressure: hypotension
   c. Elevated pulmonary artery or capillary wedge pressure
   d. Low cardiac output
   3. Presence of S_3 or S_4
   f. Presence of peripheral edema
3. Lungs
   a. Abnormal arterial blood gases
   b. Presence of cyanosis
   c. Respiratory rate and effort: tachypnea, shortness of breath, and dyspnea
   d. Presence of crackles
4. Kidneys
   a. Urinary output: reduced
   b. Abnormal levels of blood urea nitrogen, creatinine, and serum electrolytes

Knowing pattern

Assess what patients know about their heart problems and ways it has been treated in the past. Ask what they know and what their perceptions regarding pacemakers, their function, and insertion procedure are. Determine whether there are misconceptions regarding this information. Ask if patients are disturbed by any part of the therapy. Query patients regarding their expectations of the pacemaker. Note whether patients ask questions about the illness, treatment, and prognosis, which indicate readiness to learn.

Feeling pattern

Within the Feeling Pattern, assess for discomfort or pain. Have patients describe the onset of the discomfort, its location, duration, quality, and radiation. Ask about activities associated with the discomfort, and explore factors that precipitate and alleviate pain.

Nearly all patients faced with a major heart problem have some degree of anxiety. The degree depends on the severity of the illness, patients' perceptions of the illness, and their past experiences with illness. Assess patients' psychophysiologic manifestations of anxiety and fear (e.g.,

verbalizations of feeling jittery, distressed, frightened, or overexcited). Determine whether patients verbalize anxiety related to self-concept or a threat of death. Investigate symptoms and behaviors consistent with anxiety (e.g., elevated heart rate or blood pressure, cool extremities, darting eye movements, and startle reflex to normal sounds).

Moving pattern

Determine how the illness has affected patients' daily activities. Ask patients if they have noticed fatigue or decreased strength or endurance in normal activities. Explore activities that they can no longer do and patients' responses to activities. Ascertain whether patients have trouble falling or remaining asleep and whether their social activities have changed because of the illness.

Perceiving pattern

Assess patients to determine how they perceive themselves, their illness, and their ability to exert control over the current situation. For example, patients might verbally or nonverbally express an actual or perceived change in body structure or functioning. Determine what pacemaker insertion means to patients and families. Ask patients about the severity of their illness and their attitudes and feelings about the future. Note whether they view the pacemaker as a solution to their problems and whether they perceive loss of control over the situation.

Valuing pattern

Assess patients' cultural and spiritual practices. Determine whether religion is important and whether it provides support. Note whether patients show excessive concern for the meaning of life and death or regard their illness as a form of punishment. Evaluate how the family reacts when a member is ill.

Relating pattern

Assess patients' relationships with others. Determine whether the families and friends support the patients. Note whether patients believe that a pacemaker insertion will affect the families and their relationships with others.

Choosing pattern

Evaluate how patients cope with the stress. Ascertain their usual methods of dealing with stress. Determine patients' levels of compliance during past and current medical regimens. Note whether patients appear motivated or willing to comply with the future requirements of good pacemaker care.

Nursing diagnoses

The most commonly occurring human responses anticipated for a person requiring temporary cardiac pacing are indicated by the following nursing diagnosis:

1. High risk for decreased cardiac output related to bradydysrhythmias and delay in the insertion of the temporary pacing system
2. High risk for anxiety related to cardiac disorder and impending temporary pacemaker insertion
3. High risk for ventricular tachydysrhythmia related to the insertion of temporary cardiac pacing lead
4. Symptomatic, potentially symptomatic, or high risk for bradydysrhythmia or tachydysrhythmia necessitating temporary cardiac pacing related to (state cause)
5. High risk for fluid volume deficit related to bleeding due to the transvenous, epicardial, or transthoracic lead insertion
6. High risk for impaired gas exchange related to pneumothorax due to the insertion of a transvenous lead via the right subclavian vein or the insertion of a transthoracic endocardial lead
7. High risk for impaired physical mobility related to activity restrictions
8. High risk for infection related to percutaneous lead placement
9. High risk for microshock related to the presence of the temporary pacing lead
10. High risk for pacemaker malfunction related to (state cause)
11. High risk for bleeding related to the removal of the temporary pacing leads

For each of these diagnoses the patient outcomes, nursing prescriptions, and evaluation criteria are outlined with a discussion of the factual information that supports the plan and implementation of care.

NURSING DIAGNOSIS 1   **High risk for decreased cardiac output related to bradydysrhythmias and a delay in the insertion of the temporary pacing system (exchanging pattern)**

PATIENT OUTCOMES	NURSING PRESCRIPTIONS	EVALUATION
Patient will not experience signs and symptoms of decreased cardiac output such as decreased arterial pressure, loss of consciousness, abnormal arterial blood gas levels, and decreased urinary output. If hemodynamic instability occurs, patient will respond to appropriate therapy.	Monitor for signs and symptoms of decreased cardiac output such as systolic blood pressure less than 90 mm Hg, change in level of consciousness, abnormal arterial blood gas levels, and urinary output less than 30 ml/hr. Initiate therapy to maintain or achieve hemodynamic stability. For bradydysrhythmias administer atropine and isoproterenol and assess for ventricular irritability For tachydysrhythmias administer digitalis, perform synchronized cardioversion, and administer lidocaine.	Patient did not experience decreased cardiac output as defined by decreased arterial pressure, loss of consciousness, abnormal arterial blood gas levels, and decreased urinary output. Hemodynamic instability did not occur.

Plan and intervention for decreased cardiac output

The type of life support needed before the insertion of the temporary pacemaker depends on the patient's condition. The patient with symptoms outside the hospital should be kept warm and supine until transportation to the hospital. The person should not be left unattended. Heart rate is monitored continuously. If signs of cerebrovascular insufficiency appear, such as loss of consciousness, seizure, or apnea, cardiopulmonary resuscitation (CPR) is initiated. Oxygen, intravenous access, and drugs can be added to the regimen when the patient reaches a life-support facility such as an ambulance or emergency room.

In the life-support area, if a bradydysrhythmia is present, 0.5 mg of atropine can be given intravenously at 5-minute intervals to increase heart rate (usually 2 to 3 doses). If this is unsuccessful, an isoproterenol infusion is the next alternative, using 1 mg in 500 ml of 5% dextrose and water (a 2% drug solution). This can be administered at a rate of 2 to 20 micrograms (μg)/minute and titrated according to heart rate, as necessary. The nurse should be prepared to manage ventricular irritability that can occur with this sympathomimetic agent. Lidocaine should be used only when the ventricular irritability could be lethal and when the isoproterenol produces an intrinsic rhythm that can sustain the patient. Lidocaine, procainamide, or bretylium can suppress not only undesirable ventricular ectopy but also life-sustaining ventricular escape rhythms. Any other agents that depress mental, respiratory, or cardiac function (such as sedatives and narcotics) should be avoided until the patient is supported by a temporary pacing system.

The person with a symptomatic rapid heart rate requires the same support before reaching the acute care facility that a person with a bradydysrhythmia would require. In addition, the origin of the rapid heart rate must be determined (e.g., supraventricular or ventricular). Pharmacologic treatment then can be initiated. If digitalis toxicity has been ruled out as a cause of supraventricular dysrhythmia, it can be administered intravenously at doses of 0.125 to 0.25 mg until a total of 1 mg is reached. Adequate digitalization is characterized by a reduction in heart rate. If digitalis is ineffective or cannot be administered, synchronized cardioversion is the next treatment of choice before a temporary pacing lead can be positioned for overdrive therapy. The nurse watches for signs of symptoms of congestive heart failure and reduced cardiac output, which can occur with rapid heart rates. If the tachydysrhythmia is ventricular, lidocaine can be given intravenously in a bolus of 50 mg. If this is unsuccessful, cardioversion is required (see Appendix D). The nurse watches for signs of cardiac decompensation.

Arterial oxygenation, arterial pressure, and fluid and electrolyte balance are maintained as needed to help the myocardial cells respond to the electrical stimulation of the pacemaker and keep the threshold within normal limits. If the patient does not respond to pharmacologic and other intervention, advanced cardiac life support must be continued and a temporary pacing system installed as rapidly as possible.

NURSING DIAGNOSIS 2	**High risk for anxiety related to cardiac disorder and the impending temporary pacemaker insertion (feeling pattern)**	

PATIENT OUTCOMES	NURSING PRESCRIPTIONS	EVALUATION
Patient will verbalize an understanding of the dysrhythmia and its cause and treatment, the insertion of the temporary pacemaker, the amount of discomfort there may be and ways it will be managed, places the patient will go after the procedure, ways the patient will feel with the temporary lead in place, and the type of activity restrictions there will be.	Teach about the dysrhythmia and its cause and treatment, the temporary pacemaker insertion procedure, the local anesthesia and analgesia used, places the patient will go after the procedure, ways the patient will feel with the temporary lead in place, and restriction of the affected extremity.	Patient verbalized an understanding of the dysrhythmia and its cause and treatment, the insertion of the temporary pacemaker, the amount of discomfort there may be and ways it will be managed, places the patient will go after the procedure, ways the patient will feel with the temporary lead in place, and types of activity restrictions there will be.
Patient will participate in relaxation techniques and will not exhibit signs and symptoms of severe anxiety related to the disorder and the impending pacemaker insertion.	Assess patient's ability and willingness to participate in relaxation sessions before and during the pacemaker insertion. Use a short head-to-toe muscle relaxation script (see Chapters 5 and 13). Use guided imagery to "walk" patient through the procedure. Assess patient's level of anxiety before and after sessions.	Patient participated in relaxation sessions and did not exhibit signs and symptoms of severe anxiety related to the disorder and the pacemaker insertion.

Plan and intervention for anxiety

Persons faced with the diagnosis of a cardiac disorder and the need for pacing typically express fears of dying, pain, and incapacitation. The future is suddenly uncertain. Fear, panic, and dread can rob the patient of oxygen and cell substrates critically needed during this time of stress. The three most effective interventions are emotional support, education, and relaxation techniques. Reflective listening, good eye contact, and supportive touching as seems appropriate are effective. As physical care is being administered, careful and simple explanations of the diagnosis and its treatment should be given, even if patients are unconscious and receiving advanced life support. The temporary pacemaker insertion procedure is explained step by step. The nurse tells the patients where they are and that they are ill but that the medical team is taking care of them. It also may help to say, "We will take good care of you, and we will not leave you alone." Patients should be told where their families are and reassured that their families will be allowed to visit soon. Touching the person during this time helps confirm that a caring person is present. The touch should be firm and purposeful. Touch should be used in the same manner with each contact to help patients identify the nurse, especially if they are semiconscious or unconscious.

Patients with less-severe symptoms should be given an appropriate explanation of the reasons that they need temporary pacing, the way it works, and the length of time that they may need it. Their questions should be answered directly and simply. They also must be oriented to their immediate environment, including the way the ECG monitor works, their medications and persons who will be taking care of them. Patients' families also must be considered. Someone should be assigned to see that they have a private place to stay while patients are being cared for and that they are given frequent factual information.

Patients who participate in relaxation sessions before and during pacemaker insertion may experience less anxiety and some sense of control over their situation. If patients are willing to participate, the nurse can use a short head-to-toe relaxation script (see Chapter 13) to induce the relaxation response and then use guided imagery to augment the information pertaining to the pacemaker insertion procedure. An effective therapy for some patients involves suggesting that they escape to a place of comfort and peace (e.g., fishing pond, beach, or the mountains) during the procedure (see Chapter 5).

NURSING DIAGNOSIS 3   **High risk for ventricular tachydysrhythmia related to the insertion of the temporary cardiac pacing lead (exchanging pattern)**

PATIENT OUTCOMES	NURSING PRESCRIPTIONS	EVALUATION
Patient will not develop ventricular tachycardia or ventricular fibrillation. If ventricular tachycardia or ventricular fibrillation occurs, patient will respond to appropriate therapy.	Closely evaluate patient's cardiac rhythm during lead insertion. Have emergency drugs and defibrillator available.	Patient did not develop ventricular tachycardia or ventricular fibrillation.

Plan and intervention for ventricular tachydysrhythmias

The nurse must be prepared to treat the ventricular tachydysrhythmias that can occur during ventricular transvenous lead placement, particularly in patients with AMI. Lidocaine or similar agents may not prevent ventricular dysrhythmias, and sympathomimetic drugs may increase the likelihood of them.[68] Damage may occur to the pulse generator, lead, or both (despite claims to the contrary by manufacturers) if defibrillation is performed after the lead

has been inserted and connected to the pulse generator. Therefore disconnect the pulse generator from the lead before defibrillation. Reconnect quickly to provide pacing. In addition, tissue damage at the electrode tip can occur if the defibrillation current enters the lead and exits at the electrode-myocardial interface. Such damage alters the threshold to pacing and can occur even with the pulse generator disconneted. Be prepared to replace or reposition the lead after defibrillation (see Table 16-4).

NURSING DIAGNOSIS 4 **Symptomatic, potentially symptomatic, or high risk for bradydysrhythmia or tachydysrhythmia necessitating temporary cardiac pacing related to (include cause) (exchanging pattern)**

PATIENT OUTCOMES	NURSING PRESCRIPTIONS	EVALUATION
Patient will improve symptomatically or will not develop symptoms and will be stable hemodynamically as a result of pacing.	Assess patient's response to pacing.	Patient improved symptomatically as a result of pacing.
Arterial blood pressure will stabilize at a level to provide adequate systemic perfusion within 2 hours of initiation of pacing.	Monitor arterial blood pressure carefully during the first 2 hours.	Arterial blood pressure returned to an adequate level within 2 hours of initiating pacing.
Cardiac output will increase on initiation of pacing.	Evaluate adequacy of patient's cardiac output.	Cardiac output increased immediately on initiation of pacing.
Patient will be alert.	Evaluate patient's level of consciousness and alertness.	Patient was alert after initiation of pacing.
Urinary output will be at least 30 ml/hr.	Measure patient's hourly urinary output.	Urinary output was greater than 30 ml/hr.
Arterial blood gas levels will return to normal.	Analyze results of patient's arterial blood gas levels.	Arterial blood gas levels returned to normal.
Patient will not experience anginal pain.	Assess for chest pain.	Patient did not experience anginal pain.
Signs and symptoms of congestive heart failure will improve.	Assess for signs and symptoms of congestive heart failure.	Signs and symptoms of congestive heart failure improved.

Plan and intervention for symptomatic bradydysrhythmias and tachydysrhythmias

The most reliable means of temporary pacing is through the use of a transvenous lead inserted into the right ventricle. This can be accomplished in several different ways. With a balloon-tipped lead, stable pacing can be obtained in a fairly short time without the use of fluoroscopy (see p. 491).

Another insertion technique that can be used if the patient has an intrinsic cardiac rhythm involves the use of an ECG machine and intracavitary electrograms. The distal electrode of the lead is connected to the V lead of the ECG machine with an insulated alligator clip wire. The ECG machine should be electrically isolated; a battery-operated one is ideal. With the limb leads connected in the usual manner, the machine is turned on to the V setting. As the lead is advanced through the venous system toward the heart, the ECG tracing will indicate the location of the tip. Fig. 16-7 shows the appearance of the electrogram when the lead tip is touching the right ventricular endocardium. Note the deep S wave and the elevated ST segment.

In extreme emergencies during CPR the *transthoracic endocardial* lead can be used. This lead is inserted by closed-chest puncture through an intercostal space (fourth or fifth) or by a subxiphoid approach (preferred because there is less risk of lung puncture). A percutaneous introducer is inserted into the right or left ventricle until blood is aspirated from the chamber. The flexible, J-shaped lead is then threaded through the introducer. After it is in the chamber, the lead reforms into its J shape, ideally with the tip on the endocardial surface. An experienced physician should be able to insert this lead within 1 minute.[67]

CPR can continue throughout most of the procedure except during the introducer placement. The lead should be connected to the pulse generator before insertion. Some of these leads have an electrode at the tip and a second electrode a few centimeters proximal to the tip. This second electrode will have contact with the myocardium to complete the pacing circuit. Some transthoracic leads require a separate terminal pin that has to be inserted into the tissue near the insertion point and then connected to the positive pacemaker terminal. It is mandatory to be familiar with the lead before it is used in an emergency. If pacing is not obtained when the lead is first inserted, despite a high output setting, attempt to reposition the lead until capture is seen. Resuscitation must continue after 1 minute. Repeated failures to obtain capture may be secondary to the physiologic state of the myocardium. If pacing is obtained, the transthoracic system should be replaced with a transvenous system as soon as possible. The hazards involved in the use of a transthoracic lead are possible pneumothorax secondary to lung puncture and intrapericardial bleeding secondary to puncture of a coronary artery or vein.

If the patient is relatively stable, fluoroscopy should be used to insert a transvenous lead. This can be done in the patient's bed if it is radiolucent, in a nearby treatment

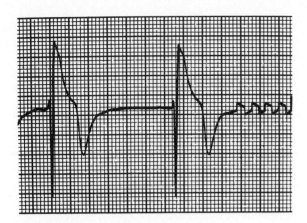

FIG. 16-7   Ventricular intracavitary electrogram with a 1-mV calibration (shown as an amplitude of 3 mm).

room, or in the cardiac catheterization laboratory. During lead insertion, all medications and equipment for advanced cardiac life support should be readily available. Care should be taken to maintain skin and field sterility, even during an emergency. A 3-minute povidone-iodine scrub followed by a povidone paint is recommended. A simple drape and sterile gloves and masks are essential. During CPR, if a transthoracic lead is inserted, a quick povidone paint can be done. If the patient is alert or sensitive to painful stimuli, local infiltration with 1% lidocaine should be carried out in the affected area.

Before connection, especially in emergencies, the pulse generator or *pacing system analyzer* (PSA) controls should be set on the following values so that pacing can be initiated quickly:

1. *Rate:* 60 to 80 ppm, depending on patient's anticipated needs
2. Output: 10 mA (20 mA for temporary epicardial or transthoracic leads) (This value can be reduced after patient threshold has been determined.)
3. Sensitivity: 0.5 mV (or lowest setting possible)
4. Pulse duration: 1 msec, if available
5. Mode: VVI, if available
6. AV interval: 250 msec, if using AV sequential pacing

A PSA is actually an external temporary pacemaker with rate and output controls. In addition, this instrument can measure and digitally display R- and P-wave values and lead resistance. The PSA is used most frequently to analyze a newly inserted pacing lead.

Usually the distal electrode of the lead is connected to the negative terminal of the pacemaker. Thresholds are generally lower in this arrangement. The proximal electrode is then connected to the positive terminal to complete the circuit. The nurse should be familiar with the operation of the pulse generator terminals and how the lead is secured in them. Proper placement and tightening can help prevent

disconnection and loss of pacing. The lead should be connected directly to the pulse generator or to a bridging cable designed for such use. The use of alligator clip wires to connect the lead to the pulse generator should be avoided because they do not provide a secure connection.

To determine the pacing threshold for the system, the output setting must be manipulated. While watching the ECG monitor during adequate pacing, the nurse slowly dials the output control down from 10 mA. At the point where pacing is lost, the nurse slowly begins to turn the output control back up toward 10 mA. The point at which pacing returns is the threshold. With acute endocardial pacing the threshold ideally should be less than 1 mA at 1 msec pulse width. Higher thresholds are seen in epicardial pacing because of tissue injury secondary to lead placement and because of the lead's large electrode area and resultant low current density. Initial threshold measurements of 10 to 15 mA at a pulse width of 1 msec are common.[15] This threshold rises during the next 2 to 3 days after insertion. After identifying the milliampere threshold value, the output dial should be turned up to a value at least 2.5 times the threshold. This setting will ensure that pacing is not lost when the threshold begins to rise. If the temporary pulse generator has an adjustable pulse duration, this value can be manipulated for threshold control along with output, if needed.

The next step in providing adequate pacing is to determine the sensitivity needed if the patient has an intrinsic rhythm. An electrogram can be obtained to determine the size of the cardiac potential seen by the electrode of endocardial and epicardial leads. One way that this can be done is by recording the electrogram with an ECG machine. The patient is connected to the machine in the usual manner, but the V lead is attached to the distal terminal of the pacing lead with an alligator clip wire. (The patient is not connected to the pacemaker at this time.) This procedure can be performed only if the patient's intrinsic rhythm is life sustaining. With the machine on the V-lead setting, an electrogram is recorded. The tracing is centered on the paper, and a 1 mV calibration signal that can be used for comparison when measuring the QRS complex obtained from the electrogram is added (Fig. 16-7) (see p. 498).

An alternative to this procedure when the patient has severe bradycardia is the use of the PSA that can measure the QRS complex and quickly return to pacing. Some of the newer temporary pulse generators also can quickly measure the QRS seen by the pacing lead. The QRS complex should be at least 4 to 5 mV but may be as large as 15 mV if the lead has been adequately placed in or on the right ventricle. Small QRS complexes can occur if the lead is touching the wall in an area of fibrosis or ischemia or if the endocardial lead is not touching the endocardium; further wedging may remedy this. If the signal is smaller than the capability of the sensing mode of the pulse generator,

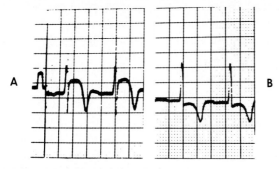

FIG. 16-8   Intracavitary electrogram of lead perforation into the pericardial sac. **A,** Proximal electrode electrogram with an elevated ST segment, suggesting contact with the endocardium. **B,** Distal electrode electrogram showing a positive complex with an inverted T wave typical of an epicardial signal.

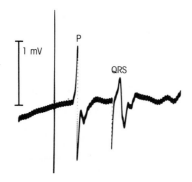

FIG. 16-9   Atrial intracavitary electrogram from the atrial appendage. The biphasic P wave is larger than the negative QRS complex.

the lead may need to be moved, although this is no guarantee that a larger QRS will be found. The QRS complex will have a characteristic deep S wave and elevated ST segment if the electrode is in contact with the endocardium (Fig. 16-7). If the electrogram from the lead tip shows a positive complex with a flat ST segment or inverted T wave, perforation may have occurred into the pericardial sac or the left ventricular area (Fig. 16-8). If this is suspected, the lead should be pulled back and repositioned until the

S wave is obtained with the elevated ST segment. With an adequate QRS, greater than 4 mV, the sensitivity control can be set on 2 mV to provide a margin of safety for sensing. Correctly placed epicardial leads usually provide adequate R and P waves for sensing. Because they cannot be repositioned after the chest has been closed, a temporary transvenous system should be available if there are severe sensing and capture problems.

Temporary atrial leads usually are not inserted in emergency situations but are used in the epicardial form after cardiac surgery or are inserted endocardially in nonemergency situations for atrial or AV sequential pacing. The P wave should be measured, if present. The technique is the same as that for the R wave. Fig. 16-9 shows an electrogram from the right atrial appendage; the P wave is a biphasic narrow complex measuring approximately 1 mV. When recording from the atrium, the QRS is typically about the same size or smaller than the P wave but is negative. Threshold and P and QRS measurements should be taken daily until the temporary unit is removed or replaced. The values obtained should be recorded on the nursing care plan and in the daily assessment notes.

After insertion of a transvenous lead, anteroposterior and lateral chest x-ray examinations should be done to confirm electrode position. If the lead has been placed in the right ventricle, the x-ray film will show that the lead is well to the left of the sternum in an anteroposterior view and is pointing anteriorly in the lateral view. The ventricular lead that is pointing posteriorly probably has been placed in the coronary sinus. Atrial J leads also should point anteriorly. This initial x-ray film should be kept with the patient so that follow-up studies can be compared with it. Any film ordered for lead placement evaluation should be made in the overpenetrated mode to ensure good visualization of the lead.

After pacing has been established, the nurse monitors vital signs and cardiac function to determine the effectiveness of therapy. Depending on the patient's hemodynamic status, arterial pressure, cardiac output, level of consciousness, neurologic signs, urinary output, presence or absence of angina, ventricular irritability, and signs and symptoms of congestive heart failure are monitored. More invasive monitoring can be discontinued as the patient stabilizes.

NURSING DIAGNOSIS 5 **High risk for fluid volume deficit related to bleeding due to the transvenous, epicardial, or transthoracic lead insertion (exchanging pattern)**

PATIENT OUTCOMES	NURSING PRESCRIPTIONS	EVALUATION
Patient will not develop bleeding at the lead insertion site.	Monitor insertion site for signs and symptoms of hematoma formation or decreased arterial perfusion.	Patient did not develop bleeding at the lead insertion site.
Hematoma formation will not occur. Decreased arterial perfusion distal to the hematoma will not occur.	Apply manual pressure to insertion site. Assess arterial pulses distal to insertion site.	There was no hematoma formation. There was no change in arterial perfusion distal to the point of insertion.
Patient will not develop bleeding into the pericardial sac related to the insertion of a temporary epicardial or transthoracic endocardial lead resulting in pericardial tamponade as indicated by decreasing blood pressure, rising venous pressure, pulsus paradoxus, and distant heart sounds.	Monitor for signs and symptoms of intrapericardial bleeding, including decreasing blood pressure, rising venous pressure, pulsus paradoxus, and distant heart sounds.	Patient did not develop bleeding into the pericardial sac resulting in pericardial tamponade as indicated by decreasing blood pressure, rising venous pressure, pulsus paradoxus, and distant heart sounds.
Patient will not develop a hemothorax related to subclavian puncture (during transvenous lead insertion) or internal mammary artery puncture (during transthoracic lead placement) as indicated by a fall in blood pressure, diaphoresis or pallor, rise in respiratory rate and effort, and chest discomfort.	Monitor for signs and symptoms of hemothorax, including a fall in blood pressure, diaphoresis, or pallor, rise in respiratory rate and effort, and chest discomfort.	Patient did not develop a hemothorax as indicated by a fall in blood pressure, diaphoresis and pallor, rise in respiratory rate and effort, and chest discomfort.

Plan and intervention for fluid volume deficit related to bleeding due to lead insertion

For several hours after the insertion of any transvenous lead, the site of entry is monitored for bleeding. Initially manual pressure should be applied, followed by a pressure dressing. In addition, arterial pulses are checked distal to the insertion point. Bleeding into the tissues surrounding the point of entry could cause enough swelling to impinge on arterial flow.

The placement of epicardial leads can result in bleeding from the myocardium. This bleeding is usually minimal but can be significant. The blind insertion of a transthoracic lead into the right or left ventricle can result in the puncturing of a coronary artery or vein. The nurse monitors patients for signs of intrapericardial bleeding and cardiac tamponade, such as a fall in arterial pressure, rising venous pressure, distended neck veins, decreasing intensity of heart sounds, and pulsus paradoxus. Pericardiocentesis may be necessary. Intrapericardial bleeding can also occur if an endocardial lead migrates and perforates the pericardial sac and would be treated in the same way. After bleeding is controlled in this situation, the lead can be repositioned.

Hemothorax can occur with subclavian vein puncture and in transthoracic puncture in which the internal mammary artery is inadvertently lacerated. Patients receiving temporary pacing leads via these routes should be monitored for signs and symptoms of fluid volume deficit from intrathoracic bleeding such as falling arterial pressure, dyspnea, increased respiratory rate, diaphoresis, restlessness, and chest pain. Many practitioners routinely order a chest x-ray study after these procedures to detect bleeding into the chest. These types of punctures can lead to disastrous bleeding. The nurse should be prepared for the insertion of a chest tube and surgical intervention.

If significant bleeding is evident into the chest or pericardium, clotting studies should be performed. If these are abnormal, the patient can be treated with an infusion of fresh frozen plasma to control the bleeding. Patients receiving temporary pacing leads of any type should not receive anticoagulant therapy unless absolutely necessary. If the patient receives such therapy, the preceding measures must be stringently observed. Blood pressure is monitored closely.

NURSING
DIAGNOSIS 6 **High risk for impaired gas exchange related to pneumothorax due to the insertion of a transvenous lead via the subclavian vein or the insertion of a transthoracic endocardial lead (exchanging pattern)**

PATIENT OUTCOMES	NURSING PRESCRIPTIONS	EVALUATION
Patient will not develop signs and symptoms of impaired gas exchange related to pneumothorax as indicated by shortness of breath, decreased arterial oxygen pressure (Pao_2), absence of breath sounds over the affected lung, cyanosis, chest x-ray film showing pneumothorax, and chest pain.	Monitor for signs and symptoms of pneumothorax, including shortness of breath, decreased Pao_2, absence of breath sounds over the affected lung, cyanosis, chest x-ray film showing pneumothorax, and chest pain. Be prepared to treat with oxygen and chest tube insertion.	Patient did not develop signs and symptoms of impaired gas exchange related to pneumothorax as indicated by shortness of breath, decreased Pao_2, absence of breath sounds over the affected lung, cyanosis, chest x-ray film showing pneumothorax, and chest pain.

Plan and intervention for impaired gas exchange

In the case of a subclavian lead insertion, the nurse monitors for pneumothorax during pacemaker insertion and for several hours after the procedure. The lung can be punctured during subclavian or transthoracic lead insertion, causing a pneumothorax and impaired gas exchange, which require a chest tube for reexpansion of the lung. The signs and symptoms are a rapid onset of shortness of breath, chest pain, tachypnea, restlessness, hypotension, cyanosis, absence of breath sounds over the affected lung, and a chest x-ray film showing puncture. The nurse should be prepared to assist in thoracentesis or chest tube insertion or to prepare the patient for thoracotomy. Respiration is supported as needed, including the administration of oxygen. As with any subclavian puncture, injury to the brachial nerve plexus also can occur. The patient is observed for signs of weakness in the affected arm. The patient will also complain of arm pain.

NURSING
DIAGNOSIS 7 **High risk for impaired physical mobility related to activity restrictions (moving pattern)**

PATIENT OUTCOMES	NURSING PRESCRIPTIONS	EVALUATION
Patient will participate in activities to prevent complications of immobility, including range of motion exercises, isometric exercises of the lower extremities, deep breathing exercises, and shifting weight from side to side.	Implement therapies to prevent complications of immobility; instruct on range of motion exercises, isometric exercises of the lower extremities, deep breathing exercises, and shifting weight from side to side. Apply antiembolism stockings and pressure-relieving pads and appliances to bed. Assist patient with repositioning and daily care activities.	Patient participated in range of motion exercises, isometric exercises of the lower extremities, deep breathing exercises, shifting weight from side to side.

Plan and intervention for impaired physical mobility

Nursing measures to prevent complications of immobility should be initiated as soon as possible after the insertion of the pacing system and the stabilization of the patient. The measures used depend on the condition of the patient. Some groups recommend that the patient with a temporary transvenous lead be confined to lying supine and keeping the affected extremity straight. These measures are used to prevent lead displacement. The smooth-tipped temporary lead is prone to displacement secondary even to the dynamics of systole. Any traction on the lead that could occur during flexion of the affected extremity could also pull the lead out of a position. Such patients should be instructed to flex the unaffected extremities once or twice hourly. The patient should also perform isometric tightening of calf and thigh muscles to promote venous circulation in both lower extremities. Under close supervision, this should be done even by patients with femoral vein insertions to prevent thrombophlebitis. Antiembolism stockings also can be used. If the patient cannot perform the exercises alone, the limbs are put through range of motion. The alert patient is coached to breathe deeply several times each hour to prevent pulmonary complications. Coughing is avoided if possible because it can cause lead displacement.

Patients who are vulnerable to skin breakdown should have protective devices such as foam pads or alternating pressure mattresses put on their beds. Shifting patients' weight from side to side with small pillows can help prevent problems and can promote comfort. Patients with an immobilized arm or leg need assistance with eating, bathing, and using the bedpan or urinal.

NURSING
DIAGNOSIS 8   **High risk for infection related to percutaneous lead placement (exchanging pattern)**

PATIENT OUTCOMES	NURSING PRESCRIPTIONS	EVALUATION
Patient will not develop an infection.	Initiate appropriate infection control measures and monitor for signs and symptoms of infection.	Patient did not develop infection.
Patient will not experience increasing pain at insertion site.	Apply antibacterial ointment and sterile dressing to insertion site.	Patient did not experience increasing pain at insertion site.
Patient will not experience redness at insertion site.	Change sterile dressing daily.	Patient did not experience redness at insertion site.
Patient will not experience swelling.	Assess for pain, redness, swelling, or purulent drainage.	Patient did not experience swelling.
Patient did not have purulent drainage from insertion site.	Culture drainage and tip of lead on removal.	Patient did not have purulent drainage from insertion site.
Patient did not have elevated temperature.	Assess patient's temperature.	Patient did not have elevated temperature.

Plan and intervention for infection

To prevent infection, lead insertion and care should be done using sterile technique. It is recommended that a antibacterial ointment (such as povidone-iodine) be applied to the insertion site before the initial dressing application. Care after insertion varies from institution to institution. Daily sterile dressing changes, a 3-minute scrub with povidone-iodine, and application of a antibacterial ointment are advisable. The site is examined for infection (purulent drainage, redness, or swelling). If drainage is seen, it should be cultured, and the alert patient is instructed to report increasing discomfort at the insertion site. The nurse closely monitors the patient's temperature; any elevation should direct suspicion to the pacing lead.

If the lead is removed because of infection, the tip is sent for culture. The infection rate is high, especially with brachial and femoral vein insertions. Infection can take the form of local cellulitis, thrombophlebitis, or both. Embolism related to the presence of a pacing lead in a vein is rare.[54] The frequency of infection begins to increase after 3 days. In most cases, if pacing is needed over 5 to 7 days and the prognosis indicates it, a permanent system is implanted. The temporary pacemaker then is removed 24 hours later. Infections usually clear without elaborate therapy after the lead has been removed. Blood cultures may be advisable with appropriate antibiotic coverage. Patients with endocardial leads are susceptible to infective endocarditis (see Chapter 13).

NURSING
DIAGNOSIS 9 **High risk for microshock related to the presence of the temporary pacing lead (exchanging pattern)**

PATIENT OUTCOMES	NURSING PRESCRIPTIONS	EVALUATION
Patient will not develop atrial or ventricular tachydysrhythmia.	Prevent microshock by maintaining electrical safety. Insulate all exposed parts of the lead. Wear rubber gloves when handling pacemaker terminals or the lead and when changing batteries. Use nonelectric beds. Avoid applying 2 different line-powered electrical devices to the patient at one time. Disconnect pacemaker from the lead during defibrillation.	Patient did not develop atrial or ventricular tachydysrhythmia.
Patient will verbalize understanding of the rationale for not touching other electrical equipment while a temporary pacemaker is in place.	Instruct patient to avoid contact with all other electrical equipment.	Patient verbalized an understanding of the rationale for not touching other electrical equipment while a temporary pacemaker is in place.

Plan and intervention for microshock

Electrical safety is extremely important in the care of the person with a temporary pacing system because the electrically conductive lead is in intimate contact with the myocardium. Even a small amount of stray electrical current, static electricity, or current from a short-circuited electrical device entering the lead and then the myocardium during the vulnerable period of the cells can elicit a tachydysrhythmia in the atrium or ventricle. This precipitation of a tachydysrhythmia is called *microshock*.

The threshold to fibrillation is fairly high in the healthy heart, but factors such as ischemia or drug toxicity can reduce the threshold and broaden time of vulnerability.[84] Older temporary pulse generators have terminals that are exposed. The nurse insulates with a rubber glove all exposed parts of the lead's external electrode at the terminals. Newer pulse generators are made with terminals that conceal the lead and the electrically active parts of the pacemaker inside the case. Additional protection may not be needed unless it is likely that the pacemaker will become wet. Guidelines in the user's manual should be followed for each pacemaker. No type of pacing lead should ever be inserted into the patient and left uncovered or unattached to a pulse generator. If pacing is not needed immediately after insertion of the lead, the external lead terminal is insulated in a rubber glove and secured with tape. Then the glove and lead are taped to the patient. Only battery-powered pacemakers should be used.

When handling the pacemaker terminals and the lead, the nurse wears rubber gloves to prevent static electricity

from the body entering the patient through the lead.[82] The wires should never be crossed or taped together. These maneuver could generate small amounts of current that could enter the wire and the heart.

It is ideal to have the patient in a nonelectric bed. If this is not possible, the electrical bed should be checked thoroughly by the biomedical engineer for proper grounding and integrity of the electrical components before use. The nurse instructs the patient to avoid using bed controls, or places the control box in a rubber glove to insulate it. The patient's call light can also be insulated in this manner.[10] If a malfunction of the bed is suspected, it should be unplugged and then inspected by the engineer, or the patient can be removed to another bed if the condition allows.

The entire patient area should be on a unipotential grounding system to prevent potential differences between monitors, ECG machines, and respirators and thus prevent stray electrical current from traveling through these devices and into the patient. In the unipotential grounding system, the grounding wires from all electrical outlets in the area are connected to the same ground below the building foundation. This reduces the likelihood of an electrical potential developing and current flow between any two pieces of electrical equipment.

All equipment around the patient area should be checked routinely by the biomedical engineer for proper functioning and grounding. The leakage current of an ECG machine connected to a pacing lead (during the recording of an electrogram) should not exceed 10 mA.[54]

The nurse should avoid applying two different line-powered electrical devices to the patient at the same time. Again, a potential difference between them could produce stray current that could enter the patient. For example, the monitor cable is disconnected from the monitor before the patient is connected to an ECG machine. Lamps connected to the bed should be disconnected and not used. No electrical device should touch the metal bed frame and the nurse should not touch the pacemaker or lead while touching an electrical device.

The patient is taught not to touch the monitor or an electrical device such as a line-powered radio while the temporary pacemaker is in place. Male patients should use rechargeable electric razors rather than line-powered ones. It is best not to allow these devices in the patient's room. Nurses alert others to these precautions with a sign over the patient's bed that reads, "Temporary pacemaker—electrical precautions in effect." Patient units caring for persons with temporary pacemakers should have policies and specific guidelines for preventing microshock.

External pacemaker batteries are not replaced while the pacemaker is in use on a patient, except when the pacemaker circuitry provides a brief continuation of pacing during battery changes.[54] The nurse wears rubber gloves during this procedure. It is preferable simply to replace the pulse generator with one having new batteries already in place.

The use of electrocautery on a person with a temporary pacemaker can cause inhibition of pacemaker output, and if the cautery current somehow reaches the pacing lead, it can enter the myocardium and elicit a tachydysrhythmia.[27] Cautery should not be used, or the guidelines listed in Table 16-4 must be carefully followed.

The currents used in defibrillation can cause permanent damage to the pulse generator if it is connected during delivery of the shock, and the presence of the pacing lead can allow current to enter the myocardium and cause tissue damage.[3] The pacemaker should always be disconnected from the lead during defibrillation and reconnected when pacing is needed (see Table 16-4).

NURSING DIAGNOSIS 10   High risk for pacemaker malfunction related to (state cause) (exchanging pattern)

PATIENT OUTCOMES	NURSING PRESCRIPTIONS	EVALUATION
Patient will verbalize an understanding of the rationale for actions taken to prevent pacemaker malfunction.	Initiate measures to prevent pacemaker malfunction.	Patient verbalized an understanding of the rationale for actions taken to prevent pacemaker malfunction.
Patient will not bend the affected extremity.	Instruct patient not to bend the affected extremity.	Patient did not bend the affected extremity.
Patient will comply with activity restrictions.	Instruct patient about activity restrictions. Secure lead at its exit point with tape. Secure pulse generator to patient with tape and Velcro straps. Assist patient with daily activities.	Patient complied with activity restrictions.
Patient will not experience pacemaker malfunctions, including failure to pace with the pacing artifact present, failure to pace with the pacing artifact absent, failure to sense, oversensing, or runaway pacemaker.	Monitor for signs of pacemaker malfunction, including failure to pace, failure to sense, oversensing, and runaway pacemaker. Initiate appropriate therapy at the first sign of malfunction.	Patient did not experience pacemaker malfunctions, including failure to pace with the pacing artifact present, failure to pace with the pacing artifact absent, failure to sense, oversensing, and runaway pacemaker.

Plan and intervention for temporary pacemaker malfunction

Prevention of lead displacement

Measures can be taken to prevent lead displacement and resultant failure to capture. The external course of the pacing lead should be properly secured to prevent inadvertent traction on the lead and subsequent displacement within the paced chamber and loss of capture. If the femoral vein has been used, the lead should be sutured to the skin at the point where it leaves the body. In addition, it can be taped to the skin with the external part of the lead lying in the inguinal fold. This prevents the lead from being pushed or pulled if the leg is flexed and then straightened. The pulse generator then should be secured to the thigh with tape or a Velcro strap so that its weight cannot pull on the lead. For patient comfort, place a folded dressing pad under the pacemaker before securing it to the extremity. If the brachial vein has been used, the lead should be taped along the bend of the elbow after suturing. The limb then can be placed on a well-padded arm board with the pacemaker taped to it. Leads with subclavian or transthoracic insertions also should be sutured and taped. The pulse generator can be secured to the patient's chest or waist.

Instruct alert patients not to bend the involved limb. Patients with subclavian insertions should not use the arm or shoulder on the affected side. Patients with femoral insertions are kept in bed with the head of the bed never raised over a 30-degree angle. A light restraint on the ankle may help to remind forgetful or sleeping patients not to bend the leg. Patients with brachial, subclavian, or jugular placement are allowed out of bed in some situations. For safety, they probably should be confined to sitting in a chair when out of bed. It is advisable that patients who depend on pacemakers be kept in bed regardless of the vein used. Transfers of patients from bed to stretcher or bed to bed should be avoided because displacement of leads can occur easily during these moves. If transfer is essential, such as to an operating room table, patients should be moved by an adequate number of people while remaining passive. The patient is never lifted from the bed by the underarms if a temporary transvenous lead is in place from any insertion site. Instead a draw sheet and two or more persons are used. Most external pulse generators are equipped with a protective face plate to prevent inadvertent movement of the controls or turning off of the unit. This face plate is used at all times.

Temporary epicardial pacing wires also may be sutured in place as they leave the body and carefully looped and taped down to prevent dislodgement. When not in use, they should be placed in a plastic tube provided by the manufacturer to prevent the Keith needle terminal from puncturing the patient. Insulate the tube with a sterile glove to prevent fluids or extraneous electrical current from touching the lead.

Monitoring

Another important element in the management of pacemaker malfunction is ECG monitoring for immediate detection of a problem. After a temporary system has been installed, take a complete 12-lead ECG to determine the best lead to use for continuous monitoring. In most instances leads II, III, V_1, or the Marriott-modified V_1 (MCL_1) are the most useful because there is usually a deep S wave that is easily counted by the monitor rate meter. In monitoring the pacemaker rate, the QRS complex rather than the pacemaker artifact must be counted, and the artifact must be clearly visible in the lead chosen. In most

instances the temporary system is a bipolar one in which the pacing artifact or spike is small and does not interfere with rate determinations on the rate meter or computer analyzer. If the system is unipolar, however, a lead must be found in which the artifact is smaller than the QRS complex, or double counting by the rate meter will occur. If atrial pacing is present, a lead in which the paced P wave can be seen is used; this is usually II, III, V_1 or MCL_1.

It is essential to detect any loss of pacing or sensing. If technicians are not available to continuously observe the ECG monitor, the rate alarm system must be used to detect loss of pacing. Rate limits are kept closely set and always in operation. Loss of pacing and asystole can occur without warning. Nurses must be familiar with the appearance of capture versus noncapture beats and never leave the patient unmonitored. A patient who must be transported to another part of the hospital should be accompanied by a portable cardiac monitor and a nurse. Patients with temporary pacing systems should never be placed in an unmonitored minimal care area.

Diagnosis and correction of malfunction

Several features of the temporary pacing system make it vulnerable to failure. Because part of the transvenous lead is external and often inserted in or near an extremity, patient motion can cause displacement. Also, this type of pacing lead is relatively rigid to facilitate insertion. This rigidity increases the risk of perforation into and through the myocardium and subsequent loss of capture. The smooth, nonflanged tip of the lead, which allows easy removal when it is no longer needed, also predisposes the lead to displacement. In addition, temporary endocardial leads inserted transthoracically are displaced easily by external cardiac massage and normal cardiac systolic dynamics. No one can depend on this type of lead for long-term (over an hour) temporary pacing. Temporary tied-on epicardial leads are fairly secure and rarely displaced. Finally, with all types of leads, there is a hand-tightened connection between the pulse generator and the lead where inadequate contact could cause loss of pacing.

Loss of pacing may not occur completely at first; it may be heralded by occasional loss of capture with the patient having no symptoms. However, the pacemaker-dependent patient develops symptoms fairly rapidly if pacing ceases abruptly and completely. In most instances the original symptoms, such as seizure or loss of consciousness, return.

The immediate actions to take in the case of the dependent patient with symptoms are critical. The nurse should rapidly confirm that the patient's symptoms result from a loss of pacing rather than other causes of the symptoms by checking the ECG monitor. A peripheral pulse is checked at the same time to make certain that it is not a monitor malfunction such as a loose ECG electrode. The nurse reassures the patient that there is a problem but that measures are being taken to remedy it. Next, while calling

TABLE 16-3
Temporary Pacemaker Malfunctions

Malfunction	Cause	Diagnosis	Correction
Failure to pace with pacing artifact present	Lead displacement (transvenous)	Abnormal or changing ECG axis	Reposition lead.
	High threshold	Rise in output needed to elicit capture	Reposition lead.
	Loose or broken connection	Pacing restored after connections are tightened	Check and tighten all connections between pulse generator and lead at least every 2 hours. Replace defective equipment.
	Lead fracture	X-ray films or flat electrogram recording	Replace lead. If only one wire in a bipolar lead is broken, make system unipolar to maintain pacing until lead is replaced.
Failure to pace with pacing artifact absent	Inhibition	Return of pacemaker function when asynchronous mode is activated	Remove source of inhibition. If electrocautery is needed, turn pacemaker to asynchronous mode.
	Battery exhaustion	Intermittent loss of output and fall in rate	Replace the pulse generator; then replace the old batteries. Keep a battery usage log.
	Circuitry failure	Loss of pacing with no other distinguishable cause	Replace the pulse generator. Label and submit the defective unit for repairs.
Failure to sense	Oversensing	Pacemaker sensitivity set too high	Reduce until normal pacing returns.
	Lead displacement	Electrogram showing reduction in size of R wave and loss of electrode contact with endocardium	Be prepared for loss of capture. Avoid competition with intrinsic beats. Reposition lead.
	Small R wave secondary to fibrosis or AMI	Electrogram showing R wave magnitude less than sensing ability of pacemaker	Reposition lead
Runaway pacemaker	Circuitry component failure	ECG with pacing artifacts at the upper rate limit (150 to 180 ppm), which are intermittent regardless of rate control setting	Replace the pulse generator. Label and submit the defective unit for repairs.

for emergency equipment and personnel, the nurse immediately increases the pacemaker output setting to its highest point (usually 20 mA) to restore capture if the loss of pacing has resulted from a simple rise in threshold. If this does not remedy the situation all connections between the pulse generator and the lead are quickly tightened. Loose connections are the most frequent cause of failure to pace, and they are preventable by routine nursing care. If tightening fails to restore pacing, the nurse turns the patient into the left lateral recumbent position. This may restore lead contact with the endocardium if displacement of a transvenous lead has occurred. These actions must be carried out in less than 1 to 2 minutes in the patient with symptoms. Afterward, the nurse may need to initiate CPR. Atropine or isoproterenol can be given to accelerate the intrinsic rhythm. If the isoproterenol does restore an acceptable rhythm, the nurse monitors for ventricular irritability. While supporting the patient with resuscitative measures, the nurse must define the loss of pacing and

correct it. Failure to pace can be categorized into two forms: (1) with the pacemaker artifact present or (2) with the pacemaker artifact absent (see Table 16-3).

Failure to pace with the pacing artifact present

If the electrical pacing circuit is intact and complete from the negative terminal of the pulse generator to the positive terminal through the lead, there will be a pacing artifact on the ECG. If, however, the current cannot reach the myocardial cells or if the cells cannot respond to it, myocardial capture will not occur. The most frequent causes of failure to pace with the artifact present are lead displacement and a high threshold in the electrode area.[65]

Lead displacement. Lead displacement usually occurs only with transvenous and transthoracic endocardial leads. Only a small amount of displacement is needed to cause loss of capture (Fig. 16-10). The diagnosis of lead displacement can be made using the 12-lead ECG (if capture is intermittent), intracavitary electrograms, and chest x-ray

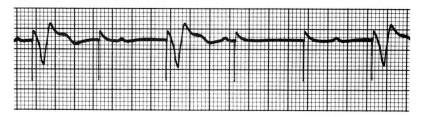

FIG. 16-10   Intermittent failure to pace with the pacing artifact present (loss of capture) secondary to lead displacement.

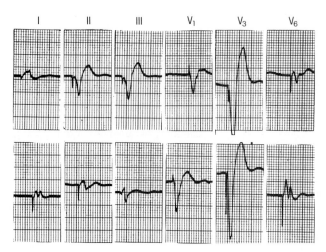

FIG. 16-11   Frontal plane axis shift secondary to lead displacement toward the pulmonary outflow tract. Note the axis shift in leads II and III from one day (*top*) to the next (*bottom*).

studies. Displacement of a ventricular lead toward the right ventricular outflow tract may cause an immediate loss of capture. The ECG axis shifts from the normal superior to an inferior axis because of the change in the site of origin of the ventricular depolarization (Fig. 16-11). As the lead migrates farther out the tract into the pulmonary artery, it is less likely that capture will continue because of the loss of proximity to excitable tissue. Intermittent loss of capture is seen, and finally, if movement continues, pacing is completely lost. Correction must begin with detection of the initial sign of occasional loss of capture. If the lead displaces into the right atrium, capture may take place there, producing paced P waves without ventricular pacing. If there is no AV conduction, ventricular asystole may occur, or a ventricular escape rhythm may take over at a slow rate.

With endocardial ventricular lead displacement and perforation into the pericardial sac, sensing may not continue with loss of capture; the results depend on the position of the lead in relation to the myocardial tissue. Other signs of this type of displacement are chest wall or diaphragmatic pacing because of the proximity of the lead to these tissues and a pericardial friction rub. The presence

of the lead in the pericardium can be confirmed with an echocardiogram. The patient may be the first to detect a change and may feel intercostal muscle pacing. This may be picked up by palpation, observation, or auscultation of a loud pacemaker sound caused by precordial muscle contraction elicited by the pacemaker. Diaphragmatic pacing is detected by palpation. (Diaphragmatic pacing can occur without perforation and can be remedied by reducing output or repositioning the lead tip if necessary.) All extraneous pacing of muscles will be seen at the rate set on the pacemaker. On the chest x-ray film, the lead will be too far anterior on the lateral view and possibly too far to the left on the anteroposterior view. The patient may complain of dull central chest pain when there is perforation into the pericardial sac. The intracavitary electrogram recorded from the distal electrode will show a positive R wave and loss of elevated ST segment (Fig. 16-8). An electrogram from the proximal electrode may also be positive. Perforation also can occur into the left ventricle, through the intraventricular septum, and into the left ventricular cavity. Pacing will not be lost as long as the electrode tip is touching excitable tissues.

There are signs of the migration, so loss of pacing can be prevented. The first sign is a shift in the ECG axis. Usually with pacing in the right ventricular apex the QRS complex produced has a LBBB configuration, and the pacing spike is followed by a deep S wave in leads II, III, and V₁. When the electrode and lead migrate into the septum and tissue of the left ventricle, the QRS complex begins to look like that of a RBBB, and the pacing spike is followed by an isoelectric or positive complex in the same lead (Fig. 16-12). In addition, with right ventricular pacing, the second heart sound is paradoxically split; with left ventricular pacing, it is widely split as in RBBB.

Atrial transvenous lead displacement is common because the atrial chamber lacks trabeculae in which to wedge and anchor the lead. A temporary J-shaped lead can be placed into the right atrial appendage to increase stability. However, any device on the atrial lead that would hold it securely in the appendage would make the lead difficult to remove after it was no longer needed. Loss of atrial pacing is indicated by a loss of P waves and QRS complexes, usually without warning.

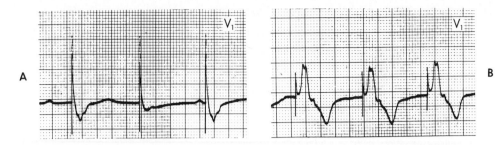

FIG. 16-12 Lead migration into the left ventricular myocardium. These are two V₁ ECG recordings from a patient with a temporary right ventricular endocardial lead. **A**, This recording was taken shortly after lead insertion. **B**, This recording was taken 6 hours later. The RBBB configuration suggests lead perforation into the left ventricular musculature or coronary sinus.

Lead displacement is remedied by repositioning. When the first signs and symptoms begin, preparations must be made for definitive treatment because pacing can be completely lost in a short time. The nurse must be prepared with pharmacologic support. It may be advisable to soak the exterior portion of the pacing lead near the insertion point with povidone-iodine–saturated sterile gauze pads for 15 to 30 minutes before repositioning. If this is not possible in the patient with severe symptoms, repositioning should still proceed. In the case of perforation into the pericardial sac, hemopericardium and cardiac tamponade rarely occur unless the patient has a concomitant coagulation disorder or is on anticoagulant therapy.

High threshold. An area of fibrosis or ischemia has a higher threshold to pacing than normal myocardial tissues. Care should be taken with the initial lead insertion not to position the electrode tip in such an area. Sensing also may be impaired. Repositioning the lead must be done until an area of normal threshold is found. Some groups[19] also have advocated the use of glucocorticoids to lower the threshold when repositioning cannot be done or has been unsuccessful. If the lead has been placed and the thresholds are normal initially (i.e., less than 1 mA) but suddenly rise enough to cause loss of capture even at an output of 20 mA, myocardial infarction at the electrode site can be suspected, although it is unusual. Rising thresholds also can be the first sign of lead displacement.

In the case of temporary epicardial pacing wires, the threshold to pacing, which is usually higher than endocardial thresholds, normally rises to levels beyond the capability of the pulse generator after 7 to 10 days of use. This may be caused by the infiltration of scar tissue into the area where the leads have been sutured.[87] Thresholds should be recorded daily on this pacing system. When they are rising, the decision must be made regarding whether to implant a permanent pacing system before the temporary one fails because of rising thresholds.

Two less frequent causes for failure to pace with the pacing artifact present are battery depletion and a break in the lead insulation. If the battery for the pulse generator is on the verge of exhaustion, it may continue to produce an output and thus artifact, but the current delivered is below the myocardial threshold and loss of capture is seen. When a break in the lead insulation occurs, current is diverted from the normal pathway down the lead and into the heart. The current is still present to make an ECG artifact, but not enough reaches the myocardial cells to produce depolarization. This diverted current may produce muscle contraction or a pricking sensation where it exits the lead.

Failure to pace with the pacing artifact absent

Complete interruption anywhere within the pacing circuit causes loss of pacing and disappearance of the pacing artifact from the ECG (Fig 16-13). The most frequently seen causes of this form of malfunction are loose or broken connections, lead fracture, inhibition of pacemaker output, battery exhaustion, and circuitry failure.

Connections. The most common yet preventable cause of an absent pacing spike is loose or broken connections between the lead and the pacemaker. Occasionally the artifact appears and disappears with manipulation of the external system. Simple routine checking of the terminals and bridging cable connections can prevent malfunction. This procedure should be carried out at least every 2 hours, depending on how active the patient is. Pacemakers and cables with failing or unreliable connection points should be repaired or replaced.

Lead fracture. Pacemaker lead fracture also causes continuous or intermittent loss of the artifact, and occasionally the spike may diminish in size. While the symptomatic patient is being supported pharmacologically, the lead should be examined externally and internally. If the fracture is in the internal portion of the lead, the diagnosis of suspected break must be made with the intracavitary or epicardial ECG recording, if the patient has an intrinsic cardiac rhythm. X-ray film may or may not show a fracture and cannot be trusted.

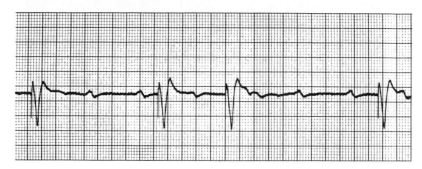

FIG. 16-13 Intermittent failure to pace with the pacing artifact absent secondary to a loose connection between the lead and the pulse generator.

Both wires within a bipolar lead should be evaluated. A complete fracture in the wire produces a flat-line recording. A partial break reveals small QRS complexes or a pattern that looks like alternating current (AC) interference. Occasionally with a partial fracture, the electrogram shows "make-break" artifacts that appear as sudden, extreme shifts in the ECG baseline. A recording from the proximal electrode or the other epicardial wire is also made. This wire may also break; if so, the recording will be a flat line.

If only one of the two wires within the bipolar lead is fractured, the intact one can be used to pace until a new lead or permanent system is installed. Pacing with one wire requires the creation of a unipolar system by connecting the intact lead to the negative terminal of the pacemaker. To complete the circuit, an ECG electrode plate is placed on the skin of the extremity nearest to the lead insertion point. The nurse ensures good contact with the skin by putting conductive paste or a saline-soaked gauze pad under the electrode plate. The place is secured with tape. Surgical or hypodermic needles have been tried in place of a plate, but because of their small size, the current density is high at the point of entry into the tissue and causes painful or annoying muscle contractions.[65] The positive pacemaker terminal is connected to the plate with an alligator clip wire. The pacing system then is functional and is operated in the usual manner. This makeshift unipolar system should be replaced with a new bipolar lead if the patient needs pacing for longer than 1 or 2 days.

Inhibition of pacemaker output. Inhibition of pulse generator output producing a failure to pace can occur when the sensing circuit is activated by extraneous *electrical interference.* Such interference can come from inside or outside the body. External sources can be oscillating magnetic fields and 60-cycle interference from sources such as line-powered electrical razors,[23] electrocautery, diathermy, and some telemetry equipment. Intermittent loss of pacemaker output also has been blamed on lead fracture in which case the connection between the two ends of the fractured lead intermittently touch each other, creating a small amount of current that can inhibit the pulse generator. Newer external pacing units are less susceptible to electrical interference, but inhibition still can occur, especially with electrocautery. When electrocautery must be used, the pulse generator is set in the asynchronous (fixed-rate) mode where sensing cannot take place. This can be done to maintain pacemaker output when inhibition is suspected. Careful attention must be paid to competition between the pacemaker and the patient's intrinsic rhythm if fixed-rate pacing is used.

Inhibition is a possibility when a ventricular endocardial pacing lead is displaced into the atrium. If P waves are present and the pacemaker is sensitive enough to sense them, pacemaker inhibition will occur. Inhibition also can occur if the lead is in the coronary sinus. In this case the tip of the lead may be near enough to the ventricular myocardium to pace and at the same time be near enough to the atrium to sense P waves and inhibit the pacemaker. If there is no AV conduction or intrinsic ventricular rhythm, the patient will develop symptoms. Repositioning of the lead is required. This type of inhibition also can occur with pacing in the DVI mode, when two temporary endocardial pacing leads are used, one in the atrium and one in the ventricle. If the atrial lead slips into the right ventricle, its electrical output can inhibit ventricular output and cause loss of pacing. If this situation is suspected, the atrial lead from the pulse generator is quickly disconnected.

Another situation that can cause inhibition is T-wave sensing, or oversensing. If the T wave is of sufficient magnitude and falls within the alert period of the pacemaker, it can be sensed. This causes pauses in pacemaker output and has been called *oversensing*. T-wave sensing may not occur after intrinsic beats when the wave's morphologic traits differ from those of paced T waves (Fig. 16-14). T-wave sensing can be suspected when pauses are seen intermittently on the ECG or when the paced rate falls below that set on the control.[5,8] This pacemaker-induced dysrhythmia can be mistaken for lead fracture or impending pulse generator failure. Decreasing the sensitivity on the pacemaker remedies this harmless problem. If the pace-

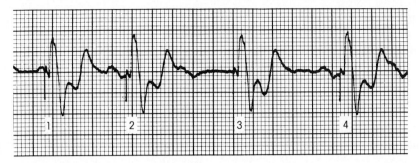

FIG. 16-14 T-wave sensing or oversensing in a temporary pacemaker with the sensitivity setting at 1 mV and a refractory period of 250 msec. The interval between complexes 1 and 2 is correct for the set rate of 70 ppm. The spike-to-spike intervals between complexes 2 and 3 and between 3 and 4 are prolonged. Decreasing the sensitivity to 2 mV eliminated the oversensing and resulted in slowing of the rate.

maker is sensitive enough and its refractory period short enough, it may also be inhibited by its own normal afterpotential wave if it persists beyond the refractory period. This situation is controlled in the same way as T-wave sensing. R-wave sensing can occur in atrial pacing, in which the refractory period is short and is managed in the same way.

Battery exhaustion and circuitry failure. When battery depletion is the cause of loss of the pacing spike, failure to pace may initially be intermittent. Most external pulse generators soon will be equipped with long-lasting lithium batteries, but there still will be a need to monitor battery life indicators and battery test systems, and it still will be wise to keep a log of pacing time on each pulse generator. It should be a routine to check the pulse generator's battery life indicator every 8 hours. Many institutions change short-life batteries after each patient use, but this is not a solution with longer lasting batteries. Nurses should be familiar with the power source of the pacemakers in use. Premature battery failure in temporary pacemakers is unusual, but it can occur. Replacement batteries and pulse generators must always be readily available in the patient care area. Prompt replacement of the pacemaker is also the solution for a suspected circuitry failure, although this type of failure is also rare.

Failure to sense

Ordinarily, when a PVC or other intrinsic beat occurs within the alert period (250 to 300 msec after the spike), a demand pacemaker will recycle and start timing for the next beat. If an intrinsic beat is not sensed, the pacemaker will fire an impulse as though the intrinsic beat had not occurred (Fig. 16-15). If the intrinsic cardiac complex is too small, less than the sensitivity setting on the pacemaker, it will not be seen by the pacemaker. This can be remedied by increasing the sensitivity. For example, if the intrinsic beat is 2 mV and the sensitivity is set at 3 mV, sensing will not occur until the sensitivity is adjusted to 2 mV or

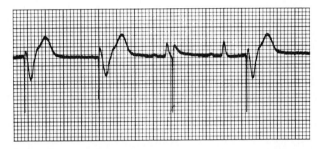

FIG. 16-15 The pulse generator failed to sense and recycle with the occurrence of the intrinsic QRS complex (third complex), despite the fact that it occurred well into the pacemaker's alert period.

less. If the intrinsic beats are smaller than the beats for which the unit can be set, the lead must be repositioned to an area where the beats are seen having greater magnitude. In some instances, only PVCs are not sensed because of reduced voltage or because they vary in slew rate. Premature beats occurring in the left ventricle may arrive late in the right ventricle and lead tip, causing the pacemaker to fail to recycle. This is called *pseudofailure to sense.*

The hazard of loss of sensing is that the pacing impulse could fall within the vulnerable period (second half of the T wave) of the ventricles after a nonsensed beat and could cause a tachydysrhythmia such as ventricular tachycardia or fibrillation. With atrial pacing, atrial tachydysrhythmias also can be induced but are not as life threatening as ventricular ones. In practice, this hazard probably is not present in every patient. In the healthy myocardium, it takes at least 20 mA of current in the vulnerable period to elicit ventricular fibrillation. However, many patients in need of pacing may have digitalis toxicity or an area of ischemic cells. The patient could also be hypoxemic or have electrolyte disturbances. All of these factors can reduce the threshold to fibrillation and extend the vulnerable period, thus making loss of sensing dangerous. Failure to sense is often a precursor of failure to pace, especially when it is caused by lead displacement. Until definitive measures can be taken, the immediate steps to take if loss of sensing is seen include checking the unit's sensitivity setting and making it as sensitive as possible. Next, the patient is placed in the position where adequate sensing was last seen. The left lateral or left lateral recumbent position may help. After this, the pacing rate is increased to override the intrinsic rhythm. If possible, the pacemaker is turned off but not disconnected. If PVCs are not being sensed, they are suppressed with drugs. The pacemaker output is decreased if possible; the less current, the less danger there is of eliciting a dysrhythmia. While preparations are made to reposition the lead, making the system unipolar can increase the sensing ability by increasing the circuit dipole size (see pp. 510 and 513).

Definitive measures for a sensing failure can be taken when the cause is determined. The most frequent causes of loss of sensing are lead displacement and an R wave too small for the pacemaker to sense. It may help to take an intracavitary electrogram to measure the patient's R wave that the pacemaker is not sensing. The nurse should anticipate the loss of capture when the loss of sensing occurs.

Runaway pacemaker

Any pacing system, temporary or permanent, is capable of circuitry component failure that produces a runaway pacemaker. In this malfunction the timing clock, which governs the rate of the regular electrical impulses of the pacemaker, fails, and impulses begin to fire at a rapid rate. Theoretically this rate could be fast enough to threaten the life of the patient. Fortunately a device that prevents the runaway rate from exceeding an upper limit of usually 150 to 180 ppm has been developed. (Check each manufacturer's manual for the specific rate.) The pacemaker, as with units used for overdrive pacing, can be set at a rate faster than the upper rate limit, but in the event of malfunction, it will not exceed the upper rate limit.

A runaway pacemaker is suspected when the paced rate rises to the upper limit despite the setting on the rate control. This increase may be intermittent initially. In the event of a runaway malfunction the pulse generator must be replaced. The defective unit should be labeled to prevent its inadvertent use and then sent for repairs.

NURSING DIAGNOSIS 11   **High risk for bleeding related to removal of the temporary pacing leads (exchanging pattern)**

PATIENT OUTCOMES	NURSING PRESCRIPTIONS	EVALUATION
Patient will not develop bleeding or hematoma formation at the transvenous lead insertion site.	Prevent bleeding and hematoma formation at the insertion site. Apply pressure to site with sterile gauze pads after lead removal. Assess site for swelling at frequent intervals during the first 24 hours.	Patient did not develop bleeding or hematoma formation at the transvenous lead insertion site.
Patient will not develop intrapericardial bleeding or cardiac tamponade after removal of the temporary epicardial or transthoracic lead.	Assess for signs and symptoms of intrapericardial bleeding and cardiac tamponade at frequent intervals during the first 24 hours after removal. These include decreasing blood pressure, narrowing pulse pressure, rising venous pressure, pulsus paradoxus, and distant heart sounds. Be prepared for pericardiocentesis.	Patient did not develop intrapericardial bleeding or cardiac tamponade after removal of the temporary epicardial or transthoracic lead.

Plan and intervention for bleeding related to lead removal

Usually before lead removal, the temporary pacemaker is turned off for 24 hours. Then if it is fairly certain that temporary pacing will no longer be needed, the lead is removed. For the temporary transvenous system, sutures are clipped, sterile gauze pads are placed over the insertion point, and the lead is slowly pulled out. Some practitioners recommend watching lead removal on the fluoroscope to make certain the entire lead is brought out. If this is not possible or practical, the lead should be examined after it has been withdrawn to see that no part has been left in the venous system. This rarely occurs with the construction of pacing leads now in use. Next, pressure is applied over the insertion point for 3 to 5 minutes with sterile gauze pads. Then the opening is checked for bleeding. The nurse observes the surrounding tissues for swelling, which may indicate internal bleeding from the puncture wound in the vein. If bleeding is not apparent, a sterile pressure dressing is placed over the site. The nurse should be certain to leave a small window in the elastic dressing tape to allow visualization of later bleeding. This dressing is removed after 24 hours. Subcutaneous bleeding and hematoma forma-

tion still can occur during the first 48 hours but are rare after the first 12. If such bleeding is suspected, the nurse notifies the physician. A pressure dressing is reapplied and the patient kept in bed until the problem resolves. Such bleeding can occur more easily in patients who have had anticoagulant therapy or who have a coagulation disorder.

Temporary epicardial or transthoracic leads are simply pulled out with gentle traction. Patients should be observed for intrapericardial bleeding and tamponade after removal. As soon as the danger of bleeding has passed, the patient is ambulated again, if it is appropriate.

SECTION III
Permanent pacing

COMPONENTS OF THE PERMANENT SYSTEM

The permanent pulse generator is a self-contained unit designed to withstand the corrosive environment of the body fluids and to cause no harm to the tissue around it. These objectives have been met by placing the pacemaker mechanism within a hermetically sealed case made of titanium or a similarly inert metal. The shape of the pulse generator is designed to avoid tissue erosion and to allow patient comfort. Also, in unipolar pacing in which the metal case around the pulse generator acts as the electrically active anode of the circuit, it is designed to avoid areas of high current density that occur at corners or acute angles. The ideal shape is cornerless, oval, or round.[72]

Permanent pulse generators can be unipolar or bipolar and programmable. The unipolar pulse generator has one opening to accommodate the pacing lead, which is also the terminal for the negative pole of the circuit (Fig. 16-16). The current flows from the terminal of the pulse generator, through the lead, to the electrode touching the endocardium or myocardium, where it stimulates myocardial contraction. The current dissipates throughout the tissues of the body. This dissipation eventually causes the current to return to the metal case on the pulse generator (buried in the tissues), which acts as the positive pole of the electrical circuit. Thus the negative-to-positive terminal flow seen in all electrical circuits is complete.

The bipolar pacemaker differs from the unipolar in that there are two terminal openings (one positive and one negative) on the pulse generator to which the bipolar lead is connected. The bipolar lead has two terminal pins and two electrodes at the tip in contact with the heart. When the bipolar system is connected, the lead terminal pin connected to the distal lead electrode is plugged into the negative pulse generator terminal, and the proximal lead elec-

trode is plugged into the positive pulse generator terminal. Pacing current flows from the pulse generator, through the negative terminal, and down the lead to the distal electrode and into the myocardium. The current then dissipates and finally reaches the proximal lead electrode. This electrode conducts the current back through the lead where it enters the positive terminal of the pulse generator to complete the electrical circuit. Without the negative-to-positive current flow, the electrical circuit would be inoperative. As with temporary systems, electrical impulses generated by the myocardium are picked up by the lead electrode and conducted up the lead and into the pulse generator where they enter the sensing circuit. Opinions vary as to whether a unipolar or bipolar system is the best. Some of the advantages and disadvantages of each follow:

1. Unipolar systems can have better sensing abilities in some cases because of the larger circuit dipole (area of active sensing in the tissue that acts as an antenna to pick up impulses from the myocardium)[5,25] (Fig. 16-16). However, this also can make the system more vulnerable to electromagnetic interference from myopotentials and outside sources.
2. Unipolar leads are in most instances smaller in diameter than bipolar. This can be important for the patient with small veins.
3. Unipolar pacing systems produce a larger pacing artifact than bipolar because of the size of the dipole. This makes the evaluation of the ECG easier.
4. Chest or abdominal wall muscle pacing can occur with unipolar systems, depending on the location of the pulse generator. In unipolar pacing the metal case around the pulse generator is electrically active; that is, it is the negative pole of the circuit. In some pulse generators, there is enough current flow around the case to stimulate underlying muscles.

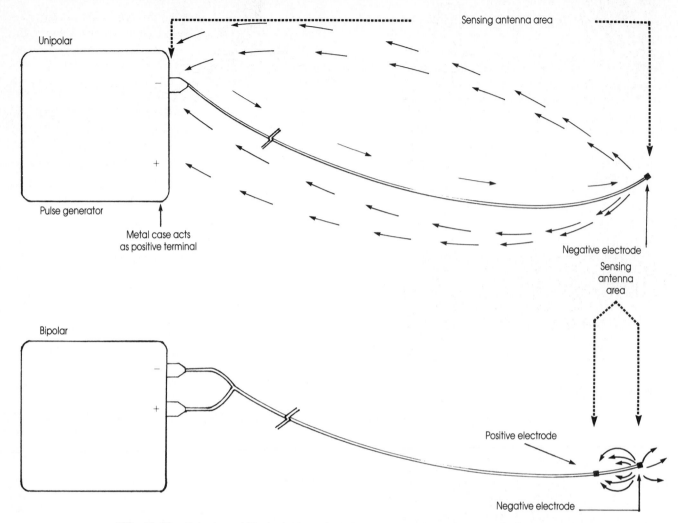

FIG. 16-16 Unipolar and bipolar leads, pulse generators, and their circuits, illustrating the sensing antenna areas.

PROGRAMMABILITY

Pacemaker programming is the noninvasive transmission of information from an external programmer to the internally implanted pacemaker to change a parameter or function. The programmer receives input from the operator, and transmits coded messages to the pacemaker through an energy link. The pacemaker must receive and decode this energy signal, as well as energy entering its sensing antenna area (between the negative and positive electrodes), and decide whether a valid programming message has been sent. If it is valid, the instructions from the programmer are sent to the pacemaker's control circuitry.[41]

Nearly all pacemakers are now programmable, which allows manipulation of vital parameters to meet the patient's pacing needs without surgical replacement of the pacemaker. Heart rate can be increased to augment cardiac output or override dysrhythmias, whereas lowering the paced rate can allow an intrinsic cardiac rhythm to pre-

dominate. Programming to a shorter pulse width can conserve battery life. Bidirectional telemetry programming allows two-way communication with the pacemaker. The pulse generator transmits its present settings of programmable parameters to a display screen, along with the R and P wave sensed by the distal electrode and the intracavitary electrogram. Other parameters on which the pacemaker is capable of giving data are real-time paced rate, lead resistance (useful in the diagnosis of lead fracture), and battery conditions. (See Table 16-7 for information on programming in the management of permanent pacemaker malfunction.)

The engineering techniques of programming are complicated. One technique involves using pulsed-electromagnetic fields that open the pacemaker reed switch and allow coded directions into the pacemaker circuitry for evaluation and decoding.[41] The pattern of coded directions is designed in such a way that it is unlikely to be duplicated by accident. Such duplication could lead to inadvertent programming. Each manufacturer has its own programming system and programmers. User's manuals must be reviewed and should be available for reference.

Some of the difficulties that can occur during programming include (1) a malfunction in the pacemaker or programmer that produces an incorrect rate or an output that results in the loss of pacing, (2) pauses in output during programming that may be significant in the pacemaker-dependent patient because cardiac output falls during the pause, and (3) a sudden loss of power in the programmer, which may render the operator unable to return the patient from a slow rate or a low output being used in a test procedure. These risks make it important to have more than one operational programmer for any pacemaker.

PERMANENT PACING LEADS

The construction of the permanent pacing lead is similar to that of the temporary lead. They differ in that the permanent lead is designed to stay within the body and the chamber in which it is placed.[12,22,39,72] It also must be flexible, durable, tolerated by the body, and capable of providing low thresholds. Several methods for endocardial anchoring have been developed over the last 10 years. These include flange-, tine-, mesh-, and fin-tipped devices for passive lead fixation and spring-released barbs, screw-in, and clamp-tipped leads for active fixation. Various types have their advantages and disadvantages and thus are indicated in different situations. Leads designed to lower acute and chronic thresholds are the steroid-eluting and mannitol-tipped leads.[57,63]

In general, transvenous pacing is the preferred method of permanent pacing because implantation of an epicardial system requires the stress of general anesthesia and a thoracotomy. However, epicardial systems are indicated in the following situations:

1. In patients with repeated episodes of endocardial exit block[17]
2. For repeated lead displacements
3. With cardiac surgery when leads can be placed before incisional closure in cases in which the need for pacing is known or strongly anticipated
4. In children because of their rapid growth and small venous systems

These leads commonly are sutured to or screwed into the right ventricle near the septum, avoiding coronary vessels, or on the lateral left ventricle between the left anterior descending and circumflex coronary arteries. Areas of surface fat deposition are avoided.

POWER SOURCES

Except for the nuclear type, which is no longer used, all pulse generators are now made with lithium batteries, which vary in their cathodal material. Lithium is used for increased longevity to spare the patient repeated replacements and to obtain reliable pacing. Some lithium-powered pacemakers have lasted 8 to 10 years; yet others have failed after only 18 to 24 months.[28]

ELECTROMAGNETIC INTERFERENCE

Pacemakers have been vulnerable to electromagnetic interference (EMI) since the first demand function was introduced. Electromagnetic signals from within or outside the body can enter the pacemaker through its sensing circuit antenna. After a signal reaches the pacemaker, a device called the *band-pass filter* allows it to enter the pacemaker's circuitry if the signal is of a predetermined size and frequency. This technique increases the pacemaker's ability to discriminate between EMI and legitimate cardiac signals. After the signal has passed through the band-pass filter, the pacemaker must then decide whether it is a legitimate programming signal, whether it is an R wave or P wave, or whether it is extraneous interference. The decoding circuit analyzes the strength and modulation characteristics of the incoming signal and reacts in one of the following ways:

1. If the signal matches the pulse generator's programming access code, the signal is sent to the control circuitry, where it can change a pacing parameter so that reprogramming could conceivably take pace. The result could be loss of capture because of a change in output or a serious drop in rate.
2. If the signal has the amplitude and wave-form configuration of an R wave, P wave, or extrasystolic beat, the pacemaker will inhibit its output or trigger output with the signal for the duration of the signal. As long as the interference lasts in that form, the pulse generator continues to recycle with it. Persons with a pacemaker inhibited by sensing and who have little intrinsic cardiac activity may begin to have symptoms if the interference lasts long enough. Pacemakers triggered by extraneous signals may increase the paced rate, and patients will experience tachycardia.
3. If the signals do not resemble programming or intrinsic beats and they are strong enough, the pacemaker will put itself into an asynchronous mode or noise rate; that is, it will fire impulses at a fixed rate until the source of the signals is removed. This fixed-rate function could cause *competition* between the pacemaker and patient if the patient has an underlying rhythm.

Most signals in a patient's environment are of low intensity and do not exceed the sensing threshold of the pacemaker or resemble the access code of the programming circuit. There also are factors that insulate the pacing system from extraneous signals, such as the air, patient's skin,

TABLE 16-4

Electromagnetic Interference in the Clinical Environment

Source	Effect	Management
Static electricity	Inhibition of temporary pacemaker can occur.	Wear rubber gloves when handling PG; do not touch PGL when touching any electrical device; insulate PGL in rubber glove; maintain all devices; do not change PG batteries when connected to patient.
Diathermy	Inhibition triggering (I/T) can occur; heating of permanent PG case can lead to tissue burns and component damage.[a]	Avoid; monitor PG if diathermy is used distant to PGL.
Ultrasound	No studies are available, but it may be all right at a distance from PGL because it uses sound waves.[b]	Avoid; monitor PG if ultrasound is used distant to PGL.
Cautery (superficial and surgical)	I/T, inadvertent reprogramming, induced dysrhythmias secondary to current, and reversion to fixed rate pacing can occur.[c] Effects vary with type of cautery, settings, current pathway, and the pacemaker type.	Know programmed values before procedure. Return pathway must be perpendicular to PGL. Ground pad placed to make current flow away from PGL and be as close to active tip as possible.[d] Ground pad well covered with conductive jelly. Program PG to fixed rate; consult manufacturer; do not use magnet over PG unless recommended (reprogramming can still occur); evaluate after procedure. Apply current for no more than 1 sec at 10-sec intervals.[e] Monitor heart with stethoscope and palpate pulse; cautery will interfere with ECG. Keep patient away from other electrical devices during procedure. Keep programmer-analyzer with patient for evaluation and reprogramming. Keep replacement temporary PG available.
Defibrillation	Circuitry damage, tissue damage at lead tip, and inadvertent reprogramming can occur.[f]	Know programmed values for comparison. Use anterior-posterior paddles if possible. If anterior paddles are used, place them perpendicular to and 4 inches away from PGL if possible. Use lowest setting on defibrillator, depending on dysrhythmia (200 to 300 W/sec for first 2 shocks).[g] Disconnect temporary PGL before shock and quickly reconnect. Keep programmer analyzer available for evaluation. Monitor patient for 24 hours because tissue damage at tip may cause rise in threshold; component failure can occur later after defibrillation.

[a]Data from Hardage M, Marbach JR, and Windsor DW: In Barold SS, editor: Modern cardiac pacing, Mount Kisco, NY, 1985, Futura Publishing Co, Inc.

[b]Data from Warnowicz-Papp MA: Clin Prog Pacing Electrophysiol 1:166, 1983.

[c]Data from Domino KB and Smith TC: Anesth Analg 62:610, 1983, and Goldberg ME, McSherry RT, and O'Connor ME: Anesth Analg 63:541, 1984.

[d]Data from Lerner SM: Anesth Analg 52:705, 1973.

[e]Data from Domino KB and Smith TC: Anesth Analg 62:610, 1983, and Lerner SM: Anesth Analg 52:705, 1973.

[f]Data from Alyward P, Blood R, and Tonkin A: PACE 2:462, 1979; Barold SS and others: PACE 1:514, 1978; Lau FYK, Bilitch M, and Wintraube HJ: Am J Cardiol 23:244, 1969; Palac RT and others: PACE 4:163, 1981; and Taube MA, Elsberry DD, and Exworthy KW: PACE 2:A103, 1979.

[g]Data from McIntyre K and Lewis J: Textbook of advanced cardiac life support, Dallas, 1981, American Heart Association.

[h]Data from Gibson TC and others: Chest 63:1025, 1973.

[i]Data from Adamec R, Haeflinger JM, and Killsch JP: PACE 5:146, 1982; Marbach JR and others: Radiat Oncol Biol Phys 4:1055, 1978; Parsonnet V and others: Circulation 68:227A, 1983; and Pourhamidi AH: Chest 84:499, 1983.

[j]Data from Heldner FJ, Linhart JW, and Poole DO: Radiology 92:148, 1969; and Walz BJ and others: JAMA 234:72, 1975.

[k]Data from Erlebacher JA and others: Am J Cardiol 57:437, 1986; Fetter J and others: PACE 7:720, 1984; Westerholm C: J Thorac Cardiovasc Surg 8:1, 1971; and Young D: Impulse 10:3, 1978.

[l]Data from Hardage M, Marbach JR, and Windsor DW: In Barold SS, editor: Modern cardiac pacing, Mount Kisco, NY, 1985, Futura Publishing Co, Inc, and Zimmerman BH and Faul DD: Diagn Imag Clin Med 53:53, 1984.

[m]Data from Erikson M, Schuller H, and Sjolund B: Lancet 1(8077):1319, 1978; and Fujiwara H and others: Chest 78:96, 1980.

[n]Data from Sylven C and Levander-Lindgren M: PACE 2:645, 1979, and Wicks JM, Davison R, and Belic N: Chest 74:305, 1978.

[o]Data from Langberg J and others: PACE 10(5):114, 1987.

[p]Data from Cooper D and others: PACE 11(11):1607, 1988.

Source	Effect	Management
Electroconvulsive therapy	No studies are available; it is probably safe because current is applied briefly between two distant electrodes and the area of current diffusion is small; repeated shocks could cause damage.[h]	Monitor ECG during procedure; evaluate pacemaker immediately thereafter; consult manufacturer if there are problems.
Radiation therapy and positron emission tomography	Component damage has been reported by some;[i] no damage has been reported by others.[j]	Shield PGL with lead; do not place PG directly in beam,[a] evaluate PG afterward; some patients have required moving the PG to an unaffected location.
Nuclear magnetic resonance (NMR) and magnetic resonance imaging (MRI)	Locking of reed switch, inadvertent reprogramming, disruption of output and rate control, and patient discomfort due to pull on PG have been reported;[k] heating of PG case can occur;[a] some groups report that the procedure is safe.	Many NMR and MRI facilities will not receive pacemaker patients. Patients should be kept away from magnetic area, 30 feet from device.[l] There is a need for more studies.
Transcutaneous nerve stimulators (TENS) and acupuncture	I/T occurs because of the use of pulsed electric current.[m]	Monitor patient carefully; evaluate after use or avoid altogether.
Phrenic or vertebral nerve stimulators	I/T can occur.[n]	Careful implantation is done, keeping receiver stimulator at least 10 cm from PGL; bipolar pacing is done if possible; monitor during use.
Lithotripsy (renal and hepatic)	I/T and damage to PGL can occur.	May be safe when water level is below PGL and pacemaker has been programmed to asynchronous mode (DDD to VOO) with machine output synchronous with pacemaker.[o] Avoid in VVIR units[p] in which damage to sensor can occur.
Dental scalers	I/T can occur if handle is held near PGL.[a]	Program to fixed rate; dentist needing pacemaker may benefit from bipolar system.

TABLE 16-5

Electromagnetic Interference in the Work Place

Source	Effect	Management
Magnets: Large mechanic's magnets, Lifting magnets, Magneto magnets	There is reversion to fixed rate pacing and the possibility of inadvertent reprogramming.	Refer for employment counseling if patient is operator or is in close proximity to magnets.
Electrical cables (greater than 10,000 amp) found in electrolytic reduction plants	I/T can occur.	Refer for employment counseling; bipolar or triggered modes with monitoring may be tried.
Alternating welding currents (arc and resistance welders)	I/T can occur.	Same as above.
Radio, TV, and radar transmitters	I/T and inadvertent reprogramming can occur.*	Same as above.
Power tools and assembly line robots	I/T can occur if the motor is in close proximity to PGL.	Same as above.
Induction furnaces	I/T can occur.	Same as above.
Electric generating plants and substations	I/T can occur.	Same as above.
Computer mainframe rooms	No studies are available, but there probably are no effects.	Monitor patient in the area.

*Data from D'Cunha GF and others: Am J Cardiol 31:789, 1973, and Picker BA and Goldberg MT: Br Med J 2:504, 1969.

TABLE 16-6
Pacemaker Electromagnetic Interference in the Home and Outdoor Environment

Sources	Effects	Management
Appliances (line-powered): Hair dryer Shaver Tools Mixer TV Computer Heating pad Welding iron Massager	There is no effect if appliances are used normally and kept in proper working order. Inhibition/triggering (I/T) can occur if device is placed directly over pulse generator and lead (PGL), turned on and off repeatedly,* or has a malfunction.	Use properly, keep in good working order. Use nonelectric shaver for underarms. Do not place device over PGL.
Microwave oven Remote control devices: TV VCR Garage door opener Toys Alarm systems	Microwave ovens are safe. No effect reported.	Reassure patient of safety.
Spark-ignited engines: Mower Car Trimmer Chain saw	There is no effect if used properly, with engine kept away from PGL (6 to 12 inches).* I/T can occur if PGL is close to machine.	Avoid placing PGL over coil area of engine. If patient wants to work on car engines, consider triggered pacemaker.
Radio transmitters: Ham radios CBs	It is safe if broadcast is within the guidelines of Federal Communication Commission (FCC). I/T is possible if PGL is near antenna area.	A triggered pacemaker could be considered or monitor pacemaker during use of equipment and program to triggered mode. Bipolar pacing can also be used.
Metal detectors: Airport security Stores Libraries	Reversion to fixed rate pacing has been reported.† Metal PG case may trigger alarm. Hand-held detector wand could cause I/T.	Tell patient that no ill effects have been reported because patient is within the alarm field for a short time. Instruct patients to show pacemaker ID at security gate.
Touch-activated switches: Elevators Some TVs Radios Some keyboards	I/T has been reported.‡	Tell patient that contact with device is brief enough that there may not be a clinical problem.
Commercial or military TV, radio transmitters, or radar	No changes have been reported if patient stays outside fenced or restricted areas.§ I/T could occur if patient operates this equipment. Studies are unavailable on mobile TV transmitting equipment.	Reassure patient and instruct patient to stay outside fenced area.
Electrical installations, substations, generating plants	I/T and reversion to fixed-rate pacing‡ occurs if patient is inside work area.	Same as above.
Police radar	There are no reports of ill effects.	Reassure patient of safety.

*Data from Cordis Corporation: Cordis Sequicor III Manual, Miami, 1983, The Cordis Corp.
†Data from Palac RT and others: PACE 4:163, 1981, and Smyth and others: JAMA 221:162, 1972.
‡Data from Irnich W, deBakker JMT, and Bisping HJ: Pace 1:52, 1978.
§Data from D'Cunha GF and others: Am J Cardiol 31:789, 1973; Picker BA and Goldberg MT; Br Med J 2:504, 1969; and Yalteau RF: N Engl J Med 283:1447, 1970.

body tissues, and titanium or other metal case of the pulse generator. These factors and the pacemaker's filtering abilities help to make ordinary appliances and devices safe. However, patients should still be instructed that interference can occur in certain situations (Tables 16-4, 16-5, and 16-6).

Another common source of interference is the body itself. High-frequency electrical impulses from skeletal muscles, called *myopotentials,* near a unipolar pacemaker are capable of disrupting function because their frequencies and amplitudes can be within the sensitivity range of the pacemaker and resemble R and P waves.[48] Bipolar pacemakers are affected almost never because of their small sensing area. Chest muscles are the most frequent source of myopotential interference, but interference from the contraction of the diaphragm or abdominal muscles has also been seen in abdominal implants.[6] Most pacing systems have been designed to ignore myopotentials, but occasionally one, especially one with high sensitivity, will react. The incidence is especially high in DDD systems.[14,32,35] Every patient should be tested within the first few months of implant to determine whether muscle activity causes inhibition.

MODES OF PERMANENT PACING

After the decision has been made to pace permanently, the best mode of pacing for the patient must be determined. This will be based on the patient's dysrhythmia, its cause, the status of the conduction system, the functional status of the myocardium, and the patient's need for variable increases in heart rate.

Ventricular pacing

Most patients requiring cardiac pacing are given VVI systems.[58] Simple ventricular inhibited pacing is sufficient to meet most patients' needs, and the system can be implanted in most medical facilities. The *VVI mode* paces in the ventricle, senses in the ventricle, and responds to incoming intrinsic signals in the inhibitory mode. The *VVT mode* is used less often but functions in the same way except that it fires a pacing impulse into a sensed QRS complex (i.e., it is triggered). Ventricular pacing can be unipolar or bipolar. This mode of pacing is indicated in patients with sick sinus syndrome who are frequently prone to atrial tachydysrhythmias such as atrial fibrillation. These persons also have been found to have a high incidence of AV node disease. Such factors make atrial pacing impractical or impossible. Patients with second- or third-degree AV heart block also usually are given VVI or VVT systems if their cardiac output is adequate and their myocardium is capable of compensating for the loss of AV synchrony.

Physiologic pacing

Cardiac output is maintained and enhanced by increasing the heart rate and augmenting the inotropic state and by the contribution that atrial systole makes to ventricular filling. The diseased heart may reach the point at which the compensatory reserves have been nearly exhausted. The loss of AV synchrony and a fixed rate, as occurs in ventricular pacing, may not be tolerated by these patients. They may have severe fatigue, poor exercise tolerance, and uncontrollable congestive heart failure, a condition known as *pacemaker syndrome.* To relieve this situation, new forms of pacing have been created. One of these modes is physiologic pacing, so named because it attempts to duplicate the normal pacing and conduction system of the heart, in hopes of maximizing cardiac output. The modes considered to be in the physiologic group are AAI-AAT, VDD, DVI, DDD, and rate responsive systems.[70,73] The objectives of these models are to restore AV synchrony and thus optimal cardiac output, to control atrial tachydysrhythmias, and as in the case of rate-responsive pacing, to allow the pacemaker to increase its rate based on patient need during activity.

Atrial demand pacing (AAI and AAT) is indicated in patients with isolated sinus bradycardia when there is no indication of AV node disease.[7] The pacemaker stimulates the right atrium, and the impulse is conducted through the atrial myocardium, into the AV node, and to the ventricles. The pulse generators used are sensitive enough to sense small (usually less than 3 mV) P waves and be inhibited or triggered by them. The refractory period must be longer in atrial pacing (i.e., 440 msec) than with ventricular pacing (i.e., 300 to 350 msec) to prevent sensing the resultant QRS complex. It is advisable to test AV node conduction periodically to detect the beginnings of AV block.

AV physiologic pacing requires the implantation of two leads, which has created difficult engineering problems. Some examples of these problems are how to sense P waves in the atrium and yet not sense both natural and artificial ventricular activity from the atrial lead and how to design the pacemaker to manage retrograde AV conduction after ventricular activity.

The first AV systems were in the VAT mode, which was originally the best solution to the need for sinus rate–controlled AV synchronous pacing in patients with AV heart block and normal atrial function. The pacemaker functioned like an AV node. A more recent type is *VDD pacing* in which pacing occurs in the ventricles, sensing is in the atria and ventricles, the response to sensing is inhibition in the atrium, and triggering and inhibition are in the ventricle (Fig. 16-17). This provides sensing for PVCs and conducted beats but still enables sinus control of the heart rate.

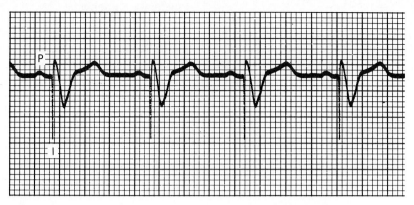

FIG. 16-17 Normal VDD pacing. The intrinsic P wave occurs and is sensed by the pacemaker; there is a delay, and the pacemaker fires a pacing impulse (*I*) into the ventricle.

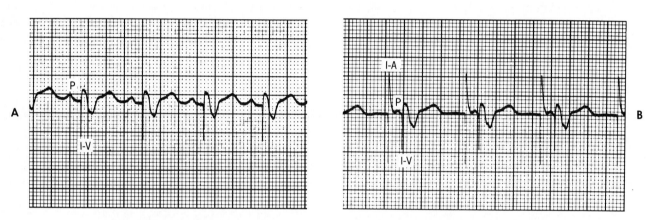

FIG. 16-18 Normal DDD pacing. **A,** When the patient's sinus rate is faster than the programmed lower rate limit of the pacemaker, the DDD system acts like a VDD system. In this case, the P wave is sensed, and an impulse (*I-V*) is fired into the ventricle, producing a paced QRS complex (VDD pacing). **B,** The sinus rate has dropped below the programmed lower rate limit of the pacemaker, causing an impulse (*I-A*) to be fired into the atrium that produces a P wave. Because this pacemaker-induced P wave was not conducted to the ventricle, the pacemaker fired an impulse into the ventricle (*I-V*) (DVI pacing). If a normal or paced beat is conducted to the ventricle, the ventricular component of the pacemaker would be inhibited.

The next AV pacemaker mode to be developed was the *DVI,* which is indicated for patients with poor SA node function and complete AV heart block, requiring AV synchrony. Pacing occurs in the atria and ventricles, sensing is only in the ventricle, and the response to sensing is inhibition. The major drawback to the DVI pacing system is that is does not sense in the atrium so that the heart rate is fixed and unable to accelerate with body needs. Paced rate, mode (DVI, VVI, or DOO), ventricular output, ventricular sensitivity, and AV delay are the programmable parameters in most of the currently available units.

The DDD, or *universal pacing system,* is indicated for patients who need occasional atrial pacing. The system comprises two leads and is capable of pacing in the atria and ventricles (Fig 16-18, *B*) and sensing in both cham-

bers. Its response is inhibition in the atria with the occurrence of a sensed P wave, inhibition in the ventricles after a sensed R wave or PVC, and triggering in the ventricle after a nonconducted sensed P wave (Fig. 16-18, *A*). The functions are performed through the use of a complex series of timing periods.

DDD pacemakers are capable of responding to atrial tachydysrhythmias, such as sinus tachycardia, supraventricular tachycardia, and atrial flutter. If the sinus or atrial impulses are of sufficient magnitude to be sensed by the atrial channel and when the programmed upper rate limit of the pacemaker is reached and exceeded by the intrinsic cardiac mechanism, it begins to block the firing of impulses into the ventricle. The ventricular impulse will be fired at a ratio of 1 (atrial beat) to 1 ventricular paced impulse, or

3:1, 4:1, and so on, depending on the atrial rate. This blocking mechanism is similar to that seen in the AV node's response to SVT or atrial flutter. Theoretically, the pacemaker can track the atrial rate as fast as that allowed by the total refractory period. The total refractory period is the sum of AV delay (e.g., 120 msec) and the postventricular atrial refractory period (e.g., 220 msec), or 340 msec. This total would allow the pacemaker to follow the atrial rate up to 180 bpm and block appropriately to maintain a correct ventricular rate. If the pacemaker cannot sense the atrial flutter waves, it reverts to its lower rate limit and fires at a fixed rate into the atrium and then into the ventricle. When examining the ECG produced by the DDD system, it helps to remember that the pacemaker provides what patients need when they need it.

Rate-responsive pacing

Up to 50% of all patients requiring cardiac pacing may have sinus node dysfunction that limits the usefulness of these forms of physiologic pacing because heart rates are unable to increase in response to the need for increased cardiac output.[66] To assist persons who need to accelerate their heart rates but who cannot because of sinus node disease, variable-rate or rate-responsive pacing has been developed.

Studies have been performed to determine the ideal sensor to detect the need for increased pacing rate. Among the factors investigated are the QT interval,[11,13] end-systolic volume, ejection time, respiratory rate, muscle noise,[29,48] blood temperature, mixed venous blood oxygen saturation,[75] blood pH, right ventricular pressure, and blood flow velocity. The most reliable sensor has been the activity-driven types that sense muscle movement through the use of a piezo crystal that, when bent or deformed, produces small electrical signals that can be fed into the pacemaker rate control center. This type of sensor responds rapidly to the onset of exercise and when it ceases.[4]

The rate-responsive feature is programmable to adapt to the patient's needs, which are usually determined during treadmill exercise testing. The programmed options that affect the operation of the activity sensing portion of this pacemaker are slope, threshold, reaction time, and recovery time. These units are available in VVI and DDD modes.[44] Patients have to be carefully evaluated before implantation to determine whether they would benefit. In the future, rate modulation sensors may be discovered for circadian variations in metabolism, fever, emotions, body position, and anemia to simulate the natural rate control of the heart.[48]

Antitachycardia or burst pacing

When a patient fails to respond to or cannot tolerate pharmacologic control of SVT, antitachycardia pacemakers can be used. Rapid bursts of electrical stimuli delivered into the atrial myocardium can terminate tachydysrhythmias.[52] In general, these pacemakers function as a normal DDD pacing system in the absence of SVT. Their pacing cycles differ in that they have a tachycardia-detection window after ventricular output. The SVT is detected followed by a short burst of stimuli. An automatic AV block occurs in the pacemaker to prevent an increase in ventricular rate. These units are programmable to meet individual needs. Electrophysiologic studies are performed before implantation to determine consistency with which the rapid stimulation terminates the dysrhythmia, as well as output and duration. These patients require the same preoperative and postoperative care as other pacemaker patients. They are asked to keep records of the frequency that the antitachycardia function responds.

In the near future, ventricular antitachycardia pacing systems will be incorporated in the implantable cardioverter-defibrillator to provide control of most ventricular tachydysrhythmias.

INDICATIONS FOR PERMANENT PACING

Patients who have required temporary pacing for the alleviation of symptoms related to bradydysrhythmia or tachydysrhythmia, regardless of cause, for over 4 to 6 days probably are candidates for permanent pacing. When evaluating patients' histories and ECGs, emphasis is placed on the following dysrhythmias that are indications for permanent pacing:

1. Asymptomatic sinus pauses longer than 2.5 seconds
2. Asymptomatic sinus bradycardia with rates less than 40 bpm (except for trained athletes)
3. Symptomatic second-degree AV heart block of either type
4. Asymptomatic second-degree AV block and bifascicular block combined
5. Anterior MI with first-degree AV block and RBBB with left anterior hemiblock, even if this occurred in the acute phase of the MI and resolved (sudden death occurs in 28% of these cases within the first year)[55]
6. Asymptomatic complete AV block when the rate is less than 40 bpm or if the block is below the AV node or intranodal area[55] and congenital heart block with rates less than 50 bpm
7. Hereditary, idiopathic, or drug-related prolongation of the QT interval (persons who are prone to syncope and sudden death)[36]
8. Carotid sinus hypersensitivity with bradycardia
9. Vasovagal bradycardia with syncope

Nursing process

Case study. Mr. R. received a permanent transvenous unipolar VVIR pacing system on the day after his admission. The rate-responsive (muscle-activity-sensing type) pacemaker was chosen because of the patient's lifestyle and age. The lead was inserted through the right subclavian vein, and the pulse generator was implanted in a subcutaneous pocket on the right anterior chest wall. At the time of insertion, the intrinsic R wave was measured at 8 mV, with the threshold to pacing at 1.0 mA at an output of 5 mV and a pulse duration of 1 msec. The permanent pacemaker was programmed to a rate of 60 ppm, sensitivity of 1 mV, an output of 5 mV, and pulse duration of 1.0 msec. The activity-sensing component was temporarily programmed to a motion sensitivity of medium, a rate response of 7, and an upper limit of 150 ppm. Reprogramming of these values was planned for later, when the patient would be ambulatory.

The following day his temporary system was removed. About 4 days after surgery the patient was discharged, to return in 4 days for suture removal, further instruction, and pacemaker testing and reprogramming.

Nursing assessment

Persons who are awaiting the implantation of a permanent pacing system require the same monitoring and physical care cited in Section II. The challenge to nurses is the emotional preparation of persons receiving a permanently implanted life-sustaining device. The way patients are prepared will affect their adaptation, compliance to the medical regimen, and therefore the effectiveness of the pacing therapy.

Feeling pattern

Assess the patient for pain or discomfort, especially if there is a temporary pacing system in place or any invasive monitoring equipment. Have the patient describe the onset, location, duration, and radiation of the pain or discomfort. Determine whether the patient can ascertain what precipitates or relieves the pain.

Assess the patient for signs and symptoms of anxiety related to the implantation of a permanent pacemaker (elevated heart rate or blood pressure, tremulousness, difficulty sleeping, and cool extremities). Ask about past experiences with surgery. Note whether the patient verbalizes anxiety concerning potential pain, change in body image, or body functions.

Knowing pattern

Assess patients knowledge regarding permanent pacemakers. Ask whether they know how the function of the pacemaker relates to their symptoms and diagnosis. Ascertain whether they know other persons with permanent pacemakers and whether they have misconceptions about pacing. Identify concerns about the implantation procedure. Recognize when they demonstrate readiness to learn.

Perceiving pattern

Assess patients' perceptions of themselves and the diagnosis that has precipitated the need for permanent pacing. Ask what permanently implanted devices mean to the patients and their families. Also evaluate their attitudes about the future and the possible effectiveness of the therapy. Determine whether they feel a loss of control.

Relating pattern

Assess the patients' relationships with others. Note whether supportive family members and friends are nearby. Ascertain whether patients feel that the permanent pacemaker will change relationships. Ask whether patients are concerned about how the pacemaker will affect their roles at home, at work, or in social situations.

Choosing pattern

Determine how patients are coping with their concerns and the stress of the situation and impending surgery. Ascertain their usual approach to stress. Assess for degree of compliance to past medical regimens. Note whether patients verbalize motivation and willingness to comply to the requirements of permanent pacemaker care. Explore whether the patients require nursing assistance at home.

Moving pattern

Assess how the permanent pacemaker and surgery may affect patients' daily activities. With a knowledge of how the prepacemaker symptoms changed endurance ability to perform self-care, explore how the pacemaker will affect these factors.

Nursing diagnoses

The most common human responses anticipated for a patient requiring permanent cardiac pacing are indicated by the following nursing diagnoses:

1. Symptomatic or high risk for symptomatic bradydysrhythmia or tachydysrhythmia requiring permanent pacing related to (include cause)
2. High risk for anxiety related to impending pacemaker surgery
3. High risk for permanent pacemaker malfunction related to the newly implanted pacing lead and pulse generator
4. High risk for infection related to presence of a foreign body in the tissue (the pulse generator and lead)
5. High risk for impaired physical mobility of the affected extremity related to restricted activity and incisional discomfort
6. High risk for impaired gas exchange related to the thoracotomy for permanent epicardial lead placement
7. High risk for noncompliance to the medical regimen related to inadequate knowledge about the pacemaker

For each of these diagnoses, the patient outcomes, nursing prescriptions, and evaluation criteria are outlined with a discussion of the factual information that supports the plan and implementation of care.

NURSING
DIAGNOSIS 1
Symptomatic or high risk for symptomatic bradydysrhythmia or tachydysrhythmia requiring permanent pacing related to (include cause) (exchanging pattern)

PATIENT OUTCOMES	NURSING PRESCRIPTIONS	EVALUATION
Dysrhythmia and its cause will be identified.	Enter identified dysrhythmia into the nursing care plan. Assess the effects of the dysrhythmia on hemodynamic status.	Dysrhythmia and its cause were identified.
Patient will verbalize an understanding of the need for a permanent pacemaker and pacemaker function in relation to patient's dysrhythmia and symptoms.	Reinforce the physician's teaching regarding the need for a permanent pacemaker and pacemaker function in relation to patient's dysrhythmia and symptoms.	Patient verbalized an understanding of the need for a permanent pacemaker and pacemaker function in relation to patient's dysrhythmia and symptoms.

Plan and intervention for bradydysrhythmias or tachydysrhythmias requiring permanent pacing

The discovery of a bradydysrhythmia or tachydysrhythmia requiring permanent pacing can be made in several ways. An ECG precursor to a potentially symptomatic dysrhythmia can be found during routine physical examination. The patient may be totally unaware of this problem or may have intermittent symptoms and be admitted for continuous monitoring to determine the cause. The patient also may have had an AMI with a dysrhythmia, which necessitates temporary pacing or cardiac surgery that resulted in the need for pacing. Accurate ECG monitoring is maintained for all patients. Dysrhythmias are documented as they occur, and the nurse notes the patient's symptoms relating to the dysrhythmias. The nurse also assesses the effect of the dysrhythmia on arterial blood pressure, the patient's exercise tolerance, the central nervous system status as reflected by the level of consciousness, and other parameters appropriate for the particular patient.

The physician should inform the patient of the need for permanent pacing and the rationale on which this decision has been based. In the information given, the patient's symptoms should be related to how the pacemaker will work within the body to relieve those symptoms. The patient who has had no symptoms will need to know that the condition eventually will produce symptoms such as dizziness and syncope that could be hazardous if they have a sudden unpredicted onset.

NURSING
DIAGNOSIS 2
High risk for anxiety related to impending pacemaker surgery (feeling pattern)

PATIENT OUTCOMES	NURSING PRESCRIPTIONS	EVALUATION
Patient will verbalize an understanding of the way the pacemaker will be implanted, the type of anesthesia that will be used, places the patient will go after surgery and the reasons, the type of analgesia that will be used for postoperative discomfort, the type of activity restrictions that will be imposed after surgery, and the way the pacemaker will feel.	Instruct patient about the way the pacemaker will be implanted, the type of anesthesia that will be used, places the patient will go after surgery and the reasons, the type of analgesia that will be used for postoperative discomfort, the type of activity restrictions that will be imposed after surgery, and the reasons and the way the pacemaker will feel.	Patient verbalized an understanding of the way the pacemaker will be implanted, the type of anesthesia that will be used, places the patient will go after the surgery and the reasons, the type of analgesia that will be used for postoperative discomfort, the type of activity restrictions that will be imposed after surgery, and the reasons, and the way the pacemaker will feel.
Patient will participate in relaxation techniques and will not exhibit signs and symptoms of severe anxiety related to the diagnosis, need for pacing, and the impending surgery.	Instruct patient in relaxation techniques and evaluate level of anxiety before and after relaxation sessions.	Patient participated in relaxation techniques and did not exhibit signs and symptoms of severe anxiety related to the diagnosis, need for pacing, and surgery.

Plan and intervention for anxiety

Comprehensive nursing intervention and patient education play an important part in reducing anxiety and promoting adaptation to chronic illness. It is ideal for the same person or persons to provide patient education. The information given should emphasize the resumption and maintenance of wellness and normal living.

Patients exhibit varying reactions to the idea of having a permanent life-sustaining device implanted. Those who have had symptoms usually welcome a solution to their discomforts and limitations. Most patients are depressed to some degree over the fact that they have a permanent condition requiring such treatment and view it as an indication that they are aging. Many have stated, "I felt as though it was the beginning of the end for me," "I guess I'm just an old man now," "I am too young for this," or "When your heart goes, that's it." The health care team's objective should be to assist the patient in achieving a positive and realistic attitude. The following facts can promote this process:

1. The need for a pacemaker is not confined to the elderly. The patient should be made aware of the cause of the disorder.
2. Even if the disorder is part of the aging process, the pacemaker will eliminate the symptom-producing bradycardia.
3. A person's life is prolonged with the use of a pacemaker and also improved by the elimination of the symptoms related to the dysrhythmia.
4. Life can be completely normal with a pacemaker. Restrictions placed on the patient are minimal and allow for the continuation of vocation and in most instances hobbies, caring for a home, traveling, and having babies. The person may be limited by other conditions but not by the pacemaker itself. It is helpful to give the patient examples of other persons who have pacemakers and live normal lives.

The use of relaxation sessions and guided imagery are useful techniques in reducing preoperative anxiety (see Chapter 5 and p. 484).

Teaching plan

In general, the objectives of a teaching plan for a person undergoing the initial pacemaker implant follow:

1. Reduction of the patient's fears concerning the impending surgery
2. Promotion of positive and realistic thinking about recovery and the lifestyle thereafter
3. Promotion of compliance to long-term pacemaker follow-up monitoring

These objectives are met through the use of direct person-to-person teaching, written information, and continuous assessment, provision of information, and reassessment of the patient's needs.

The following nursing actions help nurses to prepare patients for a permanent pacemaker implant; they can be tailored to fit individual needs:

1. Describe to the patients how they will be prepared for surgery, based on institutional procedures. Most patients want to know when they will be taken to the operating room and where their families can wait. Tell them who will be caring for them in the operating room.
2. Instruct patients about the anesthesia that will be used. The surgeon and anesthesiologist also should tell patients what to expect. Reassure patients that their comfort benefits everyone.
3. Briefly describe the surgical procedure itself. Emphasize information that will reduce fears. For patients receiving transvenous implantations under local anesthesia, explain that the operation is not considered dangerous, their condition will be well monitored throughout, the operation will last from 1 to 2 hours, and if a local anesthetic is used, pressure but usually no pain will be felt in the operative area. For patients having epicardial leads inserted, explain the thoracotomy, general anesthesia, recovery room, and endotracheal tube. Also explain that the heart will not be stopped when applying the epicardial leads because many patients ask this question. Determine how much patients want or need to know about the operation. Answer all questions with as much information as appropriate.
4. For the postoperative stage, tell patients that transvenous pacemaker surgery usually does not produce a terribly painful wound and that, if the operation is done with local anesthesia, the person will not feel ill afterward. Explain that there will be soreness of the area after surgery, but this will pass quickly, and analgesia will be ordered. For patients receiving a thoracotomy for epicardial lead implant, tell them to expect chest tubes after the operation. Explain why these are necessary and when they will be removed, and describe breathing exercises and pain management. Warn patients receiving a ventricular pacemaker that they may be more aware of their heartbeat immediately after implantation (because of a change in the origin of ventricular depolarization) but that the feeling will not be permanent. Tell them that they also may feel the pacemaker "turn on and off." Explain the demand function, and instruct patients that this feeling will disappear with time. Instruct patients on activity restrictions imposed during the first 24 to 48 hours after implantation. Tell them how to assist in preventing lead displacement by remaining passive during transfers from bed to bed, by not using the affected extremity for the first 24 hours, and by remaining

in bed for the first 24 hours. Reassure them that the nursing staff will assist them as needed and that they will be under constant monitoring and attendance.

5. When discussing recovery, explain that eventually the pacemaker will not be felt under the skin during normal activities. (Approximately 90% of my patients have stated that they were not aware of it unless they touched the pulse generator.) Show patients a pulse generator and lead if they want to see it. Eliminate misconceptions about the construction and size of the pacemaker before surgery. Tell patients that the pulse generator usually is not visible under clothing. Teach patients that no one needs to know that they have one unless told. Tell patients that how the pulse generator will appear depends on the patient's weight (amount of subcutaneous fat to cover the pacemaker) and the size of the pulse generator. (Some younger men are concerned about the appearance.) Do not give false reassurances. Tell patients that only time will tell the outcome. Tell women that they can request that the pacemaker be buried under the breast, making it nearly invisible, especially if the cephalic or subclavian vein is used for lead insertion. Encourage patients to discuss these concerns with the physician and nursing staff.

Patients can view the pacemaker as an artificial limb or organ; yet they may feel that they have no control of it as they would an artificial limb. They may feel that the heart, the supporter of life, is now being governed by a mechanical device that can fail.[85] Their acceptance will be influenced by their support systems, home and work environment, past experiences with illness, and how well the pacemaker improves their symptoms. Inform patients of the support that will be available after surgery for follow-up care, for monitoring, and for information. Support groups with other pacemaker recipients may help for some persons.

Patients who are alert and at ease may be interested in written information. The same information also should be provided for families. If literature is given, it should be discussed in subsequent visits.

Some practitioners suggest having a well-adjusted pacemaker recipient visit the prospective patient before surgery. The patient may find it helpful to talk with someone who has been through the experience. The Mended Hearts program of the American Heart Association is a good example of the way that patient-to-patient preparation can work. The person who visits new patients must be chosen wisely; he or she should be well adjusted and must understand the objectives of the visit. The patient's permission should be obtained before the visit.

Patients' families must be included as much as possible. They also will have questions and fears that must be man-aged. For patients who are confused, heavily sedated, or unable to communicate, brief explanations of what will take place should be given just before surgery. It is well known that many comatose patients can hear and remember what has been said and done to them. Families should be informed that patients have been told.

Patient literature

Written materials are a necessity, not a luxury. The anxiety and stress that patients experience with an illness will change their lives permanently and can alter their ability to remember verbal information. They will need to refer to a handbook for information. Materials that correlate with specific needs of particular patients can be developed. Such literature must be comprehensive and cover the entire experience of having a permanent pacemaker. Because patients vary in comprehension and reading abilities, some practitioners prepare more than one form of the information using different reading levels. An edition in large type for the visually handicapped is also valuable. Practitioners in certain areas of the country may find pacemaker literature written in Spanish, French, or another language to be useful. The following is an outline of a patient booklet:

1. An introduction to cardiac pacing, when it was first developed, how many people have them, and the age span of those people
2. The anatomic structure of the natural pacing system of the heart
3. Disorders of the natural pacemaker, and their causes and symptoms
4. The function of the artificial pacemaker, its makeup, the way it works, and its power source
5. The programmer and the way it works
6. The way the pacemaker is implanted, anesthesia, postoperative care, and the way patients may feel after surgery
7. Life after the implant, activities and restrictions, and follow-up care needed
8. Electromagnetic interference, signs and symptoms of malfunction, patients' perceptions of what malfunction may be like, signs and symptoms of infection, and procedures to follow if they appear
9. Battery end-of-life indicators and pulse generator replacement procedures
10. Patient profiles (stories about other persons of all ages and lifestyles)
11. The name of the manufacturer, type of pacemaker, date of implant, and an area to keep a record of programming

This information can be designed for atrial, ventricular, DDD, rate-responsive, and antitachycardia pacemakers. Correct medical terms should be used with adequate definitions in the text. The overall tone should be positive, emphasizing how normal life can be with the pacemaker.

Such information must be continually updated with new developments in pacing and revised from patient suggestions or experiences.

Techniques of permanent pacemaker implantation

It is important to be familiar with the surgical techniques of pacemaker implantation. The most widely used approach is the transvenous insertion. Another approach is the transthoracic epicardial method.

Transvenous implantation. Ideally the transvenous procedure is performed in the operating room, where sterility of the operative field can be ensured. Patient's are allowed nothing by mouth after midnight the night before the surgery. The skin is shaved and prepared the night or morning before the procedure. After they are in the operating room, patients are placed on a radiolucent table and connected to a multichanneled ECG monitor, preferably with a paper printout. An intravenous line is inserted, and indirect monitoring of blood pressure or any other appropriate vital sign is initiated. It is ideal to have an anesthesiologist or nurse anesthetist monitoring vital signs throughout the procedure. This person also can assist patients in tolerating the local anesthetic with words of encouragement and light sedation, if necessary.

The skin then is prepared with shaving and a standard scrub and paint with povidone-iodine or a similar agent. Most initial transvenous implants are done on the right side of the chest, using the cephalic vein for lead insertion. The pulse generator then is placed subcutaneously on the chest wall just below the clavicle. If the patient requests, the insertion can be done on the left side if it is a single-lead ventricular system. It is difficult to insert an atrial lead from the veins on the left side because the lead has to negotiate curves in the venous system to reach the superior vena cava and right atrium. These leads usually are inserted through the external jugular or right subclavian vein.

Patients are told that the local anesthetic (compare it with that used in dentistry) will involve a needle puncture and burning sensation when the medication is injected. The nurse reassures them that numbness will develop quickly after that. The injection of lidocaine is usually extensive and can be uncomfortable for the first few minutes until the medication is fully effective. Local anesthesia is somewhat frightening; patients may be concerned about whether the entire operative area has been effectively anesthetized, or whether pain will be felt. If patients are apprehensive at this stage, mild sedatives such as diazepam or promethazine can be given. Constant reassurance and monitoring for signs of discomfort are important. Patients who are extremely frightened or who cannot cooperate should receive a general anesthetic if possible.

After the anesthetic has taken effect, an incision approximately 15 cm in length is made transversely just below the clavicle to allow the subclavican vein to be used for lead insertion. A percutaneous introducer is used after a

dissection is made in the subclavicular area. The introducer is inserted between the clavicle and the first rib into the vein in the same direction as with any subclavian puncture. Care must be taken to avoid inadvertent damage to the subclavian artery or the apex of the right lung. After venous blood is aspirated, the lead is threaded through the introducer and into the heart. Another alternative for lead insertion is the use of the cephalic vein. If the internal or external jugular vein is used, the patient must be informed before surgery to expect an additional incision at the base of the right side of the neck. For a two-lead procedure, the cephalic and the subclavian are used unless the surgeon can place both leads in one vessel or a single-pass AV lead is used.

Fluoroscopy is used to place the lead in a desirable position in the right atrial appendage or right ventricular apex. Patients are told that they may feel their hearts beating irregularly during this period and not to be concerned. PACs or PVCs can occur as the lead touches the endocardial surface. These beats are usually benign in the relatively healthy myocardium and will stop when the lead is stabilized. Treatment usually is not necessary. It is important, however, to be prepared with drugs and a defibrillator for the occurrence of any life-threatening dysrhythmia.

To confirm that an adequate lead position has been obtained, intracavitary electrograms and myocardial threshold studies are performed in the unipolar or bipolar mode, depending on the mode of the permanent pacemaker. Electrograms, performed when patients have an intrinsic rhythm rapid enough to allow a period without the temporary pacemaker, records the P and R wave sensed by the lead tip. It is ideal to do the recording on the ECG monitor to visualize the wave itself and to measure it on the pacing system analyzer for a numeric calculation of its size. The recorded P wave should be at least 1 mV in height to allow adequate sensing by the pulse generator (Fig. 16-9). The intracavitary QRS complex should be at least 5 mV in height.[71] Characteristically it will be a mostly negative complex, but it may also be biphasic. All complexes should be consistent in morphologic traits from beat to beat, and in the ventricle the ST segment should be elevated, indicating good contact with the endocardium. The slew rate also can be obtained using an optic recording system or pacing system analyzer designed for that measurement.

Myocardial thresholds are then obtained in milliamperes, volts, or both, using the pacing system analyzer. Ideally thresholds at several pulse widths should be recorded. At a minimum the anticipated pulse width of the pulse generator to be used should be set on the pacing system analyzer to determine the voltage setting at which capture is obtained. Threshold should be less than 1 mA (or 0.5 mV) at 1 msec pulse width in acute lead placement, depending on the type of electrode on the lead.[72] Atrial thresholds are slightly higher.

After threshold measurements, it is determined whether diaphragmatic pacing occurs with ventricular pacing by turning the pacing system analyzer to the output to be used in the permanent pacemaker, usually 10 mA (5 mV) at a pulse width of 1 msec. The surgeon's hand then can be placed over the diaphragm of the patient to detect contraction of the muscle with pacemaker output.

If the P or R wave is too small for sensing, the thresholds are too high, or diaphragmatic pacing is present, then the lead must be repositioned until all parameters are acceptable. This can be done in minutes, or it may take over an hour. The patient is warned of the possibility of delays. After the best possible position is obtained and documented, the pulse generator pocket is made by separating the subcutaneous tissues from the general pectoral muscle for an area slightly larger than the pulse generator. Because the local anesthesia may not have covered this entire area, this procedure can be painful if additional lidocaine is not administered.

While the subcutaneous pocket is being made, the pulse generator is prepared for implantation. While the pacemaker is held within the sterile field, its parameters are tested by connecting it to a pacing system analyzer via a sterile cable designed for that use. The analyzer will indicate the pacemaker's output, sensitivity, rate, pulse width, refractory period, and other specialized data, depending on the unit used. Usually each manufacturer has its own pacing analyzer to be used with its pacemakers for preinsertion evaluation. This is especially important when evaluating the new pacemaker's sensitivity, a parameter that is measured in several different ways. The pacemaker can also be programmed at this time to meet the patient's needs for parameters such as output, rate, sensitivity, refractory period, pulse width, and AV delay, depending on the thresholds and intracavitary electrogram. Most pulse generators are packaged with nominal settings that will adequately pace most patients with normal thresholds, but these values still may need adjustment for some patients.

After the subcutaneous pocket has been made and good hemostasis obtained, the pulse generator is connected to the lead, with particular attention paid to seating the lead end in the pulse generator terminal. The set screw is tightened, and the connection is sealed properly to prevent body fluids from entering the terminal compartment. The lead and pacemaker are then slipped into the pocket and the pocket adjusted to accommodate the equipment without being too tight or too loose. The pulse generator is sutured to the underlying muscle in two places to prevent it from

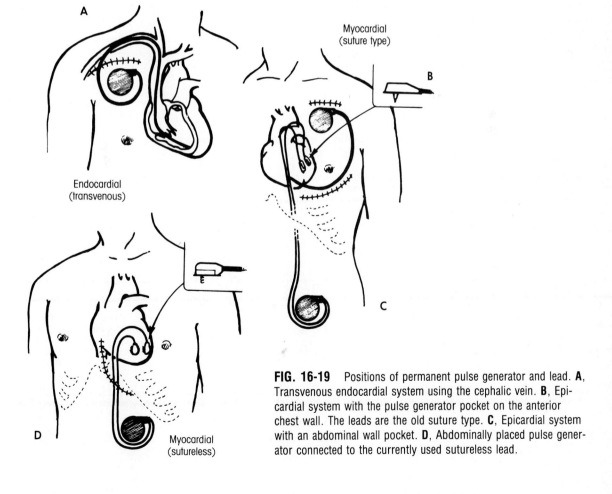

FIG. 16-19   Positions of permanent pulse generator and lead. **A,** Transvenous endocardial system using the cephalic vein. **B,** Epicardial system with the pulse generator pocket on the anterior chest wall. The leads are the old suture type. **C,** Epicardial system with an abdominal wall pocket. **D,** Abdominally placed pulse generator connected to the currently used sutureless lead.

slipping and from flipping over in the pocket. The lead is coiled within the pocket to prevent formation of acute angles that could cause a lead fracture or damage to the tissues.

A bipolar pacemaker begins to function immediately on insertion of the lead into the pacemaker terminal. A unipolar system must have the pulse generator's metal case (the anode) in contact with the body tissues to work (i.e., when the pulse generator is slipped into the pocket or placed in the open wound). The pacemaker's function is carefully monitored as the wound is being closed. If problems in capture and sensing are seen, they may be corrected with reprogramming. The wound is closed after an irrigation with antibiotic solution. Wound drains are usually avoided because they could be sources of infection.[71] The final positions of the pulse generator and lead are shown in Fig. 16-19.

A sterile pressure dressing is applied to help prevent bleeding into the new pocket. The temporary pacemaker is left in place to provide pacing if problems develop within the first 24 hours. Patients are transferred to the recovery room if there has been sedation or general anesthesia. If alert, patients can usually be transferred directly to a monitoring unit.

Epicardial implant. If a simple ventricular system is planned, the permanent epicardial pacing system is installed through a left anterior thoracotomy at the fourth or fifth intercostal space. A larger posterolateral thoracotomy is usually performed if an atrial lead is needed.[72] The pericardium is opened, and the surface of the myocardium is evaluated for lead placement. An area devoid of surface vessels and fat and away from the apex of the heart should be used for the ventricular lead. Atrial leads usually are placed on the superior region of the right atrium. Screw-on, sutureless leads are used most frequently with a two-turn, corkscrew-shaped electrode for the thin-walled atrium or a larger three-turn electrode for the ventricular myocardium. After the lead or leads are placed, the R and P waves are measured if the patient has an intrinsic rhythm. As with endocardial pacing, the P wave should be greater than 1 mV and the R wave greater than 5 mV for adequate sensing. Unipolar or bipolar thresholds are obtained and should be less than 1 mA at 1 msec. The thresholds are generally higher initially with myocardial placement of the lead because of tissue injury. This effect lasts only a short time. The pulse generator can then be tested and programmed.

Connection of the pacemaker to the lead is the same as that described for the endocardial system. The subcutaneous pocket is made on the anterior chest wall (under the breast if desired) with the lead brought out through the thoracotomy and buried subcutaneously up to the pocket (Fig. 16-19, *B*) or on the abdominal wall just above or below the waist, depending on the patient. (This area should be determined before surgery with the patient wearing a belt so that the belt area will be avoided for implant. [Fig. 16-19, *C*]). The thoracotomy is closed, and standard chest drainage is used. A dry, sterile pressure dressing is applied, and the patient is transferred to the recovery room and then the intensive care unit.

NURSING DIAGNOSIS 3	**High risk for permanent pacemaker malfunction related to the newly implanted pacing lead and pulse generator (exchanging pattern)**	
PATIENT OUTCOMES	NURSING PRESCRIPTIONS	EVALUATION
Patient will not experience pacemaker malfunctions, including failure to pace with the pacing artifact present, failure to pace with the pacing artifact absent, undersensing, oversensing, diaphragmatic or phrenic nerve pacing, chest or abdominal muscle pacing, pacemaker syndrome, runaway pacemaker, change in paced rate, muscle inhibition, or pacemaker-mediated tachycardia.	Initiate measures to prevent and detect pacemaker malfunction. Maintain ECG monitoring, frequently assessing cardiac rhythm. Instruct patient about activity restrictions for the first 24 to 48 hours. Monitor for signs and symptoms of malfunction. Initiate appropriate therapy at the first sign of malfunction.	Patient did not experience pacemaker malfunctions, including failure to pace with the pacing artifact present, failure to pace with the pacing artifact absent, undersensing, oversensing, diaphragmatic or phrenic nerve pacing, chest or abdominal muscle pacing, pacemaker syndrome, runaway pacemaker, change in paced rate, muscle inhibition, and pacemaker-mediated tachycardia.

Plan and intervention for pacemaker malfunction

After implantation, all permanent pacemaker patients should be placed in an intensive care unit or another appropriate ECG monitoring unit for continuous monitoring to detect early pacemaker malfunction. In the new system, lead displacement is the most frequent problem seen, even though the frequency has been reduced in recent years through the use of active-fixation endocardial leads. Activity restrictions imposed on the patient for 24 to 48 hours after surgery are designed to prevent endocardial lead displacement that could be caused by body motion, especially movement of the upper extremity nearest the point of the lead insertion. Even with strict adherence to the restrictions, displacement occurs, probably because of less-than-optimal placement and the normal dynamics of cardiac systole. Displacement with screw-in epicardial leads is rare.

Lead displacement produces loss of capture on the ECG, and there is failure to pace with the pacing artifact present. Loss of capture may be continuous or intermittent. Increasing the pacemaker output through reprogramming may help. Regardless, the lead will need to be repositioned. The chest x-ray film rarely helps in diagnosing this problem because displacement is usually not great enough to show on the film. The temporary pacemaker can be used to maintain the pacemaker-dependent patient until the lead is repositioned. When it is used, it is set on the asynchronous mode (VOO, AOO, or DOO) to prevent inhibition by the permanent pacemaker output; the nurse watches for ectopy because the temporary pacemaker does not sense

it. To manage this situation, the paced rate is increased to override ectopic beats. The nurse should be prepared to manage tachydysrhythmia.

The definitive treatment for lead displacement is repositioning. Patients may be anxious and perhaps angry about having additional surgery. The nurse explains the way that the incision will be reopened after a local anesthetic has been administered and that discomfort will be no greater after the second procedure.

Pacemaker-mediated tachycardia is a malfunction or pacemaker-produced dysrhythmia seen only in DDD systems. This tachycardia occurs when the patient has retrograde conduction from the ventricle to the atrium even though antigrade conduction is not intact. After each ventricular paced beat, there is retrograde conduction. If this impulse falls outside of the postventricular refractory period, it will be sensed in the atrium, causing another ventricular impulse to be fired after the AV delay. The rate of the cycle is limited by the upper rate limit of the pacemaker, usually 150 ppm.

Because each ventricular-paced beat produces a retrograde-conducted beat into the atrium, which then produces another ventricular beat, the tachycardia is persistent. An acute episode can be terminated by the application of the pacemaker's magnet over the pulse generator. After this, reprogramming the postventricular atrial refractory period to a time greater than it takes to conduct the retrograde beat will permanently eliminate the dysrhythmia. See Table 16-7 for information concerning other malfunctions.

TABLE 16-7
Complications and Malfunctions of Permanent Pacemakers

Complication or malfunction	Causes	Diagnosis	Treatment
Failure to pace with artifact present (loss of capture)	Lead displacement (can occur up to 2 to 3 months after implant)	Diagnosis is assumed with loss of capture in early postoperative period; x-ray film is of little help unless displacement is gross.	Replace lead using active fixation type.
	High threshold (exit block) resulting from fibrosis or ischemia at lead tip	Diagnosis is assumed if loss of capture occurs in late postoperative phase, or there is AMI. Invasive lead threshold studies can make definitive diagnosis.	Programming: increase pacemaker output (and/or pulse width). If programming is unsuccessful and the problem appears to be permanent, replace lead and/or use high-output pulse generator. For repeated episodes use epicardial leads.

Continued.

TABLE 16-7

Complications and Malfunctions of Permanent Pacemakers—cont'd

Complication or malfunction	Causes	Diagnosis	Treatment
Failure to pace with artifact absent			
Intermittent	Electromagnetic interference from sources within and outside body	Isometric exercise test demonstrates muscle inhibition in patient with chest wall implant. Patient may have history of symptoms when near potential source of electromagnetic interference.	Programming: decrease pacemaker sensitivity; if possible, change to bipolar or use triggered mode (VVT or AAT). Replace pulse generator and lead with bipolar system. Tell patient to avoid source of outside interference if possible. During electrocautery, program pacemaker to VOO, AOO, or DOO (Table 16-4).
	Incomplete lead fracture	Lead resistance is increased and R or P wave size decreased on electrogram; x-ray study confirms diagnosis.	Replace or repair lead.
	T wave sensing	Characteristic ECG with pauses in output equal to escape interval from T wave to next pacing artifact is seen.	Programming: decrease sensitivity to level in which oversensing is eliminated.
Continuous	Complete lead fracture	There is high lead resistance, flat electrogram, and fracture seen on x-ray film.	Replace or repair lead.
	Broken or loose connection between lead and pulse generator.	Diagnosis is assumed if there is no activation of the pulse generator with use of the magnet.	Repair connection or pulse generator, depending on type of damage.
	Pulse generator battery failure	Diagnosis is assumed if there is no activation of pacemaker on ECG with use of magnet. Battery condition indicators from interactive programmer (battery impedance and output) will be low.	Replace pulse generator
Undersensing	Reduced size of intrinsic R or P wave sensed from lead tip, less than the millivolt-sensitivity capability of pacemaker	On ECG, there is no recycling of pacemaker by intrinsic beats. On electrogram R or P wave measurements are less than the millivolt-sensitivity capability of pulse generator.	Programming: increase sensitivity; increase rate to override nonsensed intrinsic beats; if ectopy is present, treat pharmacologically to suppress. Reposition lead to obtain larger R or P wave on electrogram, or use pacemaker with greater sensitivity according to size of R or P wave on electrogram.

TABLE 16-7

Complications and Malfunctions of Permanent Pacemakers—cont'd

Complication or malfunction	Causes	Diagnosis	Treatment
Oversensing of T wave, QRS complex, or afterpotential	Short refractory period or excessively high sensing capability of pulse generator	There are pauses in output or a continuous slowing of set rate of pacemaker; distance from oversensed wave or complex to next pacemaker artifact is equal to normal escape interval.	Programming: decrease sensitivity or increase refractory period.
Pacemaker-mediated tachycardia	In the DDD pacemaker, retrograde conduction sensed by the atrial channel; after AV delay another impulse fired into the ventricle and the cycle repeats at a rate limited by the upper rate limit of the system	ECG shows rapid rate equal to the upper rate limit. Magnet over the pulse generator terminates the tachycardia and puts the pacemaker into DDD mode.	Reprogram postventricular atrial refractory period to a time greater than that needed for conduction to the atrium. If it takes 300 msec for the retrograde impulse to produce a P wave, program to 325 msec.
Diaphragmatic or phrenic nerve pacing	Tip of a ventricular lead placed too close to diaphragmatic portion of right ventricle Tip of atrial lead too close to phrenic nerve Pulse generator output too high	Diaphragmatic contractions at pacemaker rate are occurring, with pacemaker artifact. Fluoroscopy will show the diaphragm contracting with pacemaker output.	Programming: decrease pacemaker output until contractions cease but capture is maintained or decrease paced rate if patient has adequate intrinsic rhythm. If these measures fail and patient is uncomfortable, reposition lead.
	Perforation of lead tip through myocardium to close proximity with diaphragm or phrenic nerve	If perforation has occurred into pericardial sac, there may be a friction rub and positive echocardiogram.	
Chest or abdominal muscle stimulation around the pulse generator in unipolar pacing systems (muscle twitch)	High pacemaker output or high current density	Reducing pacemaker output with programming may stop twitching.	Programming: reduce pacemaker output and pulse width to level above that needed to maintain capture; change polarity to bipolar; reduce paced rate if patient has adequate intrinsic cardiac rhythm.
	Lead fracture or break in lead insulation (current leaks out of lead into muscle)	X-ray film may show lead fracture; patient may complain of pinprick sensation.	Replace or repair fractured lead.
	Flipped pulse generator (in unipolar pacemakers with posterior covering on anodal metal case) (see p. 527)	On x-ray film, pacemaker identification letters appear backward.	Reposition pulse generator in pocket, and use two-point sutured fixation of pulse generator to chest or abdominal wall muscle. Instruct patient not to "twiddle" pacemaker.
	Low threshold to muscle pacing	Inappropriate muscle pacing occurs at low pacemaker output in absence of any of preceding problems.	Use bipolar pacing system in sensitive patients or commercially prepared boot for unipolar pulse generator metal case to insulate electrically active anode from underlying muscle.

Continued.

TABLE 16-7

Complications and Malfunctions of Permanent Pacemakers—cont'd

Complication or malfunction	Causes	Diagnosis	Treatment
Pacemaker syndrome (symptomatic reduction in cardiac output)	Loss of AV synchrony in VVI or VVT pacing, reducing cardiac output (see p. 519)	Symptoms are weakness, decreased exercise tolerance, and persistent unmanageable congestive heart failure.	Programming: increase paced rate if there is no intrinsic rhythm; decrease paced rate if there is adequate intrinsic cardiac sinus rhythm. If programming is unsuccessful, replace pacing system with physiologic one.
Runaway pacemaker	Component failure	Paced rate will accelerate to upper rate limit of pulse generator, usually 140 to 150 ppm; this may be intermittent. Patient may report dizziness or syncope and sensation of rapid heart rate.	Replace pulse generator.
Change in rate or other parameter	Incorrect programming	Reprogramming with new programmer returns pacemaker to normal function.	If necessary replace pulse generator if reprogramming is unsuccessful.
	Phantom or inadvertent programming by electromagnetic interference	Same as above.	Same as above.
	Spontaneous self-reprogramming (rare)	Same as above.	Same as above.
	Programmer malfunction such as power failure	Same as above.	Same as above.
	Pacemaker circuitry failure	Attempts at reprogramming fail.	Replace pulse generator.
	Reed switch malfunction	Pacemaker fails to sense intrinsic beats or remains in magnet rate after removal of magnet.	Replace pulse generator.
	Pacemaker battery exhaustion	Battery information (impedance and current) from interactive programmer is abnormal.	Replace pulse generator.
Muscle inhibition	Myopotentials inhibiting pacemaker output (see pp. 519 and 537)	Pectoral muscle isometric test is positive. Patient may report dizziness during activities requiring use of arms such as lifting windows or pushing up in bed.	Reprogram to lower sensitivity if possible (e.g., from 0.5 mV to 2 mV). Reprogram to triggered mode if pulse generator is capable (only with single-chamber pacing systems). Reprogram to bipolar mode if possible. Instruct patient to avoid activities that produce symptoms. Replace system with bipolar or triggered one if problem is severe and not remedied by any of preceding steps.

NURSING
DIAGNOSIS 4
High risk for infection related to the presence of a foreign body in the tissue (pulse generator and lead) (exchanging pattern)

PATIENT OUTCOMES	NURSING PRESCRIPTIONS	EVALUATION
Patient's surgical wound will not develop redness, soreness, drainage, or swelling.	Monitor for signs and symptoms of surgical wound infection and initiate appropriate infection control measures.	Surgical wound did not develop redness, soreness, drainage, or swelling.
Patient will not have an elevated temperature.	Assess temperature every 4 hr.	Patient did not have an elevated temperature.
There will be no bleeding in incision or pulse generator pocket.	Assess incision and pulse generator pocket at frequent intervals during the first 24 to 48 hours. Maintain pressure dressing during that time.	There was no bleeding in the incision or pulse generator pocket.

Plan and intervention for infection

Pacemaker wound infection can be prevented, and strict asepsis in the operating room, hemostasis, and careful postoperative care are primary factors in this prevention.[18] The initial sterile pressure dressing applied in the operating room should be left undisturbed for at least 24 to 48 hours to help prevent wound and pocket bleeding. Such bleeding can delay healing and increase the likelihood of infection. The nurse monitors for bleeding through a small window cut in the elastic pressure tape. Bleeding is especially likely in patients who inadvertently receive anticoagulants before surgery or who have a coagulation disorder. The surgeon is notified if bleeding is noted or suspected by visible bleeding or swelling. Reoperation may be required if further pressure does not stop the flow.

The first sign of a wound infection is an elevated temperature if the wound is still under a dressing. The temperature is monitored at least every 4 hours, and the physician is notified of an elevation. Prophylactic antibiotics usually are given. They are administered on a rigid schedule at even intervals to obtain and maintain adequate blood levels. If an infection is suspected, the dressing must be removed and the wound inspected, cultured, and left open to air. If infection does occur, the pacing system may have to be removed; the patient is prepared for this procedure.

After the initial dressing has been removed, the patient is observed for signs of infection such as redness, swelling, and drainage. This continues throughout hospitalization and the first few weeks after implant. The nurse instructs the patient to observe for these signs at home and to report them to the nurse or physician. The patient is told to keep the incision dry until the sutures are removed on the seventh to tenth postoperative day. It is also advisable for women who have a chest wall or submammary implant to wear a brassiere during the day to provide support for the breast and tissues around the incision and the subcutaneous pocket to promote proper healing. The patient may be more comfortable with a light, sterile gauze pad over the incision and the pulse generator area when wearing the brassiere.

NURSING
DIAGNOSIS 5
High risk for impaired physical mobility of the affected extremity related to restricted activity and incisional discomfort (moving pattern)

PATIENT OUTCOMES	NURSING PRESCRIPTIONS	EVALUATION
Patient will not experience a frozen shoulder.	About 48 hours after surgery, assist patient in using the affected extremity normally.	Patient did not experience a frozen shoulder.
Patient will not experience undue weakness of the affected extremity.	Administer analgesics as necessary.	Patient did not experience undue weakness of the affected extremity.
Patient will verbalize understanding of the rationale for range of motion exercises.	Teach and demonstrate range of motion exercises.	Patient verbalized understanding of the rationale for range of motion exercises.

Plan and intervention for impaired physical mobility of the affected extremity

With transvenous lead implantation the upper extremity on the operative side is kept immobile for 24 to 48 hours after surgery to prevent traction on the lead and possible lead displacement. This immobility and incisional discomfort (which also affects patients with a thoracotomy) can lead to self-imposed immobility of the shoulder and elbow joints. Such immobility then can cause a *frozen shoulder* characterized by joint stiffness and pain and muscle weakness of the extremity. After this complication occurs, physical therapy is required to relieve it. To prevent this problem, the nurse instructs patients to begin using the extremity in a normal manner, except for the restrictions listed in the box on p. 537, after 24 to 48 hours have passed after the implant. Some patients require nursing assistance to regain joint mobility. Analgesia should be used when necessary to decrease incisional pain and facilitate use of the limb. By the time patients are discharged, or 3 to 5 days after surgery, they should be able to raise their arms over their heads. Normal performance of activities of daily living is encouraged. The range of motion of the extremity is evaluated during each follow-up visit to the clinic or office for the first 6 months. The patient is told that the incision and subcutaneous pocket will be sore for the first 3 to 4 weeks, with gradually decreasing discomfort thereafter. Aching postoperative pain will disappear during the first week.

NURSING DIAGNOSIS 6	**High risk for impaired gas exchange related to the thoracotomy for permanent epicardial lead placement (exchanging pattern)**	
PATIENT OUTCOMES	NURSING PRESCRIPTIONS	EVALUATION
Patient will not experience pneumonia, pneumothorax, or incisional or intrathoracic bleeding.	Assess patient for signs and symptoms of inadequate gas exchange. Monitor chest tube drainage and incisional bleeding. Assess patient's respiratory status. Implement measures to promote adequate gas exchange.	Patient did not experience pneumonia, pneumothorax, or incisional or intrathoracic bleeding.
Patient will maintain adequate gas exchange as evidenced by lung reexpansion, normal breath sounds, normal arterial blood gas levels, and normal respiratory rate and character.	Facilitate coughing, turning, and deep breathing. Administer analgesics as necessary. Administer oxygen, humidity, and intermittent positive pressure breathing as ordered. Perform endotracheal suctioning as needed. Elevate head of the bed and have patient ambulate when appropriate.	Patient did maintain adequate gas exchange as evidenced by lung reexpansion, normal breath sounds, normal arterial blood gas levels, and normal respiratory rate and character.

Plan and intervention for impaired gas exchange related to thoracotomy

After patients have been extubated and stabilized after an epicardial lead placement, they will be transferred to the intensive care unit for postoperative care and pacemaker monitoring. To prevent pulmonary and wound complications after the thoracotomy, the amount and character of the chest drainage are monitored. The surgeon is notified about unusual bleeding. Closed-chest drainage is maintained until the lung has reexpanded and drainage has stopped. The nurse also monitors for incisional bleeding and observes respiratory rate and character. Arterial blood gas measurements are obtained as indicated. The patient's chest will be sore, so coughing and deep breathing will be painful. The nurse administers analgesia, as ordered, at regular intervals for the first 24 hours to give the patient comfort and to enable the patient to cough, turn, and deep breathe adequately. These activities promote reexpansion of the lung and drainage of secretions. Secretions are suctioned if the patient is unable to remove secretions. The nurse also checks breath sounds frequently to determine the efficiency of these procedures. Respiratory depression may occur after the administration of analgesics. If it occurs, the nurse consults the physician for dosage assistance and elevates the head of the bed to increase respiratory capacity (no more than 30 degrees if the patient has a femoral temporary pacing lead). The nurse administers oxygen, humidity, and intermittent positive pressure breathing treatments as needed, based on breath sounds assessment. Patients are instructed regarding the use of

incentive breathing apparatus. The patient should ambulate as soon as possible. The patient in instructed to expect intercostal pain and soreness for up to 6 months. This can be relieved with oral analgesics and local heat applications.

NURSING DIAGNOSIS 7	**High risk for noncompliance to the medical regimen related to inadequate knowledge about the pacemaker (choosing pattern)**

PATIENT OUTCOMES	NURSING PRESCRIPTIONS	EVALUATION
Patient will verbalize an understanding of: Rationale for pacing Dependability of the pacemaker and lead Rationale for continuing medical follow-up visits Activities allowed and activities not recommended Signs and symptoms of malfunction and procedures if they appear Longevity of the pacemaker and its end-of-life indicators Facts about electromagnetic interference	Instruct patient regarding: Rationale for pacing Dependability of the pacemaker and lead Rationale for continuing follow-up visits Activities allowed and activities not recommended Signs and symptoms of malfunction and procedures if they appear Longevity of the pacemaker and its end-of-life indicators Facts about electromagnetic interference.	Patient verbalized an understanding of: Rationale for pacing Dependability of the pacemaker and lead Rationale for continuing follow-up visits Activities allowed and activities not recommended Signs and symptoms of malfunction and procedures if they appear Longevity of the pacemaker and its end-of-life indicators Facts about electromagnetic interference.

Plan and intervention for noncompliance

Immediately after surgery

The nurse continues to gather data about the patient's recovery, reaction to the surgery, and adjustment to being a pacemaker recipient. Clues about the patient's real feelings may begin to be evident if they were suppressed preoperatively. All information obtained then will be used in formulating further teaching plans.

The patient's and family's questions should be answered simply. More detailed teaching probably should not begin before the third or fourth day after the operation. The patient does not remember all material presented during the acute phases of an illness. Factors that contribute to this are fear, discomfort, grief, the hospital environment, sedation and analgesia, and physiologic changes that affect the central nervous system. The nurse may have to repeat information.

When the patient is ambulatory, and is comfortable, and is ready, detailed discharge instructions can be given. Written materials should be presented to the patient. The literature can be given to the family if the patient cannot read or is blind. This patient should be told that the nurse will verbally review everything in the book. Patients and families may be given several booklets to share as needed.

Patients are instructed to read at their leisure. Questions that arise from the reading can be reviewed in the planned

teaching sessions. These sessions should be designed to give patients information needed for the first few days at home.

Patients should expect to be tired and somewhat weak for the first month with gradual improvement over the next few months. They are told that, after this time, they may begin to feel better than they have in some time because of improvement in heart function.

Patients can expect to notice the pulse generator under the skin for the first 6 months with gradual lessening until it is only felt when touched. Patients who have had palpitations or have felt the pacemaker turn on and off postoperatively (not all do) are told that this may continue for the first month and then it gradually disappears.

Patients should expect to be conscious of the pacemaker for the first month or so (not all are). Many people take 1 to 6 months or more to begin to trust the device. This is especially true of patients who have had syncopal episodes before implant. Many patients are also concerned that they may damage the pacing system with activities of daily living. This is one reason for allowing patients to handle a pulse generator and lead so that their durability can be seen. Patients are encouraged to forget the pacemaker and go about their business and to remember it only enough to avoid activities not allowed and to keep follow-up appointments.

The signs and symptoms of pacemaker malfunction are reviewed. Patients must be reassured that malfunction is an exception rather than the rule. They must also be told that, even with total pacemaker failure, they will not die. Many patients worry that they will die in their sleep if the pacemaker fails, and most are hesitant to discuss this matter with the physician or nurse. They have stated, "I was afraid to ask," or "I wasn't sure if I wanted to know the truth." Explain that there will be warning symptoms such as dizziness, weakness, shortness of breath, or simply a return of the original symptoms. There will be time to get medical help. Most malfunctions are detected during routine evaluations, and the patient is unaware that something is wrong.

The symptoms of wound and pocket infection are reviewed. Patients are instructed to call the nurse or physician as soon as one of these signs or symptoms appears. This complication is rare.

The nurse reviews activity restrictions for the first month. This information is in the patient handbook and must agree with the cardiologist's or surgeon's instructions. These restrictions usually are no driving for the first 4 weeks (sudden turning of the steering wheel to avoid an accident may dislodge the pacing lead or put stress on a thoracotomy incision), and, for example, no lifting, golfing, or bowling for the first month. The patient should take walks and short trips in the car.

Facts about electromagnetic interference should be reviewed. Usually if interference occurs, the pacemaker rate will slow, causing momentary dizziness. Therefore patients are instructed to simply move away from the device and notify the physician if they become dizzy in the vicinity of electrical equipment. Patients are warned to weigh "facts" given by well-meaning friends and relatives. Most misinformation given by others concerns electromagnetic interference. Patients have been told not to go through automatic doors, use hair dryers, travel on buses, or use garage door openers. When questions arise that are not answered satisfactorily by the literature, patients should call the physician or nurse. Patients should be encouraged to rely on one source of information concerning pacemakers.

Before discharge, patients should be given pacemaker identification cards. These may be temporary but contain information on the date of implant, pacemaker and lead model and serial numbers, all programmed parameters, and the physician's name and telephone number. Some manufacturers then send patients permanent cards with these facts imprinted and an area for reprogramming records to be kept. Patients should try to keep these records with them at all times. It is also recommended that a Medic-Alert appliance be worn in case of an emergency.

A week after surgery

Patients should return for suture removal and a pacemaker evaluation 7 days after implantation. They should come prepared to ask questions and be accompanied by a family member. During each follow-up visit, patients and families are encouraged to tell how they feel about their progress and recovery. This will indicate how the patients are progressing towards resolution of this crisis. The nurse looks for nonverbal clues such as signs of tension and anxiety.

Information about battery longevity should be reviewed again. With pacemaker failure, most patients say that their greatest fear is that of unpredicted battery exhaustion. Although the manufacturer guarantees the power source for a certain number of years, it may not last that long. The nurse explains the end-of-life indicators for the pacemaker, specifically that the pacemaker will inform the physician when the battery is beginning to wear out. The programmed rate will decrease a specific number of beats in a prolonged, stepwise manner, long before the battery is completely depleted. The nurse points out the value of routine pacemaker evaluations to detect such indicators. It is also important to explain that it is not the paced rate that changes in most pacemakers but the magnet rate. Patients who do not want to be bothered with office visits sometimes try to rely on counted pulse rates. A routine ECG at the internist's office also will be unable to demonstrate end-of-life indicators. Accurate interval counter magnet rates and examinations using the pacemaker's programmer analyzer are needed for correct evaluation.

Patients can be instructed to take their pulses. Daily pulse monitoring is not always necessary, although many persons do it to relieve anxiety. Taking pulses gives patients short-term assurance and a feeling of control over their situations. Pulse-rate monitoring in lithium or nuclear pacemakers needs to be done only once a week or when patients have symptoms that seem like they could be caused by pacemaker malfunction. If the pulse is irregular or below the pacemaker's set rate, patients may be having only uncountable (nonpalpable) intrinsic beats. If this occurs with symptoms, the physician should be called. Most patients are relieved to know that pulse-generator replacement is an easier procedure than the initial implant.

A month after surgery

When the patient returns for a pacemaker evaluation 1 month after surgery, it is time to discuss safe and unsafe activities. Opinions vary regarding activities that should be permanently avoided. The main objective of restrictions is to prevent lead fracture and damage to the pulse generator. The box lists restricted activities suggested by several practitioners. Patients can be given the full rationale behind these restrictions to enable them to make the decision.

Patients should be encouraged to join a cardiac exercise program designed to condition the patient without damaging the pacing system. An exercise prescription should be designed by the cardiologist who is most aware of the patient's underlying cardiac disease and the condition of

**ACTIVITY RESTRICTIONS
WITH PERMANENT PACEMAKERS**

Mowing the lawn with anything but a riding lawn mower
(The vibrations from the handle of a push or self-
propelled mower can travel up the arms of a person
with a transvenous system and cause thrombosis of
the vein containing the lead, usually the subclavian.
Such a thrombosis could cause permanent venous
congestion of the affected extremity.*)

Lifting anything over 25 pounds

Using an axe (situation in which the tool is lifted over
the head and dropped on the item being cut)

Participating in contact sports such as football, rugby,
or basketball

Using an air hammer

Firing a rifle from the affected side (The recoil could
damage the pulse generator or lead.)

Serving overhand in tennis

Diving head first into water

*Data from Smyth N: Personal communication, 1987.

the myocardium. At a minimum, persons who are unable to participate in formal exercise should be encouraged to return to normal activities and try to include a daily walk.

Patients should be instructed to inform their dentists that they have a pacemaker; these patients will require prophylactic antibiotics before and after tooth extraction or oral surgery to help prevent infection within the heart where the pacemaker lead is placed and touches the heart valves. Other procedures such as dental x-ray studies are safe. Patients also should inform the pacemaker follow-up physician if they are going to have other surgery. Reprogramming and a postoperative pacemaker evaluation may be needed.

Long-term follow-up monitoring

The objectives of long-term pacemaker monitoring follow:

1. Detection of pacemaker malfunction
2. Detection of complications of the surgical wound and pacemaker pocket
3. Reprogramming of the pacemaker as the patient's needs change
4. Identification of the patient's education and support needs for well-being
5. Checking for end-of-life indicators

6. Gathering of data on pacemaker function and longevity for research

During the first year after permanent pacemaker implantation, it is advisable to evaluate the patient and pacing system at least every 3 months. Thereafter examination every 6 months may be sufficient unless the patient has a complicated physiologic or antitachycardia pacemaker. Patients should be monitored by telephone every 3 months in between office visits. In the future, pacemaker analyzers may be available for use at home by the patient. Such a unit is in the developmental stages and is being designed to analyze the patient's ECG for pacemaker or intrinsic rate, capture, and sensing.[28] Appearance of a warning light will alert the patient to contact the physician.

Pacemaker testing

A lead-II ECG rhythm strip is taken for visualizing the pacemaker spike, P waves, frontal plane axis and capture. Then, using an internal counter and the programmer-analyzer, the paced rate, magnet rate, impulse-to-impulse interval, and the pulse duration are measured. Changes in any of these values can represent battery decline, misprogramming, or other malfunction. When measuring the *magnet rate*, the magnet, provided by the manufacturer is used to prevent damage to the reed switch.[26] This rate is used as the *end-of-life indicator* for most pacemakers. A change in this value predicts battery exhaustion and the need for pulse generator replacement. The precise behavior of the pacemaker at this point varies from unit to unit.[17] Pacemakers with bidirectional telemetry also provide information on battery strength, lead resistance, and P or R wave magnitude.

To evaluate the underlying cardiac rhythm (i.e., in the absence of pacing), the pacemaker can be turned off for a few seconds while the ECG is recorded. This is usually done using the programmer-analyzer to reprogram the pacemaker to a rate low enough to allow the underlying rhythm to predominate.

Most patients should be tested for *muscle inhibition* if the pacemaker has an inhibitory function (AAI, VVI, DVI, or DDD). Patients are instructed to perform isometric maneuvers of the upper extremities as the ECG records. Patients who have a positive test should have their pacemakers reprogrammed, if possible, to a triggered or bipolar mode or a reduced sensitivity. If the pacemaker cannot be programmed to eliminate the inhibition, patients are instructed to avoid activities using both arms or the pacemaker arm alone, such as lifting up windows, lifting heavy boxes or suitcases, or applauding. The pacemaker pocket, old surgical incision, and the course of the lead should be examined for signs of erosion or infection.

KEY CONCEPT REVIEW

1. Bradydysrhythmias resulting from failure of the SA node occur because:
   a. The SA node is the only structure within the heart capable of self-excitation.
   b. Other tissues of the heart can neither generate a rate equivalent to that of the SA node nor respond to the directions of the autonomic nervous system as well as the SA node.
   c. Any impulse produced by tissues other than the SA node cannot reach the ventricles.
   d. Failure of the SA node depresses myocardial function.

2. Which of the following factors renders the conduction system vulnerable to dysfunction?
   a. The system has no mechanism for excitation other than the SA node.
   b. The structures are in close proximity to the cardiac skeleton and AV valves.
   c. The conduction system responds to circulating catecholamines.
   d. The tissues depend on high concentrations of extracellular sodium.

3. Which of the following is not a symptom commonly seen with bradydysrhythmias?
   a. Syncope
   b. Chest pain
   c. Central cyanosis
   d. Dizziness

4. Which one of the following is a currently accepted indication for temporary cardiac pacing?
   a. Asymptomatic sinus bradycardia with a rate less than 65 bpm
   b. Anterolateral or anteroseptal AMI
   c. Any AMI with second- or third-degree block, increasing PR interval, widening QRS complex, or shifting axis
   d. Asymptomatic slow junctional rhythm

5. Myocardial threshold to pacing can vary with which of the following factors?
   a. The length of the pacing lead
   b. The current density and duration
   c. The type of power source in the pulse generator
   d. The sensitivity setting on the pulse generator

6. Which of the following is not a complication of temporary epicardial pacing?
   a. Infection at the lead insertion site
   b. Cardiac dysrhythmias
   c. Intrapericardial bleeding
   d. Ventricular perforation

7. In the temporary pacing system, the *first* action to take in the event of a confirmed loss of pacing is:
   a. Call the physician.
   b. Check and tighten all connections between the lead and pulse generator.
   c. Increase the pulse generator output.
   d. Turn the patient to the left lateral recumbent position.

8. Which one of the following factors does not *directly* lower a person's threshold to fibrillation, making a loss of pacemaker sensing hazardous?
   a. Electrolyte imbalance
   b. Fluid overload

   c. Digitalis toxicity
   d. Myocardial ischemia

9. Which one of the following is a currently accepted indication for permanent cardiac pacing?
   a. Asymptomatic sinus bradycardia with rates greater than 40 ppm
   b. Asymptomatic second-degree heart block
   c. Vasovagal bradycardia with syncope
   d. Sinus pauses less than 2.5 seconds

10. The power source for pacemakers with the greatest longevity is:
    a. Mercury-zinc
    b. Alkaline batteries
    c. Lithium iodine
    d. Nickel cadmium

11. Of the following elements, which is most likely to interfere electromagnetically with permanent pacemaker function?
    a. Microwave ovens
    b. Automatic door openers
    c. Antitheft devices
    d. Electrocautery

12. Which procedure should not be used in the management of the patient with a permanent programmable pacemaker who requires electrocautery during surgery?
    a. Program the pacemaker to a fixed rate mode just before surgery.
    b. Program it to a triggered mode.
    c. Use short-duration bursts of low-current cautery and monitor pulse rate.
    d. Place a pacemaker magnet over the pacemaker's reed switch to produce a fixed-rate mode during the cautery.

ANSWERS

1. b	3. c	5. b	7. c	9. c	11. d
2. b	4. c	6. d	8. b	10. c	12. d

REFERENCES

1. Adamec R, Haeflinger JM, and Killsch JP: Damaging effects of therapeutic radiation on programmable pacemakers, PACE 5:146, 1982.
2. Adams D and others: The cardiac pacemaker and ultrasonic scalers, Br Dent J 152:171, 1982.
3. Alyward P, Blood R, and Tonkin A: Complications of defibrillation with permanent pacemakers in situ, PACE 2:462, 1979.
4. Anderson KM and Moore AA: Sensors in pacing, PACE 9(6):954, 1986.
5. Barold SS and Gaidula J: Evaluation of normal and abnormal sensing functions of demand pacemakers, Am J Cardiol 28:201, 1971.
6. Barold SS and others: Inhibition of a bipolar demand pacemaker by diaphragmatic potentials, Circulation 56:679, 1977.
7. Barold SS and others: Reprogramming of an implanted pacemaker following external defibrillation, PACE 1:514, 1978.
8. Berman N: T-wave sensing with a programmable pacemaker, PACE 3:657, 1980.

9. Bernstein AD and others: The NASPE/BPEG generic pacemaker code for antibradyarrhythmia and adaptive rate pacing and antitachyarrhythmia devices, PACE 10:794, 1987.
10. Birdsall C: How do you manage epicardial wires, Am J Nurs 86(3):252, 1986.
11. Bloomfield P and others: Long-term follow-up of patients with the QT rate adaptive pacemaker, PACE 12(1):111, 1988.
12. Bobyn J and others: Comparison of a porous-surfaced with a totally porous ventricular endocardial pacing electrode, PACE 4:405, 1981.
13. Boute W, Gebhardt U, and Begemann MJS: Introduction of an automatic QT interval driven rate responsive pacemaker, PACE 11(11):1804, 1988.
14. Breivik K and Ohm O: Myopotential inhibition of unipolar QRS inhibited (VVI) pacemakers assessed by ambulatory Holter monitoring of the electrocardiogram, PACE 3:470, 1980.
15. Breivik K and others: Clinical and electrophysiological properties of a new temporary pacemaker lead after open heart surgery, PACE 5:600, 1982.
16. Butrous GS and others: Interference with the pacemakers of two workers at electricity substations, Br J Int Med 40:462, 1983.
17. Byrd C: Permanent pacemaker implantation techniques. In Samet P and El-Sherif N: Cardiac pacing, ed 2, New York, 1980, Grune & Stratton, Inc.
18. Choo M and others: Permanent pacemaker infections: characterization and management, Am J Cardiol 48:559, 1981.
19. Chung E: Drugs and electrolyte balance which may alter pacemaker function, Impulse 11:11, 1978.
20. Cooper D and others: Effects of extracorporeal shock wave lithotripsy (renal) on cardiac pacemakers and its safety in patients with implanted cardiac pacemakers. PACE 11(11):1607, 1988.
21. Cordis Corporation: Cordis sequicor III manual, Miami, 1983, The Cordis Corp.
22. Cornacchia D and others: Clinical evaluation of VDD pacing with a unipolar single-pass lead, PACE 12(4):604, 1989.
23. Crystal R, Kastor J, and DeSanctus R: Inhibition of discharge of an external demand pacemaker by an electric razor, Am J Cardiol 27:659, 1971.
24. D'Cunha GF and others: Syncopal attacks arising from erratic demand pacemaker function in the vicinity of a television transmitter, Am J Cardiol 31:789, 1973.
25. Decaprio V, Hurzeler P, and Furman S: A comparison of unipolar and bipolar electrograms for cardiac pacemaker sensing, Circulation 56:750, 1977.
26. Dodinot B: The perfect magnet guide, Stimucoeur Med 9(3):282, 1981.
27. Domino KB and Smith TC: Electrocautery induced reprogramming of a pacemaker using a precordial magnet, Anesth Analg 62:610, 1983.
28. Dreifus L and others: Long-term monitoring of patients with implanted pacemakers, Heart Lung 11:417, 1982.
29. Dulk KD and others: The Activitrax rate responsive pacemaker system, Am J Cardiol 61:107, 1988.
30. Erikson M, Schuller H, and Sjolund B: Hazards from transcutaneous nerve stimulation in patients with pacemakers, Lancet 1(8077):1319, 1978.
31. Erlebacher JA and others: Effects of magnetic resonance imaging on DDD pacemakers, Am J Cardiol 57:437, 1986.
32. Fetter J and others: The clinical incidence and significance of myopotential sensing with unipolar pacemakers, PACE 7:871, 1984.
33. Fetter J and others: The effects of nuclear magnetic resonance imagers on external and implantable pulse generators, PACE 7:720, 1984.
34. Fujiwara H and others: The influence of low frequency acupuncture on demand pacemakers, Chest 78:96, 1980.
35. Gaita F and others: Holter monitoring and provocative maneuvers in assessment of unipolar demand pacemaker myopotential inhibition, Am Heart J 107:927, 1984.
36. Gann D, El-Sherif N, and Samet P: Indications for cardiac pacing. In Samet P and El-Sherif N, editors: Cardiac pacing, ed 2, New York, 1980, Grune & Stratton, Inc.
37. Gibson TC and others: Pacemaker function in relation to electroconvulsive therapy, Chest 63:1025, 1973.
38. Goldberg ME, McSherry RT, and O'Conner ME: Electrocautery and pacemaker reprogramming, Anesth Analg 63:541, 1984.
39. Goldreyer B and others: A new orthogonal lead for P-synchronous pacing, PACE 4:638, 1981.
40. Halprin JL and others: Myopotential interference with DDD pacemakers: endocardial electrographic telemetry in the diagnosis of pacemaker related arrhythmias, Am J Cardiol 54:97, 1984.
41. Hardage M and Barold SS: Pacemaker programming techniques. In Barold SS and Mugica J: The third decade of cardiac pacing, NY, 1982, Futura Publishing Co, Inc.
42. Hardage M, Marbach JR, and Winsor DW: The pacemaker patient in the therapeutic and diagnostic device environment. In Barold SS, editor: Modern cardiac pacing. Mount Kisco, NY, 1985, Futura Publishing Co, Inc.
43. Hauser R and Susmano A: After potential over-sensing by a programmable pulse generator, PACE 4:391, 1981.
44. Hayes DL and others: A shorter hospital stay after cardiac pacemaker implantation, Mayo Clin Proc, 63(3):236, 1988.
45. Heldner FJ, Linhart JW, and Poole DO: Irradiation of a pulmonary tumor with an overlying cardiac pacemaker, Radiology 92:148, 1969.
46. Irnich W, deBakker JMT, and Bisping JH: Electromagnetic interference in implantable pacemakers, PACE 1:52, 1978.
47. Johnson DL: Effect on pacemakers of airport weapons detectors, Can Med Assoc J 110:778, 1974.
48. Kubisch K and others: Clinical experience with the rate responsive pacemaker, Sensolog 703, PACE 11(11):1829, 1988.
49. Langberg J and others: The effects of extracorporeal shock wave lithotripsy on pacemaker function, PACE 10(5):114, 1987.
50. Lau FYK, Bilitch M, and Wintraube JH: Protection of implanted pacemakers from excessive electrical energy of DC shock, Am J Cardiol 23:244, 1969.
51. Lerner SM: Suppression of a demand pacemaker by transurethral electrocautery, Anesth Analg 52:705, 1973.
52. Lister JW and others: Rapid atrial stimulation in the treatment of supraventricular tachycardias, Chest 63:995, 1973.

53. Marbach JR and others: The effects on cardiac pacemakers of ionizing radiation and electromagnetic interference from radio-therapy machines, Radiat Oncol Biol Phys 4:1055, 1978.

54. McIntyre K and Lewis J: Textbook of advanced cardiac life support, Dallas, 1981, American Heart Association.

55. Mond H: The bradyarrhythmias: current indications for permanent pacing. I. PACE 4:432, 1981.

56. Ormerod D and others: Design and evaluation of a low threshold porous tip lead with a mannitol coated screw-in tip (sweet tip), PACE 11(11):1784, 1988.

57. Palac RT and others: Delayed pulse generator malfunction after DC countershock, PACE 4:163, 1981.

58. Parsonnet V, Bernstein AD, and Calasso D: Cardiac pacing practices in the United States in 1985, Am J Cardiol 62(1):71, 1988.

59. Parsonnet V, Furman S, and Smyth N: Implantable cardiac pacemaker status report and resource guideline, Circ Suppl 50:A21, 1974.

60. Parsonnet V, Furman S, and Smyth N: A revised code for pacemaker identification, PACE 4:410, 1981.

61. Parsonnet V and others: Optimal resources for implantable cardiac pacemakers, Circulation 68:227A, 1983.

62. Picker BA, and Goldberg MT: Inhibition of demand pacemaker and interference with monitoring equipment by radiofrequency transmissions, Br Med J 2:504, 1969.

63. Pirzada FA, Moschitto LJ, and Diorio D: Clinical experience with steroid-eluting unipolar electrodes, PACE 11(11):1739, 1988.

64. Pourhamidi AH: Radiation effect on implantable pacemakers, Chest 84:499, 1983.

65. Proctor D, Fletcher RD, and DelNegro A: Temporary cardiac pacing: causes, recognition and management of failure to pace, Nurs Clin North Am 13:409, 1978.

66. Rickards AF: Rate-responsive pacing. In Barold SS, editor: Modern cardiac pacing, Mount Kisko, NY, 1985, Futura Publishing Co, Inc.

67. Roberts J and others: Emergency transthoracic pacemaker, Ann Emerg Med 10:600, 1981.

68. Sclarovsky S and others: Ventricular fibrillation complicating temporary ventricular pacing in acute myocardial infarction, Am J Cardiol 48:1160, 1981.

69. Secemsky SI and others: Unipolar sensing of abnormalities: incidence and clinical significance of skeletal muscle interference and undersensing in 228 patients, PACE 5:10, 1982.

70. Smyth N: Atrial programmed pacing, PACE 1:104, 1978.

71. Smyth N: Techniques of implantation: atrial and ventricular, thoracotomy and transvenous, Prog Cardiovasc Dis 23:435, 1981.

72. Smyth N: Personal communication, 1987.

73. Smyth N, Keshishian J, and Proctor D: Atrial pacing thresholds: a twelve-year experience. In Meere C, editor: Proceedings of the sixth world symposium on cardiac pacing, PACE 2:A110, 1979.

74. Smyth N and others: Effect of an active magnetometer on permanently implanted pacemakers, JAMA 221:162, 1972.

75. Stangel K and others: Physical movement sensitive pacing: comparison of two "activity"-triggered pacing systems, PACE 12:103, 1988.

76. Sylven C and Levander-Lindgren M: Normally functioning inhibited pacemaker concomitant with vertebral nerve stimulator, PACE 2:645, 1979.

77. Taube MA, Elsberry DD, and Exworthy KW: Physiological effects of DC defibrillation on pacemaker function. In Meere C, editor: Proceedings of the sixth world symposium on cardiac pacing, PACE 2:A103, 1979.

78. vanGelder LM and El Gamal MIH: Myopotential interference inducing pacemaker tachycardia in DVI programmed pacemakers, PACE 7:970, 1984.

79. Walz BJ and others: Does radiation therapy affect pacemaker performance? JAMA 234:72, 1975.

80. Warnowicz-Papp MA: The pacemaker patient in the electromagnetic environment, Clin Prog Pacing Electrophysiol 1:166, 1983.

81. Westerholm C: Threshold studies in transvenous cardiac pacemaker treatment, Scand J Thorac Cardiovasc Surg 8(Suppl):1, 1971.

82. Whalen R and Starmer C: Electric shock hazards in clinical cardiology, Mod Con Cardiovasc Dis 26:7, 1967.

83. Wicks JM, Davison R, and Belic N: Malfunction of a demand pacemaker caused by phrenic nerve stimulation, Chest 74:305, 1978.

84. Wiggers C and Wegria R: Ventricular fibrillation due to single localized induction and condenser shocks applied during the vulnerable phase of ventricular systole, Am J Physiol 128:500, 1940.

85. Wingate S: Levels of pacemaker acceptance by patients, Heart Lung 15(1):93, 1986.

86. Yalteau RF: Radar-induced failure of a demand pacemaker, N Engl J Med 283:1447, 1970.

87. Young D: Pacemaker implant in children and adolescents, Impulse 10:3, 1978.

88. Zimmerman BH and Faul DD: Artifacts and hazards in nuclear magnetic resonance imaging due to metal implants and cardiac pacemakers, Diagn Imag Clin Med 53:53, 1984.

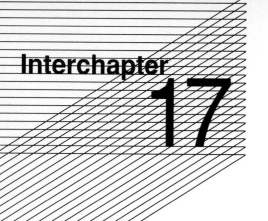

Going Fishing During a Cardiac Catheterization

Frequently, patients mentally rehearse the events surrounding their procedures, treatments, and surgery. Much of this mental rehearsal can involve negative imagery, anxiety, and fear. Patients can be taught to rehearse such situations positively, however, and replace anxiety and fear with healthy responses.

Guided imagery is one strategy that nurses can combine with traditional teaching to help patients gain a feeling of control over the event. Since it is impossible to experience fear and relaxation at the same time, guided imagery can be used to elicit positive physiologic and behavioral responses. Patients can be guided in mentally rehearsing the experience and seeing themselves as doing well and being relaxed before, during, and after the event. The image of the outcome is most important (see Awakening the Inner Healer, p. 484).

An example of this is Mr. B., a 64-year-old IBM executive who was about to undergo a cardiac catheterization. During his assessment, the following dialogue took place:

Nurse: Mr. B., how are you feeling about your cardiac catheterization?

Mr. B.: I'm scared to death. I keep having these ideas about how awful it's going to be. All I've ever seen really is stuff on television. It looks scary.

Nurse: I would like to share some positive ideas with you, as well as a few skills that you can use during the procedure to help you get through it more easily. Would you be interested?

Mr. B.: You bet. What do I need to do?

Nurse: Let me ask you a few questions. Tell me about where you like to relax. What is the most perfect and quiet place that comes to your mind which makes you feel calm and happy?

Mr. B.: That's easy. My brother and I have some property in southern Colorado.

It has a pond with beavers and big rainbow trout. Boy, I'd sure like to go fishing up there soon.

Nurse: That's perfect. Let me guide you in some basic relaxation skills that you can use during your cardiac catheterization. Then I'll use the information you just gave me about the beaver pond. Okay?

Mr. B.: I'm ready

The nurse prepared the room, closed the drapes and the door, placed the bed at a 30-degree angle, and assured that the patient was in a comfortable position. She then guided Mr. B. in a 15-minute imagery session that incorporated relaxation, as well as right and left brain teaching, to prepare him for his cardiac catheterization (see The Right and Left Brains, p. 38). The script included going through the mechanics of the procedure, his feelings during the procedure, and then going to his special beaver pond. The following script was used:

Nurse: Mr. B. with your eyes closed and your body relaxed and lying still, travel ahead in time to the morning of your cardiac catheterization. It is 7:00 AM and you are awake and feeling refreshed, relaxed, and confident about this procedure. Use these first few alert, awake moments to feel the relaxation from the top of your head to the tip of your toes. (At this point, a general head-to-toe relaxation script is used. See Chapter 13, box on p. 414).

(Following the head-to-toe relaxation script): It is now time for you to get on the stretcher and go to the cardiac catheterization laboratory. You look forward to this day. You will know information soon that will help you make decisions about your continued recovery. As you ride down the hall, use this time to focus on breathing in and out and feeling very relaxed. See yourself entering the door behind the x-ray department. The cardiac catheterization room

is on your left. As you enter the room, you are greeted by two nurses you know and you are delighted to see them this morning. As you move onto the cardiac catheterization table, feel the security of that table as the nurses place a strap over your legs and arms to help you maintain this position. At this time, the nurses begin to prepare you for the procedure by connecting ECG leads to your chest to monitor your heart. They will wash and shave the catheter insertion sites. Continue to use this time to concentrate on your breathing and achieve a deeper state of relaxation.

You hear the cardiologist entering now. She greets you and makes you feel comfortable by her confidence and caring. Your physician begins by numbing your skin in your groin area for your comfort during the procedure. When the physician injects the contrast media to see your heart on x-ray, you may feel "hot flashes" or a burning sensation or a sense of nausea. Use this time to remember your diaphragmatic deep breathing techniques. Whenever the physician wants you to participate in the procedure by coughing or deep breathing to clear the contrast media from your heart, you will be able to come back to the room quickly and follow her directions. But until that time, go to your special place.

At this point you feel in control of the situation. You feel confident and relaxed. Allow yourself to go to southern Colorado. You haven't been there in a long time. It feels so good to be back. Smell the mountain air, the pine trees so fresh and strong. Look at the different trees—the aspens as their leaves quake in the sun, the magical tall blue spruces with their unmistakable color. See the chipmunks and squirrels playing.

Today seems special. You are walking down the path that leads to the beaver pond. You hear twigs and leaves snap and crunch as you step on them. You feel balanced while you walk. This walk is relaxed and you have nothing to do today except watch the beavers play and maybe catch some trout.

As you get to the edge of the pond, see the beavers playing. They look at you. They seem to say hello. Two are in the water. They are closer to you than they ever have been before. Neither you nor the beavers are afraid. Feel yourself with your fishing pole and bait in hand. You start to fish for the first time in a long while. Feel the excitement of that first cast. It seems perfect. You get a bite, but the trout is just playing with your line. The pond water is clear and as you pull in your line, you can see two trout following it. Feel that sense of going with the flow. If you catch a trout, fine; if you don't, that is fine also.

As you continue your fishing, you hear the physician tell you that everything is going well. She asks you to cough and you do so. Then you continue your image; you again bring it back into full clear, focus, adding more details—the colors, the smells, the environment, what you are doing, and what the beavers are doing. Now focus your concentration on this image for the next few minutes. (Allow 5 minutes while the patient continues to image in an alert relaxed state with eyes closed.)

The next thing you hear is your physician telling you that the procedure is over and it went very well. She briefly tells you that she has found out the information that you both need to know. She tells you she will give you the details in a few hours.

You feel relieved that the procedure went well. Now you are back in bed where you will remain for the next 4 to 6 hours. You remember not to move the leg where the catheter was inserted or to flex or hyperextend it. You feel thirsty from the contrast media. This is normal and the nurses give you fluids. Also, you feel the need to urinate frequently. Feel yourself successfully using the urinal while in bed. Give yourself a pat on the back for staying calm and relaxed and playing an important role in making the procedure go well.

Now begin to feel the muscles around your eyes become less heavy. Begin to lighten your arms and legs and start to move slowly and gently. And when you are ready, just open your eyes and look around. (Mr. B. was instructed to practice these exercises a few more times on his own before his cardiac catheterization. The nurse did one more session with him and was available to answer any questions.)

Following his cardiac catheterization, Mr. B. reported catching one of the biggest trout that he had ever caught while on the cardiac catheterization table. He also stated that the relaxation and imagery techniques helped him tremendously to get through the procedure. He said that he felt relaxed during the procedure and in control of the situation. He reported using these same skills before and after his coronary artery bypass surgery several weeks later.

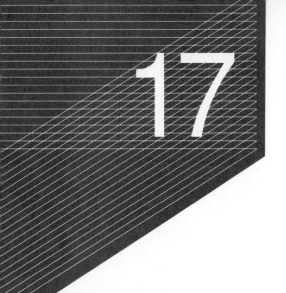

17

The Person Undergoing Cardiac Surgery

Marguerite R. Kinney
Mary Sue Craft

LEARNING OBJECTIVES

1. Examine the major indications for cardiac surgery.
2. Analyze the major criteria for selecting candidates for cardiac surgery.
3. Describe the preoperative evaluation of a patient undergoing cardiac surgery.
4. Develop a plan for preoperative patient and family teaching.
5. Evaluate the major detrimental effects of cardiopulmonary bypass.
6. Discuss the complications of cardiac surgical procedures.
7. Describe the nursing diagnoses and postoperative plan of care for an adult undergoing cardiac surgery.

Over 25 years, there have been important achievements in the surgical management of patients with heart disease. Notable technical and scientific advances in cardiac surgery include the hospital environment; surgical procedures; myocardial management; the science of comparing and predicting; and the support systems (i.e., cardiopulmonary bypass).[49] In 1987, 332,000 patients received coronary artery bypass grafts, whereas 43,000 experienced valvular surgery.[3] Growing numbers of patients with recurrent sustained supraventricular and ventricular tachycardia are undergoing successfully a variety of ablation procedures.

Myocardial revascularization was pioneered in the 1940s by Vineberg, who implanted the internal mammary artery into the myocardium. A more direct approach to revascularization was introduced in 1967 by Favalaro and his colleagues, who grafted the saphenous vein to a coronary artery, restoring blood flow to ischemic myocardium. The procedure gained great popularity because of low operative risk and prolonged and improved quality of life in selected subgroups of patients.[52] More recently, the internal mammary artery has demonstrated superior long-term patency when compared with the saphenous vein graft and is expected to further improve survival and reduce cardiac-related morbidity and need for reoperation.[76]

Valvular surgery was introduced in 1957 when Lillehei and, independently, Merendino successfully repaired incompetent mitral valves. Only a few years later the first prosthetic heart valve, a ball-in-cage prosthesis, was introduced by Starr. Aortic valve allografts and valved extra-cardiac conduits soon emerged along with techniques for preservation. Today several types of tilting disk valves are available, and all mechanical valves have excellent durability. Continuous anticoagulant therapy, however, is required to minimize thromboembolism. The search continues for an improved valve design that will be flexible for any location, will not require anticoagulant therapy, and will be functional for long periods of time.

A number of surgical procedures have been developed since the late 1970s to treat selected patients with refractory supraventricular or ventricular dysrhythmias. Variable results related to survival and relief of the tachycardia, as well as undesirable side effects of the procedures, prompt continued investigation into surgical therapies for these tachydysrhythmias.[13,73]

Even though operative procedures have been well developed and patients can be selected carefully for surgery, perioperative care remains a critical part of the overall outcome and demands knowledgeable nursing management.

PREOPERATIVE PHASE

Indications for surgery

Myocardial revascularization

Myocardial revascularization is commonly used as treatment for coronary artery disease. Subsets of patients who are likely to benefit from revascularization have been identified, including patients with left main coronary artery disease, certain groups of patients with three-vessel coronary disease, and those with severe angina who are unresponsive to medical therapy.[102]

Although myocardial revascularization was initially performed as an elective procedure for chronic stable angina, there are additional urgent and emergency complications of coronary artery disease for which it may be the preferred treatment.[90] Complications requiring surgery include acute myocardial infarction and cardiogenic shock, as well as unstable angina, failed percutaneous transluminal coronary angioplasty (PTCA), or failure of thrombolysis. Emergency operations are performed as soon as the patient can be brought to the operating suite, and urgent operations are those performed within 24 hours of the decision that surgery is necessary.

Although definitions of *stable angina* vary, it is generally defined as angina that has been present longer than 6 weeks without a significant change in frequency, duration, or severity of symptoms over the previous 4 to 6 weeks.[24] In these patients, surgical revascularization may result in relief of symptoms, may have some impact on the rate of nonfatal infarction, and decreases mortality rates except in patients at low risk.

Early surgical myocardial revascularization may be performed in patients with persistent or recurrent angina after myocardial infarction because of the high rate of reinfarction and mortality, especially in patients with non–Q-wave infarction and multivessel disease.[54] Although surgical intervention in this group of patients has a high mortality rate, the rate of survival has improved over the last several years.[23] The presence of cardiogenic shock complicating myocardial infarction indicates that at least 40% of the normal myocardial muscle mass is not functioning and is associated with an operative mortality rate of 20% to 60%.[90] Disadvantages of early myocardial revascularization in patients with persistent angina after myocardial infarction include increased risk of hemorrhage, hemodynamic instability, high costs, and the emotional trauma of undergoing a surgical procedure soon after an acute myocardial infarction.

Unstable angina is characterized by abruptness of onset and an unpredictable clinical course. Myocardial revascularization produces immediate relief of angina in these patients, and the rate of late nonfatal myocardial infarction is low. In addition, late survival is similar to that in patients with chronic stable angina who undergo myocardial revascularization.[45] However, perioperative myocardial injury and low cardiac output after surgery occur more frequently in these patients than in those undergoing revascularization for chronic stable angina.[20]

Between 5% and 6% of patients undergoing PTCA require myocardial revascularization, about half because of coronary dissection or acute closure. In patients requiring emergency myocardial revascularization, the hospital mortality rate ranges from 0% to 11%, with an average rate of 6%.[93]

Patients who have received thrombolytic therapy and are left with severely obstructed coronary lesions are candidates for myocardial revascularization. Advantages to early surgical treatment in these patients include preventing the effects of rethrombosis, treating postinfusion angina, providing more-adequate blood flow to the infarct zone to allow optimal recovery of function, and preventing infarction resulting from occlusion of diseased vessels other than the acutely infarcted vessel.[4]

Valvular surgery

Mitral valve disease. Timing of operation for valvular heart disease is an important feature of medical management. In mitral stenosis, the timing of the operation is influenced by the operative procedure to be performed (i.e., valve replacement or commissurotomy). Mitral commissurotomy is successful when the opening snap is prominent and calcification of the valve is not present on fluoroscopic examination.[50] For these patients, moderate symptoms (i.e., the New York Heart Association's functional class II or III) and a severely stenosed valve are indications for surgery. An additional indication for surgery, especially in young women, is the occurrence of acute paroxysmal nocturnal dyspnea or pulmonary edema with at least moderate mitral stenosis. Finally, surgery may be recommended when there is a significant increase in pulmonary vascular resistance, even if symptoms are not present.[50] Mitral valve replacement is usually reserved for patients experiencing more severe symptoms (i.e., the New York Heart Association's functional class III or IV).[50]

Aortic valve disease. In patients who have symptoms and a peak pressure gradient across the aortic valve of 50 mm Hg or more, surgery is generally recommended. The presence of severe left ventricular hypertrophy and increasing pulmonary venous hypertension are indications that urgent operation is needed.[50] Some patients with moderate aortic stenosis may undergo myocardial revascularization and have the aortic valve replaced at the same time. Patients with significant aortic incompetence who are experiencing symptoms are generally advised to undergo replacement. Patients with no symptoms may also undergo surgery if left ventricular enlargement is present.[50] In patients with mitral and aortic valve disease, replacement of both valves may be required if patients are in the New York Heart Associaton's functional class III or if left ventricular enlargement becomes significant.[50]

Dysrhythmias

The primary indication for surgical intervention in patients with recurrent ventricular tachycardia or supraventricular tachycardia is refractoriness to medical therapy.[13,50] The decision to operate is based on the status of left ventricular function, and the only absolute contraindication to surgery is prohibitive left ventricular dysfunction.[12]

Patient selection for cardiac surgery

Cardiac surgical mortality rates are influenced by many factors, including the physiologic status of the patient, severity of associated noncardiac disease, and severity of the cardiac disease.[44] Risk stratification techniques based on a number of factors are being developed to predict operative mortality rates and aid in patient selection.[74] Some authors believe that total body function is a larger determinant of the postoperative course than cardiac function.[44]

Severity of cardiac disease is best determined by the left ventricular ejection fraction. An ejection fraction of 50% or greater is considered good, 30% to 49% is fair, and less than 30% is poor.[17] Although the Coronary Artery Surgery Study identified poor left ventricular function as an independent risk factor for myocardial revascularization, others have not found that this factor independently predicts operative mortality rates.[69] The physiologic status of the patient and severity of associated noncardiac disease are indicated by variables such as age, gender, peripheral vascular disease, obesity, dependency on dialysis, catastrophic states (e.g., acute renal failure), reoperation, and presence of diabetes or hypertension.

The profile of the candidate for cardiac surgery has changed as patients have become older and sicker. Although age is no longer a contraindication for surgery, older patients are at greater risk for sepsis secondary to prolonged mechanical ventilation or poor wound healing.[46] As many as 40,000 coronary *reoperations* are performed annually in the United States,[27] in which operative mortality and perioperative infarction rates are high for certain subgroups of patients.[69] In patients who undergo myocardial revascularization 8 to 12 years after the initial operation, the procedure is more hazardous and the results less satisfactory because of age and changes in anatomic structure, collateral circulation, left ventricular function, and the general condition of the patient.[27] Changes in collateral and antegrade coronary flow make intraoperative myocardial protection more difficult, and the presence of atherosclerotic grafts may cause intraoperative embolization of graft debris.[27] Other perioperative complications for this group of patients include postoperative bleeding requiring reentry and neurologic complications.

Preoperative assessment
Human response patterns

Exchanging pattern. A major determinant of operative outcome is the performance of the cardiovascular, pulmonary, renal, neurologic, gastrointestinal, hematologic, and metabolic subsystems. Therefore preoperative assessment of the Exchanging Pattern addresses factors that may influence subsystem performance so that necessary preparations for postoperative support can be made.

Cardiovascular system. Evaluation of the candidate for cardiac surgery is a systematic process beginning with the history and physical examination and proceeding to adjunct studies such as exercise testing, left ventricular function studies, echocardiography, and coronary angiography. Exercise testing is useful in assessing functional capacity and anginal threshold, detecting significant coronary artery disease (i.e., 50% or greater reduction in luminal diameter), and identifying patients at increased surgical risk. Left ventriculography assesses global ejection fraction and regional wall motion abnormalities, such as hypokinesis, akinesis, and dyskinesis. In addition, the severity of mitral valvular insufficiency can be estimated. The final exercise stage achieved and left ventricular function are the most important independent predictors of postoperative survival.[101] Echocardiography offers essential information about structure and function of valve leaflets and for estimating valve orifice size. Coronary angiography permits visualization of sites of disease and assessment of vessel suitability for anastomosis. All of this information helps in planning postoperative management of the cardiovascular subsystem.

Pulmonary system. Preexisting abnormalities of pulmonary structure and function may complicate the postoperative course of patients undergoing cardiac surgery.[51] Common pulmonary complications include continued respiratory insufficiency or failure, adult respiratory distress syndrome, infections, and complications secondary to prolonged intubation.[1] Patients at increased risk for developing these complications include those who are elderly, obese, or heavy smokers and those with preexisting lung or valvular heart disease. Although preoperative pulmonary function testing does not allow precise prediction of the likelihood of postoperative pulmonary complications, testing provides a quantitative assessment of the severity of primary pulmonary disease.[65] Pulmonary function is judged to be adequate if the vital capacity and flow rates are 80% or more of their predicted values; indices below 50% of predicted values indicate the possibility of important postoperative pulmonary complications.[65]

Renal system. Preexisting chronic renal disease and chronic congestive heart failure increase the risk of developing acute renal dysfunction and renal failure in the early postoperative period.[1] Preoperative assessment of renal function includes urinalysis and blood urine nitrogen (BUN) and creatinine level measurement. A creatinine clearance test may be obtained if the BUN or creatinine levels are abnormal.

Neurologic system. Neurologic complications after cardiac surgery occur in only 1% to 5% of patients and primarily include peripheral neuropathic conditions, strokes, encephalopathic problems, and coma.[1] A number of factors are associated with the risk of stroke or transient ischemic attack (TIA), including the presence of carotid bruit, previous stroke or TIA, previous myocardial infarction, and history of congestive heart failure. Thus the history and physical examination are important components of preoperative neurologic assessment. Although the presence of a carotid bruit implies an increased risk for neurologic complications, its absence does not imply a decrease in the risk. Carotid stenosis greater than 50% has been detected by ultrasound examination when no bruit was present on physical examination.[1]

Gastrointestinal system. Because even mild preexisting liver disease increases the risk of acute hepatic failure after cardiac surgery,[51] it is important that liver function be assessed before surgery. In addition, gastroduodenal ulceration is more likely to occur in patients with a history of prior ulceration and should be treated prophylactically.

Hematologic factors. A baseline hematologic examination and coagulation profile are necessary to identify patients most prone to postoperative bleeding abnormalities. Baseline laboratory tests include a complete blood count, platelet count, prothrombin time, and partial prothrombin time. Additional studies may be necessary if abnormalities are detected.

Metabolic system. Several endocrine disorders may complicate the postoperative course, including diabetes mellitus, thyroid disease, and adrenal insufficiency. These conditions must be detected and controlled before surgery.

Choosing pattern. The physician's recommendation that surgery is the preferred treatment for the patient's cardiac disease is based on a risk-benefit analysis, taking into account the patient profile and risk stratification. This risk-benefit analysis should be explained to the patient and significant others so that an informed decision can be made. The patient must understand that disability and death may occur, that a change in lifestyle is mandatory, and that continued follow-up will be required.[20]

Coping. Although a profile of patients and families at differential risk for ineffective coping is not available, a presurgical assessment could include all or part of the following components: past medical history, past psychological history, major stress areas and coping styles, coping strategy for heart surgery, extent and availability of support systems, present level of anxiety and depression, possibility of a latent death wish or suicidal ideation, and extent to which the patient needs to control the environment.[77] For example, patients and families can be asked to relate strategies that they have found useful in coping with stressful situations in the past. Information seeking, direct action (e.g., prayer), turning to others, and relaxation techniques are coping strategies used by patients anticipating cardiac surgery.[47] Nursing care should be planned to support these strategies; such care includes preoperative teaching, providing time for prayers or meditation, or techniques chosen by the patient and significant others for coping with the stressful event (see Chapter 5).

Knowing pattern. Diagnostic-Related Groups (DRGs) have had a major impact on the time available for preoperative instruction of cardiovascular surgical patients. As a result, many health care institutions admit patients on the day before surgery or the day of surgery. Despite the subsequent reduction in hospital stay, patient acuity and educational needs have increased.

Anxiety related to lack of knowledge of cardiovascular surgery is an expected response for patients and families. Patients with moderate anxiety levels tend to ask more questions, tolerate a higher level of anxiety, and are more receptive to biopsychosocial assistance.[21,81] Concise and clear information regarding all phases of cardiac surgery may assist patients and their families in dealing with anxiety, regardless of the level of anxiety.

Preoperative teaching

In establishing an effective preoperative teaching program, the nurse may use an individualized or group method. Although individualized instruction is considered optimal in establishing a good nurse-patient rapport, the present nursing shortage limits nursing time. As a result, group teaching has become the norm. Group teaching promotes a sense of camaraderie among patients. An alternative or supplement to either method is preadmission instruction. Information may be conveyed via written materials, audiocassette tapes, videotapes, or telephone information systems. The content of the preoperative materials may be organized into several areas.

The anatomic, physiologic, and pathophysiologic aspects of the patient's cardiovascular disease should be reviewed. Use of pictures, cardiac models, and flip charts assist in the description of the coronary artery circulation, blood flow through the heart, and valvular function. The more common risk factors associated with the patient's disease should also be covered. Risk factors such as hypertension, smoking, hypercholesterolemia, diabetes mellitus, obesity, lack of exercise, family history of heart disease, age, sex, stress, and tension may complicate the patient's postoperative course.

The preoperative routine care components and their rationale should be stressed with the patient and family members. During this phase of hospitalization, a variety of procedures and activities occur. Laboratory studies, diagnostic procedures, and physical examinations will be performed. In addition, the patient will undergo a comprehensive surgical preparation involving a preoperative shave and shower with antibacterial soap, sleeping medication, nothing by mouth after midnight, and preoperative medications. The number of activities during this phase can be extremely overwhelming for the patient. Therefore emotional support is essential during preoperative instruction.

Patients receive information about the intraoperative phase from the surgeon, anesthesiologist, and nurse. General expectations regarding the surgical procedure are expressed by the surgeon. The anesthesiologist in turn reviews the medications and invasive equipment to be used during the operation. However, the nurse frequently must clarify and expand the information provided by the surgeon and anesthesiologist. A discussion regarding the sensations to be experienced in the operative suite (e.g., cold room temperature), operative procedure, and expected length of operation must be conveyed. Potential complications of cardiopulmonary bypass may be reviewed at this time (see Table 17-1).

The immediate postoperative routine is then described. A review of the various equipment (endotracheal tube, urinary catheter, hemodynamic lines, chest tubes, electrocardiogram [ECG], and intraaortic balloon pump [IABP]) should assist the patient and family in coping with postoperative sensations. For the patient, these sensations include the incisional discomfort (sternotomy and leg), noise and light levels in the critical care unit, pulmonary toilet techniques, and communication techniques. The family is equally subject to sensory overload. Reduction of anxiety may be accomplished by reviewing the location of the waiting room and critical care units, visiting hours, available resources (e.g., chaplain and social worker) and by describing the patient's expected immediate postoperative appearance (e.g., pale, edematous, and surrounded by equipment).

One facet of preoperative teaching may be performed weeks before surgery. Certain medications require gradual tapering or discontinuation to allow more effective and safer management of the patient during and after surgery. Thus patients need to understand the rationale for tapering or discontinuing these medications. In particular, digoxin, diuretics, β-adrenergic blocking agents, vasodilators, calcium channel blocking agents, and anticoagulants must be monitored carefully.

Digoxin and dysrhythmias

Digoxin usually will be discontinued 24 to 48 hours before surgery. Preoperative digitalization is a significant cause of dysrhythmias during the operation. Dysrhythmias are precipitated by digitalis excess, which can cause potassium flux and hypokalemia.[68,71] Patients generally do not react adversely to the temporary withdrawal of digoxin because they are confined to bed. An exception is the patient who is in atrial fibrillation or atrial flutter with a rapid ventricular response who may not tolerate digoxin withdrawal.

Diuretic agents

The electrophysiologic properties of the heart are most significantly influenced by the potassium ion. Imbalances in potassium levels are the most frequent cause of dysrhythmias in the clinical setting. Hypokalemia accentuates digitalis excess during and after surgery, so the nurse should watch for it carefully, particularly in patients receiving chronic diuretic therapy. As a general rule, the diuretic therapy is discontinued preoperatively, but the potassium therapy is continued to ensure adequate body supplies.[68,84]

β-Adrenergic blocking agents and vasodilators

The drug most frequently used today in the management of angina pectoris is propranolol (Inderal).[88] Propranolol is a myocardial depressant that decreases heart rate and myocardial contractility. There are many anesthetic implications for patients who are taking propranolol and undergoing myocardial revascularization. The concept of the critical balance of myocardial oxygen supply and demand play a role in ensuring the proper therapeutic drug level before and during the operation. Because heart rate is one of the prime determinants of oxygen demand,[94] propranolol decreases myocardial oxygen demand. Coronary blood flow determines myocardial oxygen supply, which is in turn influenced by the patency of the coronary arteries. Factors causing hypoxemia generally decrease oxygen supply to the myocardium. Managing the patient medically is primarily directed at reducing the oxygen demand rather than increasing the coronary blood flow, which is the object of myocardial revascularization.

Evidence suggests that in the preoperative management of patients having myocardial revascularization, propranolol should be continued until 24 to 48 hours before the operation.[8,94] Data indicate that the effects of propranolol are completely eliminated within 48 hours after the drug is discontinued.[8] Some surgeons continue the drug until 24 hours before the operation,[10,67] depending on the state of the patient. For patients experiencing angina pectoris, tapering the dosage or even continuing propranolol until the operation may be indicated. Ideally this plan prevents perioperative infarction during the induction period.[31,94] Abrupt withdrawal of large doses of propranolol can produce an increased incidence of infarction, ventricular dysrhythmias, and severe angina pectoris.[71,94]

Vasodilator drugs work with propranolol in the management of ischemic heart disease to keep the supply and demand balanced. Nitroglycerin, a vasodilator, reduces the preload. Nitroprusside reduces the preload and afterload and lessens cardiac work, thereby reducing myocardial oxygen consumption. Also, it is recommended in some institutions that nitroglycerin ointment (2%) be readily available in the operating room.

Patients with angina pectoris may also be receiving *calcium channel blocking agents*. Such drugs are used to dilate coronary arteries, enhance collateral blood flow, and reduce myocardial oxygen demand. They have also been used experimentally to preserve the myocardium during cardiopulmonary bypass.

Anticoagulants

Anticoagulants are discontinued to prevent bleeding problems during and after the operation and to allow the coagulation status to return to normal. Clotting profiles are monitored preoperatively, and usually warfarin (Coumadin) is discontinued at least 3 to 4 days before the procedure. Besides warfarin, all antiplatelet drugs, such as aspirin, dipyridamole (Persantine), and sulfinpyrazone (Anturane), are stopped. Problems with hemostasis during and after the operation can be attributed to vitamin K deficiencies, the use of salicylates, and inherent blood dyscrasias.[94]

PERIOPERATIVE PHASE

Adult cardiovascular surgical patients have unique biopsychosocial assessment and interventional needs. Awareness of these needs enables perioperative health care professionals to anticipate or confirm patient problems. Use of the Unitary Person Framework can assist in identifying and providing the specific needs of each patient. Attention to the Exchanging Pattern is crucial because of the intricate techniques used in cardiac surgery.

Aggressive hemodynamic monitoring is essential for assessing the demands that cardiac surgery places on myocardial function. The myocardium, particularly the left ventricle, is subject to dysfunction secondary to sudden alterations in afterload from the anesthetics, catecholamine release, and volume status.[21] Manifestations of such dysfunction include hypotension and low cardiac output. Detection of these states is accomplished by continuous ECG and intraarterial, intraatrial, central venous, and pulmonary artery pressure monitoring.

Cardiopulmonary bypass

Components of cardiopulmonary bypass

Cardiopulmonary bypass (CPB) is used during intracardiac surgical procedures. The purposes of CPB are to provide adequate tissue perfusion, oxygenation, and a dry, quiet operative field.[30] Three main structural elements are necessary to achieve extracorporeal circulation, including a pump, an oxygenator with reservoir function, and plastic circuitry.

CPB is accomplished by large-bore catheters diverting blood from the right atrium or from the superior and inferior venae cavae. The venous blood is drained into a reservoir positioned below the level of the patient's right atrium. A second, smaller reservoir collects blood from the operative field. Both reservoirs contain filters to reduce the quantity and size of emboli. Oxygenation of the blood is accomplished via the oxygenator. After oxygenation, filtration, dilution, and temperature alterations, the blood is returned to the patient via a single catheter inserted into the ascending aorta or femoral artery.

There are four types of oxygenators: 1) vertical screen, 2) disk, 3) bubble, and 4) membrane.[47] The stationary vertical screen oxygenator is no longer in use but was used extensively in the early years of cardiac surgery.[39] The disk oxygenator, developed by Bjork in 1948, used a series of stainless-steel disks coated with fiber and silicon. Although relatively atraumatic to blood cell components, the device required a large priming volume.[28] The bubble oxygenator and the membrane oxygenators are the two types presently used in intracardiac surgery (Fig. 17-1).

The *bubble oxygenator* has a large surface area for gas exchange. The blood and oxygen flow together to form a column of froth. The froth is then converted back into a liquid by direct contact with an antifoaming agent. The transfer of oxygen is related to the length of the bubble path and the size of the bubbles. If a higher rate of gas flow is required to cause the transfer of oxygen, an increase in turbulent blood flow, and subsequently an increase in the hemolysis of the blood cells occurs.[47]

In contrast with the bubble oxygenator in which a direct blood-gas interface exists, the *membrane oxygenator* causes gas exchange by diffusion across a nonporous, semipermeable membrane.[47] Oxygen diffuses from the gas compartment through the membrane into the blood. The reverse occurs for carbon dioxide.

Advantages of membrane oxygenators over bubble oxygenators are minimal to no microbubble production, no requirement for defoaming agents, decreased potential for air emboli, decreased platelet destruction, decreased free hemoglobin production, and improved hemostasis after longer periods of CPB.[47] Disadvantages of the membrane oxygenator are an increased cost of operation, preparation time, and amount of priming volumes.

Two types of pumps are used in cardiac surgery: a nonocclusive roller pump and an impeller centrifugal rotating cone pump. Each is capable of delivering only nonpulsatile blood flow that is maintained at a basic rate of 2.5 L/min/m² for an optimal mean arterial pressure of 55 to 60 mm Hg.[30] Although used in essentially all intracardiac surgeries, CPB devices may have a variety of detrimental effects (Table 17-1). The effects are related to the pump, as well as the methods used in their operation, including hemodilution, hypothermia, and anticoagulation.[30,48]

Hemodilution

Cardiopulmonary bypass machines were once primed with fresh, heparinized blood. This prime not only depleted blood bank stores but also significantly increased the incidence of hepatitis.[47] In addition, patients tended to suffer from *homologous blood syndrome,* which is characterized by hepatic congestion, portal hypertension, coagulopathic conditions, pulmonary congestion, renal failure, and cerebral insufficiencies.[47]

Currently, most CPB machines are primed with a combination of colloidal and crystalloid fluids. The fluids actively reduce the patient's serum hematocrit to approximately 25%.[16] Although a hematocrit near 20% will allow an adequate myocardial oxygen supply, this level would be grossly insufficient in the event of bleeding, hyperthermia, hypotension, or acute myocardial infarction.[47] By decreasing the hematocrit, the colloidal osmotic pressure and the oxygen-carrying capacity of the blood are reduced.

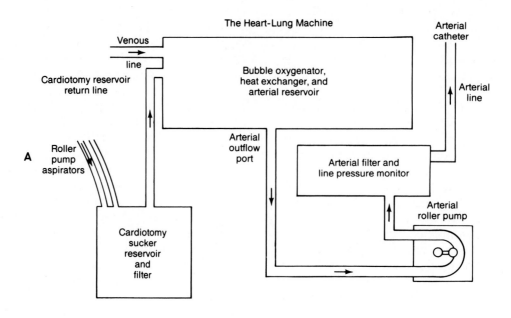

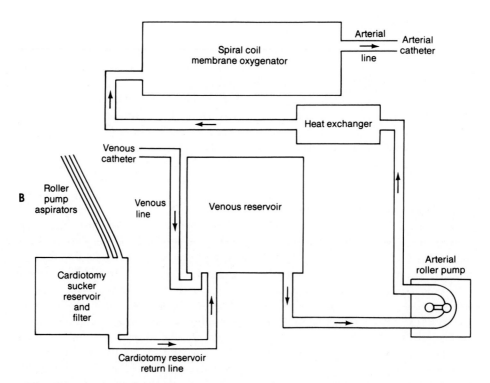

FIG. 17-1 **A,** Diagram of CPBP set up with a bubble oxygenator. **B,** Diagram of a CPBP set up with a membrane oxygenator.

Modified from Edmunds L and Stephenson L: Cardiopulmonary bypass for open heart surgery. In Glenn W, editor: Thoracic and cardiovascular surgery, East Norwalk, Conn, 1983, Appleton & Lange.

TABLE 17-1
Effects of Cardiopulmonary Bypass

Effects	Contributing factors	Effects	Contributing factors
CARDIOVASCULAR SYSTEM		**FLUID AND ELECTROLYTE BALANCE**	
Perioperative myocardial infarction	Inadequate myocardial protection and emboli	Interstitial edema	Increased extravascular fluid and organ dysfunction
Low cardiac output after surgery	Alteration in colloidal osmotic pressure, left ventricular dysfunction, and hypoperfusion injury	Intravascular hypovolemia	Decreased interstitial volume, bleeding, and interstitial edema
Increased afterload	Catecholamine release	Hypokalemia	Dilution, polyuria, intracellular shifts of potassium ions
Hypertension	Elevated renin, angiotensin, and aldosterone levels	Hyperkalemia	Potassium cardioplegia and increased intracellular exchange of glucose and potassium
PULMONARY SYSTEM		Hyponatremia, hypocalcemia, and hypomagnesemia	Dilution
Respiratory insufficiency	Alterations in colloidal osmotic pressure, interstitial pulmonary edema, decreased perfusion, and alterations in ventilatory patterns	**ENDOCRINE SYSTEM**	
		Water and sodium retention	Increase in antidiuretic hormone
Atelectasis	Complement activation, emboli, and alveolar-capillary membrane damage	Hypothyroidism	Increased levels of thyroxine (T_4) and decreased levels of triiodothyronine (T_3) and thyroid-stimulating hormone
NEUROLOGIC SYSTEM		Hyperglycemia	Depressed insulin response
Cerebrovascular accident	Cerebral emboli		
Transient motor deficits	Decreased cerebral blood flow	**IMMUNE SYSTEM**	
Cerebral hemorrhage	Systemic heparinization	Infection	Exposure to multiple pathogens and decreased complement and immunoglobin levels
GASTROINTESTINAL SYSTEM			
Gastrointestinal bleeding	Hormonal stress and coagulopathic conditions	Postperfusion syndrome	Release of anaphylactic toxins
Intestinal ischemia or infarction	Emboli and decreased perfusion	**HEMATOLOGIC FACTORS**	
Acute pancreatitis	Pancreatic vasculature emboli	Bleeding	Blood cell hemolysis, heparin rebound, and reduction in platelet count
RENAL SYSTEM			
Acute renal failure	Decreased renal blood flow, microemboli, and myohemoglobin release		

Adapted from Stewart S: The physiologic effects and nursing implications of cardiopulmonary bypass, unpublished master's thesis, Boston, 1985, Boston University.

However, hemodilution also reduces the viscosity of the blood, decreases hemolysis of the blood cell components, lowers systemic vascular resistance, and promotes postoperative diuresis.[61]

Hypothermia

Systemic hypothermia is used to lower the patient's metabolic and oxygen needs by as much as 50%.[61] Temperatures of 28° to 32° C are used for most intracardiac surgical procedures. Cooling is accomplished by convection (operative suite temperature), by cold (0° to 4° C) cardioplegia, and by the heat exchanger of the CPB machine.

Hypothermia causes an increase in blood viscosity, alters the coagulation factors and platelet function, and shifts the oxyhemoglobin curve to the left. Subsequently, clotting mechanisms and tissue oxygenation are altered. Rewarming is performed on completion of cardiopulmonary bypass and is continued during transfer to the critical care unit.

Anticoagulation

Total hemostatic paralysis is essential during cardiac surgery.[18] The goal of anticoagulation therapy is to achieve sufficient hemostatic paralysis so that thrombogenesis does not occur during exposure of the blood to the foreign surfaces of the CPB machine. An activated clotting time (ACT) of 400 seconds is considered adequate. Inadequate heparinization can result in fibrinolysis and possibly the precipitation of disseminated intravascular coagulation (DIC).[18]

The patient is heparinized fully before insertion of the bypass catheters. The conventional heparin dose is 300 units/kg and may be administered rapidly as a bolus through a central line. A disparity may exist between desired clinical effects and actual results because of the patient's weight, distribution of fluid volume, preoperative anticoagulation status, age, hemodilution, and hypothermia.[18] Individual titration of the heparin dose is often required.

Heparin is reversed on the completion of the CPB. Protamine sulfate is used to neutralize the anticoagulant effects of heparin. Most centers consider a dose ratio of 1 to 1.3 mg of protamine per 100 units of heparin as sufficient. Idiosyncratic reactions have been observed with protamine injections, and reactions range from systemic and intraatrial hypotension to catastrophic pulmonary vasoconstriction.[62] Catastrophic reactions to protamine are more prevalent in patients with allergies to fish[59] and in persons with insulin-dependent diabetes who use neutral protamine Hagedorn (NPH insulin).[22,58] Slow, dilute infusions of protamine are least likely to cause catastrophic changes when compared with a bolus administration of the drug.[36]

Heparin rebound is a phenomenon in which heparin is inadequately neutralized by protamine sulfate because of protamine's rapid elimination from the body. Bleeding can then recur.[18] The incidence ranges from 0% to 50%.

Myocardial protection

Myocardial preservation is achieved by maintaining the balance between oxygen supply and demand. If the balance is altered, myocardial ischemia or infarction results. Myocardial oxygen demand is affected by heart rate, preload, afterload, and contractility. Oxygen supply is affected by oxygen saturation, hemoglobin, oxygen delivery, and coronary blood flow. Ischemia results from any intervention that increases oxygen demand or decreases oxygen supply.

Myocardial protection during cardiac surgery is accomplished by intermittent cross-clamping, hypothermia, and cardioplegia.[22] These techniques are particularly important during interruption of coronary blood flow, such as myocardial revascularization or aortic valve surgery.

Intermittent cross-clamping of the aorta provides a quiet, bloodless operative field and is relatively simple. The intermittent reperfusion allows normalization of high-energy compounds and elimination of metabolic wastes.[22] Disadvantages include increased bypass time, increased intervals of ventricular fibrillation, and a release of endogenous catecholamines.

Myocardial hypothermia is accomplished by cold blood solution or topical hypothermia to achieve a myocardial temperature between 10° to 20° C.[22] Topical cooling of the heart is performed by iced saline slush placed in the pericardial sac. A cold, high potassium and low sodium *cardioplegia solution* injected into the aortic root proximal to the aortic cross clamp rapidly cools the coronary arteries. Buffering agents are added to neutralize the ischemic acidosis. Other components have been proposed for a more effective cardioplegic solution and may be of additional benefit.[22] Total ischemic periods may safely range from 80 to 120 minutes, with a normal ischemic period of 10 to 12 minutes per graft.

Anesthesia

The health status and type of cardiac surgery to be performed determine the anesthetic needs of a patient. Cardiac anesthesia must provide analgesia, unconsciousness, muscle relaxation, attenuation of the stress responses, and optimal myocardial function.[38,78,96] A combination of inhalation agents, intravenous agents, and muscle relaxants are used to achieve such effects. The side effects of each agent are mostly dose dependent; the severity of the side effects are diminished when the agents are used in combination.[38] One side effect common to all anesthetic agents is the potential for depressed myocardial function.[21]

Anesthesia for myocardial revascularization

Patients undergoing myocardial revascularization require anesthetics that minimize discrepancies between myocardial oxygen supply and demand. Differences in supply and demand result from a reduced coronary artery blood flow, the degree of cardiac failure, and the responses to the stress of surgery.

Myocardial oxygen consumption is reduced by the use of β-blockers (e.g., propranolol) for reduction of the heart rate; vasodilators (e.g., morphine sulfate, nitroglycerin, and nitroprusside) for afterload and preload reduction; and adequate anesthesia. Adequate anesthesia is maintained by intravenous narcotics (e.g., morphine sulfate, fentanyl, and sufentanil) supplemented by benzodiazapines (e.g., diazepam, lorazepam, and midazolam) and low-dose inhalation agents (halothane, enflurane, and isoflurane).[96] Paralysis is achieved by using a depolarizing agent (e.g., succinylcholine) or a nondepolarizing agent (e.g., pancuronium and vecuronium).

Coronary steal is a phenomenon that can result from a variety of anesthetic agents.[6,7,96] The phenomenon involves coronary vasodilation that diverts coronary blood flow from regions of borderline perfusion and limited coronary reserve toward regions already adequately perfused; the condition can involve the diversion of blood flow from one coronary artery branch to another or diversion from the subendocardium to the subepicardium.[9,29,67] The coronary arteriolar vasodilation that results leads to the "steal" and potential regional myocardial ischemia. Isoflurane can produce coronary steal. This drug acts in direct contrast to nitroglycerin, which dilates the collateral coronary circulation.

Anesthesia for valvular heart surgery

Valvular dysfunction results in excessive volume or pressure in one or both ventricles. Dilation and hypertrophy of the ventricles and myocardial dysfunction can result.

The anesthesiologist maintains optimal cardiac function by manipulating the patient's heart rate, preload, afterload, and contractility. Most of the agents used for myocardial revascularization are appropriate for use with patients undergoing valvular surgery. Inhalation agents are the exception because of their severe myocardial depressant effects. Fentanyl remains the preferred primary anesthetic agent.

Anesthesia for surgical treatment of dysrhythmias

Anesthesia for patients undergoing surgical treatment of dysrhythmias is centered around the avoidance of tachycardia and severe inotropic depression.[55] Maintenance of volume status and avoidance of histamine-releasing agents (e.g., morphine sulfate and pancuronium [Pavulon]) assist in reducing the incidence of tachycardia and myocardial depression. Barbiturates and narcotics are recommended for these cardiac patients, and inhalation agents should be used with caution.[72]

Anesthetic agents and their doses need to be chosen based on patients' physical status and associated medical conditions. Many patients with medically intractable dysrhythmias have coronary artery disease and congestive heart failure.[72] These patients are prone to myocardial infarctions and low cardiac output after surgery. For this reason, the maintenance of coronary perfusion pressure and myocardial oxygen supply is critical. Use of halothane, enflurane, and opiates can maintain adequate coronary perfusion.

Surgical procedures
Myocardial revascularization

Surgical myocardial revascularization is accomplished using reversed saphenous vein coronary artery bypass grafting, internal mammary artery (IMA) bypass grafting, or intraoperative balloon-catheter dilation. The decision of which method to use depends on the availability and adequacy of the saphenous veins and internal mammary artery, number of vessels to be bypassed, prior surgical procedures, and patient condition.[16] Frequently, the greater saphenous vein is used because of its expendability, ease of procurement, adequate proportions, and relative durability.[89] Other venous grafts include the lesser saphenous, internal mammary, cephalic, or basilic veins.

Advantages of using the IMA include a longer duration of patency (84% patent at 10 years) than the saphenous vein (52% patent at 10 years), one anastomosis site, excellent proportions, and avoidance of a leg incision.[27,89] Disadvantages include limitation of the IMA for use on the anterior epicardial surface vessels only, requirement of extensive dissection to obtain the artery, prolongation of operative time, and higher incidents of bleeding and pulmonary dysfunction after surgery.[27] Other possible arterial grafts include the radial, ulnar, gastroepiploic, and inferior epigastric arteries.

As the median sternotomy is made, the saphenous vein is visualized, ligated into 20-cm segments, and tested for leakage with saline or heparinized plasma-lyte. To decrease postoperative leg discomfort, nerves that surround the vein are carefully preserved. After patency is ensured, the direction of the veins is reversed because of the valves and the vein graft is then anastomosed to the distal portion of the stenotic coronary artery and to the ascending aorta (Fig. 17-2). If the internal mammary artery is to be used, it is dissected from the chest wall and prepared in a similar manner (Fig. 17-3). Sequential bypass grafting is often done for multiple lesions of a single artery and for diagonal branches of the anterior descending coronary artery.[41] Sequential grafting involves one graft vessel supplying more than one coronary vessel.

Certain pathologic and anatomic conditions limit the ability to achieve *total revascularization*.[66] Diffuse distal disease, for example, frequently occurs in vessels that are too small or that are inaccessible for grafting. The result may be obstruction of flow to relatively small but important

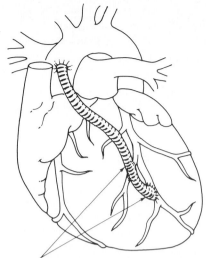

One saphenous vein, two anastamoses

FIG. 17-2   Aortocoronary artery saphenous vein "sequential" bypass graft.

From Kinney MR, Packa DR, and Dunbar SB: AACN's clinical reference for critical-care nursing, ed 2, St Louis, 1988, The CV Mosby Co.

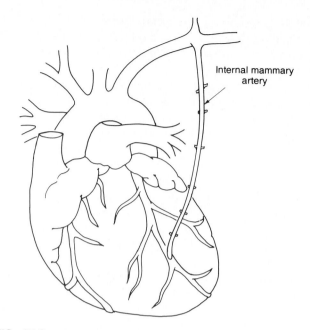

Internal mammary artery

FIG. 17-3   Internal mammary artery coronary bypass graft.

From Kinney MR, Packa DR, and Dunbar SB: AACN's clinical reference for critical-care nursing, ed 2, St Louis, 1988, The CV Mosby Co.

arteries. In this situation, intraoperative balloon-catheter dilation may be of assistance. *Intraoperative coronary angioplasty* is indicated in patients with multiple segmental coronary artery lesions that are too difficult to bypass.

The procedure involves visualizing the specific lesion, measuring the diameters of the lesion and the adjacent normal vessel with graduated probes, and selecting an appropriately sized balloon. The balloon catheter is purged with normal saline and then deflated. The balloon is then passed through an arteriotomy and across the lesion. After the balloon is in position, it is inflated to 7 to 10 atmospheres of pressure for 30 seconds. Coronary angioplasty is considered successful if the probe that calibrated the size of the normal artery proximal to the lesion can be passed through the dilated vessel. Intraoperative angioplasty is not to be used to dilate arterial anastomoses, diseased coronary arteries for the purpose of accepting a bypass graft, or proximal lesions. In the latter, intraoperative angioplasty can cause embolization of debris to the distal coronary region.[66]

On completion of the myocardial revascularization, CPB is gradually discontinued. Care is taken to evacuate all air from the left ventricle, aorta, and vessels before cessation of CPB. Anterior and posterior mediastinal chest tubes, as well as a pleural chest tube (with an IMA graft), are inserted. Intraatrial pressure lines and epicardial pacing wires are sutured into place, and the sternum is then wired with stainless steel sutures; the skin is approximated, and a sterile occlusive dressing is applied.

Valvular surgical interventions

Dysfunction of the valves can result from acquired or congenital causes (see Chapter 12). The dysfunction can be related to a narrowing of the valve orifice (stenosis), improper closing of the valve leaflets (regurgitation), or a combination of the two. Repair or replacement of the valve is considered when the patient exhibits symptoms.

Characteristics of a perfect cardiac valve include durability, optimal hemodynamics, minimal hemolysis, antithrombogenic properties, resistance to infection, quietness during movement, low cost, and ease of insertion.[100] Although the perfect valve does not exist, numerous valves have been developed to perform as physiologically normal as possible. Replacement valves are classified as biologic or mechanical. Biologic valves include allografts (e.g., pulmonic valve), homografts (e.g., cadaver aortic valve [Fig. 17-4]), or heterografts (e.g., porcine and bovine [Fig. 17-5]). Mechanical valves tend to be of the caged-ball or tilting-disk variety (Fig. 17-6).

Valvular replacement. Selection of the appropriate replacement valve is made after examining a variety of variables. The patient's age, socioeconomic status, activities of daily living, significant medical history, compliance, and cardiac anatomic features determine the choice of a valve prosthesis.[100] The need for anticoagulation therapy and valve durability are the two most important considerations in choosing a valve prosthesis. Biologic valves rarely require anticoagulation therapy; yet durability after 10 years is not reliable despite valvular preservation with glutaral-

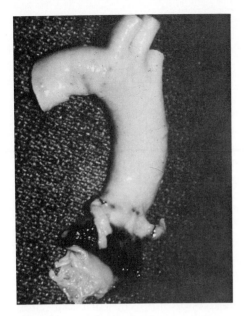

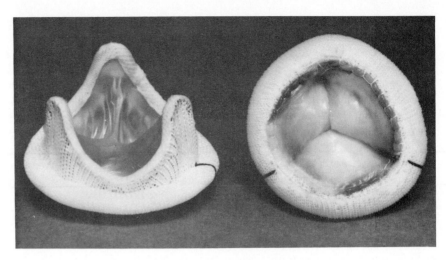

FIG. 17-5   Carpentier-Edwards porcine valve, mitral position.
From Kinney MR, Packa DR, and Dunbar SB: AACN's clinical reference for critical-care nursing, ed 2, St Louis, 1988, The CV Mosby Co.

FIG. 17-4   A cadaver aortic valve and aorta. Note the innominate left carotid and left sub-clavian branches of the aorta. Also note ligated main coronary arteries.
From Rafalowski M: Cardiac valve replacement: the homograph, Focus Crit Care 17:111, 1990, Courtesy Cryolife, Inc.

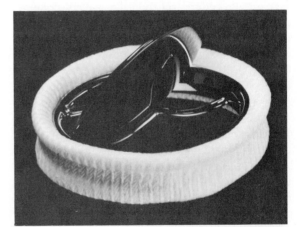

FIG. 17-6   Prosthetic replacement valves. **A,** Starr-Edwards, model 1260. **B,** Bjork-Shiley, spherical disk valves, aortic position. **C,** St. Jude medical heart valve, aortic position.
From Kinney MR, Packa DR, and Dunbar SB: AACN's clinical reference for critical-care nursing, ed 2, St Louis, 1988, The CV Mosby Co.

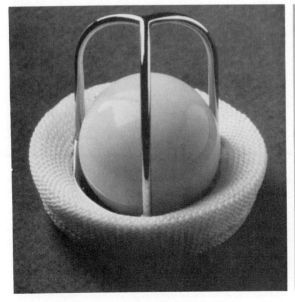

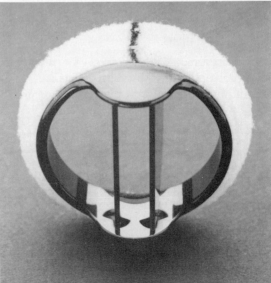

dehyde. Conversely, mechanical valves require anticoagulation therapy, but their durability usually exceeds 10 years.

A standard median sternotomy is performed in preparation for the valve replacement. After the patient is on CPB, systemic cooling and myocardial protective techniques are initiated. The diseased valve is excised, taking care in the debridement of the annulus to avoid subsequent systemic emboli.[21] Next, sutures are placed around the annulus and into the valve replacement in a simple, horizontal mattress fashion, or a figure-of-eight fashion. The valve is then pushed into position, and the sutures are tightened. The sutures may be reinforced with Teflon pledgets to decrease the incidence of perivalvular leaking. The patient is then weaned from CPB, and the sternum is closed.

Valvular repair. Alternatives to valvular replacement include annuloplasty, commissurotomy, and valvuloplasty. Reparative procedures are performed based on the pathologic condition of the valve.[80] Generally, less diseased valves can be repaired.

Annuloplasty involves the plastic reconstruction of the valve leaflets and annulus using a multiple-point fixation to a flexible ring.[80] Procedures on the valve leaflets alone may be indicated in certain conditions such as ruptured chordae tendineae. Annuloplasty is recommended for incompetent valvular function. The procedure is more commonly performed on the mitral and tricuspid valves.

A *commissurotomy* may be a closed (without cardiopulmonary bypass) or open procedure. The former method is infrequently used in the United States but is still commonly performed in other countries. The procedure is used for stenotic valves that are not heavily calcified and essentially involves the excision of the valve leaflets to create a larger valvular opening.

Valvuloplasty is another procedure used for stenotic valves. In this reparative procedure, a dilator or balloon is used to "open" or "dilate" the valve's atherosclerotic obstruction[21] (see Chapter 12).

Surgical ablation interventions

Surgical therapy has become a viable alternative for patients with medically refractory dysrhythmias.[98] Patients are referred for surgical intervention when they exhibit recurrent, sustained supraventricular or ventricular tachydysrhythmias.

The precise location of the dysrhythmia is identified by preoperative catheter electrode mapping and by intraoperative direct mapping. The former is done in the cardiac catheterization laboratory. Catheter electrodes are placed in the right and left ventricles and in the coronary sinus. The tachydysrhythmia is induced and documented by electrocardiograms.[63] If multiple morphologic dysrhythmias are induced, then each must be mapped separately.[99] The greater the number of distinct foci located, the less likely that ablation will be a success. Intraoperative direct mapping is more precise. The endocardial or epicardial surface

may be mapped in the attempt to identify the foci of the dysrhythmia. While the patient is on normothermic partial or total CPB, the tachydysrhythmias are induced.

Surgical interventions for tachydysrhythmias include myocardial revascularization, endocardial resection, and ablation.[87,99] The surgical approach is via a median sternotomy and requires partial or total cardiopulmonary bypass, depending on the intervention.

Localized *endocardial resection* has resulted in the ablation of reentrant ventricular tachydysrhythmias.[35] Electrophysiologic studies indicate that the origin of sustained ventricular tachydysrhythmias lies near the edge of the endocardial scar. The success rate with this procedure is approximately 85%.[56] A second method involves encircling endocardial resection with complete removal of the endocardial scarring.[56]

Ablation therapy is useful in treating supraventricular dysrhythmias like Wolff-Parkinson-White (WPW) syndrome, in which the accessory atrioventricular connection is ablated. Ablation therapy can be accomplished by cryoablation and electrode catheter ablation.[99] *Cryoablation* involves the freezing of a specific region of myocardial tissue to $-80°$ C. This technique is particularly useful in patients with foci located near the conduction system or the papillary muscles of the mitral valve. Resection of these areas could result in complete heart block or mitral valve dysfunction. *Electrode catheter ablation* requires one catheter as the cathode and an external paddle as the anode. From 200 to 300 joule shocks are delivered to the cathodes to ablate the focus. Both ablation therapies can be used in patients with left ventricular dysfunction.

Complications of surgical procedures

Ideally, cardiovascular surgery would have a hospital morbidity and mortality rate near zero. Most health care institutions have low rates despite the elevation in patient acuity. Still, certain cardiovascular surgical procedures have risks and potential complications.

Complications of myocardial revascularization

Potential problems of myocardial revascularization include perioperative infarction, graft occlusion, and progression of the atherosclerotic disease. Each may occur despite meticulous attention to preoperative and intraoperative patient care management.

The incidence of perioperative infarction is 2% to 4% for patients who have undergone myocardial revascularization.[51] The incidence has decreased over the years secondarily to improved preoperative medical management, anesthetic techniques, and use of cardioplegia. Perioperative infarctions can result from graft obstruction caused by thrombosis, sclerosis, or coronary artery spasms.[51]

Graft occlusion and failure of the graft can occur immediately or over time. Research studies have demonstrated that bypass grafts remain patent 6 to 12 months after surgery in up to 85% of patients.[26] Vein graft occlusion that occurs before 12 months after surgery is attributed to faulty procurement of the vein, manipulation of the donor vein, inadequate anastomosis, or bypassing a severely diseased vessel that will be unable to remain patent. The patency of the bypass grafts has correlated well with the relief of angina pectoris. Patients returning with recurrent angina within the first 12 months display subintimal hyperplasia of the grafts. The hyperplasia is thought to occur from poor preparation of the donor graft or the influence of systemic pressures on the vein grafts.[26]

Complications of valvular surgery

Valvular surgery is not a curative procedure. As such, complications may arise. The majority of valve prostheses used can cause similar complications.

Thrombogenicity of prosthetic valves is a continuing and challenging disadvantage of their use, despite advances in prosthetic valve design and anticoagulant therapy. The incidence of thromboembolic complications is similar among that of all mechanical valve designs in use. Anticoagulation is achieved by starting warfarin (Coumadin) 2 days after surgery. The most serious risk of using warfarin is hemorrhage, in particular cerebrovascular hemorrhage. Patients' prothrombin time is maintained at 30 to 35 seconds. However thromboembolic events still occur in 0.2% to 2.2% of patients with prosthetic valves.[21] The incidence tends to be higher for prostheses in the mitral versus the aortic position. Signs and symptoms associated with a thromboembolic event include fatigue, paresthesia, dyspnea, alterations in speech patterns, and cerebrovascular accidents. Less than 1% of events are fatal.[51]

Turbulent flow through the prosthetic valves can traumatize the red blood cells and lead to hemolysis. The severity of hemolysis is proportional to the type of prosthesis used and the site of the valve repair or replacement. Smaller prosthetic valves and valves in the aortic position can cause increased hemolysis.

Dysfunction of the prosthetic valve secondary to mechanical failure can occur suddenly, leading to a life-threatening event. Valve failing may be noted in patients who complain of new or worsening angina pectoris, dyspnea, or congestive heart failure or who demonstrate increased hemolysis. Valvular dysfunction can occur from periprosthetic leakage at the suture line, thrombotic obstruction, fibrous growth on the valve leaflets, or deterioration of the valve materials. If dysfunction is life threatening, reoperation is essential. Severe congestive heart failure, decreased tissue perfusion, and hypotension are indications of severe valvular dysfunction.

Valve endocarditis is another potential complication[97] (see Chapter 13). Endocarditis can occur in the first 60 days after surgery (early) or later in convalescence. Early endocarditis has been attributed to an extracardiac infec-

tion, mostly due to staphylococcal infection. *Streptococcus* organisms have been identified as the major cause of late events. The overall incidence of prosthetic valvular endocarditis is 2%, and it is higher in black patients, patients who experience longer cardipulmonary bypass times, and patients who have a history of native valvular endocarditis. Conditions predisposing to late endocarditis are urinary tract infections, dental procedures, upper airway diseases, and minor surgical procedures. Complications of this disease include embolization of the large arteries, annular abscess, calcification and cuspal rupture of the prostheses, and generalized infection.

Complications of surgical ablation

Unsuccessful resolution of dysrhythmias can occur after surgical ablation therapy. The mortality rate within 30 days of operation is approximately 9%.[98] The overall success rate associated with ablation therapy is 85%. Additional complications are similar to those of other intracardiac surgeries.

Nursing process: immediate postoperative phase

Case study. Mr. J., a 70-year-old man, was admitted to the hospital for evaluation of recurrent chest pain. About 10 years earlier, he had received saphenous vein grafts (SVGs) to his left anterior descending (LAD) and circumflex coronary arteries and had done well, returning to work and his usual recreational activities of golf, tennis, and fishing. The present chest pain was characterized as abrupt in onset and unpredictable in its course. Coronary angiography revealed complete occlusion of the LAD graft and 50% occlusion of the circumflex graft. In addition, the right coronary artery was shown to be 75% occluded. Reoperation was recommended. Mr. J.'s preoperative nursing data base is shown in Fig. 17-7.

Although the events in the operating room play a primary role in predicting patient outcomes, patient care in the immediate postoperative period is crucial to surgical success. The immediate postoperative period is one of high risk for cardiac dysrhythmias, organ-system failure, and sudden death. Diligent and astute nursing management is required to prevent complications and promote recovery. Before the patient's arrival in the critical care unit, the necessary supplies and equipment are made ready, with careful attention to calibration procedures. Calculations of body surface area, kind and amount of intravenous fluids to be infused, type and time of laboratory determinations, and drug dosing regimens are available to the admitting nurse.

The admission of the patient is a systematic process requiring the placement of ECG leads for monitoring rate and rhythm, the connection of chest tubes to the drainage or suction apparatus, the coupling of cardiac and arterial catheters to the proper transducer, and the placement of

Text continued on p. 564.

HOLISTIC CARDIOVASCULAR ASSESSMENT TOOL*

Name _J.L.J., Sr._   Age _70_   Sex _Male_

Address _P.O. Box 1771 Birmingham, AL 35226_   Telephone _661-9222_

Significant other _EJ (wife)_   Telephone _661-9222_

Date of admission _6/21_   Medical diagnosis _Unstable Angina Pectoris_

Allergies _None known_

Nursing Diagnosis

COMMUNICATING ▪ A pattern involving sending messages

(Read,) (write,) (understand) English (circle) _____

Other languages _none_

Intubated _no_   Speech impaired _no_

Alternate form of communication _none_

Impaired verbal communication

KNOWING ▪ A pattern involving the meaning associated with information

Current health problems _return of chest pain_

Previous illnesses/hospitalizations/surgeries _____
CABG × 2 10 years ago

History of the following problems: Knowledge deficit

    Heart _CABG × 2 10 years ago_

    Peripheral vascular _post CABG_

    Lung _No_

    Liver _No_   Kidney _No_

    Cerebrovascular _TIA 1 yr ago_   Rheumatic fever _No_

    Thyroid _No_

    Other _None_

Current medications _Questran_
                Ascriptin

Risk factors	Present	Perceptions/Knowledge of
1. Hypertension	No	Watches BP closely
2. Hyperlipidemia	Yes	Knows cholesterol level and tries to control it below 200 mg/dl
3. Smoking	No	Quit with surgery 10 yrs ago
4. Obesity	No	
5. Diabetes	No	
6. Sedentary living	No	
7. Stress	No	
8. Alcohol use	No	
9. Oral contraceptives	n/a	
10. Family history		

Perception/knowledge of illness/test/surgery _Recalls information from previous_
surgery, especially endotracheal tube

Expectations of therapy _To resume life style as before_

Misconceptions _Expects postop course to be uneventful as before_

Readiness to learn _____

    Requests information concerning _how long he will be intubated_

    Educational level _masters degree (educator)_

    Learning impeded by _nothing noted_

*Adapted from: Guzzetta C et al: Clinical assessment tools for use with nursing diagnoses, St Louis, 1989, The CV Mosby Co.

FIG. 17-7   Example of a cardiovascular assessment tool for the patient undergoing cardiac surgery.

Orientation
Level of alertness _Awake_
Orientation: Person _Yes_   Place _Yes_   Time _Yes_
Appropriate behavior/communication _Yes_

Altered thought processes

Memory
Memory intact: Yes _X_ No _____ Recent _X_   Remote _X_

VALUING ▪ A pattern involving the assigning of relative worth
Spirituality or religious preference _Baptist_
Important spiritual or religious practices _Daily Bible reading, prayer_
Spiritual concerns _States he is "ready to go if God calls"_
Cultural orientation _Unremarkable_
Cultural practices _None expressed_

Spiritual distress

RELATING ▪ A pattern involving establishing bonds
Role
Marital status _Married (50 years)_
Age & health of significant other _68 years, good health_

Number of children _4_   Ages _48, 46, 43, 40_
Role in home _Partner with wife in making decisions_
Financial support _Income adequate_
Occupation _Retired high school principal_
Job satisfaction/concerns _Enjoys retirement_
Physical/mental energy expenditures _Nonstressful lifestyle_
Sexual relationships (⟨satisfactory⟩ /unsatisfactory) _____
Physical difficulties/effects of illness related to sex _Resumed sexual activity after previous operation until recent onset of angina_

Altered role performance
   Parenting
   Sexual dysfunction
   Work

Altered family processes
   Parental role conflict

Altered sexuality patterns

Socialization
Quality of relationships with others:
Patient's description _close to family and small circle of longtime friends_
Significant other's description _Same_
Staff observations _Same_
Verbalizes feelings of being alone _No_
Attributed to _n/a_

Altered socialization
   Impaired social interaction

Social isolation

FEELING ▪ A pattern involving the subjective awareness of information
Comfort
Pain/discomfort: Yes _X_   No _____
Onset _variable_   Duration _variable_
Location _substernal_   Quality _severe_   Radiation _L. arm_
Associated factors _Sometimes on exertion, but not always_
Aggravating factors _Sometimes exertion_
Alleviating factors _Sometimes rest, TNG_
Objective manifestations _Sometimes SOB_

Pain/chronic
⟨Pain/acute⟩

Emotional Integrity/States
Recent stressful life events _none_

Verbalizes feelings of _uncertainty_
Source _impending surgery_

Physical manifestations _None_

Anxiety
Fear
Grieving
   Dysfunctional
   Anticipatory

Continued.

MOVING ▪ A pattern involving activity
Self-care
 Ability to perform self-care (specify level) _independent_
 Specify deficits _None, except with chest pain_
 Discharge planning needs _coronary rehabilitation_

Self-care deficit
 (Level 0-4)
 Feeding
  Impaired swallowing
 Bathing/hygiene
 Dressing/grooming
 Toileting

Activity
 Limitations of movement (specify level) _None_

 Limitations in activities _None until recurrence of pain_

 Verbal report of fatigue _Recent onset_
 Exercise habits _Golf 2 × week, tennis 1 × week prior to chest pain_

Impaired physical mobility
 (Level 0-4)
Activity intolerance
 Fatigue

Rest
 Sleep/rest pattern _Unremarkable_
  Sleep aids (pillows, meds, food) _None_
  Difficulty falling/remaining asleep _No except when awakened by chest pain and SOB_

Sleep pattern disturbance

Recreation
 Leisure activities _fishing, golf, tennis_
 Social activities _church, retirees club_

Diversional activity deficit

Activities of Daily Living
 Home maintenance management
  Size & arrangement of home (stairs, bathroom) _one level_
   _____ Safety needs _none_
  Home responsibilities _routine repairs_

Impaired home maintenance
 management

 Health maintenance
  Health insurance _BC/BS, Medicare_
 Regular physical check-ups _sees cardiologist q 3 months_

Altered health maintenance

PERCEIVING ▪ A pattern involving the reception of information
Body image/Self-esteem
 Perception of self and situation _"an old guy making it pretty well"_

 Description of body structure/functioning _"good for age"_

Self-esteem disturbance
 Chronic low
 Situational low
Body image disturbance

Meaningfulness
 Verbalizes hopelessness _No_
 Verbalizes loss of control _No_

Hopelessness
Powerlessness

Sensory/Perception
 History of restricted environment _No_
 Vision imparied _No_ Glasses _Yes_
 Auditory imparied _No_ Hearing aid _No_
 Kinesthetics impaired _No_
 Gustatory impaired _No_
 Tactile impaired _No_
 Olfactory impaired _No_

Altered sensory/perception
 Visual
 Auditory
 Kinesthetic
 Gustatory
 Tactile
 Olfactory

 Reflexes: Biceps R _2+_ L _2+_   Triceps R _2+_ L _2+_
  Brachioradialis R _2+_ L _2+_   Knee R _2+_ L _2+_
  Ankle R _2+_ L _2+_   Plantar R _2+_ L _2+_

EXCHANGING* ▪ *A pattern involving mutual giving and receiving
Circulation

Cerebral
  Neurologic changes/symptoms __*None*__   Altered cerebral tissue
  Complaints of syncope __*No*__   perfusion

Pupils   Eye Opening
  L 2 ③ 4 5 6 mm   None (1)
  R 2 ③ 4 5 6 mm   To pain (2)   Fluid volume
  Reaction: Brisk __*X*__   To speech (3)   Deficit
  Sluggish _____ Nonreactive _____ (Spontaneous) (4)   Excess
  Retina __*No AV nicking*__

Best Verbal   Best Motor
  Mute (1)   Flaccid (1)
  Incomprehensible sound (2)   Extensor response (2)   Decreased cardiac output
  Inappropriate words (3)   Flexor response (3)
  Confused conversation (4)   Semipurposeful (4)
  (Oriented) (5)   Localized to pain (5)
                   (Obeys commands) (6)

Glasgow coma scale total __*15*__   Altered cerebral tissue
                                 perfusion

Peripheral   Altered peripheral tissue
                                 perfusion

  Arterial pulses: A = absent   B = bruits   D = Doppler
   +3 = bounding   +2 = palpable   +1 = faintly palpable
  Carotid   R __*2+*__ L __*2+*__   Popliteal   R __*2+*__ L __*2+*__
  Brachial R __*2+*__ L __*2+*__   Posterior tibial R __*2+*__ L __*2+*__   Fluid volume
  Radial   R __*2+*__ L __*2+*__   Dorsalis pedis R __*2+*__ L __*2+*__   Deficit
  Femoral R __*2+*__ L __*2+*__   Excess
  BP: Sitting   Lying   Standing
      R __*130/80*__ L _____   R __*130/80*__ L _____   R __*140/90*__ L _____

  A-Line reading _____ *0* _____   CVP ____ *0* ____
  Venous pulse __*Normal*__   Jugular venous distention R ___ L ___
  Peripheral veins __*No pain or tenderness; healed old saphenous vein incision*__
  Skin temp __*warm*__   Color __*pink*__   Cyanosis __*0*__
  Capillary refill __*normal*__   Edema __*0*__
  Clubbing __*0*__

Cardiovascular
  PMI __*5th ICS MCL*__   Pacemaker __*0*__   Altered cardiopulmonary
  Apical rate & rhythm __*65, NSR*__   tissue perfusion
  Heart sounds/murmurs __*gr 2/6 SEM, 2nd ICS, LSB*__
  Dysrhythmias __*0*__
  Cardiac output __*n/a*__   Cardiac index __*n/a*__   Decreased cardiac output
  PAP __*n/a*__   PAWP __*n/a*__
  IV fluids __*0*__
  IV medications __*0*__   Dysreflexia

  Serum enzymes __*n/a*__

Physical Integrity
  Tissue integrity __*Normal*__   Impaired skin integrity
    Skin: Rash __*0*__   Lesions __*0*__   Impaired tissue integrity
    Petechiae __*0*__   Bruises __*0*__   Disuse syndrome
    Abrasions __*0*__   Surgical incision __*healed median sternotomy*__   Infection
                                       Altered protection

Continued.

Oxygenation

Complaints of dyspnea __yes__ Precipitated by __chest pain__
Orthopnea __No__
Rate __22__ Rhythm __Reg__ Depth __Normal__   Ineffective breathing patterns
Labored/(unlabored)(circle) Use of accessory muscles __No__
Chest expansion __normal__ Splinting __No__   Ineffective airway clearance
Cough: Productive/nonproductive __No__
Sputum: Color __n/a__ Amount __n/a__ Consistency __n/a__   Impaired gas exchange
Breath sounds __Normal__   High risk for aspiration
Arterial blood gases __n/a__
Oxygen percent and device __n/a__
Ventilator __n/a__

Physical Regulation

Immune
    Lymph nodes enlarged __No__ Location __n/a__   Infection
    WBC count __normal__ Differential __normal__   Hypothermia
                                                          Hyperthermia
                                                          Altered body temperature
Temperature __98.6° F__ Route __Oral__   Ineffective thermoregulation
                                                          Altered protection

Nutrition

Eating patterns
    Number of meals per day __3__   Altered nutrition
    Special diet __Low fat__   More than body
    Where eaten __Home__   requirements
    Food preferences/(intolerances) __spicey foods__   Less than body
    Food allergies __None__   requirements
    Caffeine intake (coffee, tea, soft drinks) __Coffee × 2; tea × 2 glasses__
    Appetite changes __None__
    Presence of nausea/vomiting __n/a__
    Condition of mouth/throat __good, full dentures__   Impaired oral mucous
                                                               membranes
    Height __72"__ Weight __170 lbs__ Ideal body weight __178 lbs__   Altered nutrition
                                                               More than body
                                                                 requirements
Current therapy   Less than body
    NPO __n/a__ NG suction __n/a__   requirements
    Tube feeding __n/a__   High risk for aspiration
    TPN __n/a__
Labs
    Na __138__ K __4.2__ Cl __98__ Glucose __110__
    Cholesterol __210 mg/dl__ Triglycerides __190 mg/dl__ Fasting __yes__
    Hct __14__ Hgb __42__
    Other

Elimination

Gastrointestinal/Bowel   Altered bowel elimination
    Usual bowel habits __bran cereal__   Constipation
    Use of (laxatives,) enemas, and/or suppositories __occasional__   Perceived
    Alterations from norm __None__   Colonic
    Abdominal physical exam __unremarkable__   Diarrhea
                                                               Incontinence
                                                             Altered GI tissue perfusion
Renal/Urinary
    Usual urinary pattern __Up at night × 1__   Altered urinary elimination
    Alteration from norm __None__   Incontinence
    Bladder distention __No__   Retention
    Color __Normal__ Catheter __n/a__   Altered renal tissue perfusion
    Urine output: 24 hour __n/a__ Average hourly __n/a__
    BUN __23__ Creatinine __1.2__ Specific gravity __n/a__
    Urine studies __None__

CHOOSING ■ A pattern involving the selection of alternatives
Coping

Patient's ability to cope __*good*__

Family's ability to cope/give support __*good*__

Patient's acceptance of illness __*good*__

Patient's adjustment to illness __*good*__

Ineffective individual coping
 Defensive coping
 Ineffective denial
 Impaired adjustment

Ineffective family coping
 Disabled
 Compromised

Judgment

Decision making ability:
  Patient's perspective __*good*__
  Other's perspective __*good*__
Ability to choose from alternatives __*good*__

Decisional conflict

Participation

Compliance with past/current health care regimen __*Has complied with regimen for years and done well*__

Willingness to comply with future health care regimen __*Expects to continue regimen*__

Noncompliance

Health seeking

Express desire to seek higher level of wellness __*yes—wants to resume active lifestyle*__

Health seeking behaviors

Prioritized nursing diagnoses/problem list:
1. __*pain, acute r/t myocardial oxygen demand/supply mismatch*__
2. _____
3. _____
4. _____
5. _____
6. _____

Signature __*Marguerite R. Kinney, RN*__   Date __*2/2*__ the urinary catheter with the temperature probe. The mechanical ventilator is connected to the endotracheal tube, and the adequacy of ventilation is ensured. Pacing wires are connected to a temporary pacemaker. A complete verbal report from the anesthesiologist or nurse anesthetist will alert the admitting nurse to any important intraoperative events, such as inappropriate blood pressure levels; disturbances in rate, rhythm or conduction; or electrical or pharmacologic interventions.

When the admission procedures have been completed, attention is turned to the systematic collection of data to evaluate the adequacy of performance of the cardiovascular, pulmonary, renal, neurologic, gastrointestinal, hematologic, and metabolic subsystems. Analysis of data serves as the basis for formulating nursing diagnoses according to the human response patterns of the Unitary Person Framework. In the initial postoperative period, the Exchanging Communicating, Feeling, and Moving Patterns are of primary significance, whereas the remaining patterns become more significant after the initial 24 hours.

Case study, cont'd. Mr. J. underwent a second myocardial revascularization using the left IMA to revascularize the LAD coronary artery. The right coronary artery and left circumflex artery were revascularized using the right greater saphenous vein. An IABP was placed prophylactically in the operating room (before the procedure) and was continued until the next morning. The operative course was uneventful except for some minor bleeding, which responded to infusions of fresh frozen plasma, platelets, and packed red blood cells. Aminocaproic acid (Amicar) was prophylactically administered in the initial postoperative period to limit further bleeding.

The initial cardiac index was 1.80 L/min/m² and required manipulation of preload, afterload, and contractility parameters. Preload was augmented by initiating autotransfusions within the first postoperative hour and continued 10 hours to maintain a left atrial pressure of 12 mm Hg. Afterload, reflected by Mr. J.'s initial systolic blood pressure of 165 mm Hg, was reduced by low doses of sodium nitroprusside (Nipride) to maintain a systolic blood pressure of 110 to 120 mm Hg. Asynchronous atrial epicardial pacing at a rate of 100 per minute further optimized the patient's cardiac output. On removal of the IABP the following morning, Mr. J.'s cardiac index was 2.20 L/min/m².

Oliguria was present in the first 3 hours after surgery and was effectively treated with low doses of dopamine and furosemide (Lasix). Mr. J. experienced some respiratory insufficiency as indicated by hypercapnia and hypoxia. Treatment included alterations in ventilatory rate and tidal volume, sedation, and vigorous pulmonary toilet therapy. Interventions were effective, and Mr. J. was extubated the following morning with a Pao₂ of 100 mm Hg, a Paco₂ of 38 mm Hg, and a pH of 7.45. Oxygen therapy (6 L via nasal cannula) was continued.

Mr. J., however, experienced considerable pain despite adequate analgesia and responded to the pain with shallow respirations, which contributed to the development of bilateral lower lobe atelectasis. He subsequently became febrile, with a peak temperature of 38.4° C on the second day. All cultures (blood, sputum, wound, and urine) were negative. The increased temperature was judged to be secondary to the atelectasis. Respiratory treatments (albuterol), incentive spirometry, and regularly scheduled analgesics were prescribed, and Mr. J. was then transferred to the intermediate care unit on the third postoperative day. The remainder of his postoperative course was unremarkable, and Mr. J. was discharged on postoperative day 10.

Nursing assessment
Exchanging pattern

The patient who is recovering normally from cardiac surgery will not experience restlessness, agitation, or anxiety; will be oriented and lucid with appropriate behavior; and will breathe without labor or an excessively rapid rate. In addition, the eyes and skin will appear normal, and the pulse will be full, even though it may be rapid.[50]

A subsystem analysis approach leads to therapeutic decisions that take into account present performance, adequacy of performance, and used and unused reserves of each subsystem.[51] Low cardiac output with secondary subsystem dysfunction (i.e., low cardiac output syndrome) is the most frequent cause of poor surgical outcome in the immediate postoperative period.[64] The mortality rate increases as the number of failing subsystems increases. When more than four subsystems fail to perform adequately, the mortality rate approaches 100%.[64]

Cardiovascular subsystem. Cardiac performance is very important in the early postoperative period and is influenced by the following factors:
1. The presence of preexisting heart disease
2. Myocardial injury (i.e., ischemia, edema, and infarction) during CPB
3. The presence of residual abnormalities such as valvular incompetence or occlusive coronary artery disease
4. Impairment in myocardial contractility as a sequela of CPB
5. Hypovolemia, which is related to volume replacement in the operating room, the presence of vasodilation with rewarming, and the chest-drainage and blood-infusion ratio
6. Left ventricular afterload
7. The presence of dysrhythmias, which may be related to the presence of metabolic acidosis, electrolyte imbalances, or drug toxicity

Cardiac performance is considered normal when the cardiac output is adequate for the metabolic needs of the patient. Although the normal range for cardiac index is 2.5 to 4.4 L/min/m², an index of 1.6 in the early hours after surgery and 2.0 the next morning are acceptable.[50]

A number of parameters assist in the evaluation of cardiac performance. Measure cardiac output directly using the indicator-dilution or thermodilution method. Although seriously ill patients require direct measurement of cardiac output, often at frequent intervals, indirect measurement, using pedal pulses and color and temperature of the skin, may be appropriate for patients recovering normally.

Peak systolic, diastolic, and mean arterial pressures are measured with an indwelling catheter, usually placed in the radial artery. Although the arterial pressure is not a good indicator of cardiac performance in the early postoperative period, it is useful in alerting the nurse to a possible decrease in cardiac output. Generally speaking, a mean arterial pressure of 85 to 95 mm Hg is desirable. However, after revascularization procedures the systolic blood pressure may be maintained at 100 to 110 mm Hg for SVGs, whereas IMA grafts may require systolic blood pressures of 120 to 130 mm Hg in the first 6 hours after surgery to maintain flow through the graft and prevent spasm. Right and left atrial pressures indicate the filling pressures for the right and left ventricles, which ideally should be maintained at 10 to 12 mm Hg and 12 to 14 mm Hg respectively. Cardiac rate and rhythm can affect cardiac output and may require pacing for maximizing the contribution to cardiac performance. Assess fluid balance by comparing the volume of drainage from the chest tubes and urinary catheter with intake.

Pulmonary subsystem. Also assess the adequacy of the pulmonary system especially when the patient begins to recover from anesthesia and surgery. Pulmonary performance is influenced by many factors, including preexisting pulmonary disease, duration of CPB, the patient's general health status, and adequacy of the cardiac repair.

All patients who have undergone cardiac surgery are subject to intraoperative and postoperative conditions that could lead to pulmonary insufficiency if they are not assessed and managed properly. Such conditions follow:

1. Depressed central nervous system caused by the effects of anesthetic agents and narcotics
2. Critical changes in hemodynamics causing decreased cardiac output or congestive heart failure
3. Effects of CPB such as hemodilution (which decreases the oxygen-carrying capacity of the cells) and destruction of red blood cells
4. Destruction of surfactant leading to alveolar collapse (Surfactant may decrease because of hypothermia or prolonged administration of 100% oxygen, inadequate humidity, or inappropriately high or low tidal volumes.)
5. Pneumonia
6. Atelectasis
7. Hemothorax resulting from inadequate drainage from pleural chest tubes
8. Pneumothorax resulting from inappropriately high tidal volumes and airway pressures of the ventilator or incorrect placement of central venous lines

Initial ventilator settings follow:
1. Tidal volume (TV): 10 to 15 cc/kg
2. Fractional inspired oxygen concentration (FiO$_2$): 60%
3. Intermittent mandatory ventilation: 10
4. Positive end-expiratory pressure: up to 4

A series of arterial blood gas analyses will assist in determining pulmonary performance. Be alert for agitation or restlessness because it indicates the need for modification of the tidal volume.

Renal subsystem. Patients with preexisting renal disease or low cardiac output, those experiencing lengthy periods of CPB, and those receiving selected antibiotic therapy are at risk for inadequate renal performance. Urinary output is a good index of renal function and should be at least 20 ml/hr/m^2 or 500 ml/24 hr/m^2. BUN and creatinine levels are also useful indicators of renal performance, as is the urine specific gravity which should be 1.016 to 1.022.

Neurologic subsystem. Although neurologic dysfunction is uncommon, assess the adequacy of the neurologic system. Be alert for seizures, visual field defects, hemiplegia, athetoid movements, psychotic behavior, and changes in intellectual performance because they indicate diffuse or localized neurologic deficits.

Gastrointestinal subsystem. Gastrointestinal complications after cardiac surgery may be related to low cardiac output, emboli, or antibiotic therapy. The type and amount of drainage, as well as signs of abdominal distention, are important indicators of gastrointestinal performance.

Hematologic subsystem. Some degree of bleeding can be expected in all patients after CPB because of abnormalities in clotting factors.[51] Continuously monitor chest tube drainage. The criteria for reoperation may help in determining the need for reexploration to achieve hemostasis. Suggested criteria include 150 cc/hour for 3 hours or 100 cc/hr for 12 hours. If a bleeding diathesis is suspected, clotting studies are necessary to identify the specific clotting factor that is deficient.

Metabolic subsystem. Some metabolic acidosis and alkalosis is expected in the early postoperative period. Metabolic acidosis, reflected in a base deficit of greater than 2 milliequivalents (mEq)/L, is related to the washout of areas of the microcirculation that were poorly perfused or not perfused during CPB.[50] Mild metabolic alkalosis is probably related to the sodium load present in the banked blood and should correct itself.[51]

Body temperature is the result of the interaction of a number of metabolic and physiologic processes and, although initially low, is generally normal (37° C) within 4 to 6 hours.[51] Varying degrees of hyperthermia are nearly always present in the first 48 hours after surgery.

Therapeutic hypothermia is used in cardiovascular surgery for the preservation of the myocardium, reduction of metabolic needs, and the provision of a quiet operative field.[70] Rewarming occurs centrally by means of the CPB until a nasopharyngeal temperature of 37° C is achieved and maintained for several minutes. When patients arrive in the critical care unit after cardiovascular surgery, their body temperatures are between 32° and 36° C; they typically require rewarming. Normalization of body temperature (37° C) occurs over 4 to 6 hours. During this period, shivering, a compensatory mechanism against total heat loss, can occur. Shivering is effective only 11% of the time in reducing total heat loss[37] and can increase the loss of body heat.

Shivering associated with postoperative rewarming is an undesirable physiologic stressor to an already compromised cardiopulmonary system. Possible sequelae of postoperative shivering include augmentation of metabolic demands as much as 500%, dental damage, wound dehiscence, disruption of surgical repairs, and the production and accumulation of lactic acid.[15,82,83,88,103] Various interventions have been studied for their effectiveness in reducing myocardial oxygen consumption and metabolic demands exacerbated by shivering.[42,70,82,103]

Recognition of the shivering phenomenon is the first step toward therapeutic intervention. Holtzclaw[33,34] noted a mandibular "hum" preceded the onset of visible vigorous shivering. The "hum" is palpated along the mandibular jaw line.

Infection. Infection is the most prevalent noncardiac complication occurring after cardiac surgery.[1] Sepsis must be detected and treated promptly. Elevations in temperature and white blood cell counts are normal in the early days after surgery, but an elevation in temperature or in white blood cell count after the third day should warrant an examination for evidence of infection. If the temperature exceeds 39.4° C, samples for blood cultures and a white blood cell count should be obtained.

Communicating pattern

Normally verbal communication can be assessed by speech (e.g., rate of speaking and effort to produce speech); the content of the speech (e.g., word choice and syntax); and the fluency of speech. Because speech is not possible when the patient is intubated, it is necessary to focus on other cues to evaluate the patient's ability to send, receive, and comprehend messages.

Patient response or reaction to spoken words and to the environment provides information about the state of wakefulness or alertness. As the effects of the anesthesia dissipate, patients should open their eyes when their name is called and follow sounds with their eyes. Comprehension is evaluated by asking patients to perform simple motor acts such as squeezing the hand or wiggling toes. When patients are awake and alert, they can begin to use alternative methods of communication, which are taught in the preoperative preparation session (see Nursing Diagnosis 11).

Feeling pattern

Pain. Pain in the early postoperative period emanates from a number of sources, including the damaged tissue (skin, muscle, and nerves); prolonged positioning on the operating room table; intubation; intravenous lines and irritating infusions; and chest tubes, a nasogastric tube, an indwelling urinary catheter, and other drains. IMA grafting is particularly painful.[41] In addition, pain can be aggravated by anxiety, the inability to communicate, and fear of the surroundings.[79] Control of pain is important not only because of patient comfort but also because it can contribute to confusion, delirium, and other undesirable states.

A purely objective measure of pain intensity is not possible because pain is multidimensional, subjective in nature, and encompasses physical and affective components.[17] Instruments for rating pain intensity include verbal descriptor scales and visual analogue scales that have been adapted for use in critical care settings. Patient behaviors that might indicate the presence of pain include facial expression and posturing. Although pain is expected in the postoperative period, assessment and relief are important components of nursing care.

Moving pattern

The contributions of sleep to the maintenance of optional physiologic and psychologic functioning are well documented.[86] Additionally, the detrimental effects of altered sleep patterns on ventilation, immunocompetence, and pain perception have been described.[19] However, environmental and situational factors can cause a loss of sleep in the early postoperative period while the patient is in the critical care unit. Continuous monitoring and therapies, loss of day-night orientation, noise level, discomfort or pain, and anxiety or fear contribute to the interruption of sleep. These factors can be more easily controlled in the intermediate care unit and warrant attention by the nursing staff.

Nursing diagnoses

The most common human responses anticipated for a patient after cardiac surgery are indicated by the following nursing diagnoses:

1. Decreased cardiac output related to mechanical, electrical, or cellular alterations
2. High risk for impaired gas exchange related to surgery, anesthesia, postoperative pain, and immobility
3. High risk for impaired renal function related to hemodynamic instability, fluid imbalance, and physiologic effects of cardiopulmonary bypass
4. High risk for impaired neurologic function related to surgery, drugs, and environment
5. High risk for impaired gastrointestinal function related to low cardiac output, hypoxemia, emboli, or antibiotic therapy

6. High risk for altered fluid and electrolyte balance related to the stress response of surgical trauma, the physiologic effects of cardiopulmonary bypass, and extravascular fluid shifts
7. High risk for impaired hematologic function related to inadequate hemostasis, incomplete neutralization of heparin, and coagulation abnormality
8. High risk for infection related to interruption of host defenses and placement of invasive devices
9. Altered body temperature related to physiologic effects of cardiopulmonary bypass, anesthetic agents, and ambient room temperature

10. Pain related to tissue trauma, immobility, operative maneuvering, and presence of invasive devices
11. Impaired verbal communication related to intubation and medications
12. Sleep pattern disturbance related to environmental factors, nursing care demands, and medications

For each of these diagnoses, the patient outcomes, nursing prescriptions, and evaluation criteria are outlined with a discussion of the factual information that support the plan and implementation of care.

NURSING
DIAGNOSIS 1 **Decreased cardiac output related to mechanical, electrical, or cellular alterations (exchanging pattern)**

PATIENT OUTCOMES	NURSING PRESCRIPTIONS	EVALUATION
Patient will achieve an adequate cardiac output as demonstrated by mean arterial pressure of 80 mm Hg, left atrial pressure between 10 and 20 mm Hg, warm and dry extremities with good capillary refill and no severe vasoconstriction, palpable and full pulses, urine output greater than or equal to 20 ml/hr/m², no clinically significant bradycardias or tachycardias, and normal mentation.	Evaluate patient's cardiac output by assessing mean arterial and left atrial pressures; skin temperature, moisture, and capillary refill; peripheral pulses, urine output, cardiac rhythm, and mentation.	Patient achieved an adequate cardiac output as demonstrated by mean arterial pressure of 80 mm Hg, left atrial pressure of 15 mm Hg, warm and dry extremities with capillary refill of less than 2 seconds and no severe vasoconstriction, palpable and full pulses, urine output of greater than or equal to 20 ml/hr/m², normal sinus rhythm, and normal mentation.
If alterations in cardiac output occur, patient will respond to treatment to maintain preload, afterload, myocardial contractility, heart rate, and cellular requirements.	If alterations occur, augment preload by instituting volume replacement; reduce afterload by administering vasodilator drugs (e.g., nitroprusside or nitroglycerin infusions); augment contractility by administering drugs to improve ventricular function (e.g., dopamine and dobutamine), being prepared to augment ventricular function with mechanical assistance (e.g., IABP, Hemopump, and ventricular assist devices); identify and treat clinically significant dysrhythmias (see Appendix B) and be prepared to institute cardiac pacing; assess for signs of perioperative acute myocardial infarction (e.g., new ECG changes) and institute treatment to maintain tissue and cellular needs.	Patient responded to treatment to maintain preload, afterload, myocardial contractility, heart rate, and cellular requirements.

Plan and intervention for decreased cardiac output

When the performance of the cardiovascular subsystem is inadequate for the patient's metabolic needs, improvement in cardiac output may be achieved by manipulating preload, afterload, contractility, and heart rate and by improving tissue oxygen levels.[51] Preload can be augmented by increasing fluid volume. If the contractility or compliance of the left ventricle is diminished or if the wall thickness of the left ventricle is unusually great, a left atrial pressure of up to 20 mm Hg may be desirable.[51] Right atrial pressure may need to be augmented to 18 mm Hg.

Afterload reduction with intravenous nitroprusside can maintain the sytemic arterial pressure to between normal and 10% above normal.[51] Care must be taken to avoid coronary hypoperfusion and further reduction of cardiac output. In patients with severe, long-term mitral valve disease, cardiac performance may be limited by right ventricular dysfunction associated with an elevated pulmonary arterial pressure. Reduction of right ventricular afterload with vasodilators may improve cardiac performance.

The heart rate can be optimized with atrial, ventricular, or sequential pacing or with pharmacologic agents. Failure of these efforts to normalize cardiac output may require administration of catecholamines or insertion of the IABP. The IABP may be the preferred treatment when electrical instability or myocardial necrosis is present (see Chapter 11).[51] Dopamine is begun at low doses and may be increased up to 15 micrograms (μg)/kg/min as needed. Dobutamine can be added in similar dosages. Isoproterenol

has a favorable effect on pulmonary vascular resistance and may be useful in improving right ventricular function.[51]

Determining the appropriate measures needed for optimizing the cardiac output can be a challenge for the nurse caring for the patient after cardiac surgery. Inadequate intravascular blood volume resulting from operative losses, administration of diuretics, and "third spacing" can be compounded by the various effects of cardiopulmonary bypass (Table 17-1). Knowledge of fluids, vasoactive medications (Table 17-2), and mechanical assist devices is essential in choosing effective therapeutic interventions. A sample cardiac output worksheet is provided to facilitate the coordination of the interventions (Figure 17-8).

Maximizing a patient's cardiac output depends on a stable heart rate and adequate stroke volume. A slow heart rate can be treated with temporary atrial or atrioventricular epicardial pacing. Tachycardias are treated according to the cardiac rhythm. Medications, cardioversion, and overdrive pacing may be used to control the rhythm and rate.

Stroke volume components include preload, afterload, and contractility. Preload reflects diastolic filling and is monitored in the clinical setting by the left and right atrial pressures, pulmonary artery wedge pressure (PAWP), pulmonary artery diastolic pressure, and indirectly by systolic blood pressure. These components may be affected by pharmacologic agents (e.g., vasodilators), temperature alterations, and hemoglobin. A low preload requires appropriate treatment. As noted in the box, the type of fluid to be administered depends on the patient's hemoglobin. A

 TABLE 17-2
Vasoactive Medications

Medication	Heart rate	Preload	Afterload	Contractility
Atropine	↑ *	— *	—	— or ↓ *
β-blockers	↓ ↓	↑	— or ↑	↓
Digoxin	— or ↓	—	— or ↑	↑
Dobutamine	— or ↑	↓	— or ↑	↑ ↑
Dopamine	— or ↑	↓	— or ↑	↑ ↑
Epinephrine	↑ ↑	↑	↑ or ↓	↑ ↑
Furosemide (Lasix)	—	↓	↓	—
Isoproterenol (Isuprel)	↑ ↑	↓	↓ ↓	↑ ↑
Lidocaine	—	—	—	— or ↓
Morphine	—	↓	↓	↑ or ↓
Nifedipine	↑	↓	↓	— or ↓
Nitroglycerin	— or ↑	↓ ↓	↓	—
Nitroprusside (Nipride)	— or ↑	↓	↓	—
Norepinephrine (Levophed)	↑ or ↓	↑	↑ ↑	↑
Oxygen	↓ or ↑	↓	↓	—
Phentolamine	— or ↑	— or ↓	↓	—
Phenylephrine (Neosynephrine)	↑	↑	↑ ↑	—
Procainamide	—	—	—	↓ or ↑
Verapamil	↑ or ↓	—	↑ or ↓	↓

* ↑, increase; ↓, decrease; —, no appreciable changes.

situation may arise in which the patient suffers from a high preload (hypervolemia). In this situation, other treatments such as diuretics and vasodilators are used.

Afterload is the amount of wall tension that the ventricles must generate to expel their blood volume. Afterload is influenced by aortic distensibility and by systemic and pulmonary vascular resistance. Formulas have been devised to calculate vascular resistance; however, monitoring systolic blood pressure and mean arterial pressure can provide information regarding the patient's afterload status. Medications are generally used to maintain an optimum afterload status (see Chapter 7). Mechanical assist devices such as the IABP or the ventricular assist device may be used to reduce afterload (see Chapter 11).

Contractility, or contractile strength, cannot be directly measured in the clinical setting. Noting the preoperative ejection fraction may provide a clue about the patient's myocardial contractility. Using a formula (Table 17-3) to

---

 PROPOSED ALGORITHM FOR THE CARE OF ADULT CARDIOVASCULAR SURGERY PATIENTS*

AFTERLOAD

Low

Vasoconstrictors
Normalization of temperature
Mechanical assist devices

High

Calcium channel blockers
Normalization of temperature
Volume
Vasodilators
Mechanical assist devices
α-blockers
Chest x-ray film for pulmonary abnormalities

PRELOAD

Low

Volume
Hemoglobin levels of less than 8.5
    Packed red blood cells
    Whole blood
Hemoglobin levels of greater than 8.5
    Colloids (albumin, hetastarch [Hespan])
    Crystalloids (normal saline, Ringer's lactate solution)

High

Diuretics
Vasodilators
Analgesics
Muscle relaxants
Oxygenation
Chest tube patency
Chest x-ray study

CONTRACTILITY

Low

Inotropics
Pacing
Mechanical assist devices
Calcium therapy
Magnesium therapy

High

β-blockers
Calcium channel blockers

HEART RATE

Low

Pacing
Normalization of temperature
Chronotropics (atropine, isoproterenol [Isuprel])

High

β-blockers
Calcium channel blockers
Digoxin
Normalization of temperature
Cardioversion
Overdrive pacing

ARTERIAL SATURATION

Low

Increase Fio_2
Positive end-expiratory pressure, continuous positive
    airway pressure
Extracorporeal membrane oxygenation
Augmentation of cardiac output
Normalization of temperature

High

Decrease Fio_2
Normalization of temperature

*Components are not presented in any particular priority.

Cardiac Output Worksheet

Pt. data	Cardiac output	Stroke volume preload	Afterload	Contractility	Heart rate	Treatment
HT/WT/BSA	Cardiac Index	LAP/RAP/PAD PAWP/SBP/Rx T/Hgb	SBP/MAP/PVR SVR/T/Rx PaO_2/$PaCO_2$	Eject. fraction SV/SVI/LVSWI	Rhythm Rx/T	Volume/Rx/Pacing IABP/VAD/O_2/Dx

FIG. 17-8   Cardiac output worksheet. *Ht*, Height; *Wt*, weight; *BSA*, body surface area; *LAP*, left atrial pressure; *RAP*, right atrial pressure; *PAD*, pulmonary artery diastolic pressure; *PAWP*, pulmonary artery wedge pressure; *SBP*, systolic blood pressure; *Rx*, medication; *T*, temperature; *LVSWI*, left ventricular stroke work index; *VAD*, ventricular assist device; *Hgb*, hemoglobin; *MAP*, mean arterial pressure; *PVR*, pulmonary vascular resistance; *SVR*, systemic vasuclar resistance; *SV*, stroke volume; *SVI*, stroke volume index; O_2, oxygen.
Courtesy Mary Sue Craft.

TABLE 17-3
Cardiovascular Function: Derived Data

Measurements	Equations	Normal values
Cardiac output (CO)	$CO = SV \times HR$	4.0 to 8.0 L/min
Cardiac index (CI)	$CI = CO/BSA$	2.5 to 4.0 L/min/m²
Stroke volume (SV)	$SV = CO \times 1000/HR$	60 to 130 ml/beat
Stroke volume index (SVI)	$SVI = SV/BSA$	45 to 85 ml/m²/beat
RV stroke work (RVSW)	$RVSW = SV \times (PAM - RAP) \times 0.0136$	
RV stroke work index (RVSWI)	$RVSWI = RVSW/BSA$	8.5 to 12 g/m²/beat
LV stroke work (LVSW)	$LVSW = SV \times (MAP - PAWP) \times 0.0136$	
LV stroke work index (LVSWI)	$LVSWI = LVSW/BSA$	35 to 85 g/m²/beat
Coronary perfusion	Coronary perfusion $= DBP - PAM$	60 to 80 mm Hg
Pulmonary vascular resistance (PVR)	$PVR = \dfrac{PAM - PAWP}{CO} \times 80$	<200 dyne-seconds-cm^{-5}
	$PVR = (PAM - PAWP)/CO$	0.2 to 1.5 mm Hg/L/min
Systemic vascular resistance (SVR)	$SVR = \dfrac{MAP - RAP}{CO} \times 80$	700 to 1200 dyne-seconds-cm^{-5}
	$SVR = (MAP - RAP)/CO$	9 to 20 mm Hg/L/min

Key: *HR*, Heart rate; *BSA*, Body surface area; *PAM*, Pulmonary artery mean pressure; *RAP*, right atrial pressure; *PAWP*, Pulmonary artery wedge pressure.

calculate left ventricular or right ventricular stroke work index can provide additional information. Poor contractility may be increased by using inotropes (e.g., dopamine or dobutamine), temporary epicardial pacing, or ventricular assist devices.

Tissue and mixed venous oxygen levels can be raised by administering packed red blood cells or whole blood, increasing the FiO_2, reducing oxygen consumption with sedation or paralyzing drugs, and by treating hyperthermia.[51]

NURSING DIAGNOSIS 2   **High risk for impaired gas exchange related to surgery, anesthesia, postoperative pain, and immobility (exchanging pattern)**

PATIENT OUTCOMES	NURSING PRESCRIPTIONS	EVALUATION
Patient will demonstrate adequate gas exchange by having an adequate respiratory rate, forced vital capacity, and tidal volume and a negative inspiratory force; good color and adequate arterial blood gas levels; lack of restlessness and no decrease in level of consciousness; normal breath sounds; and absence of signs or symptoms of complications (e.g., pneumonia, hemothorax or pneumothorax).	Evaluate adequacy of patient's gas exchange by assessing respiratory rate, negative inspiratory force, forced vital capacity, and tidal volume, noting trends in changes of ventilator settings; skin color and arterial blood gas levels; signs and symptoms of restlessness and decreased level of consciousness; breath sounds, checking endotracheal tube positioning and suctioning as needed; signs or symptoms of complications (e.g., pneumonia, hemothorax, or pneumothorax).	Patient demonstrated adequate gas exchange by having an adequate respiratory rate, forced vital capacity, and tidal volume and a negative inspiratory force; good color and adequate arterial blood gas levels; absence of restlessness and no decrease in level of consciousness; normal breath sounds; no signs or symptoms of complications (e.g., pneumonia, hemothorax, or pneumothorax).
Patient will tolerate weaning and extubation within 4 to 8 hours.	Prepare patient and assist with weaning and extubation process.	Patient tolerated weaning and extubation within 8 hours.
Patient will not experience respiratory complications after extubation.	Initiate coughing, deep breathing, chest physiotherapy, and mobilization after extubation; assess for respiratory complications.	Patient did not experience respiratory complications after extubation.

Plan and intervention for impaired gas exchange

The patient remains intubated and ventilated with a volume-controlled respirator until the effects of anesthesia have dissipated and subsystem performance is normal, usually 4 to 8 hours. Patients undergoing myocardial revascularization are not as prone to postoperative respiratory complications as patients undergoing mitral valve replacement. Some patients with mitral stenosis or regurgitation may remain intubated for longer periods after surgery. In addition, they may have more difficulty in weaning from the ventilator and may require more vigorous chest physiotherapy. This results from the increased back pressure exerted on the low-pressure pulmonary system, which occurs when the mitral valve is stenotic or insufficient. The replacement of the mitral valve may not correct the situation entirely, depending on the extent of disease. When the surgery has been successful, the hemodynamics can be corrected; however, pulmonary changes from long-term disease are usually fixed.

The nurse's responsibilities in regard to the patient's postoperative ventilatory status follow:

1. Note the presence of breath sounds bilaterally. Absence of breath sounds on the left may indicate that the endotracheal tube has slipped into the right main stem bronchus. Assess for adequate breath sounds in the bases of the lungs.
2. Assess for bilateral, equal excursion of the chest.
3. Check that the endotracheal tube is not inserted too far and resting on the carina. This may be the case if the patient is coughing and "bucking" the ventilator.
4. Note any trend in change of ventilator settings. Gradual increase in airway pressure indicates a decrease in lung compliance. (This illustrates the importance of knowing baseline ventilator settings.)
5. Monitor the patient's respiratory status with blood gas measurements per protocol until the measurements stabilize.

Although endotracheal suctioning is commonly performed during intubation, it is not a harmless procedure and thus should be performed only when necessary. A decrease in compliance, shunting, and reduction in arterial oxygen tension are undesirable sequelae of endotracheal suctioning.[5] Recommendations for suctioning procedures follow:

1. Suctioning should be accompanied by some form of supplemental oxygenation.
2. Suction flow rate, number of suction sequences, and the length of time suction is applied should be the minimum required to remove secretions.
3. The size of the suction catheter should have an external diameter small enough to allow the same flow rate of air as removed by the suction catheter.[5]

Suggested extubation criteria include:

1. Arterial oxygen pressure (PaO_2): greater than or equal to 80 mm Hg
2. Carbon dioxide pressure ($PaCO_2$): 30 to 35 mm Hg
3. FiO_2: 40%
4. Awake and alert status
5. Hemodynamic stability
6. Lack of evidence of respiratory distress
7. Negative inspiratory force: greater than −20 cm H_2O)
8. Forced vital capacity: at least 10 cc/kg

For selected patients who have undergone complex surgical procedures, additional criteria for extubation may be set.[51] Intermittent mandatory ventilation may be gradually reduced as the patient resumes spontaneous breathing. The incorporation of positive end-expiratory pressure is useful because it provides larger lung volumes and reduces the number of alveoli perfused but not ventilated and diminishes the alveolar-arterial oxygen differences after extubation.[51] It should not be used in patients with chronic obstructive pulmonary disease because it may produce a pneumothorax.

The patient's care after extubation includes a full regimen of pulmonary aerosol treatments, chest physiotherapy, and coughing and deep breathing exercises every 2 hours as tolerated. Most patients who undergo myocardial revascularization without complications are extubated the evening of the day of their surgery and placed on nasal cannula at 6 L/min of oxygen with high humidity and incentive spirometry. Blood gas determination is no longer necessary after one or two satisfactory postextubation readings if the patient remains stable and continues to improve. Chest x-ray films are taken each morning for 2 days.

All pulmonary care for these patients, from the time of admission to the critical care unit and especially in preparation for chest physiotherapy, includes careful planning for pain medication. These patients typically are given intravenous morphine sulfate as needed to facilitate good coughing. The patient's pulmonary status also improves with an increase in mobility, which begins the first morning after surgery.

NURSING DIAGNOSIS 3 — **High risk for impaired renal function related to hemodynamic instability, fluid imbalance, and physiologic effects of cardiopulmonary bypass (exchanging pattern)**

PATIENT OUTCOMES	NURSING PRESCRIPTIONS	EVALUATION
Patient will not experience major complications of impaired renal function as demonstrated by urine output of greater than or equal to 20 ml/hr/m², normal BUN and creatinine levels, urine specific gravity of 1.016 to 1.022, no red blood cells or protein after 6 to 8 days and no glucose or acetone in the urine, no weight gain or peripheral edema, normal serum potassium levels, and normal central venous pressure.	Evaluate patient for signs and symptoms of complications of impaired renal function by assessing urine output, BUN and creatinine levels, urine specific gravity, urine for hematuria and proteinuria and glucose or acetone, daily weight measurements and signs of edema, serum potassium levels, and central venous pressure.	Patient did not experience complications of impaired renal function as demonstrated by normal urine output, normal BUN and creatinine levels, urine specific gravity of 1.016 to 1.022, no red blood cells or protein after 6 to 8 days and no glucose or acetone in urine, no weight gain or peripheral edema, normal serum potassium levels, and normal central venous pressure.
If complications occur, patient will respond to appropriate therapy.	If complications occur, administer appropriate therapy, including fluids, inotropic agents to augment cardiac output, diuretics (e.g., furosemide or mannitol), and treatment for hyperkalemia.	

Plan and intervention for impaired renal function

Acute renal failure in adults after cardiac surgery is rare and is usually associated with low cardiac output. The lowering of the mean arterial pressure and the mean blood flow rate during CPB results in a diminished renal blood flow and glomerular filtration rate, as well as the release of endogenous vasoactive substances. The urine volume is a good index of renal function and should be at least 20 ml/hr/m^2 or 500 ml/24 hr/m^2. A pink color may indicate hemolysis of red blood cells (see Table 17-1). Solute secretion should maintain serum potassium levels below 5 mEq/L, BUN levels below 40 mg/dl, and creatinine levels below 1.5 mg/dl.[51] Protocols should provide for the measurement of serum potassium levels every 4 hours for at least the first 24 hours, as well as the measurement of serum creatinine and BUN levels and the patient's weight each morning for at least 48 hours.

Management of oliguria includes optimizing cardiac output, beginning diuretic therapy with intravenous furosemide and/or 20% mannitol, and starting treatment for hyperkalemia as necessary. If oliguria and hyperkalemia do not respond to treatment, dialysis should be instituted.

NURSING DIAGNOSIS 4 **High risk for impaired neurologic function related to surgery, drugs, and the environment (exchanging pattern)**

PATIENT OUTCOMES	NURSING PRESCRIPTIONS	EVALUATION
Patient will not experience neurologic complications (e.g., peripheral neuropathic conditions, strokes, encephalopathies, or coma).	Assess patient for signs and symptoms of neurologic complications.	Patient did not experience neurologic complications.
Patient will not demonstrate altered mental states as characterized by postcardiotomy delirium, depression, and disorientation.	Initiate interventions to maintain mental stability. Orient patient to time, place, person, and situation. Reduce or eliminate excessive environmental stimuli. Provide normal day-night cycles and uninterrupted sleep periods. Encourage frequent, short family visits. Assist patient in practicing relaxation techniques.	Patient did not demonstrate altered mental states, including postcardiotomy delirium, depression, and disorientation.

Plan and intervention for impaired neurologic function

Neurologic complications in adults after cardiac surgery are rare, occurring in 1% to 5% of patients.[1] Peripheral neuropathic conditions, strokes, encephalopathic conditions, and coma are primary manifestations. Peripheral neuropathic conditions generally involve the brachial plexus as a result of stretching the nerve fibers as the chest is opened. These conditions are usually short lived and resolve without treatment. Altered mental states occur in approximately 30% of patients with preexisting impairments, ranging from acute psychosis to depression.[1] Nurses should ascertain patient responsiveness and level of consciousness early in the postoperative period. Patient response to a request to wiggle the toes or open the eyes will indicate an ability to respond to a command, as well as motor capabilities. The care plan should include measures for protection if seizures occur.

Postcardiotomy delirium has been recognized as a complication of cardiac surgery and is believed to be the result of a number of physical and psychologic variables, such as age, length of CPB, cardiac output, sleep deprivation, and others. Manifestations may appear as early as the first operative day and generally consist of confusion, disorientation, inappropriate speech, perceptual distortion, and memory loss. Patients may hallucinate, exhibit emotional outbursts, or attempt to get out of bed and disconnect devices. The patient must be protected from harm. All medications must be reviewed, and the patient is sedated, usually with halperidol, 1 to 2 mg intramuscularly every 4 hours. Recovery is usually uneventful.

NURSING DIAGNOSIS 5
High risk for impaired gastrointestinal function related to low cardiac output, hypoxemia, emboli, or antibiotic therapy (exchanging pattern)

PATIENT OUTCOMES	NURSING PRESCRIPTIONS	EVALUATION
Patient will achieve adequate gastrointestinal function as demonstrated by absence of blood in nasogastric tube drainage or stool, normal bowel sounds, absence of abdominal distention, and a normal gastric pH.	Evaluate adequacy of patient's gastrointestinal function by assessing nasogastric tube drainage and stool, bowel sounds, signs of abdominal distention, and gastric pH; administer antacids as prescribed by physician.	Patient demonstrated adequate gastrointestinal function as demonstrated by absence of blood in nasogastric tube drainage or stool, presence of bowel sounds, absence of abdominal distention, and normal gastric pH.

Plan and intervention for impaired gastrointestinal function

There are two types of complications of the gastrointestinal subsystem: those affecting the liver and those affecting other components of the system. Hyperbilirubinemia associated with liver enzyme elevation in the absence of preexisting liver disease is usually associated with low cardiac output and hypoxemia; it is referred to as the *shock liver syndrome*.[1] Hyperbilirubinemia without liver enzyme elevation probably is a result of hemolysis.

The most common gastrointestinal complications that are not related to hepatitis are bleeding and ulceration. Other complications, although rare, include acute cholecystitis, acute diverticulitis, ischemic bowel, ruptured spleen, pancreatitis, and intestinal ileus.

Patients with a history of gastrointesinal problems and those who manifest blood in the nasogastric tube drainage or stool should be treated with Maalox, 15 ml every 4 hours to maintain the gastric pH above 3.5. Famotidine (Pepcid), 20 mg, may also be administered intravenously twice a day. Cimetidine (Tagamet) should be avoided because it tends to produce tachycardia and hypotension. Important side effects of antacid therapy include electrolyte disturbances (especially hypernatremia), metabolic alkalosis, hypermagnesemia, and diarrhea.[53]

NURSING DIAGNOSIS 6
High risk for altered fluid and electrolyte balance related to the stress response of surgical trauma, the physiologic effects of cardiopulmonary bypass, and extravascular fluid shifts (exchanging pattern)

PATIENT OUTCOMES	NURSING PRESCRIPTIONS	EVALUATION
Patient will not experience significant fluid or electrolyte imbalance as demonstrated by hypovolemia or decreased urinary output, hypotension or decreased right atrial pressure, metabolic acidosis or alkalosis, hypokalemia (no prolongation of the QT interval, no T-wave inversion, no ST-segment depression). If complications occur, patient will respond to the appropriate therapy.	Evaluate adequacy of fluid and electrolyte balance by assessing fluid volume and urinary catheter and chest tube drainage, blood pressure and right atrial pressure, arterial blood gas and serum potassium levels, and ECG.	Patient did not experience fluid or electrolyte imbalance as demonstrated by normovolemia and adequate urinary output, normotension and adequate right atrial pressure, absence of acidosis or alkalosis, and normal serum potassium levels.

Plan and intervention for altered fluid and electrolyte balance

Fluid administration in the first 48 hours after surgery must be precise because of the increase in extracellular fluid and total exchangeable sodium and the decrease in exchangeable potassium.[51] Fluids are administered intravenously as 5% glucose in water at a rate to deliver 500 to 750 ml/24 hours/m².[51] If the pH is less than 7.35, the base deficit is treated with sodium bicarbonate. If the pH is within normal limits and the $PaCO_2$ is less than 30 mm Hg, sodium bicarbonate is administered to treat a base deficit greater than 2.0 mEq/L.[51] For a serum potassium level less than 4.0 mEq/L, supplemental potassium is administered intravenously. For example, a 5.0-mEq bolus of potassium may be followed by an infusion of 20 mEq in a minimum of 50 ml of 5% dextrose in water, over a 1-hour period. The serum potassium level is measured again in 1 hour, and the treatment is repeated if necessary.

When the serum potassium is greater than 5.0 mEq/L, potassium chloride should be removed from the intravenous fluids and the serum potassium levels measured every hour until they are below 5.0 mEq/L. Serum potassium levels exceeding 6.0 mEq/L may be treated with 1 ampule of 50% dextrose in water and 20 units of regular insulin intravenously. The serum potassium level is measured in 1 hour and, if treatment has been ineffective, sodium polystyrene sulfonate (Kayexalate), 50 gm, in sorbital may be administered as an enema and retained for 20 minutes. The serum potassium level is again measured in 1 hour.

NURSING DIAGNOSIS 7	High risk for impaired hematologic function related to inadequate hemostasis, incomplete neutralization of heparin, and coagulation abnormality (exchanging pattern)

PATIENT OUTCOMES	NURSING PRESCRIPTIONS	EVALUATION
Patient will not experience bleeding or sequelae as evidenced by prothrombin time (PT), partial prothrombin time (PTT), platelet count, hemoglobin, and hematocrit within normal ranges; minimal chest tube drainage (less than 150 ml/hr for the first 3 hours and less than 100 ml/hr 4 to 12 hours after surgery; no evidence of systemic bleeding (e.g., gastrointestinal); and vital signs within normal limits.	Obtain per protocol PT, PTT, platelet count, hemoglobin, and hematocrit levels; report abnormal values and document therapy. Administer blood products, colloids, and crystalloid fluids as deemed appropriate Monitor chest tube drainage every hour and as necessary; report amounts that exceed protocol limits or excessive drainage that ceases abruptly (as in cardiac tamponade). Inspect incisions, intravascular insertion sites, and all drains for evidence of bleeding. Monitor vital signs for signs of hypovolemia, tachycardia, and hypotension.	Patient did not experience bleeding as demonstrated by laboratory values within normal ranges, chest tube drainage within normal limits, no evidence of systemic bleeding, and normal vital signs.

Plan and intervention for impaired hematologic function

Critical care nurses must be aware of the major causes of hemorrhage in the patient after cardiac surgery. Clinical signs and symptoms of hemorrhage include hypotension (systolic pressure of less than 90 mm Hg), tachycardia, increased chest tube drainage (over 200 ml/hour), anemia, decreased tissue perfusion, and alterations in gas exchange.

Hemorrhage in patients after cardiac surgery most commonly is due to inadequate surgery hemostasis, inadequate heparin neutralization, and alterations in coagulation (generally resulting from fibrinolysis or platelet function abnormalities). The amount of bleeding depends on the cause of the hemorrhage. Inadequate surgical hemostasis may require surgical reentry to locate the source of the bleeding. Maintenance of patient mediastinal chest tubes is essential before entry. Clot formation may occur, decreasing the capacity of the tubes to drain and thus lead to cardiac tamponade. Cardiac tamponade can result from as little as 100 ml of blood accumulated around the heart. Cardiac tamponade is diagnosed by a widened mediastinum on chest x-ray film, muffled heart sounds, narrowed pulse pressure, pulsus paradoxus, equalization of cardiac chamber pressures, electrical alternans, decreased tissue perfusion, and alterations in gas exchange (see Chapter 15).

Inadequate heparin neutralization may necessitate additional doses of protamine sulfate. Activated clotting times (ACTs) of greater than 150 seconds may increase such a condition. Alterations in coagulation are indicated by abnormal values of PT, PTT, platelet count, fibrinogen, hemoglobin, and hematocrit. Interventions should be guided by the specific coagulation deficiency (e.g., low platelet level requires platelet administration).

Even though good hemostasis can usually be achieved, approximately 10% to 20% of patients require multiple transfusions of blood products. *Autotransfusion* has provided an alternative to the transfusion of exogenous blood products. Systems presently available include the intermittent manual type and the continuous automated type. One automated system, developed at the University of Alabama at Birmingham, uses the left atrial pressure as a guide to the rate and amount of mediastinal blood infused. Desmopressin acetate, a synthetic analogue of the antidiuretic hormone, L-arginine vasopressin, is undergoing evaluation as a means of decreasing the need for platelet transfusions in bleeding patients.[95] Therapy for continued bleeding may include ε-aminocaproic acid (Amicar) when secondary fibrinolysis is suspected.[64] One pharmacologic agent undergoing clinical trial is aprotinin (Trasylol), which dramatically reduces bleeding after CPB, although the mechanisms of action are not yet fully understood.[49]

Measurement of chest tube drainage and management of tube patency are important in the initial postoperative period. Early detection of excessive bleeding and prevention of cardiac tamponade can result from well-defined chest tube management protocols. There are, however, no universal standards for chest tube management, and milking and stripping are used to facilitate drainage.[40] Potentially hazardous changes in intramediastinal pressures can be produced during chest tube manipulation. Clinical research findings suggest that chest tube manipulation should be avoided when suction and gravity produce adequate drainage,[75] and the type of manipulation should be selected based on the volume and viscosity of drainage and patient risk for bleeding.[40] For example, stripping can generate high pressures and should be reserved for use when clots are present and require evacuation. For patients with an increased risk of bleeding, the milking technique will produce lower pressures and may be preferable.[40]

NURSING DIAGNOSIS 8	High risk for infection related to interruption of host defenses and placement of invasive devices (exchanging pattern)

PATIENT OUTCOMES	NURSING PRESCRIPTIONS	EVALUATION
Patient will be free of wound infection as demonstrated by absence of tenderness, swelling, erythema, exudate and a temperature of less than 38° C.	Inspect incisions each shift. Monitor temperature. Change dressings per protocol. Administer antibiotics as prescribed. Practice good handwashing technique.	Patient remained free of infection as demonstrated by absence of tenderness, swelling, erythema, exudate, and a temperature of less than 38° C.

Plan and intervention for infection

Many factors contribute to the potential for infection in the patient after surgery including the creation of a surgical wound, the placement of devices, the hospital environment, and general level of health. Primary sites of concern for infection include the lungs because of hypoventilation and intubation, urinary tract because of the indwelling urinary catheter, surgical wounds, and sites of vascular lines.

Prophylactic antibiotic therapy is initiated on the day of surgery and is continued for 7 to 10 days. A broad spectrum antibiotic (e.g., cephapirin sodium [Cefadyl], 1 g every 6 hours) is administered intravenously until medications can be taken by mouth. Then cephradine (Anspor), 500 mg every 6 hours, may be substituted. In patients with impaired renal function, the dosage of medication and even the frequency of administration may be reduced.

If the central temperature exceeds 39.7° C (103.5° F), vigorous antipyretic measures should be initiated. Acetaminophen (Tylenol) suppository, 650 mg, is given every 4 hours for temperature above 38.4° C. Other antipyretic measures including placing ice in rubber gloves to the axillae and groin, cooling blanket, ice lavage through the nasogastric tube, and decreasing the temperature on the ventilator. The presence of malignant hyperthermia places the patient at risk for acute renal failure and DIC and is treated with dantrolene sodium (Dantrium) diluted in D_5W and given rapidly in an intravenous push.

If an infection is suspected, appropriate cultures are sent to the laboratory, and therapy is initiated. It may be necessary to consult an infectious disease specialist.

NURSING
DIAGNOSIS 9
Altered body temperature related to physiologic effects of cardiopulmonary bypass, anesthestic agents, and ambient room temperature (exchanging pattern)

PATIENT OUTCOMES	NURSING PRESCRIPTIONS	EVALUATION
Patient will maintain a body temperature within normal range as evidenced by temperature between 36° and 37° C (96.8° and 98.6° F), absence of mottling or pallor, absence of diaphoresis or shivering, and vital signs within normal limits.	Monitor core (rectal, bladder, tympanic, or pulmonary artery) temperature every 1 to 2 hours and as needed. Adjust environmental temperature by using overhead radiant heat lamps, warming blankets, and warmed intravenous fluids. Administer warm, humidified oxygen. Monitor cardiac, rhythm, rate, and pattern. Obtain a complete preoperative and intraoperative history. (Certain anesthetics and disease states are associated with temperature alterations.) Observe for signs of physiologic stability (core temperature of 36° to 37° C and warm, dry skin). Inspect the skin for erythema, pallor, or abnormal perspiration.	Patient maintained a normal body temperature as evidenced by temperature of 37.0° C; warm, dry, and pink skin, no evidence of diaphoresis or shivering; and vital signs within normal limits.

Plan and intervention for altered body temperature

Humans maintain their body temperature within a narrow range. Alterations above or below this range activate a physiologic response in an attempt to regain the core temperature. Induced hypothermia during cardiac surgery provides metabolic quiescence and myocardial preservation. However, after the patient's thermoregulatory mechanisms start to recover with rewarming and the intraoperative medications diminish in effectiveness, the situation is reversed. The patient responds by shivering, which is considered an undesirable response in the patient after cardiac surgery.

Postoperative hypothermia may be treated through the administration of heated, humidified oxygen or vasodilators or the use of overhead radiant lamps, warming blankets, and warmed intravenous fluids. Muscle relaxants have been effective in alleviating the effects of shivering.[103]

NURSING
DIAGNOSIS 10
Pain related to tissue trauma, immobility, operative maneuvering, and pressure of invasive devices (feeling pattern)

PATIENT OUTCOMES	NURSING PRESCRIPTIONS	EVALUATION
Patient will not experience severe pain as demonstrated by patient acknowledgement that pain is relieved or manageable; absence of grimacing, moaning, posturing, splinting, and other expressions of pain; resting quietly.	Monitor patient for presence of pain. Administer pain medications as prescribed. Administer medications before painful procedures. Provide comfort measures such as positioning, backrubs, and splinting of chest incision.	Patient was relieved of pain as demonstrated by patient acknowledgement that pain was not severe, absence of manifestations of pain, and patient resting quietly.

Plan and intervention for pain

Much of the responsibility for patient comfort rests with the nurse, who assesses for the presence and extent of postoperative pain, decides whether to administer a prescribed analgesic, and determines the dose and timing of administrations.[11] Pain should be anticipated and a protocol developed. A pain protocol might include morphine sulfate, 2 to 4 mg intravenously every 2 to 4 hours as necessary. Morphine can suppress respiration or cause hypotension and should be administered judiciously. Patients have reported that chest tube removal causes excruciating pain.[32] The protocol should provide for sufficient analgesic to be given at a time to ensure maximal effect. A nonnarcotic agent (e.g., acetaminophen [Tylenol]), should be administered 60 minutes before the procedure and be supplemented in 30 minutes with a narcotic. Each agent should exert its peak effect and provide maximal analgesia during removal of the chest tube. Analgesics are the most commonly used method of pain relief but may be augmented by nonpharmacologic therapies such as relaxation, distraction with music, and control of the environment.[2]

NURSING
DIAGNOSIS 11   **Impaired verbal communication related to intubation and medications (communicating pattern)**

PATIENT OUTCOMES	NURSING PRESCRIPTIONS	EVALUATION
Patient will achieve effective communication as demonstrated by use of an alternative communication technique, acknowledgment that the content of the message has been understood, and a decrease in the level of frustration (banging side rails), anger, anxiety, helplessness, and fear.	Use alternative communication technique (e.g., head-nod or eye-blink code or communication board). Confirm content and meaning of all communication attempts. Allow time for each communication interaction. Monitor behavioral manifestations of frustration, anger, anxiety, helplessness, and fear.	Effective communication was achieved as demonstrated by successful use of an alternative communication technique; patient acknowledgment that the content of the messages was understood; and reduction in behavioral manifestations of frustration, anger, anxiety, helplessness, and fear.

Plan and intervention for impaired verbal communication

Although intubation and mechanical ventilation are necessary adjuncts to therapy in the immediate postoperative period, patients have reported the inability to communicate as a major source of stress.[25,43,57] In addition, the inability of the patient to communicate verbally has been related to lack of nurse sensitivity to patient needs and failure to individualize communication between nurse and patient.[85] Commonly, patients attempt to communicate by looking at objects or people; pointing; making facial expressions; expressing emotions such as crying, withdrawing, and becoming angry; holding or touching others; or lip-speaking, if not hindered by equipment.[14]

Alternative methods of communication such as writing, communication boards, and computers have beneficial effects for patients and nurses. The selection of alternative methods of communication in the early postoperative period will be influenced by the level of patient sedation, restrictions imposed by devices, and the ease of use in the fast-paced setting.[92] Although further investigation is needed to define more precisely the alternative communication methods that are most effective with particular subgroups of patients, the nurse should place a priority on decreasing patient stress through satisfactory communication. Communication in the early postoperative period, while the endotracheal tube is still in place, may be enhanced by preoperative instruction that details communication techniques to be used and specific instructions in the use of these techniques. Such preparations may help patients overcome fear that their needs will not be understood and provide them with some sense of control over their situation.[92] Providing eyeglasses and cleansing the eyes is important for the success of these alternative techniques.

NURSING
DIAGNOSIS 12

Sleep pattern disturbance related to environmental factors, nursing care demands, and medications (moving pattern)

PATIENT OUTCOMES	NURSING PRESCRIPTIONS	EVALUATION
Patient will be free of detrimental effects of altered sleep pattern as demonstrated by patient acknowledgement of feeling rested and absence of signs of ICU psychosis.	Cluster nursing care activities to provide periods of uninterrupted rest. Minimize environmental noise and limit visitors as necessary to promote rest periods. Reduce pain and provide comfort measures. Administer sedative-hypnotics as prescribed.	Patient obtained adequate sleep as demonstrated by patient acknowledgement of feeling rested and absence of signs of ICU psychosis.

Plan and intervention for sleep pattern disturbance

Promoting sleep during the immediate postoperative period requires attention to patient comfort, environmental noise, and control of interruptions.[19] The pain management protocol should be coordinated with measures to control environmental noise, such as lowering monitor alarms, turning off unused suction and oxygen machines, and limiting extraneous talking.[60] Efficiently grouping nursing care activities can diminish interruptions of rest and sleep. Although positioning and backrubs increase patient comfort, nontraditional approaches to promoting sleep (e.g., relaxation techniques, music therapy, and guided imagery) also deserve investigation.[19]

INTERMEDIATE POSTOPERATIVE PHASE
Patient transfer to the intermediate care unit

The typical patient is transferred to the intermediate care unit after 2 to 3 days in the critical care unit. The transfer is initiated after the patient meets certain criteria, in particular a stable hemodynamic and oxygenation status.

Patients may experience some anxiety and stress before the transfer. Critical care nurses therefore must pay particular attention to patients' and their families' Knowing Patterns. Educating patients and families regarding the time of, reason for, and method of transfer is imperative. Information about the intermediate care unit, its staff, and methods of operation should also be reviewed.

Patients should be informed that their relevant past and current health care problems will be reported to the intermediate care unit staff. In addition, patients' perceptions regarding their illness and surgical outcome, expectations of the cardiac rehabilitative phase, and educational needs also should be communicated.

In most institutions, discharge teaching is intensified after the patient is discharged from the critical care unit. The quiet, slower pace of the intermediate care unit is considered more conducive to learning, as well as to the patient's emotional and physical recovery. The goals of the intermediate care unit include mobilization and education. Patient and family education needs center around medications, dietary habits, activity limitations (including resumption of sexual activity), and potential problems (see Table 17-4).

Incisional wound and skin care are reviewed with the signs and symptoms of infection. Areas requiring follow-up and reinforcement are documented and subsequently reported to the appropriate health care professional.

TABLE 17-4

Discharge Teaching Needs and Plan for the Patient after Cardiovascular Surgery

Outcome criteria	Intervention
Medication side effects	
Patient will state for each medication the following: name, dose, frequency and time of administration; special precautions and side effects and times to notify the physician.	Pharmacist or nurse will meet with the patient (optimally the day before discharge) to discuss each prescribed medication, doses, administration procedures, precautions, and side effects.
	Pharmacist or nurse will provide the patient with written materials (e.g., booklets) regarding the medications.
Patient will have a written prescription for each medication.	Physician will provide written prescriptions and a telephone number so that the patient can ask questions.
Diet and fluid plans	
Patient will state diet to follow after discharge.	Dietitian or nurse will meet individually or with a group of patients with similar dietary needs to discuss the actual diet, components of the diet, and foods to avoid or restrict.
Patient will state food groups to avoid or restrict intake (e.g., valve replacement patients are receiving warfarin sodium [Coumadin], which can be adversely affected by a high intake of green, leafy vegetables. These vegetables contain vitamin K, which can inactivate Coumadin).	Dietitian or nurse will give a resource telephone number and booklet to the patient.
Patient will state suggestions and restrictions regarding fluid intake.	Physician will provide a written diet and prescription and review any modifications with the patient.
Patient will state the importance of a daily weight measurement (same scale at same time of day).	
Patient will state when to notify the physician, specifically for weight gain or loss (especially if it is acute), decreased urine output, edema (dependent and/or generalized), changes in breathing (e.g., dyspnea), and delayed wound healing.	
Patient will state resources available if questions arise regarding the diet.	
Activity tolerance	
Patient will state recommendations regarding activities after discharge (e.g., walk 1 mile in 3 to 4 weeks).	Physical therapist or nurse will discuss recommendations and limitations regarding activity with the patient.
Patient will state limitations regarding weight bearing, lifting, stair climbing, driving, and positioning.	Physician will review with the patient any restrictions in activity beyond the typical ones.
The patient will state the signs and symptoms that indicate activity intolerance, including dyspnea, faintness or syncope, angina, severe diaphoresis, and irregular heart beats.	Physician, physical therapist, and nurse will review with the patient the symptoms of activity intolerance, persons to notify of these symptoms, and telephone numbers.
Patient will state persons to notify of symptoms of activity intolerance and telephone numbers.	Physical therapist will demonstrate the prescribed exercises and give written materials to the patient.
Patient will demonstrate the prescribed postoperative cardiovascular exercises.	
Treatments and procedures	
Patient will demonstrate the proper technique for wound care.	Nurse will demonstrate proper procedure for cleaning and maintaining wounds.
Patient will identify the materials needed and places to obtain them.	Physician and nurse will emphasize the importance of notifying the physician of signs of possible infection.
Patient will state signs and symptoms to report to physician, including drainage (of any color and quantity), swelling, openings in incisional line, fever, and discomfort or pain.	Nurse will provide a list of signs and symptoms requiring physician notification.
Discharge process	
Patient will state check out time.	Nurse will describe the discharge process and the individuals involved.
Patient will state the discharge process and individuals involved, including the pharmacist, physical therapist, nurse, physician, and dietitian.	Nurse will state mode of transport to be used and recommend appropriate clothing for patient to wear on day of discharge.
Patient will state appropriate attire for discharge required for season and physical condition.	

KEY CONCEPT REVIEW

1. All of the following are indications for urgent or emergent myocardial revascularization *except*:
   a. Failed angioplasty
   b. Acute myocardial infarction and cardiogenic shock
   c. Stable angina
   d. Failed thrombolysis
2. The best preoperative indicator of the severity of cardiac disease is:
   a. General patient condition
   b. Left ventricular ejection
   c. Extent of collateral circulation
   d. Number and degree of stenotic lesions
3. Potential detrimental effects of cardiopulmonary bypass include all the following *except*:
   a. Bleeding
   b. Infection
   c. Myocardial infarction
   d. Hypotension
4. All of the following are possible sequelae of postoperative shivering *except*:
   a. Dental damage
   b. Wound dehiscence
   c. Accumulation of lactic acid
   d. Diminished metabolic demands
5. The most prevalent noncardiac complication occurring after cardiac surgery is:
   a. Infection
   b. Intestinal ischemia
   c. Hyperglycemia
   d. Acute renal failure
6. The type of chest tube manipulation should be based on all of the following *except*:
   a. Volume of drainage
   b. Patient risk for bleeding
   c. Viscosity of drainage
   d. Number of chest tubes
7. The upper level for acceptable serum potassium in the postoperative patient is:
   a. 7.5 mEq/L
   b. 6.5 mEq/L
   c. 5.5 mEq/L
   d. 4.5 mEq/L
8. Minimally acceptable urine output in the postoperative period is approximately:
   a. 10 ml/hr/m^2
   b. 20 ml/hr/m^2
   c. 30 ml/hr/m^2
   d. 40 ml/hr/m^2
9. Inappropriate afterload may be managed in the postoperative patient by:
   a. Reducing left ventricular filling pressure
   b. Augmenting left ventricular filling pressure
   c. Reducing mean arterial pressure
   d. Augmenting mean arterial pressure
10. All of the following factors contribute to the risk for developing acute renal failure in the postoperative period *except*:
    a. Low cardiac output
    b. Duration of cardiopulmonary bypass
    c. Antibiotic therapy
    d. Adult age

ANSWERS

1. c	3. d	5. a	7. c	9. c
2. b	4. d	6. d	8. b	10. d

REFERENCES

1. Alfieri A and Kotler MN: Noncardiac complications of open-heart surgery, Am Heart J 119:149, 1990.
2. American Association of Critical-Care Nurses: Outcome standards for nursing care of the critically ill, Laguna, Niguel, Calif, 1990, The Association.
3. American Heart Association: 1990 heart and stroke facts, Dallas, 1989, The Association.
4. Anderson JL and others: Coronary bypass surgery early after thrombolytic therapy for acute myocardial infarction, Ann Thorac Surg 41:176, 1986.
5. Baun M: Suctioning. In Hill JB, Schmidt GA, and Wood LDH, editors: Principles of critical care medicine, New York, 1992, McGraw Hill, Inc.
6. Becker LC: Condition for vasodilator induced coronary steal in experimental myocardial ischemia, Circulation, 57:1103, 1978.
7. Becker LC: Is isoflurane dangerous for the patient with coronary artery disease? Anesthesiology 68:259, 1987.
8. Brehrendt DM and Austin WG: Patient care in cardiac surgery, Boston, 1980, Little, Brown, & Co.
9. Buffington CW and others: Isoflurane induces coronary steal in a canine model of chronic coronary occlusion, Anesthesiology 66:280, 1987.
10. Caralpi JJ and others: Results of coronary artery surgery in patients receiving propranolol, J Thorac Cardiovasc Surg 67:526, 1974.
11. Cohen FL: Postsurgical pain relief: patients' status and nurses' medication sources, Pain 9:265, 1980.
12. Cox JL: Patient selection criteria and results of surgery for refractory ischemic ventricular tachycardia, Circulation 79(suppl I):I63, 1989.
13. Cox JL, Holman WL, and Cain ME: Cryosurgical treatment of atrioventricular node reentrant tachycardia, Circulation 76:1329, 1987.
14. Cronin LR and Carrizosa AA: The computer as a communication device for ventilator and tracheostomy patients in the intensive care unit, Crit Care Nurse 4:72, 1984.
15. Earp JK: Thermal gradients and shivering following open heart surgery, Dimens Crit Care Nurs 8:266, 1983.
16. Edmunds L and Stephenson L: Cardiopulmonary bypass for open heart surgery. In Glenn W, editor: Thoracic and cardiovascular surgery, Norwalk, Conn, 1983, Appleton and Lange.
17. Ellis JA: Using pain scales to prevent undermedication, MCN 13:180, 1988.
18. Ellison N, Jobes DR, and Schwartz AJ: Heparin therapy during cardiac surgery. In Ellison N and Jobes DR, editors: Effective hemostasis in cardiac surgery, Philadelphia, 1988, WB Saunders Co.
19. Fontaine DK: Measurement of nocturnal sleep patterns in trauma patients, Heart Lung 18:402, 1989.
20. Frankl WS: A comparison of coronary artery bypass surgery and percutaneous transluminal coronary angioplasty in treatment of coronary artery disease. II. Mod Concepts Cardiovasc Dis 59:37, 1990.

21. Fromme GA and White RD: Support of the circulation during and after cardiac operations. In Tarken S, editor: Cardiovascular anesthesia and postoperative care, ed 2, Chicago, 1989, Year Book Medical Publishers.

22. Fromme GA, White RD, and Housmans PR: Myocardial preservation. In Tarhan S, editor: Cardiovascular anesthesia and postoperative care, ed 2, Chicago, 1989, Year Book Medical Publishers.

23. Gardner TJ and others: The risk of coronary bypass surgery for patients with postinfarction angina, Circulation 79(suppl I):I79, 1989.

24. Gersh BJ and others: Coronary bypass surgery in chronic stable angina, Circulation 79(suppl I):I46, 1989.

25. Gries ML and Fernsler J: Patient perceptions of the mechanical ventilation experience, Focus Crit Care 15:52, 1988.

26. Grondin CM and others: Comparison of late changes in internal mammary artery and saphenous vein grafts in two consecutive series of patients ten years after operation, Circulation 70(suppl I):I208, 1984.

27. Grondin CM and others: Reoperations in coronary artery disease. In Karp RB and others, editors: Advances in cardiac surgery, Chicago, 1990, Year Book Medical Publishers, Inc.

28. Gross FS and Kay EB: Direct vision repair of intracardiac defects utilizing a rotating disc reservoir-oxygenator, Surg Gynecol Obstet 104:711, 1957.

29. Gross GN and Warltier DC: Coronary steal in four models of single or multiple vessel obstruction in dogs, Am J Cardiol 48:84, 1981.

30. Guyton RA, Willians WH, and Hatcher CR: Techniques of cardiopulmonary bypass. In Hurst JW and others, editors: The heart, New York, 1986, McGraw-Hill, Inc.

31. Harrison DC: Practical guide for the use of lidocaine: prevention and treatment of cardiac arrhythmias, JAMA 69:1, 1976.

32. Heye ML: Patient pain perceptions and coping strategies used in early convalescence from coronary bypass surgery, PhD Dissertation, The University of Texas at Austin, 1989.

33. Holtzclaw BJ: Postoperative shivering after cardiac surgery: a review, Heart Lung 15:292, 1986.

34. Holtzclaw BJ: Shivering: In Hill JB, Schmidt GA, and Wood LDH, editors: Principles of critical care medicine, New York, 1992, McGraw Hill, Inc.

35. Horowitz LN and others: Ventricular resection guided by epicardial and endocardial mapping for treatment of recurrent ventricular tachycardia, New Engl J Med 302:589, 1980.

36. Horrow JC: Protamine: a necessary evil. In Ellison N and Jobes DR, editors: Effective hemostasis in cardiac surgery, Philadelphia, 1988, WB Saunders Co.

37. Horvath SM and others: Metabolic cost of shivering, J Appl Physiol 8:595, 1956.

38. Hug CC Jr: Anesthesia and the patient with cardiovascular disease. In Hurst JW and others, editors: The heart, ed 8, New York, McGraw-Hill, Inc. 1986.

39. Ionescu MI and Wooler GH: Current techniques in extracorporeal circulation, London, 1978, Butterworth & Co., Ltd.

40. Isaacson JJ, Genge LT, and Brewer MJ: The effect of chest tube manipulation on mediastinal drainage, Heart Lung 15:601, 1986.

41. Jansen KJ and McFadden PM. Postoperative nursing management in patients undergoing myocardial revascularization with internal mammary artery bypass, Heart Lung 15:48, 1986.

42. Joachimsson PO, Dystrom O, and Tyden H: Heating efficacy of external heart supply during and after open-heart surgery with hypothermia, Acta Anesthesiol Scand 31:73, 1987.

43. Jones J and others: What the patients say: a study of reactions to an intensive care unit, Intensive Care Med 6:89, 1979.

44. Jones RH: In search of the optimal surgical mortality, Circulation 79(suppl I):I132, 1989.

45. Kaiser GC, Schaff HV, and Killep T: Myocardial revascularization for unstable angina pectoris, Circulation 79(suppl I):I60, 1989.

46. Kay HR, Armenti FR, and Parr GV: Results to expect in today's older and sicker cardiac patients, Geriatrics 44:67, 1989.

47. King KB: Coping with cardiac surgery, doctoral dissertation, Rochester, NY, 1984, University of Rochester.

48. King RM and White RD: Oxygenators and hemodilution in cardiopulmonary bypass. In Tarken S, editor: Cardiovascular anesthesia and postoperative care, ed 2, Chicago, 1989, Year Book Medical Publishers.

49. Kirklin JW: Technical and scientific advances in cardiac surgery over the past 25 years, Ann Thorac Surg 49:26, 1990.

50. Kirklin JW and Barratt-Boyes BG: Cardiac surgery, New York, 1986, John Wiley & Sons, Inc.

51. Kirklin JW, Blackstone EH, and Kirklin JK: Cardiac surgery. In Braunwald E, editor: Heart disease, ed 3, Philadelphia, 1988, WB Saunders Co.

52. Kirklin JW and others: Summary of a consensus concerning death and ischemic events after coronary artery bypass grafting, Circulation 79(suppl I):I81, 1989.

53. Konopod E and Noseworthy T: Stress ulceration: a serious complication in critically ill patients, Heart Lung 17:339, 1988.

54. Kouchoukos NT and others: Coronary artery bypass grafting for postinfarction angina pectoris, Circulation 79(suppl I):I68, 1989.

55. Kumar CM: Wolff-Parkinson-White syndrome and general anesthesia: use of isoflurane and vecuronium, Br J Anaesth 58:574, 1986.

56. Landymore R, Kinley C, and Gardner M: Encircling endocardial resection with complete removal of endocardial scar without intraoperative mapping for the ablation of drug resistant ventricular tachycardia, J Thorac Cardiovasc Surg 89:18, 1985.

57. Lee DM: A recalled description of stressors encountered by the alert patient during mechanical ventilation, Masters thesis, University of Alabama at Birmingham, 1987.

58. Levy JH, Zaiden JR, and Faraj B: Prospective evaluation of risk of protamine reactions in patients with NPH insulin-dependent diabetes, Anesthes Analg 85:739, 1986.

59. Levy JH and others: Prospective evaluation of patients with fish allergies for anaphylaxis to protamine, 9th Annual Meeting of the Society of Cardiovascular Anesthesiologists, Palm Desert, Calif, May 1987, (abstract).

60. Littrell K and Schumann LL: Promoting sleep for the patient with a myocardial infarction, Crit Care Nurse 9:44, 1989.

61. Litwak R and Giannelli S: Open intracardiac operations employing extracorporeal circulation. In Litwak R and Jurado R, editors: Care of the cardiac surgical patient, Norwalk, Conn, 1982, Appleton and Lange.

62. Lowenstein E and others: Catastrophic pulmonary vasoconstriction associated with protamine reversal of heparin, Anesthesiol 59:470, 1983.

63. Mann DE and others: Importance of pacing site in containment of ventricular tachycardia, J Am Cardiol 5:781, 1985.

64. Marsh HM and Abel MD: Postoperative management of adult cardiac surgical patients. In Tarkan S, editor: Cardiovascular anesthesia and postoperative care, ed 2, Chicago, 1989, Year Book Medical Publishers.

65. McFadden ER and Ingram RH: Relationship between diseases of the heart and lungs. In Braunwald E, editor: Heart disease, Philadelphia, 1984, WB Saunders Co.

66. Mills NL and Solar RJ: Intraoperative coronary artery balloon-catheter dilatation. In Roberts AJ and Conti CR, editors: Current surgery of the heart, Philadelphia, 1987, JB Lippincott Co.

67. Moran JM and others: Coronary revascularization in patients receiving propranolol, Circulation 49(suppl II):116, 1974.

68. Mullen DC and others: Selection of patients for coronary bypass surgery, Postgrad Med 63:111, 1978.

69. Naunheim KS and others: The changing profile of the patient undergoing coronary artery bypass surgery, J Am Coll Cardiol 11:494, 1988.

70. Noback CR and Tinker TH: Hypothermia after cardiopulmonary bypass in man: amelioration by nitroprusside induced vasodilation during rewarming, Anesthesiol 53:277, 1980.

71. Ochsner JL and Mills NL: Coronary artery surgery, Philadelphia, 1978, Lea & Febiger.

72. Oliver WC and White RD: Anesthesia for electrophysiologic testing, surgical treatment of arrhythmias, and resection of ventricular aneurysms. In Tarhan S, editor: Cardiovascular anesthesia and postoperative care, Chicago, 1989, Year Book Medical Publishers.

73. Ostermeyer J and others: Direct operations for the management of life-threatening ischemic ventricular tachycardia, Thorac Cardiovasc Surg 94:848, 1987.

74. Parsonnet V, Dean D, and Bernstein AD: A method of uniform stratification of risk for evaluating the results of surgery in acquired adult heart disease, Circulation 79(suppl I):I3, 1989.

75. Pierce JD: Effects of two chest tube clearance protocols on chest drainage in myocardial revascularization surgical patients, Doctoral dissertation, University of Alabama at Birmingham, 1987.

76. Pierce WS and others: Cardiac surgery: a glimpse into the future, J Am Coll Cardiol 14:265, 1989.

77. Pimm JB: New ways to provide crisis intervention for heart surgery patients, Healing the heart: proceedings from the 3rd National Multidisciplinary Conference, The National Institute for the Clinical Application of Behavioral Medicine: Mansfield Center, 1990, p 348.

78. Pinsker MC: Anesthesia: a pragmatic construct, Anesthes Analg 85:819, 1986.

79. Puntillo KA: The phenomenon of pain and critical care nursing, Heart Lung 17:262, 1988.

80. Rackley CE, Edwards JE, and Karp RB: Mitral valve disease. In Hurst JW and others, editors: The heart, New York, 1986, McGraw-Hill, Inc.

81. Racosky M: The thoughts and feelings of patients in the waiting period prior to cardiac surgery: a descriptive study, Heart Lung 6:280, 1977.

82. Ralley RE and others: The effects of shivering on oxygen consumption and carbon dioxide production in patients rewarming from hypothermic cardiopulmonary bypass, J Anaes 35:332, 1988.

83. Rodriguez JL and others: Physiologic requirements during rewarming: suppression of the shivering response, Crit Care Med 11:490, 1983.

84. Sadler PD: Incidence, degree and duration of postcariotomy delerium, Heart Lung 10:1084, 1981.

85. Salyer J and Stuart BJ: Description of the content of the interaction between nurses and patients on mechanical ventilation, Masters thesis, University of Alabama at Birmingham, 1975.

86. Sanford SJ: Sleep and the critically ill patient. In Kinney MR, Packa DR, and Dunbar SB, editors: AACN's clinical reference for critical-care nursing, ed 2, St Louis, 1988, The CV Mosby Co.

87. Sealy WC and Selle JG: Surgical treatment of supraventricular arrhythmias. In Roberts AJ and Contis CR, editors: Current surgery of the heart, Philadelphia, 1987, JB Lippincott Co.

88. Sessler DI and others: Spontaneous post-anesthetic tremor does not resemble thermoregulatory shivering, Anesthesiol 68:843, 1988.

89. Singh RN, Sosa JA, and Green GE: Internal mammary artery versus saphenous vein graft: comparative perfusion in patients with combined revascularization, Br Heart J 50:48, 1983.

90. Spencer FC: A critique of emergency and urgent operations for complications of coronary artery disease, Circulation 79(suppl I):I160, 1989.

91. Stewart S: The physiologic effects and nursing implications of cardiopulmonary bypass, unpublished master's thesis, Boston, 1985, Boston University.

92. Stovsky B, Rudy E, and Dragonette P: Comparison of two types of communication methods used after cardiac surgery with patients with endotracheal tubes, Heart Lung 17:281, 1988.

93. Talley JD and others: Coronary artery bypass surgery after failed elective percutaneous transluminal coronary angioplasty, Circulation 79(suppl I):I126, 1989.

94. Tarhan S and Raimundo HS: Coronary circulation and anesthesia for coronary artery bypass graft surgery. In Tarhan S, editor: Cardiovascular anesthesia and postoperative care, Chicago, 1982, Year Book Medical Publishers, Inc.

95. Ware JA: Desmopressin acetate in hemorrhagic conditions, with emphasis on use after cardiopulmonary bypass. In Ellison N and Jobes DR, editors: Effective hemostasis in cardiac surgery, Philadelphia, 1988, WB Saunders Co.

96. Warner MA and Warner ME: Anesthetic agents for cardiac surgery. In Tarhan S, editor: Cardiovascular anesthesia and postoperative care ed 2, Chicago, 1989, Year Book Medical Publishers.

97. Wetstein L: Infective endocarditis. In Braunwald E, editor: Heart disease: a textbook of cardiovascular medicine, Philadelphia, 1985, WB Saunders Co.

98. Wetstein L and others: Surgical management and mapping of cardiac arrhythmias, Cardiovasc Clin 18:1:151, 1985.

99. Wetstein L and others: Surgery for ventricular tachyarrythmias. In Roberts AJ and Contis CR, editors: Current surgery of the heart, Philadelphia, 1987, JB Lippincott Co.

100. Whitman GR: Prosthetic cardiac valves, Prog Cardiovasc Nurs 2:116, 1987.

101. Wilkowski DAW and Lynn JJ: Preoperative evaluation. In Tarhan S, editor: Cardiovascular anesthesia and postoperative care, ed 2, Chicago, 1989, Year Book Medical Publishers.

102. Winslow CM and others: The appropriateness of performing coronary artery bypass surgery, JAMA 260:505, 1988.

103. Zwischenburger JB and others: Suppression of shivering decreases oxygen consumption and improves hemodynamic stability during postoperable shivering, Ann Thorac Surg 43:428, 1987.

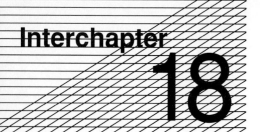

Interchapter 18

The Power of Touch

"Touch is something I do to my patients after I finish the really important things." This statement by a nurse reflects a pervasive attitude; although touching patients reflects a humane and gently caring attitude, what this nurse believes really counts is the technologic role of nurse. This attitude, however, reveals a lack of understanding of the therapeutic nature of touch.

Touch is different in all cultures. One society may view touch as necessary; another culture may view it as taboo. Awareness of personal and cultural views and reactions to touch is mandatory for the nurse.[3] There are diverse qualities of touch that serve as symbols of communication that may be invisible or intangible. Weiss[10] has defined *six tactile symbols* that create a *language* of touch: duration, location, action, intensity, frequency, and sensation. These symbols define the act of touching and not the circumstances involved. Touch can cause arousal and carry special messages.

Nurses should continue to investigate areas identified by Weiss such as (1) the response of different senders and receivers, (2) the language of touch throughout the life cycle, and (3) touch differences in the child, adolescent, adult, and elderly.

Touch is a powerful way to share presence and love from our hearts when words are meaningless.[9] Individuals are keenly sensitive to touch during dying time. Physical touch done lovingly, freely, and with joy conveys through our hands what are hearts are feeling. As a cardiovascular nurse, you touch patients all the time. How often do you touch routinely without consciously directing your touch with intention to evoke healing?

Touch is effective in decreasing the patient's anxiety and apprehension, as well as facilitating recovery. Knable[4] describes hand holding as a positive means of communication and one that seems to break down barriers. Lynch[6] studied patients in two acute care settings: a cardiac care unit and shock trauma unit. He found that human interaction and touch are extremely important in the acute care setting. In fact, the more traumatic the environment, the more important is human contact. Some patients' dysrhythmias were suppressed with touch and pulse taking, which supported the importance of this simple act.

Heidt[1] investigated the use of therapeutic touch in a controlled study of 90 volunteer subjects in a cardiovascular unit of a large medical center. She found that those patients who received therapeutic touch showed a significant decrease in anxiety compared with subjects who received only casual touch or no touch.

Heidt,[2] Krieger,[5] Macre,[7] and Quinn[8] continue to documented the importance of therapeutic touch and encourage investigation using controlled studies. Basic to the therapeutic touch is the philosophy that human beings are a continuum of life energies. Therapeutic touch involves nurses centering themselves and then sensitizing their hands to the patient's energy field. Therapeutic touch is used to assess the patient's condition and to help the patient repattern energies in a more productive manner for a higher level of wellness.

Heidt's research[2] using grounded theory indicated that the primary experience of therapeutic touch involves *opening* to the flow of universal life energy. This includes three major categories of the experience: (1) *opening intent*—allowing oneself to focus on getting the universal life energy moving again; (2) *opening sensitivity*—assessing the quality of its flow; and (3) *opening communication*—participating in a healing relationship that unblocks, engages, and enlivens its movement. Heidt[2] suggests that further research on therapeutic touch using qualitative methodologies may deepen our understanding of the inner experiences that facilitate the healing process of both patients and nurses.

Touch with intention and an openness can communicate to patients that you are a healer.[3] Some of the special moments that many patients remember that got them through the rough times are the fluffing of pillows or a straightening of sheets or eggcrate mattress, a change in position particularly to relieve bony areas, mouth care, backrubs, a foot massage, or light acupressure. They also remember being given smaller bedpans or metal equipment being warmed under warm water or a hot water bottle or receiving a warm blanket after surgery when they were shivering.

How do you touch with intention? Start your touch by centering yourself with your breath or an image of healing light surrounding you and the person. Imagine that your hands are an extension of your heart. Slowly and gently uncover only the person's body where you are touching. Then place your hands gently on the person's body. Don't be afraid to ask the person how the touch feels and if it should be done with a lighter or firmer touch. You might find that if you are tense, your hands or upper body may cramp. If so, just back off, shake your hands, do a few shoulder rolls, and use your rhythmic breathing. Again, you will know when to stop the touch. Slowly and gently remove your hands, and once again cover the person so that they feel comfortable. Bring your ritual to a close in whatever way seems right for you such as shaking your hands or washing your hands in cool water to release the energy. You will be surprised at how calm and peaceful you feel.

Encourage family and friends to participate in touch to connect them with their loved ones and make the technologic environment more human. Remember touch includes bathing, hair combing, feeding, and changing the person's position, sheets, pillows, and sheepskins. Touching also includes hugging, holding, and cuddling as powerful ways to break the illusion of separateness, loneliness, and fear. These simple acts of touching somehow seem to shake loose fear, guilt, and loneliness. These moments may evoke laughter, calmness, or tears. The emotions that come up are the ones that need to be present.

REFERENCES

1. Heidt P: Effect of therapeutic touch in anxiety level of hospitalized patients, Nurs Res 30:32, 1981.
2. Heidt P: Openness: a qualitative analysis of nurses' and patients' experiences of therapeutic touch, Image 22:180, 1990.
3. Keegan L: Touch: connecting with the healing power. In Dossey B and others: Holistic nursing: a handbook for practice, Gaithersburg, 1988, Aspen Publishers.
4. Knable J: Handholding: One means of transcending barriers of communication, Heart Lung 10:1106, 1981.
5. Krieger D: The therapeutic touch: how to use your hands to help or to heal, Englewood Cliffs, NJ, 1979, Prentice-Hall, Inc.
6. Lynch J: The single act of touching, Nursing '78 8:32, 1978.
7. Macre J: Therapeutic touch: a practical guide, New York, 1988, Alfred Knopf.
8. Quinn J: Therapeutic touch as energy exchange: testing the theory, Adv Nurs Sci 6:42, 1984.
9. Toblason SJB: Touching is for everyone, Am J Nurs, 81:728, 1981.
10. Weiss S: The language of touch, Nurs Res 28:76, 1979.

18 The Patient Undergoing Cardiac Transplant Surgery

Diane K. Dressler

LEARNING OBJECTIVES

1. Examine current trends in candidate selection and preoperative management of cardiac transplant candidates.
2. Describe how advances in recognition of rejection and immunosuppressive drug therapy have improved patient survival.
3. Discuss common psychophysiologic problems experienced after transplant surgery and appropriate interventions.
4. Evaluate nursing strategies related to monitoring for rejection, infection, and complications of immunosuppressive drug therapy.
5. Analyze common patient and family responses to the cardiac transplant experience.
6. Use research findings to assist patients in improving their quality of life after transplant.

During the last decade, cardiac transplantation has evolved into an accepted therapeutic intervention for selected patients with end-stage cardiac failure. The person who undergoes a transplant is taken through an incredible series of events. The outcome of these events is that they may move from terminal illness and class IV cardiac function according to the New York Heart Association (NYHA) to class I cardiac function with a good prognosis. This journey, however, is accompanied by physical and psychologic perils that require nursing intervention during every step. The process of transplantation demands an intense commitment from the patient, family, and transplant team if the desired results are to be achieved.

HISTORY OF CARDIAC TRANSPLANTATION

The development of cardiac transplantation technology has not always proceeded smoothly. The first successful human heart transplant was performed in 1967 by Dr. Christian Barnard in Capetown, South Africa.[18] After this event, many cardiac surgery centers began transplant programs. Between 1968 and 1970, approximately 100 heart transplants were performed in 17 countries.[70] Enthusiasm for this new surgery quickly waned when manipulation of the immune system and treatment of postoperative infection proved difficult. Patients frequently died of rejection or infection, and survival statistics were poor. A few recipients survived, a fact that encouraged further research at a few

centers. Most centers stopped their cardiac transplant programs during the 1970s and concentrated their efforts on corrective cardiac surgery.[68]

During the 1980s interest in this surgical approach to terminal heart disease was renewed. By this time, the transvenous endomyocardial biopsy technique was available to diagnose rejection at early stages when it could be most easily and successfully treated. With advances in immunology, the rejection process was better understood. The drug cyclosporine became available; it was approved for general use in 1983. Cyclosporine simplified the postoperative course of most transplant recipients and allowed earlier discharge from the hospital. During that same period, there were also advances in organ procurement and preservation, which contributed to surgical success. More recently, lower chronic steroid maintenance doses, improved diagnostic techniques for infections, new antimicrobial agents, and better patient selection criteria have continued to improve postoperative survival.

During the mid-1980s, the number of cardiac transplant procedures performed in the United States and other countries again began to rise. The Registry of the International Society for Heart Transplantation reports the number seems to be leveling off at approximately 2400 transplants per year.[33] The fact that the numbers are no longer increasing reflects the limited number of donors. The number of potential recipients continues to grow at a dramatic pace. According to the United Network for

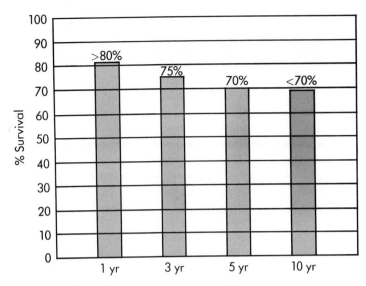

FIG. 18-1 Survival after cardiac transplantation. **Average 1-year, 3-year, 5-year and 10-year actuarial survival reported after cardiac transplantation.**

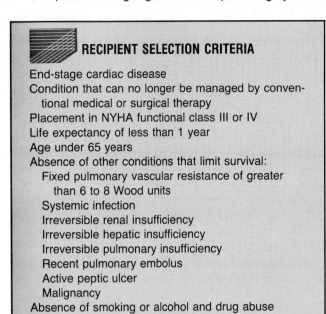

RECIPIENT SELECTION CRITERIA

End-stage cardiac disease
Condition that can no longer be managed by conventional medical or surgical therapy
Placement in NYHA functional class III or IV
Life expectancy of less than 1 year
Age under 65 years
Absence of other conditions that limit survival:
    Fixed pulmonary vascular resistance of greater than 6 to 8 Wood units
    Systemic infection
    Irreversible renal insufficiency
    Irreversible hepatic insufficiency
    Irreversible pulmonary insufficiency
    Recent pulmonary embolus
    Active peptic ulcer
    Malignancy
Absence of smoking or alcohol and drug abuse
Compliant, well-motivated patient

Organ Sharing (UNOS), there are approximately 1300 individuals waiting for a heart donor at all times.[67] Statistics vary, but between 25% and 40% of these candidates do not survive the wait for a donor.[7]

The number of transplant centers continues to rise. In the United States, 12 centers had cardiac transplant programs in 1983. This number rose to approximately 150 in 1990. This rapid rise has generated controversy related to whether all centers perform enough procedures to maintain proficiency.[33] Hospitals contend that without a transplant program they cannot be recognized as a leading center in cardiovascular surgery now that transplantation is a standard of care. Since 1987, Medicare coverage for cardiac transplant procedures has been granted to a limited number of programs approved by the Health Care Financing Administration.

Current survival statistics are shown in Figure 18-1. In a population of patients considered terminal before surgery, the 1-year survival averages 80% in U.S. centers. The 3-year survival rate averages 75%.[6] Statistics are available on a limited number of 5- and 10-year survivors. Their survival rate is reported to be approximately 70%.[33] Patients who die tend to do so during the first critical 30 days after the transplant. The most common causes of death are infection, rejection, and cardiac failure. The recipients at greatest risk are those who deteriorate in the hospital before transplant. According to the Registry, patients who require a staged transplant with ventricular assist devices or a total artificial heart may have only a 50% chance of leaving the hospital. As more sophisticated devices become available, it is thought that these "bridge-to-transplant" individuals will achieve improved survival rates.

RECIPIENT SELECTION CRITERIA

With an increasing shortage of donor organs, recipients must undergo a careful screening process to determine the need for transplant and to determine whether there are any concomitant conditions that might limit survival. As shown in the box, patients referred for evaluation are generally in the NYHA class III or IV with end-stage heart disease. Their life expectancy may be only 6 months to a year. Symptoms include fatigue, dyspnea, and weakness. They have usually experienced repeated episodes of congestive heart failure that can no longer be managed effectively through conventional treatment. They have global ventricular dysfunction with a left ventricular ejection fraction of less than 20% and sometimes as low as 5%.[50]

The majority of patients have congestive cardiomyopathy or ischemic cardiomyopathy (see Chapter 14). *Congestive cardiomyopathy* may follow a viral infection or may be idiopathic. *Ischemic cardiomyopathy* is associated with end-stage coronary artery disease. Fewer potential candidates have terminal valvular heart disease or congenital heart disease. Pediatric candidates may have congenital problems, but only 10% to 20% of children with congenital heart disease are potential candidates for transplant. Children may also develop cardiomyopathy from a viral infection.[38] Other causes of cardiomyopathy may include cancer chemotherapy or postpartum cardiomyopathy. The average age of patients referred for transplant is 43.8 years. Ages range from newborn to patients well into their 60s. About 83% of all cardiac transplant candidates are men.[33]

There are a number of absolute and relative contraindications to cardiac transplant. A patient's overall condition and other vital organs must be stable enough to withstand major surgery and the potent immunosuppressive drugs administered thereafter. Major contraindications to transplant include irreversible pulmonary hypertension (pulmonary vascular resistance greater than 6 to 8 Wood units), active infection, irreversible renal dysfunction, irreversible liver dysfunction, advanced chronic obstructive pulmonary disease, recent pulmonary embolism, active peptic ulcer disease, malignancy, diverticulitis, peripheral vascular disease, cerebrovascular disease, type I diabetes mellitus, and drug or alcohol abuse.[19,25]

The nurse begins the evaluation by taking a careful patient history and physical examination. Possible contraindications to transplant such as a history of cancer are investigated before proceeding with a full evaluation. Patients may be admitted to the hospital for the evaluation to facilitate its completion. Alternatively the evaluation can be completed on an outpatient basis for patients who are physically able to return for a series of tests and appointments. The evaluation is usually coordinated by a clinical transplant coordinator. The evaluation team may include transplant surgeons, cardiologists, an infectious disease consultant, pulmonologist, nephrologist, gastroenterologist, psychologist, psychiatrist, social worker, financial counselor, nurses, and others.

Routine preoperative blood work is done. In addition, tissue typing and screening for cytotoxic antibodies is performed. The tissue typing identifies the patient's *human leukocyte antigens* (HLAs). In cardiac transplantation the HLA typing is mainly of academic interest because there is no attempt to match donors and recipients according to their HLAs. Research continues regarding the importance of HLA matching to cardiac graft survival, but there is no conclusive evidence that it would enhance survival.

The *cytotoxic antibody* screening is carried out by mixing the patient's serum with a random panel of leukocytes containing known antigens. The leukocytes are observed for a reaction, during which they are destroyed in the presence of complement.[51] This reaction with some of the typed leukocytes indicates that cytotoxic antibodies are present in the potential recipient's serum. Candidates who have received blood transfusions or previous organ transplants or women who have had pregnancies are most likely to develop cytotoxic antibodies. Ideally a candidate's *panel for reactive antibodies* (PRA) is 0%, meaning that they have no identifiable preformed antibodies. Patients with a PRA greater than 10% will need a *prospective lymphocyte crossmatch* with a donor to test for compatibility and minimize the chance for immediate rejection of the transplanted heart.[50] A high PRA may preclude transplantation for some candidates. Patients without reactive antibodies may have transplants performed without this crossmatch procedure, facilitating organ recovery during long-distance procurement.[9]

A complete cardiac evaluation, including right and left heart catheterization and coronary angiography, is per-

formed to determine, as much as possible, the patient's diagnosis and prognosis. *Preoperative endomyocardial biopsy* has been of some value and may be useful in cases of active myocarditis or to determine a precise cause of cardiomyopathy such as amyloid heart disease.

Catheterization of the right side of the heart determines whether patients have developed high pulmonary vascular resistance (PVR) as a consequence of cardiac failure. The PVR is considered prohibitively high when it reaches 6 to 8 Wood units or a mean pulmonary artery pressure greater than 40 to 50 mm Hg. Irreversibly elevated PVR can result in acute failure of a donor heart that is not accustomed to pumping against high resistance. Attempts are made to manipulate the PVR with nitroprusside or other vasodilators when pressures are high. Some patients with high PVR may be candidates for heart-lung transplantation, depending on their age and disease process.

Coronary angiography is usually performed during the catheterization. Occasionally a patient with coronary artery disease and a low ejection fraction can be effectively treated with coronary bypass surgery rather than transplant. A ventriculogram may be done to determine the ejection fraction and analyze ventricular wall motion. Alternatively a gaited heart scan or echocardiogram is done to assess these parameters, especially in the patient with renal dysfunction.

An infectious disease evaluation is often included in the workup. An occult infection predisposes the patient to postoperative septic episodes, which may be very difficult to treat.[70] If patients have fever, positive cultures (blood, urine, or sputum), pulmonary infiltrates, or other signs of infection, they will not be candidates for transplantation until the infection is resolved. Blood is routinely analyzed to determine previous exposure to significant infections such as cytomegalovirus (CMV), Epstein-Barr virus, hepatitis, toxoplasmosis, human immunodeficiency virus (HIV), and others. These preoperative studies are particularly important in the differential diagnosis of postoperative infections because patients may have reactivation of a previous infection or may acquire a donor-transmitted disease.

Skin tests may be applied to determine immunocompetence and exposure to diseases such as tuberculosis and fungal disease. Vaccines to prevent influenza, pneumococcal pneumonia, and hepatitis may be administered. A dental evaluation is carried out to ensure that teeth are in good repair and that no teeth are abscessed.

Renal, hepatic, and pulmonary function tests are performed. If there is question of irreversible damage of these organs, specialists may be consulted for a more extensive evaluation. Patients with severe renal and hepatic dysfunction will not withstand postoperative cyclosporine therapy and will be at risk of dying from multiple organ failure. Patients with chronic obstructive pulmonary disease (COPD) are at risk of ventilatory failure and chronic pulmonary infection after surgery. Recent pulmonary embolism is a temporary contraindication because it predisposes patients to pulmonary abscess formation after transplant.[50] Patients who have recovered from pulmonary embolism can undergo transplantation.

In patients with arteriosclerosis, the evaluation may include testing for cerebrovascular disease and peripheral vascular disease. These are potential contraindications to transplant because they may limit postoperative quality of life and survival.

Careful attention is given to the patient's nutritional status. Patients with cachexia often do not survive. Obesity can also be a relative contraindication because cardiac function may improve with weight loss. Obesity can become a greater problem after surgery when the patient receives steroids. Very heavy patients also have little chance of finding a large enough donor heart.

Other medical conditions are contraindications for transplantation. Steroids are known to exacerbate peptic ulcer disease and make the management of blood glucose levels difficult in diabetic patients. Type I diabetes mellitus is considered a contraindication when patients exhibit a microangiopathic condition and other complications of diabetes.

Psychosocial evaluation is also important because cardiac transplantation requires a lifelong commitment by the patient. Prospective candidates may be interviewed by a social worker, psychologist, or psychiatrist. The major concerns are related to competence, compliance, and any problems with drug or alcohol abuse. A recipient (or parent) must understand the complicated medical regimen required after transplant. The patient must be compliant because postoperative survival depends on adherence to medications, diagnostic testing, and lifestyle modifications. Previous problems with illegal drugs or alcohol are contraindications. Psychosis also is a relative contraindication.

A patient who is well motivated is better equipped to cope with the physical and psychologic challenges of life after a transplant. A strong family support system is also a positive factor and usually indicates a positive outcome.[19]

A dilemma in transplantation is whether candidates should be excluded on only psychologic grounds. Evaluation of psychologic strengths and weaknesses is difficult in patients with low cardiac output. Their intelligence, coping ability, and personality may be adversely affected by inadequate cerebral blood flow. Their wellness behaviors may turn out to be quite different from their illness behaviors. It is necessary to interview the patient's family and the patient separately to develop a good understanding of strengths and coping abilities. Nurses play an important role in the psychosocial assessment because they can observe a candidate over time. They often detect verbal or behavioral factors important to consideration for transplant. Exclusion of patients on only psychosocial grounds is somewhat subjective and is seldom used except for severe problems that affect compliance.[19]

The financial aspects of heart transplantation cannot be ignored. The hospital financial counselor assists in determining whether the patient has insurance coverage for surgery and postoperative care. Because cardiac transplant surgery costs over $115,000, excluding drugs and diagnostic testing, financial planning must be done before the surgery.[68] To be placed on the waiting list, patients may need to have insurance coverage or a certain amount of money, depending on the center's requirements. In addition to these initial expenses the cost of medications and routine follow-up care averages $10,000 a year, necessitating the need for long-range financial planning.

Patients and their families are under a tremendous amount of stress while going through the evaluation. For some the thought of cardiac transplantation is so threatening that it has taken them months to decide to proceed with the evaluation. Patient education is extremely important throughout evaluation. The patient's clinical transplant coordinator and staff nurses are an important part of the team at this time. Before the evaluation begins, patients need to understand the diagnostic tests and consultations that will be required. They also need to know about individual problems, such as diabetes or COPD, that will receive additional attention during evaluation.

It helps for patients and families to be aware that until the evaluation is complete, the transplant team's recommendations are unknown. For some patients, transplant will be recommended. Others are told that they will probably need a transplant eventually, but that their condition does not warrant it yet. Still others are told that they will function better and for a longer period with medical therapy. Nurses may help explain test results as they become known so that there are fewer surprises at the end of the evaluation. Being "turned down" can be a devastating disappointment, to the extent that we have seen a few patients die within hours of receiving the news. Good communication can minimize disappointment so that patients are not deprived of hope.

The transplant evaluation also allows patients and families to evaluate the procedure and team. Patients need to realize that they must critically examine the option of transplant to find out whether it is what they want. They need to realize that life after transplant will never be like it was before they became ill. Potential candidates need to talk with one or two patients who have undergone transplantation to hear about their experience and their lives after transplant. Some patients choose not to go on the transplant list. It is necessary to recognize the right of patients to refuse treatment. Frequently their families pressure them to undergo transplantation. Nurses can facilitate open communication between patients, families, and the evaluation team so that everyone is satisfied that the best decision for the individual has been reached.

Nurses may also assist patients who are undergoing medical therapy to be aware that this option may afford them a satisfactory quality of life. It is posssible for some patients with cardiomyopathy to get along well on medical therapy.[69]

For patients who become transplant candidates, some continue to have difficulty accepting their diagnosis and the need for this radical surgery. Newly diagnosed and younger patients seem to have the most difficulty. They may need time to work through the losses and issues that have changed their lives. Patients who have had more illness experience appear to have less trouble accepting the situation. Eventually candidates reach the realization that transplant offers the best hope for survival. They then begin to refocus their energy into planning for surgery and life thereafter. They may list who they want to be present at the hospital during their surgery and ask whether a staff member will take pictures during the operation.

Throughout the evaluation, nurses review and clarify information, teach about life after the transplant, and promote acceptance of the diagnosis. Nurse coordinators are usually part of the patient-selection committee, which meets periodically to review information on prospective candidates to determine whether they meet the center's selection criteria. On the committee's recommendation, potential candidates are placed on the waiting list.

WAITING FOR A DONOR

When patients are placed on the transplant center's waiting list, they also are listed on the Organ Procurement and Transplantation Network. This national computerized network is based in Richmond, Virginia, and is currently managed by the United Network for Organ Sharing. Over the years, the criteria and procedure for the allocation of hearts has varied. Since 1989 there have been two categories of urgency for patients awaiting cardiac transplantation:

1. Status I: Patients in intensive care units requiring cardiac or pulmonary assistance with intraaortic balloon pumps, ventricular assist devices, total artificial hearts, ventilators, and/or inotropic agents to maintain cardiac output

2. Status II: All other patients

In addition to medical urgency criteria, hearts are distributed locally when possible to minimize the ischemic time because a short ischemic time is associated with a favorable outcome.[33] Preferably the heart will go to a recipient with an ABO-identical blood group, but if there are no local recipients with that blood group, the heart may go to a candidate with an ABO-compatible blood group. The Rh factor is not considered important in this determination. It is also necessary that there be a size match. The donor's weight should be at least 80% of the recipient's because the heart must function immediately to support the circulation. Often a larger heart is acceptable.[38] Another consideration is the lymphocyte crossmatch results. A positive donor-recipient crossmatch contraindicates transplantation. After these considerations are applied to the list of candidates, if an organ is compatible with more than one candidate, it is generally allocated to the person who has been waiting the longest.

During the waiting period, patients are discharged from the hospital when possible. They are usually assigned a pager so that they can be reached quickly if they leave their home. Candidates who live a great distance from the transplant center may have to relocate to be available for the prospective surgery.

Nursing management during the waiting period

The waiting period can be a very difficult time for patients and families. As the number of potential recipients increases, nurses have become increasingly involved in their care. Patients wait for weeks and often months, depending on the availability of donor organs. Even status I patients may wait for months while on mechanical assist devices.

Some candidates can maintain a fairly good level of activity and have few signs and symptoms of congestive heart failure. For many, however, heart failure progresses as they wait, and symptoms become increasingly difficult to control.

Decreased cardiac output

The signs and symptoms of congestive heart failure often have been a problem for patients before they become transplant candidates. As time goes on, patients become increasingly troubled by fatigue, dyspnea, cough, edema, syncope, and abdominal pain. Controlling the symptoms requires increasingly intensive medical management.[14] Digoxin, oral diuretics, and afterload-reducing agents are used first. Intravenous diuretics, administered more than once a day, may be necessary because fluid volume excess and edema tend to develop from inadequate cardiac output and renal perfusion. Respiratory insufficiency may result from pulmonary congestion. Continuous oxygen therapy may be necessary at home or in the hospital.

Inotropic agents such as dopamine or dobutamine may be added for renal perfusion and for maintenance of cardiac output. Patients requiring continuous infusion may have to stay in the hospital, but some patients requiring intermittent or continuous infusions can be managed on an outpatient basis or in the home.[17] Patients who do not require frequent intravenous inotropic agents may have to enter the hospital occasionally for therapy. Candidates may reach the point where they cannot be managed with these standard measures and may need to go to the intensive care unit for the remainder of the waiting period. It is often necessary to monitor pulmonary artery pressure and cardiac output while attempting inotropic support with other agents such as amrinone. Candidates may deteriorate to the point where mechanical support is instituted in an attempt to bridge them to transplant.[25]

Life-threatening dysrhythmias may also complicate the clinical situation in patients with end-stage heart disease.

Rhythm problems are difficult to manage because anti-dysrhythmic agents are not well tolerated because of side effects such as gastrointestinal distress or adverse effects on contractility. Some patients go through electrophysiology testing and have an automatic implanted cardioverter-defibrillator (AICD) implanted before the transplant (see Appendix D.). Although the AICD may provide essential therapy for life-threatening dysrhythmias, the resultant adhesions adjacent to the AICD patches may complicate transplant surgery.

Thrombi may form in the chambers of the dilated and poorly contracting heart or in the deep veins, placing the patient at risk of thromboembolism. Candidates may be placed on anticoagulant therapy with heparin or warfarin. Anticoagulation must be carefully monitored because many of these individuals have liver dysfunction that may lead to unstable coagulation parameters and increase the risk of bleeding. Anticoagulation is kept at a minimum to prepare for surgery.

Altered nutrition

Patients awaiting transplant frequently have abdominal problems that impair oral intake. Passive liver congestion results in abdominal pain and loss of appetite. Multiple oral medications also tend to decrease the appetite. Dyspnea and fatigue may interfere with the ability to eat. Poor nutritional status can become a problem and predisposes candidates to infection.[24] An infection may then rule out the option of transplant. A poor nutritional state also can complicate the recovery from surgery.

Nursing care is directed toward enhancing patients' nutritional status. An evaluation by a clinical dietitian helps identify patients with cardiac cachexia, anorexia, and impaired absorption. Efforts are made to supply desired foods within the sodium-restricted diet and to add vitamins and nutritional supplements as tolerated. Families are encouraged to bring food from home because patients may find it far more palatable than hospital food. Tube feedings may be indicated in patients too weak to eat. Total parenteral nutrition is usually avoided because of the risk of line sepsis.

Altered role performance

Role changes and reversals are almost inevitable in patients with end-stage heart disease.[46] Candidates frequently cannot carry out their duties in the family or community. Few are able to maintain employment. Because of increasing dependency, these patients may become irritable and self-centered. Some family relationships may become closer, whereas others may deteriorate. Patients and families are unable to plan for the future.

Some candidates may be unable to successfully adapt to the sickness role. They may demonstrate obvious personality changes and may distance themselves from their families.[30] They may also begin to distance themselves from the staff. Through their behavior and words, they withdraw, possibly because they find it painful and exhausting to maintain relationships.

An important goal of nursing care is to assist families to understand and cope with the unsatisfying interactions generated by these circumstances. Support groups and individual counseling may help. Caring for these patients may be exhausting for the staff and families.[58] As patients' conditions worsen, everyone may feel frustrated and inadequate.

High risk for ineffective coping

Patients awaiting transplant have already had to cope with their diagnosis and deteriorating health. As they wait for a donor heart, their anxiety levels may increase, and they may find it very difficult to cope with their uncertain future. As patients psychologically prepare for most surgeries, they know the date and time, so they can begin a "count down" during which they begin to feel prepared for the experience. When there is no surgery date, this process cannot begin.

Some candidates exhibit approach and avoidance behavior, asking why a heart has not been found and then leaving their home without their pager or even leaving town without notifying the transplant team.

Positive coping strategies such as seeking factual information should be encouraged. Patients may verbalize fears about receiving the heart of another. They fear that a new heart will change them physically or psychologically. Emotions are associated with the heart in literature, popular music, and conversation. Patients need to hear factual information regarding the heart as a muscular pump. Organ donation can be compared with blood transfusions in that a donor's personality, gender, and race are not relevant.

Candidates may need help with maintaining relationships with family and friends. Nurses can assist in this process by relaxing visiting restrictions to allow visits from children or even pets.

As time goes on, patients may find it difficult to maintain hope. Some may vacillate between hope and despair. They begin to fear that donors will not be located in time. Some begin a personal search, monitoring news reports for accidents that might yield a donor. Others are uncomfortable with the thought that they are waiting for someone else to die and may become clinically depressed. Their feelings regarding these issues need to be discussed openly. They also need to realize that they share these feelings with other candidates.

Specific strategies can be used to promote hope and decrease anxiety. Patients and families need to hear success stories. Visits from recovered transplant patients can be especially helpful. When possible, hospitalized candidates occasionally should be given passes to leave the hospital. To promote physical and psychological well-being, they should be encouraged to be as active and independent as possible. Participation in hobbies or projects can promote a positive self-image, although a short attention span may limit the scope of diversional activities. A care conference can help in modifying stressors and meeting individual needs. Candidates and the transplant team may experience feelings of powerlessness during the wait because neither has control over donor availability. Working together to meet patients' needs can be therapeutic.

Knowledge deficit

Preoperative teaching can be challenging for transplant coordinators and staff nurses. Patients tend to focus on the transplant and on surviving and may not place much importance on the information provided regarding life after transplant. Their low cardiac output may impair concentration and memory. Because of these factors, it is important to involve the family in the teaching and to limit the information given during any one session. For patients enduring a long wait, it is necessary to periodically review the postoperative information to avoid disastrous misconceptions after surgery.[71]

Teaching is a collaborative effort involving physicians, the transplant coordinator, staff nurses, and other team members. The outcome of this process is very important because patients' quality and length of life after surgery depend on knowledge of and adherance to the medical regimen and lifestyle modifications. The box below outlines major topics to be addressed with patients and families.

Donor selection criteria

When a donor heart becomes available, the organ procurement agency for the transplant center will notify the transplant surgeon. The heart is recovered from a heart-beating donor with a diagnosis of brain death who has been maintained on organ support systems. Often the donor is a young person who was involved in a motor vehicle or other accident that resulted in terminal brain injury. Generally the organ recovery surgery involves multiple teams recovering multiple organs, most commonly heart, lung, liver, pancreas, and kidneys. In addition, tissues such as cornea, skin, and bone may be recovered.

Potential cardiac donors are carefully screened because adequate heart function is needed immediately after implantation. As shown in the box, p. 595, donor criteria generally include an age limit of under 50.[70] There is a trend toward using older donors to maximize the use of donor organs. Donors older than 40 may have coronary angiography performed to rule out coronary artery disease.

TEACHING THE HEART TRANSPLANT CANDIDATE

Before surgery the patient and family will:
Understand the clinical condition requiring transplantation
Verbalize an understanding of the planned surgery:
  Average waiting time
  Listing of candidates according to status
  Notification of patient and family when a donor is available
  Preoperative protocol
  Orthotopic versus heterotopic transplantation
  Survival rates
  Quality of life after transplant
  Financial considerations
Demonstrate knowledge of the organ donation system:
  Evaluation of potential donors
  Definition of brain death
  Conditions that result in brain death
  Consent from donor family
  Long-distance procurement
  Possibility of canceling surgery during donor evaluation
Verbalize knowledge of postoperative care:
  Intensive care unit, usual equipment, and hemodynamic monitoring

The rejection process:
  Basic pathophysiologic condition
  Detection through endomyocardial biopsy
  Prevention through immunosuppressive drugs
  Treatment through augmented immunosuppression
  Basic action and common side effects of drugs: cyclosporine, prednisone, azathioprine, antithymocyte globulin (ATG), and OKT3
Risk of infection:
  Basic precautions taken by staff, patient, and family
  Hospital procedure for protective isolation
Awareness of late complications such as graft atherosclerosis and increased risk of cancer
Usual schedule for biopsies and clinic visits
Demonstrate knowledge of lifestyle recommendations after transplant:
No smoking
Low-cholesterol, no-added-salt diet
Exercise regimen
Lifelong medication
Close medical supervision

Often a cardiologist is involved in the donor evaluation to determine that the electrocardiogram (ECG), echocardiogram, cardiac enzymes, chest x-ray film, and other indices of cardiac function are normal. Contraindications to cardiac donation may include cardiac arrest, hemodynamic instability, prolonged hypotension, significant inotropic support, a history of cardiac disease, cardiac contusion from trauma, or extensive chest trauma. Other general contraindications to organ donation such as sepsis, positive serologic tests for transmissible disease, diabetes mellitus, or cancer other than a primary brain tumor may rule out donation.[62] The final decision regarding the suitability of the donor heart is made by the cardiac surgeon recovering the heart. Although it is a disappointment to the patient, the patient's family, and the transplant team to turn down a donor, a heart with poor wall motion or other obvious problems carries with it a high risk of failure in the immediate postoperative period.

Nurses are frequently involved in the identification and management of a multiple-organ donor. Donors are a scarce resource because few deaths result in potentially suitable donors. It is estimated that under 2000 *multiple-organ donors* become available per year in the United States.[7]

When brain death has been declared and consent has been obtained from the donor's family, an organ procurement coordinator from the local organ procurement agency will be involved in placing the organs according to national and local guidelines. During this time, careful donor maintenance protocols maintain all transplantable organs in optimal condition. Steps are taken to avoid and manage common problems such as hypotension, hypoxia, electrolyte imbalance, diabetes insipidus, hypothermia, hyperglycemia, and coagulopathic condition.[62] Aggressive fluid replacement is often necessary to maintain a systolic blood pressure above 90 mm Hg and adequate tissue perfusion because autoregulation of vascular tone may be lost. Inotropic support with vasopressors such as dopamine is often necessary, but doses of dopamine greater than 10 micrograms (μg)/kg/min may indicate poor left ventricular function.[28] Arterial blood gas levels are monitored frequently, and mechanical ventilation is adjusted to ensure adequate oxygenation of vital organs. Body temperature is regulated with warming and cooling blankets when autoregulation has been lost. Aseptic technique is strictly maintained to prevent infection in the donor. Prophylactic antibiotics are usually administered.

Because donors tend to be unstable, arrangements are made for organ recovery to take place as soon as possible. An established nursing procedure for contacting the local organ procurement organization when a potential donor is identified can greatly facilitate the process. Procurement coordinators can then assist with obtaining the consent, managing the donor, placing the organs, and coordinating the organ recovery surgery.

Donor organ procurement

The donor heart is recovered by using the techniques of other standard cardiac operations. After a median sternotomy, the heart is arrested through the infusion of cold myocardial protective solution into the aortic root. This high-potassium solution is designed to arrest and protect the heart during the ischemic period. Topical cooling is also used to lower the temperature of the heart rapidly. Adequate myocardial protection is necessary to preserve myocardial function. The high-potassium, high-glucose *cardioplegia solution* is designed to halt high-energy phosphate consumption by the myocardium, to limit myocardial edema, and to supply substrate for anaerobic metabolic respiration.[70] The rapid lowering of temperature reduces the organ's metabolic rate and oxygen demand. This increases the heart's tolerance of ischemia and anoxia.[13]

When the heart has been emptied and cooled, the inferior vena cava, aorta, pulmonary artery, and pulmonary veins are transsected. The heart is then removed from the chest.[70] After excision, the heart is further cooled by a series of iced saline washes. It is placed in a sterile plastic bag and stored in a picnic cooler surrounded by ice. This static cold preservation method is most common, but dynamic warm preservation methods and new myocardial preservation solutions are being used on an experimental basis. It is hoped that a preservation system that will extend the *ischemic time* past the 4- to 6-hour limit will be found.

With the current technology, successful heart function is associated with a short ischemic time, and most teams aim for a total ischemic time of less than 4 hours. The total ischemic time is the time elapsed from when the cross clamp is placed on the donor's aorta before infusion of cardioplegia until the time the cross clamp is opened after implantation in the recipient. Timing is facilitated by fre-

---

CARDIAC DONOR CRITERIA

Diagnosis of brain death
Age less than 50
Negative history of heart disease
Absence of heart trauma
Absence of prolonged hypotension or arrest
Absence of active infection
Absence of serologic evidence of transmissible disease
Absence of malignancy other than a primary brain tumor
Absence of diabetes
Normal clinical results of cardiac examination and echocardiogram

quent communication between donor and recipient teams and careful planning to minimize travel time. Obviously the ideal situation is to have the donor at the same institution as the recipient, but this does not happen often.

IMPLANTATION OF THE TRANSPLANTED HEART

The recipient is admitted to the hospital, if not already hospitalized, as soon as the transplant team is aware of a potential donor and is prepared for surgery and taken to the operating room. By the time the recovery team arrives in the operating room with the donor heart, the recipient has been placed on cardiopulmonary bypass. The native heart is then arrested and removed for the standard *orthotopic cardiac transplant*. As shown in Fig. 18-2, this procedure involves removing the entire native heart with exception of the upper atria, and then implanting the donor heart in the normal position. Alternatively, *heterotopic* or "piggy-back" *transplants* may occasionally be performed; these leave the native heart in place and add the second heart into the right side of the chest. Survival statistics are better with the orthotopic technique, but the heterotopic method may be considered in patients with high pulmonary vascular resistance or a mismatch in sizes between donor and recipient.[45] It may also be considered when imminent death of the recipient is anticipated unless transplant is performed.

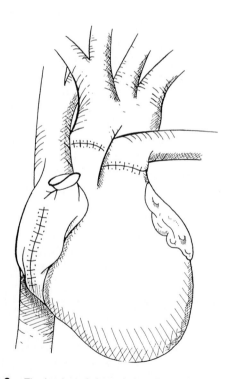

FIG. 18-2 The implanted donor heart. During orthotopic cardiac transplantation, the native heart is excised and the donor heart implanted in the normal position.

Implantation of the donor heart is performed through four anastamoses that connect the left atria, right atria, aorta, and pulmonary arteries of the donor and recipient. After the release of the aortic cross clamp, inotropic agents such as isoproterenol, dopamine, dobutamine, or epinephrine may be used to treat right-sided heart failure, improve cardiac output, and reinstitute sinus rhythm. Countershock is performed when necessary. Atrial or ventricular pacemakers may be required to maintain an adequate heart rate. The rewarming and recovery time may vary. Rapid recovery time is expected when ischemic time is short. The condition of the donor and presence of pulmonary hypertension in the recipient also affect recovery time.[70] In patients who have had previous heart surgery or a mechanical device implanted, the operation may be technically more difficult because of the presence of adhesions.

When the heart is ejecting vigorously, the patient is weaned from cardiopulmonary bypass and decannulated. Chest tubes are placed and the chest is observed for adequate hemostasis. Because catheters for hemodynamic monitoring increase the risk of infection, pulmonary artery lines may not be placed after surgery. In other patients, it will be necessary to monitor for increased pulmonary or systemic vascular resistance and decreased cardiac output and index. Inotropic support commonly includes isoproterenol to increase heart rate and contractility and decrease pulmonary vascular resistance. Low doses of dopamine and nitroprusside or other agents used to reduce afterload may also be indicated.

If the donor heart fails to function adequately, epinephrine, amrinone, or other agents may be used. Prostaglandin E_1 may be infused to dilate the pulmonary artery and thereby enhance right ventricular function. Right-sided heart failure may occur in the operating room or later and can progress to include left-sided heart failure. Occasionally a right ventricular assist device or biventricular assist devices, as well as an intraaortic balloon pump, may be required to support a failing transplanted heart. Failure of the donor heart is a very serious situation because it is rarely possible to find another donor in a short period of time. With mechanical support such as ventricular assist devices, it is possible in some instances for recovery of the transplanted heart to take place over a few days. Fortunately most hearts recover readily from the cold ischemia.

During the perioperative period, nurses provide information and emotional support to patients and families. When patients are being prepared for surgery, they need to be informed of the progress of the recovery team. The nurses also may want to review information related to intraoperative and postoperative procedures. During the surgery, families should be given periodic reports on patient status. Families are often very anxious due to the long wait for a donor and the serious and unusual nature of the surgery. Providing factual information and emotional support enhances their ability to cope with the situation. It is particularly important to explain problems such as bleeding or low cardiac output that may prolong patients' time in the operating room.

IMMEDIATE POSTOPERATIVE CARE

The recipient is taken to a private room in the intensive care unit. *Modified protective isolation procedures* are used; they usually consist of gowns, masks, and careful hand-washing. Studies suggest that strict isolation procedures offer no benefit over masks and handwashing and serve only to restrict patient accessibility and increase costs.[27,34]

Nursing care is similar to the care for other cardiovascular surgical patients. However, some problems occur more frequently in transplant recipients. In the early postoperative period, there may be instability resulting from right ventricular or biventricular failure. Myocardial depression may develop because of prolonged ischemia, inadequate preservation, or hypotension associated with bleeding. Right ventricular dysfunction may result from elevated pulmonary vascular resistance because the normal heart is not accustomed to pumping against the higher pressure.[11] In addition, the heart is denervated because the vagus nerve and other nerve connections are severed at the time of the surgery. The *denervated heart* lacks the neural feedback that normally assists in the response to hemodynamic stresses such as changes in volume. Without sympathetic innervation to provide adrenergic mechanisms that increase cardiac output, an increase in heart rate depends on the inotropic and chronotropic effects of circulating catecholamines released from noncardiac sites. Adequate preload and catecholamines are the only mechanisms available to increase heart rate and contractility.[20]

Because of these factors, careful attention is given to the hemodynamic variables of preload, afterload, and contractility. Volume is replaced as necessary. Vasoactive drugs such as isoproterenol, dopamine, and nitroprusside are adjusted carefully to maintain optimal cardiac output and index. Serial echocardiograms may be performed to assess ventricular wall motion. Because of the positive chronotropic and inotropic effects, isoproterenol is usually administered intraoperatively and continued for several days. If a thermodilution catheter is not used because of the increased risk of infection, cardiac output is monitored through serial determinations of mixed venous oxygen saturations of blood drawn from a central venous catheter.

Postoperative ECGs often show P waves originating from the donor and recipient atria because part of the native atria remain after implantation of the donor heart (Fig. 18-3). Although there are double electrical impulses, the P waves from the remnant native atria are not conducted across the suture line.[4]

Transient bradycardia may occur after transplant because of ischemia or intraoperative trauma.[11] Chronotropic drugs and atrial pacing may be used to increase heart rate to 90 to 110 beats per minute and optimize cardiac output. Occasionally, patients require artificial pacing for several weeks before the sinus node recovers. Efforts are made to avoid permanent pacemakers because of the risk of infection and potential interference of the transvenous pacing catheter with subsequent endomyocardial biopsy procedures. In addition to temporary artificial pacing, isoproterenol may be used initially. Later, patients may receive orally medications with a chronotropic side effect (e.g., theophylline).

Another potential problem is postoperative hemorrhage. Cardiac transplant recipients are at increased risk of bleeding due to many factors. Preoperative passive liver congestion and administration of anticoagulants may interfere with the production of procoagulants by the liver, resulting in inadequate postoperative hemostasis. In addition, many transplant recipients have had previous heart surgery, and the dense adhesions may increase the risk of bleeding. Meticulous hemostasis is performed in the operating room. Transfusion of blood and components is avoided unless absolutely necessary because of the risk of disease transmission. When homologous blood products are used, CMV-negative blood is preferred to avoid potential exposure to a viral syndrome that can be fatal in immunosuppressed patients. Autotransfusion of shed mediastinal blood may be used to avoid homologous transfusion.

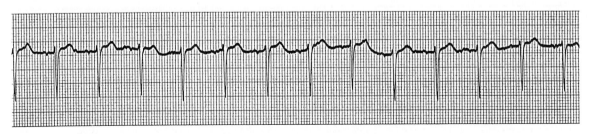

FIG. 18-3 Postoperative ECG with two P waves. The recipient ECG may show two P waves. The P waves originating from the native atria are not conducted across the suture line.

Postoperative respiratory care is a major priority so that pulmonary complications can be avoided. Preoperative restrictive deficits resulting from cardiac failure and pleural effusions are common.[11] Generalized weakness and elevated PVR may prolong the need for mechanical ventilation. When possible, patients are weaned from mechanical ventilation and extubated during the first 24 hours after surgery. After extubation, activity and vigorous pulmonary therapy are initiated. After transfer from the intensive care unit, chest x-ray studies are performed twice a week to monitor for pulmonary problems. Lung auscultation, coughing, and deep breathing exercises are performed every 2 to 4 hours.

Renal function is carefully monitored throughout the postoperative course. Prerenal azotemia is common before transplant and may be complicated by the surgery, anesthesia, and administration of cyclosporine in the perioperative period. Urine output is maintained at 30 ml/hr in adults by fluid administration and diuretics. Serum creatinine and blood urea nitrogen (BUN) levels are measured at least once a day during the first few days after surgery. Postoperative administration of cyclosporine may be withheld until renal function is well established.

As the recipient enters the recovery phase, nursing and medical management focus on the following areas:

1. Recognition of rejection
2. Administration and monitoring of immunosuppressive drug therapy
3. Prevention and recognition of infection

Attention to the detailed management of these priorities actually begins in the operating room and continues for the rest of the patient's life.

IMMUNOLOGY OF THE TRANSPLANTED HEART AND REJECTION

Because the transplanted heart is immunologically foreign to the recipient, an immune response is invoked immediately on implantation. The body's immune surveillance system recognizes foreign or mutant cells and is responsible for transplant rejection.[8] This process is directed toward specific markers or antigens present on the surface of the donor myocardial cells, as well as the blood vessels that perfuse the heart.[51]

When the immune system receives antigenic stimulation from a foreign substance, it may respond through specific or nonspecific mechanisms. As shown in Fig. 18-4, the *nonspecific immune responses* include phagocytosis by nonlymphoid white blood cells (WBCs) such as neutrophils and macrophages. The inflammatory response also is activated to bring chemical mediators and WBCs to the area where they are needed.

Specific immune responses include more sophisticated mechanisms that enable the body to develop a defense against invading organisms, toxins, or cells. *Humoral im-*

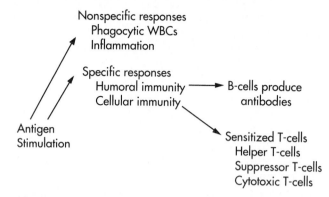

FIG. 18-4 Overview of the immune response. When confronted with a foreign substance, the immune system may respond through nonspecific or specific responses. Cellular immunity with the stimulation of small sensitized T-cells is thought to be the most important response in relation to transplant rejection.

munity involves the production of specific antibodies to destroy foreign substances. *Cellular immunity* involves the production of small, sensitized lymphocytes that can bind to and destroy invading substances or cells.[8] These two types of specific immunity result from the processing of lymphocyte precursors in different locations in the body. Lymphocytes processed in the bone marrow become *B-cells,* and lymphocytes processed in the thymus become *T-cells.* The B- and T-cells eventually become trapped in the lymph nodes, where they await stimulation by antigens.

When an antigen binds to a B-cell receptor, the cell differentiates into clones of plasma cells. These cells then become capable of producing antibodies and releasing them into the circulation. When an antigen binds to a T-cell receptor, T-cells begin to clone into small, sensitized lymphocytes with receptors that enable them to bind to antigenic cells. These T-lymphocytes are released into the circulation, where they travel to the target cells. They can then begin the process of destroying foreign cells.[8,39,70]

After transplantation of a vital organ such as the heart, the recipient's immune system recognizes the antigens on the allograft as foreign and responds through these specific immune mechanisms. T-cells play a major part in this process and may be responsible for transplant rejection.

A number of different T-cell subsets are involved in this process. *Helper T-cells* enhance both B- and T-cell responses through the release of mediators such as interleukin-2 (IL-2). *Suppressor T-cells* act to inhibit B-cell responses. *Cytotoxic T-cells* hunt and destroy cancer and other abnormal cells, including transplanted cells. Activated cytotoxic T-cells have been further defined by functional classes, depending on their cell surface markers and are referred to as *cluster differentiation (CD) 1, CD2, CD3.* The CD3 antigen is a particularly important factor in transplant rejection.[70] The identification of these markers has been important in the development of therapeutic monoclonal antibodies such as OKT3.

Many antigens on the cells of the donor heart can elicit the rejection response. The ABO antigens and HLA can stimulate the rejection response to transplanted organs. Because ABO antigens are on red blood cells (RBCs) and many other body cells, transplanted organs usually must be ABO compatible, just like blood transfusions.[51]

Other antigens capable of eliciting the rejection response are the HLA antigens. These antigens were termed *human leukocyte antigens* because they were first identified on leukocytes. The HLA system is divided into class I and class II molecules. Class I molecules are glycoproteins present on all nucleated cells and are known as *HLA-A, HLA-B,* and *HLA-C.* These molecules are the primary targets for cytotoxic T-cells. The HLA-A and HLA-B antigens are thought to be the principal antigens recognized by the recipient during graft rejection. Class II antigens, DR, DQ, and DP, also are known to participate in immunological responses.[70]

Although T-cell cytotoxicity is thought to be the most important mechanism in the destruction of a transplanted organ, other areas of the immune system are also known to contribute to the process. Antibody-dependent cell-mediated cytotoxicity, activated macrophages, and complement-dependent antibodies can contribute to the cellular damage of the transplanted organ.[18] Transplant rejection is generally classified as *hyperacute, acute,* or *chronic,* depending on the time it occurs after surgery and the pathophysiologic mechanism.

Hyperacute rejection

Hyperacute rejection can occur immediately or within hours after transplant surgery and inevitably results in rapid graft failure. It may be caused by an acute antigen-antibody reaction that takes place on the vascular endothelium of the blood vessels within the transplanted organ. The reaction induces endothelial cell damage, platelet aggregation, fibrin formation, and finally ischemic damage that results in loss of the graft.[8]

Preformed antibodies to the donor organ antigens can initiate this destructive reaction. It can occur when there is ABO incompatibility or when the recipient has developed cytotoxic antibodies. Careful ABO typing and presurgical screening for cytotoxic antibodies can minimize the chance of hyperacute rejection.[51]

Acute rejection

Acute rejection commonly occurs after transplant. Most patients have at least one episode of acute rejection, usually within the first few months after the transplant. It is more unusual but certainly possible for recipients to have an acute rejection after the first year. With advances in immunosuppressive drug therapy, acute rejection usually can be successfully treated; however rejection continues to be a major cause of death.

Acute rejection is thought to begin when macrophages and helper T-cells recognize foreign cells. As shown in Fig. 18-5, the hormone IL-1 is released and results in the pro-

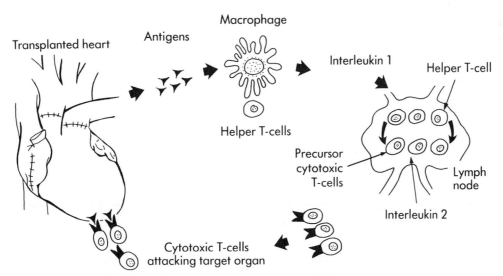

FIG. 18-5   The acute rejection process. Antigens on the transplanted cells are recognized as foreign by macrophages and precursors of helper T-cells. The interaction between these cells results in the release of IL-1, which causes helper T-cells to mature. The helper T-cells then interact with precursors of cytotoxic T-cells. Another hormone, IL-2, is released and promotes proliferation and maturation of the cytotoxic T-cells. These cells then circulate to the transplanted heart, combine with the antigens on the transplanted cells, and attempt to destroy the transplanted cells.

duction of more helper T-cells. These cells then release another hormone, IL-2, which stimulates the production of cytotoxic T-cells. These mature T-cells can combine with the antigens on the transplanted cells and cause total destruction.[51] Immunosuppressive drugs are administered to inhibit this reaction so that the transplanted organ is not destroyed.

It is not yet possible to predict which patients will have problems with acute rejection. Although a rejection episode may indicate that immunosuppression is inadequate, acute rejection can also be triggered by a viral infection.[10]

In patients receiving cyclosporine, there are few reliable signs and symptoms of rejection. Recipients may, in fact, feel well until signs of heart failure develop. Possible signs and symptoms that may occur during moderate-to-severe rejection include malaise, lethargy, fever, atrial or ventricular dysrhythmias, or a pericardial rub. Signs and symptoms of heart failure such as hypotension, dyspnea during exertion, abdominal pain from liver congestion, pedal edema, and an enlarged heart on x-ray film may be seen in some patients.[45,51] Patients are observed for signs of right-sided heart failure such as a ventricular gallop, hepatic enlargement, and jugular venous distention. Signs of left-sided heart failure such as pulmonary congestion are less commonly seen in acute rejection.

Changes in ECG and echocardiogram may accompany rejection episodes. Decreased voltage and poor R-wave progression may occur, particularly in patients who are not receiving cyclosporine. The most common dysrhythmias seen are premature atrial contractions, atrial fibrillation, and premature ventricular contractions. The echocardiogram may show right ventricular enlargement and increase in right ventricular wall thickness.[51] Wall motion abnormalities and decreased ejection fraction often become evident with severe episodes of rejection.

Because of the insidious nature of most acute rejection episodes, the most accurate diagnostic technique used for detection is *transvenous endomyocardial biopsy*. A bioptome catheter is advanced through a vein into the right ventricle (Fig. 18-6). Approximately five or six small tissue samples are taken from the right ventricular septum and sent to the pathology department for analysis. The samples are processed and examined under the microscope by the transplant pathologist and transplant physician. The specimens are rated on a scale from no rejection to mild, moderate, and severe rejection. The main histologic feature of rejection is the infiltration of lymphocytes into the myocardium.[45] Mononuclear cells stain positive with methyl green-pyronine, making them easy to identify. There may be interstitial edema and myocyte necrosis with this infiltration indicating more severe rejection. After the patient has been successfully treated for acute rejection, cardiac tissue samples will demonstrate a decrease in the inflammatory changes and positively stained lymphocytes, as well as the presence of reparative fibroblasts. This is referred to as *resolving rejection*.

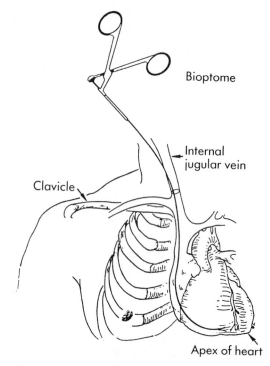

FIG. 18-6 The endomyocardial biopsy technique. The bioptome catheter is advanced into the right ventricle and biopsy specimens are obtained from the right ventricular septum.

From Murdock DK and others: Rejection of transplanted heart, Heart Lung 16(3), 1987.

Biopsies are performed weekly during the initial recovery period. Later, the time intervals between biopsies are increased. Most patients require biopsy only two to three times a year after the first year, but biopsy schedules differ considerably between institutions. Patients who have persistent problems with intermittent rejection require more frequent biopsy. When rejection is identified on biopsy, the patient is treated with augmented immunosuppression and undergoes another biopsy within a short period of time to make sure the rejection is resolving.

It may become increasingly difficult to perform biopsies on patients as the months and years go on. Problems with vascular access are common. In addition, the endocardium may develop scarring at previous biopsy sites. This may make it difficult to obtain adequate specimens. It is disappointing to patients and staff members when biopsy specimens are inadequate and the procedure must be repeated.

Many noninvasive techniques have been studied regarding their value in predicting or identifying rejection. Despite the availability of echocardiogram, magnetic resonance imaging (MRI) scanning, antimyosin antibody scans, and sophisticated immunological testing, no noninvasive test has proved reliable in diagnosing rejection, especially in patients on cyclosporine. Endomyocardial biopsy provides the only reliable way of detecting rejection at the early stages when it can be most easily treated.[5]

It is possible to have rejection even though the biopsy interpretation is negative. Sampling error can occur because the rejection process does not affect all parts of the endocardium. The diagnosis of acute rejection cannot be excluded if other signs and symptoms of rejection are present.

Treatment of rejection episodes depends on a number of factors. Patients with early rejection usually are treated more aggressively in comparison with those with late rejection. The presence or absence of signs and symptoms also can make a difference because symptomatic rejection is more virulent. Patients' rejection histories and responses to previous treatment also will affect treatment. Often patients receive high doses of steroids as the initial treatment. If the rejection is not reversed, the more powerful monoclonal or polyclonal antibody preparations are used.

Patients who are very ill with rejection are often able to respond dramatically to augmented immunosuppressive drug therapy. It is possible even for patients in cardiogenic shock to recover to the point where ventricular function is normal again.

Chronic rejection

As time goes on, most recipients are no longer threatened by acute rejection. Over the years, however, chronic rejection can begin to threaten the transplanted heart. A diffuse form of coronary artery disease characterized by intimal hyperplasia can slowly narrow the coronary arteries to the point where ischemic damage to the myocardium occurs. The distal and proximal vessels may be affected. This form of graft atherosclerosis may rapidly progress. Because of its diffuse nature, it does not often respond to percutaneous transluminal coronary angioplasty or myocardial revascularization. In other recipients, the focal type of atherosclerosis seen in ischemic heart disease may occur. This form involves lipid deposition and vessel wall calcification. It tends to occur in proximal vessels and may be treated with coronary angioplasty.[10]

Graft atherosclerosis has been seen rarely during the first year after transplant but is most commonly found later. Most reports of long-term cardiac transplant survivors report an incidence of approximately 40% to 50% at 5 years.[70] The process is generally detected through coronary angiography, which is performed yearly at many centers. Because of the diffuse nature of the atherosclerosis, it may be difficult to determine the extent of the process, and it may be underestimated on coronary arteriogram interpretation. Other indicators of the process may include dysrhythmias, myocardial infarction, congestive heart failure, impaired left ventricular function, and sudden death.[10]

Cardiac recipients do not experience angina because the heart has been denervated. Some may experience shortness of breath if myocardial ischemia occurs. Unfortunately, the first clinical indication of graft atherosclerosis may be congestive heart failure or sudden death due to myocardial infarction.[50]

The mechanism of chronic rejection is not completely understood. It is thought to be a slow immunologic response that is not controlled by present immunosuppressive drug regimens. Several studies have attempted to identify risk factors for chronic rejection.[10] There are only inconclusive results related to blood lipids, donor age, and other cardiac or immunologic factors. There have been reports of a possible association between CMV infection and graft atherosclerosis.[10] There is also evidence that the perivascular lymphocytic infiltration and vasculitis observed in endomyocardial biopsies showing acute rejection may lead to vascular changes in the coronary arteries. The immune coronary injury may then be intensified by coronary artery disease risk factors such as elevated serum cholesterol and triglyceride levels frequently associated with steroid and cyclosporine therapy.[10]

Control of coronary artery disease risk factors through the use of dietary restriction of cholesterol and antilipid agents may be recommended. Control of hypertension and elimination of smoking may help minimize the risk. The use of antiplatelet agents such as aspirin and dipyridamole has become accepted preventive therapy.

Retransplantation may be the only option for patients with diffuse graft atherosclerosis. The lower survival rates reported with second cardiac transplants and the lack of available donors for patients awaiting their first transplant limit the application of this option.

IMMUNOSUPPRESSIVE DRUG THERAPY

The goal of imunosuppressive drug therapy is to prevent rejection without oversuppressing the immune system and allowing for infection to occur. This delicate balance is not easy to achieve in all recipients. Rejection and infection remain major causes of morbidity and mortality after cardiac transplantation.

Lifelong immunosuppressive drug therapy is necessary after cardiac transplantation because the body's immune system never develops complete tolerance of the transplanted organ. Chemotherapeutic immunosuppressive agents continue to be the cornerstone of prevention and treatment of acute rejection. *Triple therapy* with cyclosporine, prednisone, and azathioprine is the most common maintenance regimen. This particular combination of agents reduces the incidence and severity of rejection and lowers the rate of infection.[11]

No one immunosuppressive drug protocol is used in all transplant centers, particularly regarding initial therapy. Some centers use *induction therapy,* which involves the routine administration of monoclonal or polyclonal antibodies during the early postoperative period. Other centers reserve these agents for *rescue therapy* to treat rejection episodes.

Greater immunosuppression is required early after the transplant compared with later in almost all recipients. This is because over time patients develop some degree of tolerance of the allograft, possibly because of the gradual emergence of suppressor mechanisms.[56] Recipients are maintained on combination protocols rather than single-drug regimens because of the effectiveness of these protocols and because of the toxic effects that would be associated with high doses of any agent.

Azathioprine

Azathioprine (Imuran) is a purine antagonist antimetabolite that is converted to 6-mercaptopurine in the liver. First used to treat renal transplant rejection in 1961, it is toxic to rapidly dividing cells, especially those in lymphoid tissue.[70] Because of this action, the drug inhibits the production of lymphocytes responsible for rejection. Azathioprine is used with cyclosporine and prednisone to *prevent* rejection and is not used to treat rejection. It may be given intravenously initially and later changed to an oral route of administration. Recipients commonly receive 1 to 2 mg/kg daily as part of their immunosuppressive drug regimen.

Side effects include increased risk of infection, liver toxicity, nausea, and vomiting. Most common, however, is bone marrow suppression, which is usually manifested by a drop in the WBC count to less than 4000 per mm^3.[38] The dose of azathioprine is adjusted to keep the WBC count above 4000 to 5000 per mm^3. Routine monitoring of the complete blood count is essential to detect bone marrow suppression and minimize susceptability to infection.

Corticosteroids

Steroids, in the form of prednisone, were added to azathioprine in 1962 to form a more effective immunosuppressive protocol. They remain an important part of immunosuppression for cardiac transplant patients and are used for *prevention* and *treatment* of acute rejection. In addition to the antiinflammatory effects, the mechanism of action in acute rejection includes sequestration of circulating lymphocytes and monocytes in lymphoid tissue and interference with the production of the mediators IL-1 and IL-2.

Intravenous methylprednisolone sodium succinate (Solu-Medrol) is commonly given intraoperatively followed by lower or tapering doses of methylprednisolone or prednisone. Some programs continue a maintenance dose of prednisone indefinitely, lowering the daily dose during the first year to approximately 0.1 to 0.2 mg/kg. Some programs are attempting to manage patients without maintenance steroids. It is reported that patients who have been successfully weaned from steroids do not have an increased incidence of rejection and may have a lower rate of infection, as well as fewer side effects and long-term

complications related to chronic steroid use.[42] In patients who are more prone to rejection, small doses of prednisone are continued. It may be more difficult to withdraw steroids in women and in patients who have had prior heart surgery.[57] Initial treatment with monoclonal antibody OKT3 or ATG may enable withdrawal of steroids from a larger number of patients.

In addition to preventive therapy, steroids are usually the first line of defense used against acute rejection. A 3-day course of prednisone, 100 mg per day, may be used to treat mild-to-moderate rejection. A 3-day course of intravenous methylprednisolone, 1000 mg per day, may be used to treat moderate or early rejection. Studies of patients on cyclosporine show that augmented doses of steroids can reverse the majority of rejection episodes.[70] Augmentation of steroid therapy results in hyperglycemia in diabetic recipients, which can be difficult to manage.

Corticosteroids can cause many early and long-term side effects and complications; many can seriously affect transplant recipients. Patients have an increased appetite, a tendency toward excessive weight gain, and often develop a Cushingoid appearance. It is possible to develop steroid-induced diabetes and gastrointestinal distress or ulcers. Over time, the skin can become fragile and bruise easily. Skin lesions such as acne or warts may develop. Osteoporosis is a complication of steroid therapy and can place patients at risk for fractures and other skeletal complications such as aseptic necrosis of the hip joints. Children who take steroids may have slowed growth. Some patients have muscle weakness that limits exercise tolerance. Others may develop cataracts. Mood swings and occasionally even psychosis have been associated with steroid therapy.[38,57] When all these possible effects are added to the increased risk of infection, it is obvious why all efforts are made to maintain patients on the lowest possible dose.

Antithymocyte and antilymphocyte preparations

ATG was first used clinically in 1967 to destroy cytotoxic T-cells and reduce cell-mediated rejection. This agent is an antiserum containing antibodies that recognizes T-cells and destroys them through complement-dependent lysis. It is produced by injecting human T-cells into a horse, rabbit, or goat. The animal then produces immunoglobulin G (IgG) antibodies, which can be separated from the serum and processed so that they will be tolerated in human use.[52] The resultant globulin can be administered intramuscularly or intravenously with appropriate premedication to prevent anaphylaxis or other hypersensitivity reactions. After the preparation is administered and begins to circulate, the antibodies attach to lymphocytes, promoting opsonization by the reticuloendothelial system and depleting the T-cells from the circulation.

ATG is a *polyclonal antibody* with a limited percentage of each dose specific for human T-cells. It can be used as initial therapy with other agents to *prevent* acute rejection.

It can also be used as *rescue therapy* to treat an episode of acute rejection. Only antithymocyte gamma globulin (ATGAM), an ATG derived from horse antisera, is available for commercial use. Other ATGs are available from private laboratories and are used under experimental protocols.

ATG may be given intramuscularly for 3 to 5 days, or it may be administered intravenously for up to 14 days. Severe muscle pain, leg edema, and fever commonly follow intramuscular administration. Other clinical side effects may accompany intramuscular or intravenous administration. Shaking chills, bronchospasm, urticaria, rash, thrombocytopenia, leukopenia, arthralgias, and serum sickness are possible reactions.[65] Previous exposure to animals (i.e., patients who have raised rabbits may be sensitized to rabbit ATG) may predispose patients to a reaction. Skin testing may be done before the first dose to identify these individuals. Late complications may include infection and lymphoma. It is also possible for patients previously treated with ATG to become refractory to treatment if the same type of ATG is used again.

OKT3 is a newer agent that works in much the same way as ATG. It is a *monoclonal antibody* produced by hybridization techniques that join antibody-producing B-cells with mouse myeloma cells. The hybridoma is then generated by innoculating mice with human T-cells. Antibodies that react with T3 cell surface antigens are produced. This results in the opsonization and elimination of these activated cells from the circulation.[60] In addition, OKT3 interferes with T-cell antigen recognition, making it more difficult for active T-cells to identify the target organ.

OKT3 is given intravenously for 10 to 14 days. It may be used as *initial therapy* or may be reserved for *treatment* of rejection. The administration of the drug may be accompanied by a symptom complex that includes fever, chills, nausea, vomiting, headache, diarrhea, and arthralgia. These symptoms are most commonly associated with the first dose of OKT3 and normally last only 24 to 48 hours. The reaction may be caused by the release of lymphokines and T-cell lysis.[60] Premedication with corticosteroids, acetaminophen, and diphenhydramine can decrease or alleviate symptoms. Patients with volume overload may be at risk for pulmonary edema when OKT3 is given, but this adverse reaction has mainly been seen in renal transplant recipients. Hypotension has been reported in cardiac recipients receiving OKT3.[37] Because of the potential for adverse reaction, patients usually are monitored in the intensive care unit for the first few days of OKT3 therapy. Afterward the course of treatment for stable patients usually is conducted on the regular nursing unit or in the outpatient department.

After OKT3 is given, there is rapid depletion of T-cells from the circulation. In some centers, the effectiveness of therapy is monitored by daily T-cell counts. Because patients may develop antibodies to OKT3, which might make them refractory to future treatment, an OKT3 antibody titer may be analyzed 30 days after treatment.

Studies continue to explore whether monoclonal or polyclonal antibody therapy should be used in all patients initially. It is expensive and may increase the risk of infection. Most sources feel that induction therapy delays the onset of the first rejection episode until after the heart has recovered from the ischemia and surgical wounds have healed.[56] It also may decrease the overall incidence of graft rejection and allow the use of lower maintenance immunosuppressive drugs. In addition, in patients with renal dysfunction, cyclosporine use can be minimized or eliminated during the early postoperative period.[50]

Cyclosporine

Cyclosporine (Sandimmune) is a fungus-derived metabolite that was introduced as an immunosuppressant in 1978 and became available for commercial use in 1983. It is used with other immunosuppressive agents to *prevent* rejection. The addition of cyclosporine to immunosuppressive drug regimens is thought to be one of the major reasons cardiac transplantation has become so successful. Patients receiving cyclosporine have fewer rejection episodes, shorter hospitalizations, and better survival when compared with patients who received only conventional therapy consisting of azathioprine and prednisone.[50] Because patients receiving cyclosporine require lower doses of prednisone, there is also less risk of infection and a lower incidence of side effects associated with high doses of steroids.

Some centers give a preoperative dose of cyclosporine, whereas others begin it after surgery. Immediately after surgery, some patients may receive cyclosporine as a continuous intravenous infusion. The drug is usually administered orally because of the greater potential for nephrotoxicity associated with intravenous administration. Oral preparations include the traditional liquid form and the newer capsule form.

Individual doses of cyclosporine are adjusted according to serum or blood levels of the drug or its metabolites. There are a number of different tests on the market to measure cyclosporine levels. Some of the most commonly used tests include the Sandoz monoclonal and polyclonal radioimmunoassay tests, the Abbott TDX system, and the high-performance liquid chromatography (HPLC) method.

The mode of action of cyclosporine is thought to be selective inhibition of T-cells. The drug is believed to interfere with the early activation of mediators of T-cells such as the acquisition receptors for IL-1 and IL-2.[32] Through this action, cyclosporine suppresses the T-cells responsible for graft rejection by interfering with their production at the early stages of antigenic stimulation. T-cells do not proliferate and consequently cytotoxic T-cells are not produced. The selective inhibition of T-cell production is a major advantage of cyclosporine because the goal of immunosuppressive drug therapy is accomplished without affecting the other areas of the immune system such as B-cells, macrophages, or neutrophils.

Long-term evaluation of patients on cyclosporine has shown that nephrotoxicity is the most common serious complication. Patients who have been receiving cyclosporine tend to have serum creatinine levels between 1.5 and 2.5 mg/dl and sometimes higher. Cardiac recipients also have a 60% to 90% incidence of arterial hypertension, which may require a multidrug regimen.[1] Other complications may include hepatotoxicity, hirsutism, tremors, paresthesias, headache, and gum hyperplasia.

Hyperuricemia and gouty arthritis have been associated with cyclosporine use in transplant recipients.[41] Episodes of gout may be severe and may lead to the development of polyarticular disease and tophi. The management of this problem is complicated by the transplant patient's renal insufficiency, immunosuppressive drug regimen, and susceptibility to infectious complications. Treatment may include careful use of nonsteroidal antiinflammatory agents with close monitoring of serum creatinine levels. Colchicine may be used with close monitoring of the WBC count. Use of allopurinal may not be an option because of the interaction with azathioprine, which can lead to profound leukopenia. For some patients, intraarticular steroid injections may be helpful.

Because of the potential for nephrotoxicity, cyclosporine may be withheld after surgery until renal function has been stabilized. Cyclosporine levels are monitored for the rest of the patient's life—to avoid serum levels higher than those considered therapeutic.

Cyclosporine interacts with many other drugs. Increases or decreases in concentration levels and additive nephrotoxicity have been described.[16] Because of this, the transplant team must be informed when changes are made in the patient's drug regimen. Often a cyclosporine test should be done to determine the effect that new drugs or discontinuing drugs have on serum levels. Other physicians, nurses, and patients need to be aware of these concerns so that cyclosporine levels are not allowed to shift to dangerously high or dangerously low levels.

Future immunosuppression

Present immunosuppressive drug therapy has problems. The drug regimens are to some extent nonspecific, predisposing the patient to infectious and other complications. It has been said that transplant recipients trade one chronic condition (end-stage heart disease) for another (chronic immunosuppression). It is assumed that the length and quality of life achieved through this trade will be beneficial for the recipient.

Research related to new immunosuppressive techniques and drugs continues. Immunoabsorption techniques in which preformed antibodies are removed from

recipients may allow greater tolerance and may even allow transplant across ABO barriers and interspecies barriers in the future. The use of anti-IL-2 antibodies is one form of monoclonal antibody investigation that attempts to block the recipient's response to activation antigens or even to the donor's specific HLA antigens.[61] A technique such as this could eliminate nonspecific therapy for recipients. Finally new chemotherapeutic agents that have fewer toxic effects are being investigated for clinical use. There have been reports of success with the investigational agent FK-506 in organ transplant recipients.[2] Patients need to know that research continues to find new protocols that will further increase the success of cardiac transplantation and recipients' quality of life.

PREVENTION AND RECOGNITION OF INFECTION

Prevention of infection has been a major goal of care since the first cardiac recipient died of infection. There has been a significant reduction in infection rates and the overall severity of infections for many reasons. Immunosuppressive drugs are kept at a minimum. Diagnosis of infection has been facilitated by new techniques, and treatment has become more effective with the availability of new broad-spectrum antibacterial, antifungal, and antiviral agents.

Infections in transplant recipients range from minor problems such as oral herpes to life-threatening problems such as pneumonia or meningitis. Transplant recipients' decreased cellular immunity puts them at risk for certain opportunistic infections or infections from organisms that might not threaten immunocompetent individuals. The specific organisms involved are listed in the box and include bacterial, viral, fungal, and parasitic infections.[36] Immunosuppressive drugs also affect other parts of the immune system. Steroids impair neutrophil chemotaxis and activity and reduce reticuloendothelial function. Azathioprine reduces neutrophil function and number and may also impair B-cell function.

The timing of infections is somewhat predictable. Bacterial pathogens seen in all surgical patients are most likely to cause infection during the first month after surgery. Infections seen between 1 and 4 months after surgery tend to involve opportunistic pathogens such as CMV. After this time, a mixture of conventional and opportunistic infections can occur.[36] Patients who have had augmented immunosuppression for rejection are at greatest risk. Those who are hospitalized are at risk for nosocomial infection.

Pulmonary infections tend to be most common in heart transplant recipients. However, infections have been documented at many sites, including the transplanted heart. The high incidence of pulmonary infection is attributed to preoperative pulmonary abnormalities such as congestive heart failure, endotrachial intubation, and general disability. Infection is suspected when a patient has fever, cough, sputum production, shortness of breath, malaise, or a chest x-ray film showing infiltrates. Attempts are made to obtain a rapid diagnosis through sputum gram stain and culture, endotracheal aspiration, bronchoscopy with bronchoalveolar lavage, transbronchial biopsy, or even open lung biopsy. Antimicrobial agents are begun while the team awaits for culture results. The patient's history can be helpful in the diagnostic process because certain clinical signs are associated with some types of infections. Severe symptoms that develop rapidly over 24 hours suggest a bacterial or noninfectious process such as pulmonary embolism. A subacute process can indicate viral infection. A very insidious pulmonary infection can indicate fungal infection.

In addition to pulmonary infection, central nervous system (CNS) infections can be problematic. Clinical features that suggest CNS infection include headache, focal neurologic deficits, seizures, and altered mental status with or without fever. Computed tomography (CT) scan, MRI scan, and lumbar puncture may be performed during the diagnostic process.

Common gastrointestinal infections include thrush, stomatitis, esophagitis, and lower gastrointestinal infection caused by *Candida albicans,* herpes simplex, CMV, and *Aspergillus* organisms. Endoscopy with biopsy and culture may be performed. Hepatitis resulting from hepatitis B, hepatitis C, CMV, or herpes simplex may also be seen.

Cutaneous infections are common in transplant recipients and can become unusually severe and prolonged. Herpes simplex and varicella zoster virus are treated intravenously with acyclovir. A mild herpes simplex infection may be treated with oral acyclovir. Cultures and a biopsy may be performed to identify the organism.

CMV is the most frequent and important viral infection in patients who have had organ transplants. The infection can occur as a primary infection or as reactivation of a latent infection. Primary infections usually are serious and are most likely to occur in a seronegative recipient who has received an organ from a donor who was seropositive for CMV.[48] Blood products can also transmit the virus. Patients may develop fever with leukopenia, which can progress to pneumonitis, hepatitis, gastritis, retinitis, and myocarditis. The infection also suppresses cellular immunity, increasing susceptibility to a superinfection. Diagnosis is made by culture or a fourfold increase in antibody titer. Asymptomatic shedding of the virus is common in transplant recipients, making a diagnosis of CMV disease difficult.

The antiviral agent *ganciclovir* has recently been released for commercial use and is the only known drug to be effective against CMV. Prevention of the infection is of primary importance. When it is necessary to administer blood products, CMV-negative products should be used. The use of *prophylactic hyperimmune globulin* in CMV-negative recipients who receive CMV-positive organs may be recommended.

Active infection with *Epstein-Barr virus* has been associated with lymphomas and other lymphoproliferative syndromes after transplant. Some of these syndromes are reversible when immunosuppression is reduced.[48]

Another infection that threatens transplant patients is *toxoplasmosis.* Patients may become infected by reactivation of a latent infection or transmission of the infection via the donor organ. Diagnosis is made through seroconversion or an increased serum titer. Clinical findings may be indicative of infection in the CNS, heart, or lungs. Intracranial lesions may be observed on CT or MRI scans. A biopsy may be needed for definitive diagnosis. After diagnosis, the patient is usually treated with pyrimethamine and sulfadiazine.[36]

Recognition of infection in immunosuppressed transplant recipients can be difficult for many reasons. The signs

---

COMMON INFECTIONS IN CARDIAC RECIPIENTS

BACTERIAL INFECTIONS
Early

Escherichia coli
Enterococci
Klebsiella organisms
Pseudomonas organisms
Serratia organisms
Staphylococcus organisms
Streptococcus organisms

Late

Legionella organisms
Listeria organisms
Mycobacterium organisms
Nocardia organisms
Salmonella organisms

VIRAL INFECTIONS

CMV
Herpes simplex
Epstein-Barr virus
Varicella zoster virus

FUNGAL INFECTIONS

Aspergillus organisms
Cryptococcus organisms
Histoplasmosis
Coccidioimycosis
Blastomycosis
Candida organisms

PARASITIC INFECTIONS

Pneumocystis organisms
Toxoplasmosis

of infection may be subtle. Steroids may mask fever and other signs of inflammation. Infections caused by opportunistic organisms may cause nonspecific symptoms. Laboratory values, particularly the complete blood count, may be unrevealing or even misleading because of the effects of immunosuppressive drugs. The clinical situation may be complicated by coexisting rejection. And even the interpretation of cultures and treatment plans can be difficult because multiple infections may coexist.[36] Because infections can rapidly become life threatening, transplant recipients may need to be hospitalized for diagnosis and treatment when such infection is suspected.

Strategies to *prevent infection* begin before surgery. Donors are screened carefully for transmissible disease. After surgery, recipients are mobilized early to prevent pulmonary infection. Invasive tubes and lines are discontinued as soon as possible to decrease the number of access routes for organisms.[26] Meticulous care of incisions and intravenous sites is performed. The number of individuals caring for the patient is kept to a minimum.

There is a trend toward using less *protective isolation* in organ recipients, mainly because it has not been valuable in preventing infections.[27,31] Many centers follow the Centers for Disease Control recommendations for the severely compromised patient, which include a private room, thorough hand washing with an antiseptic agent, and wearing of masks. Some sources recommend masks only for persons with upper respiratory tract infection, although it is felt that anyone with signs or symptoms of infection should not interact with an immunosuppressed patient.

Perioperatively prophylactic antibiotics are administered to prevent complications such as mediastinitis, pneumonia, and line sepsis. During the early postoperative period, nystatin (Mycostatin) may be prescribed orally to prevent thrush. Long-term prophylaxis with sulfamethoxazole and trimethoprim is advocated by some to prevent pneumocystic infection. Oral acyclovir may also be given prophylactically to prevent viral infections. Transplant recipients with a positive tuberculin skin test may be given isoniazid for an indefinite period of time. Using the lowest effective doses of immunosuppressive drugs remains an important strategy.

LONG-TERM CONSIDERATIONS

Most patients progress rapidly after cardiac transplant surgery. Many are able to transfer from the intensive care unit after 4 or 5 days. Recipients remain in the hospital an average of 2 weeks. After discharge, patients who do not live in the local area usually will be asked to stay near the transplant center for a few weeks.

As recipients prepare to leave the hospital, plans are made for outpatient management, and teaching is begun. During the evaluation period, all candidates are informed of the lifelong commitment required of them. Most do not remember the specifics of care after transplantation. As teaching is begun regarding follow-up care, patients and families may feel overwhelmed. They need to be informed that teaching and instructions will continue during frequent outpatient appointments. Written information is also very helpful, and most transplant centers have a booklet that outlines the major facts patients need to know.

A typical medical regimen for cardiac transplant follow-up care is shown in Table 18-1. Endomyocardial biopsies are done on an outpatient basis after discharge from the hospital. Recipients usually are hospitalized 1 to 2 days for yearly checkups, which often include coronary angiography and other tests such as 24-hour urine determination of creatinine clearance.

Clinic visits are carried out monthly at the transplant center or with the recipient's local physician and include labwork plus a patient history and limited physical examination. Patients are carefully questioned regarding symptoms. Blood pressure, heart rate and rhythm, and body weight are measured. The recipient's skin and mucous membranes are inspected for signs of skin cancer or infectious lesions. Lymph nodes are examined for swelling, which could suggest lymphoma. Heart and lung auscultation is performed, and the patient is examined for signs of heart failure such as peripheral edema, liver enlargement, or jugular venous distention.

Problems are investigated promptly and thoroughly because even trivial complaints may indicate serious problems. For example, the onset of headaches may be the first sign of an occult infection causing a brain abscess. The most common reason for readmission to the hospital is infection.[1] When problems are suspected, patients are referred to specialists (e.g., infectious disease, pulmonary medicine, and nephrology) experienced in the care of

TABLE 18-1
Routine Follow-Up Care for Heart Recipients

Test	Frequency
Endomyocardial biopsy	Weekly for 4 weeks
	Every 2 weeks for 1 month
	Monthly for 3 months
	Every 3 months until 1 year
	Every 4 to 6 months indefinitely
Coronary angiography	Yearly
Complete blood count, chemistry panel	Monthly with clinic visits
Cyclosporine level	Monthly with clinic visits
Echocardiogram	Every 6 months
Chest x-ray study	Every 6 months

transplant patients. In addition to the common transplant-related problems, they may develop other problems that affect patients with diagnoses of cardiovascular problems, such as pulmonary emboli, myocardial infarction, and cerebrovascular accident. A wide variety of diagnoses need to be considered when a transplant patient develops symptoms.

Recipients need to know that diligent self-monitoring and reporting of problems is extremely important. Those who do not live locally need to know that they must inform the transplant team when they are having problems, even if the problems are being managed by local physicians. Close collaboration is essential in ensuring that problems are managed along transplant center protocols. Decisions regarding all interventions, including changes in medications, need to involve the transplant team. If recipients require major interventions such as surgery, it is often recommended that they have it done at the transplant center. This allows the transplant team to monitor the immunosuppressive drugs and other transplant concerns.

A number of considerations in long-term management need to be addressed over time with every cardiac recipient. These include the management of hypertension, hypercholesterolemia, nutritional management, exercise and activity recommendations, recognition of malignancy, and issues related to quality of life.

Management of hypertension

Hypertension is a major clinical problem in cardiac transplant recipients. It occurs in almost all cardiac transplant patients receiving cyclosporine, even if they have no other conventional risk factors for hypertension.[64] The hypertension may be severe and can be refractory to multiple drug regimens.

The pathophysiologic mechanisms that lead to hypertension in cardiac recipients are not completely understood. Over time cyclosporine may cause chronic injury to the renal microvasculature, which may in turn cause hypertension.[64] Corticosteriods also may contribute to the development of hypertension. Another consideration is that no autonomic feedback exists between the peripheral and central circulation, and the heart is unable to respond to changes in afterload through the usual mechanism of sympathetic stimulation. Because of this lack of communication, systemic vascular resistence tends to remain high, even when cardiac output is normal. All of these multifactoral mechanisms may contribute to hypertension.

Attempts to minimize hypertension include using the lowest possible doses of cyclosporine and prednisone. Different classes of antihypertensive drugs are commonly used. Diuretics may be prescribed to reduce the increased plasma volume that has been described in patients receiving cyclosporine. However, caution must be used because the nephrotoxicity of cyclosporine therapy can be increased by

excessive diuresis, causing alarming increases in BUN and serum creatinine levels if dehydration occurs. Calcium antagonists may be used, but they tend to elevate cyclosporine levels and may cause peripheral edema in some recipients. Angiotensin-converting-enzyme inhibitors are prescribed for some patients and have not been associated with additive renal toxicity in patients receiving cyclosporine.[64] It is often necessary to try different agents or combinations of agents to achieve reasonable control of blood pressure.

Doses of antihypertensive agents may have to be altered because cardiac transplant patients lack the normal nocturnal decrease in blood pressure seen in normal individuals. In addition, early morning blood pressure measurements are often highest, with afternoon blood pressures reading considerably lower. Because of this phenomenon, a larger dose of medication may be indicated at bedtime to enhance 24-hour control.

The risks of poor blood pressure control include ventricular hypertrophy and eventual decline in ventricular function, plus the increased risk of stroke and myocardial infarction. Because of this, a goal for cardiac recipients is to aim for a blood pressure under 140/90 mm Hg.

Management of hypercholesterolemia

Hypercholesterolemia is a problem commonly seen in cardiac transplant recipients. Increases in serum cholesterol and triglyceride levels occur over time. These are well-known risk factors for coronary artery disease, and reductions in serum cholesterol levels diminish the progression of coronary artery disease. However, there is conflicting evidence regarding the relationship of elevated serum lipid levels to the development of graft atherosclerosis.[10] Increases in total cholesterol and low-density lipoprotein levels are found in cardiac recipients. This atherogenic lipid profile may contribute to the development of accelerated atherosclerosis in these individuals. It has been suggested that the interaction between hypercholesterolemia and immune-mediated endothelial injury may predispose patients to the development of this problem.[63]

High blood lipid levels are to some extent related to immunosuppressive drug therapy. Increased serum cholesterol levels are seen in patients on corticosteroid therapy, including those receiving steroids for other diseases. Cyclosporine also elevates serum cholesterol levels, possibly because of hepatotoxicity, which results in defective low-density lipoprotein clearance.[63] New drug regimens with lower-maintenance steroids or no-maintenance steroids may have a favorable effect on blood lipid levels. Transplant recipients on steroid-free regimens do not seem to have the lipid elevations seen in patients on triple therapy.[57]

In addition to the reduction of steroids, conventional means of lowering serum cholesterol levels are recommended. Patients are advised to maintain their ideal body weights through dietary restriction and reduced intake of cholesterol and saturated fats. Administration of cholesterol-lowering agents may be necessary. Cholestyramine, niacin, gemfibrozil, and lovastatin may be used. There were some early reports of lovastatin being associated with rhabdomyolysis in patients receiving immunosuppressive drugs, but this complication has now been shown to be very rare.[43] Antiplatelet agents such as aspirin and dipyridamole may also be added to the drug regimen to prevent graft atherosclerosis.[10]

Nutritional management

Nutritional management is an important part of the overall long-term goal of maintaining optimal health and preventing graft atherosclerosis. Besides the problem with hypercholesterolemia, patients receiving steroids tend to have an increased appetite and a tendency toward obesity. It is possible for them to gain excessive amounts of weight during the first year after the surgery. Although they may have been somewhat cachectic preoperatively, they can rapidly gain weight to the extent that they are 20% to 50% above their recommended weight. This can seriously affect body image and self-esteem.

Steroids have other effects on nutritional status. These agents alter carbohydrate, protein, and lipid metabolism. The changes in carbohydrate metabolism can cause Cushing's syndrome and nonketotic diabetes. Protein metabolism is also affected, and the increased catabolism can result in muscle wasting, thinning of the skin, dissolution of vertical bone matrix, and poor wound healing. Fat distribution is altered, resulting in loss of subcutaneous fat from the extremities and excessive deposition in the dorsal and ventral fat pads, the supraclavicular area, and the abdominal wall. The antagonistic effect of prednisone on vitamin D metabolism upsets body calcium balance, augmenting osteoporosis.[55]

During the immediate postoperative period, some centers restrict fresh fruits and vegetables because they have aerobic gram-negative bacilli on their surfaces. As centers have moved away from strict protective isolation, most have eliminated this restriction. Fresh fruits and vegetables are no longer considered dangerous unless the patient is neutropenic.[55]

As recipients recover from surgery, nutritional support is provided to meet the increased requirements of wound healing and accelerated protein losses from steroid therapy. The diet most commonly ordered before discharge is low-cholesterol, 4-gram-sodium restriction, with limited concentrated sweets. These restrictions may be extended to include a diabetic diet for recipients with preoperative diabetes or steroid-induced diabetes. Diet instruction stresses food planning and preparation, as well as guidelines to use when dining out. In addition, recipients are cautioned to avoid meat that is not thoroughly cooked or food that may be spoiled.

Because patients are discharged soon after surgery, the opportunities for diet instruction may be limited. Many recipients need outpatient follow-up if the goals of dietary management are to be met. This can be provided when they return to the transplant center for diagnostic testing.

Exercise and activity recommendations

During the early years of cardiac transplantation, it was not known how the denervated heart would respond to activity and exercise. It is now evident that recipients may enjoy an active lifestyle and that many recipients are capable of athletic achievements and demanding occupations. Regular exercise is an important part of the recovery process. A structured exercise program helps the recipient attain and maintain cardiovascular and cardiopulmonary conditioning. An added benefit is that exercise is thought to slow the atherosclerotic process that can occur in the transplanted heart. Exercise is also important to prevent osteoporosis.

When planning an exercise program for cardiac transplant recipients, the denervated state and subsequent abnormal cardiac responses need to be taken into consideration. Table 18-2 outlines the physiologic and functional effects of cardiac denervation. Heart rate changes in response to shifts in posture and the Valsalva maneuver are absent. Reinnervation does not occur after surgery, and therefore these changes are permanent.[66]

Denervation is not thought to have much affect on resting heart function. After initial recovery of the heart from perioperative ischemia, resting hemodynamic measurements are normal. Heart rate is usually higher than normal because of the absence of vagal tone, and cardiac output and index tend to be at the lower range of normal.

With exercise, there is definitely a different response pattern. There are several nonneural mechanisms responsible for increasing cardiac output. Increased venous return increases end-diastolic volume and pressure through the Starling mechanism. Heart rate and stroke volume increase because of circulating adrenal catecholamines. The response time of the adrenal medulla is slower than direct sympathetic heart stimulation, accounting for the delayed increase in heart rate and blood pressure. There may also be other reflex and humoral mechanisms involved in the response to exercise. The role of atrial natriuretic peptide, a hormone secreted from the atria and known to be elevated in cardiac transplant recipients, is being investigated as a mediator of increased cardiac output.

In addition to these delayed reactions, there is evidence that, at all levels of oxygen consumption, cardiac output may remain lower in transplant recipients compared with normal individuals. Cardiac output increases in the appropriate direction during exercise but may remain at a lower level for any workload. Peak exercise levels in cardiac recipients may be somewhat below normal.[66] Regardless of

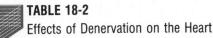

TABLE 18-2
Effects of Denervation on the Heart

	Normal	Denervation
Loss of sympathetic innervation	Sympathetic fibers release norepinephrine and acetylcholine, leading to: Increased conduction through sinoatrial and atrioventricular nodes Increased heart rate Increased stroke volume Immediate response to exercise	Without direct stimulation, response to stress and exercise depends on other mechanisms. Muscle activity increases venous return to heart, increasing cardiac output. Later, heart rate and cardiac output increase from circulating catecholamines. There is delayed response to exercise. When preload is decreased, orthostatic hypotension occurs resulting from a lack of compensatory increase in heart rate.
Loss of parasympathetic innervation	Parasympathetic fibers (including vagus nerve) inhibit conduction through atrioventricular node.	Faster resting heart rate (usually 90 to 100 beats per minute) occurs. Valsalva maneuver, carotid massage, and atropine have no effect on heart rate.
Loss of pain receptors	Angina is present during cardiac ischemia.	There is no angina.

these findings, 80% to 90% of cardiac recipients achieve the NYHA class I level of functional capacity.[46] Some have been able to participate in physically demanding sports such as soccer and running marathons.

Most cardiac recipients benefit from a structured cardiac rehabilitation program. With exercise training, maximal oxygen consumption is increased by 20%. After patients have been conditioned by exercise training, their heart rates do not slow to a lower baseline rate like they do in conditioned people with innervated hearts.[66] Rehabilitation is an important part of the recovery from surgery, especially because recipients are often deconditioned from prolonged bed rest. Physical therapy is begun in the intensive care unit, and the patient is progressed to the cardiac rehabilitation department as soon as possible.

An exercise program for cardiac recipients needs to include several key guidelines. Because of the delayed physiologic response to exercise, a warm-up period is particularly important to ensure that the patient has adequate circulating catecholamines. Before exercise, patients should be encouraged to perform arm, thoracic, and lower-extremity exercises (e.g., marching in place and flexing ankles) for 10 to 15 minutes. Recipients have reported that they become short of breath and have difficulty completing activity if they attempt sudden exertion such as running up a flight of stairs. With warm-up exercise, this problem is minimized. A cool-down phase after strenuous exercise is also recommended. The pace should be slowed for 10 to 15 minutes before the activity is stopped, and a cool-

down exercise such as seated stretching can be used. After completion of the rehabilitation program, cardiac recipients can participate in many forms of exercise using these same guidelines.

The patient's drug regimen should also be considered when an exercise program is designed. Drugs that block the central effects of catecholamines such as propranolol or other β-blockers may limit exercise capacity in some recipients.[45] Patients on long-term prednisone therapy may be at risk for hip-joint problems, and certain activities such as jogging may not be the best choice for exercise. Other forms of exercise are particularly important to these individuals because regular exercise helps decrease muscle wasting and osteoporosis associated with steroid therapy.

Other lifestyle recommendations

The lifestyle recommendations outlined so far aim to minimize cardiac risk factors, prevent graft atherosclerosis, and maintain health. These recommendations would not be complete without discussing guidelines for smoking and alcohol consumption.

Recipients must understand before surgery that smoking in any form is prohibited for the rest of their lives. Smoking increases the risk of coronary artery disease, lung cancer, COPD, and life-threatening pulmonary infections.

Patients also must understand that alcohol is a drug that can interfere with immunosuppressive medications, particularly cyclosporine. Even moderate drinking places the patient at risk. There have been reports of heavy drinking leading to nonfatal and fatal episodes of rejection. Adolescent males may be at particular risk.[59] All patients suspected of having alcohol problems need immediate intervention.

Recognition of malignancy

Organ transplant recipients have an increased risk of malignancy compared with the normal population. Cardiac recipients seem to be at particular risk, with the incidence of malignancy reported to be as high as 10%.[44] The most common forms of malignancy are lymphomas and carcinoma of the skin, but other malignancies are also seen. The increased incidence of malignancy is thought to be due to impaired immunosurveillance of mutant cells arising from somatic mutation or viral infection. The cardiac transplant recipient may be more susceptible to oncogenic viruses such as Epstein-Barr virus.[23] Recipients need to have routine physical examination and screening for malignancy. Patients are advised to avoid excessive ultraviolet radiation and to check their skin and mucous membranes for unusual growths. They are also instructed to palpate cervical, axillary, and inguinal areas for swollen lymph nodes.

Issues related to quality of life

Cardiac transplantation offers the best hope for survival of patients with end-stage cardiac disease. After surgery, their lives usually change dramatically. Most have endured a long wait, during which they have had increasing signs and symptoms of cardiac failure. They needed intensive medical management from complicated drug regimens to mechanical assist devices. Within a day or two after the transplant, recipients may remark that they already feel better and can breathe easier, despite recent thoracic surgery.

However, multiple problems may be encountered from rejection, infection, or complications from the immunosuppressive drugs. As with all new medical technologies, it is important to look at the quality of life that these individuals have.

Quality of life is a difficult phenomenon to assess. There is still no precise definition of *quality of life,* and there are still no precise tools to measure it.[69] When quality of life is explored in relation to health issues, it is common to look at individuals' functional capacity, their perceptions of health, and the signs and symptoms they experience. Measuring the objective aspects such as exercise tolerance and return to work are more easily accomplished than measuring the subjective aspects such as satisfaction with life.

Regarding physical functioning, most recipients demonstrate excellent functional capacity.[15] As recovery progresses, most patients feel that their family relationships, roles, and social lives can return to normal.

An ongoing problem is that many cardiac transplant patients are unable to return to work. Before the transplant, more than 90% of candidates are unable to work. In the United States, approximately 30% of cardiac transplant recipients return to work after the surgery.[46] Many more would like to do so but have problems finding a job because of concerns related to medical insurance. The system of private insurance in the United States also may diminish opportunities for employment. Potential employers fear future medical disability and high health insurance costs. The situation is in contrast to European countries and Australia where more than 60% of recipients return to fulltime work, and an additional number are able to work parttime.[40,53] For the patients unable to return to employment outside the home, their financial status and role function continue to be adversely affected. For many cardiac patients, employment may be the most significant factor in their positive health perception.[35] Nurses, social workers, and other members of the transplant team need to act as patient advocates to promote return to work for heart transplant recipients. Personal conversations and letters describing the current health status and good prognosis of an individual can have a favorable impact on prospective employers.

Nurses and members of other disciplines have used various tools to assess quality of life. These tools examine patient perceptions, including their symptoms and attempts to evaluate their emotional adjustment, social roles, life satisfaction, and future outlook.[46]

Lough and others[47] studied the impact of symptom frequency and related symptom distress on heart transplant recipients' perceived quality of life. Their subjects included 75 patients between the ages of 19 and 60. They used the Quality of Life Scale developed by Young and Longman and two scales they developed to measure symptoms, the Transplant Symptom Frequency Scale and the Transplant Symptom Distress Scale. More than 20% of patients reported symptoms such as changed facial appearance, changed bodily appearance, pain (from osteoporosis), overeating, fatigue, lack of sleep, decreased interest in sex, and warts. The symptoms that occurred most frequently did not cause the most distress. Impotence and decreased interest in sex were found to be the most distressing, followed by changes in facial and bodily appearance. The postoperative event found to be most distressing was rejection. It had previously been thought that only the first rejection episode was distressing to patients.

Despite the symptoms experienced, 89% of the subjects reported their quality of life to be good to excellent, and 82% had good-to-high levels of life satisfaction. Recipients did not seem to perceive the symptoms as having much impact on their quality of life. The authors suggest that an *adaptation to symptoms,* in which recipients try to make the symptoms as invisible as possible, occurs. They concluded that nurses and physicians need to be sensitive to the likelihood that common problems may be distressing and provide a comfortable atmosphere in which to discuss them. Potential candidates also need to be aware of postoperative symptoms so that a realistic view can be promoted.

Research done by Mishel and Murdaugh[49] gives nurses further insight into the adaptation process that recipients and their families go through as they adjust to life after transplant. The authors used the grounded theory approach to study the process that heart transplant families use to manage the unpredictability of their lives. They interviewed 20 subjects in a support group who were family members of heart transplant patients. A process called "redesigning the dream" was identified to describe family adjustment to heart transplant. When families and patients enter the transplant program, they have a dream that life will return to normal after the transplant. Their attitudes and beliefs change as they actually go through the experience. After transplant, they begin to realize that the patient is vulnerable to infection, rejection, and other problems. They are able to suppress these feelings of vulnerability and view the future positively, but this balance is upset when a complication occurs or when they hear about problems with another recipient. Eventually these patients and their families realize that a new lifestyle that recognizes patients' vulnerability and unpredictable future must be structured.

Other quality-of-life studies have reported conflicting findings regarding physical and psychosocial functioning after cardiac transplantation. Waldren and others compared the quality of life of 24 transplant recipients with 20 similar patients who were treated medically.[69] They used three questionnaires and physiologic indicators to assess quality of life. Both groups were similar in psychosocial functioning, with the medical group reporting greater dysfunction in social activities compared with the transplant group. Both reported activity limitations, with the medical group limited by shortness of breath and the transplant group limited by fatigue and weakness. Both took the same number of medications (13 to 16 per day) and had the same low return-to-work rate (17% to 20%). There were more unexpected hospital days in the transplant group. On psychologic tests, both groups scored high on anxiety, depression, and hostility. The authors concluded that the anticipated emotional benefits of heart transplantation were not seen in this study population. They point out that with advances in medical therapy, patients with stable heart failure can now function quite well and that although transplant may increase survival, it may not improve quality of life over medical therapy.

Packa[54] studied quality of life after cardiac transplant in 22 recipients between the ages of 22 and 60. The McMaster Health Index Questionnaire was used to assess physical and psychosocial functioning. The Cantril Self-Anchoring Scale was used to rate patients' perceptions of quality of life. Subjects reported that their greatest improvement in quality of life was in physical functioning, but benefits were also seen in social and emotional func-

tion. Recipients felt that emotional adjustments to changes in lifestyle, body image, and self-esteem were most difficult. Some reported that it took them a year to regain the perception of being normal. About 95% of subjects considered their lives to be good and considered themselves to be happy or pretty happy.

These studies related to the quality of life after transplant may vary in results, but all point out the emotional adaptation and adjustments that patients and families need to make after transplant. The possibility of improving the quality of life after transplant poses a challenge to physicians, nurses, and transplant patients.

The challenge to physicians and medical researchers relates to potential improvements in immunosuppressive techniques. The possibility of decreasing or discontinuing steroids may decrease the number of symptoms and long-term complications experienced by patients. There is hope that monoclonal antibody technology may someday eliminate nonspecific immunosuppressive drug therapy. The search for a noninvasive alternative to endomyocardial biopsy continues and could eliminate the need for frequent invasive testing. Research also continues regarding the inhibition of graft atherosclerosis.

Nurses and physicians must continue to collaborate to promote a good quality of life for cardiac transplant recipients. It is already possible to predict that certain patients would have poor quality of life and rule them out during the evaluation phase. Through selection criteria, patients who would not benefit from transplant are identified. For example, a diabetic patient with peripheral vascular disease and neuropathic, nephropathic, and retinopathic conditions would not have improved quality of life after transplant. As discussed earlier, exclusion of patients on psychologic grounds is a difficult issue. Brennan and others[12] found that the presence of a preoperative personality disorder and a poor medical course postoperatively predicted a poorer quality of life. A personality disorder was associated with a potential for noncompliance. Only through future study will researchers identify patients most likely to benefit from transplant technology. For example, Aravot and others[3] report that cardiac transplant recipients over the age of 60 are able to achieve the same physical benefits and good quality of life as younger recipients.

Recipients' quality of life can be enhanced by thorough preoperative teaching and counseling. It is particularly important to review information related to postoperative care during the waiting period because patients and their families may forget important information over time. Because the role of the clinical transplant coordinator has developed, much more can be done in terms of patient teaching.

Nurses need to take an active role in recognizing and helping patients adapt to life after transplantation. As recipients experience complications or drug side effects, their expectations for the future are forced to change. They need to come to terms with their vulnerability if they are to be satisfied with their lives. Those who focus on medical problems and life's unknowns are at risk of having a poor quality of life. Recipients who cope best are those who focus on the joy of being alive.[47] Their family, work, or continued good health may be excellent motivators. Nurses can help patients to anticipate, understand, and cope with the life changes brought about by the transplant. The goal is to give them hope for the future and support them in their efforts to achieve a healthy adaptation.

In addition to physicians and nurses, cardiac recipients need to be available to assist other patients. *Transplant support groups* may have a positive effect on patients and families. Recipients can visit pretransplant patients to encourage hope and a realistic view of life after surgery. Patients can provide one another with emotional support. They can exchange valuable information regarding ways to cope with problems. Spouses and other family members may find it valuable to talk with family members of another transplant patient. Of course, these relationships have some degree of risk. When a member of a support group suffers a major complication or dies, it can be emotionally devastating to other group members. However, the positive aspects of group interaction far outweigh the negative, and most transplant centers encourage recipients to participate in a support group.

Nursing process

Case study. Mr. J. was a 40-year-old man with idiopathic cardiomyopathy. He was married and the father of four boys whose ages ranged from 10 to 19. Because Mr. J. was 6 feet tall and weighed 185 pounds, the search for a suitable donor took a long time. During the waiting period, Mr. J. had been unable to work at his job in a factory. The family depended on his disability pay and the money his wife earned working the evening shift in the housekeeping department of their local hospital. Mr. J. and his family endured a number of cardiac crises requiring emergency intervention during the waiting period. After waiting more than a year, Mr. J. underwent a successful transplant.

He had a smooth postoperative course and was discharged from the hospital 8 days after surgery. His family documented the occasion with snapshots of Mr. J. and the hospital staff. During the next few months, things did not go as easily for Mr. J. He had two asymptomatic episodes of mild rejection diagnosed by endomyocardial biopsy. These episodes were resolved with augmented steroid therapy. His blood sugars were consistently high. Steroid-induced diabetes was diagnosed, and Mr. J. was started on insulin. He and his family coped with these minor setbacks well. He continued to exercise and returned to work 2 months after surgery.

About a month later, Mr. J. noticed he wasn't feeling as well. While at work, he stopped to see the company nurse who found his heart rate to be 140. He called the transplant center and admitted that he was also short of breath. He was instructed to come to the hospital immediately and was admitted for an endomyocardial biopsy. As expected, the biopsy showed moderate-to-severe rejection changes. Mr. J. was treated with intravenous doses of methyprednisolone for 3 days. During that time, he continued to be intermittently short of breath. He went into uncontrolled atrial fibrillation, which was treated with digoxin and calcium channel blockers. He was hypotensive at times but did not have any major hemodynamic instability

associated with the episode of rejection. A repeat biopsy showed that the rejection was not resolving. The decision was made to treat him with the monoclonal antibody, OKT3. He was transferred to the intensive care unit for observation during the first 3 days of treatment. He tolerated the drug well and was able to transfer back to be monitored on the intermediate care unit for the last 7 days of OKT3. The next biopsy showed that the rejection was resolving.

Mr. J. and his wife were greatly relieved to hear the rejection was resolving, but they were frightened by what had happened. The rejection episode and associated symptoms took them by surprise. They had assumed that after he returned to work things would return to "normal" except for the routine postoperative monitoring. They expressed some anger at the number of complications he had experienced and the number of medications he now needed to take. Some long conversations with Mr. J.'s nurses and transplant coordinator were needed to help him and his family cope with the situation and adjust to the unpredictability of life. By the time Mr. J. left the hospital, he was feeling better physically and emotionally.

Nursing assessment

The purpose of a conceptual framework is to describe, explain, predict, and control the outcomes of nursing practice. The holistic Unitary Person Framework is used as a guide for nursing assessment and care provided to patients when they enter the hospital with a medical diagnosis such as acute transplant rejection. The Unitary Person Framework guides the collection of data and formulation of nursing diagnoses (see Appendix A for the Transplant Assessment Tool).

The response patterns that are most important to assess in patients suffering acute rejection include Exchanging, Choosing, Perceiving, Relating, and Knowing. The Exchanging Pattern involves patients' mutual giving and receiving. Collect data to assess cardiovascular status, hemodynamic variables, and potential for complications related to diagnostic procedures and augmented immunosuppressive drug therapy.

The Choosing Pattern involves patients' selection of alternatives. Examine patient and family problem-solving methods and decision-making ability. Identify indications of ineffective coping such as overt expressions of anxiety or hostility.

The Perceiving Pattern involves the reception of information by patients and families. Assess the effects of illness and surgery on self-concept. Body-image disturbance is common in transplant recipients, so carefully assess for signs of distress related to changes in body appearance.

The Relating Pattern pertains to the establishment of bonds and support systems. Assess the effects of illness on role function within and outside of family life. Multiple role changes are commonly forced on transplant patients and families before and after surgery, increasing the potential for altered role performance during hospitalization. Assess patients' adaptation to new or renewed roles in the community, at work, or within the family.

The Knowing Pattern deals with individual meanings associated with information. Assess patients' knowledge of the nature of their health problems, the treatment regimens, and their prognoses. Identify misconceptions and problems pertaining to the complicated treatment regimen.

Nursing diagnoses

The most common human responses anticipated for patients with acute rejection after cardiac transplantation are indicated by the following nursing diagnoses:

1. Decreased cardiac output related to acute rejection
2. High risk for infection and altered protection related to immunosuppression
3. High risk for injury related to endomyocardial biopsy
4. High risk for impaired renal and hepatic function related to cyclosporine
5. High risk for altered fluid, electrolyte, and glucose balance related to corticosteroid therapy
6. High risk for bone marrow suppression related to azathioprine
7. High risk for injury related to antilymphocyte preparations
8. High risk for ineffective individual and family coping related to anxiety and fear
9. High risk for body image disturbance related to side effects of corticosteroids
10. High risk for altered role performance related to continuing health problems
11. Knowledge deficit related to self-care after cardiac transplant

For each of these diagnoses, the patient outcomes, nursing prescriptions, and evaluation criteria are outlined with a discussion of the factual information that support the plan and implementation of care.

NURSING
DIAGNOSIS 1 **Decreased cardiac output related to acute rejection (exchanging pattern)**

PATIENT OUTCOMES	NURSING PRESCRIPTIONS	EVALUATION
Patient will maintain adequate cardiac output as evidenced by normal *hemodynamic* parameters (systolic blood pressure greater than 90 mm Hg, right atrial pressure of 10 to 15 mm Hg, and pulmonary artery wedge pressure of 12 to 15 mm Hg); urine output level greater than 30 ml/hour; normal sinus rhythm and heart and breath sounds; absence of signs and symptoms of right-sided heart failure (peripheral edema, abdominal pain, nausea, vomiting, jugular venous distention, and liver tenderness) and of left-sided heart failure (dyspnea, pulmonary edema, and hypotension); adequate peripheral pulses; warm, dry skin with good capillary refill; and normal or near-normal left ventricular ejection fraction on echocardiogram.	Evaluate patient's cardiac output by assessing hemodynamic parameters (systolic blood pressure, right atrial pressure, and pulmonary artery wedge pressure), urine output, cardiac rate and rhythm, heart and breath sounds, signs and symptoms of right- and left-sided heart failure, peripheral pulses, moisture and temperature of skin and capillary refill, and ventricular ejection fraction.	Patient maintained normal cardiac output as demonstrated by normal hemodynamic parameters, urinary output, sinus rhythm, and heart and breath sounds; absence of signs and symptoms of right- and left-sided heart failure; adequate peripheral pulses; warm, dry skin with capillary refill in less than 2 seconds, and normal left ventricular ejection fraction.
Patient's endomyocardial biopsy will show resolving rejection.	Assess for signs and symptoms and biopsy indications of resolving rejection.	Patient demonstrated resolving rejection as evidenced by biopsy.

Plan and intervention for decreased cardiac output

The majority of rejection episodes are recognized by endomyocardial biopsy rather than signs and symptoms because there is not a defining pattern of signs of rejection in patients receiving cyclosporine. Occasionally patients develop signs and symptoms, and when possible symptoms of rejection are recognized, they require urgent endomyocardial biopsy. The signs and symptoms of rejection are often vague. When recipients are not feeling well and there are no obvious signs of infection, it may be necessary to perform a biopsy before pursuing another diagnosis.

Rejection may be easily resolved with augmented immunosuppression. In many instances, there are no detectable hemodynamic abnormalities despite histologic evidence of rejection. Occasionally patients have severe rejection and become hemodynamically compromised; these patients may develop cardiogenic shock. Because of this possibility, all patients being treated for rejection must be closely observed. When recipients become unstable, they are transferred to the intensive care unit and treated as any other patient in cardiogenic shock. They may need inotropic support, the intraaortic balloon pump, and ventilatory support. Because acute rejection is an acute event, it is possible for the transplanted heart to recover completely from a severe rejection episode. Recipients with biventricular failure who have become critically ill may recover to the point of having normal cardiac function after resolution of the rejection episode.[51]

NURSING
DIAGNOSIS 2 **High risk for infection and altered protection related to immunosuppression (exchanging pattern)**

PATIENT OUTCOMES	NURSING PRESCRIPTIONS	EVALUATION
Patient's exposure to virulent organisms will be limited.	Limit patient exposure to virulent organisms by implementing protective isolation: washing hands before and after patient contact, using masks for individuals with respiratory infections and for performing invasive patient procedures, changing all drainage containers daily, closing door of private patient room, asking patient to avoid having plants and flowers in room, damp-dusting the room periodically, letting patient have no contact with visitors experiencing respiratory infections, transferring patient to floor as soon as possible.	Patient's exposure to virulent organisms was limited according to unit policy.
Patient's first lines of defense will remain intact.	Maintain patient's first lines of body defense by using strict aseptic techniques when inserting, maintaining, and discontinuing invasive tubes and lines, instituting routine culture procedures, using low pressure for tracheal suctioning.	Patient's first lines of body defense were maintained.
Patient will be free of signs and symptoms of infection as demonstrated by body temperature less than 37° C (99° F); WBC count of 4000 to 10,000/mm³; absence of shaking chills, cough, sore throat, sinus congestion, headache, urinary tract symptoms, or diarrhea; absence of redness, swelling, erythema, or warmth at intravenous sites; absence of redness or white patches on mucous membranes; absence of vaginal discharge or symptoms; and absence of skin lesions.	Evaluate patient for signs and symptoms of infections by assessing temperature and WBC count; observing for chills, cough, sore throat, sinus congestion, headache, urinary tract symptoms, or diarrhea; identifying redness, swelling, erythema, or warmth at intravenous sites; assessing for redness or white patches on mucous membranes; checking for vaginal discharge or symptoms; observing for skin lesions.	Patient was free of signs and symptoms of infections.
Chest x-ray film will be free of infiltrates, lesions, or cavitations.	Evaluate current chest x-ray film.	Patient demonstrated no evidence of infection on chest x-ray film.
CT scan of head and spinal fluid taps will be negative.	Evaluate findings from CT scan and spinal fluid taps.	Patient's CT scan and spinal fluid taps were normal.

Plan and intervention for infection and altered protection

The hospital is one of the most dangerous places for an immunosuppressed patient. There is risk of exposure to pathogenic organisms affecting other sick patients, and just spending time in the hospital can change patients' normal flora to pathologic. Some of these hospital organisms may be resistant to antibiotics.

Infections are most common during the first weeks and months after surgery.[39] Transplant recipients may be anergic before transplant as demonstrated by skin testing. The higher doses of immunosuppressive drugs and induction therapy with ATG or OKT3 also increase susceptibility to infection. In addition, recent surgery and poor nutritional status of these individuals adds to the risk.[29]

Thorough handwashing before and after patient contact is thought to be the most important strategy to prevent transmissible infection. However, in immunosuppressed patients, studies have shown that infection is usually derived from endogenous flora and organisms in the environment. Usual precautions for immunosuppressed patients include private rooms with the door closed to prevent infection transmission, masks for all persons with upper respiratory tract infections who must enter the room, and masks for nurse and patient when a central line must be entered.[29] Specific guidelines for isolation vary between institutions.

In addition to carrying out the institutional recommendations for protective isolation, a number of strategies can be used to limit the recipient's exposure to organisms. Most obviously, visitors and staff with signs of infection should not come in contact with the patient. Staff members taking care of immunosuppressed patients should not be assigned to other patients with known or potential infection.

Careful housekeeping procedures can also provide a safer environment for immunosuppressed patients. Changing all containers such as suction containers daily and periodic damp-dusting decrease the number of organisms.

Plants and flowers should be avoided because the soil and water contain organisms such as *Pseudomonas*.[22]

All intravenous catheters, endotracheal tubes, urinary catheters, and chest tubes bypass the body's normal protective barriers and are potential sources of infection. They must be inserted under strict sterile conditions, maintained aseptically, and discontinued as soon as possible.

Trauma to mucous membranes is carefully avoided because intact mucous membranes protect the body from invading organisms. If suctioning is necessary, it is done cautiously with low suction pressure. Rectal temperature measurements and enemas are avoided.

Because the hospital environment and particularly the intensive care unit environment are also considered risk factors, another strategy that limits exposure to pathogens is transfer of the recipient from the intensive care unit as soon as possible. There is also a trend toward early discharge from the hospital for this same reason. More care is being delivered to recipients in the outpatient department. For example, patients with moderate acute rejection who need intravenous methylprednisolone for a few days may receive treatment in the outpatient department.

Pulmonary assessment and vigorous pulmonary care are priorities because the most common site of serious infection in cardiac transplant recipients is the lungs.[36] Any sign of cough, fever, chills, elevated WBC levels, or infiltrate on chest x-ray film is carefully investigated. When infection is confirmed, antimicrobial agents are started immediately. Patients are also closely observed for signs of respiratory insufficiency or septic complications.

In patients receiving corticosteroids, the inflammatory response is suppressed, and there may be few signs of infection. Thus nurses must be diligent in observing for subtle signs such as malaise. Patients are questioned daily regarding urinary tract symptoms and other insidious symptoms of infection. Incisions and invasive line sites are closely observed. Specimens are sent for routine cultures and viral cultures when indicated, and results are promptly reported to the physician.

NURSING DIAGNOSIS 3	**High risk for injury related to endomyocardial biopsy (exchanging pattern)**	
PATIENT OUTCOMES	NURSING PRESCRIPTIONS	EVALUATION
Patient will have no complications related to endomyocardial biopsy as demonstrated by stable blood pressure and heart rhythm after the procedure; no evidence of bleeding, swelling, or pain at the biopsy site; normal breath sounds and absence of dyspnea and fever.	Evaluate patient for complications related to endomyocardial biopsy by assessing blood pressure and heart rhythm; biopsy insertion site for bleeding, swelling, or pain; breath sounds for evidence of dyspnea; and temperature Administer analgesics for discomfort as needed. Spend time with patient before and after reporting of biopsy results.	The patient had no complications related to endomyocardial biopsy as demonstrated by stable blood pressure and heart rhythm; absence of bleeding, swelling, or pain at biopsy site; normal breath sounds and absence of dyspnea and fever.

Plan and intervention for injury related to endomyocardial biopsy

Cardiac transplant recipients go through multiple endomyocardial biopsy procedures to screen for acute rejection and to assess the response to treatment of acute rejection. Right-sided heart catheterization with measurement of pulmonary artery pressures and cardiac output is also usually performed. The bioptome catheter is often advanced through the right jugular vein into the right ventricle (Fig. 18-6). Alternative sites include the femoral and subclavian veins. Sites may be rotated if scarring occurs.

Preparing patients for endomyocardial biopsy is similar to preparing them for other invasive vascular procedures.[21] If the patient is anticoagulated with warfarin, the medication should be withheld a few days before the procedure and a prothrombin time assessed. Often a sedative medication is ordered before the procedure; otherwise patients usually have nothing by mouth. An antibiotic may be administered prophylactically. A scrub to the biopsy site may be ordered. The procedure is usually performed by a cardiologist or cardiovascular surgeon and may be carried out in the catheterization laboratory or in the operating room, depending on institutional protocol. Blood for testing may also be drawn during the procedure to avoid repeated venipuncture. Patients may complain of mild discomfort during or after the procedure and may require oral analgesics. They may be quite anxious while waiting for the results.

Postprocedure nursing care includes site observation, frequent vital sign measurement, and maintenance of bed rest with the head elevated for several hours. Patients are usually admitted through the outpatient department the morning of the biopsy and discharged the same day.

Complications after a biopsy are rare because it is a venous rather than arterial procedure. Cardiac and respiratory assessments are performed every 15 minutes to 1 hour immediately after the procedure to observe for complications such as cardiac tamponade, hemothorax, or pneumothorax. A chest x-ray study may be ordered if a complication is suspected. Bleeding at the site is usually easily resolved with the application of pressure.

Occasionally patients may have atrial or ventricular ectopy during or after the procedure. Atrial fibrillation also is a possible complication. Patients may have a low-grade fever within a day after the biopsy if there has been hematoma formation or other traumatic complications.

After histologic analysis, patients are informed of the biopsy results by their physician or transplant coordinator. The diagnosis of rejection may be emotionally traumatic to patients and families. They need to be reassured that rejection is a common phenomenon that is almost always effectively treated with medication. In particular, when patients have been compliant, they need to know that the rejection episode is not their fault; rather it is the physiologic result of their immune system recognizing the transplanted heart.

NURSING
DIAGNOSIS 4   **High risk for impaired renal and hepatic function related to cyclosporine (exchanging pattern)**

PATIENT OUTCOMES	NURSING PRESCRIPTIONS	EVALUATION
Patient will maintain adequate renal and hepatic function as demonstrated by adequate urine output, stable body weight and physiologic intake and output, stable BUN level (less than 30 mg/dl) and serum creatinine level (less than 2 mg/dl), therapeutic serum or whole-blood cyclosporine levels, normal serum potassium levels, normal liver function studies, and systolic blood pressure under 140 mm Hg and diastolic blood pressure under 90 mm Hg.	Evaluate patient's renal and hepatic function by assessing urinary output, body weight and physiologic intake and output, BUN and creatinine levels, serum or whole-blood cyclosporine levels, serum potassium levels, liver function studies, and blood pressure.	Patient maintained normal renal and hepatic function as demonstrated by normal urinary output, stable body weight and physiologic intake and output, stable BUN and creatinine levels, therapeutic serum or whole-blood cyclosporine levels, normal serum potassium levels, normal liver function studies, and systolic blood pressure of 120 mm Hg and diastolic blood pressure of 80 mm Hg.

Plan and intervention for impaired renal and hepatic function related to cyclosporine

Renal and hepatic function are monitored closely in patients receiving cyclosporine because of the potential for toxicity. It is not unusual to see elevated BUN and serum creatinine levels and abnormal liver function, as well as hypertension, in patients receiving cyclosporine. Nurses caring for these patients must be aware of individual patients' normal laboratory values and interpret new values in reference to them. Many transplant centers use flow-sheets to facilitate this process.

When transplant recipients are hospitalized, it is important to monitor these values because patients may be receiving diagnostic testing or medications that can be nephrotoxic. Any diagnostic test involving the administration of contrast material may stress the kidneys. Medications such as antibiotics and nonsteroidal antiinflammatory drugs also may stress kidneys that have been damaged by chronic cyclosporine therapy. Besides monitoring laboratory determinations, nurses monitor daily weight measurements and maintain careful intake and output records.

Laboratory values outside of the recipient's normal range need to be reported promptly to the physician. In addition, patients need to be taught home blood pressure monitoring so that determinations outside the acceptable range can be reported and the response to diuretics and other antihypertensives can be monitored.

NURSING DIAGNOSIS 5	High risk for altered fluid, electrolyte, and glucose balance related to corticosteroid therapy (exchanging pattern)	
PATIENT OUTCOMES	**NURSING PRESCRIPTIONS**	**EVALUATION**
Patient will have balanced intake and output, stable body weight without excessive weight gain, normal serum electrolyte and blood glucose levels, and absence of edema.	Assess patient's intake and output. Weigh patient daily. Adjust oral intake and administer diuretics as ordered. Assess patient's serum electrolyte levels. Assess patient's blood glucose levels. Institute dietary restrictions and administer oral agents or insulin as ordered. Assess patient for signs of dependent edema.	Patient maintained a balanced intake and output, demonstrated stable body weight, demonstrated normal serum electrolyte and blood glucose levels, and exhibited no signs of dependent edema.

Plan and intervention for altered fluid, electrolyte, and glucose balance related to corticosteroid therapy

Patients receiving corticosteroids need to be observed for early and late complications related to these agents. A sudden weight gain and the presence of edema may indicate fluid retention. Intravenous fluids and oral intake may need to be adjusted, and diuretics are administered. Patients who were under fluid and sodium restrictions before surgery may be very discouraged to find out that these restrictions still apply after surgery. As patients recover and steroid doses are decreased, there is less tendency towards fluid retention, and fluid restrictions are usually not indicated.

The most common electrolyte imbalance seen in transplant recipients is hypokalemia resulting from the effects of steroids. Patients may require potassium replacement, even if they are not receiving diuretics.

Persistent elevations in blood glucose levels are seen in some patients receiving steroids. In patients with a preoperative diagnosis of diabetes controlled by diet or an oral agent, it may not be possible to manage the blood sugar level without insulin. Other patients with no history of hyperglycemia may develop this problem while receiving steroids. They may require insulin therapy for a few months or be managed with dietary restrictions and an oral agent. As steroids are tapered, the need for insulin or oral agents often ceases, and patients may require no further treatment for hyperglycemia.

NURSING
DIAGNOSIS 6 **High risk for bone marrow suppression related to azathioprine (exchanging pattern)**

PATIENT OUTCOMES	NURSING PRESCRIPTIONS	EVALUATION
The patient will have a WBC count greater than 4000/mm³.	Assess patient's WBC count. Withhold azathioprine if a significant drop in WBC is found; notify the physician. Monitor patient for WBC count of less than 4000/mm³. (Drug may need to be discontinued.)	Patient maintained a normal WBC count.
Patient will have a normal platelet count, hemoglobin level, and hematocrit.	Monitor patient's platelet count (and assess for signs of thrombocytopenia), hemoglobin level, and hematocrit.	Patient maintained a normal platelet count, hemoglobin level, and hematocrit.

Plan and intervention for suppression of bone marrow related to azathioprine

Patients receiving azathioprine (Imuran) usually do not have symptoms related to drug toxicity. However, it is common for the drug to cause laboratory abnormalities indicating bone marrow depression. The complete blood count is monitored frequently when patients are hospitalized and checked every month or every other month during outpatient visits. It is most common to see a decrease in the number of WBCs because neutrophils have a short survival when compared to other blood cells and are the first to be affected by drugs that depress the bone marrow. The hospitalized patient's dose of azathioprine is usually withheld until the results of the complete blood count are known. Because it is a long-acting drug, it does not matter whether it is administered at the same time each day. When a significant drop in the WBC count occurs, it may be necessary to withhold the drug for a few days to a week until the WBC count rises into the normal range. The drug may have to be discontinued in some recipients with chronically low WBC counts. Allowing the WBC to fall below 4000/mm³ increases susceptibility to infection.

If bone marrow depression is severe, the platelet count may drop, and the patient may develop signs of thrombocytopenia such as petechiae, easy bruising, nosebleeds, or prolonged bleeding time. A fall in hemoglobin and hematocrit may also be observed.

Azathiopine also can cause liver toxicity in some recipients. Liver function tests should be performed periodically, and patients should be assessed for abdominal pain or jaundice.[38] Occasionally patients will develop gastrointestinal distress after taking the medication, so they prefer to take it with food. Other rare reactions include mouth sores and hair loss.[39]

High risk for injury related to antilymphocyte preparations (exchanging pattern)

PATIENT OUTCOMES	NURSING PRESCRIPTIONS	EVALUATION
Patient will tolerate ATG or OKT3 therapy without evidence of adverse reaction as demonstrated by absence of dyspnea, wheezing, or cyanosis; normal arterial blood gas levels or pulse oximetry; blood pressure within normal range; body temperature of less than 38° C (101° F); absence of nausea, vomiting, or diarrhea; absence of headache or seizure activity; and with ATG, minimal pain at injection sites, absence of rash or leg edema, absence of leukopenia or thrombocytopenia, and absence of late reaction indicating serum sickness (fever, arthralgia, and myalgia).	Evaluate patient's tolerance to ATG or OKT3 therapy by assessing pulmonary status for evidence of bronchospasm or pulmonary edema, arterial blood gas levels or pulse oximetry results, blood pressure, temperature, observing for nausea, vomiting, or diarrhea or headache or seizure activity; and with ATG, assessing for pain at injection site, rash or leg edema, leukopenia or thrombocytopenia, and serum sickness. Administer acetaminophen, diphenhydramine, or steroids for adverse reactions. With ATG, administer ultrasound treatments or heating pads before and after intramuscular injections. Use a local anesthetic and Z-track injection technique and have the patient ambulate.	Patient tolerated antilymphocytic agents and demonstrated no adverse reactions.

Plan and intervention for injury related to antilymphocyte preparations

ATG and OKT3 are potent agents used for prevention and treatment of acute rejection. During the beginning of a course of these drugs, patients may experience a cluster of symptoms including fever, chills, nausea, vomiting, diarrhea, headache, and arthralgia.[60] Usually these symptoms do not last longer than 24 to 48 hours. They are thought to result from the physiologic response to T-cell lysis and the release of lymphokines. Patients are usually premedicated with acetaminophen, diphenhydramine, and steroids for the first few doses of intravenous ATG or OKT3 to minimize the potential for adverse reaction.

With the initial doses, vital signs and temperature are measured every 15 minutes for 2 hours and then at increasingly longer intervals. Pulmonary and vital sign assessment is done to evaluate for bronchospasm. Pulse oximetry or arterial blood gas tests may be performed, especially if respiratory distress is observed. Pulmonary edema has been reported to occur in patients with volume overload who receive OKT3.[60] There have been other rare reports of seizure activity and hypotension. Because of the potential for serious adverse reactions, patients are usually observed in a critical care unit for the first few doses. Later doses may be administered on an outpatient basis.

Daily weight and intake and output measurements are performed. Symptoms of nausea, vomiting, diarrhea, or headache are treated with antiemetic and analgesic medication.

In patients who receive ATG, there are additional considerations. Skin testing may be ordered before the first dose is given. Because most of these agents are experimental, the patient may need to sign a permit before the first dose. The complete blood count is monitored for leukopenia or thrombocytopenia. Patients may have considerable inflammation and pain at injection sites when ATG is given intramuscularly. This pain can be minimized by ultrasound treatments or by application of heating pads before and after administration. Mixing a local anesthetic with the serum before injection, using Z-track injection technique, and having the patient ambulate frequently also help minimize discomfort. For 2 or 3 weeks after the administration of ATG, the patient should be observed for late signs of serum sickness such as fever, arthralgia, and rash.[65]

NURSING
DIAGNOSIS 8   **High risk for ineffective individual and family coping related to anxiety and fear (choosing pattern)**

PATIENT OUTCOMES	NURSING PRESCRIPTIONS	EVALUATION
The patient and family will cope effectively with complications related to transplant.	Provide patient and family with information and skills to facilitate development of coping behaviors.	Patient and family demonstrated effective coping behaviors.
Patient and family will verbalize an understanding of the physiologic processes that lead to complications.	Teach the physiologic processes leading to complications.	Patient and family verbalized an understanding of the physiologic processes leading to complications.
Patient and family will verbalize an understanding of the drug side effects that cause complications.	Teach the side effects of medications that cause complications.	Patient and family verbalized an understanding of the side effects of medications that cause complications.
Patient and family will appropriately express feelings of anxiety, fears, aggression, and hostility.	Allow patients and families to verbalize feelings and frustrations related to complications.	Patient and family appropriately expressed feelings of anxiety, fear, aggression, and hostility.
Patient and family will develop skills to reduce anxiety, fears, aggression, and hostility.	Teach patient and family problem-solving, decision-making, assertive communication, and relaxation skills.	Patient and family demonstrated problem-solving, decision-making, assertive communication, and relaxation skills to reduce anxiety, fear, aggression, and hostility.

Plan and intervention for ineffective individual and family coping

Patients and families cling to a dream that life will return to normal after the transplant. The reality of the situation is that many patients develop episodes of rejection, infection, or complications related to the immunosuppressive drugs. When these complications occur, it may be very difficult for patients and families to cope effectively with them.

Patients and families need to receive help as they struggle to adapt to the ups and downs of life after transplantation. They need to hear that these complications are common and that other transplant patients have experienced and survived these same problems. It may help to review with them the physiologic processes that predispose them to complications. They need to be informed about what (if anything) they personally can do to assist in their recovery and maintain health in the future. For example, patients have some control over excessive weight gain but little control over steroid-induced diabetes.

It usually helps for patients to have a physician or nurse spokesperson to promote consistent communication and develop a continuous relationship. With large families, it can be effective to have them appoint a family spokesperson who is responsible for relaying information to the rest of the family. Families usually cope better when they feel they have a role in patients' care. They should be involved when possible in care planning and in patient education.

When the family visits and is invited to express their feelings and concerns to a health professional, privacy should be provided. Their level of anxiety and fear needs to be assessed with their knowledge of the situation. For some families, therapeutic discussions with a nurse are helpful and adequate. Others need to be referred to a professional counselor to achieve positive adaptation. Some patients are so depressed by fears of future complications that they may need to see a psychiatrist. As patients and families are helped to integrate their feelings of vulnerability into their lives, most can feel positive about the future and again focus on the joy of being alive.

Occasionally patients and families have difficulty coping with the donor's death. A type of *survivor's guilt* can occur. They may be compulsive in their attempts to obtain information about the donor. Recipients may imagine that they are assuming some of the donor's supposed characteristics or personality traits. A few ask for their donor's birthdate so they can celebrate their "other birthday." Nurses should encourage patients and families to discuss these feelings. Anonymous thank you letters and cards may be channeled through the transplant coordinators to the donor's family. Patients and families may feel better if there is some communication, but direct communication is generally discouraged. Donor families may also have a need to find out how the recipient is doing. Nurses can be instrumental in assisting families with these delicate communications so that they can move on to look at the future.

NURSING
DIAGNOSIS 9   **High risk for body image disturbance related to side effects of corticosteroids (perceiving pattern)**

PATIENT OUTCOMES	NURSING PRESCRIPTIONS	EVALUATION

Patient will adapt to a change in body image.
  Patient will verbalize feelings of changed facial and body appearance.
 	
Patient will verbalize steps that can be taken to minimize changes.
	Assist patient to adapt to changes in body image.
	  Provide opportunities for the patient to express feelings of loss and distress about changes in facial and body appearance.
	  Teach patient about steps that can be taken to minimize changes, including that changes will decrease over time as steroids are tapered, dietary counseling will assist in minimizing weight gain and fluid retention, and regular exercise can minimize weight gain and promote feelings of well-being.
		Patient demonstrated adapation to changes in body image.
		  Patient appropriately expressed feelings of loss and distress about changes in facial and body appearance.
		  Patient correctly listed the steps that can be taken to minimize changes, including verbalizing that changes will decrease over time as steroids are tapered, participating in dietary counseling, and participating in a regular exercise program.

Patient will verbalize own strengths in appearance and functions.	Assist patient to recognize personal strengths in appearance and functions.	Patient recognized and verbalized own strengths in appearance and functions.

Plan and intervention for body image disturbance

Although patients are informed about the potential for changes in facial and bodily appearance, most do not think this will happen to them. Some recipients have minimal changes in appearance, whereas others may change considerably. For some patients, Cushingoid changes are extremely upsetting and damage their self-concept and sense of well-being. Weight gain, moon face, acne, warts, increased bodily and facial hair growth, fragile and easily bruised skin, a protuberant abdomen, and thin extremities may occur during the first year after the transplant. Patients will say things such as "I want my old face back" or "I hate my face." Younger patients and women seem to be most sensitive to the changes.

In addition to the physical changes, patients may be simultaneously dealing with mood swings and other challenges such as lifestyle changes or rejection episodes. They should be encouraged to verbalize their feelings related to all problems. In addition to discussing them with staff nurses, they may need to talk with the clinical transplant coordinator, a clinical nurse specialist, a social worker, a psychologist, or a psychiatrist. Nurses can assess the severity of the problem and facilitate communication with the most appropriate sources of help. Often a team approach involving a number of health professionals works well.

Patients struggling to accept their appearances need to know that these side effects often decrease over time, especially when steroids are tapered. For example, patients may develop acne over the upper body a few months after transplant, but it rarely persists over time and usually improves over the next few months as the steroid dose is reduced. Dietary counseling can help minimize the effects of steroid therapy. A regular exercise program can help minimize weight gain, muscle wasting, and fat deposition.

Sharing concerns with other transplant patients can also be very effective because they have a unique understanding of patients' feelings. Nurses can facilitate communication between transplant patients within support groups on an informal basis.

NURSING
DIAGNOSIS 10   **High risk for altered role performance related to continuing health problems (relating pattern)**

PATIENT OUTCOMES	NURSING PRESCRIPTIONS	EVALUATION
Patient will work to reestablish role in the family.	Assist patient in reestablishing role in family. 　Explore and clarify patient's perception of role performance in family. 　Discuss how current changes in health status will affect family dynamics. 　Facilitate family meetings to clarify role expectations. 　Involve family in clarifying expectations and in giving feedback.	Patient successfully reestablished preillness role in family.
Patient will resume preillness social relationships.	Assist patient in resuming preillness social relationships. 　Discuss how current health status will change roles regarding social, religious, and community activities. 　Facilitate discussions allowing patient to verbalize anxiety and fears regarding resumption of social activities. 　Use relaxation, guided imagery, and role rehearsal in preparing for return to social activities.	Patient resumed preillness social relationships with community group.
Patient will work toward resuming occupational role.	Assist patient in reestablishing occupational role. 　Facilitate discussions to evaluate options regarding return to work. 　Assist patient in identifying strength and weakness. 　Explore options for role changes, occupational alternatives, and necessary adjustments. 　Use supportive guidance for determining priorities. 　Foster communication and problem-solving skills. 　Refer patient to social worker to assist with medical benefits. 　Refer to appropriate occupational counselor.	Patient returned to fulltime work.

Plan and intervention for altered role performance

The main role of most cardiac transplant recipients before surgery is the sick role. Usually patients have been increasingly dependent on other family members, often lacking the stamina to perform even simple household tasks.[46] Social activities may have ceased, and almost all have stopped work or school outside the home.

After the transplant, adaptations need to be made as the recipient attempts to resume preillness roles. For some families, this is quickly and easily accomplished; for others, there may be difficulty perceiving patients as well persons. Families need to reestablish relationships, and this radical change in family dynamics can lead to marital stress and strain on all relationships within the family. Most families slowly adjust and eventually reestablish relationships.[46] An added stressor on young families is the question of reproduction. Female recipients may be advised to avoid *pregnancy* because of the unknown effects of immunosuppressive drugs on the fetus. Patients with familial cardiomyopathy may be advised against bearing children. Health professionals need to address these concerns in younger recipients.

Most recipients resume social activities with friends, religious institutions, and community organizations. Initially they may encounter insensitive persons who treat them as a curiosity and make inappropriate remarks. Patients may need to talk over these incidents so that they do not move toward social isolation. Rather they need to see that a major reason for having transplant surgery was to continue to be active and involved and do the things they want to do yet in life.

Returning to work presents a great challenge to transplant recipients. Some ceased work years before transplant and no longer have any connections with an employer. Others feel that technology has changed so much they would no longer be capable of doing their jobs without extensive training. Many fear that returning to work will result in an overall lowering of their financial status because of a loss of disability payments and Medicare coverage.

Some recipients previously worked in physically demanding or hazardous positions that would not be appropriate after surgery. For example, a patient receiving long-term steroid therapy is at risk for fractures and would no longer be suited to a physically demanding job that requires heavy lifting.

Despite all these obstacles, it is certainly possible for many heart recipients to return to work. The patients who seem to return to work most easily are those who worked up until shortly before the transplant and have a job waiting for them, but others may be able to find fulltime or part-time employment. Patients need positive encouragement to at least explore options for returning to work. Social workers can be helpful in avoiding gaps in medical benefits as patients make the transition from medical disability to employment. Nurses may be able to facilitate the process by assisting with the completion of forms and letters describing the patient's prognosis, any limitations, and the medical plan of care for the future. Having the individual go in person to talk with the previous or potential employer can be effective because some have misconceptions about transplant recipients being attached to machines or other reservations. Seeing the individual's healthy appearance can have a positive effect.

NURSING
DIAGNOSIS 11   **Knowledge deficit related to self-care after cardiac transplant (knowing pattern)**

PATIENT OUTCOMES	NURSING PRESCRIPTIONS	EVALUATION
Patient will demonstrate knowledge and assume responsibility related to self-care.	Assist patient to assume responsibilitiy for self-care.	Patient assumed responsibility for self-care.
Patient will verbalize an understanding of each content area in the discharge heart transplant teaching plan (see the box, p. 624).	Provide consistent teaching regarding content areas outlined in the discharge heart transplant teaching plan (see the box, p. 624).	Patient verbalized an understanding of the content of the discharge heart transplant teaching plan (see the box, p. 624).
Patient will participate in health care decisions.	Provide opportunities for the patient to participate in health care decisions.	Patient participated in health care decisions.
Patient will demonstrate compliance with lifestyle recommendations.	Evaluate patient compliance regarding medications, prevention of infection, prevention of rejection, maintenance of body weight, diet, activity and exercise program, stress management, and follow-up medical care.	Patient demonstrated high compliance regarding medications, prevention of infection, prevention of rejection, maintenance of body weight, diet, activity and exercise program, stress management, and follow-up medical care.
Patient will recognize and report health problems.	Teach patient health problems to recognize and promptly report.	Patient verbalized health problems to recognize and promptly report.

Plan and intervention for knowledge deficit

Teaching begins during the preoperative phase and continues throughout patients' lives. Recipients and their families need to possess a large amount of information to carry out their medical regimen. It is unrealistic to think that this teaching can be completed in the immediate postoperative period before discharge. During the early recovery period, nurses and other members of the transplant team must concentrate on the information patients need to have in the early recovery period. Because patients return frequently for postoperative testing, a broad teaching plan that includes the information needed over time (see box) is devised. The clinical transplant coordinator usually is responsible for providing much of the information after discharge from the hospital. The clinical dietician, staff nurses, cardiac rehabilitation nurses, and others may also be involved in long-term teaching. The main topics that need to be covered and reinforced periodically relate to rejection, recognition and prevention of infection, side effects and complications of drug therapy, and lifestyle recommendations.

Providing patients with factual information enables them to actively participate in health care decisions. With this information, patients are able to assume responsibility for themselves and are more likely to comply with medical regimens and lifestyle recommendations. Recognizing and reporting problems is a key goal of the teaching plan because problems must be addressed before they progress and become life threatening. Education does not, however, ensure compliance. Nurses may be the first to identify compliance problems. It is imperative that these problems are addressed and a plan implemented because noncompliance in this case can be life threatening.

Transplant recipients and families are viewed as partners in quality patient care. With the transplant team and the patient's personal physician, they complete the team effort necessary to maintain survival and quality of life after cardiac transplant.

DISCHARGE HEART TRANSPLANT TEACHING PLAN

Prior to discharge the patient and family will:

Demonstrate accuracy related to self-administration of medications:
Cyclosporine
Azathioprine
Prednisone
Other prescribed medications

Verbalize information related to immunosuppressive drugs:
Common side effects
Timing of doses
Laboratory measurement of cyclosporine levels
Adequate supply of medication

Verbalize strategies to prevent infection:
Avoidance of people with infection
Careful dietary choices

Verbalize signs and symptoms of infection and when to call physician:
Fever above 100° F
Respiratory symptoms (e.g., cough and sore throat)
Gastrointestinal symptoms
Cutaneous lesions

Verbalize strategies to prevent rejection:
Taking medication exactly as directed
Notifying transplant team of change in medications

Avoiding alcohol and over-the-counter drugs

Verbalize possible signs and symptoms of rejection:
Hypotension
Dysrhythmias
Symptoms of congestive heart failure

Accurately record vital signs and weight daily:
Record keeping
Knowledge of acceptable parameters

Maintain body weight within normal parameters:
Verbalize guidelines for low-cholesterol, no-added-salt diet
Balance intake with activity

Demonstrate compliance with activity and exercise recommendations:
Progressive cardiac rehabilitation
Expectations regarding return to work and normal activities

Demonstrate an understanding of routine follow-up care:
Laboratory work and office visits
Endomyocardial biopsy schedule
Yearly heart catheterization

Verbalize satisfaction with lifestyle after transplant:
Management of emotional problems
Daily stress management such as relaxation, music therapy, and imagery

KEY CONCEPT REVIEW

1. The transplant candidate with a high PRA is at risk for:
   a. CMV infection
   b. Hyperacute rejection
   c. Chronic renal insufficiency
   d. Hepatic failure

2. A cardiac transplant candidate's pulmonary vascular resistance is evaluated to avoid:
   a. Lifelong pulmonary hypertension
   b. Postoperative respiratory failure
   c. Right ventricular failure of the donor heart
   d. Postoperative pulmonary emboli

3. A complication of brain death commonly seen in donors is:
   a. Diabetes insipidus
   b. Diabetes mellitus
   c. Hypertension
   d. Hyperventilation

4. Efforts are made to keep the ischemic time of the donor heart below:
   a. 4 hours
   b. 6 hours
   c. 8 hours
   d. 12 hours

5. The diet most commonly ordered for cardiac recipients is:
   a. 1800-calorie ADA
   b. Low purine
   c. 2-gram sodium
   d. Low cholesterol, no added salt

6. Acute rejection of the transplanted heart can be most accurately detected by:
   a. Echocardiogram
   b. Endomyocardial biopsy
   c. ECG
   d. Coronary angiography

7. In recipients receiving azathioprine (Imuran), it is important to closely monitor:
   a. Serum K levels
   b. Sedimentation rate
   c. Uric acid level
   d. WBC count

8. Adverse reactions in patients receiving a course of OKT3 are most often seen:
   a. On day 1
   b. On day 10
   c. 2 weeks after therapy
   d. 4 weeks after therapy

9. Common side effects of cyclosporine include:
   a. Bone marrow depression and hypercalcemia
   b. Bradycardia and hypotension
   c. Nephrotoxicity and hypertension
   d. Osteoporosis and fluid retention

10. An important strategy that the hospital staff can use to prevent infection in transplant recipients is:
    a. Wearing gowns, hats, and gloves
    b. Not allowing fresh fruit in the patient's diet
    c. Using sterile linen
    d. Thorough handwashing

11. Nursing research indicates that successful adaptation to life after transplant involves coping with:
    a. Probable social isolation
    b. Frequent venipuncture
    c. The unpredictability of their condition
    d. Limited cardiac function

12. Recipients who seem to be most satisfied with their quality of life are those who focus on:
    a. Drug side effects
    b. The joy of being alive
    c. Perioperative family stress
    d. Returning to work

ANSWERS

1. b.	3. a.	5. d.	7. d.	9. c.	11. c.
2. c.	4. a.	6. b.	8. a.	10. d.	12. b.

REFERENCES

1. Achuff SC and Augustine SM: Outpatient management of the heart transplant patient. In Baumgartner WA, Reitz BA, and Achuff SC, editors: Heart and heart-lung transplantation, Philadelphia, 1990, WB Saunders Co.

2. Altman LK: New drug shows stunning success in organ transplant operations, The New York Times, p A1, Oct 18, 1989.

3. Aravot DJ and others: Cardiac transplantation in the seventh decade of life, Am J Cardiol 63(1):90, 1989.

4. Augustine SM: Nursing care of the heart and heart-lung transplant patient. In Baumgartner WA, Reitz BA, and Achuff SC, editors: Heart and heart-lung transplantation, Philadelphia, 1990, WB Saunders Co.

5. Baughman KL: Monitoring of allograft rejection. In Baumgartner WA, Reitz BA, and Achuff SC, editors: Heart and heart-lung transplantation, Philadelphia, 1990, WB Saunders Co.

6. Baumgartner WA: Comparative results and future implications of heart transplantation. In Baumgartner WA, Reitz BA, and Achuff SC, editors: Heart and heart-lung transplantation, Philadelphia, 1990, WB Saunders Co.

7. Baumgartner WA: Evaluation and management of the heart donor. In Baumgartner WA, Reitz BA, and Achuff SC, editors: Heart and heart-lung transplantation, Philadelphia, 1990, WB Saunders Co.

8. Bellanti JA: Immunology III, Philadelphia, 1985, WB Saunders Co.

9. Bollman RM: Cardiac transplantation without a prospective crossmatch, Transplant Proc 17(1):209, 1985.

10. Borkon AM: Morbidity following heart transplantation. In Baumgartner WA, Reitz BA, and Achuff SC, editors: Heart and heart-lung transplantation, Philadelphia, 1990, WB Saunders Co.

11. Borkon AM and Augustine SM: Immediate postoperative management of the heart transplant recipient. In Baumgartner WA, Reitz BA, and Achuff SC, editors: Heart and heart-lung transplantation, Philadelphia, 1990, WB Saunders Co.

12. Brennan AF and others: Predictors of quality of life following cardiac transplantation, Psychosomatics 28(11):566, 1987.

13. Cameron DE and Baumgartner WA: Organ preservation in cardiac and cardiopulmonary transplantation, part 1, Transplant Management 1(2):3, 1989.

14. Cardin S and Clark S: A nursing diagnosis approach to the patient awaiting cardiac transplantation, Heart Lung 4(4):500, 1985.

15. Christopherson LK: Cardiac transplantation: a psychological perspective, Circulation 75(1):57, 1987.

16. Cockburn ITR and Krupp P: An appraisal of drug interactions with Sandimmune, Transplant Proc 21(5):3845, 1989.

17. Collins JA and others: Home intravenous dobutamine therapy in patients awaiting heart transplantation, J Heart Transplant 9(3):205, 1990.

18. Cooper DKC and Lanza RP, editors: Heart transplantation, Boston, 1984, MTP Press Ltd.

19. Copeland JG and others: Selection of patients for cardiac transplantation, Circulation 75(1):2, 1987.

20. Dietz RR: Characteristics of the transplanted heart in the radionuclide ventriculogram, J Heart Transplant 5(2):116, 1986.

21. Dressler DK: Current trends in heart transplantation. In Kern LS, editor: Cardiac critical care nursing, Rockville, Md, 1988, Aspen Publishers, Inc.

22. Dressler DK: Infection in the immunosuppressed patient. In VonRueden KT and Walleck CA, editors: Advanced critical care nursing, Rockville, Md, 1989, Aspen Publishers, Inc.

23. Duncan C: De novo cancer in transplant recipients, Transplantation Today 2(1):32, 1985.

24. Frazier OH and others: Nutritional management of the heart transplant recipient, J Heart Transplant 4(4):450, 1985.

25. Futterman LG: Cardiac transplantation: a comprehensive nursing perspective. I. Heart Lung 17(5):499, 1988.

26. Futterman LG: Cardiac transplantation: a comprehensive nursing perspective, II. Heart Lung 17(6):631, 1988.

27. Gamberg P, Miller JL, and Lough ME: Impact of protective isolation on the incidence of infection after heart transplantation, J Heart Transplant 6(3):147, 1987.

28. Goldsmith J and Montefusco CM: Nursing care of the potential organ donor, Crit Care Nurs 6(2):25, 1985.

29. Griffin JP: Nursing care of the critically ill immunocompromised patient, Crit Care Nurs Q 9(1):25, 1986.

30. Gutkind L: Many sleepless nights, New York, 1988, WW Norton & Co., Inc.

31. Guttendorf B and others: The impact of protective isolation on the incidence of early infection of adult heart transplant patients, Circulation supplement II 78(4):11, 1988.

32. Harwood CH and Cooke CV: Cyclosporine in transplantation, Heart Lung 4(4):529, 1985.

33. Heck CF, Shumway SJ, and Kaye MP: The registry of the international society for heart transplantation: sixth official report—1989, J Heart Transplant 8(4):271, 1989.

34. Hess N and others: Complete isolation: is it necessary? J Heart Transplant 4(4):458, 1985.

35. Hiatt DP, Peglar M, and Borgen FH: Patterns of perception of health in cardiac patients, Psychosom Res 28:87, 1984.

36. Horn JE and Bartlett JG: Infectious complications following heart transplantation. In Baumgartner WA, Reitz BA, and Achuff SC, editors: Heart and heart-lung transplantation, Philadelphia, 1990, WB Saunders Co.

37. Hosenpud JD and others: OKT3-induced hypotension in heart allograft recipients treated for steroid-resistant rejection, J Heart Transplant 8(1):159, 1989.

38. Hutchings SM and Monett ZJ: Caring for the cardiac transplant patient, Crit Care Clin North Amer 1(2):245, 1989.

39. Imperial FA, Cordova-Mangibas L, and Ward CR: Cardiac transplantation, Crit Care Clin North Am 1(2):399, 1989.

40. Jones BM and others: Psychological adjustment after cardiac transplantation, Med J Aust 149:118, 1988.

41. Kahl LE, Thompson ME, and Griffith BP: Gout in the heart transplant recipient: Physiologic puzzle and therapeutic challenge, Am J Med 87:289, 1989.

42. Katz MR and others: Are steroids essential for successful maintenance of immunosuppression in heart transplantation? J Heart Transplant 6(5):293, 1987.

43. Kuo PC and others: Lovastatin therapy for hypercholestremia in cardiac transplant recipients, Am J Cardiol 64:631, 1989.

44. Lanza RP and others: Malignant neoplasms occurring after cardiac transplantation, JAMA 13:1746, 1983.

45. Levett JM and Karp RB: Heart transplantation, Surg Clin North Am 65(3):613, 1985.

46. Lough ME: Quality of life for heart transplant recipients, J Cardiovasc Nurs 2(2):11, 1988.

47. Lough ME and others: Impact of symptom frequency and symptom distress on self-reported quality of life in heart transplant recipients, Heart Lung 16(2):193, 1987.

48. Love KR: Donor-transmitted infections, Cardiac surgery: state of the art reviews, 3(3):639, 1989.

49. Mishel M and Murdaugh CL: Family adjustment to heart transplantation: redesigning the dream, Nurs Res 36(6):332, 1987.

50. Muirhead J: Heart and heart-lung transplantation, Nurs Clin North Am 224(4):865, 1989.

51. Murdock DK and others: Rejection of the transplanted heart, Heart Lung 16(3):237, 1987.

52. Najarian JS: Immunological aspects of organ transplantation, Hosp Prac 17(10):65, 1982.

53. Niset G, Coustry-Degre C, and Degre S: Psychosocial and physical rehabilitation after heart transplantation, Cardiology 75:311, 1988.

54. Packa DR: Quality of life of adults after a heart transplant, J Cardiovasc Nurs 3(2):12, 1989.

55. Ragsdale D: Nutritional program for heart transplantation, J Heart Transplant 6(4):228, 1987.

56. Renlund DG, O'Connell JB, and Bristow Mr: Early rejection prophylaxis in heart transplantation: is cytolytic therapy necessary? J Heart Transplant 8(3):191, 1989.

57. Renlund DG and others: Feasibility of discontinuation of corticosteroid maintenance therapy in heart transplantation, J Heart Transplant 6(2):71, 1987.

58. Riether AM and Boudreau MZ: Heart transplant impact on CCU nurses, Am J Nurs 88(11):1521, 1988.

59. Ring WS: Pediatric transplantation, paper presented at the meeting of The Minneapolis Heart Institute, Tucson, Ariz, Feb 28 to March 3, 1990.

60. Rogers KR, Sinnott JT, and Ferguson JE: Using OKT3 to reverse cardiac allograft rejection, Heart Lung 18(5):490, 1989.

61. Shapiro ME: Use of anti-IL-2 receptor monoclonal antibodies for immunosuppression, Transplant Management 2(1):3, 1990.

62. Soifer BE and Gelb AW: The multiple organ donor: identification and management, Ann Intern Med 110(6):814, 1989.

63. Stamler JS, Vaughan DE, and Rudd MA: Frequency of hypercholesterolemia after cardiac transplantation, Am J Cardiol 62:1268, 1988.

64. Starling RC and Cody RJ: Cardiac transplant hypertension, Am J Cardiol 65:106, 1990.

65. Tatum AH, Bollinger RR, and Sanfilippo F: Rapid serological diagnosis of serum sickness for antithymocyte globulin therapy using enzyme immunoassay, Transplantation 38(6):582, 1984.

66. Traill TA: Physiology and function of the transplant allograft. In Baumgartner WA, Reitz BA, and Achuff SC, editors: Heart and heart-lung transplantation, Philadelphia, 1990, WB Saunders Co.

67. United Network for Organ Sharing: UNOS update 5:10, October 1989.

68. United States General Accounting Office: Heart transplants: concerns about costs, access, and availability of donor organs, U.S. General Accounting Office, Washington, DC, 1989.

69. Waldren JA and others: Heart transplantation may not improve quality of life for patients with stable heart failure, Heart Lung 18(5):497, 1989.

70. Young JB and others: Heart replacement for terminal cardiac disease: cardiac transplantation and mechanical sustenance of the cardiovascular system, Baylor Cardiology Series 12:4, 1989.

71. Zehr P: Assessing patient knowledge of essential transplant concepts, research presented at the meeting of the North American Transplant Coordinators Organization, Washington, DC, July 1989.

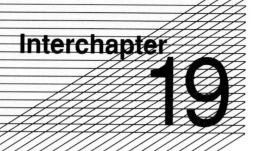

Interchapter 19

Bringing Healing into Technology

Have you ever thought of the hospital or clinic in which you work as an unchangeable, monolithic structure completely outside the influence of you or others? What visions have you had about bringing healing qualities into modern hospitals, clinics, and outpatient facilities? What can be done to reduce the fear and apprehension that patients and families feel on entering them? What can be done to blend technology and healing? The following examples can serve as models.

Planetree, a 13-bed medical-surgical unit in San Francisco Pacific Presbyterian Medical Center[4] has achieved national prominence among hospital administrators and designers for its philosophy and design. At Planetree, the staff is selected carefully; only those nurses and physicians committed to the Planetree philosophy work on the unit. The nurses station is in full view of the patients and is open to them. Patients can read their own medical charts and may add their own observations, responses, and feelings. The Planetree staff goes to great lengths to answer questions and dispel the mysteries surrounding the patient and family. Each patient can request a survey of the pertinent medical literature from the Planetree library, giving him or her a chance to read about the illness. Nurses are available to interpret anything that is not clear. Planetree has created a nurturing environment with carefully selected colors, lighting, fabrics, carpet, furniture, art, and curved walls. There is a piano and an art program, and patients may choose pictures for their walls from an "art cart." The intrusive, jarring hospital items and clutter, such as chart racks, linen charts, bandage carts, and technologic equipment, are kept in storage and brought out when needed.

Visiting hours at Planetree are at the discretion of the patient. A patient lounge and comfortable surroundings encourage family and visitors to stay near. Family and friends are taught how to participate in patient care before, during, and after hospitalization. Patient and family can also cook for themselves in the unit's kitchen, and a nutritionist assists them in the best foods for recovery.

Planetree illustrates how changes can occur as a result of creativity, ingenuity, and sharing of ideas with colleagues and management. Moreover, it models a philosophy, an environment, and a health care team approach that enhances the healing and well-being of patients, families, and staff

Next time you go into a patient room, imagine that you are the patient. What is nurturing in the environment? What takes your energy away? What does the art look like? What would it take to develop an "art cart" for your unit? Are beds placed near windows for viewing nature? If there are rooms with no windows, is it possible to get a poster or picture of nature to hang on the wall? Patients with a view of nature have been shown to have shorter postoperative hospital stays, take less pain medication, have fewer complications, and give fewer negative evaluations of nurses.[5]

What kind of clutter stands in patient areas that could be organized or stored differently? Is your nurse's station behind a glass wall? Does it convey the unspoken message that patients must stay away? If the nurse's station is cold and isolated, what can be done to change its image?

Music, a long-neglected therapy in medical settings, can be a solace in the hospital or clinic. Properly selected music should be played throughout the hospital corridors, patient rooms, family units, cafeterias, and elevators. Studies have demostrated the power of music to enhance healing. An example is that the incidence of anxiety and complications can be reduced when a patient listens to a music cassette of choice following acute myocardial infarction.[2] The use of music to enhance healing and relaxation is applicable to all patients during medical and surgical procedures. Patients can be given the choice of bringing their own music and audiocassette recorders to the procedures or they can check out this equipment from the unit's audiocassette library if one is available (see Chapter 5). The music played by the patient is unobtrusive to the staff or other patients when it is channeled to the patient via the audiocassette headphones. Music selections are also important to consider for nursing stations and lounges, and for the medical or surgical team as they perform their procedures. Properly chosen music can decrease tension and help with focused concentration.[3]

Behavioral anesthesia is a technique used by nurses, nurse anesthetists, anesthesiologists, and surgeons before, during, and after anesthesia induction. It incorporates the precise use of drugs and other anesthesia agents with simultaneous use of psychological agents—touch, music, communication signals, gestures, nonverbal gesturing that conveys love and caring and positive suggestions. Some examples of these positive suggestions are "You will awake with minimal pain" "You will have complete healing" "You will be back at work in 6 weeks." It is well documented that patient healing is enhanced with the use of behavioral anesthesia.[1]

Our challenge is to use behavioral anesthesia to lessen the anxiety and fear surrounding the procedure or surgery. We can assist patients in choosing positive suggestions and how to use them in their healing. We also can have available or can make customized preoperative and postoperative audiocassette tapes for patients to use before, during, and after procedures and allow uninterrupted periods for practice sessions.

One of the greatest gifts nurses can give patients is the use of biobehavioral interventions—relaxation, music therapy, and imagery—that assist patients in accessing their inner healing resorces. The important qualities for the nurse are a presence of healing, active listening skills, and serving as a facilitator. Details of each intervention are discussed in Chapter 5.

REFERENCES

1. Bennett HL: Behavioral anesthesia, Advances 2:11-21, 1985.
2. Guzzetta CE: Effects of relaxation and music therapy on patients in a coronary care unit with presumptive acute myocardial infarction, Heart Lung 18:609-616, 1989.
3. Guzzetta CE: Music therapy: hearing the melody of the soul. In Dossey B and others: Holistic nursing: a handbook for practice, Gaithersburg Md, 1988, Aspen Publishers.
4. Planetree: The new industry standard for satisfying customers, Hosptial Entrepreneurs' Newsletter 4 (2), July, 1988.
5. Ulrich RS: View through a window may influence recovery from surgery, Science 224:420-421, 1984.

19

The Person Participating in Inpatient and Outpatient Cardiac Rehabilitation

Ursula K. Anderson

LEARNING OBJECTIVES

1. Define three important topics to be included in an inpatient cardiac education program for patients and families.
2. Name at least three key members of an inpatient cardiac rehabilitation team.
3. Describe three role components of a nurse involved with a multidisciplinary program for inpatients and their families.
4. Examine the three components of a comprehensive rehabilitation program.
5. Write the formula for 1 MET.
6. Discuss two evaluation methods for measuring readiness to learn.

7. Describe an effective evaluation method to measure rehabilitation success.
8. Explore three contraindications to exercise for a cardiac patient.
9. Explain two expected physiologic effects of a β-adrenergic blocking drug in an exercising cardiac patient.
10. Describe three types of candidates for an outpatient cardiac exercise program.
11. Evaluate the benefits and hazards of performing an exercise test on a myocardial infarction patient or cardiac surgery patient in relation to rehabilitation.

12. Outline the three components of an exercise prescription.
13. Explain the important reasons for including warm-up and cool-down periods as part of an exercise session.
14. Explain three objectives for discussing sexual considerations with patients with coronary artery disease and their partners.
15. Investigate the resources in your community available to the cardiac patient and family members.

Everyone has heard the depressing statistics. Sometimes the statistics take on a personality—a patient cared for, a relative, or perhaps even ourselves. According to the American Heart Association, over 67 million Americans alone are predicted to have heart disease or other blood vessel diseases.[20] Cardiovascular disease causes nearly 50% of all deaths in the United States every year. Yet the disease is not well understood by the public. Most individuals have never heard of coronary artery disease (CAD), and few realize that it is a chronic, slowly progressive disease that must be dealt with for the rest of the person's life. Close family and friends of CAD patients are also affected. For many, their lives are never the same again.

Heart disease is costly in financial terms, as well. Americans spend approximately $94.5 billion on cardiovascular illness, diagnosis, and treatments every year.[20] The amount keeps rising significantly every year, and this sum does not include the money lost due to absences from work and community service.

In the last two decades there has been a dramatic decline in the number of deaths resulting from CAD partly because of better technology and nursing care techniques and a rising awareness by the public that CAD risk factors exist and must be modified. Because more persons survive an initial cardiac event now than ever before, the natural progression of nursing and medical care is focused on these survivors and their families.[7] A formal or structured rehabilitation program starts in the coronary care unit soon after stabilization, continues through the convalescent period, and reaches completion in the outpatient program. It has brought improved physical and psychologic health by dealing with the entire patient—body, mind, and spirit. In many cases the person emerges from the rehabilitation process in better health than before the cardiac event. Ideally, what has been learned in cardiac rehabilitation will become a way of life to stabilize the disease process.

Cardiac rehabilitation is an exciting field in which to practice nursing. Nurses can make a significant contribu-

	PHASES OF CARDIAC REHABILITATION
PHASE I	Inpatient activities; anywhere from 4 to 12 stages; patient should be at 3 to 5 METs at discharge.
PHASE II	Begins 2 to 6 weeks after the cardiac event; training phase; patient exercises 3 to 5 times a week under supervision for up to 12 weeks; patient should be able to perform at 10 METs or greater at the end of this phase.
PHASE III	Begins at the end of the training phase and continues for patient's lifetime; patient maintains the level of training by exercising 3 times a week; stress tests usually done at yearly intervals to measure effectiveness and to amend the exercise prescription.

tion to these persons, many in the prime of life, by helping them to recover and resume living in a productive way with a new zest for living.

There is still some disagreement among health professionals engaged in cardiac rehabilitation regarding the exact definition of the phases of rehabilitation. Therefore it is better to state specifically which part of the rehabilitation process is being addressed. The box defines the phases referred to in this chapter.[41]

HISTORIC DEVELOPMENT

Cardiac rehabilitation is not really a new health approach. The physicians of the eighteenth century considered the therapeutic value of physical activity in the management of patients with myocardial infarction (MI). In 1937 an Israeli named Viktor Gottheimer described the basic principles followed today in cardiac rehabilitation.[24] In 1952 Levine and Lown wrote of their success with a program involving armchair sitting and gradual mobilization for the acute MI patient.[27] Most of their colleagues continued to follow a rigid program of 6 weeks of hospitalized bed rest, a private room setting, and a sedentary existence when the patient returned home. They generally made invalids of the survivors of MI. Retirement and no sexual activity were the usual prescriptions for these patients.

It was not until the late 1960s that Hellerstein and Wenger began to actively promote a "new" program of early mobilization for cardiac patients.[24] At first, other professionals thought that these two physicians were endangering patients' lives. However, when the Hellerstein and Wenger patients had fewer complications, shorter hospitalizations, and less invalidism and hypochondriasis,

others began to take notice of the program. The marvelous results continued to impress others. When operating on patients who had actively exercised under the outpatient rehabilitation program, surgeons marvelled at the strength and appearance of their myocardial tissue.

Initially physicians used only the physical exercise portion of rehabilitation. They gradually realized the importance of treating the whole patient and accepted the need for an educational component so that the patient and family would be able to cooperate better with the treatment regimen. *The patient was gradually recognized as an active partner in the process.* This approach was supported by nurses and others who dealt with the patient daily for long periods, and they brought their expertise to bear in the rehabilitation process. Cardiac rehabilitation is becoming more generally accepted throughout the country, but there is still much more work to be done. Some physicians are still not convinced that the process is necessary and are reluctant or resistant to order it for their patients.

Some benefits of cardiac rehabilitation are a shortened hospital stay, better emotional and spiritual recovery, and better compliance with new lifestyle recommendations to reduce CAD risk factors. Patients viewed as active members of the team feel less helpless and play an active role in their recovery. The complications frequently seen as a result of prolonged bed rest and inactivity are rare today where cardiac rehabilitation is practiced. The key components of exercise, education, and psychosocial counseling provide an ideal program for patients and families.

DEFINITION AND GOAL

Cardiac rehabilitation is "the process of actively assisting the known cardiac patient to achieve and maintain an optimal state of health."[7] The rehabilitation goals and process are defined by *both* the patient and rehabilitation team.

The patient must want to achieve the goals of cardiac rehabilitation through behavioral modification because the process must continue for the rest of the person's life. Far too often, the team, family, and other staff members define the goals without involving the patient in their decision. Goals must be defined jointly by all involved persons. The team must respect the patient's wishes and goals, whether they entirely approve or not. Each person must be free to make informed choices about matters that affect health. Nurses need to be certain that the patient has the correct facts and the encouragement to implement the decisions. Patients should have a good understanding of the problem, the treatment, and illness management to cooperate with the management of health.

DESIRABLE NURSING ATTRIBUTES

Cardiac rehabilitation nursing is not an entry level nursing position. The nurse specialist needs special training and

**COMMON REQUIREMENTS FOR THE
CARDIAC NURSE SPECIALIST**

Two or more years of cardiac critical care nursing experience
Exercise physiology course and background
In-depth knowledge of cardiovascular nursing
Certification in advanced life support
Certification in basic life support (ideally at instructor level)
Advanced physical assessment skills
Advanced dysrhythmia interpretation skills
Patient teaching experience
Understanding of and intervention skills in psychologic reactions
Coordinator skills with other multidisciplinary staff
Personal malpractice insurance
Complete familiarity with exercise equipment
Certification in defibrillation and administration of intravenous medications and infusions
Up-to-date knowledge of cardiac rehabilitation
Achievement of American Academy of Sports Medicine competency for health personnel who participate in cardiac exercise training
Middle management skills and experience
Effective written and oral communication skills

Data from American College of Sports Medicine: Guidelines for graded exercise testing and exercise prescription, ed 5, Philadelphia, 1987, Lea & Febiger.

nursing background to function independently. Some common requirements for the cardiac nurse specialist are outlined in the box.

The nurse is concerned not only with current observations but also with the patient's social and physical life, before the cardiac event, as well as the patient's ability to achieve change after the rehabilitation process. The nurse should be person-oriented and practice a healthful lifestyle that follows cardiac rehabilitation principles, demonstrate a willingness to tolerate slow results to nursing interventions, and have zest for living that is infectious to patients and families.

The nurse must have excellent technical and interpersonal skills. The ability to assess physical and emotional responses to cardiovascular deficits is a requirement because the nurse may be the only health professional initially available to the patient. The nurse needs good communication and management skills for inpatient and outpatient phases. Finally, the nurse must be skilled in adult learning principles, use of audiovisual aids, and assessment of learning readiness. Above all, the nurse must be objective and nonjudgmental in approaching cardiac patients and families. Not all patients will accept the nurse's suggestions

and teaching. The nursing role in cardiac rehabilitation is to assess the patient's needs, be a good listener, present the facts clearly, make recommendations, and help the patient repattern behavior for better health.

Continued education is important in this fast-moving, rapidly changing field. The nurse must keep abreast of new information and communicate this information to other health care professionals and patients and their families. A peer group may not exist in the nurse's institution, so the nurse may have to form a support group to exchange ideas and learn from others in the rehabilitation field.

METs

Metabolic equivalents of a task (METs) are a common way to measure the workload of various activities on the cardiovascular and pulmonary systems. The term is frequently used for the rehabilitation of pulmonary and cardiovascular patients. It is also used to measure the aerobic exercise ability and performance of healthy individuals who are participating in an exercise program for endurance training. The formula for a MET follows:

$$1 \text{ MET} = 3.5 \text{ ml O}_2/\text{kg body weight}/\text{minute}$$

Lying quietly at rest is approximately equal to 1 MET of energy expenditure. Climbing a flight of stairs is equal to 3.5 to 4 METs. Sexual intercourse with one's usual partner in comfortable positions and surroundings is usually equal to about 3.5 to 4 METs of energy requirement. The sedentary adult should be able to perform at least 10 METs of work.[7]

An *exercise* or *stress test* is used to measure a person's ability to perform work. With the use of a treadmill or ergometric bike the workload is changed every few minutes according to one of several accepted protocols available for the purpose (see Chapter 6). Each protocol stage is approximately equal to a stated number of METs, based on research. These MET numbers are approximately the average energy expenditure, measured by testing the O_2 content of the air expired by the subject during the test, and using the weight of the person.

INPATIENT CARDIAC REHABILITATION: PHASE I Candidates

Eligible patients should be started on the hospital's cardiac rehabilitation program as soon as possible after stabilization in the critical care unit to achieve the best results. For many patients this is the second or third day after admission or surgery. Because the time needed for hospitalization is declining, the team should maximize the use of time with the patient and family.[32] A specific method of case finding is needed to reach these patients as soon as possible. Frequently nurses in the coronary care unit notify the team of upcoming patients at a weekly meeting. Other institutions use a member of the team, usually the nurse specialist, who initiates daily rounds on all the units where possible candidates may be located.

Potential rehabilitation candidates include patients who have experienced AMI, surgical myocardial revascularization, and percutaneous transluminal coronary angioplasty (PTCA) and patients with stable angina pectoris, congestive heart failure, cardiac valve replacements or disorders, cardiac transplants, and with artificial pacemakers or automatic implantable cardioverter-defibrillators.

Team formats

The box lists the ideal team composition for inpatient rehabilitation. Note that not all these team members are required initially for success of the program. Generally, in places where the rehabilitation process is formalized, the team organizes by one of two formats. *Interdisciplinary teams* use health professionals with different abilities to focus on the various aspects of the cardiac patient's recovery. The members continue to report to their own department heads and are paid out of the various departments' budgets or cost centers if computerized. One person, usually the nurse specialist, coordinates their work. By regular communication and formal meetings they share insights and information to ensure that all are familiar with the goals for the various patients referred to them.

Under the *direct team format,* all team members report to one head, usually a cardiologist or nurse specialist. One benefit of this format is that all report to a single person who is oriented to cardiac rehabilitation and evaluates the team members accordingly. The direct team format is less cost effective because all salaries come out of a single budget. This method is more commonly seen in an outpatient program organization, although it may be seen in hospitals that have a high volume of patients and sufficient reimbursement to cover the salary costs.

Method of referral and advancement

The referral process should be written in a procedure book format, and copies should be posted in a visible place on all units where the patients are usually found. Some hospitals have automatic referrals of certain groups of patients and do not require that each patient's physician order rehabilitation. It is recommended that a health team professional screen these patients so that patients who are inappropriate for the rehabilitation process are excluded. Most hospitals require a physician's written order, and many insurance programs will not cover the costs of rehabilitation unless specifically ordered by a physician.

Advancement or reversal of the stages of the program can be done by the team or by a physician's written order, depending on the institution's policies and the physician's wishes. The patient's current stage should be part of the care plan or other suitable patient record and verbally stated at the end of each shift report.

IDEAL TEAM COMPOSITION FOR REHABILITATION

Cardiac patient and family
Attending physician or cardiac surgeon
Primary nurse and associate nurses
Cardiac rehabilitation clinical nurse specialist
Cardiologist consultant
Physical therapist
Occupational therapist
Social worker
Vocational rehabilitation counselor
Dietitian
Leisure counselor
Chaplain
Liaison for the Visiting Nurse Association or public health nurse
Outpatient cardiac exercise clinic staff or representative
Psychologist or psychiatric clinical nurse specialist

Psychosocial component

The diagnosis of heart disease fills most patients and family members with anxiety and despair. Nurses are best prepared to help the patient and family psychologically adjust to their heart disease in terms of future plans and activities.

Because the goal of cardiac rehabilitation is to enable patients to attain their highest level of wellness and work ability, the nurse must consider the patient's psychologic status. Permitting the patient to wear street clothes, if desired in the later stages of the rehabilitation program, can bolster self-esteem and reduce the sick role image. Allowing the patient to have some control over routines and personal care can reduce the frequently seen dependency, depression, and anger.

Stigma of heart disease

The diagnosis of heart disease in our culture places a stigma on individuals. The public is frequently unaware of all the new advances in the treatment of heart disease. Too frequently, the public's image is the same one true in the 1940s—the person is considered an invalid, not a good candidate for promotion or continued employment, or unable to hear any bad news or deal with daily stress.

Many choose not to be around a person who has cardiac illness because they fear that the person may die suddenly. Former patients relate how the conversation stops abruptly when they state that their recent hospitalization was caused by an MI, cardiac surgery, or cardiac transplantation. They sense that people take a few steps backward and leave the conversation as soon as possible. The cause of the fear is that heart disease is usually not visible and seems to strike suddenly with little or no warning. People may fear that they, too, may also be at high risk for heart disease, or that it may in some way be contagious.

Myths and misconceptions about heart disease

People believe many myths about the heart and heart disease.[43] Anyone who teaches cardiopulmonary resuscitation (CPR) classes to laypersons will hear comments from otherwise well-educated people that persons should be given brandy (when unconscious!) or that the human heart has a certain finite number of beats. Once that number is used up, death will occur suddenly. Hearts are thought to be weak, mysterious organs. Some people are not even sure where the heart is located.

Some patients think that an MI means that there is a clot in a major blood vessel leading into or out of the heart. Another frequently heard opinion is that an MI causes a hole in the heart and that blood leaks out of the hole.

After the physician has told the patient that an MI has occurred, the nurse should assess the patient's understanding of the MI. The nurse determines whether the patient knows anyone else who has *recently* suffered from the same problem and asks how that person is progressing. A patient who has known several persons who have recovered and resumed most or all of their activities will feel more hopeful than the patient who knows several friends who died from an MI. It is important to identify these feelings early in the rehabilitation process. Knowing more about the emotional state of the patient makes a tremendous difference in how well the nurse can assist the patient and family with recovery.

Skills in psychologic assessment and intervention are a necessity for any health professional who deals frequently with patients who have cardiac disorders. Because heart disease seems to strike with little or no previous symptoms, patients are fearful of the next attack and wonder whether they will survive. Patients are interested in learning early in the convalescent period about what might have caused the cardiac problem so that other cardiac events may be avoided or mitigated.

Assigning blame

Frequently there is no variation from daily routine when a cardiac problem occurs. Many persons are asleep when they are stricken. They scrutinize their life to find some reasonable explanation for the problem. This is a natural reaction—attempting to relate events to factors that can be controlled. The concept of CAD as the most common culprit is usually dismissed by patients and their loved ones. They prefer to think that the cause of the problem was their spouse, their boss, cutting the lawn, moving heavy furniture, cleaning the attic, shoveling snow, or the food they ate. They believe that if they avoid the person or activity that "caused" the attack, it will never happen again.

Other patients will intellectually accept their heart disease, but they are not able to deal with the fact that the disease cannot be cured. They will ask why the health profession cannot cure them so that they can resume their previous (and frequently unhealthy) lifestyles. It is more desirable to think that extraneous sources are totally responsible for heart disease than controllable risk factors.

Changing lifestyles

There is still an incomplete understanding of the cause of heart disease. The public has great faith in the ability of health professionals to cure any illness. Many persons who have had myocardial revascularization truly believe that the disease has been cured.[1] They then see no need to make any lifestyle changes, such as not smoking, modifying fat intake, and exercising aerobically. Some patients are even openly hostile when referred to a cardiac rehabilitation program if they have been under the impression that surgery would take care of the problem. It is an immediate responsibility of the nurse to explain the situation to them.

Understandably, the idea of making difficult changes in lifestyles with no guarantee of success is unpalatable to many patients. Family life sustains substantial changes in many cases. The roles that the patient previously held will need some adjustments, at least initially. Life patterns or means of employment may need revision. Their loved ones constantly worry whether an MI will happen again. Many spouses awaken at night frequently just to hear whether their partner is still breathing. Much of this worry and indignation remains hidden from the casual observer. When a nurse asks, however, they admit their concerns. If they do not deal with psychologic issues during hospitalization, they will keep their feelings to themselves and hinder the recovery process.

Studies show that up to 88% of MI patients were depressed or anxious 6 months to 1 year after the event.[16] Studies of partners and other family members show that they too suffer from the event.[16,44,53] Frequently spouses state that they have to deal with angry outbursts, serious changes in personalities, and guilt (usually expressed by wives) that they were responsible for their partner's illness. Any deviation from prescribed medication schedules, smoking cessation mandates, or dietary noncompliance causes them to feel angry and guilty. Many keep silent, fearing that confrontations will result in new illness or death. There usually is a scarce number of self-help groups to assist these partners with adjustments to their spouses' heart disease.

Many spouses fear sexual activity because of their lack of knowledge about the true cardiac workload during sexual intercourse. This reluctance is usually interpreted by patients as rejection and reinforces the belief that they are no longer desirable. This deepens the depression, tension, and anger, leading some couples to break up or seek companionship elsewhere.

Educational programs help to dispel fear and replace it with hope for a good future. Tensions are reduced, and the energy that patients used for fear can be applied in learning new adaptation skills. Patients are frequently surprised to learn that most persons are able to return to work, at least part-time, in 2 or 3 months. Those who have had successful PTCA or pacemaker procedures are usually able to return to work within weeks after hospitalization. Jobs that require heavy physical labor or are extremely stressful may require that the person delay return for a longer time or seek another position. This knowledge can help patients and families to begin to plan for the future.

The most common psychologic reactions to heart disease are anxiety, depression, grief, anger, shock and disbelief, denial, and sexual aggressiveness.[4] The nurse should assess the current and past psychologic states. It is important to learn about past psychologic illnesses and coping mechanisms used during past crises.

Supporting family and friends

Family and friends should be assessed by the nurse as possible sources of strength in the rehabilitation process (see Chapter 3). The patient who is unable to state the name of someone to notify in an emergency is in great need of a support system, and a team member may need to fill that gap. The team can effectively encourage family and friends to help during the convalescent period. Sometimes an explanation of the patient's new behavior is necessary because many patients act in ways that baffle family and friends. After the family understands that behavioral changes are a common way of dealing with the news of cardiovascular disease, they can try to help the person to regain lost self-esteem or emotional equilibrium.

Family groups organized by the nurse, psychologists, or social workers who are skilled in group meeting techniques let family and friends verbalize fears and anger without the patient being present. They are also a source of support, not only from the health professional but also among the members.[5] Usually a 30-minute meeting once or twice a week is enough to help these persons. Until they gain support for themselves, they cannot be expected to exert effort toward the patient's rehabilitation.

Cultural implications

Cultural ties can be quite strong and warrant nursing assessment. Patients who are first- or second-generation members of a particular culture usually retain the beliefs and needs of that culture. If nurses are unfamiliar with these beliefs, especially those concerning heart disease, they should learn as much as possible before proceeding with the rehabilitation. Family members can help; books written for the health professional also are available.[54]

Cultural beliefs about health, especially cardiovascular health, differ. Sometimes the patient will need translation of spoken instructions or literature. The family may need transportation to appointments because many immigrants are not permitted to drive if they have recently arrived in the United States. The patient may consider hospital food inedible because of differing tastes or beliefs regarding the diets of ill persons. Religious preferences also might affect the patient's needs. After these barriers have been broken, the patient can begin to understand the purpose of cardiac rehabilitation. Then the team can help the patient and family to adapt to the illness and convalescence.

In certain cultures, such as Filipino, Korean, Gypsy, Native American, Vietnamese, Indian, and Middle Eastern, it is the custom to have many family members and friends spend a lot of time with the patient.[9,33,46] This is an important part of convalescense. Nurses might consider only the number of visitors and believe they are keeping the patient from getting rest. However, observation reveals that the patient is usually quietly listening or sometimes even sleeping peacefully while family members chat with each other. When possible, the nurse arranges for a private room so that patients of other cultures will not be disturbed by the visitors. Flexibility in visiting rules will permit the needed support for the patient to regain health. The family's needs are also met because they are able to visit and assist the patient as their culture demands. Rehabilitation should be individualized to meet the patient's needs, not the institution's needs.

Social and financial needs

Social service is "any work intended to promote the welfare of the sick, homeless, or destitute."[55] The social needs of patients frequently go unheeded because many patients do not directly express these needs without some skilled evaluation by a nurse or a social worker. The earlier the appropriate person is alerted to the patient's needs, the better the need can be met before discharge. A seemingly chance remark, made during a bath or other treatment, may be a clue that patients need help.

Many persons endure much because they do not know that help is available or they are too proud to ask for it. Education about their health problems is not assimilated because of anxiety. If education attempts do not succeed, frequently the cause is an unresolved social problem. Planning for some of these problems may involve the social worker, the visiting or home health care nurse, or the dietitian. The nurse should be familiar with the varying skills and job descriptions of the different team members. Many hospitals now have patient advocates who assist the patient with any nonmedical or nonnursing needs.

Many patients begin to worry about finances soon after admission. They are very aware of the cost of a hospital stay, especially one that includes a stay in a critical care unit. The sooner that their minds can be relieved of this worry, the better the recovery process will be. Most people do not mind being asked whether finances are a problem for them or their family. Many people do not purchase health insurance or have no insurance because of unemployment. They may be unaware that Medicaid or other partial or complete financial help is available. They might worry about how they will pay the bill or if the hospital will ask them to leave before they are ready for discharge.

This worry may be compounded if the person has no sick leave available or thinks that a new job may have to be found. Exploring alternatives with a financial aid officer or social worker can lift some of the burden.

If the possibility of getting a new job is valid, a referral to a vocational rehabilitation worker at the state level may help. Some states offer job aptitude testing, job retraining, or schooling and also may provide a stipend to help with expenses. Sometimes the outpatient rehabilitation exercise training can be partially or completely paid for by vocational resource funds. Frequently patients who have not spoken with their physicians assume that return to work is out of the question. The nurse should speak to the physician to ascertain whether the patient really needs to change jobs before making the referral.

The nurse may learn that the patient lives alone, has few interested family members, has no pets or friends, or is retired from work. These circumstances have been identified as psychologic risk factors for heart disease.[59] The nurse can tell the patient about social contacts available in the area. Many communities have day care centers for elderly persons, and some will even pick up and return the patient to the home. Other centers have lunch or dinner available with social contact opportunities.

Many community groups are looking for volunteers who have the skills that the patient may have to offer. The local chapters of the American Heart Association frequently have "heart clubs" for these patients and their families and friends. There may also be pacemaker clubs, Mended Hearts Clubs for those who have had heart surgery, diabetic clubs, and ostomy clubs. If the person is retired, there might be a retired persons group in the area. Many of these clubs arrange for the person to be transported to the meetings and other social outings. It is helpful to identify the patient's interests and barriers that the patient feels are a hindrance to joining group activities. Certainly persons should not be forced to take part but may benefit from knowing what is available. A person may need to learn new social skills to make life more rewarding.

Pet therapy is a relatively new and exciting technique. Through contact with puppies and kittens and other small animals, elderly and chronically ill persons can generate social skills and feelings. Volunteers take the animals to nursing homes and schools for special children to visit with the residents and share the animals. Cardiac patients may be interested in volunteering for this work. It requires little time and effort, yet is very rewarding to the residents and volunteers.

Frequently patients are not aware that they will probably need assistance with household work. Many are not initially permitted to resume driving, shopping or doing the laundry and cleaning. After this has been discussed, the team should help the patient plan for assistance, if needed. The social worker usually has a list of household cleaning persons and community resources to help patients temporarily.

If cost is a problem, patients may be eligible for financial assistance to cover a part-time homemaker until they are able to do these tasks. Some homemakers will also do the shopping and can prepare food if needed. This service should also be considered for patients whose spouses will not or cannot assist with these chores. Too often spouses cause patients to feel guilty, and patients then resume heavy work or other previous role requirements before the healing is complete. All patients should be aware that arm work dramatically increases heart work because of a rise in blood pressure. Therefore chores such as dusting and vacuuming are not permitted in the early weeks of recovery.[14]

Invalid aids such as portable toilets, walkers, canes, and other types of equipment, as well as oxygen and prescriptions, may need to be obtained or rented before patients go home. The job of the nurse and other team members is to assist with arrangements that patients cannot make themselves.

Sometimes a patient becomes ill far from home. The nurse, social worker, or other team members then need to help the patient arrange to return home. Flying is usually much less taxing to the patient than being driven in a car and is usually permitted immediately after discharge. Air ambulances, private aircraft, or accompanied flight on an airliner might be necessary. Usually the patient is financially responsible for the charges. Airlines will provide transportation to the gates in the airport if given advance notice. They will also arrange for the patient to have a private waiting area in some airports and will permit the patient to board first and obtain extra seating if necessary to accommodate patient health needs such as casts or an extra seat to raise the legs. A number of special diets are also available with advance notice.

Aircraft usually are pressurized only to about 5000 feet of altitude pressure. Usually this is no problem for a patient who is relatively inactive during the flight. Some airlines have extra oxygen available, but this should be ascertained before the flight. To prevent stasis and phlebitis, the patient should be encouraged to move about the cabin of the aircraft every 1 to 2 hours, conditions permitting.

Spiritual needs

Belief system. Learning that one has had cardiac illness or will need heart surgery triggers much soul-searching. "I can't believe that I've been so ill," is a remark that nurses and other health team members frequently hear. It may be the first time that patients have been seriously ill. It may be difficult for the patients to be dependent on others. This usually causes most patients to begin to examine their philosophy of life and personal religious beliefs. Being confronted with their mortality and the reality of death is the source of much anxiety in patients and families. They may require much nursing, medical, and counseling assistance to help them resolve feelings.

Many staff persons think of the chaplain only for patient religious needs and are not aware of the other special skills that a hospital chaplain can use in the rehabilitation of these patients and families. Many have had extensive education in stress management and crisis intervention.

Changing relationships. It is a common response for patients who have learned of their heart disease to begin to examine relationships in their lives and to resolve to change some of them. Some may grow closer to their spouses. Others find that their spouses offer little support, or they may even be abandoned by them. Friends may become important for the first time. Others may realize that their lives have been barren of important relationships and that few care about them. This is a sobering experience, and many patients begin to despair. These persons need assistance in evaluating priorities and deciding what changes they want to make.

The Chinese symbol for crisis represents danger and opportunity. Some patients develop new philosophies and rearrange priorities, whereas others crumble or show no apparent change. Many persons find that they are never the same afterward. It is said that even though it takes 6 weeks to recover physically from an MI or heart surgery, it may take a year or longer to recover spiritually and psychologically. Patients may find that priorities change overnight.

Active listening. The nurse can help the patient and family by using good listening skills. Actively listening to what a patient is saying is a skill that can be learned. The patient needs to sort out feelings and beliefs during the convalescent period. There may be much self-recrimination about the past and what could have been done better. It helps to remind these patients to plan for the life ahead.

The nurse also needs to be comfortable with periods of silence as the patient progresses. Active listening differs from merely hearing what the patient is saying. Active listening involves analyzing what is said and what is *not* said. This process can be used while the nurse is performing personal care, carrying out procedures, or administering medications. It is not always necessary that the nurse say much while listening because it is highly therapeutic merely to give the patients the opportunity to express thoughts and fears. Often a solution then becomes apparent to the patient.

Spouses and family members may also undergo the same process of soul-searching and evaluating priorities and beliefs. The shock of seeing their loved one so ill in a critical care unit may initiate intense feelings and evaluation of current needs. Although it may be painful, change must occur. The nurse, social worker, or chaplain can help these persons regain control as they struggle with the ideas of mortality and chronic illness.

Physiologic component
Negative effects of bed rest

Exercise, a gradual return to daily activities, and a walking program are initiated to prevent or counteract the negative effects of bed rest and inactivity. Before the late 1960s bed rest was enforced for at least 6 weeks. When permitted to get up, patients had weak muscles and tight joints and were frequently candidates for thromboembolic phenomena.

The heart muscle, like other muscles, does not benefit from inactivity. Patients who are confined to bed for longer than a few days frequently develop orthostatic hypotension when they first rise. The dizziness and sometimes syncope are due to the inability of the cardiovascular system to adjust to the force of gravity. After a few minutes the patient recovers as the body slowly compensates for the change in position.

Studies have shown that it takes only a day or so of bed rest for the body to begin to decondition[8,34] and for the cardiovascular system and other body systems to lose some of their abilities to function. Muscles begin to atrophy, and joints tighten, losing flexibility. This makes the patient more prone to injuries such as muscle tearing with exercise or other movement. Pulse rate is elevated in response to a minimal workload. Pulmonary function studies show decreased vital capacity and a decreased lung volume. Pneumonia becomes a hazard, especially to patients who smoke, are elderly, or have a preexisting lung disease such as chronic pulmonary fibrosis or chronic obstructive pulmonary disease. Atelectasis reduces the amount of lung tissue available for oxygenation, further complicating the condition.[34]

Patients should be involved in a gradual exercise program as soon as possible and should sit in a chair at the bedside as soon as they stabilize.[57] The criteria for stabilization are stable blood pressure, relieved or controlled pain, minimal dysrhythmias, and satisfactory pulmonary oxygenation. During the stabilization period, nursing care should include instruction and careful monitoring of *active* or *passive range of motion exercises* to keep muscles and joints as flexible and strong as possible. Simple and easily performed leg exercises should be done at least every 2 hours while the patient is awake. For example, ankle dorsiflexion can reduce leg vein stasis and phlebitis. Patients should be carefully questioned about a history of embolization or phlebitis. If the patient has such a history, nursing care must include vigorous precautions to minimize the problems.

Goals in the exercise component

Most programs suggest similar goals within the exercise component of cardiac rehabilitation program:[7,14]

1. Maintain the range of joint motion and muscle function that the patient had on admission.
2. Prevent the problems associated with bed rest and inactivity.
3. Gather appropriate information on the patient's remaining cardiovascular response to exercise.
4. Observe and report adverse responses to exercise.
5. Encourage patient and family confidence about exercise safety.

6. Establish and promote a habit of regular, monitored exercise.
7. Reinforce goals established for each patient and family.

The inpatient exercise component is geared to prevent and deal with the problems associated with bed rest and has little or no endurance training effect. As a result of being more active early in the hospitalization period, many patients have less depression and exhibit fewer symptoms of invalidism.

Nursing assessment

The primary nurse or cardiovascular nurse specialist should identify rehabilitation problems and formulate patient outcome criteria. This assessment is different from that done on admission or that commonly done during each shift. It is vital to set mutual goals for the physiologic component of rehabilitation. Key assessment points follow:

1. What was the patient's level of activity before hospitalization?
2. What type of exercise did the patient do regularly?
3. What type of work does the patient perform?
4. What is the patient's perception of the purpose of cardiac inpatient exercise?
5. What is the design of the patient's living quarters?
6. What types of leisure activity does the patient do?
7. What goals does the patient want to achieve before discharge and afterward?
8. What does the patient want to learn?
9. What does the patient know about the disease?
10. Who is the patient's support system?
11. Who can help the patient after discharge?
12. Is the patient literate?

Physical therapy assessment

The physical therapist, if involved in inpatient rehabilitation (phase I), investigates body function, muscle strength, and preexisting problems such as residual damage from strokes, degenerative diseases such as arthritis, and previous injuries to muscles and joints. The therapist then can plan an exercise program for the patient's specific needs. Occasionally a patient previously diagnosed as having arthritis or bursitis may actually have cardiac disease with associated symptoms caused by angina pectoris. After the cardiac surgery or other cardiac event, the physical therapist evaluates whether joint dysfunction continues to be a valid diagnosis.

If a patient uses a cane or walker, the nurse or therapist should have a friend or family member bring it in so that the therapist can evaluate whether the patient is using the aid correctly. The patients also find personal equipment easier to use. If the patient has a prosthesis, it should be available for use with the exercises, and its use is evaluated by the therapist. The patient benefits from these evaluations and is able to exercise better and walk as a result.

Nursing diagnoses

Nursing diagnoses derived from the assessment are written on the team care plan. Other health professionals can then support or observe for psychophysiologic symptoms or needs. The diagnostic categories for formulating nursing diagnoses applicable to cardiac rehabilitation are outlined in the box.

FREQUENTLY ANTICIPATED NURSING DIAGNOSES WITH CARDIAC REHABILITATION PATIENTS

EXCHANGING PATTERN

Decreased cardiac output
Altered nutrition

RELATING PATTERN

Altered role performance
Altered family processes
Sexual dysfunction
Social isolation

VALUING PATTERN

Spiritual distress

CHOOSING PATTERN

Ineffective coping (individual and family)
Impaired adjustment
Noncompliance
Health-seeking behaviors

MOVING PATTERN

Fatigue
Impaired functional performance
Activity intolerance
Sleep pattern disturbance
Self-care deficit
Impaired home maintenance management
Diversional activity deficit
Altered health maintenance

PERCEIVING PATTERN

Powerlessness
Self-esteem disturbance

KNOWING PATTERN

Knowledge deficit

FEELING PATTERN

Anxiety
Depression
Dysfunctional grieving

Inpatient stages

Most inpatient rehabilitation programs are structured into several stages that gradually increase the intensity of exercise and range of permitted activities. These stages are numbered so that the higher the number, the more patients are permitted to do and the more intense the exercises. The number of stages varies according to the institution but generally ranges between 4 and 12. The first stage usually begins with patients lying down to do simple arm and leg exercises. If patients tolerate this stage, they advance gradually to exercising while sitting and then finally standing during the exercises. Many hospitals now include stair climbing in the final stages before discharge. Because many patients live in multistoried homes or apartment buildings, stair climbing in the hospital can give them and staff members information to determine whether this activity will be harmful after discharge.

Exercise usually begins at the 1 MET level and gradually progresses to about 3.5 to 4 METs before discharge. Usually 4 METs is the greatest amount of energy required by convalescent activities immediately after discharge. The physical therapist or nurse monitors patient performance of these exercises by checking the pulse and blood pressure before beginning exercise. The pulse is usually checked by patients or health team members during each exercise set, and blood pressure and pulse are checked after the exercises are completed. It is recommended that patients repeat the exercises two more times during the day by themselves, unless an adverse response is observed during the monitored session.

The data should be carefully recorded on a flow sheet so that exercise responses can be compared over time. In some hospitals, patients are also given recording sheets to note the pulse response and other comments while independently exercising. The exercises are numbered on the instruction sheet and on the response sheet so that patients can be consistent. These response recording sheets make it easier to note whether the arm or leg exercises are tolerated and whether the pulse increases above the established limits, usually 20 to 30 beats above the resting level.

Patients, if permitted to exercise independently during the day, should be carefully instructed, both verbally and in writing, about their pulse limits, warning signs to report, times to avoid exercises, and ways to space the exercise within their schedules. This material is also reviewed frequently by rehabilitation team members with patients and families to be sure there is no misunderstanding. Patients should be told the purpose behind the exercises so that they will be able to cooperate better with their program.

Patients are reminded that if adverse responses occur, they should stop exercising and call the nurse immediately so that their condition can be assessed and their blood pressure, pulse, and ECG can be evaluated. Warning symptoms include anginal pain or discomfort, palpitations, dizziness or syncope, unusual fatigue, and dyspnea.

Not all patients are capable of completing the total number of phase I inpatient stages before discharge. Patients spend differing amounts of time in each stage according to their recovery rate and their cardiac disease and reserve.

In a four-stage program, patients spend an average of 2 days at each stage. When there are more stages, patients spend less time on each stage, according to their condition. Any setback in patients' progress usually causes them to feel depressed. It is important to support patients and families and to remind patients that people heal at different rates, that this type of setback has happened to others, and that progress may begin again soon. The physician or rehabilitation team will allow patients to attempt the next stage when medication has been adjusted or when the heart has had more time to heal.

If possible, spouses or friends or family members should be present during exercise sessions so that they can see patients safely performing the permitted exercises and activities. Families find this very reassuring, and they begin to feel that patients are on the way to recovery. Families should be involved in the exercise program so that they can understand the purpose of the exercises and monitor patients' appearance.

Exercise

Excellent detailed discussions on exercise can be found in several texts.[2,7,14]

Breathing techniques. Rhythmic breathing should be performed regularly during exercises, and patients should be reminded to refrain from holding their breaths because it may result in a Valsalva response and cause slowing of the pulse and an initial rise in blood pressure, with adverse or even fatal results.[25] During the first days in the critical care unit, patients should be taught to do *rhythmic diaphragmatic breathing*. This helps to increase the relaxation response and reduces the probability of pneumonia. Patients should inspire slowly through the nose and breathe out through pursed lips. It is sometimes easier for patients to understand the directions if the nurse compares the expiratory exercises to that of blowing out a match or candle. If patients are unable or unwilling to do this, they can be told to yawn and to breathe out through pursed lips. During waking hours, patients should do at least two sessions, of five deep breaths each, every hour while confined to bed. Because syncope or dizziness can be caused by a low carbon dioxide level, patients should avoid taking more than five deep consecutive breaths. Many patients have difficulty remembering events while hospitalized, so the nurse should remind them of these instructions as needed. This is especially true for surgical patients.

Arm exercise. Arm and leg exercises are included in the inpatient and outpatient phases of rehabilitation because patients need to use both in many daily activities. Studies have shown that when only arms or only legs are exercised there is a tendency for a decrease in strength in the unexercised limbs.[15,34] Use of the arms causes a greater increase in pulse and blood pressure response, especially if the arms have not been exercised in a regular program before surgery.[59] This increased response causes a greater cardiac oxygen demand, which may cause angina pectoris or dysrhythmias. By training at even very low levels, a patient's arm strength and muscle agility can be maintained at least at the preillness levels.

Pulse-taking. Patients are taught to take a radial or carotid pulse reading during independent exercise and to assess response in medications that alter pulse rates, such as digoxin and propranolol. Instructions are discussed on p. 644. Patients should check the pulse in the same position that they will be performing the exercise. For example, if the exercises are to be done standing, the pulse is checked in the standing position.

The pulse should be checked for a full minute before exercising and then counted for 10 or 15 seconds and multiplied by 6 or 4 after each exercise set and at the end of exercise. The reason for the short counting time after exercise is to be certain that the correct pulse rate during exercise is recorded. The pulse rate declines quickly after exercise, and a shorter pulse-counting time is needed to correctly note the exercise response.

Pulse parameters for exercise during phase I (inpatient phase) depend on the patient's needs and the team guidelines and physician instructions. Generally, the pulse should not exceed 30 beats above the resting rate with exercise. If the patient is taking a calcium-channel blocking or β-adrenergic blocking medications, the parameters have to be adjusted. Usually, the patient is told not to exceed 15 beats above the resting pulse in this situation. The patient should wait at least an hour after eating and bathing before exercising. This prevents placing an extra workload on a healing heart. The patient should also wait an hour after tiring procedures and visitors for the same reason.

Drug effects. As previously noted, any β-adrenergic blocking agent or calcium-channel blocking medication changes the body's response to exercise because of the action on the sympathetic nervous system or the cardiac muscle cell's calcium channel activity. This usually results in a slower resting and exercise pulse, a lower systolic blood pressure, lower diastolic pressure, and a very blunted response to exercise in general.

When patients are given these medications, the nurse should notify the rehabilitation team so that they can readjust exercise parameters. Patients should be told the purpose of the medication, changes to expect, and the new pulse parameters that should not be exceeded. Patients should be prepared for the sometimes drastically lower pulse so that they will not be alarmed.

Blood pressure response. The blood pressure should be measured before and after each exercise session, and the patient's appearance is noted during exercise. These observations are recorded to maintain a comprehensive record, to assess when the patient is ready to progress to the next stage, and to evaluate the effect of medications on the cardiovascular response to exercise.

The blood pressure should rise with exercise, and the diastolic pressure should stay the same or drop slightly. With phase I exercise the systolic pressure should never exceed 200 mm Hg at any time because of the needs of the healing myocardium. Blood pressure varies among individuals, but the response should be similar from session to session. If the systolic pressure falls more than 15 mm Hg during the exercise session or if the diastolic pressure rises more than 10 mm Hg, the patient should stop exercising and be reevaluated by a nurse and physician. Frequently these responses indicate that the myocardium is decompensating and the patient may be in jeopardy. Sometimes this response indicates that the patient is hypovolemic because of overuse of diuretics or other causes. Such a patient should be reevaluated before exercising again.[2]

Ministress test. A lower-level walking (ministress) test is ideally performed a few days before discharge to determine whether the patient will have problems with activities after discharge.[1,15] The ministress test has been found helpful in the prognosis of problems or mortality in the first year after an MI.[51] The test also boosts the patient's morale and confidence by proving that the prescribed activity is safe to do. Often a patient is pleasantly surprised by the results of the test.

The patient is usually asked to walk on a treadmill until a preset heart rate (usually around 120 to 130 beats per minute) is achieved, has symptoms that require the test to be stopped, or is able to achieve safely a workload equal to 4 METs. If the patient is unable to achieve the desired heart rate or MET level because of symptoms of ischemia or dysrhythmias, therapy can usually be instituted and the test repeated before or soon after discharge. However, occasionally a patient needs immediate referral for angiography and possible surgery or PTCA to correct the problem. The test also gives the patient and physician specific data needed for accurate advice on postdischarge activity, exercises, and walking programs. If possible, the partner should observe the test for reassurance that the patient is doing well and is capable of exercise and activity.

Walking program. Walking specified distances is also a part of the inpatient program. Placing signs in the hospital corridors helps patients know how far they have walked so that they can stay within their limitations. Because deconditioning can occur when exercise and walking are omitted for even a few days, exercises should continue on weekends when staffing tends to be lower. A nurse or therapist should accompany the patient who climbs stairs in case of complications.

Educational component

Education is one of the most important components of the cardiac rehabilitation program. In the short time available the health team must try to teach the patient and family about the cardiac disease, the appropriate coping methods, and the important role of exercise. This component is frequently treated casually, and education is given "if I have time." Some nurses may not like to teach, are unsure of what to teach, or are unaware of how to assess learning readiness or use audiovisual aids. The patient is frequently given written materials that may not be appropriate and then is told to ask questions. Several health members may give the patient conflicting information, and there is frequently no list of standardized information that should be taught. Only by making one nurse primarily responsible for each patient's educational program can there be some assurance that the patient will receive the necessary preparation for discharge.

Each patient and family are unique. The primary nurse must assess and plan for individual needs and appropriateness of topics. The time that the patient remains in the hospital also influences the priority of topics to teach. Finally, the psychologic state influences how much and when the patient will learn. Before teaching, the nurse should carefully investigate what the patient already knows about the subject and what the patient believes is important to learn. After this is known, the nurse can plan the progression of the education.

Effects of anger and depression on learning

If there is deep depression, energy for learning will be unavailable until the depression is treated. The nurse should support such patients and refer them to a psychologist, psychiatric nurse specialist, or psychiatrist if the depression does not respond or is severe. Meanwhile, families can be taught much of the curriculum while the nursing plan deals with relieving the depression. If patients are angry, the cause of the anger is frequently the heart disease diagnosis. Anger can be reduced by education, according to the situation.

If the patient or family is denying the event, there is no stimulus to learn because the patient does not feel vulnerable to heart disease. The nurse should never directly confront the patient because denial is a psychologic mechanism that protects the patient or family until the psyche is ready to cope (see Interchapter 10). Taking charts into the patient's room to show laboratory tests or progress notes will not help and may even hinder patient readiness or emotional stability.

Sometimes it helps for "deniers" to attend a group "meeting" (never a class) with other cardiac patients. Seeing that others were having difficulty dealing with cardiac disease may enable them to feel more comfortable. It becomes acceptable to have heart disease because the others did not look mortally ill. In a few days these patients are usually eager to learn and begin to participate in the educational program. This technique may help even if the unit is short staffed because it requires little time (usually sessions last 30 minutes) and patients seem to learn faster

in a group. They frequently adjourn to each others' rooms to continue discussion. Families enjoy the meetings and frequently already know one another from the critical care unit waiting room.

Teaching barriers

The nurse will encounter various difficulties when trying to teach in a hospital environment. Hospitals make bad classrooms. Some common teaching barriers follow. In addition to these problems, the nurse needs to evaluate readiness to learn, learning handicaps, and cultural influences.

1. Environmental: noise, visitors, telephones, televisions and VCRs
2. Drug effects, especially of diazepam, propranolol, diuretics, pain medications, and steroids
3. Sleep deprivation
4. Lack of energy because of depression, congestive heart failure, and drugs such as propranolol
5. Lack of staff availability when the patient is ready to learn
6. Sensory deprivation, such as when a patient in a private room is confined for a prolonged period (especially a cardiac transplant patient)
7. Loneliness
8. Poor sight, hearing ability, or incomplete language comprehension

Interpreting medical terminology

One of the most valuable functions that a teaching health professional can perform is to help patients and families understand correctly what has been told to them. Frequently a physician may have explained the problem in unclear medical language. The patient might be reluctant to ask more questions.

In one case, for example, an older man, although recovering from an MI, became profoundly depressed, made out a will, and generally lost the desire to live. At one point he mentioned that he had leukemia. It seems that a house officer had been discussing this patient's laboratory values on rounds and remarked that the man had developed leuko*penia* in response to a drug. The man wrongly interpreted this as leukemia because he had never heard of leukopenia. Obviously, it is most important to have patients explain their understanding of the problem. The nurse should also try to think in lay terms and to use words familiar to the patient.

Session structure

The nurse should not present too much information at one time; 15- or 30-minute sessions suffice. Repetition should be built into the presentation, especially for surgical patients, and patients should be given time to ask questions. The most important information should be presented in the beginning of the session or at the end. Studies have shown that people remember more material presented at these times.[40] Finally, the nurse should evaluate the amount of information learned and chart appropriately the topic presented, the audiovisual aids used, and the response with recommendations for future teaching sessions.

Cultural effects on learning

Cultural attitudes affect exercise performance, self-image, dietary preferences, the role of the spouse, and beliefs about the role of the person who has heart disease.[43] Cultural background should be considered in the teaching instructions.

An *interpreter* should be present unless nurses and patients speak the same languages. Although patients might be able to understand the nurse, they might not be able to express their thoughts correctly in English. Some common mistakes that nurses and others frequently make when using an interpreter for patient teaching follow[46]:

1. Assuming that the interpreter understands the material correctly
2. Speaking directly to the interpreter instead of to the patient
3. Speaking too fast and not allowing time for translation
4. Maintaining eye contact with the interpreter instead of with the patient
5. Assuming that the interpreter is equally facile in both languages

The nurse should face the patient and have the interpreter sit beside the patient, also facing the nurse. The interpreter can also explain to the nurse any related customs before the teaching session so that faux pas are avoided. This will increase the nurse's credibility with the patient and family members.

The patient might not be literate in the primary language. In this case the nurse can rely heavily on pictures, demonstrations, and models of body parts. Another person who can read in the patient's language may be able to assist. If the subject of the teaching session involves intimate topics, some cultures prefer that a nurse of the same sex as the patient teach these topics. The best way to determine this is to ask someone familiar with the culture. The greatest amount of teaching and learning is accomplished through verbal communications. Any language barrier can significantly reduce learning.

Teaching session program content

Basic anatomic, physiologic, and pathophysiologic aspects. Patients should be taught basic anatomic structure, physiologic function, and pathophysiologic information appropriate to their cardiovascular disease.

All MI patients should understand that a small part of the cardiac muscle has been damaged and needs to heal like any other injury to the body. This is vital if patients are to comply with activity restrictions because many believe that the entire heart is involved. A cardiac model that illustrates an MI is helpful. If a model is not available, a picture or drawing may help. Some people want to know the location of the infarction; others are content to know only a little information. Patients might use the word *massive* when talking about their MI. This is a lay term and not a medical term, usually having the connotation of poor prognosis. Reminding patients that an MI is usually about the size of a dime can have a calming effect.

Angina pectoris identification and management. Many people think that angina is merely a manifestation of the aging process and do not appreciate that this is the same disease that causes MI. Many do not manage their disease correctly, take their medications sporadically, if at all, and describe their problem as "a touch of angina." They need to learn the same material as other cardiac patients with emphasis on how to control and recognize symptoms.

Patients with angina pectoris should learn the purpose of medications and the importance of regular medication schedules. The route of the medication should be clarified. In one case, a patient was taking sublingual medications orally and noted that the medication did not control her symptoms. She had not understood the meaning of the word *sublingual* and was too proud to ask. This underlines the importance of using familiar language when discussing health matters with patients. Patients need special emphasis on the concept that the reduction in symptoms does not mean that the disease is cured or better but that the medication is controlling the symptoms and that patients should continue to take it.

Many anginal patients are unfamiliar with the use of nitroglycerin or other sublingual nitrates in anticipation of an anginal attack. Patients who use the transdermal-patch nitroglycerin should not use a patch for acute angina attack relief because the drug in this form takes about 20 minutes to take effect.[17]

Inform them that nitroglycerin tablets lose potency 4 to 6 months after opening and they are sensitive to heat, light, and air. The date on the vial is the *shelf life date*, which does not include opening the vial and exposing the pills to air. It is equally important to review this teaching material with patients who have been treated for angina in the past because they may have received information that is now outdated or they may have never been told about such problems. The best way to determine whether patients need reinforcement is to ask them to describe their disease and medications. The nurse should ask open-ended questions such as, "Please tell me what you have already been told about your illness and medications so that I don't go over material that you already know." If the nurse asks, "Do you know about your illness?" patients may state that they do, but the nurse still does not know exactly *what* is known.

Warning signs of MI and access to the emergency medical system. Many patients die outside the hospital after suffering MIs (many because they delayed seeking help). This topic should be discussed in depth with all cardiac patients and families before discharge, and families should be taught CPR if possible. They should be familiar with the warning signs of infarction and ways to get help if they are at home, at the office, or at a favorite vacation area. Many patients become frustrated with the inability of medical personnel to describe specific symptoms. There is confusion about the wide variety of symptoms that other patients have had, and it is upsetting to learn that symptoms may differ during a second attack.

Many patients are relieved to know that nitroglycerin will not relieve the pain of infarction and can be used to help differentiate between anginal attacks and MI. According to the physician or institutional policy, patients are told to take up to three sublingual nitroglycerin tablets 3 to 5 minutes apart. If little or no relief occurs in response to the nitroglycerin, the patient should immediately call for the emergency medical system (EMS). If possible, co-workers or family members can make the call for patients and then be ready to signal paramedics when they approach the patients' locations.

Patients should be given a printed card with the EMS emergency number for each telephone in the home and office. Patients and families should be taught to tell the dispatcher an ambulance is needed for a possible heart attack, the address where patients are, any identifying landmarks, and the phone number of the location in case the EMS personnel are unable to locate it. The EMS should be called first, before calling the physician, spouse, or other friend or relative. Patients and families should understand that the EMS personnel will not rush patients immediately to the hospital but will administer needed therapy to stabilize them first.

In areas where there is still no functioning EMS system, appropriate plans for getting patients into the emergency system should be worked out *in advance.* Patients associated in some way with the military should consider the relative distance of military and civilian hospitals. Otherwise they might attempt to get to a military clinic or hospital far from home, thus risking death or further myocardial tissue damage due to the delay in receiving help.

Cardiac healing process. Few people are aware that, after infarction, there is scar formation (fibrosis) that takes about 6 to 8 weeks to develop completely. Cardiac patients generally feel well after the initial pain is gone and need some explanation about the reason for gradual return to activities. If this process is equated to scar formation after a surgical procedure or childbirth, patients are better able to understand.

Test procedures. Patients may receive little or no information from physicians about the purpose of evaluation tests. In addition to the purpose of the test, cardiac patients need to know what they will *hear, see,* and *feel* during the test. They also appreciate knowing the time involved in the test.[31] This information needs to be extended to the families so that they will not fear that something untoward has taken place. Some tests require that additional clothing

be brought from home. An example is a stress test (*exercising cardiogram* is a preferable word to use with patients because stress is perceived by them to be a major contributor to the cardiac event). Shoes that tie and shorts or loose-fitting pants are needed. Patients need to know the reasons that meals are delayed or that they should not smoke before a test.

Any pictures of the equipment can dispel anxiety about what to expect. If patients are scheduled for tests, ask them what the test will mean and what they expect to assess understanding. Talking with other patients who have had the procedure with no adverse problems can reinforce teaching and usually will reassure patients and families about the experience.

If nurses have not recently observed a procedure that will be described to the patient, they should arrange to accompany another patient who will be having the same procedure or call the laboratory or place of the test to find out what the test involves. Changes are made periodically, and knowing about them will reduce the credibility gap.

Risk factor modification. Risk factors play a large role in the development and continued disease process of CAD.[16,30] Instruction about CAD risk factors and modification of them is one of the most important topics that nurses can teach patients and families. Many Americans are still ignorant of CAD risk factors, their origin, and the facts about modification (see Ornish, p. 5).

Both patients and families need to be included because many cardiovascular diseases are hereditary. One study noted that spouses of MI patients have an increased risk of developing CAD.[30] Patients should be taught to review the CAD risk factors with their biologic children; they have an increased risk if one parent has a manifestation of CAD before the age of 60. The nurse or other health professional who teaches risk factor modification must believe in the modification and should be a model of healthy living.

When patients ask what caused their heart attacks, a good answer is CAD. This provides an entry into discussion about the disease, which patients usually have never heard of, and of the risk factors that may have contributed to its formation. After this is known, a checklist can be given to patients to note risk factors present in their lives and situations. Patients can then decide, with the nurse's assistance, risk factors that can be changed and the order in which to proceed.

Some patients may decide that they do not wish to change anything. The nurse's role is to provide information and facilitate change. As long as the nurse is sure that patients have the correct information, the decision that they make must be respected. Support of modification should be continued because some patients who initially are against any modification may later decide to stop smoking, lose weight, join an exercise program, or decrease some of the stress in their lives. Having a former graduate of the inpatient program return for a group or individual discussion can work wonders. Patients can see the person looks well, has returned to work, and can discuss frankly problems encountered during hospitalization.

After patients have identified risk factors present in their situations and have indicated ones that they are willing to change, the nurse should assist them in working out a plan to achieve this goal. When patients say that they plan to stop smoking, the nurse should ask how they are going to do it. Patients who have plans are much more likely to succeed than those who have the intention but no real plan.

The nurse should make available to patients a list of community resources or classes for those who wish to stop smoking. Lung associations, hospitals, and other local groups have programs, usually free or with little cost to patients. If spouses smoke, they should also try to quit because it increases patients' difficulty. Pointing out that passive smoking can be a hazard to patients sometimes will make spouses also willing to try to quit.

Stress is the factor that many patients like to credit with the highest rating for causing their heart disease.[44] There are many self-regulation therapies available for modification of and dealing with stress that require neither medications nor a physician's order (see Chapter 5). They help control the harmful effects of catecholamines, which increase the workload of the already stricken cardiovascular system. Exercise also is an excellent way to treat stress while improving cardiovascular fitness.[8]

Sometimes patients have many risk factors and decide to stop smoking, lose weight, control high blood pressure, change the diet dramatically, and begin exercise programs all at once. Patients are usually more successful (and suffer less stress) if they modify one risk factor at a time. After control in one area has been achieved, another risk factor can be modified. Concentrate on the major risk factors, pointing out that not smoking, controlling lipid levels in the blood, and treating high blood pressure (seldom a problem after an infarction) are much more important initially than is losing weight. Of course, each situation must be measured individually. The control of one factor will give patients confidence to try modification of another.

Pulse-taking. Pulse taking is taught early in hospitalization. Instructions should include ways to locate the pulse, length of time to palpate it, suitable pulse parameters not to be exceeded, and times to take the pulse. This can be a difficult procedure for patients to learn. Have patients use the dominant hand to feel for the pulse; the fingertips seem to be more sensitive in the dominant hand. The nurse should palpate both radial pulses and select the strongest pulse for patients to palpate.

Some patients with cardiac disease also have some degree of peripheral arterial disease or may have undergone tests that interfered with arterial flow, making the radial pulse difficult to palpate. Patients who have diabetic peripheral neuropathic disease frequently are unable to palpate the radial pulse despite a variety of approaches because of the destruction of nerves in their fingers. Spouses or friends should be taught the technique, or the patient can buy a pulse-meter.

Written instructions with good illustrations of the techniques are important. If the patient is willing, the nurse can mark an X over the radial pulse site for independent practice. Another hint for patients who have difficulty palpating the pulse is to have them bend the wrist back. This brings the radial artery closer to the surface. Patients can also simultaneously place the index, middle, and ring fingers over the radial pulse. If the carotid pulse is used, patients should be cautioned not to press firmly so that they will not occlude blood flow to the brain, possibly resulting in syncope.

Medications. Up to 50% of all cardiac patients do not use their medications as prescribed. As soon as possible the nurse should begin to discuss medications with patients. If the institution policy permits, patients' self-medication should be monitored in the hospital. If there is any doubt that patients take medications correctly, a referral to the Visiting Nurse Association or a home health care nurse should be explored. All patients should be able to state the medication name, dosage, frequency of administration, route, purpose, major side effects, any major interactions with food or drugs (including over-the-counter drugs), and considerations for storing the medication (such as refrigeration or avoiding plastic containers for nitroglycerin). Patients should plan with the nurse the best times to take the medication. This schedule should be given in writing. The nurse should not automatically use hospital medication schedules but should plan for times convenient for the patient's lifestyle.

The hospital medication record can be used as a discharge medication teaching aid with medication times highlighted in some manner. The times for medication should interfere as little as possible with patients' lifestyles to ensure better compliance. The nurse should try to schedule as few medication times as possible because taking medications at various times can be confusing and disruptive to patients. If there is too much disruption, patients may omit doses. Patients should also be instructed about what to do if a dose of medication is omitted (see Appendix C). Antidysrhythmic drugs, antibiotics, antianginal drugs, anticoagulants, and steroids are examples of drugs that should be scheduled around the clock (6-12-6-12) instead of four times a day to ensure adequate blood levels.

If pulse-taking is part of medication monitoring, patients or others should be aware of pulse limitations and times to notify the physician. While β-adrenergic blocking drugs, digitalis products, or other pulse-altering medications are used, the nurse should check with the physician for specific pulse limits for patients' needs. Patients should also be instructed on what to do if unable to reach the physician. This should be in writing.

Patients can be given index cards with a sample of the medication (when possible) taped to the corner. On the card, all information that the patients will need to know about a particular medication is listed. Many drug companies and the American Medical Association can provide preprinted cards or other information about the medication. Ideally, all medication teaching should be completed before the day of discharge because patients seem to remember little of what they hear on that day.

Activities. Probably nothing generates more questions and anxiety than the topic of activities before and after discharge. Many patients and families still have the notion that cardiac disease equals disability and resign themselves to quitting their jobs and moving bedroom furniture downstairs. Too often, questions about activity are answered in general terms, such as, "Take it easy for a few weeks," which is of no help at all. They need specifics, such as not to lift more than 30 pounds of weight or to limit stair-climbing to five times a day. Because patients' needs and abilities differ and physicians have different expectations, the nurse can find out from the physician the definition of "take it easy." Patients can be encouraged to write lists of activities about which they are concerned so that they can get the information needed when the physician visits.

In some hospitals, activity information is standardized, but with a community hospital there may be up to 200 different physicians with varying standards for return to activity. Most physicians prefer that patients avoid driving for a few weeks after discharge, and most patients are unaware of this restriction. This can be a problem if spouses do not drive or if there are others who depend on the patients' driving. If this is the case, the social worker can arrange transportation for outings such as grocery shopping or physician or clinic visits. This may take time, so the earlier the worker is aware of the problem, the better.

If there are restrictions to activity in the hospital, the patient should be told the reason for the restriction and when it may be possible to resume the activity. A patient who is unaware of the reasons will be more likely to "cheat" when there is less supervision. Occasionally a patient is reluctant to be active at all, usually because of misunderstanding or fear based on another's experiences. Discussion with the patient may elicit this information. After the reason for the reluctance is known, the nurse or physician can address the specific fear. The patient will then feel more comfortable about resuming activity.

Some patients might use activity restrictions and heart disease as weapons against the family or others. These patients may have been caretakers of others for years. They feel that the family owes them for the sacrifices made, and this is a way to receive "payment." For example, patients might have an angina attack when daughters go out on a date, or spouses might decide that heart disease is the excuse to suspend sexual intercourse that has been unsatisfying. Such feelings require professional treatment. Therapy can provide more appropriate ways of expressing hostility and stating needs and feelings in a constructive man-

ner. The behavior pattern may have been established for a long time and be beyond the ability of nonpsychologic professionals to treat. As with other teaching topics, activity guidelines should be in writing.

To prevent an overprotective family, spouses or close family members should be present when activities are discussed. Patients also need to know that overprotectiveness frequently is an expression of concern for them. It can be exasperating for patients when families forbid activities that the physician or team member has deemed acceptable. Family meetings, without patients present, allow family members to express fears.

Patients may need to be encouraged to make exercise a regular part of their routine. By concentrating on the effects that patients and others can notice, such as clothes fitting better, feeling better,[23] and frequently gaining a more youthful appearance, the nurse may be able to generate interest in regular exercise (see the box, p. 646). Patients need not think that the exercise must cause a great deal of pain and sweating. If they know that low-level, prescribed exercise can be beneficial, patients may be more interested to try it.

The names of nearby cardiac rehabilitation programs that provide supervised exercise can be given to patients, who can ask the physician to prescribe the program. Supervised programs are better than health club settings because they provide teaching, reinforcement of risk factor modification, and support. Staff members are experts in detecting untoward dysrhythmias, adverse responses to exercise, and increase of congestive heart failure symptoms.[7,15]

Sexuality. Most patients are sexually active or plan to be in the future. This is a primary concern for them and their partners. Until recently, however, little or no information was given to them about this very important part of daily living after a cardiac event or cardiac surgery. It is said that a cardiac patient asks three questions on admission to a coronary care unit: "Will I live? Will I work? Will I make love again?"

Many patients are unaware of normal sexual demands on the cardiovascular system. Some may need a review of sexual organs and functions. Many patients and partners are reluctant to bring up the subject, and when nothing is said, they wrongly assume that sexual activity is forbidden. Until the 1960s, cardiac patients were told never to resume intercourse or any other type of sexual activity. The medical profession did not have any research data about the sexual workload on the cardiovascular system of an average, middle-age cardiac patient. The few studies that were done showed that the heart rate rose to 180 beats per minute at orgasm of healthy, young adult men. Not until Masters and Johnson began to do clinical research on the true demands of sexual expression in older persons did the medical profession begin to assemble data on these patients.

The results of this research showed that the average cardiac patient having intercourse with the usual partner

BENEFITS OF A REGULAR AEROBIC EXERCISE PROGRAM

PHYSIOLOGIC BENEFITS

Lower systolic blood pressure and pulse rate while performing a task
Lower rate of breathing and increased pulmonary capacity
Better efficiency and lower perceived effort at a task
Increased peripheral blood flow
Enhanced blood volume and red cell mass
Lowered incidence of embolic and thrombotic phenomena
Improved tolerance and adaptation to heat and cold
Reduced bone mineral loss
Improved flexibility of joints and muscles
Ability to eat more food with less weight gain
Improved bowel function and regularity
Stimulation to develop collaterals around an arterial obstruction
Less problem with hemoconcentration

SOCIOECONOMIC BENEFITS

Better enthusiasm for life and living
Less illness and absence from work
Better chance of surviving a second MI
Reduced inappropriate hospitalization and shorter hospital stay when necessary

BIOCHEMICAL BENEFITS

Better intake of needed vitamins, minerals, and other desirable elements in the diet
More concern for proper nutrition
Increase in high-density lipids and reduced low-density lipids
Reduction in total serum cholesterol
Increased fibrinolysis and reduced platelet adhesion
Increased insulin effectiveness
Reduced serum triglyceride levels
Reduced problem with cardiac dysrhythmias
Reduced inappropriate catecholamine response to stress

PSYCHOLOGIC BENEFITS

Improved self-image
Reduced depression
Improved confidence in ability to exercise and be active
Better sleep and relaxation patterns
Improved sexual responses and libido
Better stamina

---

in a comfortable room had a heart rate of only 120 beats per minute during the usual 15 seconds of orgasm.[37,42] This is comparable to climbing one or two flights of steps or other similar activity requiring 3.5 to 4 METs.[35] This is certainly in marked contrast to previous beliefs. As yet, the information on women and sexual activity demands is minimal.

Another unspoken sexual fear of many patients is that they will die during intercourse. The chance of this is very small. Studies show that there is only a slight increase in the incidence of death for men while having intercourse with illict sexual partners.[35] It is important to address this issue with all patients.

Patients should be approached on the issue of sexual expression in their lives if they have not mentioned the subject before discharge.[42] It is important to be very objective in discussions, even if patients engage in sexual activities of which the nurse does not personally approve. Spouses should not be included in the initial conference because the usual sexual partner of this patient may not be the spouse. Only with patients' permission should the topic be discussed with another.

Heterosexual person's needs. After a review of the physical responses to sexual activity (the pulse will quicken and there may be increased perspiration, a rise in blood pressure, and an increased respiratory rate) the nurse should describe the physical effects of intercourse because patients and partners will have an increased awareness of physical effects after a cardiac event or cardiac surgery. The nurse should never give a list of *dont's,* because the activity should be pleasurable and free of many restrictions.

Patients and partners should be rested, wait an hour after heavy meals, plan to be free from distractions, plan rest periods afterward, and choose positions that are comfortable. Any clothing that is worn should be loose and comfortable. Formerly, patients were told to use positions in which the patient is lying supine or lying on the side. Sitting in a chair so that the feet reach the floor was also recommended. However, research has shown that there is a difference of only 2 beats per minute when the patient is in the superior position.[37] Some cultures may disapprove of a position that places the man underneath, so this recommendation may generate more anxiety and consequently more cardiac workload. Recommending a usual, comfortable position is better for the patient and partner.[27] The nurse or other health professionals should not assume that patients over 50 are not sexually active.

Masturbation and oral-genital contact are usually permitted early in the convalescent period, even if other sexual intercourse activities are not permitted. However, the physician will need to advise the patient when these activities are safe because all cardiovascular illnesses are different in various patients.

Homosexual person's needs. The patient who is homosexual has many of the same needs for information as does the heterosexual person. Men who are homosexual may practice anal intercourse, which can cause increased cardiac workload because of vagal stimulation. Many heterosexual couples also engage in anal intercourse, so this information should be available to all persons. The physician should be consulted before the couple resumes anal intercourse, especially if there is a continuing problem with dysrhythmias. Female homosexuals usually practice oral-genital stimulation, which has no major adverse effects on the cardiovascular system.[30]

It is important that the nurse be objective and sensitive when discussing sexual practices with these patients. Privacy should be provided so that partners can feel free to discuss questions and concerns. Patients are not seeking acceptance of their lifestyle, but rather information with which they can make the best decisions about their lives and health.

Effects of drugs on sexual response. Some patients may be accustomed to using alcohol or other recreational drugs when engaging in sexual activities. Alcohol is a cardiac depressant, and usually physicians recommend only a glass of wine or a single cocktail before sexual activity. The patient should not attempt intercourse when intoxicated because the workload of the heart is increased. It is important to remind patients that beer *is* alcohol and that a can of beer is equal to an ounce of other liquor. The physician may have specific reservations about the use of any alcohol, and patients should ask the physician for specific guidelines, especially if other drugs being taken may be affected by alcohol use.

Patients should not smoke tobacco or marijuana before sexual activities because of the adverse cardiovascular effects of these drugs[29,35,50] Both also reduce the amount of oxygen carried by the blood because of their carbon monoxide content. They also may increase the preload on the heart, and marijuana increases the afterload in susceptible patients.

Some patients use amyl nitrate in conjunction with intercourse in the belief that the drug can increase the intensity of orgasm. Amyl nitrate is packaged in small ampules that are broken under the nose and inhaled. Patients may refer to these as "poppers." They should be told of the adverse effect on the cardiac output, which can be fatal to someone with cardiovascular disease.[11]

Medications such as any of the β-adrenergic blocking drugs, many antihypertensives, and some vasodilators can disrupt sexual responsiveness and performance. These medications usually blunt or block the response of the sympathetic nervous system. The patient should be aware that, if a problem is noted, there are usually many other types of medications that can be used without the same

adverse effect. It is unethical to deny that these side effects do occur in some patients. Usually a patient can accept this information without becoming unduly focused on the side effects. Under no circumstances should the patient stop taking these medications without the physician knowing because some cause serious problems, even reinfarction, if they are suddenly withdrawn.

If patients use sublingual nitroglycerin or intradermal paste, they should not expose their partners to the unpleasant side-effects of nitrates, such as flushing or headache. Patients should not deeply kiss their partners after using nitroglycerin tablets under the tongue. If the paste is used before intercourse or at bedtime, the area should be covered with plastic wrap. The patient may also want to place the paste on the leg or arm instead of the chest.

Fears related to sexual activity. In addition to the fear of dying while having sexual intercourse, the patients and partners may have other fears that can be eased with correct information in many cases. Study of these patients reveals that many substantially reduce the frequency of sexual activity after recovery from MIs, cardiac surgery, or PTCA.[29] The major reasons for this decrease or cessation of sexual activity are impotence, loss of libido, cardiac symptoms, and depression. Even when information is made available to patients and their partners, discussion does not always prevent an overall reduction in sexual activity.[31] It may be that these patients have also had a "mind infarction," which results in permanent changes in their personalities or those of the sexual partner. They seldom seem to be able to completely resume the personalities that they had before the event.[16] Thus the nurse should not feel that the educational session was not a success if patients report that they have trouble with sexual expression.

Many patients are not aware that sexual expression also includes being close to each other, caressing, touching, kissing, and providing close body contact. For those few who cannot resume intercourse for some reason, suitable alternative expressions should be explored so that this important aspect of life will not be neglected while awaiting recovery. Patients who report complete impotence may benefit from referral to a urologist or gynecologist for a complete physical examination. Some may have sexual dysfunctions that are beyond the scope and ability of the nurse. These patients should be referred to a competent practitioner in the area of sexual dysfunctions. Many persons with diabetes or peripheral vascular disease are permanently impotent due to occlusion or destruction of pelvic vascular vessels. These persons may be unaware of the new advances in the treatment of this type of impotence. Some are able to resume intercourse after appropriate urologic surgery or treatment.[58]

Food planning. Food can cause many problems for the patient and staff. Cultural beliefs and preferences can complicate the problem. For many patients food is one of the few pleasures left. In the hospital, food provides a break in the tedium of the daily routine. Some patients imagine that they have ordered sumptuous foods and are naturally disappointed when the food arrives and does not meet their expectations. Others express anger about their food instead of their illness. Complaints about food should be investigated because they may actually represent other concerns.

As a rule, most inpatients are not particularly interested in learning about diet changes. This may be related to the denial of some of the aspects of newly diagnosed chronic heart disease. Established dietary habits are difficult to change, sometimes because of the emotional connotations that food has to many people. It is certainly difficult for patients to think about changing habits that have brought much pleasure. A better approach for the nurse and other health professionals might be to delete the word *diet* from any teaching that is done about food. *Diet* in our culture denotes deprivation. A better phrase is *food plan,* which removes any idea of giving up favorite foods while stressing a definite system of food intake.[56]

Unless the patient has definite signs of fluid or sodium retention problems, it is probably not necessary to restrict the sodium below 4 g a day.[56] Some physicians still routinely order 1 g sodium diets for all patients admitted to the coronary care unit, without any planning for the person's individual needs. Thus it becomes the nurse's responsibility to guide the diet prescription by making information available to the physician and questioning any dietary prescription that seems irrelevant to the patient's condition or needs.

Before undertaking the diet instruction, the dietitian should conduct *food preference interviews* to discover patients' usual diet and food preferences. The dietitian can also ascertain the current level of knowledge that patients and food preparers (if different) have about the basic food groups and body needs. After this is done, the dietitian can modify the menu to provide food that patients are more likely to eat and enjoy while hospitalized. If patients do not eat properly, healing will be slowed. Patients do not usually realize that, even though they are not very active, they still have definite caloric needs. Severe reducing diets, such as 800- to 1000-calorie diets, have no place during the acute hospital phase and should be started only when patients are fully healed and are outpatients. Of course, medical supervision and supplementation of vitamins are needed for patients on this type of diet restriction.

Diet instruction should not be started until the food plan that the patient will follow after discharge is known. It makes no sense to instruct patients about a 2-g sodium, 1500-calorie restricted diet if the physician will order a no-added-salt, 2000-calorie diet on discharge. The dietitian and nurse should *jointly* plan the instruction so that information is consistent. The nurse should not put the entire burden on the dietitian or feel there is no need to augment and reinforce the teaching. Appropriate audiovisual aids should be chosen. Pictures or models of foods, labels, and packaging can be used to measure the patient's understanding. The food preparer, if not the patient, should also be

present during lessons. Family members should understand why the patient is eating less of one food group and more of another. This may encourage them to make some changes in the way they eat.

Most patients need more information about data on the labels of various foods and way to interpret the amount of an ingredient present in foods. Many people do not realize that ingredients are listed in order of the amount found in the food. It usually is not necessary for patients to buy large amounts of special foods (low sodium, low sugar) because these tend to be more costly and usually are not needed if they check labels and make substitutions when necessary. Patients need help in interpreting the polyunsaturated/saturated fats ratio found on many packages.

If patients eat frequently in restaurants, a collection of menus can help them plan in advance what to order to stay within the food plan limits. If possible, other family members can also be present to reinforce the teaching at a later date.

A food-tasting session can be conducted for patients and food preparers to illustrate that the diet need not include only boring, tasteless food. Many believe this, based on the institutional food received in many hospitals. Recipes should be available near the food being tasted so that people can have an immediate awareness that usually only a little modification of favorite recipes is needed. Patients can also decide which of the foods presented are tasty to them, saving them the cost of preparing recipes that do not appeal to them. The fewer changes that have to be made, the more likely persons are to incorporate those changes in the future.

Dietitians can work with the person who prepares the food so that favorite cultural foods can be modified, if necessary, to comply with the new food plan. Conversion can be easy. The family can bring favorite foods into the hospital for the patient who is unable to eat traditional American foods. Dietitians should be notified of this food so that they can account for the patient's daily intake of prescribed dietary components.

Several days should be devoted to food instruction and practice if the diet is to be changed. The nurse and dietitian should remember that community resources are available to assist the patient after discharge, when readiness to learn about the diet usually occurs. The American Heart Association is a source of much diet information, and many chapters also have a dietitian available at no charge to help persons with heart disease. A home health care nurse or a member of the Visiting Nurse Association is available in most hospitals through the social service department. This person will make the necessary arrangements *once the referral is made*. A notation should be placed on the care plan or chart along with the liaison member's name and phone number so that additional information can be communicated quickly.

Preparation for cardiac surgery. If it is known that a patient will need cardiac surgery or PTCA, the nurse should begin to teach the families and patients as soon as they indicate readiness. Most patients enter the hospital only 1 day before surgery[48] so there is little time to teach them about what to expect. The anxiety and confusion on the preoperative day usually render patients unable to remember much about what is said. Therefore the nurse should start while patients are recovering from the cardiac event that necessitated admission to the hospital.

If possible, the hospital should have some type of preoperative classes or tours during the week of admission. Some hospitals place a new preoperative patient in a room with a patient who has had the same procedure and is about to be discharged. Many patients comment favorably about this practice.

Patients may be very fearful of surgery or a procedure that deals directly with the heart. Many cardiac surgery patients are less fearful when they learn that surgeons will be working on the surface of the heart and not in the interior. Other patients may not wish to know much about the surgery. The best approach is to cover the basic information and then wait for patients to exhibit more curiosity and ask more questions.[28]

In many centers the patient and family are oriented to the intensive cardiovascular surgical unit the night before surgery. Sometimes the unit is extremely busy, and certain scenes might upset the patient and family. On those days it may be better to show slides of the unit and take the family to the area of the hospital where the unit is located so that the family can find it the next day (see Chapter 17).

PTCA. Patients who are having PTCA will need an explanation of the procedure and information about the anticoagulation therapy used during and after the procedure (see Chapter 9). They should realize that the procedure is a treatment and not a cure for CAD and that follow-up care is necessary. These patients are also candidates for outpatient rehabilitation exercise and education.

OUTPATIENT REHABILITATION: PHASES II AND III
Purpose and goals

Ideally, outpatient programs that continue rehabilitation should emphasize physical training and lifestyle management of CAD risk factors, which are accomplished through education and behavioral modification techniques. The patient and famiy must understand from the beginning that the commitment is lifelong.[7] Otherwise, the rehabilitation benefits will be lost (see p. 631).

The goals of outpatient rehabilitation are much the same as those of inpatient programs, with a difference in the intensity of physical training. The program goal is for the person with cardiovascular disease and family to achieve the highest level of wellness possible. Education about how to achieve wellness continues; the exercise component assumes greater prominence as the patient makes

the body more efficient and learns about normal physical responses. The final goal is renewed confidence so that the patient feels comfortable exercising alone or with other "normal" persons in a gym or spa setting. If this can be achieved, the patient has been truly rehabilitated.

Candidates

Most outpatient programs are structured to deal with several categories of patients with cardiovascular disease[38]:
1. Patients 2 to 6 weeks after an MI or myocardial revascularization surgery
2. Patients with stable angina pectoris
3. Patients who have had PTCA

Some centers also accept persons who have had artificial cardiac valve replacements or who are at unusually high risk for the development of CAD.[38]

To enter the program, patients usually need permission from the physician, exercise tests (preferably symptom limited), copies of procedures performed, and a modest battery of laboratory tests to determine whether there is significant renal involvement, electrolyte imbalance, anemia, or uncontrolled blood sugar levels. Diabetic patients generally can participate once the blood sugar level is controlled. If they use insulin, they are instructed to inject the insulin in a site other than their arms or legs on exercise days. The increased blood flow to these muscles will enhance the absorption of insulin and might lead to an insulin reaction or, depending on the type of insulin, a diabetic coma response later in the day.[26] Some diabetic persons control the disease better after an exercise training program because exercise frequently reduces the need for extraneous insulin.[47]

The patient is examined by clinic personnel before being admitted to the program. The nurse or physician may note other physical problems that preclude exercise or require modification of the exercise prescription. A physical therapist or exercise physiologist can be a valuable addition to the clinic staff because they are experts in detecting and treating disabilities of the muscles, joints, and nerves. These persons should also be familiar with the inpatient rehabilitation process to ensure continuity. A thorough assessment of the patient's nine human response patterns is also performed (see Cardiovascular Rehabilitation Tool in Appendix A).

Staff rotation for continuity

Staff rotation allows wider experience in treating cardiac inpatients and outpatients. Frequently staff members know the patient from the inpatient center. This enhances the patient's trust and learning retention in the outpatient area. If the clinic has separate inpatient and outpatient staffs, there should be some provision for regularly scheduled meetings so that there is continuity and communication between staffs.

Hospital-based versus community-based programs[6,16]

Hospital-based programs can use facilities of the hospital, such as ECG station, laboratory, and emergency department with minimal time and effort. These programs usually can treat patients who have more complicated cases or who have minimal physical functioning. They tend to be more structured and treat fewer patients at each session. Typically, four to eight patients per session is the maximum. Adherence to these programs is frequently better, perhaps because an absence is readily noticed and the patient is immediately contacted about problems.[21] Patients and families who are uneasy about exercising after cardiac surgery or infarction may feel safer in a hospital-based program because of the immediate availability of sophisticated medical assistance.

Community-based programs are usually conducted in a gym or community center.[6] The groups range from 10 to more than 50 persons. Typical programs use a walking-jogging format, and some have a swimming pool or other exercise facilities, depending on availability and philosophy of the staff. Generally a cardiologist, exercise physiologist, and one or more nurses and other ancillary personnel are present. More independent patient participation is common, and patients may be responsible for recording their own exercise responses, doing warm-up and cool-down exercises, and reporting adverse symptoms. Education sessions are conducted before or after the exercise sessions.

ECG monitoring may be done for a few sessions initially, and further monitoring, usually by telemetry, is done at the discretion of the staff. Because of the setting and the type of exercises done, a minimal MET level (usually 5) of achievement on the graded exercise test is usually required. Some centers also have an age limit, but excellent results can be achieved by persons older than 65. The best course is individual evaluation rather than limitation by age. The physician, nurse, other staff, and the patient should collectively decide which type of setting will achieve best results and produce the greatest patient satisfaction and safety.[13]

Types of exercise programs and protocols

Exercise modalities include treadmills, exercise bikes, arm exercise devices, rowing machines, step-climbing (usually to a metronome pace) and other types of aerobic activities. Other programs use the walking-jogging approach. Some programs train only legs, and others train both arms and legs. Studies[15] have substantiated that training of both arms and legs is needed. Training effect cannot be transferred from the legs to the arm. Because patients use both arms and legs in daily activities, it is important not to neglect arm training. Arm training can also reduce cardiac workload because usually arm activities cause the greatest increase in pulse and blood pressure and therefore cardiac oxygen demand.[7,8,45]

Each program has an individual protocol for achieving patient fitness. They may be very specific, or they may permit leeway for exercise prescription. Some protocols divide patients according to the maximal *safe* level that the patient achieved on the admission graded exercise test. It is vital that the test be done when the patient is taking *all medications* that will be used when the patient is exercising because performance can change dramatically when medication is changed or omitted. The exercise prescription will be based on these data. If the medication is altered or stopped, the staff must decide whether the patient needs another graded exercise test to evaluate the new physical state before continuing with the exercise program.

There is currently no significant evidence that either continuous or interval training is preferable.[8] Persons with cardiac disease seem to prefer the intermittent method, which includes the warm-up period, an exercise period, a walk period of 2 minutes, another exercise period, another walk period, and so on until the end of the exercise session, when the cool-down is done. The continuous method includes the warm-up period, the exercise period, and the cool-down period. The intermittent method is more suited to a program in which the patient moves from the one modality to another following the 2-minute walk break. The choice of method is made by the physician and other health staff personnel associated with the program.

Most programs begin with a 2- to 3-month training program that requires patients to come to the clinic three times a week. There may also be an exercise or walking program on the days that exercise at the clinic is not done. Patients are taught the importance of doing warm-up and cool-down exercises to reduce injuries and to allow the cardiovascular system to prepare for the additional work load of exercise. Patients are also taught pulse-taking if they do not already know the exercise pulse method (p. 644).

After the patient has completed Phase II, graded exercise testing is again done to measure improvement (which in many cases is substantial). The patient then has two options, depending on the situation and finances. (Some insurance programs will not cover the costs after the first 3 months.) The patient can continue at the center, perhaps one or two times a week while exercising at home one or two times a week. The patient can continue this for 3 months and then reduce the visits to the center once every other week while exercising at home three to five times a week. At this point many physicians perform another graded exercise test and, unless there are unresolved problems, the patient is discharged from the clinic.

The exercise should continue for patients' lifetimes. Graded exercise testing and exercise modification are done annually. Most patients show the greatest improvement in their exercise capacity within Phase II. After this is achieved, most patients reach a plateau for maximal capacity, so fewer changes in the exercise prescription are necessary. Thus home exercise programs can be prescribed as a second option for those patients who do not choose to continue at the center after they have completed their Phase II sessions.

Contraindications to exercise

After patients have been screened, specific contraindications to exercise must be noted and treated.[19] Patients who have asthma that worsens with deep inspiration probably should not exercise. Patients who have moderate-to-severe arthritis or other joint disability may find that some forms of exercise may worsen the condition. Patients should be evaluated individually for the extent of the disability. Patients with severe neurologic disability may not be candidates. One program had excellent success with a person who suffered a polio attack in his 30s and later had an MI. Although he could walk with great difficulty using canes and braces, he exercised by using arm training alone and did very well.

Severe claudication may be a contraindication to exercise, although many individuals have reported improvement by exercising to the point of pain, resting, and exercising again. Trained leg muscles need less oxygen to work, and exercise builds collateral blood vessels, so the patient may be able to walk farther without discomfort.[39]

It is vital to screen patients for neck injury or disease, back problems, and knee problems. Many times, with some modification of the exercise prescription or routine, these patients will do well, but they must be watched closely for exacerbation of injury or disability. After cardiac surgery, patients may experience shoulder problems because of positioning and the surgical techniques used during the operation.

Severe pulmonary disease may be a contraindication, depending on the result of the graded exercise test. Many patients have been heavy smokers and need a more-gradual introduction to the exercise sessions. A pulmonary function test is recommended. Renal disease may preclude exercise, depending on the instability of the patients' conditions. Patients who are on dialysis or have had a kidney transplant, however, can usually benefit from such a program with no adverse effects. Because exercise will decrease the blood supply to the kidney, patients with renal disease will need further evaluation before exercise begins. Finally, patients unwilling to come regularly for exercise sessions should not be forced to attend.[21] Sometimes fears that are holding persons back can be uncovered, but for some individual programs of walking or other activities may be better.

Each clinic usually has a written list of contraindications and expectations, and if there are questions about whether a patient should exercise, the clinic staff should make the decision because they are responsible for the patient while in the program.

Exercise complications

Not all symptoms of major and minor complications appear immediately.[7,19] It is important to tell patients that the occurrence of symptoms does not necessarily mean that they will have to leave the program. Many persons conceal symptoms if they believe that they will be asked to leave.

Common adverse symptoms during exercise are angina pectoris or muscular skeletal discomfort, a gallop rhythm (S_3) signaling possible cardiac failure, unusual dyspnea, loss of coordination, dizziness or syncope, unusual fatigue or muscle soreness, and dysrhythmias. These dysrhythmias are varied, but premature ventricular contractions are commonly seen in most patients. The nurse who monitors patients in an outpatient setting will have to adjust to the fact that not all premature ventricular contractions are treated. If they increase with exercise, occur in bursts of ventricular tachycardia, or are multiformed, exercise is halted, the patient is cooled down and is evaluated by the physician before being permitted to exercise again. Patients should be closely questioned about antidysrhythmic medications. Sometimes forgetting a dose or taking a dose later than usual increases premature ventricular contractions. Determining the blood level of the medication may be indicated to evaluate whether it is in the therapeutic range. Often the medication is increased or changed to regain control of the dysrhythmia. Sometimes eliminating caffeine from the diet will be the decisive factor. Patients may be helped by advising them to switch from their usual cup of coffee in the morning to a low-caffeine drink.

Other dysrhythmias commonly seen are premature atrial contractions, junctional premature beats, paroxysmal atrial, junctional, or ventricular tachycardia, bundle branch blocks, wandering pacemakers, heart blocks, and ST-segment depression. Each clinic has a protocol for the staff to follow in the event of any of these problems. Although rare, MI may occur during or after exercise. This fact is usually mentioned in the consent form that the patient signs before beginning the program.

After exercise, the following untoward effects may occur, and the patient should be told specifically what to do if certain problems occur:

1. Insomnia
2. Weakness and fatigue
3. Muscle cramping or muscle tears
4. Nausea, vomiting, and diarrhea
5. Joint swelling and soreness
6. Sprains
7. Increase or change in anginal pattern
8. Dysrhythmias, especially if patient previously had none
9. Loss of circulation in a limb or digit

If the patient does report one of these symptoms, the clinic nurse must decide whether the problem requires a physician's intervention or if the exercise prescription should be modified. If the patient does see a physician, it is important that the nurse have written or direct phone communication from the physician that the patient may resume exercise. Any change of medication should be noted in the patient record and the exercise prescription modified if necessary.

Exercise prescription

The prescription of exercise for a particular patient is written in accordance with the clinic protocol. In many states the exercise prescription must be written by a physician, but a nurse specialist or exercise physiologist may modify the prescription if the modification is within the protocol guidelines. Nurses frequently write an initial exercise prescription recommendation, which is then reviewed by the cardiologist or other physician in charge of the clinic.

The exercise prescription has *three components:* frequency of exercise, intensity of exercise effort, and time or duration of the exercise. Patients' target heart rates and progression of exercise are also noted on the prescription. These components are different for each patient because they are based on individual graded exercise testing data. Patients tend to compare the exercise target pulse on their exercise prescriptions. There should be no competition between patients, and the nurse needs to intervene if it occurs. Patients should be reminded that each person has a unique exercise level; a lower target heart rate does not mean that those persons have more severe cardiac disease.

The patient typically attends the clinic three to five times a week. It has been demonstrated that exercise less than three times a week will not produce the desired effect.[13] More than five times a week, except for a trained athlete, is not recommended due to increase in overuse muscle and joint injuries.[45]

Intensity of exercise is controlled by the settings on the machines used, such as the speed and percentage of incline of the treadmill. In other programs that use jogging or walking, the intensity is determined by time and speed.

Duration of exercise specifies the amount of time that the patient spends on each modality or the time that the patient will walk or jog. A usual beginning is 12 to 18 minutes of total exercise, excluding the warm-up period (usually 5 to 10 minutes) and the cool-down period (usually 5 to 10 minutes or until the patient is within 10 to 20 beats of the beginning pulse rate). Cardiac transplant patients require a minimum of 10 minutes for warm up and cool down due to the denervation of their hearts. As the patient continues with the program, the exercise time is gradually increased with the intensity of the exercise. It is a good idea to review the exercise prescription after each exercise session in response to the patient's performance that day.

Patients' *target heart rates* play a very important role in exercise prescriptions. In most clinics, exercise is graded in accordance with patients' ability to reach and sustain the target heart rate with little difficulty. This target heart rate is usually 65% to 85% of the maximal safe pulse rate achieved on the graded exercise test. The clinic protocol determines which formula to use to calculate the target heart rate. A common formula is to take 65% to 85% of the maximal heart rate achieved on the graded exercise test. Thus if patients achieved a pulse rate of 160 on the exercise stress test, the target heart rate for exercise achievement would be 65% to 85% of 160, or 104 to 136 beats per minute. Patients should also be asked to grade their perceptions of the exercise difficulty via the Borg scale before any changes are made in the exercise prescription.[18]

Some clinics require the achievement of a MET level percentage along with or instead of the target heart rate. Excellent results have been achieved using the target heart rate and patient perception of exercise difficulty.[8,18,45] Many clinics now use these parameters instead of METs.

Education

Education plays a role equal to that of exercise in an outpatient rehabilitation program (see p. 640). Each patient and family member should be evaluated to determine the level of understanding of cardiac disease, exercise training, cardiac surgery and testing, medications, way to get help, recognition of the signs of MI, and diet. Risk factor modification should be continued in the clinic.

Education can be accomplished individually by having the patient watch films before or after exercise, or it can be done in informal or formal group discussion. An evening family meeting with a speaker on some topic of interest, followed by a question-and-answer period, can be very helpful and will involve the family in the rehabilitation process.

For many patients a contracting approach is helpful.[49] Patients indicate changes they are willing to make or goals they want to achieve by the end of the outpatient sessions. A suitable plan is delineated by patients, and progress is measured by objectives that can be achieved and measured. This involves patients and gives the nurse insight into patient expectations. Changes can then be suggested as the rehabilitation progresses.

Progress communication

The physician must be kept aware of the patient's progress at the rehabilitation clinic. Summary letters to each physician who has a patient in the program are helpful. These letters summarize the patient's exercise and education progress. Any adverse effects are immediately reported to the patient's physician by phone, and the clinic cardiologist should also be notified. In addition, a copy of the exercise flow sheet could be included with the letter and a copy placed in the patient record. When the patient leaves the clinic program, a progress summary should be placed at the front of the chart so that it is easily available for future research or consultation.

Financial considerations

Many patients do not have enough insurance coverage or financial resources to meet the expenses of the rehabilitation sessions. The costs range from nothing (if patients are in a research grant study) to $35 or more per session, depending on the type of program and the cost of the equipment. The state rehabilitative service department may offer assistance, depending on the state policies and requirements for eligibility. Some hospitals admit certain patients on the basis of need in return for federal or state reimbursement. Finally, a service group or volunteer group might be willing to contribute to the support of a needy patient.

Many insurance plans cover up to 80% of the cost of the programs after a deductible is met. Many third-party organizations are completely independent from each other, so the expenses that one group (called a *plan*) covers may not be covered by another plan. It is the patient's responsibility to learn what the health insurance will cover. Persons in the military or their dependents may be eligible for military outpatient programs, and some Veterans Administration hospitals have programs for those who qualify.

Research

No research has shown definitely that exercise training reduces the incidence of future MI in patients known to have CAD.[12,45] Because of this, some physicians and insurance providers do not feel that formal exercise training should be prescribed or covered by insurance. The chances of serious complications and death seem to be reduced if another MI occurs in a patient who maintains this training.[45] Some professionals consider exercise training something that patients can do on their own without professional supervision. However, an editorial[12] in the *Journal of Cardiac Rehabilitation* inquired, "Have we been asking the right questions?" As the editorial points out, rather than asking about the reinfarction rate (only 3% in the population tested) and "the possibility that exercise will alter the late prognosis of the postcoronary patient," perhaps we should be asking, "What are the patients' objectives? Are they seeking an increase in longevity or an attainment of happiness for their remaining years?" Many patients enter an exercise program and attain a support group, find answers to questions about heart disease, reduce mild depression by stimulating hormones that counter depression, and enhance return to normal daily life and the work place. The increase in confidence and compliance frequently seen in this patient group must be considered. Such qualities are more difficult to measure, but if these are what the patient is seeking, they may have more relevance in research studies than the incidence of longevity or reinfarction.

Another consideration is to study programs that have a high rate of adherence and compare them with programs in which adherence is low.[12] Perhaps this is where the research should be directed as American health professionals enter the fourth decade of outpatient cardiac rehabilitation.

KEY CONCEPT REVIEW

1. Three important topics to be included in the inpatient cardiac education program for families and patients are:
   a. Activities, medications, and sexuality
   b. Injection techniques, foot care, and medications
   c. Warning signs of infarction, activation of the EMS, and jogging
   d. Prognosis, exercise training, and pet ownership
2. Key members of an inpatient rehabilitation team are:
   a. Nurse, vocational rehabilitation specialist, and chaplain
   b. Physician, physical therapist, and pharmacist
   c. Occupational therapist, nurse, and dietitian
   d. Nurse, physical therapist, and patient and family
3. A contraindication for inpatient exercise is:
   a. Occasional premature ventricular contractions
   b. Continued anginal-type of pain
   c. Rise in systolic blood pressure with exercise
   d. Fourth heart sound
4. A *usual* candidate for an outpatient exercise program is the:
   a. Aortic valve replacement patient
   b. Unstable angina patient
   c. MI patient 3 to 6 weeks after hospitaliation
   d. Hypertensive patient
5. An expected effect of a β-adrenergic blocking drug on the patient's exercise response is:

   a. Low diastolic blood pressure
   b. Low resting and exercise pulse
   c. Elevated preload
   d. High systolic blood pressure
6. The component of the exercise prescription that states the amount of exercise that the patient should perform is the:
   a. Intensity
   b. Frequency
   c. Duration
   d. Target heart rate
7. One reason for performing a ministress test before discharge after an MI is to:
   a. Gain data for an outpatient exercise prescription
   b. Obtain functional data for discharge planning
   c. Measure the achievement of exercise training
   d. Screen the patient for possible CAD
8. The formula for a MET is:
   a. 2.5 ml O_2/kg/minute
   b. 1.5 ml O_2/kg/minute
   c. 3.5 ml O_2/kg/minute
   d. 5 ml O_2/kg/minute
9. Which of the following patients would not be a candidate for an outpatient program?
   a. Patient with insulin-dependent diabetes
   b. Patient with peripheral vascular disease

   c. Patient who has undergone PCTA
   d. Patient with unstable angina
10. Phase I cardiac rehabilitation refers to the:
   a. Maintenance period
   b. Exercise training period after discharge
   c. Inpatient program
   d. Period immediately after discharge
11. A patient is usually taught to respond to a suspected angina attack by:
   a. Calling the physician immediately
   b. Stopping activity, taking three nitroglycerin tablets 3 to 5 minutes apart, and calling the EMS if no relief is obtained
   c. Driving to the emergency department
   d. Taking a propranolol tablet as needed
12. A cardiac patient who is noted by the primary nurse to be very happy and relaxed during the inpatient phase may be experiencing:
   a. Anger
   b. Depression
   c. Denial
   d. Regression

ANSWERS

| 1. a | 3. b | 5. b | 7. b | 9. d | 11. b |
| 2. d | 4. c | 6. a | 8. c | 10. c | 12. c |

REFERENCES

1. Allen J, Becker D, and Swank R: Factors Related to Functional Status after Coronary Artery Bypass Surgery, Heart Lung 19:337, 1990.
2. American College of Sports Medicine: Guidelines for graded exercise testing and exercise prescription, ed 5, Philadelphia, 1987, Lea & Febiger.
3. Anderson U: After the ICU: how do the patients feel? In Noble M, editor: The ICU environment: directions for nursing, Reston, Va, 1982, The Reston Publishing Co.
4. A baffling coronary puzzle, Time, p 42, Jan 12, 1981.
5. Baker KG: Group sessions as a method of reducing anxiety in patients with coronary artery disease, Heart Lung 8:180, 1979.
6. Berra K: YMCArdiac therapy: a community-based program for persons with coronary artery disease, J Cardiac Rehab 1:354, 1981.
7. Comoss P, Burke E, and Swails S: Cardiac rehabilitation: a comprehensive approach, Philadelphia, 1979, JB Lippincott Co.
8. Curtis A and Davis P: Exercise physiology in cardiac rehabilitation, CVP Aug-Sept 1980, p 19.
9. DeGracia R: Cultural influences in Filipino patients, Am J Nurs 79:1413, 1979.
10. Dehn M: The effects of exercise, Am J Nurse 80:435, 1980.
11. DeMoya D and DeMoya A: Effects of amyl nitrate "poppers," RN June 1980, p 101.
12. Editorial, J Cardiac Rehab 2:21, 1982.
13. Fardy P and others, editors: Cardiac rehabilitation: implications for the nurse and other health professionals, ed 2, St Louis, 1988, The CV Mosby Co.
14. Ferguson R and others: Coronary blood flow during isometric and dynamic exercise in angina pectoris patients, J Cardiac Rehab 1:21, 1981.
15. Froelicher V: Exercise and coronary heart disease, J Cardiac Rehab 1:277, 1981.
16. Gentry D and Williams R Jr: Psychological aspects of myocardial infarction and coronary care, ed 2, St Louis, 1979, The CV Mosby Co.
17. Gever L: Administering drugs through the skin, Nurs 82, March 1982, p 88.
18. Gutmann M and others: Perceived exertion–heart rate relationship during exercise testing and training in cardiac patients, J Cardiac Rehab 1:52, 1981.
19. Haskell W: Cardiovascular complications during exercise training of cardiac patients, Circulation 57:920, 1978.
20. Heart facts 1990: National Center, Dallas, 1989, American Heart Association.
21. Hoepfel-Harris J: Improving compliance with an exercise program, Am J Nurs 80:449, 1980.
22. Johnson B: Influence of environmental factors on exercise and activity of cardiac patients, Cardiovasc Nurs 18:7, 1982.
23. Kaplan J: Exercise—a serious report on the astonishing benefits physical exercise can bring to your mind, Glamour, May 1978, p 248.
24. Kellerman J: Cardiac rehabilitation: reminiscences, international variations, experiences, J Cardiac Rehab 1:53, 1981.
25. Kinney M and others: Comprehensive cardiac care, ed 7, St Louis, 1991, Mosby–Year Book, Inc.
26. Koivisto V and Felig P: Effects of leg exercise on insulin absorption in diabetic patients, N Engl J Med 298:79, 1978.
27. Levine SA and Lown B: "Armchair" treatment of acute coronary thrombosis, JAMA 148:1365, 1952.
28. Lovvorn J: Coronary artery bypass surgery: helping patients cope with postoperative problems, Am J Nurs 82:1073, 1982.
29. Mann S and others: Effects of M.I. on sexual activity, J Cardiac Rehab 1:187, 1981.
30. Maroc J: Coronary artery disease risk factors. In Fardy P and others, editors: Cardiac rehabilitation: implications for the nurse and other professionals, ed 2, St Louis, 1988, The CV Mosby Co.
31. McHugh N, Christman N, and Johnson J: Preparatory information: what helps and why, Am J Nurs 82:780, 1982.
32. McNeer J: Hospital discharge one week after acute myocardial infarction, JAMA 298:1978.
33. Meleis A: The Arab-American in the health care system, Am J Nurs 81:1180, 1981.
34. Meyer G: Exercises for the inpatient. In Fardy P and others, editors: Cardiac rehabilitation: implications for the nurse and other health professions, ed 2, St Louis, 1988, The CV Mosby Co.
35. Moore K, Folk-Lighty M, and Nolen M: The joy of sex after a heart attack: counseling the cardiac patient, Nurs 77, June 1977, p 53.
36. Miller P Sr: Health benefits of and adherence to the medical regimen by patients with ischemic heart disease, Heart Lung 11:332, 1982.

37. Nemec E: Heart rate and blood pressure responses during sexual activity in normal males, Am Heart J 92:274, 1976.

38. Newell J: Physical training after heart valve replacement, Br Heart J 44:638, 1980.

39. Ogawa T and others: Peripheral circulatory changes after physical conditioning in coronary artery disease patients, J Cardiac Rehab 1:269, 1981.

40. Patient education in practice, pub no 351, Washington, DC, 1981, American Society of Internal Medicine.

41. Proceedings of the Cardiac Rehabilitation Workshop Conference, Chicago, April 24-25, 1980, J Cardiac Rehab 2:73, 1982.

42. Puksta N: All about sex . . . after a coronary, Am J Nurs 77:602, 1977.

43. Reitz N: Considerations in health education. In Fardy P and others, editors: Cardiac rehabilitation: implications for the nurse and other health professionals, ed 2, St Louis, 1988, The CV Mosby Co.

44. Rudy E: Patients' and spouses' causal explanations of a myocardial infarction, Nurs Res 29:352, 1980.

45. Shaw L: Effects of a prescribed supervised exercise program on mortality and cardiovascular morbidity in patients after a myocardial infarction, Am J Cardiol 48:39, 1981.

46. Smith S and del Bueno D: How to get through to a refugee patient, RN, Jan 1981, p 43.

47. Soman V: Increased insulin sensitivity and insulin binding to monocytes after physical training, N Engl J Med 301:1200, 1979.

48. Stanford J: Who profits from coronary artery bypass surgery? Am J Nurs 82:1068, 1982.

49. Steckel S: Patient contracting, St Louis, 1982, The CV Mosby Co.

50. Synthesis Communications, Inc: Sex and the heart patient, New York, 1977.

51. Theroux P and others: Prognostic value of exercise testing soon after myocardial infarction, JAMA 301:341, 1979.

52. Toth J: Effect of structured preparation for transfer on patient anxiety on leaving the coronary care unit, Nurs Res 29:28, 1980.

53. Tyzenhouse P: Myocardial infarction: its effect on the family, Am J Nurs 73:1012, 1973.

54. Washington International Center, Meridian House International: There is a difference, ed 2, Washington, DC, 1980, Fontana Lithograph, Inc.

55. Webster's Dictionary, Chicago, 1979, Consolidated Book Publishers.

56. White B: Adaptation to salt, Unpublished lecture at the Catholic University of America, April 1982.

57. Winslow E and Weber T: Progressive exercise to combat the hazards of bed rest, Am J Nurs 80:440, 1980.

58. Wood R and Rose K: Penile implants for impotence, Am J Nurs 78:234, 1978.

59. You are how you live (editorial), The Washington Post, Feb 9, 1982.

APPENDIX
A

Various Cardiovascular Assessment Tools

Anita P. Sherer

The Holistic Cardiovascular Assessment Tool discussed in Chapter 3 facilitates the difficult transition from a medical to a holistic nursing assessment and allows nursing diagnoses to be generated easily.

The cardiovascular patient population is a large and diverse group with a variety of nursing care needs. Because nurses encounter cardiovascular patients in a variety of clinical settings, the focus of their assessment changes with the setting. To address this changing focus, several variations of the Holistic Cardiovascular Assessment Tool are included in this Appendix. These include the Holistic Cardiovascular Assessment Tool, the Cardiovascular Rehabilitation Assessment Tool, the Transplant Assessment Tool, and the Cardiovascular Screening Tool. Each tool is used in a case study to model the process of a holistic assessment.

The Holistic Cardiovascular Assessment Tool (Fig. A-1) is used to assess Mr. B.F., who has been admitted to the progressive care unit. Mr. B.F. is 52 years old and has been diagnosed with congestive heart failure and hypertension.

The Cardiovascular Rehabilitation Assessment Tool (Fig. A-2) focuses on a patient being admitted to the outpatient cardiac rehabilitation program. Mr. C.F., a 49-year-old patient, is recovering from myocardial revascularization.

The third case study uses the Transplant Assessment Tool (Fig. A-3) to assess Mrs. E.L., a 29-year-old cardiomyopathy patient who is recovering from cardiac transplantation 2 weeks before.

The Cardiovascular Screening Tool (Fig. A-4) is used to assess a same-day admissions patient. Mr. A.D. is scheduled for cardiac catheterization this morning. He is 52 years old and is diagnosed with new onset of angina.

We encourage you to use these tools and evaluate their effectiveness in your clinical setting. You may add, delete, or change the assessment parameters according to the needs of your patient population. For further information regarding these tools and others see Guzzetta CE and others: *Clinical assessment tools for use with nursing diagnoses*, St Louis, 1989, The CV Mosby Co.

HOLISTIC CARDIOVASCULAR ASSESSMENT TOOL*

Name _B.G._   Age _52_   Sex _M_

Address _4063 Sixty-third St., Pelzer, S.C._   Telephone _232-4059_

Significant other _L.G._   Telephone _W-245-5666_

Date of admission _3/26_   Medical diagnosis _Congestive Heart Failure, Hypertension_

Allergies _NKA_

Nursing Diagnosis

COMMUNICATING ■ A pattern involving sending messages

(Read,) (write,) (understand) English (circle) _____

Other languages _none_

Intubated _no_   Speech impaired _stutters when anxious_

Alternate form of communication _none_

Impaired verbal communication

KNOWING ■ A pattern involving the meaning associated with information

Current health problems _"The doctor says my heart is bad" Describes DOE and PND x2 weeks c̄ chest pain or palpitations_

Previous illnesses/hospitalizations/surgeries _HTN diagnosed 1 year ago. Treated in the outpatient clinic_

History of the following problems:

Heart _CHF, aortic stenosis_

Peripheral vascular _no_

Lung _pneumonia 10 yrs ago_

Liver _no_   Kidney _no_

Cerebrovascular _no_   Rheumatic fever _(m) since childhood_

Thyroid _no_

Other _no_

Current medications _Lasix 20 mg po qd, Micro K 10 po qd, Calan SR 240 mg po q am, Vasotec 5 mg po qd_

(Knowledge deficit)

Risk factors	Present	Perceptions/Knowledge of
1. Hypertension	⊕	"I know my blood pressure is high"
2. Hyperlipidemia	⊕	"The doctor said to watch my cholesterol"
3. Smoking	⊖	
4. Obesity	⊕	"I've been trying to lose weight"
5. Diabetes	⊖	
6. Sedentary living	⊕	Job requires walking/lifting "I walk enough @ work"
7. Stress	⊕	"I get upset about my job sometimes"
8. Alcohol use	⊕	1 pint/day of vodka—does not perceive as excessive
9. Oral contraceptives	⊖	
10. Family history		Father died when pt age 12 of ? etiology. Mother—alive c̄ heart disease

Perception/knowledge of illness/test/surgery _"The doctor told me before that I had high blood pressure, but I didn't know there was something wrong c̄ my heart."_

Expectations of therapy _"to get me better, so I can go back to work"_

Misconceptions _unclear about HTN, its effect on heart, need for meds_

Readiness to learn _"I want to know what I need to do"_

Requests information concerning _HTN, CHF, diet, meds_

Educational level _high school_

Learning impeded by _none_

*Adapted from: Guzzetta C et al: Clinical assessment tools for use with nursing diagnoses, St Louis, 1989, The CV Mosby Co.

FIG. A-1 The Holistic Cardiovascular Assessment Tool.

Orientation
Level of alertness _Alert_
Orientation: Person _√_   Place _√_   Time _√_
Appropriate behavior/communication _yes_

Memory
Memory intact: Yes _√_ No _____ Recent _yes_   Remote _yes_

VALUING ■ A pattern involving the assigning of relative worth
Spirituality or religious preference _Baptist_   Spiritual distress
Important spiritual or religious practices _Church on Sundays_
Spiritual concerns _none_
Cultural orientation _Black American_
Cultural practices _family important, gets together c̄ friends most evenings and has a few drinks_

RELATING ■ A pattern involving establishing bonds
Role
Marital status _married_   Altered role performance
Age & health of significant other _wife 50, good health_   Parenting
                                                                             Sexual dysfunction
Number of children _1_   Ages _daughter—30 single_   Work
Role in home _provider_
  Financial support _his income, wife—beautician_
  Occupation _Shipping/receiving clerk in a glass factory_   Altered family processes
    Job satisfaction/concerns _worked there 10 yrs—likes it_   Parental role conflict
    Physical/mental energy expenditures _requires heavy lifting, walking_
  Sexual relationships ((satisfactory) /unsatisfactory) _____   Altered sexuality patterns
  Physical difficulties/effects of illness related to sex _____
    "I get tired/SOB lately"

Socialization
  Quality of relationships with others: Altered socialization
    Patient's description _"I have a good family—my wife takes good care of me"_   Impaired social interaction
    Significant other's description _good relationship_
    Staff observations _good positive interactions_
    Verbalizes feelings of being alone _none (lonely in hospital)_   Social isolation
    Attributed to _hospitalization_

FEELING ■ A pattern involving the subjective awareness of information
Comfort
  Pain/discomfort: Yes _____ No _√_
    Onset _—_   Duration _—_   Pain/chronic
    Location _—_ Quality _—_ Radiation _—_   Pain/acute
    Associated factors _—_
    Aggravating factors _—_
    Alleviating factors _—_
    Objective manifestations _Pt's only symptom is SOB c̄ activity, no pain or discomfort_

Emotional Integrity/States
  Recent stressful life events _none except hospitalization and symptoms_

  Verbalizes feelings of _anxiety_   (Anxiety)
    Source _"I'm worried about my heart—I hope I'll be OK"_   Fear
                                                                            Grieving
    Physical manifestations _fidgets when discussing diagnosis and stutters more_   Dysfunctional
                                                                            Anticipatory

Altered thought processes

Continued.

MOVING ▪ A pattern involving activity

Self-care

Ability to perform self-care (specify level) __*independent*__

Specify deficits __*none*__

Discharge planning needs __*Arrangements to ensure prescriptions filled and follow-up visits*__

Self-care deficit
  (Level 0-4)
Feeding
  Impaired swallowing
Bathing/hygiene
Dressing/grooming
Toileting

Activity

Limitations of movement (specify level) __*none*__

Limitations in activities __*SOB c̄ walking, climbing stairs*__

Impaired physical mobility
  (Level 0-4)

Verbal report of fatigue __*c̄ activity*__

Activity intolerance

Exercise habits __*walks on job, no regular regimen*__

Fatigue

Rest

Sleep/rest pattern __*6-7 hours/night*__

Sleep aids (pillows, meds, food) __*none*__

Difficulty falling/remaining asleep __*no*__

Sleep pattern disturbance

Recreation

Leisure activities __*works in yard; wood working*__

Social activities __*visiting c̄ friends, church*__

Diversional activity deficit

Activities of Daily Living

Home maintenance management

Size & arrangement of home (stairs, bathroom) __*1-story rancher style*__
_____ Safety needs __*none*__

Home responsibilities __*yard work*__

Impaired home maintenance
  management

Health maintenance

Health insurance __*BC/BS*__

Altered health maintenance

Regular physical check-ups __*2 visits last year, had difficulty getting appointment and meds ran out before pt saw physician*__

PERCEIVING ▪ A pattern involving the reception of information

Body image/Self-esteem

Perception of self and situation __*"I hope I'm gonna be OK"*__

Self-esteem disturbance
  Chronic low
  Situational low
Body image disturbance

Description of body structure/functioning __*"I know my heart's bad now—I gotta do better—take care of it"*__

Meaningfulness

Verbalizes hopelessness __*no*__

Hopelessness

Verbalizes loss of control __*no*__

Powerlessness

Sensory/Perception

History of restricted environment __*no*__

Altered sensory/perception

Vision imparied __*no*__ Glasses __*no*__

  Visual

Auditory imparied __*no*__ Hearing aid __*no*__

  Auditory

Kinesthetics impaired __*no*__

  Kinesthetic

Gustatory impaired __*no*__

  Gustatory

Tactile impaired __*no*__

  Tactile

Olfactory impaired __*no*__

  Olfactory

Reflexes: Biceps   R __2+__ L __2+__   Triceps R __2+__ L __2+__
           Brachioradialis R __2+__ L __2+__   Knee   R __2+__ L __2+__
           Ankle   R __2+__ L __2+__   Plantar R __2+__ L __2+__

EXCHANGING ▪ **A pattern involving mutual giving and receiving**

Circulation

Cerebral   Altered cerebral tissue

Neurologic changes/symptoms __*none*_____   perfusion

Complaints of syncope __*no*_____

Pupils   Eye Opening

     L 2 ③ 4 5 6 mm   None (1)

     R 2 ③ 4 5 6 mm   To pain (2)   Fluid volume

     Reaction: Brisk __✓__   To speech (3)   Deficit

     Sluggish _____ Nonreactive _____   (Spontaneous) (4)   Excess

     Retina __*no AV nicking*_____

Best Verbal   Best Motor

     Mute (1)   Flaccid (1)

     Incomprehensible sound (2)   Extensor response (2)   Decreased cardiac output

     Inappropriate words (3)   Flexor response (3)

     Confused conversation (4)   Semipurposeful (4)

     (Oriented) (5)   Localized to pain (5)

                              (Obeys commands) (6)

Glasgow coma scale total __*15*_____   Altered cerebral tissue

                                     perfusion

Peripheral   Altered peripheral tissue

                                     perfusion

     Arterial pulses: A = absent   B = bruits   D = Doppler

     +3 = bounding   +2 = palpable   +1 = faintly palpable

Carotid   R __*2+*__ L __*2+*__   Popliteal   R __*2+*__ L __*2+*__

Brachial   R __*2+*__ L __*2+*__   Posterior tibial   R __*2+*__ L __*2+*__   (Fluid volume)

Radial   R __*2+*__ L __*2+*__   Dorsalis pedis   R __*2+*__ L __*2+*__   Deficit

Femoral   R __*2+*__ L __*2+*__   (Excess)

BP: Sitting   Lying   Standing

        R __*190/120*__ L __*190/120*__   R __*188/114*__ L __*186/114*__   R __*184/112*__ L __*184/112*__

        A-Line reading __*0*_____   CVP __*0*___

Venous pulse __*Normal a and v waves*__ Jugular venous distention R ⊖ L ⊖

Peripheral veins __*no pain or tenderness*_____

Skin temp __*warm*__ Color __*adequate*__ Cyanosis __*none*_____

Capillary refill __*<2 sec*_____ Edema __*2 + ankle/pedal edema bilaterally*__

Clubbing __*none*_____

Cardiovascular

   PMI __*5th ICS @ Anterior Axillary Line*__ Pacemaker __*no*__   Altered cardiopulmonary

   Apical rate & rhythm __*regular—100*_____   tissue perfusion

   Heart sounds/murmurs __*S₁ S₂ S₃ 2/6 systolic ⓜ in aortic region c̄ radiation to carotids*__

   Dysrhythmias __*ST c̄ occ PVC's*_____

   Cardiac output __*0*_____ Cardiac index __*0*___   (Decreased cardiac output)

   PAP __*0*_____ PAWP __*0*___

   IV fluids __*D5W @ KVO*_____

   IV medications __*Lasix 40 IV × 1 dose*_____   Dysreflexia

   Serum enzymes __*pending*_____

Physical Integrity

Tissue integrity __*intact*_____   Impaired skin integrity

   Skin: Rash __*no*_____ Lesions __*no*_____   Impaired tissue integrity

   Petechiae __*no*_____ Bruises __*no*_____   Disuse syndrome

   Abrasions __*no*___ Surgical incision __*no*_____   Infection

                                       Altered protection

Continued.

Oxygenation

Complaints of dyspnea _yes_ Precipitated by _activity, occasionally @ rest_
Orthopnea _yes_
Rate _24_ Rhythm _regular_ Depth _deep_
Labored/(unlabored)(circle) Use of accessory muscles _none_
Chest expansion _symmetrical_ Splinting _none_
Cough: Productive/nonproductive _Productive—occasional_
Sputum: Color _yellow_ Amount _moderate_ Consistency _thick_
Breath sounds _bibasilar crackles_ ¹⁄₄ ↑
Arterial blood gases _pH 7.47 pCO₂ 29 mm Hg PO₂ 97 mm Hg HCO₃ 22 mM_
Oxygen percent and device _room air_
Ventilator _no_

Ineffective breathing patterns

Ineffective airway clearance

(Impaired gas exchange)
High risk for aspiration

Physical Regulation

Immune
Lymph nodes enlarged _no_ Location _no_
WBC count _7.1 × 10³/μL_ Differential _Bands 0% Neut 58% Eos 1%_
Baso 1% Lymph 26% Mono 4%
Temperature _98.8° F_ Route _Oral_

Infection
Hypothermia
Hyperthermia
Altered body temperature
Ineffective thermoregulation
Altered protection

Nutrition

Eating patterns
Number of meals per day _2-3_
Special diet _"I watch my salt"_
Where eaten _home for dinner, lunch out_
Food preferences/intolerances _none_
Food allergies _none_
Caffeine intake (coffee, tea, soft drinks) _2-3 cups of coffee/day, 4 glasses iced tea/day_
Appetite changes _none_
Presence of nausea/vomiting _none_
Condition of mouth/throat _normal_

Height _6'0"_ Weight _225 lbs_ Ideal body weight _184_

Current therapy
NPO _no_ NG suction _no_
Tube feeding _no_
TPN _no_
Labs
Na _145 mEq/L_ K _4.8 mEq/L_ Cl _103 mEq/L_ Glucose _126 mg/dl_
Cholesterol _292 mg/dl_ Triglycerides _222 mg/dl_ Fasting _no_
Hct _48.6%_ Hgb _15.8 g/dl_
Other _

(Altered nutrition
More than body
requirements)
Less than body
requirements

Impaired oral mucous
membranes
Altered nutrition
More than body
requirements
Less than body
requirements
High risk for aspiration

Elimination

Gastrointestinal/Bowel
Usual bowel habits _bowel movement qd_
Use of laxatives, enemas, and/or suppositories _no_
Alterations from norm _none_
Abdominal physical exam _abd lg, soft, nontender, nondistended, ⊕ BS x 4 quads_

Renal/Urinary
Usual urinary pattern _Voids 7-8 x/day_
Alteration from norm _none_
Bladder distention _no_
Color _clear yellow_ Catheter _no_
Urine output: 24 hour _pending_ Average hourly _300-400 cc each void_
BUN _14 mg/dl_ Creatinine _1.0 mg/dl_ Specific gravity _
Urine studies _urinalysis and urine C & S ⊖_

Altered bowel elimination
Constipation
Perceived
Colonic
Diarrhea
Incontinence
Altered GI tissue perfusion

Altered urinary elimination
Incontinence
Retention
Altered renal tissue perfusion

CHOOSING ▪ A pattern involving the selection of alternatives
Coping
  Patient's ability to cope ___*"I handle things OK" "I do what I gotta do"*___   Ineffective individual coping
  _____   Defensive coping
  Family's ability to cope/give support ___*My wife—she helps me a lot"*___   Ineffective denial
  _____   Impaired adjustment
  Patient's acceptance of illness ___*"I know I got a bad heart now—I didn't know it*___
  ___*was bad before."*_____   Ineffective family coping
  Patient's adjustment to illness ___*"I gotta do what ya'll say—I gotta take care of myself"*___   Disabled
  _____   Compromised

Judgment
  Decision making ability:
    Patient's perspective ___*good*_____   Decisional conflict
    Other's perspective ___*good*_____
  Ability to choose from alternatives ___*"I make my own decisions"*___
  _____

Participation
  Compliance with past/current health care regimen ___*poor R/T inadequate*___   (Noncompliance)
  ___*knowledge, poor follow-up*_____
  Willingness to comply with future health care regimen ___*good—need to ensure*___
  ___*follow-up*_____

Health seeking
  Express desire to seek higher level of wellness ___*"I want to get better"*___   (Health seeking behaviors)
  _____

Prioritized nursing diagnoses/problem list:
1. ___*Decreased cardiac output R/T cardiomegaly, lung congestion, peripheral edema*___
2. ___*Knowledge deficit R/T inadequate knowledge of diagnosis and treatment regimen*___
3. ___*Activity intolerance R/T shortness of breath and fatigue*___
4. ___*Altered health maintenance R/T inadequate follow-up care*___
5. ___*Altered nutrition: more than body requirements R/T obesity*___
6. ___*Anxiety R/T diagnosis and prognosis*___

Signature ___*Anita P. Sherer, RN*_____   Date ___*3/26*_____

CARDIOVASCULAR REHABILITATION ASSESSMENT TOOL*

Name _C.A._   Age _49_   Sex _M_

Address _22 Twenty-second St., Cleveland, Ohio_   Telephone _345-1200_

Significant other _R.A. - wife_   Telephone _345-8729 (W)_

Date of admission _3/21_   Medical diagnosis _Coronary Artery Bypass Surgery 2/5_

Allergies _NKA_

Nursing Diagnosis

COMMUNICATING ▪ A pattern involving sending messages

(Read,) (write,) (understand) English (circle) _____

Other languages—read, write, understand (circle) ____—____

Speech impaired by dyspnea _no_   Other ____—____   Impaired verbal

Alternate form of communication _none_   communication

Difficulty expressing self verbally _no-expresses self well_

Inconsistent statements and/or behavior _no_

KNOWING ▪ A pattern involving the meaning associated with information

Cardiovascular history _CAD diagnosed 2 years ago by cardiac catheterization. Having more angina past 2 months → cath showed 3 vessel disease → CABG ×4 on 2/5_

Previous illnesses/hospitalizations/surgeries _HTN, appendectomy as a child_

Other health problems _none_

(Knowledge deficit)

Current medications

Drug	Dosage	Times taken	Side effects
Maxide	T̄	8A	"I don't know—bad I guess
Lopressor	50 mg	8A-6P	if you don't take it?"
ASA	T̄	8A	"bleeding?"
Persantine	50 mg	8A-12N-6P	"bleeding?"

Difficulties taking medications _none_

Method of organizing medications _puts meds for day in bottle and carries c̄ him_

Patient's perceived risk factors _HTN, ↑ cholesterol, stress, lack of exercise_

Actual risk factors:

Hypertension: Diagnosed when _4-5 yrs_   Normal BP range _140-150 / 80-90_

    Controlled by _meds_   Regular BP checkups _yes_

    Low sodium diet _yes_   Exercise habits _walking-only fair compliance_

    Learning needs _exercise regimen_

Hyperlipidemia: At present _yes_   Past history _yes_

    Cholesterol _230 mg/dl_ Triglycerides _1200 mg/dl_ HDL ____—____ LDL ____—____

    Dietary habits _↓ fat, ↓ cholesterol_   Knowledge of diet _good_

    Exercise habits _See above_   Learning needs _how to follow diet more closely when traveling_

Smoking: At present: _no_   Past history _no_

    Packs/day ____—____ Number of years ____—____ When stopped ____—____

    Previous attempts to quit ____—____ Complicated by ____—____

*Adapted from Guzzetta C et al: Clinical assessment tools for use with nursing diagnoses, St Louis, 1989, The CV Mosby Co.

FIG. A-2   The Cardiovascular Rehabilitation Assessment Tool.

Plans for cessation ___—_____   Knowledge deficit
Learning needs ___—_____
Obesity: (Yes)/no __✓_____ Recent weight changes __*lost 5 lbs.*___
  Previous dieting methods _↓ *food intake*_____ Problems _*hard when traveling*_
  Description of daily intake _*no breakfast, small lunch, large dinner*___
  Learning needs _*how to balance meals*___
Diabetes: Type __*no*_____ Controlled by ___—_____
  Most recent fasting glucose ___—_____ Regular checkups ___—__
  Glucose monitoring method ___—_____ ADA diet ___—__
  Degree of diabetic control _____—
  Learning needs ___—___
Sedentary living: Exercise habits _*only fair compliance*__
  Type __*walking*_____ Frequency _*3 × week*____ Duration _*2-3 miles*_
  Method of monitoring exercise tolerance _*pulse taking*__
  Learning needs _*how to follow regimen more closely*_
Stress: Patient's description of stressors: Home ___—___
  Work _*yes*_____ Social ___—___ Other ___—__
  Present/past management methods _*"try to leave problems @ work"*_
  Effectiveness _*good*_____ Knowledge of other methods _*good*___
  Learning needs _*minimal-managing well*_
Alcohol use: _*socially*____ Drinks/day ___—_ Type _*beer*__
  Present/past excessive usage _*2-3 beers/wk only*_
  Plans for cessation _*none*_____
  Assistance/support available _*not required*___
  Learning needs _*none*____
Oral contraceptives: Type ___—_____ How long taken ___—__
Family history of cardiovascular disease, diabetes _*Strong family hx of CAD,*_
*MJ's, HTN, CVA*___
Educational level _*4 years college*__
Understanding of disease _*adequate knowledge of CAD, CABG*_
Expectations of treatment _*"a chance to start over-to keep my heart healthy"*_
Rehabilitation goals _*help to comply better c̄ exercise, diet*_
Misconceptions _*none*___
Learning needs _*diet, exercise, weight loss, meds*_
Preferred method of learning _*reading, films, discussion*_
Readiness to learn as indicated by questions _*yes*___
  Eye contact _*yes*_____ Body language _*yes*___
  Learning impeded by _*none*_____   Altered thought
Memory intact: Yes/no _*yes*____ Recent _✓___ Remote _✓___   processes

VALUING ▪ A pattern involving the assigning of relative worth
Spirituality or religious preference _*Presbyterian*___   Spiritual distress
Important spiritual or religious practices _*Church on Sundays*_
Spiritual concerns _*none*___
Cultural orientation _*White Caucasian*__
Cultural practices _*none specified*__

RELATING ▪ A pattern involving establishing bonds
Role
  Marital status _*married*_____   (Altered role performance)
  How long married/divorced/widowed _*25 years*__   Parenting
  Age and health of significant other _*47 c̄ hx HTN*_   Sexual dysfunction
  Number of children _*3*____ Ages _*son 23, daughter 21, son 19*_   (Work)
  Role in home _*main provider*___

Continued.

Financial support _his and wife's income, wife-secretary_

Occupation _mechanical engineer, currently part-time_   Altered family processes

    Job satisfaction/concerns _not totally satisfied with his work, quite stressful,_   Parental role conflict

    lots of travel

    Physical/mental energy expenditures _more mental energy than physical work_

Sexual relationships ((satisfactory)/unsatisfactory)   Altered sexuality

    Physical difficulties/effects of illness related to sex _minimal since surgery d/t_   patterns

    healing process-not concerned

Socialization
                                                                     Altered socialization

Quality of relationships with others _good_   Impaired social

    Patient's description _good-"no problems"_   interaction

    Significant other's description _good-"we take care of each other" (wife)_

    Staff observations _positive interaction_

Verbalizes feelings of being alone _none_   Social isolation

    Attributed to _—_

FEELING ■ A pattern involving the subjective awareness of information
Comfort
                                                                             (Altered comfort)

Pain/discomfort: Yes _✓_ No _____

    Patient's perception of etiology of pain: Angina _—_

    Incisional _Yes_   Other _—_

    Frequency _rare_   Duration _short_   Pain/chronic

    Location _sternum_ Quality _minimal_ Radiation _no_   (Pain/acute)

    Associated factors _none_

    Aggravating factors _arm movements_

    Alleviating factors _rest_

    Objective manifestations _no evidence @ present_

Emotional Integrity/States
Recent stressful life events _surgery, working part-time & giving responsibilities to_   (Anxiety)

someone else, concerned about mother's health   Fear

Verbalizes feelings of _worry, anxiety_

    Source _job, mother_

                                                                 Grieving

    Physical manifestations _facial expression, frown, grimace_   Dysfunctional

                                                                    Anticipatory

MOVING ■ A pattern involving activity
Self-care
                                                                Self-care deficit

Ability to perform ADL's: Independent _✓_ Dependent _____   (Level 0-4)

Specify deficits _none_   Feeding

                                                                 Impaired swallowing

                                                                   Bathing/hygiene

                                                                   Dressing/grooming

                                                                    Toileting

Activity
Limitations of movement _minimal difficulty with raising arms over head_   Impaired physical

                                                                    mobility (Level 0-4)

Limitations in activities _"I get very tired—I have to take breaks when I'm doing_   (Activity intolerance)

things to rest"   (Fatigue)

Verbal report of fatigue/weakness interfering with exercise _fatigue since surgery_   Fatigue

Favorite sports activities _basketball, tennis_

Rest
Hours slept/night _6-8 hours_   Feels rested: Yes/No _Yes_   Sleep pattern disturbance
Sleep aids (pillows, medications, food) _none_
Difficulty falling/remaining asleep _none_

Recreation
Leisure activities _reading, playing c̄ computer_   Diversional activity
Social activities _visiting friends/family_   deficit

Activities of Daily Living
Home maintenance management
  Size and arrangement of home (stairs, bathroom) _2 story c̄ 10 steps to_   Impaired home maintenance
upstairs   Safety needs _none_   management
  Home responsibilities _yardwork, pays bills_

Health maintenance
  Health insurance _Yes BC/BS_   Altered health
  Regular physical check-ups _Yes_   maintenance

PERCEIVING ▪ A pattern involving the reception of information
Self-esteem/body image
  Perception of self and situation _With his strong family hx of CAD & high lipid levels,_   (Self-esteem disturbance)
"I'm just not sure what chance I have"   Chronic low
  Effects of illness/surgery on self-concept _"I hope the surgery will give_   (Situational low)
me a second chance"
  Patient's description of own strengths/weaknesses _"I'm a positive person"_
"I worry too much sometimes"   Body image disturbance
  Patient's perception of health/illness _"I hope I'll get better"_   Personal identity
  Patient's perception of lifestyle changes _"I can do them"_   disturbance

Meaningfulness
  Verbalizes hopelessness _No_   Hopelessness
  Verbalizes loss of control _Yes R/T above_   (Powerlessness)
  Verbalizes grief related to loss of health _Yes_

Sensory/Perception
  Sensory/perceptual deficits: Specify _none_   Altered
                    sensory/perception
                    Visual
  Glasses _no_   Hearing aid _no_   Auditory
                    Kinesthetic
                    Olfactory
                    Gustatory
                    Tactile

EXCHANGING ▪ A pattern involving mutual giving and receiving
Circulation
  Cerebral
    Level of alertness _Alert, oriented × 3_   Altered cerebral tissue
    Neurologic changes/symptoms _none_   perfusion
    Appropriate exam _negative_

Continued.

Peripheral
    Jugular venous distention: Yes _____ No __✓__ R __—__ L __—__
    Pulses _*2+ radials, 2+ pedals, 2+ posterior tibial*_
    Skin temperature _*warm*_   Color _*pink*_
    Capillary refill _*<2 sec*_   Clubbing _*none*_
    Edema _*1-2 + Ⓛ pedal/ankle*_   Claudication _*none*_

    Altered peripheral
        tissue perfusion

Cardiovascular
    PMI _*5th ICS @ MCL*_   Pacemaker _*no*_
    Apical rate and rhythm _*regular 86*_
    Heart sounds/murmurs _*S₁, S₂*_
    Dysrhythmias _*SR č ectopy*_
      BP: R _*140/84*_ L _*142/80*_ Position _*Sitting*_

    Altered cardiopulmonary
        tissue perfusion

    Decreased cardiac output

    Fluid volume
      Deficit
      Excess

Physical Integrity
    Tissue integrity _*intact*_   Surgical incision _*median sternotomy*_
    Abnormalities: Specify _*and Ⓛ leg incision from groin to foot healing well*_

    Impaired skin integrity
    Impaired tissue
      integrity
    Infection

Oxygenation
    Respiratory pattern _*Respirations deep, easy   Rate 20*_
    Abnormalities _*none*_
    Breath sounds _*clear bilaterally*_

    Ineffective airway
      clearance
    Ineffective breathing
      pattern
    Impaired gas exchange

Nutrition
    Eating patterns
      Number of meals per day _*2-3*_   Where eaten _*60% home 40% out*_
      Special diet _*low cholesterol, low fat/low sodium*_
      Food preferences/intolerances/allergies _*none stated*_
      Caffeine intake (coffee, tea, soft drinks)
      *4 cups coffee/day, 4 soft drinks/day*
      Appetite changes _*none*_
    Height _*71"*_ Weight _*190 lbs*_ Ideal body weight _*165-175 lbs*_
    Body fat measurements _*not measured yet*_

    (Altered nutrition
      More than body
        requirements)
    Less than body
      requirements

Elimination
    Bowel
      Abnormal bowel patterns _*none*_

    Altered bowel
      elimination
    Altered GI tissue
      perfusion

    Urinary
      Abnormal urinary patterns _*none*_
      Pertinent lab values _*negative*_

    Altered urinary
      elimination
    Altered renal tissue
      perfusion

CHOOSING ▪ A pattern involving the selection of alternatives
Coping
    Patient's ability to cope _*having a difficult time dealing c̄ dietary & exercise changes*_

    (Ineffective individual
      coping)

Family's ability to cope/give support _family supportive, wife tries to encourage him_

Patient's acceptance of illness _"I've accepted that this is the way it's gonna be"_

Family's adjustment to illness _Good adjustment—Strong support_

Patient's affect _good, pleasant, cooperative_
Physical manifestations _body language suggests nervousness_
Coping mechanisms used _rationalization_
Adequacy of social support available _wife, children supportive_

Defensive coping
Ineffective denial
Impaired adjustment
Ineffective family
  coping
Disabled
Compromised

Participation
Compliance with past/current health care regimen _good re: medications, fair re: diet, exercise_
Willingness to comply with future health care regimen _good-wants to change_

Noncompliance

Health Seeking
Express desire to seek higher level of wellness _Voices desire to be healthy again_

(Health seeking behaviors)

Judgment
Decision making ability:
  Patient's perspective _good_
  Other's perspective _(wife) "makes good decisions"_
  Ability to choose from alternatives _"I think about the options, pick one, and don't look back"_

Decisional conflict

Prioritized nursing diagnoses/problem list:
1. _Knowledge deficit R/T risk factor modifications_
2. _Activity intolerance R/T fatigue post open heart surgery_
3. _Altered role performance R/T work d/t part time hours post surgery_
4. _Ineffective individual coping R/T lifestyle changes imposed by disease process_
5. _Acute pain R/T sternal incision & (L) leg incision_
6. _Powerlessness R/T perceived loss of control over disease process_
7. _Altered nutrition: More than body requirements R/T obesity_
8. _Health seeking behaviors R/T risk factor modifications_
9. _____
10. _____

Signature _Anita P. Sherer, RN_   Date _3/21_

TRANSPLANT ASSESSMENT TOOL*

Name _E.L._ _____ Age _29_ Sex _♀_

Address _4220 Spring St., Summer, N.C._ _____ Telephone _451-3062_

Significant other _W.L._ _____ Telephone _W-451-8092_

Date of admission _4/1_ _____ Medical diagnosis _S/P Heart transplant 2 weeks ago_

Allergies: _Sulfa_ _____

Nursing Diagnosis

COMMUNICATING ▪ A pattern involving sending messages

(Read,) (write,) (understand) English (circle) _____

Other languages _No_ _____

Communication barriers _None_ _____ Impaired verbal

Alternate form of communication _None_ _____ communication

KNOWING ▪ A pattern involving the meaning associated with information

Current health problems _Cardiac transplant 2 weeks ago. Chronic immunosuppression_

Previous illnesses/hospitalizations/surgeries _Congestive cardiomyopathy diagnosed 2 yrs p̄_
birth of child. Required therapeutic abortion 6 mos prior to transplant d/t inability to carry child
to term

History of the following diseases:

(Knowledge deficit)

Heart _Congestive cardiomyopathy_

Peripheral vascular _No_

Lung _No_

Liver _No_ _____ (hepatitis?) Kidney _No_

Cerebrovascular _No_ _____ Rheumatic fever _No_

Thyroid _No_

Rejection of transplant _No_

Drug abuse _No_ _____ Alcoholism _No_

Current medications _Cyclosporine 200 mg bid_
Prednisone 10 mg bid
Imuran 100 mg qd
Aspirin 81 mg qd

Nephrotoxic medications _Cyclosporine_

Risk factors for heart disease:

	Present	Perceptions/Knowledge of
1. Hypertension	⊖	
2. Hyperlipidemia	⊖	
3. Smoking	⊖	
4. Obesity	⊕	_Verbalizes understanding of risk factors and the_
5. Diabetes	⊖	_need to control/modify risk factors_
6. Sedentary living	⊕	
7. Stress	⊕	
8. Alcohol use	⊖	
9. Oral contraceptives	⊕	
10. Family history	_Father died age 38 c̄ MI. Mother age 64 living c̄ HTN and Breast Cancer_	

Perception/knowledge of illness/tests/surgery _Verbalizes knowledge of treatment regimen_ Knowledge deficit
and follow up post transplant

Expectations of therapy _Wants to return to work, "more able to do things c̄ my son"_

Misconceptions _Recovery will be quick and life will return to normal_

Readiness to learn _Good, motivated_

Requests information concerning _medications_

Educational level _high school_

Learning impeded by _—_

*Adapted from Guzzetta C et al: Clinical assessment tools for use with nursing diagnoses, St Louis, 1989, The CV Mosby Co.

FIG. A-3 The Transplant Assessment Tool.

Orientation

Level of alertness __Alert__

Orientation: Person __✓__   Place __✓__   Time __✓__

Appropriate behavior/communication __appropriate__

Altered thought
processes

Memory

Memory intact: Yes __✓__   No _____   Recent __✓__   Remote __✓__

VALUING ▪ A pattern involving the assigning of relative worth

Spirituality or religious preference __Baptist__

Important spiritual or religious practices __Church on Sundays, used to sing in choir__

Spiritual concerns __None stated__

Cultural orientation __Black American__

Cultural practices __Strong family ties__

Spiritual distress

RELATING ▪ A pattern involving establishing bonds

Role

Marital status __Married__

Age and health of significant other __Husband, 29, good health__

Number of children __1__   Ages __5—son__

Family relationships __close to husband, parents & extended family__

Distance from home to hospital __500 miles__

Family transportation arrangements __husband drives, owns car__

Permanent/ temporary (circle) relocation of family __staying c̄ aunt__

Financial support __Primarily husband's income__

Occupation __Was sales clerk in a department store__

  Job satisfaction/concerns __Would like to return to work__

  Physical/mental energy expenditures __not significant__

Sexual concerns __Difficulty c̄ sexual activity prior to transplant d/t fatigue, SOB and__ __whether she should consider pregnancy in the future__

(Altered role performance)
(Parenting)
(Sexual dysfunction)
(Work)

Altered family processes
Parental role conflict

Altered sexuality
patterns

Socialization

Quality of relationships with others:

  Patient's description __Good—"all this has been a strain though"__

  Significant other's description __Close—"Her being sick has been hard"__

  Staff observations __Close marital relationship—managing c̄ strain of illness__

  Verbalizes feelings of being alone __Yes__

  Attributed to __being away from home, family__

Altered socialization
Impaired social
  interaction

Social isolation

FEELING ▪ A pattern involving the subjective awareness of information

Comfort

Pain/discomfort: Yes __✓__ No _____

  Onset __with movement__   Duration __while moving__

  Location __chest incision__ Quality __sharp__   Radiation __no__

  Associated factors __none__

  Aggravating factors __movement__

  Alleviating factors __Changing positions slowly, using pillow__

  Objective manifestations __grimace c̄ movement__

Altered comfort

Pain/chronic
(Pain/acute)

Emotional Integrity/States

Recent stressful life events __Transplant, therapeutic abortion 6 mos. ago__

Verbalizes feelings of __sadness, guilt, anger__

  Source __not being able to have second child; illness__

Physical manifestations __quiet, withdrawn @ times, tearful__

Anxiety
Fear
(Grieving)
Dysfunctional

Continued.

MOVING ▪ A pattern involving activity
Self-care
Ability to perform ADL's: Independent __✓_____ Dependent _____
                             Needs assistance _____
Specify deficits _*must have frequent rest periods*_____
Discharge planning needs _*need to assess closer to discharge*_____

Self-care deficit
  (Level 0-4)
Feeding
  Impaired swallowing
Bathing/hygiene
Dressing/grooming
Toileting

Activity
Limitations of movement (specify level) _*none*_____

_____
Limitations in activities _*Good progress in cardiac rehab*_____
Verbal report of fatigue _*during ADL's at times*_____
Exercise habits _*No active regimen prior to illness*_____

Impaired physical
  mobility (Level 0-4)
Activity intolerance
  Fatigue

Rest
Hours slept/night _*6-8 hours*_____
Sleep aids (pillows, medications, food) _*3 pillows in the past*___
Difficulty falling/remaining asleep _*No*_____

Sleep pattern
  disturbance

Recreation
Social/leisure activities _*Visiting friends/family, going to the park c̄ son, church activities,*
  _*cross-stitch*_____

Diversional activity
  deficit

Activities of Daily Living
Home maintenance management
  Home responsibilities _*child care, shopping, cooking, cleaning*___
  Home maintenance management concerns _*Must determine who will assist with*_
    _*home management during her recovery*_____
Health maintenance
  Health insurance _*Blue Cross*_____
  Regular physical check-ups _*Yes—past few years*_____
  Transportation to appointments _*mother, aunt, husband*_____
  Health care regimen concerns _*Multiple biopsy procedures and clinic visits required*_
    *during the first months after transplant. Logistically difficult for out of town patients.*

Impaired home maintenance
  management

Altered health
  maintenance

PERCEIVING ▪ A pattern involving the reception of information
Self-esteem/body image
Perception of self and situation _*"I haven't been good for much this past year"*_
Description of body structure/functioning _*"My face is starting to look puffy"*_

_____

Self-esteem
  disturbance
Chronic low
Situational low
Body image disturbance

Meaningfulness
Verbalizes hopelessness _*No*_____
Verbalizes loss of control _*"Sometimes I feel I can't change all these things that have happened*_
  _*to me"*_____

Hopelessness
Powerlessness

Sensory/Perception
History of restricted environment _*ICU stay pre-transplant*_____
Vision impaired _*No*_____ Glasses _—_____
Auditory impaired _*No*_____ Hearing aid _—_____
Kinesthetics impaired _*No*_____
Gustatory impaired _*No*_____
Tactile impaired _*No*_____
Olfactory impaired _*No*_____
Reflexes: Grossly intact __✓__ Altered _____
  Biceps   R ____ L ____   Triceps R ____ L ____
  Brachioradialis R ____ L ____   Knee   R ____ L ____
  Ankle   R ____ L ____   Plantar R ____ L ____

Altered
  sensory/perception
Visual
Auditory
Kinesthetic
Gustatory
Tactile
Olfactory

EXCHANGING ▪ A pattern involving mutual giving and receiving

Circulation

Cerebral

Neurologic changes/symptoms _None_   Altered cerebral tissue
                                                        perfusion
Complaints of syncope _No_

Pupils   Eye Opening
  L 2 (3) 4 5 6 mm   None (1)
  R 2 (3) 4 5 6 mm   To pain (2)
  Reaction: Brisk ✓   To speech (3)   Fluid volume
  Sluggish _____ Nonreactive _____ (Spontaneous)(4)   Deficit
                                                             Excess

Best Verbal   Best Motor
  No response (1)   Flaccid (1)
  Incomprehensible sound (2)   Extensor response (2)   Decreased cardiac output
  Inappropriate words (3)   Flexor response (3)
  Confused conversation (4)   Semipurposeful (4)
  (Oriented)(5)   Localized to pain (5)
                                      (Obeys commands)(6)

  Glascow Coma Scale total _15_

Peripheral   Altered peripheral
  Jugular venous distention R ⊖ L ⊖   tissue perfusion

  Arterial pulses: A = absent   B = bruits   D = Doppler
        +3 = bounding   +2 = palpable   +1 = faintly palpable
  Carotid   R _2+_ L _2+_   Popliteal   R _2+_ L _2+_
  Brachial R _2+_ L _2+_   Posterior tibial R _2+_ L _2+_
  Radial   R _2+_ L _2+_   Dorsalis pedis   R _2+_ L _2+_   Fluid volume
  Femoral   R _2+_ L _2+_   Deficit
  Skin temp _warm_   Color _adequate—no cyanosis_   Excess
  Edema _2+ ankle edema_   Capillary refill _<2 sec_   Decreased cardiac output
  Clubbing _no_   Turgor _good_

Cardiovascular
  Pacemaker _none_
  Apical rate and rhythm _100_   PMI _5th ICS@ MCL_   Altered cardiopulmonary
  Heart sounds/murmurs _S1 S2 regular_   tissue perfusion
  Dysrhythmias _NSR c̄ RBBB, 2 p waves noted_   Fluid volume
  BP: Sitting   Lying   Standing   Deficit
      R _110/80_ L _108/74_ R _104/78_ L _102/74_ R _100/76_ L _102/78_ Excess
  A-Line reading _N/A_
  Cardiac index _3.01_   Cardiac output _5.3_   (Decreased cardiac output)
  CVP _5 mm Hg_ PAP _29/15/20 mm Hg_ PAWP _14 mm Hg_
  IV fluids _Heparin well_
  IV cardiac medications _none_
  Diagnostic tests _Most recent endomyocardial biopsy: negative for rejection._
     Echocardiogram—small pericardial effusion, moderate tricuspid insufficiency, LVEF—53%

Physical Integrity

Injury
  Convulsions _No_   Tetany _No_
  Dialysis access: Yes _____ No _✓_   (Altered protection)
     Fistula _—_   A-V Shunt _—_   PD cath _—_   (High risk for infection)
     Central line _—_   Current condition of access _—_
  Tissue integrity: Skin rashes _No_   Lesions _Acne—face_   (Impaired skin integrity)
  Petechiae _No_   Bruises _No_   Impaired tissue
  Abrasions _No_   Surgical incisions _sternotomy incision healing,_   integrity
     chest tube sites closed. Mouth lesions: none present. Jugular site from recent endomyocardial   High risk for disuse
     biopsy is clean & dry.   syndrome

Continued.

Oxygenation

Complaints of dyspnea _No_ _____ Precipitated by ___—___

Orthopnea _No_ _____

Rate _16_ _____ Rhythm _regular_ _____ Depth _shallow_ _____

Labored/ (unlabored) (circle) Use of accessory muscles _No_ _____

Chest expansion _symmetrical_ _____ Splinting _Yes_ _____

Cough: Productive/ (nonproductive) _____

Sputum: Color ___—___ Amount ___—___ Consistency ___—___

Breath sounds _few bibasilar crackles_ _____

Arterial blood gases _pH 7.44, PCO₂ 34mm Hg, PO₂ 98 mm Hg, HCO₃ 23 mM_

Oxygen percent and device _room air_ _____

Ventilator _n/a_ _____

Chest x-ray: _Persistent atelectasis Ⓛ base. Minimal pleural fluid bilaterally._

Ineffective airway
  clearance
Ineffective breathing
  patterns

Impaired gas exchange

High risk for aspiration

Physical Regulation

Lymph nodes enlarged _No_ _____ Location ___—___

WBC count _12.9 × 10³ μL_ Differential: PMN _90%_ ____ Mono _2%_

Eos _4%_ ____ Baso _1%_ ____ Lymph _1%_

Cytomegalovirus titer _negative_ _____

Cultures _sputum, urine, blood cultures negative_ _____

Temperature _98.6°_ _____ Route _Oral_ _____

(Altered protection)
(High risk for infection)

Altered body temperature
Hypothermia
Hyperthermia
Ineffective
  thermoregulation

Nutrition

Eating patterns

Number of meals per day _3_ _____

Special diet _Low cholesterol, no added salt_ _____

Food (preferences) /intolerances _hamburgers, fried foods_ _____

Food allergies _none_ _____

Caffeine intake (coffee, tea, soft drinks)
  Coffee 2 cups/day   6-8 glasses iced tea/day

Appetite changes _none_ _____

Nausea/vomiting _none_ _____

Condition of mouth/throat _normal_ _____

Height _5'10"_ ____ Weight _190 lbs_ ____ Ideal (dry) body weight _150 lbs_

Current therapy

NPO _No_ _____ NG suction _No_ _____

Tube feeding _No_ _____

TPN _No_ _____

IV fluids _No_ _____

Labs

Na _139 mEq/L_ ____ K _4.0 mEq/L_ ____ CL _105 mEq/L_ ____ CO₂ _24 mM_

Glucose _101 mg/dl_ ____ Ca _9.1 mEq/L_ ____ Phos _3.4 mg/dl_

Mg _2.0 mEq/L_ ____ Uric acid _5.8 mg/dl_ ____ Total bilirubin _0.8 mg/dl_

Total protein _6.4g/dl_ ____ Albumin _3.5 g/dl_ ____ Cholesterol _145 mg/dl_

Liver enzymes _SGOT—17 μ/ml, SGPT—40 μ/ml, LDH—212 U_ ____ Amylase ___—___

Hct _26%_ ____ Hgb _8.0 g/dl_ ____ RBC _2.84_ ____ Platelets _456,000_

PT _11.8 sec_ ____ PTT _30 sec_ ____ Other _Cyclosporine level—150 mg/ml_

(Altered nutrition)

(More than body
  requirements)

Less than body
  requirements

Impaired oral mucous
  membrane

Fluid volume
  Deficit
  Excess

Elimination

Gastrointestinal/bowel

Usual bowel habits _1 × /day_ _____

Alterations from normal _none_ _____

Abdominal physical examination _abd lg soft ⊕ BS × 4 quads_

Liver: Enlarged _No_ _____ Ascites _No_ _____

Altered bowel
  elimination
Constipation
  Perceived
  Colonic
Diarrhea
Incontinence
Altered GI tissue perfusion

Renal/urinary

Usual urinary pattern _6-8 X / day_

Alterations from normal _No_

Currently dialyzing _n/a_

Color _clear yellow_   Catheter _No_

Urine output: 24 hour _2800 cc_   Average hourly _90-110 cc_

Bladder distention _none_

Specific gravity _1.028_

Urine studies _negative_

Serum BUN _12 mg/dl_   Serum creatinine _1.0 mg/dl_

Altered urinary
    elimination
Incontinence
Retention
Altered renal
    tissue perfusion
Decreased cardiac output
Fluid volume
    Deficit
    Excess

CHOOSING ▪ A pattern involving the selection of alternatives

Coping

Patient's ability to cope _"I'm handling all this OK I think"_

Family's ability to cope/give support _Husband, parents supportive_

Patient's acceptance of illness _"I have to accept it—what choice do I have?"_

Family's adjustment to illness _Husband feels stressed re: illness, finances, need for wife's complex medical regimen_

Ineffective individual
    coping
Defensive coping
Ineffective denial
Impaired adjustment
(Ineffective family
    coping)

Judgment

Decision making ability

Patient's perspective _good_

Other's perspective _Husband—"makes good decisions"_

Ability to choose from alternatives _"I think about what choices I've got and just decide"_

Decisional conflict

Participation

Compliance with past/current health care regimen _Is following current treatment protocol_

Willingness to comply with future health care regimen _Demonstrates willingness_

Noncompliance

Health Seeking

Express desire to seek higher level of wellness _"I want to be normal again"_

(Health seeking behaviors)

Prioritized nursing diagnoses/problem list:

1. _High risk for decreased cardiac output R/T acute rejection_
2. _Altered protection and high risk for infection R/T immunosuppression s/p transplant_
3. _Acute pain R/T chest incision_
4. _Knowledge deficit R/T lifestyle changes imposed by disease and complex medical regimen_
5. _Body image disturbance R/T side effects of corticosteroids_
6. _Grieving R/T illness, loss of child_
7. _Altered nutrition: More than body requirements R/T obesity_
8. _Altered role performance R/T changes imposed by disease process and complex medical regimen_
9. _Impaired home maintenance management R/T need for assistance d/t complex medical regimen_
10. _High risk for ineffective family coping R/T illness, financial strain, complex medical regimen_

Signature _Anita P. Sherer RN_   Date _4/17_

CARDIOVASCULAR SCREENING TOOL*

Name _Mr. A.D._   Age _52_   Sex _M_
Address _2929 Willow St., Appleton, N.C._   Telephone _241-9560_
Significant other _Mrs. A.D._   Telephone _232-6210_
Date of admission _11/24_   Medical diagnosis _new onset of angina_
Allergies _NKA_

Nursing Diagnosis

COMMUNICATING ▪ A pattern involving sending messages
(Read,) (write,) (understand) English (circle) _____
Speech impaired: Yes _____ No _✓_

Impaired verbal
communication

KNOWING ▪ A pattern involving the meaning associated with information
Current health problems _Midsternal chest pain started 2 weeks ago c̄ activity radiates to_
(L) arm c̄ SOB—relieved c̄ rest
Medications _NTG 0.4 SL prn, Isordil 20 mg qid, Procardia 10 mg q8h_
Risk factor analysis: (designate + or −)

1. Hypertension ⊕ _×4 yrs—mild_	6. Sedentary living ⊖
2. Hyperlipidemia ⊕	7. Stress ⊕ _income concerns, 2 teenagers_
3. Smoking ⊖	8. Alcohol use ⊕ _3-4 beers qd_
4. Obesity ⊕	9. Oral contraceptives ⊖
5. Diabetes ⊖	10. Family history ⊕ _Father died 65 c̄ MI_

(Knowledge deficit)

Perception/knowledge of: Appropriate   Inappropriate
Illness/disease   ✓ _Needs more information_
Test/surgery   ✓ _"Will test make my heart stop?"_
Medications   ✓
Physical activity   ✓
Prognosis   ✓ _"What will I be able to do?"_
Misconceptions _procedure information, prognosis, illness_
Orientation: Person _✓_ Place _✓_ Time _✓_
Memory intact: Yes _✓_ No _____ Recent _✓_ Remote _✓_

Altered thought
processes

VALUING ▪ A pattern involving the assigning of relative worth
Spiritual concerns _none voiced_

Spiritual distress

RELATING ▪ A pattern involving establishing bonds
Predominant role in home _breadwinner_
   Problems _Missed work frequently lately—impacts income_
Family situation: (Stable) /unstable
Job satisfaction/concerns _painter—heavy physical work @ times_
Sexual relationships intact: Yes _✓_ No _____
Social relationships: (Functional) /dysfunctional
   Prefers to be alone/ (with family) / (with friends)

(Altered role
performance)
Altered family
processes
Altered sexuality
patterns
Impaired social
interaction
Social isolation

FEELING ▪ A pattern involving the subjective awarness of information
Presence of pain/discomfort: Yes _✓ Not @ present but earlier this am_ No _____
Onset _sudden—early am_ Location _midsternal_ Duration _5-6 min_
Quality _heaviness_ Radiation: Back/jaw/ (arm) /other _(L) arm_
Associated factors: Nausea/vomiting/headache/other _SOB_
Aggravating factors: (Activity) / (emotions) /exposure/ (eating)
Alleviating factors: (Rest) / (medication) /position change/other _NTG_
Recent stressful life events _disease process limiting work_
Verbalizes feelings of: Anxiety _✓ R/T above_ Fear _____
   Grief _____ Other _____

Altered comfort
Pain/Chronic
(Pain/Acute)
(Anxiety)
Fear
Grieving
Dysfunctional
Anticipatory

*Adapted from Guzzetta C et al: Clinical assessment tools for use with nursing diagnoses, St Louis, 1989, The CV Mosby Co.

FIG. A-4 The Cardiovascular Screening Tool.

MOVING ▪ A pattern involving activity

Ability to perform daily activities/exercise habits: Yes _____ No __✓_____   Impaired physical
    Verbal report of fatigue or weakness: Yes __✓__ No _____   mobility

Verbalizes rest/sleep as: (Restful) /not restful _____   (Activity intolerance)
    Characterized by inability to fall or remain asleep __*No*__   Sleep pattern

Verbalizes boredom over lack/decreased social/leisure activities: Yes ___ No __✓__   disturbance

Size and arrangement of home __*1 level rancher*__   Diversional activity
    deficit

Home responsibilities: Shopping _____ Cleaning _____
Cooking _____ Finance management __✓__ Transportation __✓__   Impaired home maintenance

Ability to perform activities of daily living independently: Yes __✓__ No _____   management
    Specify deficits __*None*__   Self-care deficit

PERCEIVING ▪ A pattern involving the reception of information

Verbalizes change in feelings about self due to: (Self-esteem
    Diagnosis _____ Illness __✓__ Surgery _____ Other _____   disturbance)

Verbalizes hopelessness/ (loss of control) (circle)   Body image disturbance
    Hopelessness
    (Powerlessness)

EXCHANGING ▪ A pattern involving mutual giving and receiving

Syncopal episodes: Yes/ (No)   Carotid bruits: Positive/ (Negative)   Altered cerebral tissue

Palpitations: Yes/ (No)   perfusion

Pacemaker (brand, model, mode) __*None*__   (Altered cardiopulmonary

Apical rate __*84*__ Rhythm __*regular*__ Heart sounds __S_1 S_2 S_4__   tissue perfusion)

Dysrhythmias __*SR c̄ ectopy*__   Decreased cardiac

Blood pressure: __*160/90*__ Position __*sitting*__   output

Jugular venous distention: Yes _____ No __✓__ Right __—__ Left __—__   Altered peripheral

Capillary refill __*brisk <2 sec*__ Clubbing __*no*__ Edema __*no*__   tissue perfusion

Complaints of dyspnea: Yes __✓__ No _____ Precipitated by __*exertion*__   Ineffective breathing

Rate __*20*__ Rhythm __*regular*__ Depth __*deep*__ Labored/ (unlabored)   patterns

Cough: Productive/nonproductive Describe sputum _____   Ineffective airway

Breath sounds: (Clear) /crackles/rhonchi/wheezes/other _____   clearance
    Impaired gas exchange

Eating pattern: Changed/ (unchanged)

Caffeine intake: (Coffee) / (tea) /soda/chocolate   Amount __*2 cups/4 glasses*__   (Altered nutrition)

Food allergies __*None*__   (More)/less than body

Height __*5'9"*__ Weight __*180 lbs*__ Recent weight change __*no*__   requirements

Labs: Cholesterol __*288 mg/dl*__ HDL __?__ LDL __?__ Triglycerides __*300 mg/dl*__

Gastrointestinal changes __*none*__   Altered bowel
    elimination

Urinary changes __*none*__   Altered urinary
    elimination

Skin intact: Yes __✓__ No ___ Specify: _____   Impaired skin integrity

CHOOSING ▪ A pattern involving the selection of alternatives

Verbalizes individual/family inability to problem solve/cope with illness/   Ineffective coping
surgery/situation __*Anxious "but I'm making it—want to find out what's wrong"*__

Compliance with past/current health care regimen: Yes __✓__ No _____   Noncompliance

Willingness to comply with future health care regimen: Yes __✓__ No _____   Health seeking
    behaviors

Verbalizes ability to make sound decisions: Yes __✓__ No _____   Decisional conflict

Prioritized nursing diagnoses/problem list:

1. __*Acute chest pain R/T myocardial ischemia associated c̄ activity*__
2. __*Knowledge deficit R/T procedural information, illness, and prognosis*__
3. __*Altered role performance R/T work D/t restrictions imposed by illness*__
4. __*Activity intolerance R/T chest pain c̄ exertion*__
5. __*Anxiety R/T procedure, new onset of chest pain*__
6. __*Altered nutrition: More than body requirements R/T obesity, hyperlipidemia*__
7. _____
8. _____

Signature __*Anita P. Sherer RN*__   Date __*11/24*__

APPENDIX

B

Dysrhythmias

Mary Kay Feeney

The purpose of this section is to describe the cardiac rhythms that are most prevalent in the critical care environment. These will be presented relative to their description, cause, ECG characteristics, pathophysiology, clinical signs and symptoms, hemodynamic consequences, and pertinent therapies. The cardiac rhythms will be presented in a format appropriate for the experienced clinician. Rather than identifying content by site and then applicable dysrhythmias, the dysrhythmias are organized based on the pathologic conditions producing the rhythms, with subsequent delineation by site of origin of the dysrhythmia.

All rhythms can be categorized relative to intrinsic (or inherent) myocardial activity, rhythms of excitation (tachycardias), and rhythms of depression (bradycardias). Further delineation can be accomplished by differentiating rhythms by abnormalities in impulse formation or impulse conduction.

PURPOSE OF THE CARDIAC CONDUCTION SYSTEM

The heart's primary function is to perform as a pump. This activity is served by the contractile fibers of the heart. All other heart components support the pumping action:

- Blood flow is limited to one direction by the valves.
- The smooth movement of the heart within the mediastinum and its resistance to sudden cardiac distention from severe hemodynamic stresses are facilitated by the pericardium.
- The rate of pumping and the sequences in which the cardiac chambers are activated are regulated by the tissues responsible for electrical impulse formation and conduction.

The study of cardiac rhythms focuses on the formation and conduction of the electrical impulses necessary to initiate myocardial contraction. Disturbances in the development or transmission of this electrical activity result in altered contractility and decreased cardiac output.

The determination of cardiac output can be simplified to the formula of stroke volume times heart rate. The proper function of the cardiac conduction system ensures maximum cardiac output by regulating the heart rate and factors that influence the volume ejected.

The initiation of impulses by the sinus node, which is responsive to physiologic needs, is increased or decreased depending on demand. A heart rate in the range of 60 to 120 beats per min provides the most adequate ejection of volume. Transmission of the impulse through the normal atrial conductile fibers assures that contraction proceeds from top to bottom and results in optimal atrial emptying. The delay created by the atrioventricular (AV) node provides for maximal emptying of the atria and the resultant optimal stretch of the ventricular fibers (Frank-Starling mechanism). This beneficial relationship of atrial ejection causing substantial ventricular filling is referred to as *atrial kick*. The AV node also imposes a limit on the frequency of impulses transmitted from the atria to the ventricles. This physiologic control prevents the ventricles from being stimulated at catastrophic rates in case the atria develop excessively rapid rates. The rapid conduction of the impulse through the common bundle and the left and right bundle branches permits activation of the ventricles at the apex. This rapid transmission directs the ventricular contractile force and subsequent ventricular ejection of blood toward the outflow tracts at the base of the heart.

CATEGORIES OF CARDIAC RHYTHMS

Rhythm disturbances impair cardiac output through alterations in:

1. Rate of impulse initiation
   a. Decreased formation (depression)
   b. Increased formation (excitation)
2. Rate of impulse transmission
   a. Decreased conduction (depression)
   b. Increased conduction (excitation)

Optimal myocardial stretch and volume ejection is obtained with rates ranging between 60 and 120 beats per min. A decreased rate of impulse formation (a slow heart rate) allows for an increased venous return to the chambers, which can cause excessive dilation of the ventricles. This overdistention (beyond the peak of the Starling curve) results in diminished contraction by the myofibrils, and cardiac output falls. An athlete trained for endurance events exhibits slower rates without deleterious effects because of conditioned myocardial tone. To a patient with an already dilated ventricle, however, a slight slowing of heart rate may provoke myocardial failure.

Conversely, an increased heart rate decreases diastolic filling time. The diminished venous volume per beat prevents adequate myocardial stretch and reduces myocardial contractility. Thus faster rates compromise both the volume and the force of ejection per cardiac cycle. In a patient with impaired coronary artery flow, this decrease in cardiac output occurs when an actual increase is required to meet the increased metabolic need associated with rapid rates. Therefore maintenance of the heart rate within given limits maximizes cardiac function.

Transmission of impulses through the normal conduction pathways provides for optimal sequencing of chamber contraction. The AV node, which allows transmission of impulses between the atria and ventricles, is the primary region of concern for alterations in conduction. A decrease .in the speed of transmission prolongs the interval between sequential contraction of chambers. This delay may reduce the benefit of atrial kick by supplying the extra end-diastolic volume to the ventricles at a time when ventricular contraction has already begun. Additionally, the delay in conduction may prolong ventricular diastolic filling time beyond the point where maximum effectiveness of myocardial stretch and contraction can occur. An accelerated rate of transmission permits early electrical activation of the ventricles, premature contraction of the ventricular myofibrils, a diminished preload volume for ejection, and reduction in atrial kick.

The clinical significance of rhythm disturbances can be viewed on a continuum. Extreme slowing of impulse formation or impulse transmission has greater influence on cardiac output than do rhythms that alter activity only slightly. Conversely, extremely rapid conduction or rates can have a profound impact on output. In addition, combinations of rhythm disturbances, such as excitation of impulse formation and depression of impulse conduction, are often responsible for the clinical symptoms experienced by cardiac patients. Therefore accurate interpretation of dysfunctions is mandatory for the clinician.

TERMINOLOGY

Before proceeding with the presentation of rhythm interpretation, a discussion of terminology is appropriate. Disturbances in impulse formation or conduction are most accurately termed *dysrhythmias*. However, by convention, they have been referred to as *arrhythmias*. Thus these terms are used interchangeably.

Cardiac cycles are variably referred to as *beats, contractions, cycles, conductions,* or *complexes.* Although it is perhaps the least representative because it refers to the mechanical function of the myocardium, the term *contraction* has been used most frequently. Because cardiac rhythm interpretation involves analysis of electrical activity only, the term *complex* will be used in this text.

RHYTHM ANALYSIS

Interpretation of cardiac rhythms requires the evaluation of the wave forms, their duration, and their relationship

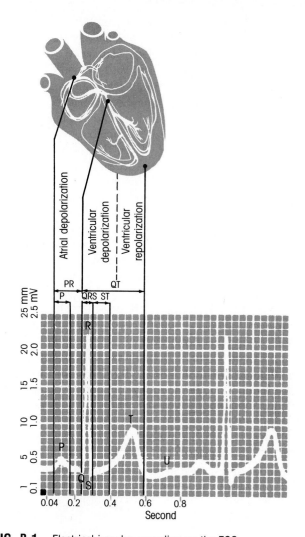

FIG. B-1 Electrical impulse recording on the ECG.
From Dossey BM, Guzzetta CE, and Kenner CV: *Critical care nursing: Body-mind-spirit,* Philadelphia, 1992, JB Lippincott Co.

to each other. A complete description of the anatomic components and electrocardiographic representations of the conduction system can be found in Chapter 6.

Components of the cardiac cycle

To review briefly, a typical cardiac cycle is composed of a P wave, QRS complex, T wave, and sometimes a U wave (Fig. B-1). Relationships of these components to each other, or to similar components in another cycle, are the investigative tools in rhythm interpretation. Although an estimate of dysfunction can be made from a monitor screen, an evaluation of any rhythm requires an imprinted tracing.

Electrocardiographic paper

The standardized 1-mm grid on the electrocardiographic paper permits analysis of cycle components. The measure-

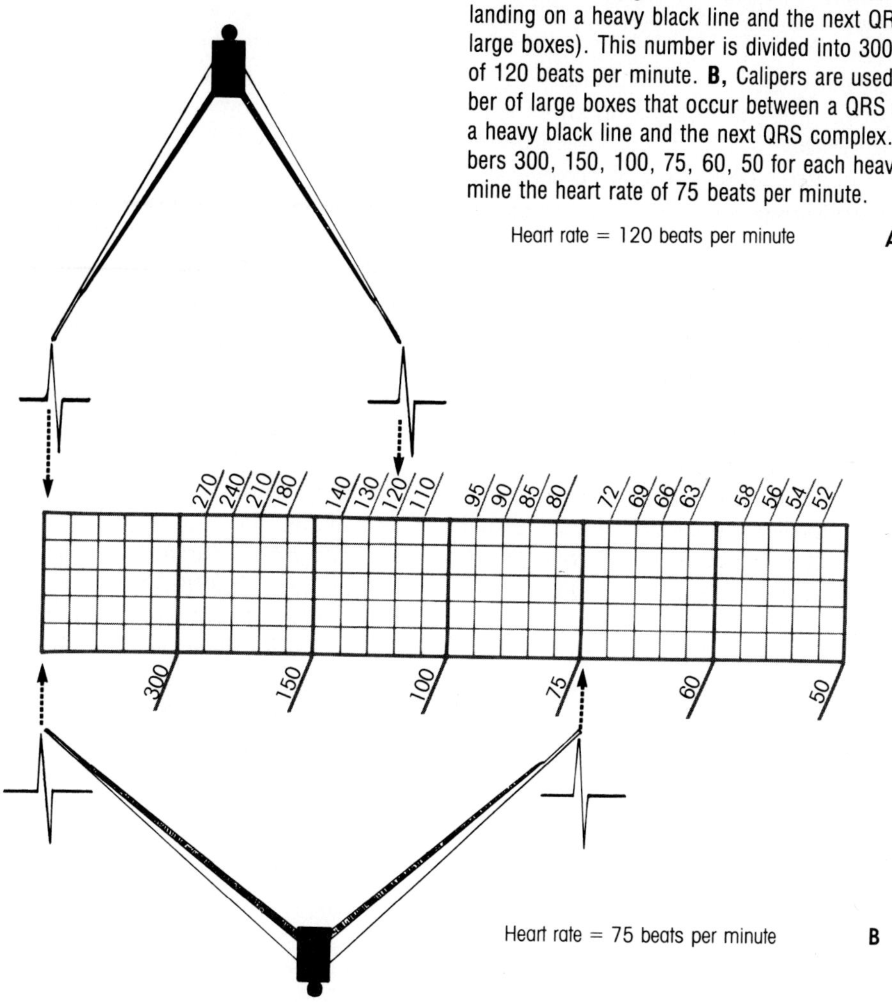

FIG. B-2 Calculating heart rate. **A,** Calipers are used to measure the number of large boxes that occur between a QRS complex landing on a heavy black line and the next QRS complex (or 2.5 large boxes). This number is divided into 300 to determine a rate of 120 beats per minute. **B,** Calipers are used to identify the number of large boxes that occur between a QRS complex that falls on a heavy black line and the next QRS complex. Count off the numbers 300, 150, 100, 75, 60, 50 for each heavy black line to determine the heart rate of 75 beats per minute.

Heart rate = 120 beats per minute   **A**

Heart rate = 75 beats per minute   **B**

ment of voltage using the vertical axis, essential for determining conditions on the 12-lead ECG, is not particularly pertinent for rhythm interpretation. The horizontal axis represents passage of time as the paper moves past the stylus at a standardized rate of 25 mm per sec. Thus each small square represents 1 mm in length and 0.04 sec in time. The larger square (or five small squares) represents 5 mm in length and 0.20 sec in time. Cycle duration is measured by evaluating the number of lines included within or between cycle events. Additionally, many brands of paper provide markers at the border, which indicate 1-sec or 3-sec time spans.

Determination of rate. Several methods can be used to evaluate the cardiac rate. All require that the reader use a specific point in a cardiac cycle and measure to the same point in the later cycle. Although both atrial and ventricular rates are determined, it is usually easier to evaluate the ventricular rate using the QRS complex.

Grid method. Determining the rate using the grid method requires counting the number of light grid lines between consecutive cycles and using a rate ruler or refer-

ence illustration. A second approach using the paper grids involves memorizing the mnemonic 300-150-100-75-60-50, which is applied to the number of heavy grid lines between complexes. With the mnemonic, if a cycle occurs at every 0.20-sec grid, the rate is 300. If two heavy lines fall between cycles, the rate is 150. Rates assigned to subsequent heavy grid lines are 100, 75, 60, and 50 (Fig. B-2, *B*).

Mathematical calculation. Another method for determining heart rate involves counting the number of heavy grid lines between cycles and dividing that number into 300 (Fig. B-2, *A*) (or divide 1500 by the number of light grid lines between cycles).

Border application. To determine rate using the border mark method, locate markers (typically found at 1-sec or 3-sec intervals) and identify a 6-sec span. Count the number of complexes within the 6-sec period and multiply this number by 10. This method is most useful for irregular rhythms.

When determining rates, it must be remembered that an inspection of only one cycle limits the generalization of the rate. Therefore if the cycling is regular, investigation of several isolated beats may be sufficient. However, if the rate is irregular, the use of the border marks may be more appropriate.

The crosshatched pattern of the ECG paper further allows determination of time intervals required for conduction through the various regions of the myocardium. The identification of intervals is best accomplished by using the lighter, 0.04-sec grid lines.

Cycle intervals

Determining durations of various cycle components reveals the amount of time required for depolarization or repolarization of myocardial regions. To measure intervals, the grid markings on the ECG paper are used (see Fig. B-2).

R-R interval. The time interval between two consecutive QRS complexes indicates the rate of ventricular depolarization. This is considered equivalent to the actual heart rate. The normal R-R interval is 0.60 to 1.00 sec (reflecting the normal heart rate of 60 to 100 beats per min).

P-P interval. The time interval between two consecutive P waves (regardless of the origin) determines the atrial depolarization rate, which may or may not be the same as the ventricular rate. The normal P-P interval is 0.60 to 1.00 sec.

PR interval. The time required for transmission of impulses through the atria and AV node is the PR interval. A normal PR interval indicates an appropriate relationship of atrial to ventricular sequencing. A PR interval that is shorter or longer than normal results in contraction of the ventricles either too early or too late and may cause inadequate ventricular contractility, abnormal closure of the AV valves and ultimately a decrease in cardiac output. The normal PR interval is 0.12 to 0.20 sec.

QRS interval. The QRS interval reflects the duration of ventricular depolarization. A normal QRS interval indicates that conduction through the ventricular tissue has proceeded within a normal timing interval, but it does not signify normal pathways. The normal QRS interval is 0.06 to 0.10 sec.

QT interval. The QT interval measures time from the onset of the QRS to the conclusion of the T wave. The QT interval thus reflects both depolarization and repolarization within the ventricles, and an alteration from normal indicates an abnormality in one of these components. Changes in the QT interval occur as a result of abnormal electrolyte levels (potassium, calcium, or magnesium) or chemical influences (drugs such as quinidine and procainamide). The normal QT interval is 0.38 to 0.42 sec and normally varies with the heart rate. A general principle to determine the value for any given QT interval is that the QT duration at normal sinus node rates should be less than 50% of the preceding R-R interval.

Lead placement

The placement of electrodes is not as crucial for monitoring cardiac rhythms as it is for diagnosis of disease states (see Chapter 6). Rather, the most important factor in determining placement of electrodes in cardiac monitoring is identifying locations that provide clear configurations for all complexes of the cycle, negligible interference from extraneous electrical activity, and sufficient room between electrodes to place defibrillator paddles in case they are needed. Avoidance of major muscle masses that can produce stylus deviation from patient movement is important. Occasionally disease processes or surgical incisions may require the nurse to be creative in the approach to lead placement.

Cardiac monitoring requires attaching a minimum of three electrodes to the patient. Two electrodes provide a recording of the electrical activity between the points of attachment, and the third electrode provides electrical grounding. Three preferred placements, all modifications of leads from the standard 12-lead ECG, are described and illustrated in Fig. B-3.

Lead I. Electrode placement for lead I provides prominent positive deflections for all complexes. The advantage to using lead I is that it supplies prominent P waves. The ground electrode (often labeled *G*) is placed on the lower left thorax. The positive (recording) electrode (labeled +) is placed on the upper left anterior chest. The negative (reference) electrode (labeled −) is placed on the right upper anterior chest surface.

Lead II. As with lead I, positions for electrodes in lead II furnish positive deflections for all complexes. However, the QRS becomes more prominent. The ground electrode is best positioned on the upper left anterior chest. The positive electrode is placed lateral to the apex of the heart

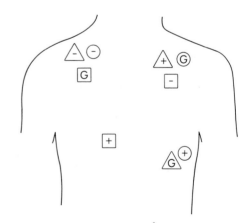

FIG. B-3 Three monitoring leads. The + indicates a receiving (positive) electrode, the − indicates the reference (negative) electrode, and *G* indicates the ground electrode. Lead I is displayed with triangles, Lead II is identified with circles, and MCL₁ is represented by squares.

(found by identifying the point of maximum impulse). The negative electrode is placed on the right upper anterior chest surface.

Lead MCL₁. The benefit of using an MCL₁ lead is the ability to differentiate the origin (right or left) of ectopic ventricular complexes or ventricular tachycardia and differentiate the type of bundle branch block. The ground electrode is placed on the upper right thorax. The negative electrode is positioned on the upper left thorax, and the positive electrode is placed in the fourth intercostal space to the right of the sternum.

The previously described lead arrangements typically provide the best cardiac activity with a minimum of interference. If interference creates false alarms on the equipment, the electrodes can be moved to decrease or increase the size of complexes. Cardiac monitoring alarm systems must always stay on. No single lead placement is appropriate for every patient, and often satisfactory interpretation of a rhythm may require manipulation and use of a secondary lead arrangement.

Systematic evaluation of cardiac rhythms

The interpretation of cardiac dysrhythmias requires developing an approach that ensures analysis of all essential components. One helpful method is presented here.

Scan strip. A quick glance at the strip often provides clues to an abnormality. Factors to consider include heart rates (too fast, too slow, regular, or irregular), configuration of complexes (such as a change in the appearance of the P wave), relationship of complexes (to others within the cycle, as well as to similar complexes in other cycles).

Determine rates. Rates for both atrial and ventricular complexes should be determined.

Determine intervals. Measurements should be made for PR, QRS, and QT intervals to ascertain whether they are within normal limits.

Interpretation. The interpretive statement for all monitor strips should include the basic or underlying rhythm, as well as any additional alteration in impulse formation or conduction. The final interpretation may include a combination of many rhythms (such as sinus rhythm with first-degree AV block and VPCs).

The following pages contain examples of rhythms that are routinely seen in the clinical setting. They are presented by site within the categories of intrinsic rhythms, rhythms of depression, and rhythms of excitation.

INTRINSIC RHYTHMS

Specialized cells within the myocardium have the inherent ability to initiate depolarization without external stimulation. The resting membrane potential and the slope of phase 4 of the action potential (refer to Chapter 6) determine which cell will assume control of the cardiac rhythm.

Of these features, the slope of phase 4 has the greatest influence on the rate at which cells initiate impulses, termed *automaticity*. The sinus node, because it has the fastest spontaneous depolarization rate (i.e., steepest slope of phase 4), is the dominant pacemaker. If the sinus node fails to form impulses or if its impulse is blocked from transmission to other tissues, cardiac standstill is prevented by automatic sites further along the conduction system that can initiate impulse formation. These distal pacemakers are usually quiescent because of depolarization originating in the sinus node. Each more distal pacemaker has an inherent rate slower than its proximal counterpart. Therefore each remains a latent pacemaker unless the site above fails to fire or conduct. Thus the myocardium has numerous subsidiary pacemakers located in the atria, the AV junction, and the ventricles. Subsidiary pacemakers may assume control for a single beat or a sustained rhythm. The prefix *idio-* is applied when a subsidiary pacemaker assumes continuous control of conduction (e.g., idioventricular rhythm).

The following rhythms, which assume control of cardiac conduction because of their inherent capacity to initiate impulses, are referred to as *intrinsic rhythms*. A description of each rhythm is followed by an example that has been labeled according to the underlying rhythm, the secondary rhythm, and specific measurable parameters such as rates and intervals.

Normal sinus rhythm

DESCRIPTION: This is a rhythm controlled by impulses initiated in the sinus (sinoatrial) node. Impulses generated by the sinus node are transmitted in a predictable sequence providing for coordinated contraction of the atria and ventricles.

CAUSES: There is normal physiologic rhythm.

ECG CHARACTERISTICS: Each cycle contains a P, QRS, and T of normal configuration. Heart rate ranges from 60 to 100 beats per minute. Changes in rate occur in response to physiologic needs regulated by the autonomic nervous system. An increase in the sympathetic nervous system output increases the rate at which the sinus node produces impulses, and a decrease in sympathetic activity slows sinus node firing (similar to a gas pedal on a car). Fluctuations in parasympathetic nervous system activity have the reverse effects. Increased parasympathetic activity slows formation of sinus node impulses, whereas decreased parasympathetic activity increases the frequency of sinus node firing (similar to a brake in a car—decreased speed with an increase in pressure on the brake).

Cycle-to-cycle intervals may vary slightly because of the influence of respiratory activity on the sympathetic nervous system (an increase in cardiac rate immediately precedes inspiration and reaches maximum at mid- to late inspiration (see Fig. B-4). A PR interval of 0.12 to 0.20 is normal, and a QRS interval of 0.06 to 0.10 is normal.

PATHOPHYSIOLOGY: There is normal rhythm.

SIGNS AND SYMPTOMS: There are none.

HEMODYNAMIC CONSEQUENCES: It provides the most advantageous rate and chamber sequencing to facilitate optimal cardiac output.

INTERVENTIONS: There are none.

Sinus arrhythmia

DESCRIPTION: Rhythm of sinus node origin wherein the phasic variations due to respiration are unusually prominent. This is not an abnormal rhythm.

CAUSES: It is generally more prevalent in young adults. It may be more pronounced in some individuals during episodes of deep inhalation and exhalation.

ECG CHARACTERISTICS: It resembles normal sinus rhythm in that typical P-QRS-T configurations and intervals, as well as rhythmicity, are present. The rate difference between the slowest and fastest cycling interval must exceed 10% (see Fig. B-5).

PATHOPHYSIOLOGY: It is a normal phenomenon but may indicate a sinus node particularly responsive to autonomic nervous system influence.

SIGNS AND SYMPTOMS: There are none.

HEMODYNAMIC CONSEQUENCES: Arterial pressure curves may vary in relation to the length of time available for diastolic filling (lower arterial pressure when the rate is highest; higher pressures during the slower phases). This same variability in intensity of pulsations is usually imperceptible when palpating peripheral pulses.

INTERVENTIONS: There are none.

Atrial escape complex and rhythm

DESCRIPTION: A beat or sustained rhythm originates from an ordinarily latent pacemaker in the atria. The intrinsic rate of firing for atrial tissue is approximately 50 beats per min.

CAUSES: It is caused by a decreased impulse formation or decreased impulse conduction from the sinus node.

ECG CHARACTERISTICS: An atrial escape beat occurs after a pause in normal cardiac activity and consists of a normal QRS complex and T wave, an abnormal P-wave configuration, and a possible change in PR interval. In the presence of sustained sinus node dysfunction, the atrial tissue can assume control of cardiac conduction and appears as a rhythm lacking rhythmicity, which has complexes resembling isolated escape complexes (see Fig. B-6).

PATHOPHYSIOLOGY: The escape mechanism is a normal action; the pathophysiology involves the sinus node.

SIGNS AND SYMPTOMS: Patients may have symptoms as a result of the pause or the increased diastolic filling time of the ventricles, and the resultant large ejection volume associated with the escape beat may be felt by the patient. A sustained atrial escape rhythm at a slow rate may produce insufficient cardiac output, and the patient may complain of lightheadedness, syncope, or angina. Heart sounds are usually normal.

HEMODYNAMIC CONSEQUENCES: Normal atrial-to-ventricular sequencing exists; therefore normal arterial pres-

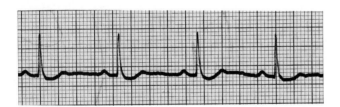

FIG. B-4 Normal sinus rhythm (rate, 68; PR interval, 0.18 sec; QRS interval, 0.08 sec).

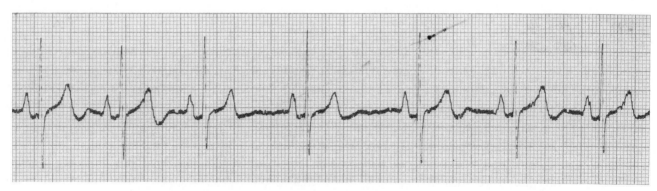

FIG. B-5 Sinus arrhythmia can be identified by the exaggerated rhythmic cycling of the rhythm (rate, 52 to 67; PR interval, 0.16 sec; QRS interval, 0.08 sec).

sures are present with atrial escape beats. However, the interruption in sinus activity that has permitted the atrial escape results in prolonged absence of output. There is usually no perceptible difference in peripheral pulse intensity.

INTERVENTIONS: There are none; investigation and treatment of the underlying sinus dysfunction are done. Administration of atropine may increase the rate of firing of the atrial cell or may resolve the underlying sinus problem.

Junctional escape beat and rhythm

DESCRIPTION: A beat or sustained rhythm originates from an ordinarily latent pacemaker in the AV junctional tissue. The intrinsic rate of firing for junctional tissue is between 40 and 60 beats per min.

CAUSES: Junctional escape activity occurs in the absence of depolarization from a higher pacemaker; this would occur when there is decreased impulse formation or decreased impulse conduction from the sinus node, failure of atrial tissue to initiate impulses, or decreased conduction at the AV node.

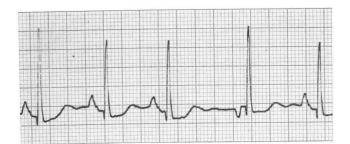

FIG. B-6 Sinus rhythm (rate, 80; PR interval, 0.16 sec; QRS interval, 0.08 sec) with a sinus pause ending with an atrial escape beat (fourth complex terminates the 0.94-sec pause; abnormal P configuration; PR interval, 0.12 sec; normal QRS complex).

ECG CHARACTERISTICS: A classic junctional escape beat is a cycle terminating a pause in normal cardiac activity that consists of a normal QRS complex and T wave but an abnormal P-wave configuration and a change in the PR relationship. The P wave may be visible before or after the QRS or often may be obscured by the more prominent QRS complex. Examination of the P wave may reveal a sinus-initiated P wave because reverse (retrograde) conduction from the junction to the atria does not always occur. The P waves may be inverted in lead II or upright in MCL$_1$. When depression of higher pacemakers is sustained, junctional tissue can assume control of cardiac rhythm, presenting a regular rhythm with each cycle exhibiting characteristics of a junctional escape complex (Fig. B-7).

PATHOPHYSIOLOGY: The escape mechanism is a normal mechanism to prevent asystole; pathophysiologic factors involve other conduction system components. Atropine may enhance the firing rate of the escape focus or may assist in resolving the underlying impulse formation or conduction problem.

SIGNS AND SYMPTOMS: Patients may have symptoms as a result of the pause, or the augmented ejection volume associated with the escape beat may be felt by the patient. A sustained junctional rhythm may be too slow to accommodate normal patient activity, and the patient thus might exhibit symptoms of decreased cardiac output.

HEMODYNAMIC CONSEQUENCES: Normal atrial-to-ventricular sequencing is absent; thus the benefit of atrial kick is lost. However, the slower rate may result in normal intensity of peripheral pulses and arterial pressure curves equal to those obtained when the patient has normal sinus rhythm. Heart sound intensity may change because of the altered relationship of atrial and ventricular contraction.

INTERVENTIONS: The main concern is investigation and treatment of the underlying sinus dysfunction. In the symptomatic patient, atropine may be effective in eliminating delays in normal impulse formation or conduction.

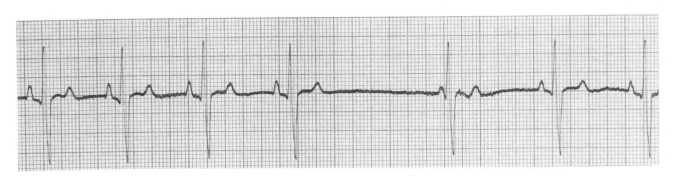

FIG. B-7 Sinus rhythm (rate, 60; PR interval, 0.14 sec; QRS interval, 0.12 sec) with a 1.76-sec sinus pause, which is terminated by a junctional escape beat (fifth complex exhibits abnormal P wave; shortened PR interval of 0.06 sec; normal interval, 0.12 sec).

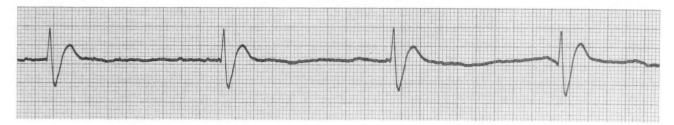

FIG. B-8 Atrial standstill (no P wave) with idioventricular escape rhythm (ventricular rate, 33; QRS, 0.18 sec).

Ventricular escape complex and rhythm

DESCRIPTION: A beat or sustained rhythm originates from an ordinarily latent pacemaker in the ventricles. The intrinsic rate of firing for ventricular tissue is between 20 and 40 beats per min. Ventricular tissue assumes control of cardiac conduction when all other mechanisms fail.

CAUSES: It is caused by absence of supraventricular impulse formation or conduction to the ventricles.

ECG CHARACTERISTICS: A cycle, terminating a pause in normal cardiac activity, consists of an abnormal and prolonged QRS. Although ventricular conduction may enter the atria through retrograde conduction, P waves are more often the result of independent sinus node activity. A sustained ventricular escape rhythm exhibits the same cycle characteristics as an isolated beat. The lower the site of this latent pacemaker within the ventricles, the more bizarre the QRS complexes and the slower the inherent rate of impulse formation (see Fig. B-8).

PATHOPHYSIOLOGY: The escape mechanism demonstrates the normal cardiac backup pacemaker activity; the pathophysiologic factors involve depression of impulse formation or conduction from superior pacemakers.

SIGNS AND SYMPTOMS: The patient usually experiences symptoms of decreased cardiac output such as syncope and angina, which result from the very slow rate of ventricular automaticity and the absence of atrial-to-ventricular sequencing. At the slower rates of ventricular firing, the patient may become unresponsive.

HEMODYNAMIC CONSEQUENCES: Normal atrial-to-ventricular sequencing is absent; thus the benefit of atrial kick is lost. Additionally, the slow rate of the ventricular escape mechanism results in prolonged absence of curves on the pressure monitor. Although each cycle thus has a longer filling time, the typical arterial curve produced is decreased as the direction of ventricular impulse transmission is altered, and normal apex-to-base contraction is compromised. Peripheral pulses are poorly palpated.

INTERVENTIONS: Initial intervention should include investigation and treatment of the underlying dysfunction of higher pacemakers. Prevention of cardiovascular collapse is of prime concern. Isoproterenol can be tried to increase the rate at which the ventricular focus initiates impulses. Additionally, epinephrine may be administered to increase the force of myocardial contraction. Atropine has no effect on the myofibrils of the ventricles (which have no parasympathetic fibers) but may accelerate formation and conduction from superior pacemakers. An artificial electronic ventricular pacemaker may be required to support the rate. NOTE: Electrical-mechanical dissociation often exists in the presence of idioventricular rhythms and should be ruled out before insertion of a pacemaker (see Chapter 10).

RHYTHMS OF DEPRESSION: IMPULSE FORMATION AND IMPULSE CONDUCTION

Optimal cardiac output relies on the normal development and transmission of impulses within the cardiac conduction system. Mechanisms that impede adjacent cells from transmitting impulses, lower the resting membrane potential, or prolong the slope of phase 4 depolarization are responsible for rhythms of depression. Depressors of depolarization (resulting in decreased impulse formation or automaticity) and transmission (impaired impulse conduction) include hyperkalemia, ischemia, hypothermia, increased parasympathetic tone, decreased catecholamine release, digitalis, quinidine, procainamide, beta blockers, edrophonium, calcium channel blockers, and acetylcholine.

Complete or intermittent interruption in impulse conduction can occur anywhere within the conduction system. Electrocardiographic evidence of impaired conduction depends on the site and severity of dysfunction. Depressed conduction from the sinus node results in cycles that exhibit pauses in the occurrence of P waves, whereas depressed impulse conduction in the AV node results in delays or interruption in the development of QRS complexes. Abnormal conduction within the ventricular bundle branches results in prolongation of the QRS complex and/or may be responsible for dissociation of atrial and ventricular activity.

Rhythms in this category will again be presented based on the site of depression, with variances in sinus activity covered first.

Sinus bradycardia

DESCRIPTION: A rhythm that exhibits normal characteristics of each cycle (respiratory rhythmicity, normal configuration of complexes, normal conduction intervals) but at a frequency below 60 per min is termed *sinus bradycardia*.

CAUSES: Sinus bradycardia can be the result of ischemia or infarction involving the sinus node or atrial tissue, or more often it represents the influence of a variety of drugs. Most often implicated are digitalis, beta blockers, calcium channel blockers, reserpine, methyldopa, and guanethidine. Severe depression of sinus firing may occur during endotracheal intubation. Sinus bradycardia can also be a normal phenomenon indicating the responsiveness of the sinus node to decreased demand for cardiac output. At rest, and particularly during sleep, many individuals may exhibit a slowing in sinus rates below 60 per min. Additionally, sinus bradycardia can be a reflection of athletic training (the improved contractile ability of the myocardium allows for a reduced resting and exercise heart rate while maintaining a satisfactory cardiac output).

ECG CHARACTERISTICS: Each cardiac cycle exhibits the typical respiratory-related rhythmicity (faster with inspiration, slower with exhalation) of sinus-initiated conduction. It is composed of a normal configuration of complexes and normal PR and QRS intervals. However, the rate of impulse initiation is decreased below the usual rate for sinus depolarization (i.e., less than 60 beats per min; see Fig. B-9).

PATHOPHYSIOLOGY: Depression of impulse formation in the sinus node occurs when the resting membrane potential becomes more negative, the threshold for depolarization is elevated, or the slope of phase 4 is reduced.

SIGNS AND SYMPTOMS: A minimal reduction in rate coinciding with a reduction in demand is well tolerated. However, if the sinus rate does not increase proportionately to demand, the individual may experience chest pain, lightheadedness, dizziness, nausea, syncope, and other symptoms of decreased cardiac output. A rate below 50 may be especially detrimental to patients with already compromised cardiac output.

HEMODYNAMIC CONSEQUENCES: Severe sinus bradycardia, with rates below 40 per min, produces a significant decrease in arterial pressures. Palpation of peripheral pulses reveals prolonged intervals between beats with increased intensity of the pulsations.

INTERVENTIONS: Nursing measures include observing the patient's tolerance to the bradycardia. Emergency management of symptomatic sinus bradycardia includes atropine, isoproterenol, and artificial pacemaker support. Drugs that increase both rate and contractility or increase peripheral vascular resistance should be used judiciously in patients with myocardial ischemia. For long-term support, a rate-responsive artificial cardiac pacemaker is appropriate (see Chapters 10 and 16).

Sinus pause or arrest

DESCRIPTION: Failure of the sinus node to generate an impulse for an extended period of time is referred to as a *sinus pause* or *sinus arrest* (prolonged episode of failure to fire).

CAUSES: Coronary artery disease producing ischemia or infarction is the usual cause of sinus arrest, especially when combined with strong vagal stimulation such as vomiting, straining at stool, or carotid hypersensitivity. Chemicals, particularly digitalis, can also depress sinus node firing.

ECG CHARACTERISTICS: A normal sinus rhythm is suddenly interrupted by complete absence of cardiac activity. The duration may be a loss of one or two beats or may continue for several seconds. The sinus pause is not equal to a multiple of the sinus cycle. Greater periods of cardiac silence are usually prevented by the development of an escape beat from a subsidiary pacemaker in the junctional or ventricular tissue (see Fig. B-10).

PATHOPHYSIOLOGY: The pacemaker cells of the sinus node fail to reach threshold because of a severe depression in the slope of phase 4 depolarization, a lower resting membrane potential, or a higher threshold.

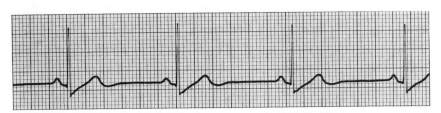

FIG. B-9 Sinus bradycardia (rate, 48; PR interval, 0.16 sec; QRS interval, 0.06 sec).

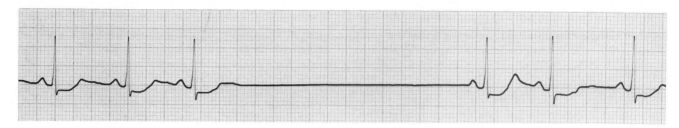

FIG. B-10 Sinus rhythm (rate, 80; PR interval, 0.18 sec; QRS interval, 0.08 sec) to sinus pause of 3.22 sec. The sinus pause is not equal to a multiple of the sinus cycle. The fifth beat is an atrial premature complex.

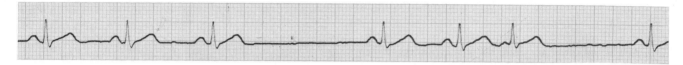

FIG. B-11 Normal sinus rhythm (rate, 68; PR interval, 0.16 sec; QRS interval, 0.10 sec) with sinus exit block (absence of a complete cycle of P-QRS-T resulting in a pause, which is a precise duplicate interval of the preceding sinus cycle). The sixth beat is a premature supraventricular complex.

SIGNS AND SYMPTOMS: The severity of symptoms depends on the duration of pacemaker silence but may include visual disturbances, lightheadedness, and syncope.

HEMODYNAMIC CONSEQUENCES: During the pause, there is no cardiac contraction, and thus no arterial pressure is generated. The subsequent beat, however, often produces a significantly increased arterial curve. Similar phenomena may be palpated peripherally.

INTERVENTIONS: Monitoring the patient for further episodes and preventing injury during episodes are the prime nursing interventions. Medications typically administered include atropine or isoproterenol. If the sinus arrest results in clinically significant symptoms (i.e., cardiac arrest), cardiac compression may be required to maintain circulation. An artificial cardiac pacemaker may be indicated if the condition is expected to persist.

Sinus exit (sinoatrial) block

DESCRIPTION: When an impulse formed in the sinus node fails to propogate into the surrounding atrial tissue, it is termed *sinoatrial*, or *sinus exit, block*.

CAUSES: Conditions that produce ischemia in the tissues surrounding the sinus node (the transitional cells) are believed to be the prime causes of the block. Sinoatrial block may be aggravated by factors that increase vagal tone such as straining, vomiting, or carotid pressure. Digitalis, because of its vagotonic action, may also precipitate an attack

in a susceptible person. Quinidine has also been implicated in production of sinoatrial block.

ECG CHARACTERISTICS: In classic sinus exit block, the pause that interrupts the sinus rhythm is a precise multiple of the usual sinus cycle. Thus measurement of the pause will demonstrate an exact multiple of the basic cycle length, with the P wave following the pause occurring at the expected cycling interval (see Fig. B-11).

PATHOPHYSIOLOGY: It is believed that the transitional cells found between the sinus node and atrial tissues are prevented from depolarizing in response to the sinus stimulus.

SIGNS AND SYMPTOMS: Patient awareness of the dysfunction depends on the duration of asystole. When several successive sinus impulses are blocked, the patient may experience visual disturbances, lightheadedness, nausea, and syncope.

HEMODYNAMIC CONSEQUENCES: Each blocked sinus impulse results in a loss of arterial pressure. If several successive sinus impulses are blocked, the patient will have no cardiac output for the duration of the pause. The pause and the subsequent greater ventricular volume may be palpable peripherally.

INTERVENTIONS: Atropine, isoproterenol, and an artificial cardiac pacemaker are recommended therapies. The patient and the rhythm should be observed closely after even one episode to ensure that prolonged absence of conduction is identified and treated quickly.

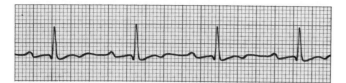

FIG. B-12 Sinus rhythm (rate, 70; QRS interval, 0.10 sec) with first-degree AV block (PR interval, 0.24 sec).

First-degree AV block

DESCRIPTION: Rhythm that presents with a consistent prolongation of the PR interval beyond the normal upper limit of 0.20 sec is known as *first-degree AV block.*

CAUSES: Factors that cause first-degree AV block include calcium-channel blocking agents, amiodarone, digitalis, enhanced parasympathetic tone, and ischemic heart disease. First-degree block also has been observed in healthy trained athletes and in the elderly population.

ECG CHARACTERISTICS: A brief glance at a cardiac rhythm strip may not identify any abnormality. However, precise measurement of the PR interval will identify a duration of greater than 0.20 sec. Usually the primary rhythm is sinus; thus there is rhythmicity related to respiratory activity (see Fig. B-12).

PATHOPHYSIOLOGY: Cellular changes that produce first-degree block result in delayed conduction velocity through the AV node or the segment of the conduction system immediately below the AV node.

SIGNS AND SYMPTOMS: Prolongation of the PR interval beyond the normal range generally produces no symptoms.

HEMODYNAMIC CONSEQUENCES: Prolongation of the PR interval has only a slight influence on the cardiac output. Typically, no discernible change is perceived when palpating peripheral pulses although the intensity of heart sounds may change.

INTERVENTIONS: Nonsymptomatic first-degree AV block requires only patient monitoring to observe for greater prolongation of the PR interval or development of higher degrees of block, which may be precipitated by vagotonic activities such as straining or vomiting. Digitalis may need to be discontinued or the dosage reduced if it was the precipitating cause.

Second-degree AV block: Mobitz type I (Wenckebach phenomenon)

DESCRIPTION: Mobitz type I second-degree AV block is a rhythm that results from intermittent conduction failure

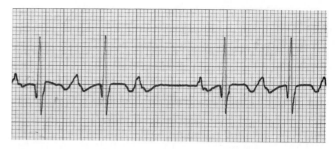

FIG. B-13 Sinus rhythm (atrial rate, 88; QRS interval, 0.10 sec) with type I (Wenckebach) second-degree AV block (grouped ventricular beats with a rate of 60; PR intervals prolong from 0.24 to 0.30 sec with the longest PR in the series preceding the dropped QRS and the shortest PR in the series following the dropped beat; ratio of P waves to QRS is 3:2).

through the AV node to the ventricles producing groupings of beats, with PR intervals becoming progressively longer throughout each series.

CAUSES: Multiple factors can produce type I second-degree AV block, including inferior wall myocardial infarction, rheumatic fever, chronic ischemic heart disease, propranolol, digitalis, aortic valve disease, mitral valve prolapse, amyloidosis, and atrial septal defect. Typically the frequency of block worsens with carotid pressure or other forms of increased vagotonic tone. When type I second-degree AV block is the result of an acute inferior wall infarction, it may be a transient phenomenon.

ECG CHARACTERISTICS: The QRS is of normal duration in each cycle if intraventricular conduction is normal. However, there is gradual prolongation of successive PR intervals until eventually an impulse fails to penetrate the AV node to activate the ventricles. After the dropped ventricular complex, the PR reverts to normal, or near normal, and the Wenckebach sequence is repeated. The longest PR interval in a series may reach 0.60 sec. The greatest increment in the PR interval typically occurs between the first two consecutive conducted beats in each series. A minimum of two consecutive beats must be conducted to determine the variance in length of PR intervals. The intermittent block of conduction into the ventricles results in grouping of beats. An additional finding in type I second-degree AV block is the shortening of the R-R interval within the series (see Fig. B-13).

PATHOPHYSIOLOGY: Type I second-degree AV block typically occurs within the AV node itself, although it can be infranodal in origin. Each successive impulse takes longer and longer to penetrate the AV node (decremental conduction) because each successive beat arrives earlier and earlier in the relative refractory period of the preceding beat.

SIGNS AND SYMPTOMS: The tolerance of type I second-degree AV block depends on the frequency with which the impulse fails to penetrate the AV node. In longer series in which the drop occurs infrequently, the individual may be unaware of the disturbance in conduction. Sequences with fewer conducted beats in the series may cause the patient to experience various signs of decreased cardiac output.

HEMODYNAMIC CONSEQUENCES: Arterial pressure is absent with the dropped beat; often the beat after the pause presents with an increase in height of the pressure curve. Peripheral pulses and heart sounds are irregular, although detection of a pattern may be difficult to perceive.

INTERVENTIONS: Type I second-degree AV block usually is transient and does not progress to a higher degree of block. Generally it is not treated, but the patient is assessed closely. If patients have symptoms, they should be treated with atropine, which is effective in diminishing the block. Additionally, patients should be cautioned to avoid vagal maneuvers, and nausea and vomiting should be vigorously treated. Patients' medication histories are reviewed to determine possible causative factors such as digitalis. Isoproterenol may resolve the blockade in acute situations. If patients experience sufficient symptomatology to limit activities of daily living, a cardiac pacemaker is considered.

Second-degree AV block: Mobitz type II

DESCRIPTION: Sinus rhythm with intermittent failure of ventricular conduction wherein consecutive conducted beats have identical PR intervals is called *Mobitz type II second-degree AV block.*

CAUSES: Type II second-degree AV block is the result of hypoxia of the conduction system at the level of the His-Purkinje system (acute anterior or anteroseptal wall infarction is often the precipitator). Other causes include sclerosis of ventricular tracts (such as Lenegre's disease) or

cardiomyopathy. If this rhythm is a complication of acute infarction, unlike type I, it usually does not resolve when the acute phase is over.

ECG CHARACTERISTICS: Intermittent failure of sinus impulse conduction into the ventricles results in absence of ventricular complexes and grouping of conducted beats. Consecutive conducted cycles within each series present with identical PR intervals that may or may not be within the normal range. Intraventricular conduction defect producing broadened QRS complexes may be present. A minimum of two consecutive beats must be conducted to determine the identical lengths of PR intervals (see Fig. B-14).

PATHOPHYSIOLOGY: The blockage is infranodal with advanced bilateral bundle branch or trifascicular block. There is apparently no relationship between the block and refractory periods of preceding beats; instead an all-or-nothing form of conduction occurs.

SIGNS AND SYMPTOMS: Infrequent dropped beats seldom produce symptoms. However, the patient may experience dizziness, lightheadedness, visual disturbances, or syncope with frequent absence of conduction. Type II second-degree AV block often proceeds without warning to third-degree AV block, producing Adams-Stokes syndrome.

HEMODYNAMIC CONSEQUENCES: Each nonconducted impulse produces a loss of conduction and an absence of arterial pressure, which may cause severe depression in cardiac output. The pauses produced by the dropped beats produce irregular heart sounds and peripheral pulses.

INTERVENTIONS: It is treated if the patient has symptoms or an acute anteroseptal infarction. Atropine and isoproterenol are administered if the lowered heart rate produces symptoms. An artificial cardiac pacemaker generally is indicated because frequently the rhythm progresses to third-degree AV block and ventricular asystole.

NOTE: The cadence of the nonconducted P wave must be identified to distinguish nonconducted P waves of atrial premature complexes from the blocked P waves of second-degree AV block. Atrial premature complexes that fail to

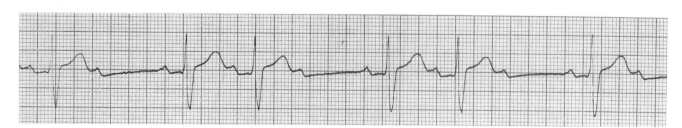

FIG. B-14   Sinus rhythm (atrial rate, 80; QRS interval, 0.12 sec) with type II second-degree AV block (consistent PR interval, 0.24 sec; ventricular rate, 54; ratio of 2:1 and 3:2).

conduct are considered physiologic conditions (the premature impulse reaches the AV node during its normal refractory period); blocked sinus P waves are considered pathologic conditions.

Second-degree AV block: advanced

DESCRIPTION: Rhythm presents with multiple nonconducted atrial beats for each QRS complex.

CAUSES: Etiologic factors of advanced second-degree AV block include sclerosis, ischemia, and infarction of the conduction tracts.

ECG CHARACTERISTICS: Two or more consecutive P waves are not followed by ventricular complexes. Cycles that include QRS complexes have identical PR intervals. P waves occur at relatively normal rates (e.g., less than 120 per min); the ventricular rate is slow (rate depends on atrial rate and frequency of conduction) (see Fig. B-15).

PATHOPHYSIOLOGY: Interruption of conduction at the AV node or infranodally can produce advanced second-degree AV block.

SIGNS AND SYMPTOMS: Weakness, lightheadedness, and fainting are often expressions of the slow ventricular rate.

HEMODYNAMIC CONSEQUENCES: Cardiac output is severely compromised because of the excessively slow ventricular rate. Heart sounds may have an increased intensity, and peripheral pulses are slow.

INTERVENTIONS: Patients should be monitored closely, and medications to support circulation and improve conduction should be administered. Atropine or isoproterenol may resolve the conduction defect, although an artificial cardiac pacemaker is generally indicated.

Third-degree AV block

DESCRIPTION: In third-degree AV block, no impulses are conducted through the AV nodal system to the ventricles, which results in independent atrial and ventricular complexes with the atrial rate greater than the ventricular rate.

CAUSES: Acute inferior or anterior infarction, sclerosis, and systemic hypoxia can cause third-degree AV block.

ECG CHARACTERISTICS: Ventricular complexes are produced by escape mechanisms within the AV junction (rates of 40 to 60 with narrow QRS complexes) or ventricles (rate less than 40 with broad QRS complexes). The atrial rate, driven by the sinus node, ranges from 60 to 100 per min, although sinus tachycardia may develop as a result of sympathetic stimulation of the sinus node in an attempt to compensate for the decreased cardiac output. Although atrial and ventricular activity are completely independent of each other (no PR relationship), P waves and QRS complexes appear at regular intervals. Thus P-P intervals are regular, and R-R intervals are usually regular (inherent firing rate of escape mechanism). Cardiac arrest, or ventricular standstill, is prevented by the escape beats from the junctional or ventricular tissues (see Fig. B-16).

PATHOPHYSIOLOGY: Disease process has resulted in complete inability of the AV node or bundles to conduct supraventricular impulses into the ventricles. The site of obstruction can be the AV node, the common bundle, or a combination of the three ventricular bundles.

SIGNS AND SYMPTOMS: The lower the site of the escape mechanism, the slower the ventricular rate and the more severe the presenting clinical manifestations, which may range from dizziness to syncope.

HEMODYNAMIC CONSEQUENCES: The slow ventricular rate and lack of AV synchrony produce a severe decrease in cardiac output. Prominent or irregular cannon *a* waves and a variance in the first heart sound may be observed because of the independence of atrial and ventricular contractions.

INTERVENTIONS: The patient must be closely monitored, and medications to support circulation and the existing escape mechanism are administered. Until medications can

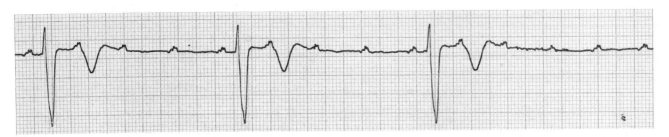

FIG. B-15 Sinus tachycardia (atrial rate, 114; QRS interval, 0.14 sec) with advanced second-degree AV block (constant PR interval, 0.20 sec; ventricular rate, 24 to 29; ratio of 4:1 changing to 5:1 conduction).

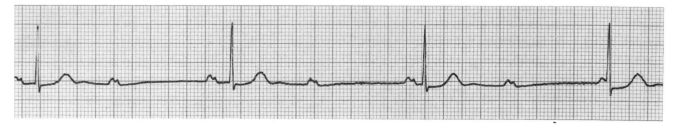

FIG. B-16 Sinus bradycardia (atrial rate, 54) with third-degree AV block (no consistent PR interval; ventricular rate, 31; QRS interval, 0.08).

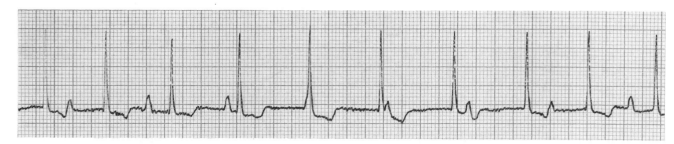

FIG. B-17 Sinus rhythm (atrial rate, 68) with AV dissociation (no consistent PR interval; ventricular rate, 78; QRS interval, 0.08 sec).

be administered, the patient should be placed in a supine position with activity restricted. If digitalis toxicity is suspected, the drug is discontinued. Drugs include atropine and isoproterenol, and an emergency artificial cardiac pacemaker is indicated.

NOTE: Third-degree AV block is a form of AV dissociation. The term *AV dissociation* simply means that the atria and ventricles are independently controlled. Thus two categories of rhythms can be described wherein unrelated atrial and ventricular activity exist: a rhythm in which the atria are activated at a rate faster than the ventricles (third-degree AV block) and rhythms in which the ventricles are controlled by a faster firing pacemaker than that controlling the atria (such as accelerated junctional rhythm and ventricular tachycardia). Fig. B-17 illustrates a rhythm wherein the atria and ventricles are beating independently, with the atrial rate slower than the ventricles (thus not third-degree AV block).

Idioventricular rhythm and ventricular bradycardia

DESCRIPTION: Idioventricular rhythm is a rhythm supported by a slow escape mechanism from the ventricle. It is also referred to as *ventricular bradycardia* and when extremely slow, may be termed an *agonal rhythm.*

CAUSES: Such severe depression is usually the result of metabolic or ischemic diseases.

ECG CHARACTERISTICS: An extremely slow idioventricular rhythm (rates from 15 to 40 per min) produces broad QRS complexes. Often there is no evidence of supraventricular impulses (P waves) (see Fig. B-18).

PATHOPHYSIOLOGY: Idioventricular rhythm implies depression of impulse formation and impulse conduction.

SIGNS AND SYMPTOMS: Because of severely depressed impulse formation and conduction, the patient is usually minimally or totally unresponsive and often exhibits respiratory depression.

HEMODYNAMIC CONSEQUENCES: Minimal cardiac output is evident because atrial-to-ventricular sequencing is absent, and the depressed myocardium often lacks adequate contractile ability. Palpation of peripheral pulses reveals infrequent weak beats.

INTERVENTIONS: Measures are initiated to increase the effectiveness of contractility and enhance impulse formation. Isoproterenol and dopamine are recommended agents. Additionally contributing factors, such as electrolyte or acid-base imbalance and hypoxia, must be corrected. Insertion of an artificial cardiac pacemaker is also indicated.

Ventricular asystole

DESCRIPTION: Complete absence of ventricular activity is known as *ventricular asystole.*

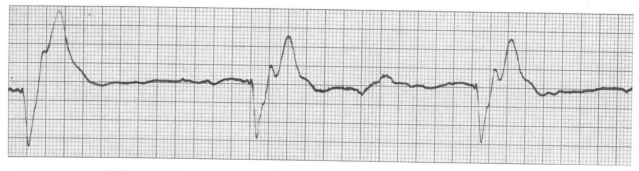

FIG. B-18   Atrial standstill (no P waves) with idioventricular rhythm (ventricular escape) (ventricular rate, 25; QRS interval, 0.24 sec).

CAUSES: Asystole is the result of severe metabolic or cardiopulmonary derangements and third-degree AV block with failure of subsidiary pacemakers.

ECG CHARACTERISTICS: Ventricular asystole is recognized by a total absence of QRS complexes, although P waves may be present. Several leads should be analyzed to differentiate asystole from fine ventricular fibrillation.

PATHOPHYSIOLOGY: Severe depression of myocardial function leads to lack of depolarization.

SIGNS AND SYMPTOMS: Lack of cardiac output rapidly produces unresponsiveness.

HEMODYNAMIC CONSEQUENCES: Asystole produces complete cardiovascular collapse with no evidence of heart sounds, peripheral pulses, or arterial pressure.

INTERVENTIONS: Cardiopulmonary resuscitation (CPR) is required until definitive therapies, including epinephrine, atropine, and an artificial cardiac pacemaker, can be initiated.

RHYTHMS OF EXCITATION: IMPULSE FORMATION AND IMPULSE CONDUCTION

Excitation of impulse formation or impulse conduction result in dysrhythmias commonly called *tachydysrhythmias* or *tachycardias*. This category additionally includes rhythms referred to as *flutter* or *fibrillation*. The site or focus of these dysrhythmias can be limited to just the ventricles, or they can be located in the sinus node, atria, or junction.

Mechanisms of excitation

The pathophysiologic factors responsible for production of tachydysrhythmias involve reentry of impulses within the myocardium or an increase in the automatic firing rate within a single cell.

Enhanced automaticity. Cells throughout the myocardium can initiate the conduction process. Such cells may be excited by a variety of disturbances resulting in enhanced automaticity. The increase in impulse formation results by increasing the slope of phase 4 spontaneous diastolic depolarization, lowering the threshold, or decreasing the resting membrane potential. When a cell fires as a result of enhanced automaticity, it can assume control for a single cycle or a series of ectopic impulses. Rhythms or complexes resulting from enhanced automaticity are also referred to as *ectopic focus dysrhythmias*.

Enhanced automaticity can be precipitated by multiple factors such as electrolyte abnormalities (hypokalemia, hypomagnesemia, hypercalcemia, or hypocalcemia), metabolic changes (hypoxemia, acidosis, alkalosis, or adrenergic stimulation from pain, excitement, or strenuous exercise), chemical influences (alcohol, drugs—digitalis and adrenergic agents such as epinephrine or dopamine), or direct myocardial injury (trauma, ischemia, infarction, or myopathy).

Reentrance. A reentrant mechanism surfaces when a portion of an advancing wave front turns back on itself, forming an electrical loop (or circus movement) and producing an additional cycle or series of cycles. This circuit is the result of abnormal wave front propagation, not enhanced impulse formation. This excitation of impulse conduction can be responsible for isolated beats or sustained tachydysrhythmias. Normally, the heart is protected from reentrant rhythms because of the uniform speed of impulse transmission through the cells and the relatively long refractory period of myofibrils.

Reentrant mechanisms may surface when the velocity of transmission or the duration of the refractory period of adjacent cells is altered. Unlike tachycardias originating from enhanced automaticity, reentry does not imply underlying systemic disease or an acute myocardial pathologic condition. Rather, the development of reentrant circuits indicates localized abnormalities that provide two pathways for conduction, permitting retrograde (reverse) conduction and the normal antegrade conduction. Often these conductile loops involve anomalous pathways that permit the abnormal transmission of impulses. Rhythms that use these pathways are grouped under the heading of preexcitation syndromes (PESs). Additionally, reentrant rhythms may result when localized dysfunction creates a unidirectional block within usual conduction fibers. Thus the antegrade impulse is blocked, but an impulse entering distally is able to travel in a retrograde direction.

Sinus tachycardia

DESCRIPTION: Sinus tachycardia is rhythm originating from the sinus node that exceeds the normal depolarization rate of 100 beats per min.

CAUSES: Sinus tachycardia typically reflects the body's need for increased cardiac output. Conditions that may provoke sinus tachycardia include exercise, stress or anxiety, fever, anemia, hypoxia, hypovolemia, hypotension, and congestive heart failure. Drugs such as atropine, epinephrine, aminophylline, isoproterenol, and dopamine may also increase the rate of sinus node firing.

ECG CHARACTERISTICS: P-initiated cycles exceed a rate of 100 beats per min (see Fig. B-19).

PATHOPHYSIOLOGY: There is none. However, sinus tachycardia may reflect underlying pathologic conditions.

SIGNS AND SYMPTOMS: The patient may complain of palpitations. In the presence of coronary artery disease, the excessive rate may cause ischemia and angina pectoris.

HEMODYNAMIC CONSEQUENCES: As the sinus rate increases, the arterial pressure curve will begin to fall because of decreased diastolic filling time and reduced stroke volume. Peripheral pulse strength may diminish as the rate increases.

INTERVENTIONS: Because sinus tachycardia is a sign of another condition, it is treated by eliminating the cause. If heart failure develops, digitalis may be helpful. Monitoring of the patient's tolerance to this rhythm is essential.

Atrial premature complex

DESCRIPTION: An early cycle that originates anywhere in the atria outside of the sinus node is called an *atrial premature complex (APC)*.

CAUSES: Multiple factors can result in enhanced automaticity or reentry of atrial fibers, including emotional stress, fatigue, excessive use of caffeine, tobacco, or alcohol, ischemia or infarction, atrial dilation, congenital defects, thyrotoxicosis, bronchopulmonary disease, myocarditis, cardiomyopathy, and various drugs such as catecholamines, digitalis, quinidine, and procainamide.

ECG CHARACTERISTICS: A complete cardiac cycle (PQRST) occurs prematurely, has a P wave with a different configuration from the sinus P wave, and has a PR interval within normal range or longer. Atrial premature complexes typically depolarize the sinus node, resulting in a resetting of its firing interval (referred to as a *noncompensatory* or *incomplete compensatory pause*) (see Fig. B-20).

PATHOPHYSIOLOGY: Enhanced spontaneous depolarization of atrial fibers typically is the precipitator of premature complexes, although reentry may also cause premature atrial activity.

SIGNS AND SYMPTOMS: The patient may experience a sensation within the chest resulting from the beat that follows the prematurity (ventricles contain extra volume

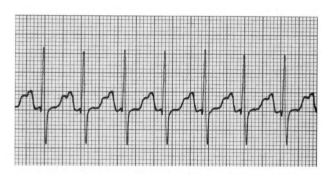

FIG. B-19 Sinus tachycardia (rate, 134, regular; PR interval, 0.14 sec; QRS interval, 0.10 sec).

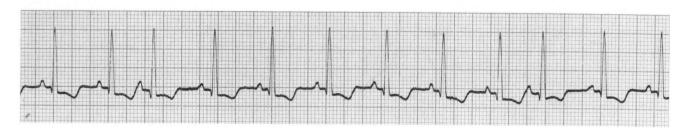

FIG. B-20 Normal sinus rhythm (rate, 96; PR interval, 0.12 sec; QRS interval, 0.08 sec) with atrial premature complexes at beats 3 and 10 (early cycle; abnormal P wave; PR interval, 0.14 sec).

because of prolonged diastolic filling after the premature beat).

HEMODYNAMIC CONSEQUENCES: The arterial curve may show a slight decline if the beat is exceptionally early. When frequent premature beats are present, the irregularity of the rhythm may be detected in heart sounds and peripheral pulses.

INTERVENTIONS: Monitoring the frequency of the APCs is the most important clinical implication because an increasing occurrence may warn of the potential for the atria to assume total control of the rhythm.

Wandering atrial pacemaker

DESCRIPTION: A rhythm produced by initiation of conduction from various sites within the atria is termed *wandering atrial pacemaker.*

CAUSES: Ischemic disease, especially of the sinus node, acute rheumatic fever and other inflammatory conditions, atrial enlargement, and digitalis toxicity have been implicated in production of wandering atrial pacemaker.

ECG CHARACTERISTICS: Cycles arising from multiple atrial sites produce P waves of varying configurations. The variable conduction from these sites results in PR intervals of different durations. Additionally, there is no established regularity of impulses causing a variance in cycle-to-cycle intervals. When these sites initiate impulses at a rate greater than 100, the rhythm is termed *multiple atrial tachycardia* (see Fig. B-21).

PATHOPHYSIOLOGY: Disease states alter the ability of the sinus node to maintain control and further produce enhanced automaticity of atrial tissue.

SIGNS AND SYMPTOMS: Unless a tachycardic rate is present, the patient may exhibit no symptoms.

HEMODYNAMIC CONSEQUENCES: Normal atrial-to-ventricular sequencing and rates within normal ranges produce normal pulses, heart sounds, and hemodynamic parameters.

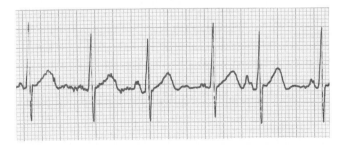

FIG. B-21 Wandering atrial pacemaker (rate, 91 to 98; P wave configuration varies; PR interval, 0.12 to 0.18 sec; QRS interval, 0.08 sec).

INTERVENTIONS: Monitoring of the altered rhythm and patient tolerance are the primary nursing functions. Correction of the underlying medical condition may or may not alleviate the rhythm.

Atrial tachycardia

DESCRIPTION: A rhythm of atrial origin that has a rate of 100 to 250 beats per min is termed *atrial tachycardia.*

CAUSES: Multiple factors can result in enhanced spontaneous depolarization of atrial fibers or activation of a reentry circuit; these factors include emotional stress, fatigue, excessive use of caffeine, tobacco, or alcohol, ischemia or infarction, atrial distention, congenital defects, heart surgery, cardiomyopathy, myocarditis, anomalous bypass tracts (PES), bronchopulmonary disease, hyperthyroidism, and various drugs such as catecholamines, digitalis, quinidine, and procainamide.

ECG CHARACTERISTICS: A rapid cycle rate with normal configuration of the QRS, an eccentric appearance to the P wave, and normal or prolonged PR interval characterize this condition. Atrial tachycardias due to enhanced automaticity typically are irregular and exhibit a slow increase in rate initially and conclude with a gradual slowing of the rate. Reentrant atrial tachycardias begin like those of increased automaticity with one premature complex. However, the cycles immediately assume a regular cadence and terminate abruptly when the tissues transmitting the reverberating impulse become less responsive to the incoming stimuli. The abrupt onset and cessation of reentrant atrial tachycardia has been termed *paroxysmal atrial tachycardia (PAT).* Excessively rapid atrial rates may result in AV block. Atrial tachycardia with 2:1 block may indicate digoxin toxicity. *Multiform or chaotic atrial tachycardia* refers to rapid rhythms exhibiting variable appearance to the P wave. The term *paroxysmal supraventricular tachycardia (PSVT)* should be restricted to the initial phase of interpretation of a narrow QRS complex tachycardia or to those situations in which the site (sinus, atrial, junctional) cannot be identified by the surface ECG (see Fig. B-22).

PATHOPHYSIOLOGY: Increased upslope of phase 4 depolarization in the atria or reentrance/circus movement phenomenon is the pathophysiologic condition found in atrial tachycardia.

SIGNS AND SYMPTOMS: The symptoms experienced by the patient are determined by the rate and general state of the patient's cardiovascular system. Individuals with a healthy myocardium, such as the young adult experiencing atrial tachycardia due to preexcitation, may complain of palpitations, lightheadedness, or stomach upset. The patient with compromised cardiac circulation, however, may additionally have complaints of angina and may experience congestive heart failure. Additionally, the decrease in car-

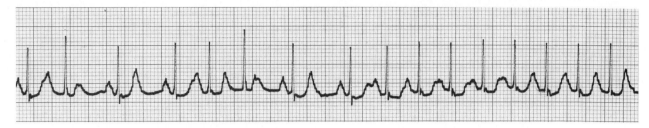

FIG. B-22 Normal sinus rhythm (rate, 98 for beats 3, 4, 7, and 8; PR interval, 0.12 sec; QRS interval, 0.06 sec); atrial premature complexes at beats 2, 5, and 6; blocked APCs follow cycles 3 and 7; and run of atrial tachycardia beginning with cycle 9 (rate, 186; PR interval, 0.14 sec; QRS interval, 0.06 sec).

diac output due to the rapid rate and failing myocardium may also cause syncopal episodes.

HEMODYNAMIC CONSEQUENCES: The arterial pressure curves reflect the effects of the increased cardiac rate and thus will diminish with greater rates. Peripheral pulses are very rapid and may be thready.

INTERVENTIONS: The treatment depends on the hemodynamic stability of the patient and the presence of underlying disease such as acute myocardial ischemia or infarction. Calcium blockers and β-adrenergic blockers are the drugs of choice for suppression of atrial tachycardia caused by enhanced automaticity. In addition, identification and reversal of the causative factors should be attempted. Sedation may be helpful in alleviating the catecholamine effects. The circuit of a reentrant rhythm can be interrupted by administration of digitalis and calcium blocking agents (prolong the refractory period) or quinidine (increases impulse transmission). Vagal stimulation through vagotonic maneuvers such as carotid sinus stimulation may be used for terminating reentrant tachycardias. Synchronized cardioversion is also effective for terminating reentrant tachycardia and is recommended for patients in unstable condition (see Appendix D). Overdrive pacing is effective in terminating all forms of atrial tachycardia. Causative factors, such as digoxin, should be investigated and treated.

Atrial flutter

DESCRIPTION: An atrial tachydysrhythmia in which the atrial rate is extremely rapid, ranging from 200 to 350 per min, is called an *atrial flutter*.

CAUSES: Typically, atrial flutter develops from factors such as mitral valve disease or chronic pulmonary disease, which cause atrial enlargement. The enlarged chamber creates intraatrial delays in conduction or alters excitability of atrial tissues.

ECG CHARACTERISTICS: Atrial flutter is conspicuous by the sawtooth or flutter (F) waves that replace typical atrial

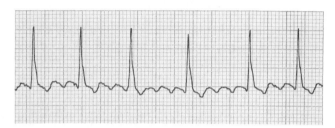

FIG. B-23 Atrial flutter (atrial sawtooth pattern; atrial rate, 355) with variable AV conduction (FR interval varies; QRS interval, 0.08 sec).

complexes. These flutter waves are regular and typically occur at a rate of 270 to 300. The rapid rate exceeds the capacity for conduction at the AV node so that transmission into the ventricles is intermittent (1:1 conduction occurs rarely and is catastrophic). The conduction into the ventricles usually exhibits a consistent ratio, although variable block may be seen. This relationship and any constant ratio should be identified as part of the rhythm interpretation. The FR interval is measured like a PR interval. When no constant relationship between atrial and ventricular complexes can be measured, conduction is said to be *variable*. If a constant FR relationship is identified, the ratio of atrial to ventricular complexes is stated (even-numbered ratios such as 2:1 and 4:1 are more common than odd-numbered ratios such as 3:1). Because of the intermittent conduction of the AV node, the ventricular rate is considerably less than the atrial rate. Interpretation of atrial flutter includes the atrial rate, the ventricular rate, and their relationship (ratio or variable) (see Fig. B-23).

PATHOPHYSIOLOGY: Although enhanced automaticity may produce atrial flutter, more often it is the result of a reentrance mechanism. It is felt that a concommittant delay in atrial conduction, or perhaps some form of sinus node dysfunction, exists.

SIGNS AND SYMPTOMS: The symptoms exhibited by the patient directly reflect the ventricular response rate. As the

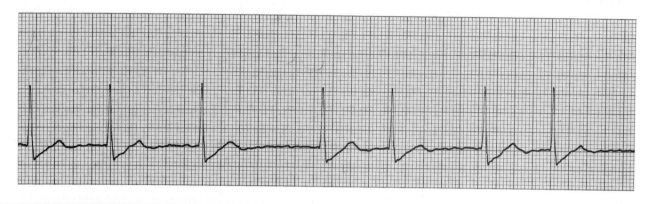

A

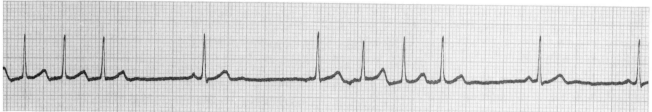

B

FIG. B-24 **A,** Controlled atrial fibrillation (no distinct P waves; ventricular rate, 60; irregular ventricular response; QRS interval, 0.08 sec). **B,** Tachycardia-bradycardia syndrome is evidenced by alternating episodes of sinus bradycardia (rate, 56; PR interval, 0.14 sec; QRS interval, 0.06 sec) and atrial tachycardia (rate, 141). An atrial escape beat (beat 5) follows a pause of 1.30 sec.

frequency of transmission through the AV node increases, the patient will experience increased discomfort in the form of palpitations, chest pain, dizziness, blurred vision, nausea, or even syncope.

HEMODYNAMIC CONSEQUENCES: The lack of consistent AV conduction will result in a variance in arterial pressure from beat to beat. The height of the curve will be higher with slower rates. Heart sounds and peripheral pulses may exhibit some irregularity in timing and intensity.

INTERVENTIONS: Vagotonic maneuvers used with atrial flutter of reentrant origin will decrease the frequency of AV conduction temporarily, which reduces the ventricular rate. Reduction in the ventricular rate can also be accomplished with the administration of digitalis. Calcium channel and β-adrenergic blockers have also proved effective in control of atrial flutter. Synchronized cardioversion is also an applicable therapy for conversion of flutter to sinus rhythm.

Atrial fibrillation

DESCRIPTION: Rhythm of atrial origin wherein impulses are generated at excessively rapid rates (may exceed 500 per minute) resulting in chaotic atrial, AV junctional, and ventricular conduction is termed *atrial fibrillation.*

CAUSES: Atrial dilation (regardless of cause), hypoxia, acidosis, electrolyte imbalance are causes of atrial fibrillation.

ECG CHARACTERISTICS: Clearly defined P waves are replaced by erratic undulations of the baseline (*f* waves) and random response of ventricular activity. Ventricular depolarization is normal if ventricular conduction follows normal pathways, which allows the QRS to have a normal configuration. Aberrant ventricular conduction may be present because of changes in repolarization that are caused by the irregular occurrence of depolarization. The ventricular rate in untreated atrial fibrillation is typically 150 to 180 beats per min (see Fig. B-24, *A*).

PATHOPHYSIOLOGY: This rhythm is believed to be the result of an altered relationship between adjacent atrial cells allowing tissues at any given moment to be in various stages of depolarization and repolarization.

SIGNS AND SYMPTOMS: A radial pulse deficit (apical rate is greater than radial rate) is typical. Variability of audible systolic blood pressure may result in erroneous pressure measurements. Patients may experience symptoms of decreased cardiac output related to the absence of atrial kick, especially when the ventricular response rate is slow.

HEMODYNAMIC CONSEQUENCES: Variance in intervals between ventricular beats allows for differences in diastolic filling and variability in arterial pressure curves. Heart sounds and peripheral pulses vary in timing and intensity. Systolic blood pressure sounds may be extremely soft between beats that are close together. In this case, care is required when the blood pressure is auscultated.

INTERVENTIONS: Management of atrial excitability includes the use of drugs such as calcium channel blocking agents, quinidine, and procainamide. Digitalis is used to decrease ventricular rate response. Electrocardioversion will disrupt chaotic atrial activity. If conversion to a regular ventricular response with a rate below 60 is observed, it may indicate development of a junctional escape rhythm resulting from digitalis toxicity–induced complete AV block. Precision is required in obtaining accurate heart rates and blood pressures because of the extreme variance in diastolic filling time. Assess patients for the development of emboli as a result of the pooling that can occur in the atria with the lack of coordinated atrial contraction. Emboli can also occur after conversion of atrial fibrillation to sinus rhythm as the atria begin to contract properly, releasing thrombi from the atrial wall.

Tachycardia-bradycardia syndrome

DESCRIPTION: Tachycardia-bradycardia syndrome develops as a result of excitation of atrial tissue and depression of impulse formation in the sinus node. Various names have been applied to this rhythm including *tachycardia-bradycardia syndrome* and *sick sinus syndrome*.

CAUSES: Ischemic and inflammatory conditions that affect the sinus node and atria are the primary causes of the tachycardia-bradycardia syndrome. Additionally, metabolic imbalance and drugs can precipitate this dysrhythmia.

ECG CHARACTERISTICS: This rhythm is characterized by alternating periods of severe sinus suppression and rapid atrial activity. The atrial component may present as atrial tachycardia, but more often atrial fibrillation is seen. The bradycardic segments are typically initiated by an extremely slow sinus rate, which may increase with subsequent beats until the rate falls within the normal range for sinus activity. However, the normal phasic variation of sinus node firing is absent (see Fig. B-24, *B*).

PATHOPHYSIOLOGY: Altered cellular function is responsible for both the atrial excitation and sinus depression.

SIGNS AND SYMPTOMS: The peripheral pulse is irregular during both the slow and the fast segments. A wide variance in blood pressure readings is typical because of this irregularity and the resultant changes in diastolic filling times. An apical-radial pulse deficit is present if the tachycardic phase is produced by atrial fibrillation. Typically the patient complains of palpitations during the tachycardic phases and may experience lightheadedness, dizziness, and visual disturbances if the bradycardic segments are extremely slow and prolonged.

HEMODYNAMIC CONSEQUENCES: The decreased height of the arterial curve reflects the typical changes seen with sinus bradycardia and atrial tachydysrhythmias. If the atrial component is fibrillation, there will be a variance in height of the curve with each complex. The intensity and timing of peripheral pulses and heart sounds will reflect the dominant rhythm.

INTERVENTIONS: Drugs indicated for atrial tachydysrhythmias, such as digitalis and quinidine, are used to treat the rapid atrial activity. An artificial cardiac pacemaker is inserted to protect against excessive slowing of the rate during the bradycardic phases.

Junctional premature complex

DESCRIPTION: A cardiac cycle occurring earlier than anticipated in which the AV junctional tissue controls atrial and ventricular depolarization through antegrade and retrograde conduction is termed *junctional premature complex*. The more appropriate term for conduction initiated in this intermediate area is *junctional,* although the term *nodal* is often used interchangeably for both escape and excitable activity.

CAUSES: Multiple factors have been implicated for producing excitable rhythms in the AV junction, including myocardial ischemic and inflammatory diseases and digitalis toxicity. Additionally, during sinus bradydysrhythmias, subsidiary pacemakers often exhibit excitation.

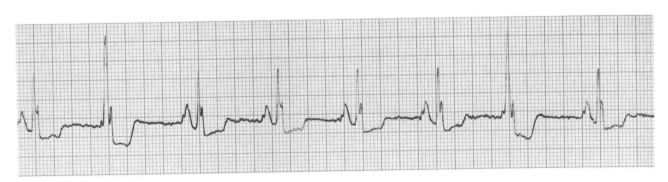

FIG. B-25 Sinus rhythm (rate, 66; PR interval, 0.16 sec; QRS interval, 0.08 sec) with junctional premature complexes at beats 2 and 7 (early cycles; no visible P wave; normal QRS configuration).

ECG CHARACTERISTICS: A premature QRS of normal configuration with an unconventional P wave that immediately precedes the QRS (PR interval is less than 0.12 sec), immediately follows the QRS (an RP relationship), or is superimposed within the QRS. The sinus cadence may be reset when retrograde conduction occurs, resulting in a noncompensatory pause after the junctional complex (see Fig. B-25).

PATHOPHYSIOLOGY: Isolated premature complexes from the junctional region are typically the result of enhanced automaticity, although reentry mechanisms may be involved.

SIGNS AND SYMPTOMS: Patients may be unaware of the junctional premature complexes, although they may complain of a strange flip-flop sensation in the chest.

HEMODYNAMIC CONSEQUENCES: The arterial curve of a junctional premature beat typically records a lower pressure because of the earlier depolarization (decreased diastolic filling time) and the absence of atrial kick (abnormal PR relationship). The degree of change in heart sounds and peripheral pulses depends on how early the junctional premature complex occurs in the cycle.

INTERVENTIONS: The primary intervention involves monitoring the frequency of the junctional premature complexes because increasing frequency may herald the development of sustained rhythm control by the junctional tissue. If the premature beats cause the patient distress, quinidine or propranolol may be used to reduce the frequency of prematurities. In the presence of congestive heart failure, digitalis may be indicated.

Accelerated junctional rhythm

DESCRIPTION: A rhythm arising from the AV junctional region that has a rate between 60 and 100 per minute is termed *accelerated junctional rhythm.*

CAUSES: Primary factors precipitating accelerated junctional rhythms are inflammatory diseases of the heart such as myocarditis and myocardial infarction, especially of the inferior wall. Patients with chronic obstructive pulmonary

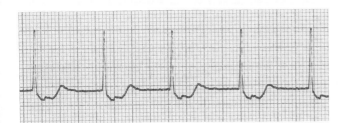

FIG. B-26 Accelerated junctional rhythm (rate, 80; no PR interval; possible RP interval, 0.12 sec; QRS interval, 0.06 sec).

disease may be susceptible to junctional acceleration. Digitalis toxicity is also often implicated.

ECG CHARACTERISTICS: Normal QRS complexes with abnormal P waves that immediately precede the QRS (PR interval is less than 0.12 sec), immediately follow the QRS (an RP interval), or are superimposed within the QRS occur at a regular rate. Retrograde conduction may be absent, resulting in AV dissociation in which the ventricular rate exceeds the rate of the sinus rhythm. Isorhythmic dissociation exists when sinus and junctional rhythms have nearly identical rates, which allow the junctional focus to assume control when the sinus node slows (see Fig. B-26).

PATHOPHYSIOLOGY: Enhanced automaticity of the AV junctional region is believed to be the usual mechanism responsible for acceleration of the depolarization rate.

SIGNS AND SYMPTOMS: Although atrial kick is lost, the patient often has no symptoms because the loss of volume per beat is compensated by the faster rate.

HEMODYNAMIC CONSEQUENCES: The arterial pressure curve may appear normal, and peripheral pulses and heart sounds exhibit no changes.

INTERVENTIONS: Care involves monitoring the patient's tolerance to the dysrhythmia, discontinuing digitalis if implicated, and administering propranolol or quinidine.

Junctional tachycardia

DESCRIPTION: In junctional tachycardia, sustained excitation in the AV junctional tissue results in a rhythm with normal ventricular conduction but altered AV sequencing, at a rate greater than 100.

CAUSES: The prime precipitators of junctional tachycardia are acute myocardial infarction, especially of the inferior wall, or a preexisting preexcitation syndrome. Junctional excitation also is a common manifestation of digitalis toxicity.

ECG CHARACTERISTICS: The QRS complexes, which have a rate greater than 100, are normal in configuration. Abnormal P waves immediately precede the QRS (PR interval is less than 0.12 sec), immediately follow the QRS (an RP interval), or are superimposed within the QRS. The cycle-to-cycle intervals are typically regular and may reach rates of 200 per min. The tachycardia has a tendency to recur in paroxysms with rapid onset and termination (see Fig. B-27).

PATHOPHYSIOLOGY: Both reentry and enhanced automaticity are implicated in the production of junctional tachycardia. The reentry circuit is typically composed of an antegrade AV nodal pathway with retrograde conduction occurring through an anomalous pathway.

SIGNS AND SYMPTOMS: The patient often complains of palpitations. Angina pectoris may be experienced by patients with coronary artery disease.

HEMODYNAMIC CONSEQUENCES: A decrease in arterial pressure is experienced because of the loss of proper AV synchrony and the decrease in filling pressure caused by the rapid rate. Peripheral pulses may be normal, but the first heart sound may be altered.

INTERVENTIONS: Suppressors of excitation and reentry, such as propranolol, verapamil, and lidocaine, are effective in converting the rhythm. Vagal stimulating maneuvers may result in conversion to sinus rhythm. In addition, electrical interventions, such as cardioversion or pacemaker overdrive, are appropriate.

Ventricular premature complex

DESCRIPTION: A premature cycle that is produced by a site within the ventricle resulting in aberrant depolarization of the ventricles without preceding atrial activation is termed *ventricular premature complex (VPC)*.

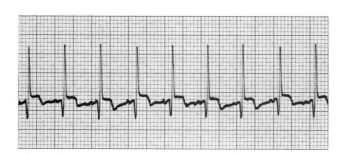

FIG. B-27 Junctional tachycardia (rate, 158; abnormal P wave configuration; PR interval, 0.06 sec; QRS interval, 0.06 sec).

CAUSES: The most common cause of ventricular premature complexes in the critical care setting is acute myocardial ischemia or infarction due to coronary artery disease. Additional conditions that can produce prematurities include hypoxia, acidosis, anesthetic agents, digitalis, adrenergic stimulation (stress, epinephrine, isoproterenol, caffeine, and nicotine), structural heart disease (mitral valve prolapse), cardiac inflammatory disease (myocarditis), cardiac trauma, disorders of the lung, metabolic derangements, and electrolyte imbalances (especially hypokalemia).

ECG CHARACTERISTICS: The primary rhythm is interrupted by an early cycle that has a wide, distorted QRS complex, altered ST segment, and T wave contour. Atrial activity does not precede the QRS complex. If retrograde conduction into the atria does not occur, a complete compensatory pause will be present (sinus rhythm cycling is not altered). In slow sinus rhythms, each P wave may be conducted, including the P wave after the premature complex. Such a premature ventricular complex is termed *interpolated*. Terms applied to ventricular premature beats that occur in patterns include *bigeminy* (every other beat is a ventricular beat), *trigeminy* (two ventricular complexes for each normal complex, although one ventricular beat for two normal complexes is erroneously called *trigeminy* as well), *doublet* or *couplet* (two ventricular beats occurring sequentially), and *triplet* (three consecutive ventricular complexes).

The waveform of premature complexes are also compared; similar configurations are called *uniform, unifocal,* or *monomorphic*. Premature ventricular beats that have dissimilar forms are referred to as *multiform, multifocal, multiphasic,* and *polymorphic*. The relationship of the premature QRS to the preceding normal complex, called the *coupling interval*, is measured to determine if a consistent interval exists. Beats with a constant, or fixed, coupling interval are felt to be more benign than premature QRS complexes

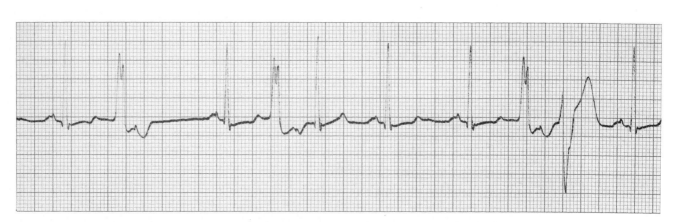

FIG. B-28 Normal sinus rhythm (rate, 75; PR interval, 0.18 sec; QRS interval, 0.10 sec) with four multiform ventricular premature complexes (beats 2, 4, 8, and 9) (variable coupling intervals; second VPC is interpolated; VPCs 3 and 4 form a couplet).

that have a variable, or unfixed, coupling interval. When an unfixed coupling interval exists, it indicates a variable relationship to the preceding beat's repolarization phase (and also its refractory period) (Fig. B-28). This concern for an unfixed relationship of ventricular premature complexes to the preceding beat is based on the increased frequency with which ventricular tachycardia is induced when a premature ventricular beat falls on the T wave of the preceding beat (R-on-T phenomenon). Occasionally patients have benign variable coupling intervals as a result of a parasystolic focus. A patient with parasystole has an automatic focus within the ventricle that will assume ventricular control at regular intervals when surrounding tissue is not in a refractory phase from the dominant pacemaker impulse. Another phenomenon, a wavefront, which is a combination of the ventricular ectopic impulse and the sinus impulse (a fusion beat), is typical in the presence of parasystole.

PATHOPHYSIOLOGY: Both enhanced automaticity and reentrance can be responsible for production of ventricular premature complexes.

SIGNS AND SYMPTOMS: The only complaint from the patient may be a thumping sensation in the chest. This sensation is not caused by the premature complex but rather by the increased volume ejected with the beat that follows the premature beat.

HEMODYNAMIC CONSEQUENCES: Arterial pressures typically show a significant decrease in the waveform with the premature complex but an enhanced height to the wave that follows the ectopic beat. The irregularity of the rhythm and the augmented ejection volume of the beat that follows the VPC may be palpated.

INTERVENTIONS: The treatment of ventricular ectopic activity depends on the cause of the excitability and the characteristics of the electrocardiogram. VPCs are treated aggressively in the following situations: frequent VPCs (greater than 6 per min), R-on-T phenomenon, multiform complexes, and triplets. In the presence of acute ischemic disease, a lidocaine bolus followed by a titrated lidocaine drip is usually initiated. If not effective, procainamide fol-

lowed by bretylium may be used. Long-term management includes the administration of a variety of drugs, often used in combination, that decrease excitability. Dilantin is indicated when digitalis toxicity is implicated. In addition, verapamil or nifedipine have been used for prematurities associated with coronary artery spasm (see Chapter 10). Correction of precipitating factors is essential.

Accelerated idioventricular rhythm

DESCRIPTION: When an area of the ventricles assumes control of ventricular depolarization at a rate greater than the intrinsic rate but less than 100 beats per min, it is termed *accelerated idioventricular rhythm.*

CAUSES: Accelerated ventricular activity in the critical care setting is most commonly the result of coronary artery disease. Additional conditions that can produce enhanced automaticity include hypoxia, acidosis, adrenergic stimulators (epinephrine and isoproterenol), structural heart disease (aneurysms, mitral valve prolapse), cardiac inflammatory disease (myocarditis), myopathies, disorders of the lung, metabolic imbalances, and electrolyte derangements.

ECG CHARACTERISTICS: Atrial and ventricular activity are completely independent. The rate of ventricular depolarization ranges between 40 and 100 per min (Fig. B-29).

PATHOPHYSIOLOGY: Ventricular excitation can result from reentrant mechanism, but more typically it is the result of enhanced automaticity.

SIGNS AND SYMPTOMS: The patient may experience symptoms of decreased cardiac output caused by the loss of atrial and ventricular sequencing. Presenting signs may be dizziness, fainting, weakness, blurred vision, gastric upset, chest pain, and congestive heart failure. However, the patient who has a rate of 60 per min or greater seldom exhibits symptoms.

HEMODYNAMIC CONSEQUENCES: Cardiac output can be severely impaired when the idioventricular rate is slow. Loss of arterial curve height reflects the independence of the ventricular activity. Peripheral pulses may feel normal. Prominent cannon *a* waves and a variance in the first heart sound may be observed because of the independence of atrial and ventricular contraction.

INTERVENTIONS: Treatment focuses on the management of the condition that has precipitated the accelerated rhythm. The administration of lidocaine is controversial and is contraindicated at rates less than 100 per min.

Ventricular tachycardia

DESCRIPTION: Repetitive beating from the ventricular tissue that assumes control of cardiac activity at a rate over 100 per min is termed *ventricular tachycardia.*

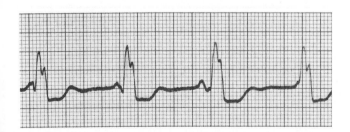

FIG. B-29 Sinus bradycardia (atrial rate, 66) with accelerated idioventricular rhythm (ventricular rate, 66; QRS, 0.14 sec) resulting in AV dissociation.

CAUSES: Multiple factors can produce sustained ventricular excitability; these include myocardial ischemia or infarction, systemic conditions resulting in acid-base imbalance, hypoxia, metabolic derangements, medications (digitalis and quinidine), electrolyte imbalance (especially extremely low potassium levels), R-on-T phenomenon, ventricular aneurysms, decreased left ventricular function, and mechanical stimulation during cardiac catheterization or endocardial pacemaker electrode insertion.

ECG CHARACTERISTICS: Ventricular complexes exhibit prolonged duration and abnormal configuration, and the ST segments and T waves are altered. The rate of ventricular depolarization surpasses 100 beats per min. Isolation of atrial and ventricular depolarization can be identified by complete independence of the two rhythms (AV dissociation). NOTE: Any broad complex tachycardia should be considered to be ventricular in origin until proved otherwise. A 12-lead electrocardiogram should be obtained if possible to assist in delineation of the ectopic focus (see Fig. B-30).

PATHOPHYSIOLOGY: Both reentrant circuits and early ventricular diastolic depolarization have been implicated in production of ventricular tachycardia.

SIGNS AND SYMPTOMS: A patient with minimal intrinsic cardiac disease may be able to tolerate extended periods of ventricular tachycardia. In addition, patients with refractory ventricular tachycardia who are receiving antidysrhythmic agents that slow the rate of tachycardia may have no symptoms. More common, poorly perfused tachycardias result in loss of consciousness or grand mal seizures, which typically develop within several seconds from the onset of the dysrhythmia.

HEMODYNAMIC CONSEQUENCES: Arterial pressure is severely compromised with the onset of ventricular tachycardia. If there is perfusion, pulses are poorly palpated, and heart sounds are muffled.

INTERVENTIONS: Cardiopulmonary resuscitation should be initiated when cardiovascular collapse occurs. Medications used to treat ventricular tachycardia include lidocaine as an emergency intervention, followed by the administration of procainamide or bretylium. Digibind is indicated in the presence of digitalis toxicity. Electrical management includes cardioversion, an antitachycardic pacemaker, and an automatic implantable cardioverter-defibrillator (see Appendix D). Specific foci can be obliterated through endocardial resection or cryothermic or laser ablation.

NOTE: An atypical ventricular tachycardia called *polymorphous tachycardia*, or *Torsade de pointes*, requires special consideration. The cause is unclear, although afterpotentials are probably responsible. It is known to be associated with the following situations: congenital Q-T prolongation, prolonged QT intervals caused by drug influence (quinidine, procainamide, disopyramide, mexiletine, amiodarone, phenothiazines), Prinzmetal's angina, electrolyte disturbances, alcoholism, hypothermia, and diffuse cerebral disturbances. The name, *Torsade de pointes*, refers to the characteristic pattern of QRS complexes appearing to twist around the isoelectric line with apices, first positive and then negative. Drug therapy includes isoproterenol (shortens the QT interval), magnesium, and propranolol (depresses excitation). Normal antidysrhythmic drugs, especially class I-a agents such as lidocaine, are not only ineffective but may worsen the situation. Cardioversion is also appropriate if the tachycardia is prolonged. In addition, an artificial cardiac pacemaker is inserted for rhythm control. However, polymorphous ventricular tachycardia is often self-limiting (see Fig. B-31).

Ventricular fibrillation

DESCRIPTION: Impulses initiated within the ventricles that are formed and scattered too rapidly to propagate in an orderly sequence causing uncoordinated ventricular contractions are termed *ventricular fibrillation*.

CAUSES: The primary cause of ventricular fibrillation is circulatory failure from a preceding episode of ventricular tachycardia. However, a single premature ventricular complex can initiate fibrillation; then it is termed *primary ventricular fibrillation*.

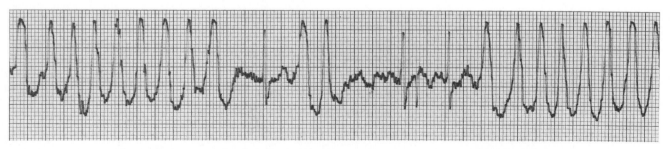

FIG. B-30 Supraventricular tachycardia (rate, 110; PR interval, 0.16 sec; QRS interval, 0.08 sec) with self-limiting runs of ventricular tachycardia (ventricular rate, 250; QRS interval varies).

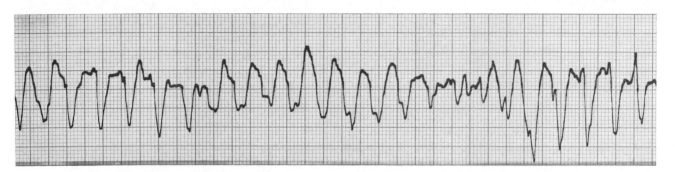

FIG. B-31 Torsade de pointes ventricular tachycardia (identified by alteration of complexes from positive to negative deflections around the baseline; ventricular rate, 180; QRS intervals greater than 0.16 sec).

ECG CHARACTERISTICS: The electrocardiogram records complete chaotic ventricular activity with no clearly identifiable QRS complexes. Often there is also no evidence of atrial depolarization (see Fig. B-32).

PATHOPHYSIOLOGY: The mechanism responsible for fibrillation is unclear, although it is thought that innumerable small portions of the ventricles are in various states of depolarization and refractoriness.

SIGNS AND SYMPTOMS: Symptoms reflect the complete absence of coordinated ventricular conduction and contraction—seizures, loss of consciousness, cyanosis, and apnea.

HEMODYNAMIC CONSEQUENCES: Ventricular fibrillation produces complete cardiovascular collapse; thus there are no heart sounds, arterial pressure curves, or peripheral pulses.

INTERVENTIONS: Cardiopulmonary resuscitation (CPR) is required until definitive therapies, including defibrillation, lidocaine, and bretylium, can be initiated. Epinephrine is administered to stimulate the myocardium to be more responsive to defibrillation. Correction of the hypoxia and acid-base imbalance that occurs in cardiac arrest often must be reversed before therapy is effective (see Appendix D).

Table B-1 delineates the dysrhythmias based on the categories of intrinsic rhythms and rhythms of increased or decreased impulse formation or conduction.

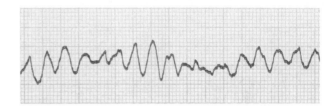

FIG. B-32 Ventricular fibrillation (no heart rate; no P waves; no QRS complexes).

REFERENCES

Benditt DG and Benson DW: Cardiac preexcitation syndrome, Boston, 1986, Martinus Nijhoff Publishing.

Benditt DG and others: Supraventricular tachycardias: mechanisms and therapies, Hosp Pract 23(8):161, 1988.

Chung EK: Manual of acute cardiac disorders, Boston, 1988, Butterworth Publishers.

Conover M: Understanding electrocardiography, St Louis, 1988, The CV Mosby Co.

Josephson ME and Wellens HJJ: Tachycardias: mechanisms, diagnosis, treatments, Philadelphia, 1984, Lea & Febiger.

Lowenstein SR and Harken AH: A wide complex look at cardiac dysrhythmias, Emerg Med 5(6):519, 1987.

Mandel WJ: Cardiac arrhythmias: their mechanisms, diagnosis, and management, Philadelphia, 1987, JB Lippincott Co.

Phillips RE and Feeney MK: The cardiac rhythms, Philadelphia, 1990, WB Saunders Co.

TABLE B-1
Summary of Dysrhythmias

Rhythm	P wave	PR interval	QRS complex	Comments	Significance
INTRINSIC AND INHERENT RHYTHMS					
Normal sinus	Precedes each QRS	0.12-0.20 sec	0.06-0.10 sec	Respiratory influence on rhythmicity of cycling	None/normal
Sinus arrhythmia	Precedes each QRS	0.12-0.20 sec	0.06-0.10 sec	Exaggerated rhythmic variance. May indicate sensitive vagal response	None/normal
Atrial escape	Precedes late QRS; aberrant configuration	May be greater than 0.20 sec	0.06-0.10 sec	Terminates a pause caused by sinus arrest, bradycardia, or block	Normal escape mechanism; indicates dysfunction of sinus node impulse formation or conduction
Junctional escape	Precedes, hidden within, or follows QRS complex; altered appearance	Shortened, not apparent, or presents as RP	0.06-0.10 sec	Terminates a pause caused by sinus arrest, bradycardia, block	Normal escape mechanism; indicates dysfunction of sinus node impulse formation or conduction
Ventricular escape	Unrelated or absent	Not applicable	Greater than 0.10 sec with aberrant configuration	Terminates a pause caused by failure of higher pacemakers or conduction	Normal escape mechanism; indicates dysfunction of sinus node or higher pacemakers or conduction
RHYTHMS OF DEPRESSION					
Sinus bradycardia	Precedes each QRS Rate less than 60	0.12-0.20 sec	0.06-0.10 sec	Not often below 40; treat with atropine, isoproterenol, pacemaker	Low cardiac output if stroke volume is limited
First-degree AV block	Precedes each QRS Sinus origin	0.21 sec or greater	0.06-0.10 sec	PR intervals can be extremely long. Observe for increased levels of block	May indicate excessive levels of drugs (especially digitalis)
Second-degree AV block	Each QRS preceded by a P wave, but some P waves are not conducted; periodic absence of QRS	Wenckebach: progressive lengthening of PR before loss of QRS; next series begins with shorter PR. Mobitz II: no alteration in PR intervals; abrupt conduction failure	0.06-0.10 sec. Usually greater than 0.12 sec	Suspect second degree block whenever "grouped beating" is observed; treat Mobitz II with atropine, isoproterenol, pacemaker; may proceed to higher degree of block	Some types may be transient after acute MI; vagal stimulation may increase frequency of block; check digitalis level
Third-degree AV block	Occur regularly, but without relationship to QRS complexes	Variable (no relationship of atria and ventricles)	Rate below 60 — usually; regular — usually; normal or prolonged and aberrant QRS	Form of AV dissociation wherein atrial rate is always greater than ventricular rate; treat with atropine, isoproterenol, and cardiac pacemaker	Syncopal episodes (Adams-Stokes syndrome), check for digitalis toxicity

	P wave/atrial activity	PR interval	QRS	Treatment	Clinical significance
Idioventricular rhythm	No atrial activity	None	0.12 sec or greater; rate less than 40	Often accompanied by mechanical dysfunction; treat with CPR, isoproterenol, pacemaker; correct cause	Indicates severely depressed myocardium (failure of normal impulse formation/conduction)

RHYTHMS OF EXCITATION

	P wave/atrial activity	PR interval	QRS	Treatment	Clinical significance
Sinus tachycardia	Precedes each QRS; Rate over 100; Respiratory variance	0.12–0.20 sec	0.06–0.10 sec	Normal response to need for increased cardiac output; treat underlying cause (anemia, anxiety, pain)	Diminished cardiac output if diastolic filling time too short; angina in presence of CAD
Atrial premature complex	Early P wave, may have distorted configuration	Greater than 0.12 sec; May be greater than 0.20 sec	0.06–0.10 sec; Normal/aberrant complex	Usually no compensatory pause; treatment usually unnecessary	Frequent APCs may forewarn of development of atrial tachycardia or fibrillation
Wandering atrial pacemaker	P waves vary in configuration; Irregular rates	Varies—usually within normal range	0.06–0.10 sec	Often asymptomatic—identified on routine ECG	May indicate extensive atrial dysfunction
Atrial tachycardia	Precedes each QRS; May be hidden in previous T wave; Rate usually over 140	Usually 0.12–0.20 sec; may be greater than normal	0.06–0.10 sec; Normal/aberrant	Produced by enhanced automaticity (irregular onset/offset) or reentrance (extremely regular); treat with digitalis; calcium blockers; vagal stimulation; overdrive pacing; cardioversion	Diastolic filling time diminished; may indicate digitalis toxicity
Atrial flutter	P replaced with saw-tooth pattern (F waves); rate usually over 300	FR interval; constant or variable; Specify atrial-to-ventricular ratio	0.06–0.10 sec; May be regular or irregular	Temporary ventricular slowing with vagal stimulation; treat with cardioversion; digitalis; quinidine; calcium channel blockers	Lack of coordinated atrial contraction; May produce congestive heart failure
Atrial fibrillation	No identifiable P waves; undulations of baseline (f waves)	No measurable PR	0.06–0.10 sec; Irregular	f waves may show better in selected leads; treat with cardioversion, digitalis; quinidine; calcium channel blockers	Often produces or results from congestive heart failure
Junctional premature complex	Precedes, hidden in, or follows QRS	Shortened, not apparent, or presents as RP interval	0.06–0.10 sec; Early—normal or aberrant	May or may not have compensatory pause; No treatment necessary	May not produce symptoms
Junctional tachycardia	Precedes, hidden in, or follows QRS; Rate over 100	Shortened, not apparent, or presents as RP interval	0.06–0.10 sec; Early—normal or aberrant	Usually an extremely regular rhythm; Treat by suppression of reentrance or automaticity; cardioversion; Accelerated rate is less than 100	Diminishes cardiac output because of rate and altered atrial to ventricular sequencing

CAD, Coronary artery disease; *COPD,* chronic obstructive pulmonary disease.

Continued.

TABLE B-1

Summary of Dysrhythmias — cont'd

RHYTHMS OF EXCITATION — cont'd

Rhythm	P wave	PR interval	QRS complex	Comments	Significance
Ventricular premature complex	Unrelated to QRS complex	Not applicable	QRS early; change in QRS and T wave appearance; usually interval is over 0.12 sec	Followed by a compensatory pause; Treatment with lidocaine or other supressor drugs	May forewarn of ventricular fibrillation Check potassium and acid-base May be normal for patient (COPD)
Ventricular tachycardia	Unrelated to ventricular complexes	Variable (AV dissociation)	Usually over 150 Aberrant configuration	Treatment: lidocaine for alert patient CPR and cardioversion for unresponsive patient Torsade de pointes — altering QRS polarity — is treated with propranolol, isoproterenol, cardioversion	Often produces syncope/loss of consciousness; check electrolytes and arterial blood gases; precedes ventricular fibrillation
Ventricular fibrillation	None	None	No well-defined complexes	No palpable pulse; no audible tones Treatment: CPR, defibrillation; lidocaine, bretylium	

APPENDIX

C

Selected Cardiovascular Drugs

Virginia Burke Karb

The following groups of cardiovascular drugs are included in this Appendix:

Analgesics (p. 708)
Antidysrhythmics (p. 711)
Antihypertensives (p. 718)
Atropine (p. 723)
β-Adrenergic blockers (p. 724)
Calcium channel blockers (p. 726)
Catecholamines and drugs for shock (p. 728)
Corticosteroids (p. 729)
Cyclosporine (p. 731)
Diuretics (p. 732)
Inotropic agents:
    Cardiac glycosides (p. 737)
    Phosphodiesterase inhibitors (p. 738)
Lipid-lowering drugs (p. 739)
Thrombolytics (p. 740)
Vasodilators (p. 741)

A standard format will be used as much as possible in presenting the material. Each group of drugs will begin with a brief narrative discussion, followed by a table listing relevant information about drugs in the group. Specific nursing considerations written as nursing prescriptions will be listed at the end.

NURSING PRESCRIPTIONS

To prevent repetition, the following nursing prescriptions should be assumed to apply as appropriate to all drugs listed in this appendix (this assumes that patients are seriously ill; modifications would be appropriate for management of chronic/stable health conditions):
• Monitor level of consciousness.
• Keep patients supine until the effects of medication can be assessed. Keep siderails up and call bell within patient's reach.
• Monitor serum electrolytes, BUN, serum creatinine, liver function tests. Reduce most drug dosages in the presence of renal impairment.
• Assess the elderly carefully. Older patients may have an exaggerated response to what would be a normal dose in younger individuals. Usually, doses are reduced in the elderly.
• Monitor intake, output, and weight.
• Assess parameters of cardiovascular functioning on a regular basis: cardiac rhythm and rate, blood pressure and pulse, heart and lung sounds, peripheral pulses, presence of edema (especially in dependent areas), jugular venous distention. See Chapters 3, 6, and 7 for more detailed guidance.
• For titrating intravenous doses based on patient response, use a microdrip intravenous set-up. Use intravenous regulators to control rate of infusion, but remember these do not replace vigilant nursing assessment. Use infusion filters as agency policy requires.
• Label all intravenous infusions carefully, and keep accurate records of drug additives to prevent inadvertent medication errors.
• Calculate dosages carefully; double-check calculations with a colleague if in doubt.
• Teach patients and families about the desired effects and common side effects of prescribed drugs; even critically ill patients can understand a simple explanation. Encourage patients to report the development of subjective or objective changes.
• Emphasize the importance of *all* prescribed therapies: all drugs, electrolyte replacements, weight loss, stopping smoking, salt restriction or other dietary changes, exercise program, relaxation techniques, support groups, and so on.

For discharge to home

• Remind patients to keep all medications out of the reach of children.
• Teach patients to keep all health care providers informed of all medications being used; this includes dentists, oral surgeons, podiatrists, nurse practitioners, and medical doctors.
• Teach patients with drug allergies or patients taking corticosteroids, anticoagulants, or other serious drugs to wear a medical identification tag or bracelet noting their allergies or chronic medications. The patient's pharmacist can assist the patient in ordering these tags.
• Emphasize to patients the importance of taking drugs as ordered, not discontinuing drugs without consultation with the physician, not sharing drugs with friends or relatives, and not self-medicating with over-the-counter drugs unless first approved by the physician. Point out to patients that the physician cannot determine the best

treatment program if the patient is erratic about following the prescribed regimen. On the other hand, the physician may be able to change drugs or dosages in response to side effects if the patient will tell the physician about new signs or symptoms.

- Review with patients what to do if a dose is missed. Patients should not double up for missed doses. A common guideline would be to take the missed dose as soon as remembered, unless within 2 hours of the next dose (for a drug ordered every 4 hours). If within 2 hours of the next dose, omit the missed dose and resume dosing with the next scheduled dose. This guideline would be 3 hours for a drug ordered every 6 hours, 4 hours for a drug ordered every 8 hours, or within 6 hours for a drug ordered every 12 hours. Specific guidelines may always be modified based on the specific health problems, drugs and doses ordered, dosing schedule, age of the patient, and ability of the patient to adhere to dosage guidelines.
- Some drugs should be taken on an empty stomach for best effect, but this often contributes to gastric irritation. Taking drugs with meals or snack will lessen gastric irritation, which may improve compliance. In addition, using mealtimes as a reminder is often a way to help patients remember prescribed drugs. Generally, encourage patients to take their drugs *consistently*, either with or without meals.

ANALGESICS

Analgesics are drugs administered to lessen or relieve pain. For the purpose of this appendix, only two groups will be discussed: aspirin and narcotic analgesics.

Acetylsalicylic acid (aspirin)

Aspirin can be classified as a nonsteroidal antiinflammatory agent. It produces analgesic, antiinflammatory, and antipyretic effects, primarily by inhibiting the synthesis and release of prostaglandins. Aspirin (but not other salicylates) also has the ability to inhibit platelet aggregation and has thus been studied for the therapeutic effect of preventing thrombosis formation.

Uses

To symptomatically treat mild-to-moderate pain, fever, inflammation, and rheumatic fever; to prevent arterial and possible venous thrombosis.

Dosage

See Table C-1.

Side effects

Most of the side effects are dose related. Tinnitus (ringing in the ears) is the most frequent sign of salicylism (mild aspirin toxicity). Hyperventilation can result from the stimulation of the respiratory center. Other side effects include hypoprothrombinemia; decreased thrombus formation, sometimes with associated gastrointestinal or cardiovascular bleeding; acid-base imbalance (usually from overdose); hypersensitivity reactions; and gastric irritation.

Nursing prescriptions

- Assess for tinnitus.
- Inspect for unexplained bleeding or bruising. Check stools for occult blood. Monitor platelet count and CBC.

TABLE C-1
Adult Dosage Guidelines for Aspirin

Use	Route	Dosage
Antipyresis, analgesia	Oral, rectal	325-650 mg (1-2 regular tablets) every 4 hr; do not exceed 4 grams daily. Rarely, higher single doses (975 mg) may be used.
	Chewing gum	454 mg (two pieces), repeated as needed, to a maximum of 3.63 grams/day. Chew pieces thoroughly for at least 15 min, then discard.
	Extended-release tablets	650 mg (1 extended-release tablet) to 1.3 grams every 8 hr, to a maximum of 3.9 grams/day. Tablet may be broken or crumbled; do not crush. Do not confuse with enteric-coated or delayed-release preparations.
Antiinflammatory	Usually oral	2.4-3.6 grams daily, administered in divided doses. May be increased to 5.4 grams daily, based on patient tolerance, response, and serum level.
Rheumatic fever	Usually oral	Initial dose: 4.9-7.8 grams/day, in divided doses every 4-6 hr. Continue dose for 1-2 weeks, then decrease to approximately 60-70 mg/kg/day for 1-6 weeks.
Antithrombosis: after TIAs	Usually oral	1.3 grams daily, in 2-4 divided doses. Do not use delayed- or extended-release forms.
Antithrombosis: after MI; with unstable angina	Usually oral	300-325 mg once daily. Doses as low as 162.5 mg (½ regular tablet) daily may be used. A dose of 325 mg every other day has been used to reduce the risk of MI in men with no history of MI. Research continues to be done; dosage recommendations may change. Do not use delayed or extended-release forms.

- Administer other anticoagulants cautiously when aspirin is being administered; monitor coagulation studies and check with physician.
- Administer oral doses with milk, snack, meals, or large volume of water (8 oz) to help lessen gastric irritation. Try switching to a different brand or film-coated, enteric-coated, or delayed-release formulations to decrease gastric irritation. Do not use the extended-release formulation for antiplatelet activity. If in doubt, consult pharmacist or physician.
- Chronic therapy may increase excretion of vitamin C and decrease blood levels of folic acid; use supplemental vitamin therapy if needed.
- Aspirin is widely used for self-medication. Instruct patients to read all drug product labels carefully because many cold remedies and other products contain aspirin. Teach patients who are to receive limited amounts of aspirin to avoid combination products that may contain aspirin. Also, trade names may be confusing; teach patients to read the list of ingredients carefully when comparing products with names like "arthritis strength" or "extra strength" to check for the amount of aspirin in each dose.
- Instruct patients to avoid the use of alcohol while on chronic aspirin therapy because both are irritating to the gastric mucosa. In some patients the combinations may contribute to an increase in gastrointestinal bleeding.
- Be wary of effervescent preparations because they may contain high levels of sodium.

Possible nursing diagnoses

Possible complication: gastric bleeding from chronic aspirin use.

Noncompliance related to gastric irritation from aspirin regimen.

Treatment of overdose

Treatment of overdose may be complicated. The problems found include acid-base and electrolyte disturbances, dehydration, hyperpyrexia, and hyperglycemia or hypoglycemia. Initially, induce emesis or perform gastric lavage (depending on patient condition), then administer activated charcoal. Care is supportive. Monitor electrolytes, blood gases, serum drug levels, and blood glucose levels.

Narcotic analgesics

Morphine is the prototype of the narcotic analgesics. Morphine is derived from opium, the sticky brown gum collected from a type of poppy. The term *narcotic* is derived from the Greek word meaning stupor; the chief characteristic of the narcotics is their ability to render the individual unreactive to pain, even though the person is conscious and the source of the pain has not been removed.

Opioid drugs act on at least three types of receptors, the mu, kappa, and sigma receptors. The *mu receptor* mediates central analgesia, euphoria, respiratory depression, and physical dependence (the classic morphine effects). The *kappa receptor* mediates spinal analgesia, miosis, sedation, and appetite regulation; it is sensitive to drugs with mixed agonist-antagonist activity. The *sigma receptor* mediates the dysphoric, hallucinogenic, and cardiac stimulant effects. Opioid drugs vary in their spectrum of activity at these three types of sites. Morphine and other opioid agonists have their main effect at the mu receptor, while buprenorphine and pentazocine exert agonist activity at the kappa and sigma receptors. The specific effects of each opioid are a result of the receptors' activity produced by the drug.

Uses

To produce analgesia. Less frequent uses include treatment of diarrhea and suppression of the cough reflex.

Dosage

See Table C-2.

Side effects

Respiratory depression; dizziness, mental clouding, sedation; rarely agitation, restlessness, delirium, and insomnia; flushing and bradycardia; visual disturbances and miosis; nausea, vomiting and constipation; urinary retention.

Nursing prescriptions

- Use of narcotics is often an appropriate patient intervention, but it should not be used to substitute for other nursing care measures: massage, distraction, deep breathing or relaxation exercises, application of heat or cold, or just being there to provide comfort to the patient.
- Monitor respiratory rate as an indicator of central nervous system (CNS) depression. If the rate is less than 12 per minute in an adult, withhold additional doses unless ventilatory support is being provided.
- Ausculate breath sounds every 2 to 4 hours. Since narcotic analgesics suppress the cough reflex, it is especially important to have patients turn, cough, and breathe deeply every 2 hours.
- Have readily available narcotic antagonists, oxygen, and resuscitation equipment in settings where narcotics are administered.
- Assess level of consciousness and mental status. Evaluate findings carefully. Restlessness may be caused by pain, hypoxia, shock, or an unusual reaction to the analgesic.
- Keep siderails up, keep a nightlight on, supervise ambulation, and discourage smoking.
- Monitor the pulse. If bradycardia develops, withhold dose and notify physician.
- Monitor pupillary response to light. The presence of pupillary constriction may indicate narcotic use when the patient is unable or unwilling to discuss drug use.

TABLE C-2
Comparison of Narcotic Analgesics

Generic name (trade name)	Equivalent analgesic dose given IM or SC (mg)	Administration/adult dosage	Comments
buprenorphine (Buprenex)	0.5	IM, IV: 0.3-0.6 mg, every 6 to 8 hr as needed	Possesses both agonist and antagonist properties. May displace opioids having only agonist activity from their receptor sites, precipitating withdrawal symptoms in patients physically dependent on those agonists.
butorphanol tartrate (Stadol)	1.5-3.5	IM: 1-4 mg every 3 to 4 hr IV: 0.5-2 mg every 3 to 4 hr	Possesses both agonist and antagonist properties. May displace opioids having only agonist activity from their receptor sites, precipitating withdrawal symptoms in patients physically dependent on those agonists. Not a controlled substance.
codeine sulfate, codeine phosphate	120	PO, IM, SC: 30-60 mg every 4 to 6 hr	
hydromorphone (Dilaudid)	1.5	PO: 2 mg every 4 to 6 hr IM, SC: 1-1.5 mg every 4 to 6 hr	
meperidine (Demerol)	75-100	PO, IM, SC, slow IV: 50-150 mg every 3 to 4 hr	
methadone (Dolophine)	7.5-10	PO, IM, SC: 2.5-10 mg, repeated every 6 hr for pain relief	Used as a replacement drug for opiate dependence or to facilitate withdrawal. Not well absorbed orally.
morphine sulfate	10	PO: 10-30 mg every 4 hr. For extended-release preparations, give total daily dose in 2 divided doses every 12 hr. IM, SC: 5-20 mg every 4 hr IV: 2.5-15 mg in 5 ml water, injected over 4 to 5 min	
nalbuphine (Nubain)	10	IM, SC, IV: 10 mg every 3 to 6 hr, maximum single dose 20 mg, and maximum daily dose 160 mg	Possesses both agonist and antagonist properties. May displace opioids having only agonist activity from their receptor site, precipitating withdrawal symptoms in patients physically dependent on those agonists. Not a controlled substance.
oxymorphone (Numorphan)	1-1.5	IM, SC: 1-1.5 mg every 6 hr IV: 0.5 mg Rectal: 5 mg every 4 to 6 hr	
pentazocine Talwin Nx Talwin Lactate	40-60	PO: 50 mg every 3 to 4 hr; maximum daily dose 600 mg IM, SC, IV: 30 mg every 3 to 4 hr; SC route is not recommended	Possesses both agonist and antagonist properties. May displace opioids having only agonist activity from their receptor sites, precipitating withdrawal symptoms in patients physically dependent on those agonists.
propoxyphene hydrochloride (Darvon, Dolene) propoxyphene napsylate (Darvon-N)	180-240 (PO only)	PO: 65 mg every 4 hr; maximum of 390 mg/day. PO: 100 mg every 4 hr; maximum of 600 mg/day.	

- Monitor intake, output, and weight. If nausea and vomiting occur, try switching to another analgesic (consult physician). If nausea occurs, it may be appropriate to administer an antiemetic concomitantly with the narcotic. Note that the peak effect of many antiemetics occurs at a different time than that of the narcotic, so often the drugs should be on different dosing schedules. Also, antiemetics may potentiate CNS depression, but they do not potentiate analgesic effects. Sedation and hypotension may be pronounced.
- Constipation may be severe. Increase fluid intake to 2500 to 3000 ml/day if not contraindicated by other health problems; increase dietary intake of fruit, fruit juices, and fiber; increase level of exercise. The use of stool softeners may be necessary.
- Urinary retention may be more pronounced in the elderly, the immobilized, and men with preexisting prostatic hypertrophy. Question patients about difficulty in voiding, pain in the bladder area, or sensations of inadequate bladder emptying when narcotic analgesics are being used. Palpate bladder for distention. Have patients void before receiving dose of analgesic.
- Caution patients to avoid the use of alcohol.
- In preparation for discharge review the action of the analgesics with the patient. If the patient is to receive a combination product (e.g., Tylox [acetaminophen and hydrocodone] or Mepergan Fortis [meperidine and promethazine]) review the actions of each drug in the compound. Warn patients to avoid other drugs that may also cause CNS depression—sleeping pills, antiemetics, antihistamines, sedatives, and so on—unless first approved by the physician.

Nursing diagnosis

High risk for altered bowel elimination: constipation related to narcotic analgesic use.

Treatment of overdose

Severe overdose, especially with narcotics administered intravenously, may result in apnea, circulatory collapse, and cardiac and respiratory arrest. Provide support as needed, especially ventilatory support. Respiratory depression produced by an opiate agonist may be treated with parenteral naloxone hydrochloride; monitor patients carefully because the naloxone may need to be repeated.

Note about addiction

The majority of patients treated with narcotic analgesics will not become addicted because their need and desire for medication will decrease as the pain lessens. *Tolerance,* however, may develop rather quickly in any person receiving an opioid for severe pain. Patients requiring continued or increasing doses of narcotic analgesics should be carefully evaluated to see if underlying physiologic or even psychologic changes are producing this need. In the rare event addiction has developed, the health care team should work together to develop an appropriate treatment plan to assist the patient in overcoming this problem.

ANTIDYSRHYTHMICS

Antidysrhythmics are drugs used for controlling cardiac dysrhythmias. These drugs have been classified according to their mechanism of action (Table C-3). The β-adrenergic blockers and the calcium channel blockers represent two classes of the antidysrhythmics but are discussed in separate sections of this appendix. The remaining drugs are discussed in the order listed in the table.

Quinidine

Quinidine, a Class IA antidysrhythmic, alters sodium ion influx and slows the rate of depolarization of cardiac cells. The excitability of cells is lowered, and conduction through cardiac tissues is slowed. Quinidine also lengthens the refractory period. Changes in the ECG include widening of the QRS and prolongation of the PR and QT intervals.

TABLE C-3
Classification of Antidysrhythmic Drugs

Generic (trade)	Class*	Comments
quinidine (Quinidex, others)	IA	
procainamide (Procan, Pronestyl, others)	IA	
disopyramide (Norpace)	IA	
lidocaine (Xylocaine)	IB	
mexiletine (Mexitil)	IB	
tocainide (Tonocard)	IB	
flecainide (Tambocor)	IC	
propafenone (Rythmol)	IC	
propranolol (Inderal)	II	Other β-adrenergic blockers would also be included in this class; they are discussed on p. 724.
bretylium (Bretylol)	III	
amiodarone (Cordarone)	III	
verapamil (Calan)	IV	Other calcium channel blockers would also be included in this class; they are discussed on p. 726.

*Class I drugs change the sodium ion influx that allows cells to depolarize. Class IA drugs slow conduction and prolong refractoriness. Class IB drugs shorten the refractory period. Class IC drugs slow conduction without changing refractoriness. Class II drugs are adrenergic blockers. Class III drugs prolong refractoriness. Class IV drugs block calcium influx.

Uses

To maintain sinus rhythm after atrial flutter or fibrillation have been converted; to control ectopic sites with premature atrial and ventricular contractions; to control paroxysmal atrial fibrillation; to treat paroxysmal ventricular tachycardia, unless associated with complete heart block. Other uses include treatment of malaria, but this will not be discussed in this appendix.

Dosage

Dosage must be individualized and based on patient's response (Table C-4).

Side effects

Side effects include dysrhythmias, especially at high doses; hypotension, especially with intravenous administration; lowered contractility; slowed conduction through the AV node and/or AV nodal block, widening of the QRS complex. Up to 40% of patients treated with quinidine develop significant side effects, especially severe gastrointestinal distress: nausea, vomiting, abdominal pain, and diarrhea; these are the most frequent reasons for discontinuing the drug. Other side effects include headache, mood changes, altered consciousness, and a variety of visual changes; rash, urticaria, and, occasionally, photosensitivity; rarely, hypoprothrombinemia, thrombocytopenia, acute hemolytic anemia, and granulomatous hepatitis; cinchonism in sensitive patients (ringing in the ears, headache, nausea, and/or changes in vision).

TABLE C-4
Adult Dosage Guidelines for Quinidine

Drug form	Dose
quinidine sulfate (Cin-Quin, Quinidex)	200-400 mg po, every 6 hr; extended-release formulations (e.g., Quinidex extentabs) should be administered every 8-12 hr
quinidine polygalacturonate (Cardioquine)	275 mg (1 tablet) every 8-12 hr or 2-3 times daily
quinidine gluconate (Quinaglute Duratabs, Duraquin, others)	324-972 mg (1-3 tablets) every 8-12 hr
quinidine gluconate IM	Initial dose: 600 mg followed by up to 400 mg every 2 hr as needed, based on evaluation of effectiveness of previous dose
quinidine gluconate IV	Dilute 800 mg (10 ml of the drug solution) in 40 ml of 5% dextrose injection; infuse at a rate of 16 mg (1 ml) per min; monitor blood pressure and ECG tracing continuously during IV infusion

Nursing prescriptions

- Monitor blood pressure, pulse, and continuous ECG tracing, especially during intravenous administration. Monitor indicators of cardiovascular functioning: intake and output, weight, heart and lung sounds, presence of edema, and jugular venous distention (see Chapters 3, 6, and 7).
- Monitor serum electrolytes because quinidine effectiveness is reduced in the presence of hypokalemia. Monitor liver function tests, complete blood count test, platelet count, and prothrombin time. Monitor serum drug levels if available.
- Oral and intramuscular routes are preferred over intravenous administration. Read labels carefully—do not confuse quinidine with quinine.
- Assess mental status regularly. Instruct patients to avoid driving or operating hazardous equipment if visual changes develop.
- Instruct patients to take doses on an empty stomach with a full glass of water 1 hour before or 2 hours after meals or snack. If gastrointestinal side effects are common, suggest that patients take doses with meals or snack. Teach patients to take drug in a consistent fashion to help ensure less fluctuation in serum drug levels.
- If photosensitivity develops, instruct patients to avoid exposure to the sun or other sources of ultraviolet light, wear a wide-brimmed hat, keep extremities covered, and use a maximum protection sunscreen on exposed skin surfaces.
- Instruct patients to report the development of right upper quadrant abdominal pain, fatigue, malaise, fever, change in the color or consistency of stools, or the development of jaundice.
- Assess for development of cinchonism (see Side Effects), and instruct patients about the symptoms of this side effect. It is recommended that a test dose of 1 tablet or 200 mg intramuscularly always precede full-dose administration to test for idiosyncrasy.
- Teach patients that extended-release tablets may be broken but should not be crushed or chewed.
- Instruct patients to report the development of a fever, sore throat, infection, unexplained bleeding or bruising (signs of possible hematologic disorders), and prolonged diarrhea because this may contribute to electrolyte imbalance.
- For missed doses (unless otherwise directed by the physician): take the missed dose as soon as remembered, if within 2 hours of the missed dose. Otherwise, omit the missed dose and resume the regular dosage schedule with the next dose. Do not double up for missed doses.

Possible nursing diagnosis

Altered nutrition: less than body requirements related to nausea, vomiting, and anorexia from quinidine therapy.

Procainamide

Also a Class IA drug, the actions of procainamide in the heart are similar to those of quinidine. Procainamide alters sodium ion influx, thereby slowing the rate of depolarization. The excitability of cells is lowered and conduction is slowed through the heart. The refractory period is lengthened, especially in the atria. Other actions include widening of the QRS and prolongation of the PR and QT intervals.

Uses

To treat ventricular tachycardia or premature ventricular contractions when lidocaine has failed; to treat paroxysmal atrial tachycardia or atrial fibrillation; to treat Wolff-Parkinson-White syndrome.

Dosage

Oral: Sustained release formulations (Procan SR; Pronestyl-SR, Procamide SR) should be used only for maintenance therapy after correct dosage with conventional tablets or capsules has been determined. For ventricular tachycardia, 1 gram loading dose, followed by 50 mg/kg/day divided into doses given every 3 hours. Omit loading dose for PVCs. For atrial fibrillation and paroxysmal atrial tachycardia, give a 1.25-gram loading dose followed by 750 mg 1 hour later, then give doses of 0.5 to 1 gram every 2 hours until dysrhythmia is controlled or toxicity requires switching to another drug. *IM*: 50 mg/kg given in divided doses every 3 to 6 hours. *IV*: Dilute before intravenous administration. Administer at a rate of 25 to 50 mg/minute. Keep patient supine and monitor ECG and blood pressure.

Side effects

Up to 60% of patients develop significant toxicity. When administered over a long time, procainamide is commonly associated with the development of a lupuslike syndrome. Signs include positive antinuclear antibody (ANA) test, arthritis, polyarthralgia, pleuritic pain, myalgia, skin lesions, and fever. Symptoms of allergic reactions include fever, rash, urticaria, agranulocytosis, pancytopenia, and nephrotic syndrome; anorexia, nausea, and vomiting; hypotension and cardiac dysrhythmias (often related to dose and route of administration); dizziness, especially in the elderly. Dizziness may also signal drug toxicity and indicate a need to evaluate the dosage.

Nursing prescriptions

- Monitor blood pressure, pulse, and continuous ECG tracing, especially during intravenous administration. Monitor indicators of cardiovascular functioning: intake and output, weight, heart and lung sounds, edema, and jugular venous distention (see Chapters 3, 6, and 7).
- Monitor serum drug levels if available. Monitor ANA test, complete blood count test, platelet count.

- Assess for development of lupuslike syndrome (see earlier discussion). Instruct patients to report the development of the symptoms listed, as well as fever, sore throat, unexplained bleeding or bruising, pallor, fatigue, or malaise because these may be signs of hematologic problems.
- Instruct patients taking sustained-release preparations to swallow the tablets whole, without crushing or chewing them.
- Instruct patients to take doses on an empty stomach with a full glass of water, 1 hour before or 2 hours after meals or snack. If gastrointestinal side effects are common, suggest that patients take doses with meals or snack. Teach patients to take drug in a consistent fashion to help insure less fluctuation in serum drug levels.
- Instruct patients to move slowly from lying to sitting or standing if hypotension is a problem. Assess elderly patients carefully for dizziness. Instruct patients to avoid driving or operating hazardous equipment if dizziness is common.
- For missed doses (unless otherwise directed by the physician), take the missed dose as soon as remembered, if within 2 hours of the missed dose (4 hours for sustained-released preparations). Otherwise, omit the missed dose and resume the regular dosage schedule with the next dose. Do not double up for missed doses.
- For best results, this drug should be taken at regular intervals around the clock. Work with patients to find an acceptable schedule for ensuring evenly spaced doses.

Possible nursing diagnosis

Possible complication: development of lupuslike syndrome related to chronic administration of procainamide.

Disopyramide

Disopyramide (Norpace) is also a Class IA antidysrhythmic and is similar to quinidine and procainamide in many ways. It slows the normally rapid depolarization of automatic cells in the heart by altering sodium ion flow across the cell membrane. This causes an increase in the action potential duration and an increase in the effective refractory period. This in turn produces a widening of various intervals on the ECG tracing, such as the QT interval. Disopyramide has little effect on α- or β-adrenergic receptors but does produce anticholinergic effects. It is a potent negative inotropic agent that diminishes myocardial contractility. Unlike quinidine and procainamide, disopyramide does not cause vasodilation, and it may set off reflex activities that increase peripheral resistance.

Uses

To treat premature ventricular contractions; to treat ventricular tachycardia (but it should not be substituted for DC cardioversion for persistent ventricular tachycardia).

Dosage

Conventional oral preparations: 100 to 150 mg every 6 hours. An alternative schedule is 300 mg as a loading dose, followed by 100 to 150 mg every 6 hours. Doses may be lower in the elderly; persons weighing less than 50 kg; or patients with hepatic or renal impairment, congestive heart failure (CHF), or cardiomyopathy. Extended-release preparations (Norpace CR): 300 mg every 12 hours.

Side effects

Side effects include precipitation of CHF or worsening of it because of the negative inotropic effects; hypotension; ECG changes—excessive widening of the QRS complex, excessive prolongation of the QT interval, bradycardia, disturbances of conduction, and asystole with toxic drug levels; anticholinergic effects in up to 40% of patients—dry mouth, urinary hesitancy, constipation, blurred vision; gastrointestinal side effects such as nausea, vomiting, bloating, anorexia; rarely, hypoglycemia; nervousness, dizziness, insomnia, fatigue, or weakness.

Nursing prescriptions

- Monitor blood pressure, pulse, and ECG tracing. Monitor indicators of cardiovascular functioning: intake and output, weight, heart and lung sounds, presence of edema, and jugular venous distention (see Chapters 3, 6, and 7).
- Monitor serum drug levels if available. Monitor serum electrolytes, serum creatinine and/or creatinine clearance, liver function tests, blood glucose levels.
- Assess for hypoglycemia. Instruct patients with diabetes to monitor blood glucose levels frequently during periods of dosage adjustment; changes in diet or insulin may be necessary.
- Teach patients to avoid the use of alcohol because this may potentiate development of hypoglycemia.
- If constipation develops, instruct patients to increase daily fluid intake to 2500 to 3000 ml (if not contraindicated by medical condition); increase dietary intake of fruit, fruit juice, and fiber and increase level of exercise as tolerated.
- If dry mouth develops, suggest that patients suck on sugarless hard candy or chew sugarless gum, suck on ice chips, and perform regular oral hygiene; but they should avoid lemon-glycerin swabs or mouthwashes that contain alcohol. Some patients may wish to try commercially available saliva substitutes.
- Assess for urinary hesitancy, difficulty in starting voiding or a sense of inadequate emptying of the bladder. Palpate bladder for distention. Suggest patients void before taking each dose of medication.
- Instruct patients to avoid driving or operating hazardous equipment if dizziness or weakness develop.
- Supervise ambulation. Keep siderails up. Discourage or, if necessary, supervise smoking. Keep nightlights on.
- If insomnia develops, work with the patient and physician to adjust dosing schedule to make the last dose of the day earlier than at bedtime.
- Teach patients to take disopyramide on an empty stomach with a full glass of water, 1 hour before or 2 hours after meals. If gastrointestinal problems are persistent, suggest patients take doses with meals or snack. Teach patients to take the drug in a consistent manner to help ensure less fluctuation in serum drug levels.
- Teach patients taking sustained-release preparations to swallow dose whole and not break, chew, or crush capsules.
- For missed doses (unless otherwise directed by the physician), teach patients to take missed dose as soon as remembered unless within 4 hr of the next dose, in which case they should skip the missed dose and resume the regular dosing schedule. Do not double up for missed doses.

Possible nursing diagnoses

Dry mucous membranes related to disopyramide side effects.

Constipation related to anticholinergic side effects of disopyramide.

Altered nutrition: less than body requirements related to chronic cardiovascular disease and anorexia as a side effect of disopyramide therapy.

Lidocaine

Like all Class I drugs, lidocaine (Xylocaine) alters sodium ion influx and thereby impairs the ability of cardiac cells to depolarize. It is relatively selective, suppressing automaticity at ectopic sites but having little effects on SA node automaticity or AV node function. Lidocaine produces minimal effects on cardiac output, arterial pressure, heart rate, or contractility, and it does not interact with adrenergic receptors. Lidocaine usually produces no changes in the ECG.

Uses

Lidocaine is used to treat ventricular dysrhythmias following myocardial infarction and to treat ventricular dysrhythmias during cardiac surgery or cardiac catheterization.

Dosage

For intravenous treatment of dysrhythmias, use only preparations marked *without preservatives* or *for cardiac dysrhythmias*. Do not use preparations containing epinephrine. Lidocaine must be diluted before intravenous administration, or a commercially prepared diluted solution should be used. Follow manufacturer's instructions or use agency dilution guidelines. Usual dilution is 1 mg/ml, although if fluid restriction is necessary, concentrations up to 8 mg/ml may be used. Administer at a rate of 1 to 4 mg/minute, with dose often titrated to patient response on the ECG tracing. Do not administer more than 300 mg in 1 hour. For emergency situations, 300 mg may be administered intramuscularly in the deltoid muscle until intravenous administration can be instituted.

Side effects

Hypotension, bradycardia, and cardiac arrest are possible. Urticaria, edema, skin lesions, or anaphylactic reactions indicate allergy. CNS side effects are dose related, with drowsiness and dizziness occurring at the upper range of normal serum concentrations. At plasma concentrations above 10 mcg/ml, confusion, coma, and seizures may occur.

Nursing prescriptions

- Patient should have continuous ECG monitoring during lidocaine therapy; monitor blood pressure.
- Monitor serum drug levels. Assess for signs of toxicity (see above).
- Question patient about previous allergic response to lidocaine before initiating therapy. Have emergency drugs and resuscitation equipment available.

Possible nursing diagnosis

High risk for dysrhythmias.

Mexiletine

Mexiletine (Mexitil) was first used as an anticonvulsant but was later found to have some antidysrhythmic properties. It is similar to lidocaine and is also classified as a Class IB drug. Mexiletine slows the sodium ion influx in cardiac tissues without involving the autonomic system. The drug shortens the duration of the action potential and shortens the effective refractory period. It does not affect the resting potential, automaticity of the sinus node, left ventricular function, systolic arterial pressure, or the QRS or QT intervals.

Uses

To treat ventricular tachycardia, either in combination with other antidysrhythmics or when lidocaine has failed. It may be as effective as lidocaine in treating ventricular ectopic activity following MI.

Dosage

200 mg, orally, every 8 hours. Increase or decrease dosage by 50- to 100-mg increments, every 2 to 3 days. Some patients may tolerate doses twice a day, while others may need doses 4 times a day.

Side effects

Side effects include possible dysrhythmias, tremors, nystagmus, diplopia, dizziness, confusion, and ataxia; gastro-intestinal distress (dyspepsia, nausea, and vomiting in up to 30% to 40% of patients); rarely, thrombocytopenia.

Nursing prescriptions

- Monitor blood pressure, pulse, and ECG tracing. Monitor indicators of cardiovascular functioning: intake and output, weight, heart and lung sounds, and presence of edema (see Chapters 3, 6, and 7).
- Monitor serum drug levels if available. Monitor CBC, platelet count.
- Monitor CNS side effects. Instruct patients to avoid driving or operating hazardous equipment if dizziness or visual changes occur; notify physician. Supervise ambulation, keep a nightlight on, and keep siderails up until effects of medication have been evaluated.
- Instruct patients to take doses with meals or snack to reduce gastric irritation.
- Inspect patients for petechiae, unexplained bruising, or bleeding.

Possible nursing diagnosis

Altered nutrition: less than body requirements related to gastrointestinal side effects of mexiletene drug therapy.

Tocainide

Tocainide (Tonocard) acts on the heart like lidocaine and is also classified as a IB antidysrhythmic. Sodium ion influx is altered, and the ability of cardiac cells to depolarize is altered. There are minimal effects on cardiac output, arterial pressure, heart rate, contractility, or ECG.

Uses

To treat ventricular dysrhythmias, including some which have not responded to quinidine, procainamide, disopyramide, or propranolol. For sustained ventricular tachy-dysrhythmias tocainide should probably be used in combination with other drugs.

Dosage

400 mg every 8 hours, orally. Dosage must be individualized to patient response.

Side effects

Dysrhythmias and cardiovascular side effects are always possible, including hypotension and bradycardia. CNS effects including lightheadedness, vertigo, paresthesias, quivering, confusion, altered mood, visual changes, or ataxia; CNS effects are usually dose related. Skin rashes are also possible.

Nursing prescriptions

- Monitor blood pressure, pulse, and ECG tracing. Monitor indicators of cardiovascular functioning: intake and

output, weight, heart and lung sounds, and presence of edema (see Chapters 3, 6 and 7).
- Assess for CNS side effects. Instruct patients to avoid driving or operating hazardous equipment if lightheadedness, vertigo, confusion, or visual changes occur, and to notify physician as these may indicate a need for dosage adjustment. Supervise ambulation, keep siderails up, and keep a nightlight on.
- Inspect patient for skin changes.
- Teach patients to take doses with meals or snack to lessen gastric irritation.

Possible nursing diagnosis

Possible complication: inability to tolerate tocainide in therapeutic doses due to intolerance of CNS effects.

Encainide

Encainide (Enkaid), the related drug flecainide, and the recently released propafenone are the Class IC antidysrhythmics. Although not identical, they are similar. Encainide alters the sodium ion influx and slows the rate of depolarization of cardiac cells. This prolongs conduction through various areas of the heart. The effect on the ECG is to prolong the QRS, QT, and other intervals.

Increased experience with this drug indicates that there is an increase in mortality associated with its use. Encainide has been withdrawn from the market.

Flecainide

Flecainide (Tambocor) is similar to encainide and is also a Class IC drug. It alters sodium ion influx, impairs the ability of the cardiac cells to depolarize, and prolongs conduction through the heart, especially in the His-Purkinje system and the ventricles.

Uses

It is used to treat ventricular dysrhythmias such as PVCs and ventricular tachycardia.

Dosage

100 mg orally every 12 hours. Dosage must be individualized. Dosage may be increased by 50 mg per dose every 4 days.

Side effects

Increased experience with this drug indicates that there may be an increase in mortality associated with its use. Flecainide use should be carefully evaluated. As with all antidysrhythmics, aggravation of dysrhythmias may develop. Changes in vision with dizziness and blurred vision may occur. Gastrointestinal side effects include nausea, metallic taste. Headache, anxiety, and ataxia may occur.

Nursing prescriptions

- Monitor blood pressure, pulse, and ECG tracing. Monitor indicators of cardiovascular functioning: intake and output, weight, heart and lung sounds, presence of edema, and jugular venous distention (see Chapters 3, 6, and 7).
- Monitor serum drug levels if available.
- Metallic taste can be very annoying. Monitor weight as an indicator of nutrition. If patient is unable to tolerate this side effect, consult physician. Remind patient not to discontinue medication without consulting physician.
- Suggest patients take ordered doses with meals or snacks to lessen gastrointestinal side effects (this probably will not decrease metallic taste).
- Instruct patients to avoid driving or operating hazardous equipment if dizziness or visual changes develop. Supervise ambulation; keep a nightlight on and siderails up.
- Taking any antidysrhythmic is very serious. With this drug, review the importance of taking the drug as ordered, of not discontinuing the drug without consultation with the physician, of not doubling up for missed doses, and of consulting the physician if new signs or symptoms develop.
- For missed doses, instruct patient to take missed dose as soon as remembered, if within 6 hours of the time it was due (assumes doses every 12 hours). Otherwise, skip the missed dose and resume the usual dosing schedule. Do not double up for missed doses.

Possible nursing diagnosis

Altered nutrition: less than body requirements related to decreased nutritional intake due to metallic taste secondary to flecainide therapy.

Propafenone

Propafenone (Rythmol) is a relatively recently developed Class IC antidysrhythmic. Like other drugs of the class, propafenone alters the sodium ion influx into myocardial cells. It decreases excitability, conduction velocity, and automaticity, with the greatest effect on the His-Purkinje system. Propafenone produces a negative inotropic effect in the heart. It has β-blocking activity equivalent to low doses of propranolol and local anesthetic activity approximately equal to that of procaine.

Uses

Propafenone is used to treat ventricular dysrhythmias, including sustained ventricular tachycardia. Because of the potential for serious side effects or mortality associated with other Class IC drugs, propafenone is not approved for other uses at this writing.

Dosage

Orally, 150 mg every 8 hours. Dose may be increased after 3 to 4 days to 225 mg every 8 hours if needed; it may be further increased after another 3 to 4 days to 300 mg every 8 hours if needed. Dosage must be individualized.

Side effects

Cardiovascular effects include new or exacerbated ventricular dysrhythmias; CHF, first, second, or third degree AV block; sinus bradycardia; and, rarely, sinus pause or sinus arrest; cardiovascular side effects may be dose related. Other side effects include angina, agranulocytosis, hypotension, joint pain, and change in taste. CNS effects include dizziness, blurred vision, headache, fatigue and weakness. Gastrointestinal effects include constipation or diarrhea, dry mouth, nausea and/or vomiting. Skin rash may occur.

Nursing prescriptions

- Monitor blood pressure, pulse, and ECG tracing. Monitor indicators of cardiovascular functioning: intake and output, weight, heart and lung sounds, presence of edema, and jugular venous distention (see Chapters 3, 6, and 7).
- Monitor serum drug levels if available.
- Instruct patients to avoid driving or operating hazardous equipment if dizziness or visual changes develop. Supervise ambulation, keep a nightlight on, and keep siderails up.
- Taking any antidysrhythmic is very serious. With this drug, review the importance of taking the drug as ordered, of not discontinuing the drug without consultation with the physician, of not doubling up for missed doses, and of consulting the physician if new signs or symptoms develop.
- For missed doses, instruct the patient to take missed dose as soon as remembered, if within 4 hours of the time it was due. Otherwise, skip the missed dose and resume the usual dosing schedule. Do not double up for missed doses.
- For dry mouth, suggest patients suck on sugarless hard candy or chew sugarless gum or suck on ice chips. Perform regular oral hygiene, but avoid mouthwashes containing alcohol because they are drying. Some patients may wish to purchase commercially available saliva substitutes; consult the pharmacist.
- Assess for constipation or diarrhea. Auscultate bowel sound. For constipation, suggest patient increase daily dietary intake of fruit, fruit juice, and fiber, increase level of exercise, and increase fluid intake to 2500 to 3000 ml per day, unless otherwise contraindicated by the medical condition.
- Altered taste can be very annoying. Monitor weight as an indicator of nutrition. If patient is unable to tolerate this side effect, consult physician. Remind patient not to discontinue medication without consulting physician.

Possible nursing diagnosis

High risk for dysrhythmias.

Propranolol

Propranolol is a Class II antidysrhythmic agent (see β-adrenergic blocking drugs, p. 724).

Bretylium

Bretylium (Bretylol) is a Class III antidysrhythmic. Its complete actions are not completely understood. It initially releases catecholamines that increase sympathetic effects, resulting in tachycardia and an increase in blood pressure. These responses diminish as peripheral adrenergic blockade predominates, resulting in hypotension. It does not prolong the PR or QT interval or the QRS complex.

Uses

Bretylium is used to treat or prevent ventricular fibrillation and to treat ventricular tachycardia in patients who do not respond to lidocaine.

Dosage

For life-threatening dysrhythmias: *Intravenous*: 5 to 10 mg/kg given undiluted (as a 5% solution) by rapid intravenous push over 1 minute. For continued suppression of dysrhythmias, continuous intravenous infusion of 1 to 2 mg/minute. *Intramuscular*: 5 to 10 mg/kg (undiluted drug) administered hourly if needed. Rotate injection sites.

Side effects

Initial side effects are temporary increases in blood pressure and possibly in the activity of ectopic pacemakers. Other dysrhythmias are always possible. Gastrointestinal effects include nausea and vomiting if administered too rapidly. CNS effects include vertigo, lightheadedness, syncope related to hypotension. Anxiety, confusion, and other psychiatric symptoms have been reported.

Nursing prescriptions

- The use of this drug is usually limited to the critical care situation. Monitor blood pressure, pulse, and continuous ECG tracing. Keep patient supine; hypotension may still be marked and will usually occur within an hour of intravenous administration.
- To lessen nausea and vomiting, slow the rate of intravenous administration.
- Keep siderails up and keep the patient supine until hypotensive effects can be evaluated and have stabilized. Do not leave patient unattended. Reorient as needed.
- Keep family informed of patient's condition.

Possible nursing diagnosis

High risk for dysrhythmias.

Amiodarone

Amiodarone (Cordarone) is the other Class III antidysrhythmic. It alters function in all cardiac tissues: it slows

SA nodal firing and AV nodal conduction time and prolongs the refractory period in the AV node, the atria, and the ventricles.

Uses

Amiodarone is used to treat refractory supraventricular or ventricular dysrhythmias. Amiodarone is not considered a first-line antidysrhythmic.

Dosage

Orally, 600 to 1200 mg, divided into three daily doses. After a week, dosage may be reduced to 200 to 600 mg, divided into three doses. Dosage must be individualized and based on the patient's response.

Side effects

Cardiovascular effects include SA node blockade, bradycardia, myocardial depression, and hypotension. Other side effects include pulmonary fibrosis or pneumonitis; tremor, headache, depression, insomnia, and hallucinations; anorexia, nausea, abdominal pain, constipation. Small corneal deposits that can impair vision may develop with long-term therapy. Crystals may be deposited in the skin, producing photosensitivity and causing a bluish tinge to the skin.

Nursing prescriptions

- Monitor pulse, blood pressure, and ECG tracing. Monitor indicators of cardiovascular function: intake and output, weight, heart and lung sounds, and presence of edema (see Chapters 3, 6, and 7).
- Assess for signs of depression: apathy, lack of interest in personal appearance, insomnia, increase or decrease in appetite.
- Assess for gastrointestinal side effects. If constipation develops, suggest patients increase fluid intake to 2500 to 3000 ml per day (if not contraindicated by the medical condition); increase dietary intake of fruit, fruit juice, and fiber; and increase level of activity.
- Warn patients about the possibility of photosensitivity. Instruct patients to avoid exposure to the sun, wear a wide-brimmed hat, keep extremities covered, and wear a maximum protection sunscreen containing zinc or titanium oxide on exposed skin surfaces.
- Warn patients about the possible skin discoloration, and instruct them to notify the physician if it begins to develop.
- Counsel patients on long-term therapy to have regular ophthalmic examinations to monitor for visual changes. Tell patients to report any subjective changes in vision.

Possible nursing diagnoses

Constipation related to chronic therapy with amiodarone.
Impaired skin integrity: photosensitivity related to chronic amiodarone therapy.

Verapamil

Verapamil is a Class IV antidysrhythmic agent (see calcium channel blocking drugs on p. 726).

ANTIHYPERTENSIVES

Treatment of hypertension is directed at lowering the blood pressure. For chronic hypertension, drug therapy is usually done through a stepped approach. *Step 1* involves encouraging weight reduction and limiting sodium intake and prescribing a diuretic (usually a thiazide) or a β-blocker. *Step 2* involves adding a sympathetic depressant or a diuretic (if not done in step 1) or giving an angiotensin-converting enzyme inhibitor with a diuretic, and a calcium channel blocker with a diuretic. *Step 3* involves adding a vasodilator or angiotensin-converting enzyme inhibitor or calcium channel blocker to the drug(s) used in step 2. *Step 4* involves substituting guanethidine for the step 2 drug. Many patients are able to achieve control before step 4 (see Chapter 8). The following groups of drugs will be discussed:

Centrally acting drugs (α_2-adrenergic agonists): clonidine, guanabenz, methyldopa.
Centrally and peripherally acting agents: rauwolfia alkaloids
Ganglionic blocking drugs: mecamylamine, trimethaphan
Neuroeffector blockers: guanadrel, guanethidine
Vasodilators: diazoxide, hydralazine, minoxidil, sodium nitroprusside
Angiotensin-converting enzyme inhibitors (ACE inhibitors): captopril, enalapril, lisinopril
α-Adrenergic blockers: phentolamine, phenoxybenzamine, prazosin, terazosin.
α-and β-adrenergic receptor antagonist: labetolol

Nursing prescriptions

- Monitor the blood pressure and pulse before the start of therapy and at regular intervals. Check the pressure in both arms and in the lying, sitting, and standing positions. For hypertensive emergencies, it may be necessary to keep the patient supine until the blood pressure is stabilized.
- Monitor intake, output, and weight.
- Encourage the patient to lose weight to ideal body weight; refer to a dietitian as needed. Some patients respond well to limiting sodium intake also.
- Encourage patients to stop smoking and limit caffeine intake.
- Some of these drugs are associated with fluid retention. Instruct patients to report weight gain in excess of 2 lb/day or 5 lb/week. Subjective signs of fluid retention include tight rings, shoes, or clothing.
- Instruct patients to avoid other drugs that may increase (e.g., sympathomimetics commonly found in cold remedies) or decrease (e.g., alcohol, barbiturates, CNS depressants) the blood pressure unless first approved by the physician.

- Review with patients the importance of continuing medications on a chronic basis. Erratic use of these medications will not produce the desired effect and may produce side effects. It is difficult for some patients to continue therapy when they do not feel symptoms associated with high blood pressure or when they experience side effects from the drugs. Encourage patients to discuss symtoms with the physician before discontinuing medications.
- Orthostatic hypotension is fairly common with antihypertensives. Symptoms include dizziness, lightheadedness, weakness, and fainting. Associated or contributing factors include long periods of standing, hot weather, hot showers or baths, ingestion of alcohol, dehydration, and exercise, especially when followed by immobility. Teach the patient to tighten calf muscles regularly while standing, or take a break to walk around frequently. Consider sitting instead of standing at work. Reduce the temperature of baths and showers. Wear support stockings; in severe cases, tailor-made waist-high stockings may be needed. Avoid the use of alcohol. Move slowly from lying to sitting. Hold on to something while moving from lying to sitting or standing. Maintain sufficient fluid intake to prevent dehydration. If hypotension is severe or persistent, consult physician: a change in drug or dose may be needed.
- Tactfully assess patients on chronic therapy for sexual dysfunction, which may cause patients to discontinue medication without notifying the physician. Question patients about changes in libido or impotence. Provide for emotional support as needed. Consult the physician about possible drug or dosage adjustments. Reinforce to patients the need to take medications as ordered for best effects.
- For intravenous treatment of hypertensive emergencies, use an infusion control device to regulate flow. Monitor the blood pressure and pulse frequently and the ECG if possible. Keep the patient supine. Raising or lowering the head of the bed may alter the blood pressure; monitor carefully. Keep siderails up. Supervise ambulation. Assess level of consciousness. Provide calm reassurance and do not leave patient unattended.

Dosage

See Table C-5.

Centrally acting drugs: clonidine, guanabenz, methyldopa

Clonidine (Catapres), guanabenz (Wytensin), and methyldopa (Aldomet) are α_2-adrenergic agonists and act as sympathetic depressants. The vasomotor center in the medulla is a major cerebral center for control of blood pressure. In the *central* nervous system, norepinephrine is the neurotransmitter for nerve tracts that ultimately decrease blood pressure. The centrally acting α_2-adrenergic agonists

prevent the reuptake of norepinephrine, so there is an increase in the CNS levels of norepinephrine. This leads to a decrease in sympathetic tone in the periphery. In the *peripheral* nervous system norepinephrine increases blood pressure.

Uses

These are used in the treatment of hypertension.

Side effects

Side effects include drowsiness, dizziness, headache, fatigue; and rarely, depression, hallucinations. Overdose may produce hypotension and bradycardia. Other side effects include constipation, which may decrease in severity with time; rashes; dry mouth, nausea, vomiting. Sodium and water retention are common with methyldopa unless a diuretic is administered concomitantly. Sexual dysfunction is possible. Methyldopa may also produce alterations in liver function tests and a positive Coomb's test.

Nursing prescriptions

- See the general guidelines for antihypertensive therapy.
- Tell patients to avoid driving or operating hazardous equipment if drowsiness or dizziness are prominent.
- Assess for constipation. Auscultate bowel sounds. Encourage patients to increase fluid intake to 2500 to 3000 ml per day (unless contraindicated by the medical condition); increase dietary intake of fruit, fruit juices, and fiber; and increase level of exercise.
- For dry mouth suggest that patients suck on sugarless hard candy or chew sugarless gum or suck on ice chips. Encourage regular oral hygiene but avoid drying mouthwashes. Some patients may wish to use a commercially available saliva substitute.
- Monitor weight. Instruct patients to monitor and record weight at home, and have them report apparent fluid retention (weight gain, tight rings, shoes, and clothing).
- For patients receiving methyldopa monitor liver function tests and Coomb's test. Instruct patients to report the development of right upper quadrant abdominal pain, fever, malaise, jaundice, and change in color or consistency of stools.
- Be alert for signs of depression: apathy, withdrawal, lack of interest in personal appearance, insomnia, change in appetite.

Possible nursing diagnosis

Constipation related to methyldopa therapy.

Rauwolfia alkaloids: reserpine, others

Rauwolfia alkaloids such as reserpine (Serpasil) deplete catecholamine stores. Since norepinephrine is the major catecholamine, this effect reduces sympathetic tone. Also, cardiac output is reduced. Depletion of catecholamine and

TABLE C-5

Adult Dosage of Selected Drugs to Treat Hypertension

Drug	Route	Dosage
CENTRALLY ACTING DRUGS		
clonidine (Catapres)	Oral	0.1 mg 2 or 3 times daily; dosage may be increased daily; maintenance doses commonly 0.2-1.2 mg daily
(Catapres-TTS)	Transdermal	1 system applied weekly; available in 100, 200, or 300 μg/day
guanabenz (Wytensin)	Oral	4 mg twice a day; may increase gradually to 32 mg twice a day or 64 mg once a day
methyldopa (Aldomet)	Oral	Initially, 250 mg 2 or 3 times/day; after 2-7 days, dose may be increased
	IV	For hypertensive emergencies: 250-500 mg in 100 ml 5% dextrose, administered over 30-60 min; maximum dose is 1 gram in 6 hr
RAUWOLFIA ALKALOIDS		
reserpine (Serpasil)	Oral	Initial dose 0.25 to 0.5 mg daily; maintenance dose 0.1-0.25 mg daily
GANGLIONIC BLOCKING DRUGS		
mecamylamine (Inversine)	Oral	Initial dose: 2.5 mg twice daily; dose may be increased by 2.5 mg every 2 days; usual maintenance dose is 25 mg/day in 2-4 divided doses
trimethaphan (Arfonad)	IV	For hypertensive emergencies: administer as a 0.1% infusion (1 mg/ml) in 5% dextrose; begin infusion at 0.5-1.0 mg/min and titrate to patient response
NEUROEFFECTOR BLOCKERS		
guanadrel (Hylorel)	Oral	5 mg twice daily, increased daily or less often; maintenance dose is 25-75 mg/day
guanethidine (Ismelin)	Oral	Initial dose is 10 mg/day; dosage may be increased every 7 days by increments of 10 mg, to a maximum daily dose of 100 mg; further increases of 25 mg/week may be made to a maximum of 300 mg
VASODILATORS		
diazoxide (Hyperstat)	IV	For hypertensive emergencies: 1-3 mg/kg to a maximum of 150 mg, administered over 30 sec; may be repeated after 5-15 min
hydralazine (Apresoline)	Oral	Initially, 10 mg 2-4 times daily; dosage may be increased by 10-25 mg daily; maximum dosage, 400 mg in 4 divided doses
minoxidil (Loniten)	Oral	5 mg once daily, increased by 5 mg twice daily after 3 days if needed; up to 40 mg/day may be given
nitroglycerin (Nitro-Bid, Nitrostat)	IV	For hypertensive emergencies: 5 μg/min; increase in 5-μg increments every 3-5 min until a clinical response is achieved, or until 20 μg/min is achieved. Consult manufacturer's insert regarding dilution; nitroglycerin migrates into some kinds of IV tubing, which affects proper dosage calculation. IV nitroglycerin requires special patient monitoring; see section on vasodilators on p. 741.
sodium nitroprusside (Nipride, Nitropress)	IV	For hypertensive emergencies: dissolve 50 mg in 250 to 1000 ml of 5% dextrose; infuse 0.5-8 μg/kg/min; solution must be protected from light and discarded after 24 hr; patients receiving IV nitroprusside require continuous monitoring
ANGIOTENSIN-CONVERTING ENZYME INHIBITORS (ACE INHIBITORS)		
captopril (Capoten)	Oral	12.5 mg three times daily; may increase up to 25 mg 3 times daily in 1-2 weeks; take doses 1 hour before meals.
enalapril (Vasotec)	Oral	Initially, 5 mg once daily; increase gradually to a maximum of 40 mg/day
	IV	For hypertensive emergencies: 1.25 mg administered over 5 min; use half that dose for patients on diuretic therapy or in renal failure
lisinopril (Prinivil, Zestril)	Oral	Initially, 10 mg once daily; increase gradually to a maximum of 40 mg/day

TABLE C-5

Adult Dosage of Selected Drugs to Treat Hypertension—cont'd

Drug	Route	Dosage
α-ADRENERGIC BLOCKERS		
phentolamine (Regitine)	IV, IM	5 mg diluted in 1 ml sterile water for injection; may be further diluted; administer IV dose over at least 1 min
phenoxybenzamine (Dibenzyline)	Oral	10 mg/day; may be increased by 10 mg every other day to a maximum dose of 60 mg/day
prazosin (Minipress)	Oral	Initially, 2-3 mg in divided doses; dosages may be increased gradually to 20-30 mg/day
terazosin (Hytrin)	Oral	1 mg/day at bedtime; may increase slowly to 5 mg if needed
α- AND β-ADRENERGIC RECEPTOR ANTAGONIST		
labetolol (Trandate)	Oral	100 mg, twice daily; maintenance doses for mild to moderate hypertension: 200-800 mg/day; for severe hypertension: 1200-2400 mg/day
	IV	For hypertensive emergencies: 20 mg or 0.25 mg/kg injected over 2 min. Additional injections of 40-80 mg may be given in 10-min intervals until blood pressure control is achieved or a total dose of 300 mg has been given; alternatively, it may be infused at a rate of 2 mg/min

serotonin stores in the CNS may contribute to mental depression and indifference.

Uses

These are used to treat hypertension and hypertensive crisis.

Side effects

Side effects include drowsiness, dizziness, depression, headaches; nightmares. Overdose may lead to hypotension, hypothermia, respiratory depression, bradycardia, excessive drowsiness, and coma. Other possible side effects are nasal congestion; sexual dysfunction; weight gain; breast engorgement; dry mouth, nausea, vomiting, diarrhea, anorexia; and bleeding.

Nursing prescriptions

- See the general guidelines for antihypertensive therapy.
- Assess for signs of depression: apathy, withdrawal, lack of interest in personal appearance, insomnia, and change in appetite.
- Caution patients to avoid driving or operating hazardous equipment if drowsiness and dizziness occur.
- For dry mouth, instruct patients to suck on sugarless candy or chew sugarless gum or suck on ice chips. Encourage regular dental hygiene. Some patients may wish to use a commercially available saliva substitute.
- Advise patients not to treat nasal congestion with over-the-counter products unless first approved by the physician.
- Monitor weight.

Possible nursing diagnosis

Dry oral mucous membranes related to drug therapy with reserpine.

Ganglionic blocking drugs: mecamylamine, trimethaphan

Ganglionic blockers such as mecamylamine (Inversine) and trimethaphan (Arfonad) inhibit the activation of the sympathetic and parasympathetic postganglionic neurons and block receptor sites for acetylcholine. The effect is to lower blood pressure by dilation of arterioles and veins. These drugs also have parasympatholytic (anticholinergic) effects, so they will produce dry mouth, blurred vision, constipation, tachycardia, and anhidrosis.

Uses

These drugs are used to treat hypertension.

Side effects

Side effects include hypotension, sedation, weakness, fatigue; anticholinergic effects (see above); sexual dysfunction and urinary retention.

Nursing prescriptions

- See the general guidelines for antihypertensive therapy.
- Warn patients to avoid driving or operating hazardous equipment if sedation is a problem.
- For constipation, instruct patients to increase fluid intake to 2500 to 3000 ml per day (if not contraindicated by medical condition); increase dietary intake of fruit, fruit juice, and fiber; and increase level of exercise.

- For dry mouth, instruct patients to suck on sugarless candy or chew sugarless gum or suck on ice chips. Encourage regular dental hygiene. Some patients may wish to use a commercially available saliva substitute.
- Assess for urinary retention. Be especially alert for this in elderly, immobilized men.
- Monitor intake, output, and weight.

Possible nursing diagnosis

Constipation related to mecamylamine therapy.

Neuroeffector blockers: guanadrel, guanethidine

Neuroeffector blockers such as guanethidine (Ismelin) and guanadrel (Hylorel) inhibit norepinephrine release and deplete norepinephrine stores. This results in a drop in blood pressure.

Uses

These are used to treat hypertension.

Side effects

Sympathetic blockade causes dizziness, weakness, lassitude, and fainting. Because parasympathetic activity is unopposed there may be a slowing of heart rate. Orthostatic hypotension is common and may be severe. Other possible side effects are diarrhea and inhibition of ejaculation. Sodium retention is common, so a diuretic is often administered concomitantly. Side effects for guanadrel are usually less severe than for guanethidine.

Nursing prescriptions

- See the general guidelines for antihypertensive therapy.
- Monitor intake, output, and weight. If diarrhea is severe or persistent, notify the physician.
- Monitor weight. Instruct patients to monitor and record weight at home and have them report apparent fluid retention as evidenced by weight gain, tight rings, shoes, or clothing.

Possible nursing diagnosis

Diarrhea related to guanethidine therapy.

Vasodilators: diazoxide, hydralazine, minoxidil, nitroglycerin, sodium nitroprusside

Vasodilators such as diazoxide (Hyperstat), hydralazine (Apresoline), and minoxidil (Loniten, Minodyl) relax arterial smooth muscle to reduce blood pressure. Nitroprusside and intravenous nitroglycerin are also vasodilators. Nitrates and nitrites are also discussed on p. 741.

Uses

These drugs are used to treat moderate to severe hypertension. Some of these drugs are used only in hypertensive emergencies.

Side effects

Side effects include hypotension, cerebral ischemia; reflex increases in heart rate and force of contraction; and anorexia, nausea, vomiting. *Diazoxide* may produce hyperglycemia, sodium and water retention, and hyperuricemia. *Hydralazine* may produce peripheral neuropathy (which can be reversed with pyridoxine therapy) and symptoms of lupus erythematosus. *Minoxidil* may produce fluid retention, pericardial effusion, ECG abnormalities (flattening of the T wave, increase in QRS peaks), and hypertrichosis. *Sodium nitroprusside* may produce disorientation, delirium, and psychotic behavior; overdosage can lead to cyanide poisoning.

Nursing prescriptions

- See the general guidelines for antihypertensive therapy.
- Monitor intake, output, and weight. Assess for fluid retention and presence of edema. Instruct patients to monitor weight and to report signs of fluid retention—weight gain, tight rings, shoes, or clothing.
- Monitor blood glucose levels, and instruct patients with diabetes to monitor blood glucose levels. Adjustments in diet or insulin may be needed.
- Assess patients taking hydralazine for symptoms of lupus: arthralgia, myalgia, dermatoses, fever, anemia, and splenomegaly. Monitor CBC.
- Treat sodium nitroprusside overdosage with amyl nitrite, followed by sodium nitrite and sodium thiosulfate (see manufacturer's instructions).

Possible nursing diagnosis

Body image disturbance related to hypertrichosis (excessive hair growth) related to minoxidil therapy.

Angiotensin-converting enzyme inhibitors (ACE inhibitors): captopril, enalapril, lisinopril

Angiotensin II, a vasoconstrictor, is formed from angiotensin I by angiotensin-converting enzyme (ACE). Inhibiting this enzyme with angiotensin-converting enzyme (ACE) inhibitors decreases the amount of angiotensin II produced, resulting in less vasoconstriction and a lowering of the blood pressure. ACE inhibitors include captopril (Capoten), enalapril (Vasotec), and lisinopril (Prinivil, Zestril).

Uses

These drugs are used to treat hypertension and congestive heart failure.

Side effects

Cardiovascular side effects are relatively rare. Possible side effects include elevated liver enzymes, hyperkalemia, proteinuria, rash, neutropenia, gastrointestinal irritation, and loss of taste.

Nursing prescriptions

- See the general guidelines for antihypertensive therapy.
- Monitor CBC, liver function tests, serum electrolytes, and urinalysis.
- Monitor intake, output, and weight. Assess for weight loss resulting from loss of taste.

Possible nursing diagnosis

Altered nutrition: less than body requirements related to loss of taste due to therapy with captopril.

α-adrenergic blocking drugs: phentolamine, phenoxybenzamine, prazosin, terazosin

Blocking the α receptors produces dilation of arterioles and veins, and this lowers blood pressure. α-adrenergic blocking drugs include phentolamine (Regitine), phenoxybenzamine (Dibenzyline), prazosin (Minipress), and terazosin (Hytrin).

Uses

These drugs are used to treat hypertensive crises, hypertension, and Raynaud's disease.

Side effects

Side effects include hypotension; dry mouth; nausea, vomiting, diarrhea; nasal congestion or stuffiness; and sexual dysfunction. *Prazosin* is associated with a "first-dose" effect: some patients react to initial therapy with marked orthostatic hypotension and fainting.

Nursing prescriptions

- See the general guidelines for antihypertensive therapy.
- Monitor intake, output, and weight. Monitor serum electrolytes.
- For dry mouth, suggest patients suck on sugarless hard candy or chew sugarless gum or suck on ice chips. Encourage regular oral hygiene but avoid drying mouthwashes. Some patients may wish to use a commercially available saliva substitute.
- Advise patients not to treat nasal congestion with over-the-counter products unless first approved by the physician.

Possible nursing diagnosis

Altered nutrition: less than body requirements related to persistent nausea and vomiting due to prazosin therapy.

α- and β-adrenergic receptor antagonist: labetolol

Labetolol (Trandate) is included with the β-adrenergic blockers, although this agent also blocks α-adrenergic activity.

ATROPINE

Atropine is the prototype muscarinic antagonist, or anticholinergic. Because atropine blocks acetylcholine, there are many effects: increased heart rate, CNS stimulation, orthostatic hypotension from ganglionic blockade, blurred vision and photophobia, dry mouth and constipation, urinary retention, bronchodilation, and flushed, dry skin. The increased heart rate is a direct result of antagonism of acetylcholine released by the vagus nerve at the SA node.

Uses

In the patient with cardiovascular disease, atropine is used to treat bradycardia. It is used to inhibit salivation and excessive secretions of the respiratory tract before surgery; to treat bronchospasm associated with asthma; to cause mydriasis and paralyze accommodation for eye examinations (administered ophthalmically); and to treat some gastric disorders.

Dosage

See Table C-6.

Side effects

CNS side effects include CNS stimulation, manifested as restlessness, irritability, disorientation, hallucinations, and delirium at toxic doses. Other side effects include orthostatic hypotension; blurred vision and photophobia; dry mouth and constipation; urinary retention; and flushed dry skin.

Nursing prescriptions

- Monitor heart rate and blood pressure.
- Assess for side effects (see earlier discussion). If used occasionally or only for resuscitation, constipation, dry mouth, and blurred vision may not be noted.
- Instruct patients with orthostatic hypotension to move slowly from lying to sitting or standing. If patients be-

TABLE C-6

Adult Dosage Guidelines for Atropine

Use	Route	Dosage
Bradycardia	IV	0.5 mg; repeat same dose at 5-min intervals if needed, to a maximum dose of 2.0 mg because this dose usually results in full vagal blockade; administer at a rate of 0.6 mg over at least 1 min
Asystole	IV, endotracheal	1.0 mg; repeat after 5 min if needed
Bronchospasm	Nebulizer	0.025 mg/kg 3 to 4 times daily
Preoperative	IM, SC	0.4 mg, 30-60 min before surgery

come dizzy, they should sit down. Avoid hot showers and prolonged periods of standing. Suggest support stockings for appropriate patients. In the hospital, keep siderails up and supervise ambulation until the patient's blood pressure is stabilized.

- For dry mouth, suggest the patient suck on ice or sugarless hard candy or chew sugarless gum. Some patients may wish to try commercially available saliva substitutes.
- Keep a record of bowel movements and auscultate bowel sounds. To help prevent constipation increase intake of fluids, especially fruit juices (if increased fluid intake is not contraindicated by other health problems); increase level of activity; and increase dietary intake of fruits and fiber.
- If blurred vision occurs, caution patient to avoid driving or operating hazardous equipment until the effects of the medication wear off.
- If photophobia develops, keep room lights dim. Instruct patient to wear sunglasses when outside in daylight.

Possible nursing diagnoses

Constipation related to chronic atropine administration.
Altered thought processes: disorientation and hallucinations related to CNS effects of atropine.
Dry oral mucous membranes related to atropine use.

Treatment of overdose

Treatment of overdose is supportive. Attach patient to ECG monitor. Induce emesis if overdose occurred because of oral ingestion and if vomiting is not contraindicated by the patient's condition. Avoid phenothiazines because they may contribute to anticholinergic effects.

β-ADRENERGIC BLOCKERS

Blocking the stimulation of the β-adrenergic receptors produces several effects in the cardiovascular system (see Table C-7). Blocking the β_1-receptors produces a decrease in heart rate and a decrease in force of contraction, which results in a decrease in blood pressure. These actions decrease the cardiac workload, which makes these drugs useful in treating hypertension and angina pectoris. Other effects of blocking β-receptor activity in the heart include decreasing the conduction velocity through the SA and AV nodes and decreasing myocardial automaticity. These actions make the β-blockers useful as adjuncts in treating some dysrhythmias. Blocking β_1-receptors also inhibits production of renin by the kidney, which in turn causes less angiotensin to be produced. This is another reason why these drugs are useful in treating hypertension. Blocking the β_2-receptors will limit the bronchiole dilation and

TABLE C-7

Adrenergic Receptors, Their Location, and the Response Produced When These Receptors Are Stimulated

Receptor	Location	Response to stimulation	Receptor	Location	Response to stimulation
α_1	Eye	Contraction of the radial muscle of the eye, producing mydriasis	β_1	Heart	Increases heart rate Increases force of contraction
	Arterioles -skin	Constriction			Increases conduction velocity
	-viscera -mucous membranes			Kidney	Release renin-->angiotensin I-->angiontensin II -->increase blood pressure
	Veins	Constriction			
	Sex organs	Contraction of uterus (female)	β_2	Arterioles -heart	Dilation
		Ejaculation (male)		-lung	
α_2	Presynaptic sympathetic neuron terminals	Inhibits further release of norepinephrine		-skeletal muscle Bronchi	Dilation
				Uterus	Relaxation
	Smooth muscles of blood vessels that determine blood pressure	Mediates vasoconstriction in response to dopamine and other catecholamines; more research is being conducted with these receptors	Dopamine	Liver Kidney	Vasodilation

A drug that *stimulates* the alpha$_1$ receptors would produce an increase in blood pressure; a drug that *blocks* stimulation of the beta$_1$ receptor might decrease the heart rate.

may compromise pulmonary function in patients with asthma. Blocking glycogenolysis and gluconeogenesis may cause problems for patients with diabetes, because it may make them prone to hypoglycemia. Because of the effects of blocking β_2-receptors, cardioselective drugs have been developed that have their effect in blocking only the β_1-receptors.

β-adrenergic blockers can be divided into two groups, nonselective and cardioselective. *Cardioselective* β-blockers block primarily the β_1-receptors of the heart, while the *nonselective* β-blockers have an effect on both the β_1 and β_2-receptors. The clinical significance of this selectivity is that nonselective agents should generally not be used in persons with a history of asthma or respiratory disease where bronchial *constriction* (i.e., blocking of bronchial dilation) may cause problems. Nonselective agents should usually not be used with patients with diabetes. Blocking glycogenolysis and gluconeogenesis may produce hypoglycemia in the patient with diabetes who depends on this process to maintain blood sugar levels.

Uses

See Table C-8.

Dosage

See Table C-9.

Side effects

Many of the side effects are obvious from study of Table C-7. Cardiovascular ones include symptoms of excessive cardiac depression, including bradycardia, shortness of breath, worsening of angina, peripheral vascular insufficiency, edema, hypotension, and heart block. Abrupt cessation of the drug may precipitate angina pectoris or lead to an MI or ventricular dysrhythmias. Other side effects include gastrointestinal irritation and impotence and decreased libido. For nonselective drugs, masking of hypoglycemia and bronchospasm may occur. Allergic reactions include skin rash, fever, sore throat, and unusual bleeding. CNS effects include dizziness, fatigue, mental depression, impaired concentration, disorientation, acute mental changes, and emotional lability. Symptoms of hypotension include dizziness, lightheadedness, weakness, and fainting. Also, for *atenolol*: CNS side effects are uncommon. *Metoprolol* may aggravate peripheral vascular insufficiency, decrease HDL cholesterol, and increase serum triglyceride levels. *Labetolol* may cause flushed face, dry mouth, and gastrointestinal disturbances; nasal congestion; increases in antinuclear antibody titer; tingling of the scalp and muscle cramps.

Nursing prescriptions

- Take the full-minute apical pulse before administering. If below 60 per minute, withhold dose and notify physician.
- Monitor the blood pressure. Monitor in lying, sitting, and standing positions.
- Monitor general indicators of cardiovascular function: intake and output, weight, heart and lung sounds, and presence of edema (see Chapters 3, 6, and 7).
- Monitor serum electrolytes, BUN, and serum glucose levels.
- Suggest that patients take doses with meals or snack to lessen gastric irritation.
- Instruct patients with diabetes to monitor blood glucose levels carefully. It may be necessary to adjust diet or insulin.
- Assess patients carefully for sexual dysfunction. Many patients are reluctant to discuss sexual difficulties, but sexual problems may cause patients to discontinue medications. Provide emotional support as needed. Remind patients not to discontinue medications without notifying physician. Remind patients to take medications as prescribed for best effect. Consult physician for changes in drug or dosage.
- Assess for signs of depression: apathy, lack of interest in personal appearance, insomnia, and change in appetite.

TABLE C-8

Uses of the β-Adrenergic Blockers

Drug	Cardio-selective	HT	AP	DYS	Other
acebutolol (Sectral)	X	X		X	
atenolol (Tenormin)	X	X	X		
betaxolol (Kerlone)	X	X			
carteolol (Cartrol)		X			
esmolol (Brevibloc)	X	X			surgical tachycardia
labetolol† (Trandate, Vescal)		X			
metoprolol (Lopressor)	X	X	X		MI
nadolol (Corgard)		X	X		
penbutolol (Levatol)		X			
pindolol (Visken)		X			
propranolol (Inderal)		X	X	X	MI, migraine, pheochromocytoma, anxiety, others
timolol (Blocadren)		X			MI, glaucoma

*HT, Hypertension; AP, angina pectoris; DYS, dysrhythmias.
†This drug blocks both α- and β-receptors.

TABLE C-9

Adult Dosages for β-Adrenergic Blockers for Selected Indications

Drug	Route	Dosage
acebutolol	Oral	For hypertension: 400 mg daily as a single dose or divided into 2 doses; maintenance is usually 200-800 mg daily; some patients may require up to 1.2 grams/day; elderly patients should not receive more than 800 mg/day
atenolol	Oral	For angina, hypertension: 50 mg once a day; after 2 weeks, dosage may be increased to 100 mg once daily if needed
	IV	Administer 5 mg by slow IV injection at a rate of 1 mg/min; can be diluted before injection; monitor blood pressure, pulse, and ECG tracing; may repeat 10 min later
betaxolol	Oral	10 mg once a day
carteolol	Oral	2.5 mg once a day
esmolol	IV	For supraventricular tachycardia: See manufacturer's instructions for correct dilution. Administer loading dose of 500 µg/kg/min for 1 min, followed by maintenance infusion of 50 µg/kg/min for 4 min. If optimum response is not obtained, repeat loading dose followed by a maintenance dose of 100 µg/kg/min. Other regimens may be used. Monitor pulse, blood pressure, and ECG tracing
labetolol	IV	For hypertensive emergencies: 20 mg by slow IV injection over 2 min; at 10-min intervals additional doses of 40-80 mg may be given. Do not exceed 300 mg. Keep patient supine and monitor blood pressure and ECG. Can be diluted for continuous IV infusion
	Oral	For hypertension, 100 mg twice daily; dosage may be increased after 2-3 days if necessary
metoprolol	Oral	For hypertension, angina pectoris: 50 mg twice daily; dosage may be increased at weekly intervals
	IV	For MI: 5 mg rapid IV injection, repeated at 2-min intervals, for a total of 3 doses. If tolerated, begin oral doses 15 min after last IV dose, 50 mg every 6 hr for 48 hr, then 100 mg twice daily. Other regimens may be used. Monitor blood pressure, pulse, and ECG during IV administration
nadolol	Oral	For hypertension, angina: 40 mg once daily; may increase dose every 3-7 days if needed
penbutolol	Oral	20 mg once a day
pindolol	Oral	For hypertension: 5 mg twice daily; gradually increase dose by 10 mg daily at 3-4 week intervals if needed
propranolol	Oral	For hypertension: 40 mg twice daily as conventional tablets; 80 mg once daily in extended-release form; increase dosage at 3-7 day intervals
		For angina: 10 to 20 mg, 3-4 times daily, or 80 mg once daily as extended-release form. Increase dose at 3-7 day intervals if needed
		For dysrhythmias: 10-30 mg 3 or 4 times daily; extended-release form not usually used
	IV	For dysrhythmias: 0.5-3 mg; may repeat after 2 min; no further doses for 4 hr. Monitor blood pressure, pulse, and ECG
timolol	Oral	For hypertension: 10 mg twice daily; increase dose by 10 mg per week if needed
		For MI: 10 mg twice daily

- Instruct patients to avoid driving or operating hazardous equipment if dizziness, lightheadedness, or disorientation develop; consult physician.
- For orthostatic hypotension, instruct patients to move slowly from lying to sitting or standing. If patients become lightheaded, they should sit down and put the head down between the knees. Hypotension is often worse in the morning and may be aggravated by long periods of standing, hot weather, hot showers or baths, ingestion of alcohol, and exercise.
- Because these drugs should not be discontinued suddenly, review with patients the importance of taking drugs as ordered. Unreliable patients may not be good candidates for therapy with β-adrenergic blocking drugs.
- Many of these drugs cross the placenta and/or are excreted in breast milk. Women of childbearing age may wish to use some form of birth control while taking these drugs. Counsel and teach women as needed. Women who do become pregnant should see the physician immediately.

Possible nursing diagnoses

Sexual dysfunction related to drug therapy with a β-adrenergic blocker.

Altered cerebral tissue perfusion: orthostatic hypotension related to drug therapy with β-adrenergic blocker.

CALCIUM CHANNEL BLOCKERS

Calcium channel blocking drugs are used in the treatment of angina, certain dysrhythmias, and hypertension. As the name would indicate, the drugs interfere with influx of calcium through specific channels on cell surfaces. Calcium activates the contractile mechanisms and must be removed for relaxation. By interfering with the entrance of calcium they cause relaxation of the muscle. Calcium channel blockers also decrease tissue oxygen requirements in the heart, and this makes them effective in treating angina. They reduce peripheral vascular resistance through vasodilation, which decreases the workload of the heart. They dilate coronary arteries by decreasing the contractility of the coronary smooth muscle, which makes them especially useful for variant angina. Calcium channel blockers also reduce myocardial contractility, which decreases the oxygen demands of the heart.

Specific drugs vary in their ability to induce coronary vasodilation versus decrease myocardial contractility. The drugs may affect AV node function and may slow conduction from ectopic pacemakers in the heart.

Uses

These drugs are used to treat angina pectoris, especially from coronary artery spasm; paroxysmal supraventricular tachycardias; hypertension.

Dosage

See Table C-10.

Side effects

Side effects include dizziness or lightheadedness; hypotension, bradycardia, or asystole, although these are usually seen with excessive doses; edema secondary to peripheral vasodilation; gastrointestinal disturbances; liver damage; rarely, bleeding and tender or swollen gums.

Nursing prescriptions

- Monitor pulse and blood pressure. When giving intravenously, monitor ECG tracing. Assess indicators of cardiovascular functioning: auscultate heart and lung sounds, monitor intake, output, and weight. Inspect for development of edema (see Chapters 3, 6, and 7).
- Be alert for bradycardia, especially if the patient is receiving other medications that also may cause bradycardia.
- Teach patients to take doses with meals or snack to lessen gastric irritation. Tell patients to take drugs consistently, either with meals or snack or without.
- If constipation develops, instruct the patient to maintain a fluid intake of 2500 to 3000 ml per day (unless contraindicated by the medical condition); increase dietary intake of fruit, fruit juice, and fiber; and increase level of exercise.
- If a dose is missed, tell patients to take the dose as soon as remembered unless within 2 hours of the next scheduled dose, in which case the forgotten dose should be omitted and the dosing schedule resumed with the next dose. Teach patients not to double up for missed doses.

TABLE C-10
Adult Dosages of Various Calcium Channel Blockers

Drug	Route	Dose
diltiazem (Cardizem)	Oral	For Prinzmetal variant angina or chronic stable angina, 30 mg every 6 hr; increase dose every 1-2 days, based on patient response; optimal dosage is often 180-240 mg/day For hypertension: 60-120 mg as the extended-release capsule (Cardizem SR) twice daily
nifedipine (Procardia)	Oral	For Prinzmetal variant angina or chronic stable angina: 10 mg 3 times daily (in the conventional liquid-filled tablet); increase if needed over 1-2 weeks to 20-30 mg 3 times daily. Doses exceeding 30 mg at one time or a total daily dose of 180 mg are not recommended. Alternatively, the extended-release formula at a dose of 30-60 mg once daily may be used. For hypertension: 30-60 mg once daily as the extended-release tablet (Procardia XL)
verapamil (Calan, Isoptin)	Oral	For Prinzmetal variant angina or chronic stable angina: 80 mg every 6-8 hr, increased as needed; usual dosages range from 240-320 mg/day
	IV	For dysrhythmias: 5-10 mg as a bolus, given over 2 min; after 30 min an additional 10 mg (0.15 mg/kg) may be given; doses may be lower or given more slowly in the elderly For hypertension: 80 mg 3 times daily; alternatively, 240 mg as the extended-release tablet (Calan SR, Isoptin SR), once daily

- Tell patients taking extended release forms (e.g., Calan SR, Cardizem SR), to swallow the dose whole, without breaking, crushing, or chewing. If scored, the medicine may be broken in half.
- Monitor liver function tests. Instruct patients to report the development of right upper quadrant abdominal pain, jaundice, fever, malaise, and change in color or consistency of stools.
- Postural hypotension may develop; it is discussed in this appendix in the section about antihypertensives, p. 718.
- Inspect gums for swelling or bleeding. Encourage regular oral hygiene and dental care if possible.

- Instruct selected patients to monitor their pulse and/or weight at home.

Possible nursing diagnosis

Possible complication: liver damage.

CATECHOLAMINES AND DRUGS FOR SHOCK

The sympathomimetic drugs stimulate the sympathetic nervous system. If they stimulate the α-receptors (see Table C-7), they will usually increase blood pressure, so they are often used to treat shock or severe hypotension. Drugs that stimulate β_1-receptors stimulate cardiac function and increase the force of contraction, which increases cardiac output and blood flow to body organs. Other β_1-effects include increasing heart rate and cardiac excitability. Stimulation of β_2-receptors relaxes smooth muscle in several

TABLE C-11
Selected Sympathomimetic Drugs, Adrenergic Receptor Site Stimulated, and Major Therapeutic Indications for Use

	Receptors stimulated					
	α		β		Dopaminergic	Indications
	1	2	1	2		
dobutamine (Dobutrex)			X			Cardiogenic shock, severe congestive heart failure (CHF)
dopamine (Dopastat, Intropin)			X		X	Shock
ephedrine	X	X	X	X		Shock, hypotension, nasal congestion, and as a bronchodilator
epinephrine (Adrenalin)	X	X	X	X		Assist in treatment of cardiac arrest, anaphylactic shock, as a bronchodilator, to prolong the effects of local anesthesia
isoproterenol (Isuprel)			X	X		Bronchospasm, shock, cardiac arrest
mephentermine (Wyamine)	X	X	X	X		Hypotension, shock
metaraminol (Aramine)	X	X	X			Hypotension, shock
norepinephrine (Levophed)	X	X	X			Hypotension, shock
phenylephrine (Neo-synephrine)	X					Hypotension, shock

TABLE C-12
Adult Dosages of Selected Sympathomimetics

Drug	Route	Dosage
		To treat shock use an infusion control device to accurately titrate dose. Monitor central venous or pulmonary artery wedge pressure and cardiac output whenever possible. Dilute for infusion as directed by manufacturer or as agency policy prescribes
dobutamine	IV	2.5-10 μg/kg/min
dopamine	IV	Initially, 1-5 μg/kg/min; increase in increments of 1-4 μg/kg/min every 10 to 30 min until desired response is obtained
ephedrine	IV, IM	For shock, hypotension: 25 mg, 1 to 4 times daily
epinephrine	IV, Intracardiac	To reverse cardiac arrest: 0.5-1.0 mg (0.5-1.0 ml of 1:1000 solution or 1-10 ml of a 1:10,000 solution)
	ET	To reverse cardiac arrest: 1 mg (10 ml of a 1:10,000 solution)
	IM, SC	To treat severe anaphylactic reactions: 0.1-0.5 mg (0.1-0.5 ml of a 1:1000 injection)
isoproterenol	IV	For shock: 0.5-5 μg (0.25-2.5 ml of a 1:500,000 dilution) per min
mephentermine	IV	For hypotension: 30 to 45 mg as a single injection or as an infusion of a 0.1% solution in 5% dextose
metaraminol	IV	For hypotension: 15-100 mg in 500 ml sodium chloride or 5% dextrose, with infusion adjusted to maintain blood pressure
norepinephrine	IV	For hypotension: 2-3 ml/min of a 0.4 mg/100 ml solution; titrate to patient response
phenylephrine	IV	For severe shock: dilute 10 mg in 500 ml 5% dextrose or 0.9% sodium chloride; begin infusion at 100-180 drops per min, and titrate to patient response

tissues; drugs in this group are used to treat asthma or to inhibit uterine contractions in preterm labor. Dopaminergic receptors are found primarily in the kidney. Stimulation of these receptors dilates the renal blood vessels, improving blood flow through the kidney. This is a desirable effect in treating shock (Table C-11).

Dosage

See Table C-12.

Uses and side effects

Stimulation of α_1-receptors is useful in stopping bleeding through vasoconstriction; treating nasal congestion through vasoconstriction of blood vessels in the nasal mucosa; and prolonging the effects of local anesthetics through vasoconstriction, which slows the blood flow to the area. Mydriasis is helpful for eye examinations and eye surgery. Blood pressure may be increased through vasoconstriction, but α_1-stimulation is usually used in conjunction with fluid and/or blood replacement and other therapies. Side effects of α_1-stimulation include hypertension, reflex bradycardia, and tissue necrosis if these agents extravasate into surrounding tissues. Stimulation of α_2-receptors is not significant for treatment of shock and hypotension.

Stimulation of β_1-receptors is helpful in treating shock and heart failure through the actions of increasing heart rate, increasing force of contraction, and increasing cardiac output. Intracardiac epinephrine is also used to stimulate the heart during cardiac arrest. Side effects of β_1-stimulation include tachycardia, dysrhythmias, and stimulation of anginal attacks.

Stimulation of β_2-receptors is useful in treating asthma and other conditions characterized by bronchospasm and in delaying premature labor. A significant side effect of β_2-stimulation is hyperglycemia. Stimulation of dopaminergic receptors produces vasodilation of blood vessels in the kidney. This action is useful in treating shock, in which a major toxicity may be renal failure due to inadequate blood flow to the kidneys.

Nursing prescriptions

(Discussion of these drugs administered via inhalation for treatment of asthma is not included in this appendix.)

- Monitor blood pressure, pulse, ECG tracing, and central venous pressure or pulmonary artery wedge pressure and cardiac output when administering these drugs intravenously.
- Monitor intake and output and daily weight.
- CNS effects of anxiety, fear, apprehension, and palpitations may be related to the drug in use, or to air hunger and the general shock process. Assess the respiratory system, listen to lung sounds. Provide calm reassurance to patients. Do not leave patients unattended. Keep siderails up.

- Inspect intravenous infusion sites carefully. Change sites if signs of extravasation develop, or the infusion rate slows without explanation. Because extravasation may result in severe vasoconstriction with tissue necrosis and sloughing, notify physician immediately of extravasation. Follow agency protocol. A typical protocol is outlined: following extravasation with dopamine (Dopastat, Intropin) or norepinephrine (Levophed), infiltrate the area with a subcutaneous injection of 5 to 10 mg of phentolamine diluted in 10 to 15 ml of normal saline solution. Some may be injected via the infiltrated intravenous system, then the intravenous system is removed.
- Read labels carefully. These drugs must often be further diluted for safe administration. Also, not all solutions are safe for intravenous use.
- Keep the patient and family informed of the patient's condition.

Possible nursing diagnoses

Possible complication: dysrhythmias.
Possible complication: hyperglycemia.
Possible complication: renal failure.
Possible complication: hypertension.

CORTICOSTEROIDS

Adrenocorticosteroids are administered for two major purposes: to replace steroids not being made by the body, as might occur following adrenalectomy or removal of the pituitary gland, or for their immunosuppressive and antiinflammatory activity. When given to replace naturally occurring steroids, the doses are generally low, and the side effects minimal to moderate. When given on a chronic basis for the antiinflammatory effect, the doses are higher and the effects more serious and widespread throughout the body.

The effects of the adrenocorticosteroids can be divided into *mineralocorticoid* effects: sodium and fluid retention with potassium loss; and *glucocorticoid* effects: protein catabolism, increasing gluconeogenesis, antiinflammatory effects, and suppression of the immune system. All adrenocorticosteroids have both glucocorticoid and mineralocorticoid effects, but they vary in the relative amount (Table C-13). When given on a chronic basis, the steroids suppress the patient's own adrenal steroids. If they are abruptly discontinued after chronic administration, the patient may not be able to produce sufficient steroids and may manifest adrenocortical insufficiency. For this reason the steroid dose is usually tapered when discontinuing the drug, to allow the patient's adrenal gland to begin producing steroids in sufficient quantities. In some patients, chronic steroid administration has occurred for so long that the patient's own adrenal glands are never able to produce steroids again, and the patient must remain on at least physiologic doses of steroid forever (see Chapter 18).

TABLE C-13

Adult Dosage and Sodium-Retaining and Antiinflammatory Properties of Selected Steroids

Drug	Activity relative to hydrocortisone*		Route	Dose
	Antiinflammatory	Sodium-retaining		
cortisone (Cortone)	0.8	0.9	Oral	25-300 mg daily
			IM	25-300 mg/day, divided into 2 equal doses
dexamethasone (Decadron)	30.0	0	Oral	0.75-9 mg/day, divided into 2-4 doses
			IV	Dexamethasone sodium phosphate: 0.5-24 mg/day; up to 40 mg every 2-6 hours may be given for massive shock
			IM	Dexamethasone acetate: 8-16 mg repeated every 1-3 weeks. Dexamethasone sodium phosphate: 0.5-24 mg/day
fludrocortisone (Florinef)	±1.0	±100	Oral	0.5 to 2 mg/day. This drug has strong mineralocorticoid activity and is not used alone when antiinflammatory effects are needed
hydrocortisone (Cortef, others)	1.0	1.0	Oral	10-320 mg/day in divided doses
			IM, IV	Hydrocortisone sodium phosphate: 15-240 mg/day as an IV infusion or by injections every 12 hr
				Hydrocortisone sodium succinate: 100 mg-8 gram/day, given as 100-500 mg doses every 2-10 hours
methylprednisolone (Medrol)	5.0	0	Oral	2-60 mg/day in divided doses
			IM, IV	Methylprednisolone sodium succinate: 10 mg-1.5 gram or higher; usual doses of 10-250 mg repeated up to 6 times daily
			IM	Methylprednisolone acetate: 10-80 mg
prednisolone (Cortalone, others)	4.0	0.8	Oral	5-60 mg/day, divided into 2-4 doses
			IV	Prednisolone sodium phosphate: 4-60 mg/day
			IM	Prednisolone acetate or prednisolone sodium phosphate: 4-60 mg daily, divided into 2 doses
				Combined suspension of prednisolone sodium phosphate and acetate: 0.25-1 ml of suspension (20-80 mg acetate and 5-20 mg phosphate forms)
prednisone (Deltasone)	3.5	0.8	Oral	5-60 mg/day in divided doses

*By custom, hydrocortisone is assigned a relative potency of 1.0 for both antiinflammatory activity and associated sodium retention. Study of the table indicates, for example, that cortisone is slightly less strong than hydrocortisone in both antiinflammatory effects and sodium retaining properties. Dexamethasone is 30 times stronger as an antiinflammatory agent, with essentially no associated sodium retention. These effects are dose related also, but the greater the antiinflammatory effect, the greater the potential for susceptibility to infection. The greater the sodium retention, the greater the possibility of fluid retention and electrolyte imbalance.

Uses

Steroids are administered for many reasons, a few of which include adrenocortical insufficiency, allergic states, collagen diseases, following organ transplant to maintain immunosuppression to help prevent tissue rejection, and for respiratory diseases. Topical, inhalation, ophthalmic, and otic uses for steroids will not be discussed in this appendix.

Dosage

See Table C-13.

Side effects

See Table C-14.

Nursing prescriptions

• Monitor blood pressure, pulse, intake, output, and weight. Inspect for development of edema. Monitor serum electrolytes, blood glucose levels, CBC, and platelets.

• Review side effects with patients and families (Table C-14). With short-term use (7 to 10 days), side effects may be minimal. With chronic use, side effects will usually develop.

• Take oral doses with meals or snack to lessen gastric irritation. Some physician prescribe antacids or H_2 receptor antagonists prophylactically to lessen the risk of ulceration.

TABLE C-14

Summary of Major Drug Actions and Toxic Reaction to Long-Term Glucocorticoid Activity at Pharmacologic Doses

Action	Toxic reaction
Gluconeogenesis	Impaired glucose tolerance and/or hyperglycemia
Stimulation of lipid synthesis	Fat deposition on trunk; produces the classic Cushingoid appearance (moon face); increases in plasma triglyceride levels
Stimulation of protein breakdown	Muscle weakness or wasting; delayed bone healing
Direct irritation and protein-wasting	Peptic ulceration of intestinal perforation
? lipid metabolism	Pancreatitis
Inhibition of growth hormone	Growth inhibition in children
Effects on calcium metabolism-->increased bone resorption	Osteoporosis or bone fractures
Varying degress of mineralocorticoid activity	Sodium retention and potassium loss
Inhibition of the immune system	Increased susceptibility to infection
Interference with normal aqueous outflow from the eye	Glaucoma
?	Mood changes or psychoses
	Cataracts

Other side effects include euphoria, vertigo. Fluid retention may contribute to development of congestive heart failure. Thrombocytopenia may develop. Also included are anorexia, constipation, nausea; acne, atrophy of the skin, bruising, ecchymoses, hirsutism, petechiae, striae. Allergic reactions are possible but uncommon. Amenorrhea or menstrual difficulties may occur in women; decreased sperm counts and motility may occur in men.

- Instruct patient to notify physician if stools become tarry in appearance or patient has "coffee ground" emesis. Check stools and vomitus for occult blood.
- If constipation occurs, instruct the patient to increase daily fluid intake to 2500 to 3000 ml (if not contraindicated by the medical condition); to increase dietary intake of fruit, fruit juice, and fiber; and to increase daily exercise.
- If weight gain is excessive, counsel about weight reduction diets; consult physician about a change in drug or dose. Other dietary modifications that may be necessary include decreasing sodium intake and increasing potassium intake; monitor serum electrolytes.
- Avoid rough handling of patients to prevent irritation and bruising of fragile skin and possible fractures of bones.

- Warn patients on long-term therapy to take doses every day as ordered, even if sick. Failure to take ordered doses, even for a few days, may result in adrenocortical insufficiency in susceptible patients.
- Teach patients not to have immunizations while taking steroids unless approved by the physician.
- Encourage patients on long-term therapy to wear a medical identification tag or bracelet.
- Instruct patients to avoid friends and associates with infections. Teach patients to notify the physician of fever, cough, sore throat, malaise, and injuries that do not heal.
- Monitor blood glucose levels. Warn patients with diabetes to monitor blood glucose levels. A change in diet or insulin may be needed.
- Instruct women to keep a record of menstrual periods. Counsel about birth control if appropriate. Caution patients to notify the physician if pregnancy is suspected.

Possible nursing diagnoses

Body image disturbance: acne (or weight gain/Cushingoid appearance or hirsutism) related to chronic steroid therapy.

Impaired skin integrity: bruising and tearing of skin related to chronic steroid therapy.

Altered protection and high risk for infection related to steroid (and immunosuppressant) therapy (see Chapter 18).

Altered electrolyte balance.

CYCLOSPORINE

Cyclosporine inhibits cell-mediated immune reactions, such as those involved in transplant rejection. The drug appears to inhibit T-lymphocytes, especially T-helper cells (see Chapter 18). It is not clear whether the drug affects B-lymphocytes. Unlike other immunosuppressive agents, cyclosporine is not myelosuppressive, so bone marrow function is retained and blood counts are not significantly altered in most patients.

Uses

Cyclosporine is used to prevent rejection of kidney, liver, heart, or bone marrow transplantation. Corticosteroids are usually administered concomitantly.

Drug administration

Measure oral doses carefully, using the graduated pipette provided. Dilute measured dose with milk, chocolate milk, or orange juice to increase palatability. Do not use a styrofoam container. Administer diluted solution immediately. See manufacturer's insert for further directions. Limit intravenous use to patients who cannot take oral doses because there is a risk of anaphylaxis. Drug concentrate for injection must be diluted before intravenous use.

Dosage

Dosage is based on serum drug levels and serum creatinine concentrations. Review manufacturer's guidelines. The usual initial oral dose in 15 mg/kg (range is 14 to 18 mg/kg) administered 4 to 12 hr before transplantation. The same dose is administered after surgery as a single daily dose for 1 to 2 weeks and is then tapered by 5% per week over several weeks to a maintenance dose of 5 to 10 mg/kg daily.

Side effects

The most significant side effect, observed in over 30% of patients, is nephrotoxicity. Increased BUN and serum creatinine appear to be dose related; clinical symptoms may include fluid retention, dependent edema, and electrolyte disturbances. Other side effects reported frequently include hypertension, tremor, seizures, headache, and other CNS effects, hirsutism, and gingival hyperplasia. Side effects reported less often include hepatotoxicity, anorexia, nausea, vomiting, diarrhea, leukopenia, anemia, thrombocytopenia, infectious complications, and hyperlipidemias. As the use of this drug in heart transplants increases, more information about the frequency and severity of side effects will become available.

Nursing prescriptions

- Have available drugs, equipment, and personnel to treat acute allergic reactions when administering this drug intravenous.
- While immunosuppression is not prominent when cyclosporine is administered alone, the patient may be susceptible to infection when cyclosporine and corticosteroids are administered concomitantly. Instruct patients to avoid contact with individuals who are sick or have infections and to avoid large crowds. Instruct patient to notify physician if fever, malaise, sore throat, or symptoms of infection develop.
- Instruct patients to avoid having any immunizations or vaccines unless first approved by the physician. Also, patients should avoid close contact with individuals who have just received the oral polio vaccine.
- Monitor CBC, serum electrolytes, BUN, creatinine clearance, bilirubin, and liver function tests.
- Monitor weight and blood pressure.
- Gingival hyperplasia may occur. When possible, encourage patients to have necessary dental care completed before starting drug therapy. Encourage regular dental examinations and teeth cleaning. Review components of good dental hygiene—regular brushing and flossing.
- Review the correct technique of drug administration with patients, and have patients give return demonstration (see drug administration, earlier, and manufacturer's instructions).
- Instruct patients to avoid getting pregnant or breast feeding while taking cyclosporine unless first approved by the physician. Instruct in methods of birth control as necessary.
- Teach patients to report the development of any new sign or symptom.

Possible nursing diagnoses

Altered oral mucous membranes (gingival hyperplasia) related to chronic cyclosporine use.

Altered protection and high risk for infections related to concomitant administration of cyclosporine and corticosteroids (see Chapter 18).

Treatment of overdose

If overdose occurs following oral ingestion, empty the stomach through emesis or gastric lavage, depending on the patient's condition. Provide supportive care as indicated. Hemodialysis and charcoal hemoperfusion are not useful. Withhold further doses until the patient's condition is stabilized.

DIURETICS

Diuretics increase the elimination of water and electrolytes through the kidneys. There are several different mechanisms for this increased water elimination. The *carbonic anhydrase inhibitors* increase sodium ion excretion by increasing elimination of bicarbonate ions. *Loop diuretics* block reabsorption of chloride and associated sodium ions, increasing salt excretion. The loop diuretics are widely used in clinical practice to treat hypertension, heart failure, and pulmonary edema. *Thiazide and thiazide-like* diuretics also block reabsorption of chloride and sodium but in a different part of the neuron than the loop diuretics. *Potassium-sparing* diuretics block the pump that exchanges sodium for potassium in a portion of the nephron. This results in an increase in sodium excretion. *Osmotic diuretics* produce a urine with a high osmotic strength so that water is excreted as it enters the tubule to dilute the urine. Osmotic diuretics will not be discussed in this appendix because their primary uses are in treating excessive intraocular or intracranial pressure.

There are many combination products available combining a diuretic with one or more other drugs. For example, Dyazide combines a potassium-wasting diuretic with a potassium-sparing diuretic (hydrochlorothiazide with triamterene), and Ser-Ap-Es combines hydrochlorothiazide with reserpine and hydralazine. It is important to read labels carefully and to learn to recognize these drugs by their generic names.

Uses

See Table C-15.

Dosages

See Table C-15.

TABLE C-15

Adult Dosages of Representative Diuretics

Drug	Use	Route	Dose
CARBONIC ANHYDRASE INHIBITOR			
acetazolamide (Diamox, Dazamide)	Intermittent diuresis	Oral	5 mg/kg daily as a single dose for 2 days, followed by 1 day without the drug. Not good for long-term use because the drug produces metabolic acidosis, which limits the continued effectiveness of the drug
LOOP DIURETICS			
bumetanide (Bumex)	Reduce edema associated with CHF, hepatic disease, renal disease; hypertension	IV, IM	0.5-1 mg, followed by repeated doses as needed each 2-3 hr; maximum daily dose is 10 mg
		Oral	0.5-2 mg daily as a single dose or divided into 2 equal doses
ethacrynic acid (Edecrin)	Same as bumetanide	IV	50 mg, or 0.5-1 mg/kg; up to 100 mg may be administered if required; dose may be repeated in 2-4 hr
		Oral	50 mg once a day; increase dose in 25-50 mg increments per day to achieve desired effect; daily dose should not exceed 400 mg
furosemide (Lasix)	Pulmonary edema	IV	40 mg, followed an hour later with 80 mg
	Hypertensive crisis	IV	100-200 mg have been used
	Edema	IV, IM	20-40 mg as a single injection; repeat if needed in hours; dosage increments made 20 mg at a time
		Oral	20-80 mg, once in the morning; dosage is increased 20-40 mg at 6-8 hr intervals if needed
	Hypertension	Oral	40 mg twice a day
POTASSIUM-SPARING DIURETICS			
amiloride (Midamor)	Edema, hypertension, hypokalemia caused by potassium-wasting diuretics	Oral	5 mg daily added to the established dosage of potassium-wasting diuretics or antihypertensives; doses above 10 mg/day are rare
spironolactone (Aldactone)	(see amiloride)	Oral	Initially, 100 mg is given for 5 days, after which dosage is adjusted. Usual range is from 25-200 mg in 1-4 doses/day
triamterene (Dyrenium)	(see amiloride)	Oral	Initially, 100 mg twice daily; lower doses may be satisfactory; daily maximum should not exceed 300 mg
THIAZIDE AND THIAZIDE-LIKE DIURETICS			
bendroflumethiazide (Naturetin)	Edema, hypertension	Oral	Range is 2.5-20 mg/day, usually given once a day; dosage is adjusted to patient response
benzthiazide (Marazide)	(as above)	Oral	Range is 50-200 mg/day; dosage is adjusted to patient response
chlorothiazide (Diuril)	(as above)	Oral, IV	500 mg-2 gram daily in 1 or 2 doses; dosage is adjusted to patient response
chlorthalidone (Hygroton, others)	(as above)	Oral	25-200 mg daily, but usual doses are 25-100 mg daily; daily dose should not exceed 200 mg
cyclothiazide (Anhydron)	(as above)	Oral	1-2 mg daily; dose may be lowered to 1-2 mg on alternate days; dosage must be adjusted to patient response

Continued.

TABLE C-15
Adult Dosages of Representative Diuretics—cont'd

Drug	Use	Route	Dose
hydrochlorothiazide (Esidrix, HydroDiuril, others)	(as above)	Oral	25-200 mg divided into 1-3 doses; dosage must be adjusted to patient response
hydroflumethiazide (Saluron, others)	(as above)	Oral	20-200 mg daily, adjusted to patient response
indapamide (Lozol)	(as above)	Oral	2.5-5 mg daily, adjusted to patient response
methyclothiazide (Aquatensin, Enduron)	(as above)	Oral	2.5-10 mg daily, adjusted to patient response
metolazone (Zaroxolyn)	(as above)	Oral	2.5-20 mg daily, adjusted to patient response
polythiazide (Renese)	(as above)	Oral	1-4 mg daily, adjusted to patient response
quinethazone (Hydromox)	(as above)	Oral	50-200 mg daily, adjusted to patient response
trichlormethiazide (Aquazide, Naqua, Triazide, others)	(as above)	Oral	1-4 mg daily, adjusted to patient response

Carbonic anhydrase inhibitors

Carbonic anhydrase inhibitors such as acetazolamide (Diamox, Dazamide) block secretion of the hydrogen ion into the renal tubule, which results in an increased excretion of bicarbonate. Sodium ions are excreted with the bicarbonate. Potassium ions are lost with the water. The diuretic action of these drugs is self-limiting because they produce a metabolic acidosis, which blocks their renal effects. These diuretics are used less often for CHF than loop diuretics or thiazide diuretics.

Side effects

CNS effects include paresthesias, sedation, depression, weakness, fatigue. Other side effects include fever, rash; blood dyscrasias including thrombocytopenia, pancytopenia, and agranulocytosis; anorexia, nausea or constipation; urinary frequency, renal colic, or stone formation; weight loss and flaccid paralysis; metabolic acidosis with continuous administration; metallic taste; photosensitivity; hyperglycemia and glycosuria.

Nursing prescriptions

- Monitor blood pressure, pulse, and weight on regular basis.
- Assess for sedation, depression, weakness, and fatigue. These may be incorrectly attributed to aging or chronic illness.
- Assess for history of allergic response to sulfonamide antibacterials, thiazide diuretics, or other sulfonamide derivatives before administering carbonic anhydrase inhibitors because cross-sensitivity may occur.
- Monitor CBC, serum electrolytes, and platelet count.
- If constipation occurs, instruct patients to increase daily fluid intake to 2500 to 3000 ml (if not contraindicated by the medical condition); increase dietary intake of fruit, fruit juice, and fiber; and increase level of exercise as needed.
- Urinary frequency may occur because of the diuretic effect; it should lessen with continued use of the drug. Teach patients to take the last dose of the day before 6 PM to reduce frequency of voiding during the night. Teach patients taking a single dose each day to take the dose in the morning, again to prevent interruptions in sleep.
- Dehydration may occur with any diuretic. Assess for thirst, decreased skin turgor, nausea, lightheadedness, weakness, increased pulse, oliguria, decreased blood pressure, and elevated hemoglobin, hematocrit, and BUN.
- Assess for signs of hypokalemia: muscle weakness, apathy, abdominal distention, and paralytic ileus. ECG changes include flattened or inverted T waves, prolonged QT interval, and a prominent U wave.
- If a potassium supplement is prescribed, teach the patient the importance of taking it as ordered. Dietary sources of potassium include citrus fruits and juices; grape, cranberry, apple, pear, and apricot juices; bananas; meat, fish, and fowl; cereals; and tea and cola beverages. Some patients with borderline low potassium levels can maintain potassium levels by increasing their daily intake of potassium-rich foods. Note that some potassium-rich foods are also high in sodium and may be contraindicated on that basis. Remind patients not to make dietary adjustments unless directed to do so. Not all patients need to increase potassium intake; for some it may be harmful.
- Instruct patients to avoid the use of alcohol, which may potentiate hypotension. Treatment for postural hypotension is discussed in the section about antihypertensives; refer to that section of the appendix.
- Assess for signs of metabolic acidosis: headache, mental dullness, rapid and deep respirations, and stupor or coma.

- Metallic taste may occur. Sucking on sugarless hard candy or chewing sugarless gum may help. Monitor weight; decreased intake may develop if the metallic taste is annoying to patients.
- Instruct patients with diabetes to monitor blood glucose levels. A change in diet or insulin dose may be needed.
- For photosensitivity, instruct patients to wear a wide-brimmed hat and long-sleeved clothing, avoid exposure to the sun, and wear a maximum strength sunscreen on exposed skin surfaces.
- Instruct patients not to switch drug brands unless approved by the physician. Different brands may not be bioequivalent.

Possible nursing diagnosis

Altered nutrition: less than body requirements related to metallic taste in the mouth resulting in loss of appetite due to acetazolamide therapy.

Loop diuretics

The loop diuretics such as bumetanide (Bumex), ethacrynic acid (Edecrin), and furosemide (Lasix) are the most powerful diuretics in clinical practice. While this makes them useful in a variety of conditions, it also means they are associated with several severe side effects.

Loop diuretics inhibit active reabsorption of the chloride ion in the ascending limb of Henle's loop in the kidney (thus the name loop diuretic). Because chloride reabsorption is blocked, reabsorption of sodium is blocked. Sodium chloride is retained in the tubule and excreted in the urine. Water accompanies the sodium chloride. Potassium ions are also excreted in higher than normal amounts.

Side effects

Excessive diuresis may lead to dehydration and electrolyte imbalance, especially hypokalemia. Gastrointestinal side effects of nausea, vomiting, and diarrhea may occur, which may also contribute to electrolyte imbalance. Blood dyscrasias may occur. Ringing in the ears may be the first sign of ototoxicity, which can progress to permanent hearing loss. CNS side effects include headaches, dizziness, blurred vision, and paresthesias. Rashes and allergy and alterations in glucose metabolism are also possible.

Nursing prescriptions

- Monitor blood pressure, pulse, and weight on a regular basis.
- Assess for sedation, depression, weakness, and fatigue. These may be incorrectly attributed to aging or chronic illness.
- Assess for history of allergic response to sulfonamide antibacterials, thiazide diuretics, or other sulfonamide derivatives before administering loop diuretics because cross-sensitivity may occur.
- Monitor CBC, serum electrolytes, platelet count, and serum pH.
- Urinary frequency may occur because of the diuretic effect; it should lessen with continued use of the drug. Teach patients to take the last dose of the day before 6 PM to reduce frequency of voiding during the night. Teach patients taking a single dose each day to take the dose in the morning, again to prevent interruptions in sleep.
- Dehydration may occur with any diuretic. Assess for thirst, decreased skin turgor, nausea, lightheadedness, weakness, increased pulse, oliguria, decreased blood pressure, elevated hemoglobin, hematocrit, and BUN.
- Assess for signs of hypokalemia: muscle weakness, apathy, abdominal distention, and paralytic ileus. ECG changes include flattened or inverted T waves, prolonged QT interval, and a prominent U wave. Hypokalemia is serious in any patient, but especially in patients who may be taking other drugs that are toxic in the presence of hypokalemia, such as the cardiac glycosides.
- If a potassium supplement is prescribed, teach the patient the importance of taking it as ordered. Dietary sources of potassium include citrus fruits and juices; grape, cranberry, apple, pear, and apricot juices; bananas; meat, fish, and fowl; cereals; and tea and cola beverages. Some patients with borderline low potassium levels can maintain potassium levels by increasing their daily intake of potassium-rich foods. Note that some potassium-rich foods are also high in sodium and may be contraindicated on that basis. Remind patients not to make dietary adjustments unless directed to do so; not all patients need to increase potassium intake, and for some it may be harmful.
- Assess for hyponatremia: muscle weakness, leg cramps, irritability, confusion, lethargy, headache, hypotension, nausea, vomiting, and abdominal discomfort.
- Assess for hypocalcemia: tingling of the fingers, toes, nose, and ears, and muscle spasms (tetany) and convulsions.
- Assess for metabolic alkalosis: mental confusion, dizziness, tetany, and convulsions. When a result of diuretic therapy, metabolic alkalosis is often related to potassium loss, and the symptoms are similar to hypokalemia.
- Instruct patients to avoid the use of alcohol, which may potentiate hypotension. Treatment for postural hypotension is discussed in the section about antihypertensives; refer to that section of the appendix.
- Instruct patients with diabetes to monitor blood glucose levels. A change in diet or insulin dose may be needed.
- For photosensitivity, instruct patients to wear a wide-brimmed hat and long-sleeved clothing, avoid exposure to the sun, and wear a maximum strength sunscreen on exposed skin surfaces.
- Assess for ototoxicity: tinnitus, reduced hearing acuity, vertigo, and sensations of full ears.

Possible nursing diagnosis

Altered electrolyte balance.

Potassium-sparing diuretics

Potassium-diuretics such as amiloride (Midamor), spironolactone (Aldactone), and triamterene (Dyrenium) prevent the exchange of sodium for potassium in the distal tubule. This action causes a small increase of sodium excretion and an accompanying potassium retention. This makes this group of diuretics unique and explains their use in combination with potassium-losing diuretics to help produce a net effect of potassium balance.

Side effects

Side effects include hyperkalemia, metabolic acidosis; confusion, headache, dizziness, weakness; nausea, vomiting, anorexia, diarrhea; and blood dyscrasias. Photosensitivity may occur with triamterene. Spironolactone may cause gynecomastia, decreased libido, and relative impotence in men, and breast soreness, altered menstrual periods, amenorrhea, or bleeding after menopause in women.

Nursing prescriptions

- Monitor serum electrolytes, BUN, and serum pH. Monitor CBC, serum glucose levels, liver function tests.
- Assess for metabolic acidosis: deep, rapid respirations, weakness, disorientation.
- Assess for hyperkalemia: nausea, colic, diarrhea, skeletal muscle spasms.
- If patients have been switched to a potassium-sparing diuretic, or a potassium-sparing diuretic is prescribed in addition to a potassium-losing diuretic, impress on patients the need to *omit* previous potassium supplements that may have been ordered; consult the physician.
- Instruct patients to avoid salt substitutes containing potassium while taking potassium-sparing diuretics.
- Urinary frequency may occur because of the diuretic effect; it should lessen with continued use of the drug. Teach patient to take the last dose of the day before 6 PM to reduce frequency of voiding during the night. Teach patients taking a single dose each day to take the dose in the morning, again to prevent interruptions in sleep.
- Dehydration may occur with any diuretic. Assess for thirst, decreased skin turgor, nausea, lightheadedness, weakness, increased pulse, oliguria, decreased blood pressure, elevated hemoglobin, hematocrit, and BUN.
- Instruct patients to avoid the use of alcohol, which may potentiate hypotension. Treatment for postural hypotension is discussed in the section on antihypertensives; refer to that section of the appendix.
- For photosensitivity, instruct patients to wear a wide-brimmed hat and long-sleeved clothing, avoid exposure to the sun, and wear a maximum strength sunscreen on exposed skin surfaces.

- Assess carefully for endocrine abnormalities in patients taking spironolactone. The development of these side effects often contributes to the patient stopping drug therapy. If side effects occur, notify the physician. Provide emotional support as needed. Remind patients not to stop therapy without first consulting the physician.

Possible nursing diagnosis

Altered electrolyte balance (hyperkalemia).

Thiazide and thiazide-like diuretics

The thiazide diuretics are outlined in Table C-15. Nonthiazides with thiazide-like actions include chlorthalidone (Hygroton), indapamide (Lozol), metolazone (Zaroxolyn), and quinethazone (Hydromox).

These drugs block reabsorption of chloride and sodium in the distal tubule. This increases excretion of sodium chloride and water. Thiazides and related drugs enhance potassium excretion by the kidneys, but this action is not required for diuresis and is one of the most troublesome side effects of these agents.

Side effects

Side effects include headaches, dizziness, vertigo, and paresthesias. Potassium depletion can cause dysrhythmias. Other side effects are orthostatic hypotension; nausea, vomiting, anorexia, gastrointestinal irritation, cholestatic jaundice; hypokalemia, hypercalcemia, hyperglycemia; increased serum cholesterol, triglycerides, and very-low-density lipoproteins (VLDL); photosensitivity; skin reactions and allergic reactions.

Nursing prescriptions

- Monitor blood pressure, pulse, and weight on regular basis.
- Assess for sedation, depression, weakness, and fatigue. These may be incorrectly attributed to aging or chronic illness.
- Monitor CBC, serum electrolytes, platelet count, and serum pH. Monitor serum glucose, serum cholesterol, triglycerides, and lipoprotein levels.
- Urinary frequency may occur because of the diuretic effect; it should lessen with continued use of the drug. Teach patient to take the last dose of the day before 6 PM to reduce frequency of voiding during the night. Teach patients taking a single dose each day to take the dose in the morning, again to prevent interruptions in sleep.
- Dehydration may occur with any diuretic. Assess for thirst, decreased skin turgor, nausea, lightheadedness, weakness, increased pulse, oliguria, decreased blood pressure, elevated hemoglobin, hematocrit, and BUN.
- Assess for signs of hypokalemia: muscle weakness, apathy, abdominal distention, and paralytic ileus. ECG changes include flattened or inverted T waves, prolonged

QT interval, and a prominent U wave. Hypokalemia is serious in any patient but especially in patients who may be taking other drugs that are toxic in the presence of hypokalemia, such as the cardiac glycosides.

- If a potassium supplement is prescribed, teach the patient the importance of taking it as ordered. Dietary sources of potassium include citrus fruits and juices; grape, cranberry, apple, pear, and apricot juices; bananas; meat, fish, and fowl; cereals; and tea and cola beverages. Some patients with borderline low potassium levels can maintain potassium levels by increasing their daily intake of potassium-rich foods. Note that some potassium-rich foods are also high in sodium and may be contraindicated on that basis. Remind patients not to make dietary adjustments unless directed to do so. Not all patients need to increase potassium intake; for some it may be harmful.
- Assess for hyponatremia: muscle weakness, leg cramps, irritability, confusion, lethargy, headache, hypotension, nausea, vomiting, and abdominal discomfort.
- Assess for hypercalcemia: thrist, polyuria, anorexia, nausea, vomiting, constipation, and altered level of consciousness.
- Assess for hypomagnesemia: confusion, hallucinations, tremors, muscle spasms, paresthesia, convulsion, and hyperactive reflexes.
- Instruct patients with diabetes to monitor blood glucose levels. A change in diet or insulin dose may be needed.
- For photosensitivity, instruct patients to wear a wide-brimmed hat and long-sleeved clothing, avoid exposure to the sun, and wear a maximum strength sunscreen on exposed skin surfaces.

Possible nursing diagnosis

Altered electrolyte balance.

INOTROPIC AGENTS

Inotropic agents increase cardiac output. For many years the cardiac glycosides represented the primary drugs of this category. Three drugs listed under the catecholamines and drugs for shock will also increase cardiac output by acting as inotropic agents: isoproterenol (Isuprel), dopamine (Intropin), and dobutamine (Dobutrex). Another group of drugs has recently been developed that will increase cardiac output, the phosphodiesterase inhibitors. The cardiac glycosides and the phosphodiesterase inhibitors will be discussed separately.

Cardiac glycosides

Digitalis (digoxin, Lanoxin) and other cardiac glycosides inhibit Na^+, K^+-ATPase and promote the accumulation within heart cells of the calcium required for contraction. This produces a positive inotropic effect on the heart, increasing myocardial contractility and cardiac output. In failing hearts, elevated ventricular end-diastolic pressure is also reduced, resulting in decreased pulmonary and systemic venous pressure. Cardiac glycosides slow conduction velocity through the AV node and prolong the effective refractory period of the AV node through three mechanisms: increased vagal activity; a direct effect on the AV node; and through a sympatholytic effect.

Uses

Cardiac glycosides are used in the treatment of heart failure; control of ventricular rate in patients with atrial fibrillation, flutter, or other supraventricular tachycardias (SVTs); treatment of recurrent paroxysmal atrial tachycardia (PAT).

Dosage

Because the half-life of these drugs may extend to a week or longer, initial doses may be higher than maintenance doses to help achieve a therapeutic serum drug level more quickly. The initial higher doses are called *loading doses* or *digitalizing doses,* and the lower chronic doses called *maintenance doses* (Table C-16).

Side effects

Side effects include increased cardiac automaticity (irregular pulse, premature ventricular contractions, or other dysrhythmias) and slowing of conduction through the AV node (bradycardia, partial or complete heart block). Stimulation of medullary centers leading to anorexia, nausea, and vomiting. Less commonly, depression, confusion, drowsiness, or headaches arise. Fatigue is a common sign of toxicity. Blurred vision, color distortion, halos, or flashing lights are common signs of toxicity. Renal failure and hypokalemia may predispose to toxicity.

Nursing prescriptions

- If patient is not being monitored, monitor the apical pulse for 1 full minute before administering the drug. If the rate is below 60 beats/minute withhold the dose and notify the physician.
- Observe ECG tracings for possible effects; prolonged PR interval, sagging ST segment, AV block, atrial tachycardia, ventricular tachycardia, or PVCs.
- Monitor serum electrolytes, especially potassium. Hypokalemia predisposes to toxicity from cardiac glycosides. Symptoms of hypokalemia include weakness, thirst, depression, anorexia, nausea, vomiting, abdominal distention, postural hypotension, and hypoactive reflexes.
- Assess for common signs of toxicity: fatigue, anorexia, nausea, vomiting, blurred vision, color distortion, halos, or flashing lights. Note that some signs of toxicity and/or hypokalemia may be incorrectly attributed to the patient's general condition (e.g., anorexia, fatigue, depression, weakness); evaluate patient carefully.
- Monitor serum drug levels, BUN, and serum creatinine. Renal failure may predispose to toxicity.

TABLE C-16

Comparison of Selected Cardiac Glycosides

Generic (Trade*) name	Route	Onset	Peak	Duration	Dose
deslanoside (Cedilanid-D)	IV	10-30 min	1-3 hr	2-5 days	0.8 mg initially, then 0.4-0.8 repeated at 4-hr intervals to a maximum of 2.0 mg
	IM				Rarely used
digitoxin (Crystodigin)	PO	1-4 hr	8-14 hr	14 days	0.8 mg initially, then 0.2 mg every 6-8 hr for 2-3 doses for rapid loading, or 0.2 mg twice daily for 4 days for slow loading; maintenance dose is 0.05-0.2 mg daily
digoxin (Lanoxin, Novodigoxin)	PO (tablets)	1-2 hr	1½-6 hr	2-6 days	10-15 µg/kg for loading dose, with 25%-35% of loading dose administered daily for maintenance, or 0.5-0.75 mg loading dose, with 0.25-0.5 mg at 6- to 8-hour intervals for 2 or 3 doses for rapid loading Maintenance dose (also used for slow loading) is 0.125-0.5 mg daily. Liquid-filled capsules have greater bioavailability than tablets; dosages are similar to IV dosages
	IV	5-30 min	1-4 hr	2-6 days	Loading dose of 8-12 µg/kg, with dose of 25%-35% of IV loading dose as daily maintenance dose, or loading dose of 0.25-0.5 mg followed by 0.25 mg 2 or 3 more times at 4- to 6-hour intervals; maintenance dose ranges from 0.125-0.5 mg daily

*Commonly encountered trade names are listed; there may be others.

• Many known drug interactions may increase or decrease cardiac glycoside levels. Monitor patient carefully.

Possible nursing diagnoses

Knowledge deficit related to new cardiac medications.
Possible complication: Glycoside toxicity related to electrolyte imbalance (hypokalemia) secondary to combination drug therapy (e.g., potassium-losing diuretic and cardiac glycoside).

Treatment of overdose

Treatment of overdose depends on the amount ingested and the severity of symptoms. Digoxin immune Fab is a specific antidote that can be used. The drug should be administered via intravenous infusion, but it can be given via intravenous injection. The dose is based on the amount of digoxin or digitoxin to be neutralized. Consult the package insert for current guidelines about dosing.

Phosphodiesterase inhibitors

The phosphodiesterase inhibitors (amrinone, milrinone, and enoximone ([enoximone is still an investigational drug]) represent a relatively new group of inotropic agents. The major effect of this group of drugs is to increase the force and velocity of systolic contraction. These drugs also cause vasodilation, which may help explain the therapeutic effects. The group of drugs appears to act directly on vascular smooth muscle but may also occur indirectly because of decreased sympathetic tone that has resulted from the improved myocardial contractility.

Uses

These drugs are used in short-term management of congestive heart failure (see Chapter 11). The drugs may be given concurrently with a cardiac glycoside because the phosphodiesterase appears to have additive effects with the cardiac glycoside. As more experience is gained with these drugs, additional indications may be approved.

Dosage

Dosage for amrinone (Inocor): 0.75 mg/kg injected directly intravenously. Maintenance dose: 5 to 10 µg/kg per minute via continuous infusion. Total daily dose, including bolus and continuous infusion doses should not exceed 10 mg/kg/day. Amrinone has been used orally, but it is associated with significant gastrointestinal side effects; as of this writing oral doses are not available for general use. Consult the manufacturer's insert for current dosing guidelines for milrinone and enoximone.

Side effects

Cardiac effects include dysrhythmias and hypotension. Administering intravenous doses slowly may reduce the in-

TABLE C-17

Lipid-Lowering Drugs, Usual Adult Dosages, Action, and Common Side Effects

Drug	Dose	Action and common side effects
cholestyramine resin (Questran, Cholybar)	4 grams 4 times/day (at meals and at bedtime) 1 chewable Cholybar = 4 gram	Binds bile acids in the intestine. Side effects: bloating, nausea and constipation, which may lessen with time. May interfere with absorption of fat-soluble vitamins, digitalis, thyroxine, and coumarin anticoagulants.
clofibrate (Atromid-S)	500 mg 3-4 times/day	Activates the enzyme lipoprotein lipase; inhibits release of VLDL by the liver. Side effects: few; some gastrointestinal upset, muscle cramps, impotence in men. Displaces several drugs from albumin, including coumarins, phenytoin, and tolbutamide. Long-term use may increase incidence of gallstones.
colestipol HCl (Colestid)	15-30 g daily in 2-4 doses, with meals	Similar to cholestyramine.
dextrothyroxine (Choloxin)	1-2 mg/day initially. May increase dose monthly. Doses vary if thyroid function is abnormal	Enhances degradation of LDL, thus lowering cholesterol. Side effects dizziness, diarrhea, altered taste. May produce symptoms of hyperthyroidism: weight loss, nervousness, insomnia, sweating, menstrual irregularities; hypersensitivity to iodine with itching, rash; aggravation of angina. Can decrease glucose tolerance in diabetics. Enhances action of coumarin anticoagulants.
gemfibrozil (Lopid)	600 mg twice/day, 30 min before breakfast and dinner	Chemically related to clofibrate. Side effects: gastrointestinal upset, rashes, increased incidence of gallstones.
lovastatin (Mevacor)	20 mg/day with evening meal	Inhibits an early step in cholesterol synthesis. Side effects: gastrointestinal discomfort, headaches, dizziness, skin rash; muscle aches or cramps, fever, tiredness or weakness, blurred vision. Changes in liver function tests. Yearly ophthalmic exams recommended.
niacin (Nicobid, Niac, Nicolar)	100 mg 3 times/day, increased to 2-6 grams daily in divided doses	Depresses synthesis of VLDL at these doses. Side effects: flushing due to vasodilator action; itching, gastrointestinal upset. Tolerance to side effects may develop with time, so dose usually started low and increased. Can aggravate peptic ulcer disease, glucose intolerance, high plasma uric acid.
probucol (Lorelco)	500 mg twice daily, with breakfast and dinner	Inhibits cholesterol synthesis. Side effects: gastrointestinal upset: diarrhea, gas, abdominal pain, nausea, vomiting. Cholesterol but not triglyceride level is decreased. Monitor patients with cardiac dysrhythmias carefully.

cidence of cardiovascular side effects. Gastrointestinal effects include nausea, vomiting, and diarrhea. Other side effects include hepatotoxicity, thrombocytopenia and allergic reactions. Consult the manufacturer's literature for current information.

Nursing prescriptions

- Although these drugs are not known for altering the heart rate, monitor the pulse and blood pressure regularly.
- Observe the ECG tracing for possible effects.
- Monitor serum drug levels, if available.
- Monitor liver function tests, platelet count, and CBC.
- Assess for possible liver toxicity: development of jaundice, right upper quadrant abdominal pain, fatigue, malaise, nausea, and anorexia.

- Assess for symptoms of thrombocytopenia: development of petechiae, unexplained bleeding, or bruising.
- As of this writing, these drugs are rarely used outside of the critical care setting. Keep patient and family informed of the patient's condition.

Possible nursing diagnosis

High risk for dysrhythmias.

LIPID-LOWERING DRUGS

Drugs to lower blood lipids are used to treat chronically elevated levels of one or more of the lipoproteins (see Chapter 8). These elevations may be genetically determined, or secondary to diabetes, obesity, alcoholism, hypothyroidism, and liver and kidney disease. Lowering elevated cholesterol and lipoprotein levels may also help reduce the risk of coronary artery disease. As a generalization, these drugs are not prescribed unless dietary changes have not been successful, because most of these drugs have annoying side effects. On the other hand, trying to maintain significant dietary changes that are markedly different from lifetime dietary patterns and preferences is difficult for most persons. The actions, dosages, and side effects of the lipid-lowering drugs are outlined in Table C-17 on p. 739.

Nursing prescriptions

- Most of these drugs should not be used during pregnancy. Counsel patients about birth control as needed. Instruct patients who become pregnant to notify the physician as soon as possible.
- Cholestyramine and colestipol powder should never be taken in dry form. Review instructions for administering drug carefully with the patient (see manufacturer's insert).
- Cholestyramine and colestipol may bind with other drugs taken concurrently. Work out an appropriate dosing schedule. Consult pharmacist as needed.
- Instruct patient in low cholesterol, low saturated fat, weight reduction, or other diets as appropriate for the patient. Provide emotional support. Consult dietitian as needed.

Possible nursing diagnoses

Diarrhea related to antilipemic therapy.
Noncompliance with antilipemic therapy related to distention and gas.

THROMBOLYTICS

Thrombolytics are drugs that promote the digestion of fibrin, thereby dissolving a clot. The discovery and use of these drugs has revolutionized treatment of acute myocardial infarction (see Chapter 10).

Uses

Thrombolytics are used to treat acute MI, acute pulmonary embolism, deep vein thrombosis, peripheral arterial occlusion, arteriovenous shunt occlusion in patients on renal dialysis.

Dosage

See Table C-18.

Side effects

Bleeding and hemorrhage are most serious. Intracranial bleeding can occur. Blood coagulation tests are altered.

Nursing prescriptions

- Monitor vital signs. Assess regularly for shock, hemorrhage, and alterations in level of consciousness. Monitor

TABLE C-18
Usual Adult Dosages of Thrombolytic Drugs

Drug	Dose	Comments
alteplase recombinant (Activase, tPA [tissue plasminogen activator])	IV: 100 mg Total: 60 mg first hr (with 6-10 mg infused rapidly over 1-2 min), then 20 mg per hr for 2 hr	Has a half-life of ±5 min
anistreplase (Eminase, APSAC)	IV: 30 units over 2-5 min	Significantly longer half-life (90 min) than other drugs in this category. Allergic reactions occur about as often as with streptokinase. Other side effects are similar to other drugs in this category. Costs about 25% less than alteplase but significantly more than streptokinase.
streptokinase (Streptase)	IV: 1.5 million IU over 1 hr; other regimens may be used Intracoronary: after patient is heparinized, 20,000 IU administered via catheter that has been threaded to occluded artery	This drug is highly antigenic; up to 30% of patients have a febrile reaction, and about 2.5% have anaphylactic reactions. Have drugs, equipment, personnel handy to treat allergic reactions. Half-life is about 23 min.
urokinase (Abbokinase)	IV: 4400 IU/kg is infused over 10 min, followed by infusion of 4400 IU/kg/hr for 12-24 hr	Less allergenic than streptokinase but very expensive. Half life is about 16 min.

blood pressure, electrocardiogram, and ordered blood work. Visually assess for bruising and bleeding. Check stools for occult blood/guaiac daily.

- Avoid venipunctures, intramuscular injections, and arterial punctures as much as possible. Tag bed (or as agency procedure dictates) to alert lab personnel and house staff to permit only experienced individuals to perform venipunctures. Apply pressure for 5 to 10 minutes after venipuncture to help stop bleeding.
- Handle patients carefully to avoid unnecessary bruising. Pad siderails.

Possible nursing diagnoses

Possible complication: hemorrhage.
Possible complication: anaphylaxis or severe allergic reaction to streptokinase.

VASODILATORS

Several groups of drugs are used to improve blood flow. These groups include the antianginal nitrates and nitrites (including intravenous nitroglycerin), the calcium channel blockers (discussed on p. 726), drugs used as peripheral vasodilators, and the drug pentoxifylline.

Nitrates and nitrites

The nitrates and nitrites relax smooth muscle. Relaxation of veins in the periphery cause blood to pool there, decreasing preload. Decreased preload results in less workload for the heart, and thus the heart requires less oxygen, helping to relieve angina. Because these drugs also affect the arteries, there is also a reduction in afterload.

Uses

Nitrates and nitrites are used to treat acute angina (see Chapter 9), as a prophylaxis for angina, CHF (see Chapter 11), and acute MI (see Chapter 10). Intravenous nitroglycerin is used to decrease myocardial ischemia following myocardial infarction.

Dosage

See Table C-19.

TABLE C-19
Typical Adult Dosages, Routes of Administration, Onset, and Duration of Action for Nitrates and Nitrites

Drug	Route/dosage form	Dose	Onset	Duration
amyl nitrate	Inhalant	0.18 or 0.3 ml, (1 ampule, crushed)	30 sec	3-5 min
erythrityl tetranitrate (Cardilate)	Sublingual (SL) or buccal	10 mg before physical or emotional stress	5 min	2 hrs
	Oral	10 mg 3 times/day, may be increased to 100 mg daily; bedtime doses for patients wtih nocturnal angina.	30 min	Variable
isosorbide dinitrate (Isogard, Isordil, Sorate, Sorbitrate)	Sublingual	2.5-10 mg	2-5 min	1-3 hrs
	Chewable	5 mg initially	2-5 min	1-3 hrs
	Oral	5-30 mg, 4 times/day	15-30 min	4-6 hrs
	Sustained release (oral)	40 mg every 8-12 hours	Slow	12 hrs
nitroglycerin (Cardabid, Nitro-Bid, Nitro-Dur, Nitroglyn, Nitrol, Nitrospan, Nitrostat, Nitrolingual spray, Transderm-Nitro, others)	IV	5 µg/min; protocols vary; see insert for dilution instructions	Immediate	Transient
	Sublingual	0.15-0.6 mg; repeat in 5 min, to a maximum of 3 tabs in 15 min	3 min	10-30 min
	Transmucosal (buccal tab)	1-2 mg 3 times/day	3 min	6 hr
	Oral, timed-release tabs or capsules	2.6-13 mg 3 times/day	Slow	8-12 hr
	Topical ointment	2% ointment contains 15 mg drug/inch. ½ inch initially. Usual: 1-2 inches every 8 hrs.	30-60 min	4-6 hrs
	Transdermal	1 patch every 24 hrs; some prefer removing patch for several hours (e.g., at night)	30-60 min	24 hrs
	Lingual spray	1-2 sprays on oral mucosa		
pentaerythritol tetranitrate (Peritrate Plateau Caps, Duotrate)	Oral	10 or 20 mg 3-4 times/day	20-60 min	4-5 hrs
	Sustained release (oral)	30-80 mg every 12 hours	Slow	12 hours

TABLE C-20

Typical Adult Dosages for Peripheral Vasodilators and the Drug Pentoxifylline

Drug	Route/Dose	Comments
cyclandelate (Cyclospasmol)	Oral: 200-400 mg, 4 times daily	Direct vasodilator. Side effects: belching, heartburn, flushing, headache, weakness, increased heart rate. Clinical effectiveness not certain.
ergot mesylates (Hydergine)	Sublingual, oral: 1 mg, 3 times/day	Produce vasodilation, which decreases blood pressure. Block α-adrenergic receptors. Side effects: marked bradycardia, sublingual irritation, nausea, and gastrointestinal upset.
isoxsuprine (Vasodilan)	Oral: 10-20 mg, 3-4 times/day IM: 5-10 mg, 2-3 times/day	Direct-acting vasodilator. Clinical usefulness questionable. Side effects: rash, flushing hypotension, dizziness, increased heart rate.
nicotinyl alcohol (Ronigen, Rycotin)	Oral: 50-100 mg, 3 times/day Timed-release: 300-400 mg every 12 hr	Direct acting vasodilator that causes pronounced flushing. Clinical usefulness questionable. See section on lipid-lowering drugs.
nimodipine (Nimotop)	Oral: 60 mg every 4 hr, beginning 4 days after hemorrhage and continuing for 21 days	Calcium channel blocker for treatment of cerebral vasospasm following subarachnoid hemorrhage. See Calcium Channel Blockers elsewhere in appendix.
nylidrin hydrochloride (Arlidin)	Oral: 3-12 mg, 3-4 times/day	Stimulates β-adrenergic receptors and also directly dilates vessels. Side effects: trembling, nervousness, weakness, dizziness, palpitations, and nausea and vomiting.
papaverine hydrochloride (Pavadur, many others)	Oral: 100-300 mg, 3-5 times/day Timed-release: 150 mg every 12 hours IV: 30-120 mg over 1-2 min IM: 30-120 mg	Relaxes smooth muscle. Depresses the heart. Used to relieve smooth muscle spasm in vascular disorders or colic; effectiveness not proven. Side effects: flushing, malaise, gastrointestinal upset, headache, excess perspiration, loss of appetite, increased heart rate. Rarely, a hypersensitivity reaction involving the liver. Symptoms include jaundice, eosinophilia, and altered liver function tests.
tolazoline hydrochloride (Priscoline)	IM, SC, IV: 10-50 mg 4 times/day	Direct-acting vasodilator. May relieve vasospastic disorders. Side effects: headache, nausea, chills, flushing, tingling of the skin, gastrointestinal disturbances. Occasionally, irregular heart function.
pentoxifylline (Trental)	Oral: 400 mg 3 times daily with meals	Not a vasodilator. Drug reduces the blood viscosity and increases the flexibility of red blood cells. These actions improve blood flow through narrowed vessels. Side effects: dizziness, headache, nausea, vomiting. May potentiate antihypertensives.

Side effects

Side effects include headache, flushing, and dizziness. Tolerance occurs with prolonged therapy. Dependence is rare clinically, but it means patients on high doses should not discontinue treatment suddenly.

Nursing prescriptions

- Assess all chest pain carefully, systematically, and thoughtfully.
- Review method of administration carefully. There are many forms available, and patients who are elderly, anxious, taking many prescribed medications, or who have had their dosages and dosage forms changed frequently are at risk for unintentionally not using the prescribed drug correctly. For a review of how to administer various dosage forms, see a basic nursing text, the manufacturer's insert, or consult the pharmacist.
- At the first sign of angina, instruct the patient to sit or lie down. This is important to help decrease the workload of the heart, but also if a nitrate or nitrite will be used because these drugs may make the patient hypotensive.
- Nitroglycerin tablets lose their potency over time and also decompose easily when exposed to moisture or light.

Review with the pharmacist and patient appropriate storage instructions.

- Instruct patients to avoid alcohol, which may potentiate the hypotensive effects of these drugs.

For intravenous nitroglycerin. Follow the manufacturer's instructions for dilution. The type of intravenous administration set (containing polyvinylchloride [PVC] or not) must be considered in determining dosage. Nitroglycerin migrates into many plastics.

During infusion, continuously monitor blood pressure and heart rate and other available data (e.g., PAWP).

Nitroglycerin administered intravenously should be used only in the critical care setting. Keep patient and family informed of the patient's condition.

Possible nursing diagnosis

Potential for injury related to orthostatic hypotension secondary to vasodilator therapy.

Peripheral vasodilation

There is a group of drugs (Table C-20) used to dilate vessels in the periphery to treat peripheral vascular disease (PVD) or to improve circulation in patients who have arteriosclerosis of cerebral vessels. There is some disagreement on the clinical value of many of these drugs because they may not alter the course of disease and may result in shunting blood away from areas with adequate circulation.

Uses

Vasospastic disorders.

Dosage

See Table C-20.

Nursing prescriptions

- Monitor blood pressure and pulse when beginning therapy or changing doses.
- Teach patient to take doses with meals or snack to reduce gastrointestinal irritation.
- Teach patients to avoid use of alcohol because it may potentiate hypotensive side effects and to avoid smoking because it causes vasoconstriction.
- Instruct patients taking pentoxifylline to avoid aspirin and aspirin-containing products while using this drug.
- Losing weight to ideal body weight may help lessen symptoms from peripheral vascular disease. Instruct patients as necessary.

Possible nursing diagnosis

Alteration in comfort: headache related to vasodilator therapy.

REFERENCES

Anistreplase for acute coronary thrombosis, The Medical Letter 32:812, 1990.

Beare PG: Calcium channel blockers: nursing care for hypertension, Crit Care Nurse 9(2):37, 1989.

Betaxolol for hypertension, The Medical Letter 32:61, 1990.

Black HR and Setaro JF: Antihypertensive treatment: monotherapy and beyond, Consultant 29(1):88, 1989.

Chernow B, editor: Essentials of critical care pharmacology, Baltimore, 1989, Williams & Wilkins.

Chernow B, editor: Pharmacologic approaches to the critically ill patient, ed 2, Baltimore, 1988, Williams & Wilkins.

Clark JB, Queener SF, and Karb VB: Pharmacological basis of nursing practice, ed 3, St Louis, 1990, The CV Mosby Co.

Curran CC: Use of cardiac glycosides in the critically ill, Crit Care Nurse 7(6):31, 1987.

Dennison RD: Understanding the four determinants of cardiac output, Nursing 90 20:35, 1990.

Dix-Sheldon DK: Pharmacologic management of myocardial ischemia, J Cardiovasc Nurs 3(4):17, 1989.

Frohlich ED: Calcium antagonists for initial therapy of hypertension, Heart Lung 18(4):370, 1989.

Gavras H: Angiotensin converting enzyme inhibition and its impact on cardiovascular disease, Circulation 81(1):381, 1990.

Karb VB, Queener SF, and Freeman JB: Handbook of drugs for nursing practice, St Louis, 1989, The CV Mosby Co.

McEvoy GK and others, editors: AHFS drug information, Bethesda, MD, 1990, American Society of Hospital Pharmacists, Inc.

Miller CL: Medications in angina, Focus Crit Care 15(4):23, 1988.

Misinski M: Role of conventional management and alternative therapies in limiting infarct size in acute myocardial infarction, Heart Lung 16(2) part 2:746, 1987.

Nagelhout JJ: AANA journal course: advanced scientific concepts: update for nurse anesthetists—Cardiac pharmacology: calcium antagonists, AANA J 56(4):367, 1988.

Propafenone for cardiac arrhythmias. The Medical Letter 32:816, 1990.

Shapiro W: Calcium channel blockers: Update on uses in ischemic heart disease, Cons 29(8):132, 1989.

United States Pharmacopeial Convention, Inc.: USPDI (United States Pharmacopeial Dispensing Information), vol 1, Drug information for the health care professional; vol 2, Advice for the patient, Rockville, MD, 1990, The US Convention, Inc.

Defibrillation, Cardioversion, and the Automatic Implantable Cardioverter-Defibrillator

Linda A. Prinkey

ELECTRICAL THERAPY*

The notion that electricity could affect life-sustaining bodily functions was first explored by Abilgaard in 1775.[12] Early researchers used electricity to induce pulselessness and fibrillation. It was not until 1900 that Prevost and Batelli discovered that stronger shocks could cause the heart beat and pulse to return.[11] The first successful human defibrillation was accomplished much later, in 1947, using specially designed internal paddles.[3]

Today, defibrillation and cardioversion are commonly used forms of cardiovascular electrical therapy. In theory these interventions cause the simultaneous depolarization of myocardial cells, which then allows normal impulse formation and conduction to resume. *Cardioversion* is the delivery of an electrical shock timed to occur approximately 10 milliseconds after the peak of the R wave. In contrast, *defibrillation* is the application of asynchronous or untimed shocks.

PRINCIPLES OF ELECTRICAL THERAPY
Equipment

The devices used to defibrillate and cardiovert are referred to collectively as *defibrillators*. In general, these devices possess the ability to deliver both synchronous and asynchronous shocks, depending on user selection. The amount of energy delivered is also controlled by the operator. Portable defibrillators use batteries as their primary power source. Other defibrillators contain AC-to-DC converters, which change the electrical power obtained from standard wall sockets to direct current. All defibrillators possess capacitors that store the selected amount of energy until it is discharged via the electrodes or paddles. Most defibrillators also offer ECG monitoring capabilities. Some models provide "quick look" ECG monitoring when the defibrillator paddles are applied to the chest. Other devices offer transcutaneous pacing capabilities in addition to defibrillation and cardioversion.

To ensure the proper functioning of defibrillators, the actual energy delivered through a 50-ohm resistance load (which simulates body resistance) should be measured by biomedical engineering personnel for each setting of stored energy. Critical care personnel should charge the defibrillator to the highest energy level and discharge it into a test load once a week. They should also perform a visual inspection and a charge/discharge test at 50 joules (J) into a 50-ohm test load daily.[7] Visual inspection includes examining the paddles for pitting and oxide film buildup. Biomedical engineering personnel and critical care staff should also check the batteries of battery-powered defibrillators according to service manual recommendations.[1] Logs recording these maintenance activities should be kept near the defibrillator.

Defibrillators deliver energy that is quantified as joules or watt-seconds:

$$\text{Energy (Joules)} = \text{Power (watts)} \times \text{Duration (seconds)}$$

However, it is the current flow that actually defibrillates.[19] The amount of current flow depends on the strength of the shock and the impedence between the defibrillator electrodes.[20] Since *transthoracic impedence* is mainly resistive, the greater the resistance, the less current is delivered.[1]

$$\text{Current (amperes)} = \frac{\text{Potential (volts)}}{\text{Resistance (ohms)}}$$

Therefore successful defibrillation depends, in part, on effective resistance reduction efforts.

Electrical resistance

The main resistance to be overcome during cardioversion and defibrillation is transthoracic impedance. The following factors affect transthoracic impedance[1]:

---

*Pages 745-751 from Dossey B, Guzzetta C, and Kenner C: Critical care nursing: body-mind-spirit, ed 3, Philadelphia, 1992, JB Lippincott Co.

- Energy delivered
- Electrode size and composition
- Interface between the electrode and the skin
- Number of shocks delivered and the time interval between them
- Patient's phase of ventilation
- Distance between electrodes

Resistance related to energy level cannot be controlled by the defibrillator operator.[14]

The optimal size for electrodes varies. Much depends on the type of electrode used. For instance, research indicates that the optimal external paddle for adults is between 10 cm and 13 cm in diameter.[17,23] The optimal size for self-adhesive defibrillator electrodes is thought to be 11 cm, although 8-cm apical electrodes used in combination with 12-cm parasternal pads have also been effective.[9,21] Paddles for infants and children should be 4.5 cm and 8 cm, respectively.[1]

The interface between defibrillator paddles and the skin is very important. This is the factor most easily affected by critical care personnel technique. First, transthoracic resistance can be reduced by applying conductive cream or gel to the paddles. Care must be taken to spread the gel or cream evenly across the paddle surface and to prevent any excess from being smeared across the chest between the paddles. Saline soaked gauze or gel pads may also be used, but electrode cream is more effective.[20] Alcohol pads should never be used because they can cause serious skin burns.

The passage of current through the chest is necessary to depolarize the critical mass of myocardium required for successful defibrillation.[26] Since electricity follows the path of least resistance, any connection between paddles created by conductive material will cause the current to flow along this connection and not through the chest. Therefore the success of cardioversion or defibrillation attempts can be affected by the care taken in applying the conductive material. Excess cream or gel can also create a shock hazard for the defibrillator operator and other rescuers if allowed to contact their bodies. Conductive gel pads and self-adhesive defibrillation electrodes can reduce this risk.

The pressure used to apply hand-held paddles to the chest also affects the electrode-to-skin interface and therefore the transthoracic resistance. Firm pressure of approximately 25 lbs per paddle is recommended.[1] Interestingly, self-adhesive pads used without the added benefit of firm pressure have been demonstrated to have comparable defibrillation success rates.[21]

Other factors affecting impedance include the number of shocks delivered, the distance between paddles, and the phase of ventilation. Transthoracic resistance is lowered by previous shocks. Decreasing the distance between paddles or electrodes and delivering the shock during expiration also reduces resistance.[1]

Electrode placement

Standard paddle or self-adhesive electrode placement consists of one electrode placed to the right of the sternum just below the right clavicle and one electrode placed just left of the left nipple with the center of the electrode in the midaxillary line (Fig. D-1). Anteroposterior positioning consists of placing one electrode anteriorly over the left precordium and the other electrode posteriorly, behind the heart. When patients have permanent pacemakers, electrodes should be positioned a minimum of 5 inches from the pacemaker generator.[1]

CARDIOVERSION
Procedure

Cardioversion, or synchronized shock, is indicated for unstable ventricular tachycardia (except for patients who are pulseless, hypotensive, or in pulmonary edema) and rapid supraventricular tachycardias (Figs. D-2 and D-3). For the device to time the shock to occur after the peak of the R wave, ECG electrodes must be applied and a monitoring

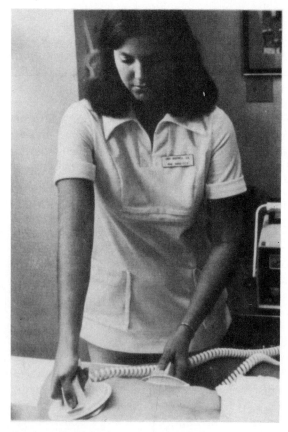

FIG. D-1 Electrode placement for defibrillation (anterior placement of electrode paddles).

From Dossey B, Guzzetta C, and Kenner C: Critical care nursing: body-mind-spirit, ed 3, Philadelphia, 1992, JB Lippincott Co.

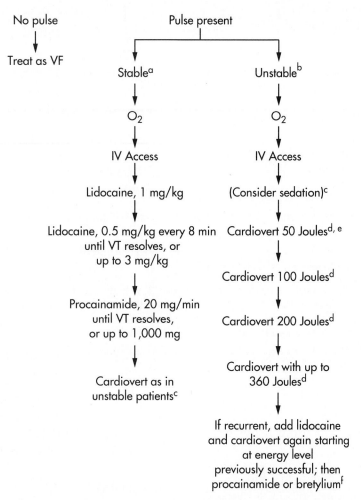

FIG. D-2 Sustained ventricular tachycardia (VT). This sequence was developed to assist in teaching how to treat a broad range of patients with sustained VT. Some patients may require care not specified herein. This algorithm should not be construed as prohibiting such flexibility. Flow of algorithm presumes that VT is continuing. VF indicates ventricular fibrillation.

aIf patient becomes unstable (see footnote b for definition) at any time, move to "Unstable" arm of algorithm.

bUnstable indicates symptoms (e.g., chest pain or dyspnea), hypotension (systolic blood pressure <90 mm Hg), congestive heart failure, ischemia, or infarction.

cSedation should be considered for all patients, including those defined in footnote b as unstable, except those who are hemodynamically unstable (e.g., hypotensive, in pulmonary edema, or unconscious).

dIf hypotension, pulmonary edema, or unconsciousness is present, unsynchronized cardioversion should be done to avoid delay associated with synchronization.

eIn the absence of hypotension, pulmonary edema, or unconsciousness, a precordial thump may be used before cardioversion.

fAfter VT has resolved, begin intravenous (IV) infusion of antiarrhythmic agent that has aided resolution of VT. If hypotension, pulmonary edema, or unconsciousness is present, use lidocaine if cardioversion alone is unsuccessful, followed by bretylium. In all other patients, recommended order of therapy is lidocaine, procainamide, and then bretylium.

From McIntyre KM and Lewis AJ: Standards and guidelines for cardiopulmonary resuscitation and emergency cardiac care, JAMA 255:2841, 1986.

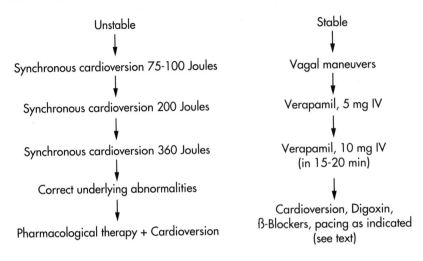

If conversion occurs but PSVT recurs, repeated electrical cardioversion is *not* indicated. Sedation should be used as time permits.

FIG. D-3 Paroxysmal supraventricular tachycardia (PSVT). This sequence was developed to assist in teaching how to treat a broad range of patients with sustained PSVT. Some patients may require care not specified herein. This algorithm should not be construed as prohibiting such flexibility. Flow of algorithm presumes PSVT is continuing.

From McIntyre KM and Lewis AJ: Standards and guidelines for cardiopulmonary resuscitation and emergency cardiac care, JAMA 255:2841, 1986.

lead that best facilitates recognition of the QRS complex must be selected. The synchronization switch must also be activated.

Patients requiring cardioversion are conscious. Because cardioversion is potentially uncomfortable, anesthesia or analgesia is necessary. Even when the cardioversion is emergent, sedation should be considered.[1] A physician skilled in airway management, preferably an anesthesiologist, should be present. In addition, a patent intravenous line should be established. Emergency drugs and equipment should also be available. The procedure is explained to the patient as conditions permit. Informed consent is obtained from patients undergoing elective cardioversion.

After all the preparations have been completed, the paddles or self-adhesive electrodes are placed on the patient's chest as described previously. The synchronizer switch is activated, the energy level is selected, and the defibrillator is charged. When the operator depresses the buttons to deliver the shock, the paddles must be held in place until the synchronizer discharges the energy. This is necessary because the energy is not released until the machine senses the appropriate portion of the QRS complex. This avoids delivering the shock during the vulnerable period of the T wave and reduces the probability of inducing ventricular fibrillation. If the patient's rhythm is cardioverted to ventricular fibrillation, the synchronizer switch should be turned off and the unit charged to 200 J. The patient should then be defibrillated immediately. If necessary, the rest of the ventricular fibrillation treatment algorithm should be implemented (Fig. D-4).

Energy levels

The energy required for cardioversion depends on the type of dysrhythmia being treated. For cardioversion of atrial fibrillation, the recommended energy level is 100 J for the first shock, 200 J for the second, and 360 J for the third. For paroxysmal supraventricular tachycardia, the recommended initial energy level is 75 to 100 J. The second and third shocks should be 200 J and 360 J, respectively. The initial energy used to cardiovert atrial flutter should be 25 J. For urgent or emergent treatment of unstable ventricular tachycardia, the initial shock should be 50 J followed by subsequent shocks of 100 J, 200 J, and 360 J, if necessary.[1]

DEFIBRILLATION
Procedure

Defibrillation, the delivery of unsynchronized shocks, is indicated for ventricular fibrillation and for pulseless ventricular tachycardia. Ventricular tachycardia associated with hypotension, unconsciousness, or pulmonary edema also requires defibrillation.[20] If the development of these conditions is witnessed, the nurse should check for a pulse.

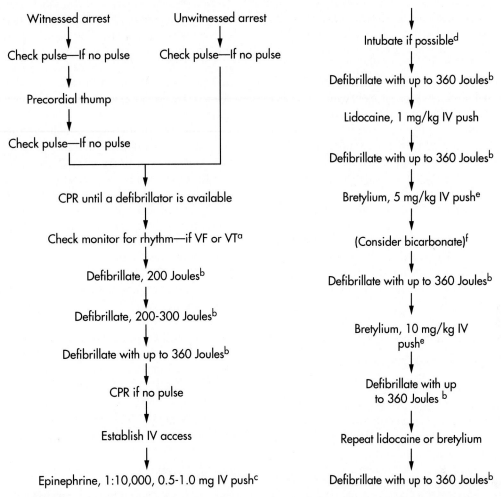

FIG. D-4   Ventricular fibrillation (and pulseless ventricular tachycardia).[a] This sequence was developed to assist in teaching how to treat a broad range of patients with ventricular fibrillation (VF) or pulseless ventricular tachycardia (VT). Some patients may require care not specified herein. This algorithm should not be construed as prohibiting such flexibility. Flow of algorithm presumes that VF is continuing. CPR indicates cardiopulmonary resuscitation.
[a]Pulseless VT should be treated identically to VF.
[b]Check pulse and rhythm after each shock. If VF recurs after transiently converting (rather than persists without ever converting), use whatever energy level has previously been successful for defibrillation.
[c]Epinephrine should be repeated every 5 minutes.
[d]Intubation is preferable. If it can be accompanied simultaneously with other techniques, then the earlier the better. However, defibrillation and epinephrine are more important initially if the patient can be ventilated without intubation.
[e]Some may prefer repeated doses of lidocaine, which may be given in 0.5-mg/kg boluses every 8 minutes to a total dose of 3 mg/kg.
[f]Value of sodium bicarbonate is questionable during cardiac arrest, and it is not recommended for routine cardiac arrest sequence. Consideration of its use in a dose of 1 mEq/kg is appropriate at this point. Half of original dose may be repeated every 10 minutes if it is used.

From McIntyre KM and Lewis AJ: Standards and guidelines for cardiopulmonary resuscitation and emergency cardiac care, JAMA 255:2841, 1986.

Finding no pulse, the nurse may administer a precordial thump (see box below). After rechecking for a pulse, the nurse initiates cardiopulmonary resuscitation (CPR) for pulselessness. When the arrest is unwitnessed, the nurse confirms pulselessness and starts CPR without first delivering a precordial thump while awaiting the arrival of a defibrillator.

After a defibrillator arrives, the nurse should check the rhythm with "quick look" paddles or by placing ECG electrodes on the patient. Paddle monitoring has the advantage of being faster; however, fine ventricular fibrillation can mimic asystole. Since confirmation of asystole requires observation of a "flat line" pattern in at least two leads,[1] ECG electrodes will need to be applied. Therefore when an unmonitored patient arrests, it is recommended that one nurse use the "quick look" paddles while another applies ECG electrodes.

If the rhythm is confirmed to be ventricular fibrillation or pulseless ventricular tachycardia, conductive material is applied to the paddles or to the chest (saline-soaked gauze or gel pads). The defibrillator is set to charge the capacitor to 200 J. While the capacitor is charging, the paddles are positioned on the chest and 25 lbs of pressure is applied. Before discharging the defibrillator, the paddle operator should ensure that all personnel have no direct or indirect contact with the patient. The paddle operator then delivers the countershock. Usually, this is accomplished by depressing the buttons located on each paddle simultaneously. In certain instances, the defibrillator is discharged by other personnel positioned at the defibrillator's controls.

If the electrical energy is delivered to the patient, the patient's chest wall muscles will contract. If the muscles do not contract, the nurse should check to ensure that the synchronizer mode is off and that the defibrillator is plugged in or has adequate battery charge levels.

After the shock has been delivered, the nurse should assess the patient's pulse and rhythm. If the patient continues to remain pulseless and in ventricular tachycardia or fibrillation, the defibrillator is set to charge to either 200 J or 300 J. The defibrillation procedure is then repeated. If pulseless ventricular tachycardia or fibrillation persists, a third shock of 360 J is delivered.

If no pulse is present after the third shock, CPR is resumed and an intravenous line is established. Epinephrine is then given. The patient also is intubated if possible. After these interventions have been completed, the patient is defibrillated with 360 J. If no pulse is established, drug therapy alternating with shocks of 360 J is initiated (Fig. D-4). The patient's pulse and rhythm are checked after each debrillation attempt.

Energy levels

Since up to 90% of adult patients in ventricular fibrillation who weigh up to 90 kg can be successfully defibrillated using 200 J,[18] this energy level is recommended for the first shock. The energy required for the second shock is more controversial. Considering the changes in impedance and the predictability of delivered energy, the second shock can be 200 J to 300 J.[1] Higher energy levels can cause dysrhythmias and myocardial damage.[25] The maximum recommended energy level is 360 J.[1]

Open-chest defibrillation requires far less energy than transcutaneous defibrillation. When specially designed sterile electrodes are placed over the right atrium and the apex of the heart, shocks starting at 5 J can be delivered. The recommended maximum energy level for open chest interventions is 50 J.[20]

The recommended defibrillation energy for infants and children is 2 J per kilogram, initially. If this level is insufficient to convert the patient's rhythm, two additional shocks of 4 J per kilogram may be given. If the second 4-J-per-kilogram shock is unsuccessful, interventions should be initiated to correct existing acidosis, hypoxemia, and hypothermia.[1]

PRECORDIAL THUMP*

MECHANISM OF ACTION

- Mechanical energy from a blow to the chest creates an electrical stimulus that can potentially depolarize the heart.

TECHNIQUE

- Raise a closed fist no more than 12 inches above the center of the patient's chest.
- Deliver a single sharp blow to the midsternal area using the fleshy portion of the fist.

GUIDELINES FOR USE

- Deliver only a single blow. Do not delay defibrillation to deliver.
- Use only in the following situations:
  1. A witnessed cardiac arrest while awaiting arrival of the defibrillator
  2. Monitored patients with ventricular fibrillation
  3. Monitored patients with asystole or marked bradycardia *and* hemodynamic instability
  4. Monitored patients with ventricular tachycardia *and* a palpable pulse *only* when a defibrillator is immediately available (precordial thump may induce ventricular fibrillation in these patients)

*The precordial thump is an ACLS technique only.
Adapted from Standards and guidelines for cardiopulmonary resuscitation (CPR) and emergency cardiac care (ECC), JAMA 255(21): 2915, 1986.

Factors affecting defibrillation outcomes

In addition to defibrillation techniques and protocols, other factors affect the success of defibrillation attempts. The duration of the ventricular fibrillation or pulseless ventricular tachycardia influences outcomes. Long periods of these rhythms decrease the chances of successful countershock.[1] Early and effective CPR can improve the chance for positive outcomes. Conditions such as acidosis, hypoxemia, hypothermia, drug toxicity, and electrolyte imbalance can make the heart more refractory to defibrillation.[1] Prompt assessment and intervention to correct these problems increase the possibility of successful resuscitation.

Other defibrillation techniques

Automatic external defibrillators (AEDs)

AEDs can be used by both medical personnel and nonmedical rescuers. AEDs have defibrillator pads that must be applied after pulselessness has been determined. After the pads are applied, the device uses preprogrammed algorithms to determine the rhythm and energy level for the shocks to be delivered. AEDs also provide messages informing the user of poor lead contact, charging activity, and when to check pulses. After the device is charged, the only way to prevent firing is to turn the machine off. Semiautomatic models inform the user of ventricular fibrillation or ventricular tachycardia and advise the user to press the defibrillation button.

It takes 6 to 12 seconds for AEDs to commit to firing. An additional 8 to 15 seconds is required to charge the capacitor. Therefore there will be approximately 15 to 30 seconds between shocks delivered by an AED if the patient remains in ventricular tachycardia or fibrillation. The unit should be turned off during CPR and when the patient is moving or having a seizure.[4]

The effectiveness and feasibility of using AEDs in the homes of high-risk patients is being studied. Initial results are disappointing. Skill retention and the emotional impact of family members with life-threatening dysrhythmias are two factors affecting home use success rates.[8]

Transtelephonic defibrillation

Transtelephonic defibrillation is another new intervention for high-risk patients. A trained family member or other individual applies self-adhesive monitor-defibrillator pads to the patient. The pads are then attached to the cables of a device that transmits the rhythm via telephone to a remote base station. Emergency personnel at the base station control the charging and discharging of the home device. These devices also offer two-way voice communication.[8]

Automatic implantable cardioverter-defibrillators (AICDs)

AICDs can be surgically placed in patients at high risk of sudden cardiac death. Unlike AEDs, AICDs do not depend on human operators to activate them. Once implanted and activated, AICDs continuously monitor the patient's rhythm. AICDs use QRS morphologic condition and/or heart rate to determine when to discharge. Depending on the model implanted, they can deliver up to four or five shocks per dysrhythmia. However, they require at least 35 seconds of a rhythm other than ventricular tachycardia or fibrillation to reactivate the defibrillation cycle.[24]

The device. The AICD system consists of a pulse generator and several lead wires. The pulse generator is larger than modern pacemakers (10.8 cm × 7.6 cm × 2.0 cm) and weighs 250 grams[24] (Fig. D-5). The generator box contains the sensing circuitry, lithium batteries, and energy storage capacitors. Newer models also have memory and programming functions. Rate sensing is accomplished via either a transvenous bipolar electrode positioned in the apex of the right ventricle or two screw-in epicardial leads placed 1 to 2 cm apart[5] on the left ventricular wall.[24] Two patch electrodes, placed over the right ventricle and the apex of the left ventricle, monitor QRS duration and defibrillate. A transvenous electrode, placed in the superior vena cava at the right atrial junction, may be used instead of the right ventricular patch (Fig. D-6).

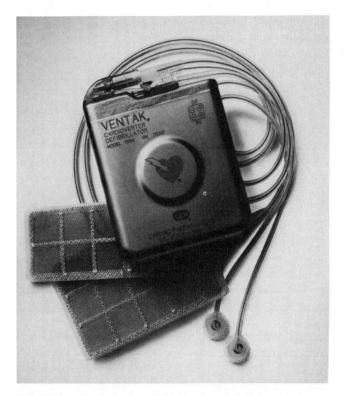

FIG. D-5 The automatic implantable cardioverter-defibrillator (AICD). This configuration consists of the pulse generator box, two epicardial screw-in leads *(right)* for rate sensing, and two patch leads *(left)* for monitoring QRS morphology and defibrillating.
Courtesy Cardiac Pacemakers, Inc.

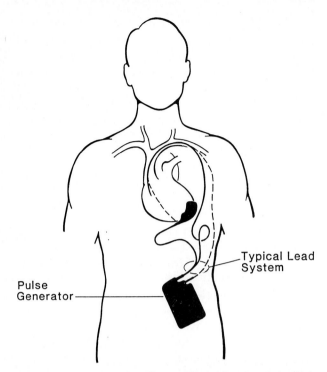

FIG. D-6 The implanted cardioverter-defibrillator. This configuration shows a transvenous rate sensing electrode *(dotted line)*, a transvenous superior vena caval electrode *(solid line)*, and a left ventricular patch electrode for monitoring QRS morphologic condition and defibrillating. The lead wires are tunneled to the abdominal pouch created for the pulse generator.

Courtesy Cardiac Pacemakers, Inc.

The AICD continuously monitors the patient's heart rate and, in most cases, QRS duration. It requires 5 to 20 seconds to recognize rhythms meeting the preprogrammed criteria for defibrillation. After the dysrhythmia is recognized, the device takes another 5 to 15 seconds to charge the capacitors and deliver the shock. Depending on the model and how it is programmed, the AICD can deliver up to 30 J per shock and up to 5 shocks.

Surgical approaches. Several different surgical techniques can be used to implant the AICD. Two features common to all of these procedures are the use of general anesthesia and the subcutaneous tunneling of lead wires to an abdominal pocket where the AICD pulse generator is inserted. When transvenous electrodes are used, they are inserted via the subclavian or internal jugular venous systems and then tunneled to the pulse generator (Fig. D-6).

The least invasive technique, the subxiphoid approach, requires a small lengthwise incision just below and to the left of the xiphoid process. Similarly, the subcostal approach provides access to the heart via an incision along the left costal margin. In both of these techniques, the pericardium is opened and the appropriate leads are attached to the epicardial surface. The main disadvantage of these procedures is limited exposure of the epicardium.[6]

When patients require concomitant open heart surgery, a median sternotomy is used. This approach allows greater visibility and access to the heart. However, it is a much more invasive procedure. The recovery period for these individuals is generally longer and is related to the extent of procedures performed.

Patients who have undergone previous cardiac surgery usually require a left lateral thoracotomy to avoid problems caused by preexisting sternotomy scar tissue. In this procedure, exposure of the cardiac surface is accomplished via an incision made in the fifth or sixth intercostal space. Patch leads can either be sutured to the outside of the pericardium or placed directly over the left ventricular apex.[6]

Regardless of the surgical approach, the lead wires are tunneled to the abdomen, where a pocket for the pulse generator is created in the subcutaneous tissue. The leads are then connected to the generator and the device is tested before the surgical incisions are closed. Testing includes inducing ventricular tachycardia or fibrillation to determine the device's effectiveness in sensing and terminating the dysrhythmia. In some institutions the AICD is then inactivated to prevent the possible delivery of inappropriate shocks during the immediate postoperative period. During the first few days after surgery, supraventricular dysrhythmias and short bursts of ventricular tachycardia can occur as a result of pericarditis, disruptions in antidysrhythmic medications, and irritability caused by mechanical manipulation of the heart during surgery.[6] The "active" or "inactive" status of the device should be clearly communicated to everyone involved in caring for these patients.

Postoperative nursing care. Postoperative care for AICD patients depends on the surgical techniques used. In general, these individuals have one or more chest tubes. Their incisions are covered with occlusive dressings for the first 24 to 48 hours and are treated according to general hospital nursing procedures. Patients also receive intravenous fluids. The type, amount, and site of fluid administration varies based on individual needs.

Depending on the institution, the surgical approach, and physician preferences, some patients may be extubated and recover from anesthesia in the postanesthesia care unit. Others may return to the critical care unit directly from the operating room and require mechanical ventilation. The duration of mechanical ventilation depends on the type of procedure performed and the patient's previous medical history, particularly history related to pulmonary disease. After patients are extubated, frequent coughing and deep breathing exercises and incentive spirometry are encouraged. Because these patients usually have a significant amount of incisional pain, premedication with the prescribed analgesics can greatly improve their comfort level and their ability to perform these exercises.

In addition to wound and pulmonary care, these patients require careful electrocardiographic monitoring. When the device is "active," careful observation and documentation of both appropriate and inappropriate shocks are important. If the device is "inactive," prompt recognition and treatment for any sustained ventricular dysrhythmias are primary concerns. Often this treatment is highly individualized and should be clearly delineated by both written and verbal communication. Staff should also be aware that external defibrillation will not harm the AICD regardless of its activation status.

Patients with AICDs and permanent pacemakers require particular attention, since pacemakers can interfere with proper AICD sensing.[6,13,15] Careful monitoring and recording of pacemaker and AICD function are important. Use of epicardial AICD rate-sensing leads and implantation of a bipolar permanent pacemaker can reduce the risks of AICD-pacemaker interaction.[13] Reducing the electrical output of the bipolar pacemaker to just above the capture threshold is also recommended.[15]

Patients usually remain in the critical care unit for approximately 24 hours and are then transferred to a telemetry nursing unit. Early mobilization and ambulation are encouraged. Often, structured cardiac rehabilitation programs are used. Before discharge, patients undergo exercise tolerance testing to estimate maximal heart rates that might occur with the performance of daily activities. Test results are used to determine whether AICD rate limits need to be adjusted. Sinus tachycardia, particularly when associated with a widened QRS complex, can trigger AICD firing if the heart rate exceeds the rate criteria. Therefore whenever possible, the rate limit should be set higher than the maximum heart rate achieved during exercise testing. In some instances, drug therapy may be necessary to control the patient's rate below the firing threshold.[6]

Electrophysiology studies are also conducted before discharge to ensure the proper functioning of the device and its effectiveness in terminating life-threatening dysrhythmias. This testing is particularly important when antidysrhythmic medications have been added or restarted postoperatively. These tests can be very anxiety provoking for patients because they know they will most likely receive at least one shock during the study.

Patient teaching. Patients diagnosed as having malignant ventricular dysrhythmias and their families often experience a great deal of fear and anxiety.[10] Because of this, it may be difficult for them to concentrate on or retain any information presented. Methods for increasing understanding include the use of varied media, simple explanations, repetition, and individualization of the teaching plan. The presence of significant others during instruction is of paramount importance. In addition, patient and family participation in an AICD support group, both before and after surgery, can be very beneficial.[2,22]

Before surgery, patients and families need to receive information concerning the pathophysiologic characteristics of the dysrhythmia, possible treatment options, AICD function, and the implantation procedure. They should also be told what to expect after surgery, including unit routines and the normal recovery course. The explanation of postoperative experiences should include a description of sensations associated with receiving a shock. Patients should be made aware that they may become dizzy or weak or lose consciousness as a result of their dysrhythmia. If they remain conscious when the AICD fires, they may feel what is often described as a blow, kick, or thump to the chest.[24]

After surgery, patients and families need to be told of planned tests and procedures. Often patients have had diagnostic procedures such as exercise tolerance testing and electrophysiology studies before. In these instances, reinforcement of previous teaching may be all that is necessary. Reinforcement of preoperative teaching concerning activity and breathing exercises may also be required.

Before discharge AICD patients and their families must receive and understand a great deal of critical information. This information includes life-saving techniques, wound care, medication and activity instructions, and an overview of follow-up care. Both verbal and written instructions should be provided. In addition, patients should be given 24-hour phone numbers for the electrophysiologist and the nurse responsible for AICD follow-up care.

Emergency medical instructions are multifaceted. Patients should be taught cough CPR.[6,16] Family members should be instructed in conventional CPR. Emphasize to patients and their families that persons touching the patient when the device delivers a shock will not be harmed but may experience a tingling sensation. Also stress the importance of wearing Medic-Alert identification and carrying the AICD emergency identification card. Whenever possible, contact should be made with the patient's local hospital and emergency medical service so that basic information concerning AICDs can be communicated. The electrophysiologist should provide the patient's primary physician with information regarding AICDs and any patient-specific concerns. Finally, patients should be told what to do when they experience a shock or shocks. Whenever a shock occurs, patients should notify the AICD nurse or the electrophysiologist. A single shock usually does not require an office visit. However, patients should be seen if two successive shocks are delivered. Stress the importance of calling for emergency medical assistance if more than two consecutive shocks occur. Patients should also keep a diary of shock occurrences, associated activities, and any prodromal symptoms.[6]

In addition to instructions concerning emergency care, patients should also receive information on proper wound care. All incisions should be observed for redness, swelling, tenderness, and purulent drainage. Any persistent temperature elevations should be reported to the physician. The pulse generator pocket should also be inspected for any persistent bruising or signs of erosion. Fluid collection in this pocket is not unusual during the immediate postoperative period and may persist for up to a month.[24] However, the pocket should not become reddened or tender. Occasionally belts or tight fitting clothing may cause discomfort over the generator pocket. Unless this discomfort is associated with signs of infection or erosion, elimination of the cause of the irritation is all that is required.

Discharge medication and activity information is more highly individualized than emergency and wound care instructions. Patients may or may not require antidysrhythmic medications. Further, the doses and combinations of these drugs vary widely. Patients should receive verbal and written information detailing the medications prescribed, their dosages, side effects, and any special precautions or follow-up required. Activity instructions are often determined by the surgical approach used. Patients with median sternotomy incisions should not drive or lift objects weighing more than 10 pounds for 4 to 6 weeks. Patients can resume sexual activity after 4 weeks.[6] They should be reassured that if a shock occurs during intercourse, it will not harm their partner. All patients should avoid activities that could result in a heavy blow to the pulse generator pocket. This type of injury can lead to pocket erosion.

Patients should also avoid strong magnetic fields such as those generated by arc welders, power plants, large running engines, and nuclear magnetic resonance imaging (see Chapter 16). Contact with these types of magnetic interference can cause inadvertent device deactivation or activation of the battery testing sequence. Frequent accidental battery testing can lead to premature battery depletion.[24] Usually, patients will hear beeps coming from the pulse generator pocket if the AICD is being affected by a magnetic field. Patients should be instructed to move away from the source of this interference immediately and to call the electrophysiologist or the AICD nurse. Patients should also be advised to contact the AICD physician or nurse if they require procedures involving electrocautery or diathermy. In these instances, the AICD can be deactivated during the procedure and then reactivated to avoid potential damage.[24]

The importance of follow-up care should be stressed to both patients and families. Regular office visits are essential to determining proper AICD function and ensuring timely battery replacement. Patients should be told that battery life varies, depending on the model implanted and the number of shocks delivered to the patient and the testing circuit. Explain that the noninvasive office tests used to assess charge time and the number of shocks delivered provide information that assists the physician in deciding the best time for battery replacement. Office visit battery checks are usually scheduled every 2 months for the first year and then monthly until the battery is changed.

As part of follow-up care, patients should be encouraged to participate in an AICD support group whenever possible. The psychosocial impact of malignant ventricular dysrhythmias and AICD implantation is significant. As patients with life-threatening dysrhythmias, these individuals express concerns regarding the well-being of other family members, alterations in family roles, changes in lifestyle, and the need for lengthy hospitalization. Often they have fears regarding cardioversion, medications, and surgery.[10] Implantation of the AICD raises additional concerns regarding the discomfort of shocks and feelings of dependence on the device.[6] Family members deal with similar issues. The ability to express these concerns to individuals with similar experiences is often helpful to AICD patients and their families. The availability of assistance from a social worker and a psychiatric liason nurse who are often associated with these support groups can also be reassuring. Most importantly, involvement in AICD support groups decreases patient and family feelings of being alone in their struggle to deal with issues surrounding sudden death survival.

REFERENCES

1. American Heart Association: Textbook of advanced cardiac life support, Dallas, 1987, The Association.
2. Badger JM and Morris PL: Observation of a support group for automatic implantable cardioverter defibrillator recipients and their spouses, Heart Lung 18:238, 1989.
3. Beck CS, Pritchard WH, and Feil SA: Ventricular fibrillation of long duration abolished by electric shock, JAMA 135:985, 1947.
4. Bocka JJ: Automatic external defibrillators, Ann Emerg Med 18:1264, 1989.
5. Brodman R and others: Implantation of automatic cardioverter-defibrillators via median sternotomy, PACE 7:1363, 1984.
6. Cooper DK, Valladares BK, and Futterman LG: Care of the patient with the automatic implantable cardioverter defibrillator: a guide for nurses, Heart Lung 16(6):640, 1987.
7. Creed JD and others: Defibrillation and synchronized cardioversion. In McIntyre KM and Lewis AJ, editors: Textbook of advanced cardiac life support, Dallas, 1981, The Association.
8. Cummins RO: From concept to standard-of-care? Review of the clinical experience with automated external defibrillators, Ann Emerg Med 18:1269, 1989.
9. Dalzell GW and others: Electrode pad size, transthoracic impedance and success of external ventricular defibrillation, Am J Cardiol 64:741, 1989.
10. DeBasio N and Rodenhausen N: The group experience: meeting the psychosocial needs of patients with ventricular tachycardia, Heart Lung 13(6):597, 1984.
11. DeSilva RA and others: Cardioversion and defibrillation, Am Heart J 100:881, 1980.
12. Driscol TE, Ratnoff OD, and Nygaard OF: The remarkable Doctor Abildgaard and countershock, Ann Intern Med 83:878, 1975.
13. Epstein AE and others: Combined automatic cardioverter-defibrillator and pacemaker systems: implantation techniques and follow-up, J Am Col Cardiol 13(1):121, 1989.
14. Ewy GA and others: Canine transthoracic resistance, J Appl Physiol 32:91, 1972.
15. Flores BT and Hildebrandt M: The automatic implantable defibrillator, Heart Lung 13(6):608, 1984.
16. Higgins CA: The AICD: a teaching plan for patients and families, Crit Care Nurse 10(6):69, 1990.
17. Kerber RE and others: Transthoracic resistance of human defibrillation: influence of body weight, chest size, serial shocks, paddle size and paddle contact pressure, Circulation 63:676, 1981.
18. Myerburg RJ and Castellanos A: Cardiac arrest and sudden cardiac death. In Braunwald E, editor: Heart disease: a textbook of cardiovascular medicine, ed 3, Philadelphia, 1988, WB Saunders Co.
19. Patton JN and Pantridge JF: Current required for ventricular fibrillation, Br Med J 1:513, 1979.
20. Standards and guidelines for cardiopulmonary resuscitation (CPR) and emergency cardiac care (ECC), JAMA 255(21):2915, 1986.
21. Stults KR and others: Self-adhesive monitor/defibrillator pads improve prehospital defibrillation success, Ann Emerg Med 16(8):872, 1987.
22. Teplitz L: Life after sudden death: the development of a support group for automatic implantable cardioverter-defibrillator patients, J Cardiovasc Nurs 4(2):20, 1990.
23. Thomas ED and others: Effectiveness of direct current defibrillation: role of paddle electrode size, Am Heart J 93:463, 1977.
24. Verseth-Rogers J: A practical approach to teaching the automatic implantable cardioverter-defibrillator patient, J Cardiovasc Nurs 4(2):7, 1990.
25. Warner ED, Dahl C, and Ewy GA: Myocardial injury from transthoracic defibrillator countershock, Arch Pathol 99:55, 1975.
26. Zipes DP and others: Termination of ventricular fibrillation in dogs by depolarizing a critical amount of myocardium, Am J Cardiol 36:37, 1975.

APPENDIX

The Person with a Near-Death Experience

Cathie E. Guzzetta

Successful cardiopulmonary resuscitation (CPR) has created an unusual phenomenon called near-death experiences (NDEs) in patients who perceive and experience events during the moment of clinical death. The recollection of NDEs by patients who survive cardiac arrest also has created new problems and important nursing implications.

Patients have described five common stages that characterize the core experience of an NDE.[8,9,10,13,14] During the *first stage,* patients may remember having a discussion with themselves during the arrest about whether they are alive or dead. Although they may decide that they are indeed dead, they frequently also report positive affective feelings such as being relaxed, comfortable, and pain free. During the *second stage,* patients may describe transcendental or out-of-body experiences such as a separation of mind and body, where the mind takes on capabilities not limited by physical dimensions.[9,15] Patients may relate, for example, that the mind, after separating from the body, positioned itself in a corner of the room to observe the resuscitation efforts. This is known as autoscopic observation. The cognitive features of this stage include accelerated thoughts and a distortion of time wherein patients relate that their sense of time, body, and space vanished. After resuscitation, patients may describe the procedures, the type and placement of equipment, personnel, and other details that could not have been known unless one was actually standing in the room and observing the situation.

One distressing component of this stage is the inability to communicate with the health team during the resuscitation. Patients often relate wanting desperately to talk to, touch, or contact caregivers to let them know that they were comfortable and pain free. Some have wanted to comfort distressed caregivers or tell them to stop the resuscitation efforts.[9]

In the *third stage,* transcendental experiences predominate. Patients may relate that their mind actually left the room and began a journey to another environment or place. Many describe their minds traveling through a long, dark tunnel characterized by a space lacking any distinctive dimensions.[12] The journey may be associated with loud noises or music.[4] At the end of this tunnel, during the

fourth stage, many patients relate that their consciousness was brought to an unbelievably bright light, a beautiful meadow, or a heavenly place. The light has been described as restful, brilliant, and extraordinarily beautiful and perceived as the beginning of a new life.[12] The mind may or may not be allowed to enter the light or the place of peace and comfort. In contrast, a few patients may perceive negative, frightening experiences, reporting sights of hell, flames, burning, strange creatures or feelings of terror, doom, loneliness, and helplessness.

During the *fifth stage,* many patients relate that their mind was allowed to enter the light and beauty. At this point, a critical decision must be made—that of whether to continue into the beyond or return to life. Some patients describe coming to a river or a dividing line that represents a border between life and death.[4,15] Patients understand that crossing the line would require that they remain in the beyond forever.[4] At this point they may experience a life review manifested by vivid panoramic images, much like a hologram, that occurs either as flashbacks or flashforwards and provides a sudden understanding of the meaning of life. Also during this stage, the mind may be met by an escort such as a dead relative, friend, or deity. The deities described depend on the patient's cultural and religious beliefs (e.g., God, Jesus, Buddha).[15] Frequently the escort urges the patient to return because it is not yet their time or because their life mission has not yet been fulfilled. A decision is then made either for them or by them to return to physical life.[12]

Although their mind may desire to remain in the light or the place of peace and comfort, patients frequently experience their minds rapidly traveling backward in the tunnel until it is reunited with the body. The reunion of mind and body may not be desired by the patient and can be associated with physical pain and emotional distress.

Case Study*

About 10 minutes into the operation.
"Her pressure is crashing!"

---

*Copyright © 1982 by Carolyn D. Henson, RN, MA. Reprinted by permission.

"What is it? What's the matter?"

At first there was a feeling of sweeping motion. It felt like my mind—the thinking and feeling part of me—quickly moved out of my body. I could see my body lying there on the table, but the real "me" hovered near my head.

It was clear that there was an emergency. The scene was frantic. People I didn't recognize were scurrying in and out of the room. I searched for my surgeon. I knew he was there, but he wasn't standing where I thought he should have been.

Initially, I joined in the frenzy. I wanted to help. I am a nurse. I wanted to tell the doctors what was happening. Frantically, I tried to approach them. I tried to speak, but nothing came out. I reached to touch them, but a barrier kept me from getting close. Then I realized that no one could see or hear me. At that moment, an extraordinary calmness came over me. I moved toward a corner of the ceiling close to a "light."

I had an euphoric feeling of peace. It was as though warmth and acceptance were being communicated to me through the light. There was absolutely no fear. I felt safe and secure. There was a sense of timelessness—as though there was no time. I wanted to linger with the thoughts and feelings I was experiencing.

I was totally unconcerned about what was happening to my body. It was like being in a room with a television set turned on, without paying attention to the images and sounds coming from the set. I was aware that the operating room drama was occurring, but my mind was totally absorbed in the intensity of the peacefulness.

I heard someone say, "I don't think she's going to make it," but the words didn't concern me. I had no thought that I was dying, or that I was going to die. I felt very much alive. I wanted to tell the doctors that there was no need for their urgency—that I liked where I was and that everything was going to be okay. I heard my surgeon say, "She's hemorrhaging. We'll have to open her up!"

I don't know how long my mind remained separated or when it rejoined my body. I remember feeling intense pain when the surgeon made the incision for the exploratory laparotomy. I remember using mental energy to help myself deal with the pain. Inhale—exhale—relax; inhale—exhale—relax . . . When I tired of the breathing exercise, I imagined myself in a very healthy state, jogging at the lake. One, two, three, four, five . . . For the past 10 years, counting had been the technique I had used to keep a steady jogging cadence. I knew when I reached 500 I had jogged about a mile.

What are they doing now? Are they doing open chest heart massage? I've got to tell them I can feel this. Move your head, Carolyn, move your head.

"She feels that! I'm going to put her under again."

The next morning.

I woke up. My chest was sore. My husband was at my side. I was in the intensive care unit. I remembered . . . "Jerry! I almost died. I could see. I was watching. I separated from my body. I was on the table, but I was watching. They did CPR." I began to drift off. I went back to the jogging trail. One-hundred-and-one, one-hundred-and-two . . .

The following days.

Physically my recovery went exceptionally well. But psychologically, I had changed. There were many adjustments to make. At first, I was elated to be alive. I wanted to share that excitement with others. I marvelled at the near-death experience. I wanted to tell others about it, even when they looked at me in disbelief—or fear.

I went to White Rock Lake daily to walk. The jogging trail felt different now, as though it were a very intimate part of me. The colors and sounds along the trail came alive. It felt like I was seeing objects and hearing sounds for the very first time.

A few weeks after the surgery, I became very depressed. The reality of my close encounter with death set in. I now had new scars that were not there before. I felt somehow "different" because of this experience. There seemed to be too much to deal with at once.

There was a need to reset priorities and eliminate the trivia. I found myself concentrating on my family, friendships, and the development of my mind. I spent time reflecting on how we get caught up in unimportant things and miss the beauty of life.

EFFECTS OF NDEs

Patients experiencing an NDE relate the event as being very real, lucid, and vivid.[12] Many are deeply affected by the experience and report a reorganization of their personal values, attitudes, and beliefs. Many believe they have been spared for a particular reason and now have a new sense of mission in life. Most of the personality changes brought on by an NDE appear to be positive[12]; patients have reported enhanced self-esteem, increased self-worth, and a heightened appreciation of life, relatives and friends, and nature.[15] Frequently, patients describe themselves as more helping, tolerant, understanding, and compassionate of others. They have reported also that they are less concerned about what others think of them and less interested in material possessions, worldly success, and social status.[6,12]

Most patients who describe this experience discuss gaining a "living spirit." NDEs have been described to be a spiritual experience that serves as a stimulus for spiritual awakening and development to understand their human existence.[12] Many patients report moving from an entirely formal, religious affiliation to one that takes on a universal spiritual orientation with a belief in a higher mode of being, the unity of all religions, and a conviction of an after-life.[12]

CHARACTERISTICS OF NDE PATIENTS

Up to 48% of persons who have come close to death are reported to have had an NDE.[5,14,17] NDEs have been documented in patients throughout the life span ranging from small children to elderly patients.[4] They also have been recorded throughout history and reported in assorted near-death incidents such as childbirth, drowning, experiencing near-lethal falls, surgery, trauma, combat, and terminal illness.[15] No correlation has been found between the occurrence of NDEs and the patient's age, sex, occupation, education, marital status, or religious background.[8]

Although not all patients experience each of the five stages of the core experience, the affective, cognitive, and transcendental characteristics are common features among diverse cultural and religious groups. The symbolic imagery experienced during the NDE may differ, however, depending on the patient's culture and religious orientation.[15] For example, the Christian patient who experiences a religious figure will use the name God while the Hindu patient will name a Hindu deity.[11]

EXPLANATIONS OF NDEs

NDEs have been explained on the basis of diverse theories. These include psychologic, physiologic, and religious theories, as well as combination theories that include components of each.[12,15] There is little data to support any one of these theories, however, and none can explain all of the stages and features of NDEs.[15]

Psychologic theories explain NDEs as a defensive mechanism for dealing with the annihilation.[1,15] The person substitutes the frightening reality of death with pleasing apparitions. The sense of peace, tranquility, and well-being associated with the experience is believed to be a stunning psychologic response to insulate the person from the trauma of the event.[1] Moreover, the out-of-body experiences may be an adaptive coping response that allows the patient to dissociate from the devastating bodily danger and watch the event as a disinterested third party.[1,15]

Physiologic theories focus on several different physical causes of NDEs.[15] One theory asserts that the cerebral anoxia occurring during the dying process is responsible for the sense of well-being, loss of critical judgment, and the hallucinations and illusions that occur with the event. Another theory asserts that the extreme anxiety associated with dying causes a stress-induced limbic lobe syndrome wherein the central nervous system produces peptides that affect behavior and create the hallucinatory events associated with the NDE. The role of some neuropharmacologic hyperactivity[15] during NDEs is supported by the occurrence of similar hallucinogenic episodes also observed with fever, exhaustion, coma, and the use of anesthetics such as ketamine or recreational drugs such as LSD.

Religious theories purport that the NDE provides proof that an after-life exists. Supporters of this theory believe the dead have returned to report this experience. Critics of such theories argue that these patients were not really dead because death is characterized by irreversible loss of brain function[15] and is a fixed and permanent state. Rather, they argue that the individual experiencing the NDE was alive but entered the early stage of the dying process, which was reversed by successful CPR.[15]

NURSING IMPLICATIONS

It is possible for any patient who has a cardiac arrest to have an NDE. There are many nursing interventions that can be used to assist these patients. During CPR, nurses can position themselves at the head of the bed, reassuring, touching, and explaining the procedures as if the patient were alert and awake.[7] It may be useful for nurses quietly to bid patients "to return" or suggest that it is "not yet their time to go."[7] Because clinically dead patients can accurately and vividly describe the resuscitative procedures and conversations, all health team members must remember that, even in the midst of the crisis, threatening or frightening language should not be used.[9]

When the patient resumes consciousness, it is important to remember not to become so preoccupied with complex physiologic monitoring equipment and postresuscitation physical care that the patient's emotional needs are abandoned. Stay with and support the patient. Assess the patient's level of anxiety, restlessness, orientation, and degree of insomnia. Note any changes in the thinking, personality, mood, attitudes, and memory that may indicate that the patient has had an NDE.[4] Slowly reorient the patient to time, place, and person.

When the patient has been stabilized, determine whether the patient wants to discuss the events before, during, or after the resuscitation.[7] Discuss the resuscitation honestly with the patient. Although not all cardiac arrest patients experience NDEs, nurses can bring up the subject as a means of opening up the discussion.[3,7] Some patients already may be familiar with the concept because it has become more widely publicized in recent years. Interestingly enough, however, most are hesitant to relate their perceptions to others for fear of being labeled as "crazy."[9] Although patients have a great need to discuss their experience,[16,18,19] they may be extremely reluctant until a member of the health team encourages them to do so. Patients frequently are relieved to learn that other survivors have had NDEs and that nurses have encountered this phenomenon before.[3,4]

Create an atmosphere that is caring, nonjudgmental, and attentive. If patients have had such an experience and desire to discuss it, begin by asking patients to discuss their perceptions. Do not pressure them to remember any events associated with the clinical death period if they are not ready to do so.[9] Identify the specific phrases, words, and symbolic imagery the patient uses to describe the experience.[7]

Many patients report extreme difficulty finding the words to describe their NDE. Many will have difficulty coping with the memory. Most will search for the meaning of the experience. Holistic techniques such as relaxation, guided imagery, and music therapy can be used to assist patients in understanding their experience, exploring their attitudes and feelings, and comprehending how the event has affected their lives.[7] These techniques can be used to help patients "relive" the experience as a means of releasing tension, fear, and anxiety. During the guided sessions, the nurse uses the patient's own words, phrases, and symbolic imagery to help in reframing and/or reinforcing the experience as a powerful event that can positively transform the patient physically and emotionally. The Nursing Care Plan that follows outlines the patient outcomes, nursing prescriptions, and evaluation criteria that can be used to guide patients through this process.[7]

NURSING
DIAGNOSIS

Ineffective individual coping related to NDE (or potential for enhanced adaptive or effective coping related to NDE)[7] (choosing pattern)

PATIENT OUTCOMES	NURSING PRESCRIPTIONS	EVALUATION
Patient will demonstrate adaptive individual coping responses as evidenced by: Their ability to discuss their perceptions with the nurse and family Their willingness to participate in relaxation, guided imagery, and music therapy sessions Their ability to explore their feelings and attitudes regarding the experience Their ability to explore and verbalize how the experience has had an impact on their life No evidence of serious behavioral, emotional, or personality problems after the event	Assist patient in achieving adaptive coping responses by offering coping support: Provide behavioral, cognitive, and emotional support. Provide reassurance, as appropriate, and confirm that others have had similar NDEs. Establish a pattern of active listening. Encourage patient to discuss their perceptions openly if they are ready to do so. Allow patient to discuss the events at their own pace without pressure to provide the details surrounding the clinical death period.[4] Identify, for patient, the adaptive coping behaviors they are already using. Assist patient in exploring their feelings regarding the NDE and focus on how the experience has had an impact on their life by using relaxation, guided imagery, and music therapy sessions: Determine patient's willingness to participate in relaxation, guided imagery, and music therapy sessions to "relive" the experience.	Patient demonstrated adaptive individual coping responses as evidenced by: Their ability to discuss their perceptions with the nurse and family Their willingness to participate in relaxation, guided imagery, and music therapy sessions Their ability to explore their feelings and attitudes regarding the experience Their ability to explore and verbalize how the experience has had an impact on their life No evidence of serious behavioral, emotional, or personality problems after the event

Adapted from Guzzetta CE: Near-death experiences. In Dossey BM, Guzzetta CE, and Kenner CV: Critical care nursing: body-mind-spirit, ed 3, Philadelphia, 1992, JB Lippincott.

NURSING DIAGNOSIS	**Ineffective individual coping related to NDE (or potential for enhanced adaptive or effective coping related to NDE)[7] (choosing pattern)—cont'd**

PATIENT OUTCOMES	NURSING PRESCRIPTIONS	EVALUATION
	Because part of NDE is influenced by patients' cultural expectations, beliefs, and attitudes, NDEs represent patient's own symbolic imagery. Using patient's NDE symbolic imagery during a relaxation and guided imagery session is therefore a powerful technique (see Chapter 5, p. 106). The symbolic imagery that emerged during the NDE may remain the same, be similar, or may take on a whole new quality during the relaxation and guided imagery sessions. The two most important aspects for the nurse to remember are that (1) the imagery is generated by patient, and (2) it is impossible to predict what will emerge for patient during guided imagery sessions when suggestions of previously experienced symbolic imagery are given.	
	Begin with a general relaxation session to induce psychophysiologic relaxation (see Chapter 13, p. 414). Soothing, relaxing music may be added to the session to enhance the relaxation and imagery process. Then combine symbolic imagery with the techniques used in the Empowering Relaxation, Imagery, and Music Scripts found in Chapter 5 (p. 119):	

Continued.

NURSING
DIAGNOSIS

Ineffective individual coping related to NDE (or potential for enhanced adaptive or effective coping related to NDE)[7] (choosing pattern)—cont'd

PATIENT OUTCOMES	NURSING PRESCRIPTIONS	EVALUATION
	Use truism: "As you take in your next breath, become aware that you are breathing air into your lungs (truism) and let yourself imagine that you are becoming very relaxed (suggestion). As the oxygen moves into your lungs (truism), imagine that you are back in the operating room (suggestion). As the oxygen fills your lungs (truism), permit the images of your out-of-body experience to come back (suggestion)." Use embedded commands: "You don't have to . . . imagine any of the experiences, Carolyn . . . if you don't want to." Use linkages: "As you feel yourself take in your next few deep breaths, allow yourself to feel the peace, calm, warmth, and sense of timelessness that you experienced during your out-of-body experience" (used to relive and confront the experience without fear). Use reframing: "Because of your out-of-body experience, your life has been changed positively. You will be able to live life more fully. Reflect on how this experience has positively changed your life . . . Now think about how this experience will positively change your life after you return home." Assist patient in explaining the NDE to the family if they so desire. Educate family about NDEs. Provide patient and family with the names of books or articles on NDEs if they desire more information.	

Patients may also fear telling spouses or close relatives about their NDEs. They may prefer to discuss such perceptions with relatives when a member of the health team is present to provide legitimacy to their story and evidence that such events have been experienced by others.[7,9] In this situation, assist patients in recounting their story to the family. Because the NDE frequently has such a profound impact on the patient's life and personality, it is important to educate relatives about NDEs and help them to understand the importance of the experience so that they can support the patient and facilitate future coping behaviors.[3,7]

For patients and families who desire more information about this phenomenon, one of many books currently available on NDEs (e.g., *Life After Life*[8]) can be suggested. Also patients can be referred to the International Association of Near-Death Studies (IANDS*), which is a re-search and teaching organization with support groups and a publication entitled *Anabiosis*.[2,13] Postresuscitation patients, especially those who demonstrate behavioral or personality changes related to NDEs such as depression, moodiness, or suicidal tendencies should be referred to the appropriate individuals for long-term counseling.[7,9,10]

Nurses may respond to the near-death phenomenon with a variety of reactions ranging from complete disbelief or total fascination to absolute acceptance. Regardless of personal beliefs, these experiences are perceived as real by patients. Thus nurses have the responsibility of assisting patients in sorting out their perceptions and coping with the experience as well as in supporting them after the experience.[16,18]

*International Association of Near-Death Studies (IANDS), Dept. N88, P.O. Box 24665, Philadelphia, PA 19111.

REFERENCES

1. Appleby L: Near death experience, Brit Med J 298:977, 1989.
2. Association for the Scientific Study of Near-Death Phenomena: Statement of purpose, Peoria, Ill, 1979, The Association.
3. Clark K: Clinical interventions with near-death experiences. In Greyson B and Flynn CP, editors: The near-death experience: problems, prospects, perspectives, Springfield, Ill, 1984, Charles C Thomas.
4. Corcoran DK: Helping patients who've had near-death experiences, Nurs 88, Nov 1988, p 34.
5. Gallup G and Proctor W: Adventures in immortality: a look beyond the threshold of death, New York, 1982, McGraw-Hill, Inc.
6. Greyson B: Near-death experiences and personal values, Am J Psychiatry 140:618, 1983.
7. Guzzetta CE: Near-death experiences. In Dossey BM, Guzzetta CE, and Kenner CV: Critical care nursing: body-mind-spirit, ed 3, Philadelphia, 1992, JB Lippincott Co.
8. Moody R: Life after life, New York, 1975, Bantam.
9. Oakes AR: Near death events and critical care nursing, Topic Clin Nurs 3:61, 1981.
10. Oakes AR: The Lazarus syndrome: care for patients who've returned from the dead, RN 41:54, 1978.
11. Osis K and Haraldsson E: Deathbed observations by physicians and nurses: a cross-cultural survey, J Am Soc Psychical Res 71:237, 1977.
12. Ramaswami S: Omega as alpha: implications of near-death experiences. In Sheikh AA and Sheikh KS, editors: Death imagery: confronting death can bring us to the threshold of life, Milwaukee, 1991, American Imagery Institute.
13. Ring J, editor: Editorial, Anabiosis 2:1, 1981.
14. Ring J: Life after death: a scientific investigation of the near-death experiences, New York, 1980, Coward, McCann & Geoghegan.
15. Roberts G and Owen H: The near-death experience, Brit J Psychiatry 153:607, 1988.
16. Rodin E: The reality of death experiences: a personal perspective, J Nerv Ment Dis 168:259, 1980.
17. Sabom MB: Recollections of death: a medical investigation, New York, 1982, Harper & Row.
18. Siegel R: Accounting for "afterlife" experiences, Psychol Today 15:65, 1981.
19. Taylor PB and Gideon MD: Cardiac arrest: a crisis for all people, Nurs 80, Sept 1980, p 42.

Index

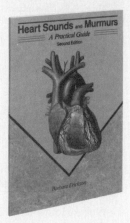
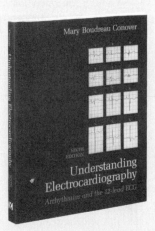
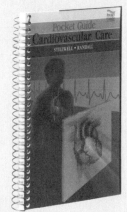

Decreased Cardiac Output

- Related to myocardial dysfunction (Chap. 7, Hemodynamic Monitoring, p. 186)
- Related to electrical factors (rate, rhythm, and conduction), mechanical factors (preload, afterload, and inotropic state), or structural factors (papillary muscle dysfunction, interventricular septal rupture, ventricular aneurysm, and ventricular rupture) (Chap. 10, The Person with Myocardial Infarction, p. 273)
- Related to mechanical factors (preload, afterload, and inotropic state of the myocardium) and electrical factors (rate, rhythm, or conduction) (Chap. 11, The Person with Congestive Heart Failure and Cardiogenic Shock, pp. 317 and 334)
- Related to mitral stenosis (or include valvular problem) (Chap. 12, The Person with Valvular Heart Disease, p. 381)
- Related to mechanical factors (preload, afterload, and inotropic state), electrical, and structural factors (Chap. 14, The Person with Cardiomyopathy or Myocarditis, p. 437)
- Related to structural factors (changes in the pericardium) (Chap. 15, The Person with Pericarditis, Pericardial Effusion, and Cardiac Tamponade, p. 471)
- Related to chronic pericardial disease (include this diagnosis only if constrictive pericarditis is present) (Chap. 15, The Person with Pericarditis, Pericardial Effusion, and Cardiac Tamponade, p. 474)
- Related to bradydysrhythmias and delay in the insertion of the temporary pacing system (Chap. 16, The Person with an Artificial Cardiac Pacemaker, p. 495)
- Related to mechanical, electrical, or cellular alterations (Chap. 17, The Person Undergoing Cardiac Surgery, p. 567)
- Related to acute rejection (Chap. 18, The Person Undergoing Cardiac Transplant Surgery, p. 613)

High Risk for Cardiac Tamponade

- Related to pericardial effusion (Chap. 15, The Person with Pericarditis, Pericardial Effusion, and Cardiac Tamponade, p. 471)

Impaired Gas Exchange

- Related to pulmonary congestion (Chap. 11, The Person with Congestive Heart Failure and Cardiogenic Shock, p. 322)
- Related to pneumothorax due to the insertion of a transvenous lead via the right subclavian vein or the insertion of a transthoracic endocardial lead (Chap. 16, The Person with an Artificial Cardiac Pacemaker, p. 502)
- Related to the thoracotomy for permanent epicardial lead placement (Chap. 16, The Person with an Artificial Cardiac Pacemaker, p. 534)
- Related to surgery, anesthesia, postoperative pain, and immobility (Chap. 17, The Person Undergoing Cardiac Surgery, p. 571)

High Risk for Injury

- Related to hemorrhage (Chap. 7, Hemodynamic Monitoring, p. 188)
- Related to thromboemboli (Chap. 7, Hemodynamic Monitoring, p. 188)
- Related to venous air embolization (Chap. 7, Hemodynamic Monitoring, p. 189)
- Related to pulmonary infarction or hemorrhage (Chap. 7, Hemodynamic Monitoring, p. 189)
- Related to cardiac dysrhythmias or conduction disturbances (Chap. 7, Hemodynamic Monitoring, p. 190)
- Related to endomyocardial biopsy (Chap. 18, The Person Undergoing Cardiac Transplant Surgery, p. 615)
- Related to antilymphocyte preparation (Chap. 18, The Person Undergoing Cardiac Transplant Surgery, p. 619)

High Risk for Microshock

- Related to the presence of the temporary pacing lead (Chap. 16, The Person with an Artificial Cardiac Pacemaker, p. 504)

High Risk for Infection

- Related to invasive monitoring (Chap. 7, Hemodynamic Monitoring, p. 187)
- Related to hemodynamic valve deformity (Chap. 12, The Person with Valvular Heart Disease, p. 387)
- Related to (include name of organism infecting cardiac valve) (Chap. 13, The Person with Infective Endocarditis, p. 406)
- Related to insufficient knowledge about illness and future prophylactic care (for valvular reinfection) (Chap. 13, The Person with Infective Endocarditis, p. 419)
- Related to percutaneous lead placement (Chap. 16, The Person with an Artificial Cardiac Pacemaker, p. 503)
- Related to the presence of a foreign body in the tissue (permanent pulse generator and lead) (Chap. 16, The Person with an Artificial Cardiac Pacemaker, p. 533)
- Related to interruption of host defenses and placement of invasive devices (Chap. 17, The Person Undergoing Cardiac Surgery, p. 576)
- Related to immunosuppression (Chap. 18, The Person Undergoing Cardiac Transplant Surgery, p. 614)

Infective or Phlebotic Vascular Complications

- Related to prolonged intravenous therapy (Chap. 13, The Person with Infective Endocarditis, p. 415)

Altered Protection

- Related to anticoagulation (emboli and bleeding) (Chap. 12, The Person with Valvular Heart Disease, p. 384)